*Rudolph's*

# PEDIATRICS

23RD EDITION

SELF-ASSESSMENT AND BOARD REVIEW

AF767061

## NOTICE

Medicine is an ever-changing science. As new research and clinical experience broaden our knowledge, changes in treatment and drug therapy are required. The authors and the publisher of this work have checked with sources believed to be reliable in their efforts to provide information that is complete and generally in accord with the standards accepted at the time of publication. However, in view of the possibility of human error or changes in medical sciences, neither the authors nor the publisher nor any other party who has been involved in the preparation or publication of this work warrants that the information contained herein is in every respect accurate or complete, and they disclaim all responsibility for any errors or omissions or for the results obtained from use of the information contained in this work. Readers are encouraged to confirm the information contained herein with other sources. For example and in particular, readers are advised to check the product information sheet included in the package of each drug they plan to administer to be certain that the information contained in this work is accurate and that changes have not been made in the recommended dose or in the contraindications for administration. This recommendation is of particular importance in connection with new or infrequently used drugs.

# *Rudolph's* PEDIATRICS

## 23RD EDITION

## SELF-ASSESSMENT AND BOARD REVIEW


**Co-Editors-in-Chief**

**Michael D. Cabana, MD, MPH**
The Michael I. Cohen, M.D., University Chair
Department of Pediatrics
Albert Einstein College of Medicine
Physician-in-Chief
The Children's Hospital at Montefiore (CHAM)
Bronx, New York

**Angelo P. Giardino, MD, PhD, MPH**
Wilma T. Gibson Presidential Professor and
Chair/Chief Medical Officer
Department of Pediatrics
University of Utah School of Medicine/Intermountain
Primary Children's Hospital
Salt Lake City, Utah

**Editors**

**Julie Stein O'Brien, MD, MS**
Associate Clinical Professor of Pediatrics
UCSF Benioff Children Hospital, San Francisco
San Francisco, California

**Brent Mothner, MD, FAAP**
Associate Professor of Pediatrics
Baylor College of Medicine
Texas Children's Hospital
Houston, Texas

**Heather C. Moore, MD**
Assistant Professor of Pediatrics and Clinic Chief
Baylor College of Medicine
Texas Children's Hospital
Houston, Texas

**Christian M. Niedzwecki, DO, MS**
Assistant Professor
Baylor College of Medicine
Texas Children's Hospital
Houston, Texas



Mc Graw Hill

New York Chicago San Francisco Athens London Madrid Mexico City
Milan New Delhi Singapore Sydney Toronto

**Rudolph's Pediatrics, 23rd Edition, Self-Assessment and Board Review**

Copyright © 2023 by McGraw Hill LLC. All rights reserved. Printed in The United States of America. Except as permitted under the United States Copyright Act of 1976, no part of this publication may be reproduced or distributed in any form or by any means, or stored in a database or retrieval system, without the prior written permission of the publisher.

1 2 3 4 5 6 7 8 9 LKV 27 26 25 24 23 22

ISBN 978-1-265-01237-3
MHID 1-265-01237-7

The book was set in Minion Pro by KnowledgeWorks Global Ltd.
The editors were Andrew Moyer and Leah Carton.
The production supervisor was Richard Ruzycka.
Project management was provided by Tasneem Kauser, KnowledgeWorks Global Ltd.
Cover photography was provided by Smiley N. Pool.

This book was printed on acid-free paper.

**Library of Congress Control Number: 2022945507**

McGraw Hill books are available at special quantity discounts to use as premiums and sales promotions, or for use in corporate training programs. To contact a representative please visit the Contact Us pages at www.mhprofessional.com.

*This book is dedicated to Alonzo deGrate Smith, MD (1890–1970) and Roland Boyd Scott, MD (1909–2002). With his appointment in 1932 to the Howard University School of Medicine, Dr. Smith was the first African American pediatrician to serve full time on an academic medical faculty in the United States. Dr. Scott was an internationally recognized pediatrician-scientist focused on the care of sickle cell disease. In addition, Dr. Scott served as Chair of the Department of Pediatrics at the Howard University School of Medicine. Drs. Smith and Scott were made to bear numerous professional indignities and clear many hurdles, despite being successful clinicians, investigators, and leaders in the pediatric academic community. They are remembered for their accomplishments, perseverance, advocacy, and leadership in the field of pediatrics.*

# CONTENTS

# CONTRIBUTORS

**Elisha M. Acosta, MD**
Assistant Professor
Department of Medicine
Transition Medicine
Baylor College of Medicine
Houston, Texas

**Ayesha Ahmad, MD**
Professor of Pediatrics
Division of Pediatric Genetics, Metabolism, and Genomic Medicine
Department of Pediatrics
University of Michigan
Ann Arbor, Michigan

**Elizabeth G. Ames, MD, PhD**
Assistant Professor of Pediatrics and Internal Medicine
Division of Pediatric Genetics, Metabolism, and Genomic Medicine
Department of Pediatrics
University of Michigan
Ann Arbor, Michigan

**Lynda Chima Aririguzo, MD, MPH**
Staff Pediatrician
Sharpstown Rookin Clinic
Legacy Community Health
Houston, Texas

**Rathi Asaithambi, MD, MPH, EdM**
Assistant Professor
Baylor College of Medicine
Texas Children's Hospital
Houston, Texas

**S. Yukiko Asaki, MD**
Assistant Professor of Pediatrics
Pediatric Cardiology and Electrophysiology
Primary Children's Hospital
University of Utah
Salt Lake City, Utah

**Kathryn Ban, MD**
Assistant Professor of Pediatrics
Section of Pediatric Hospital Medicine
Baylor College of Medicine
Texas Children's Hospital
Houston, Texas

**Alan P. Baptist, MD, MPH, FAAAAI**
Associate Professor of Medicine
Program Director
University of Michigan Allergy/Immunology Fellowship Program
Director
University of Michigan Comprehensive Asthma Management Program
Ann Arbor, Michigan

**Jennifer Benjamin, MD, MS**
Assistant Professor of Pediatrics
Baylor College of Medicine
Texas Children's Hospital
Houston, Texas

**John F. Bohnsack, MD**
Professor of Pediatrics
University of Utah Health
Salt Lake City, Utah

**Scott D. Burge, MD**
Mid-South Ear, Nose, and Throat
Germantown, Tennessee

**Antonio G. Cabrera, MD, FAAP, FACC, FAHA**
L. George Veasy Presidential Endowed Chair
Co-Director Intermountain Primary Children's Heart Center
Chief, Pediatric Cardiology
Associate Professor of Pediatrics
University of Utah Pediatric Cardiology, Department of Pediatrics
Intermountain Primary Children's Hospital
Salt Lake City, Utah

**Kristine A. Campbell, MD, MSc**
Associate Professor
Division of Child Protection and Family Health
Department of Pediatrics
University of Utah
Center for Safe and Healthy Families
Intermountain Primary Children's Hospital
Salt Lake City, Utah

**Rebecca L. Carl, MD, MSCI**
Assistant Professor of Pediatrics
Northwestern Feinberg School of Medicine
Institute for Sports Medicine
Ann & Robert H. Lurie Children's Hospital
Chicago, Illinois

**Whitney Chadwick, MD**
Clinical Assistant Professor of Pediatric Hospital Medicine
Associate Chief Medical Information Officer
Stanford Children's Health
Palo Alto, California

**Eric Chiou, MD**
Assistant Professor of Pediatrics
Department of Pediatrics
Baylor College of Medicine
Texas Children's Hospital
Houston, Texas

**Madeleine B. Chollet, MD, PhD**
Fellow in Allergy and Immunology
University of Michigan
Ann Arbor, Michigan

**Elise Coulson, MD**
Fellow in Allergy and Immunology
University of Michigan
Ann Arbor, Michigan

**Megan F. Craddock, MD**
Assistant Professor of Dermatology and Pediatrics
Baylor College of Medicine
Texas Children's Hospital
Houston, Texas

**Shailendra Das, DO**
Assistant Professor
Department of Pediatrics
Baylor College of Medicine
Texas Children's Hospital
Houston, Texas

**Adam W. Dell, MD**
Assistant Professor of Pediatrics
Division of Adolescent Medicine
University of Utah
Salt Lake City, Utah

**Colleen A. Hughes Driscoll, MD**
Assistant Professor of Pediatrics
University of Maryland School of Medicine
Baltimore, Maryland

**Sabrina Fernandez, MD**
Associate Professor of Pediatrics
University of California, San Francisco
San Francisco, California

**Amy G. Filbrun, MD, MS**
Clinical Associate Professor
Pediatrics, Pulmonary Division
CS Mott Children's Hospital, University of Michigan
Ann Arbor, Michigan

**Dana Foradori, MD, MEd**
Assistant Professor of Pediatrics
Cleveland Clinic Children's Hospital
Cleveland, Ohio

**Anisha Gohil, DO**
Assistant Professor of Clinical Pediatrics
Indiana University School of Medicine
Indianapolis, Indiana

**W. Christopher Golden, MD**
Associate Professor of Pediatrics
Department of Pediatrics
Johns Hopkins University School of Medicine
Baltimore, Maryland

**Heather Haq, MD, MHS**
Assistant Professor
Department of Pediatrics
Pediatric Hospital Medicine
Baylor College of Medicine
Texas Children's Hospital
Houston, Texas

**Fauziya Hassan, MD, MS**
Associate Professor, Service Chief
Pediatric Pulmonology, Pediatric Sleep Medicine
University of Michigan
Ann Arbor, Michigan

**Aimee O. Hersh, MD**
Associate Professor
Division of Pediatric Rheumatology
Department of Pediatrics
University of Utah
Salt Lake City, Utah

**Larissa Hines, MD, FAAP**
Clinical Assistant Professor of Pediatrics
University of Oklahoma Health Sciences Center
Oklahoma City, Oklahoma

**Galit Holzmann-Pazgal, MD**
Associate Professor
Pediatric Infectious Diseases
Baylor College of Medicine
Texas Children's Hospital
Houston, Texas

**Eva C. Ihle, MD, PhD**
Health Sciences Clinical Professor
University of California, San Francisco
San Francisco, California

**Christi J. Inman, MD, MS**
Assistant Professor
Pediatric Rheumatology
University of Utah
Salt Lake City, Utah

**Omar Jaber, MD, MPH**
Children's National Hospital
Washington, DC

**Karen E. James, MD, MSCE**
Assistant Professor
Division of Pediatric Rheumatology
Department of Pediatrics
University of Utah
Salt Lake City, Utah

**Andres Jimenez-Gomez, MD**
Pediatric Neurology, Neurodevelopmental Disabilities
Joe DiMaggio Children's Hospital
Hollywood, Florida

**Bernadette Crowder Johnson, MD**
Attending Neonatologist
Mt. Washington Pediatric Hospital
Baltimore, Maryland

**Patrick M. Jones, MD**
Memorial Hermann
Houston, Texas

**Ashley Joshi-Patel, DO, FAAP**
Assistant Professor of Pediatrics
Baylor College of Medicine
Texas Children's Hospital
Houston, Texas

**Rachael J. Keefe, MD, MPH**
Assistant Professor of Pediatrics
Baylor College of Medicine
Texas Children's Hospital
Houston, Texas

**Amaris M. Keiser, MD**
Assistant Professor of Pediatrics
Johns Hopkins University School of Medicine
Baltimore, Maryland

**Judy Lu Kim, MD**
Assistant Professor
Baylor College of Medicine
Texas Children's Hospital
Houston, Texas

**Sarah B. Kinsella, MD, CAQ, FAAP**
Sports Medicine Physician
Adjunct Assistant Professor
Department of Pediatrics
M Health Fairview Orthopedics
Blaine, Minnesota

**Cynthia R. LaBella, MD**
Professor of Pediatrics
Northwestern University's Feinberg School of Medicine
Medical Director
Institute for Sports Medicine
Ann & Robert H. Lurie Children's Hospital of Chicago
Chicago, Illinois

**Elton Lambert, MD**
Assistant Professor
Baylor College of Medicine
Texas Children's Hospital
Houston, Texas

**Grace Liao Lee, MD**
Assistant Professor of Pediatrics and Dermatology
Baylor College of Medicine
Texas Children's Hospital
Houston, Texas

**Kristen N. Lee, MD**
Medical Biochemical Genetics Fellow
Division of Pediatric Genetics, Metabolism and Genomic Medicine
Department of Pediatrics
University of Michigan
Ann Arbor, Michigan

**Frank Y. Lin, MD**
Assistant Professor of Pediatrics
Texas Children's Cancer and Hematology Centers
Baylor College of Medicine
Houston, Texas

**Huay-ying Lo, MD**
Associate Professor of Pediatrics
Baylor College of Medicine
Texas Children's Hospital
Houston, Texas

**Michelle A. Lopez, MD, MPH**
Assistant Professor of Pediatrics
Baylor College of Medicine
Texas Children's Hospital
Houston, Texas

**Priya Mahajan, MD**
Assistant Professor
Department of Pediatrics
Section of Hematology/Oncology
Baylor College of Medicine
Texas Children's Hospital
Houston, Texas

**Andrea Marmor, MD, MSEd**
Professor of Pediatrics
Zuckerberg San Francisco General Hospital
University of California, San Francisco
San Francisco, California

**Nicole L. Mihalopoulos, MD, MPH**
Associate Professor of Pediatrics
Chief, Division of Adolescent Medicine
University of Utah
Salt Lake City, Utah

**Wallis Molchen, DO**
Assistant Professor of Pediatrics
Baylor College of Medicine
Texas Children's Hospital
Houston, Texas

**Heather C. Moore, MD**
Assistant Professor of Pediatrics and Clinic Chief
Baylor College of Medicine
Texas Children's Hospital
Houston, Texas

**Brent Mothner, MD, FAAP**
Associate Professor of Pediatrics
Baylor College of Medicine
Texas Children's Hospital
Houston, Texas

**Todd D. Nebesio, MD**
Professor of Clinical Pediatrics
Indiana University School of Medicine
Riley Hospital for Children
Indianapolis, Indiana

**Hannah C. Neubauer, MD**
Assistant Professor of Pediatrics
Section of Pediatric Hospital Medicine
Baylor College of Medicine
Texas Children's Hospital
Houston, Texas

**Joslyn R. Nolasco, MD**
Associate Clinical Professor of Pediatrics
University of California San Francisco
San Francisco, California

**Stacy B. Pierson, MD, FAAP**
Assistant Professor of Pediatrics
Baylor College of Medicine
Texas Children's Hospital
Houston, Texas

**Sarah Risen, MD**
Assistant Professor
Baylor College of Medicine
Texas Children's Hospital
Houston, Texas

**Keith J. Robinson, MD**
Associate Professor and Vice Chair
Quality Improvement and Population Health
University of Vermont Larner College of Medicine, UVM Children's Hospital
Burlington, Vermont

**Anna Rueda, MD**
Assistant Professor of Pediatrics
Department of Academic General Pediatrics
Baylor College of Medicine
Texas Children's Hospital
Houston, Texas

**Brittany Schwarz, MD**
Instructor
Department of Pediatrics
Associate Program Director Neonatal-Perinatal Medicine Fellowship
Johns Hopkins University School of Medicine
Baltimore, Maryland

**Charu Jajoo Sehgal, DO**
Assistant Professor of Pediatrics
Baylor College of Medicine
Attending Physician, Complex Care Clinic
Texas Children's Hospital
Houston, Texas

**Mona D. Shah, MD, MS, MBA**
Associate Professor
Baylor College of Medicine
Texas Children's Hospital
Houston, Texas

**Julia T. Shelburne, MD**
Senior Faculty
Baylor College of Medicine
Director of Clinical Operations
Section of Pediatric Hospital Medicine
Department of Pediatrics
Texas Children's Hospital
Houston, Texas

**Martin T. Stein, MD**
Professor of Clinical Pediatrics Emeritus
Rady Children's Hospital
University of California, San Diego
San Diego, California

**Sara M. Stern, MD**
Assistant Professor
Pediatric Rheumatology
University of Utah
Salt Lake City, Utah

**Natalie C. Stork, MD**
Orthopaedics and Musculoskeletal Medicine
Children's Mercy Hospital Kansas City
Assistant Professor
Orthopaedic Surgery
University of Missouri-Kansas City School of Medicine
Kansas City, Missouri

**Padma Swamy, MD, MPH**
Assistant Professor of Pediatrics
Baylor College of Medicine
Texas Children's Hospital
Houston, Texas

**John Takayama, MD, MPH**
Professor of Pediatrics
University of California, San Francisco
San Francisco, California

**Andria Tatem, MD**
Instructor
Baylor College of Medicine
Texas Children's Hospital
Houston, Texas

**Erin M. Treemarcki, DO**
Assistant Professor
Division of Pediatric Rheumatology
Department of Pediatrics
University of Utah
Salt Lake City, Utah

**Megen Vo, MD**
Clinical Assistant Professor of Pediatrics
Division of Adolescent Medicine
Lucile Packard Children's Hospital, Stanford
Palo Alto, California

**Kristin Whitfield Van Buren, MD, MEd**
Assistant Professor of Pediatrics
Baylor College of Medicine
Texas Children's Hospital
Houston, Texas

**Sigrid F. Wolf, MD**
Assistant Professor of Pediatrics
Division of Orthopaedic Surgery and Sports Medicine
Ann & Robert H. Lurie Children's Hospital of Chicago
Chicago, Illinois

**Margaret Wood, MD, MPH**
Assistant Professor
Baylor College of Medicine
Texas Children's Hospital
Houston, Texas

**Sherry Zhou, MD, MSc**
Fellow in Allergy and Clinical Immunology
University of Michigan
Ann Arbor, Michigan

# FOREWORD

*"Give me six hours to chop down a tree and I will spend the first four sharpening the axe."*

Abraham Lincoln

In the 23rd edition of *Rudolph's Pediatrics*, the editorial team provided a comprehensive review of essentially the entire field of pediatrics spanning the development of the normal infant and child to the maturing adolescent at the threshold of adulthood. In between these life stages, the chapter authors constructed useful materials that addressed the many disorders and diseases that may affect infants, children, and adolescents. A prime objective was the consideration of the biological basis for normal and abnormal development and for the changes associated with disease. With this vast amount of background information, it may be difficult to define the role of etiological factors and the significance of various clinical observations in differential diagnosis and management.

In *Rudolph's Pediatrics Self-Assessment and Board Review*, Drs. Cabana and Giardino, along with their colleagues, follow the tradition of President Lincoln, quoted above, by focusing how best to prepare for an important board exam that certifies one as a pediatric expert. Proper preparation, akin to sharpening the proverbial axe, in part rests on the careful review and study of a series of questions designed to assist the learner/trainee in analyzing the importance of abnormal physiologic, biochemical, genetic, and other features in pediatric disorders and to highlight clinical features that aid in differential diagnosis. Pertinent questions allow the student to assess the extent of their own knowledge and may point the reader to the need for further study. Brief explanations attached to each question illustrate key points, and readers are conveniently referred to the 23rd edition of *Rudolph's* textbook for in-depth learning. Heartfelt congratulations to the authors for creating this valuable resource to help all of us evaluate our knowledge of pediatrics and thereby assure we provide children with the best care possible.

*Gordon E. Schutze, MD*
*Professor of Pediatrics*
*Baylor College of Medicine*
*Houston, TX*

# PREFACE

*Rudolph's Pediatrics,* 23rd edition, *Self-Assessment and Board Review,* builds upon the 23rd edition of the textbook, *Rudolph's Pediatrics.* Although *Rudolph's Pediatrics* is already a key resource and reference, our goal was to create a companion book that would allow readers to more easily and quickly absorb the contents presented in *Rudolph's Pediatrics.*

As a result, this book contains over 1500 questions that place the content in *Rudolph's Pediatrics* in a clinical context. While the textbook presents a general overview of different pediatric topics, this edition of the *Self-Assessment and Board Review* book actively questions the reader about the clinical application of such material in terms of the epidemiology, pathophysiology, presenting symptoms, clinical decision-making, therapeutics, and prognosis of different pediatric disorders. This book is designed for practicing pediatricians who need to quickly assess their knowledge of pediatrics, by topic. This book then gives the reader a quick reference to the pertinent sections in *Rudolph's Pediatrics* to reinforce the reader's knowledge about the topic.

We have been able to enlist an outstanding group of pediatric clinician educators who have provided a collection of challenging questions for each chapter. These questions highlight the key clinical issues from the 23rd edition of *Rudolph's Pediatrics.* Organized with the content outline issued by the American Board of Pediatrics for the in-training and certification exams, the 28 topics presented in this book also mirror the topics and chapters covered in the *Rudolph's Pediatrics* text. This feature allows readers the opportunity to focus on any one specific topic, based on their own learning needs.

We are sure that you will find this review book both comprehensive and challenging. We hope you find this book indispensable as part of your preparation and review for the Pediatric Board examination.

*Michael D. Cabana, MD, MPH*
*Bronx, NY*
*Angelo P. Giardino, MD, PhD, MPH*
*Salt Lake City, UT*

# CHAPTER 1 Preventive Pediatrics/ Well-Child Care

Sabrina Fernandez, Andrea Marmor, Joslyn R. Nolasco, Martin T. Stein, John I. Takayama, and Megen Vo

**1-1.** A 17-year-old boy presents to the emergency department after his mother found him unconscious in his car in his garage. He was last seen sitting in his car listening to music on the car radio. He regains consciousness in the emergency department and denies drug use, trauma, fever, or other infectious symptoms. His urine drug screen is negative. He says that he remembers feeling nauseated and dizzy and having a headache before he passed out. What is the most likely cause of his symptoms?

**A.** Influenza

**B.** Carbon monoxide poisoning

**C.** Marijuana use

**D.** Heroin use

**E.** Meningitis

**1-2.** A 1-year-old child presents for a routine well visit. You perform blood lead screening, and the child's lead level is found to be 6 μg/dL. The child lives in an older home, built in the 1950s, and the parents note that there is chipping paint in the window sill in the child's room. Which statement about lead poisoning is true?

**A.** Lead, like other metals including iron, serves some physiologic functions in the body.

**B.** Lead-based paint was banned in the United States in 1940.

**C.** Nervous system development can be affected at blood lead levels < 5 μg/dL.

**D.** The most common source of lead exposure in children is imported cosmetics.

**E.** The child in the vignette should receive chelation therapy.

**1-3.** A girl presents for a routine 4-year-old well-child visit. You notice that the mother and father have evidence of tooth decay. In addition, the child has some brownish discoloration and decay on examination. She is happily playing in the room with a lollipop in her mouth. Which of the following is a risk factor for development of childhood caries?

**A.** Living in a high-income household

**B.** Living in a high-altitude household

**C.** A history of bottle use in infancy

**D.** A history of dry mouth and poor salivary production

**E.** Presence of a high-arched palate

**1-4.** You are seeing a 2-year-old girl for a well-child check. She is playing around the room, and you notice a bottle of juice on the stroller. On examination of her teeth, you notice brown and white stains. Which bacteria are implicated in the pathogenesis of dental caries?

**A.** *Streptococcus pyogenes*

**B.** *Streptococcus viridans*

**C.** *Staphylococcus epidermidis*

**D.** *Staphylococcus aureus*

**E.** *Streptococcus mutans*

**1-5.** A family presents for their child's 3-year-old well-child visit. They live in a county where the water is not fluoridated. They have recently been to a dentist to get silver caps on the child's teeth. They are wondering about fluoride supplementation. Which statement about fluoride is true?

**A.** Infants should use a tiny smear of fluoridated toothpaste when they brush their teeth.

**B.** All brands of bottled water contain fluoride.

**C.** All brands of toothpaste contain fluoride.

**D.** Fluoride varnish can only be applied at a dentist's office.

**E.** Fluoride supplementation is required even when drinking water contains a fluoride level > 0.6 ppm.

**1-6.** A 10-year-old boy presents with his mother for school difficulties. He fidgets in class, gets up frequently from his chair, and frequently talks out of turn. His teachers requested that you evaluate him for attention-deficit hyperactivity disorder (ADHD). In the office, you see similar behaviors, and the mother describes difficulties with his behavior at home as well. You proceed with an ADHD assessment and find that he meets criteria for combined-type ADHD. The mother says that she will never allow him to take medicines for ADHD. She seems very adamant about this. She prefers a different approach if one is available. What is your response?

- **A.** Obtain a court order to prescribe him methylphenidate.
- **B.** Discuss complementary medicine practices such as hypnosis, meditation, and yoga.
- **C.** Prescribe him fluoxetine.
- **D.** Recommend a sleep study.
- **E.** Prescribe him a multivitamin.

**1-7.** Which statement about homeopathy is true?

- **A.** Homeopathy is a whole medical system based on the principle that herbs in high doses cure various ailments.
- **B.** Homeopathic medicines must be prescribed by a homeopathic practitioner.
- **C.** Homeopathic medicine is based on the idea that the remedy that would cause a set of symptoms in a healthy person is used to treat the same symptoms in a sick person.
- **D.** Homeopathic medicines are based on the foundation that all medications can be derived from plants.
- **E.** Homeopathic medicine practices used for children are extremely rare.

**1-8.** A 17-year-old girl presents to your office with sleep difficulty. She has trouble falling asleep even when her room is quiet and dark, with no screens visible. You recommend melatonin. Which statement about dietary supplements is true?

- **A.** Melatonin is available by prescription only.
- **B.** Dietary supplements are regulated like pharmaceutical drugs.
- **C.** Dietary supplements are rigorously studied for safety and efficacy.
- **D.** Melatonin is an effective sleep aid for many pediatric patients.
- **E.** Pediatric patients rarely use dietary supplements.

**1-9.** A 9-month-old infant presents with her parents for a well-child check. The mother was breastfeeding but has returned to work and is unable to pump. The mother and father state they switched the baby over to soy milk because they knew they were not supposed to give cow's milk until 1 year of age. The baby eats some fruit purees. The family asks you what they should be giving the baby now for the best nutrition. Which of the following do you recommend?

- **A.** Switch the soy milk to infant formula and continue solids as they have been doing.
- **B.** Continue the soy milk but add in some textured foods.
- **C.** Switch the soy milk to cow's milk and add in some iron-rich foods such as meats and leafy greens.
- **D.** Switch the soy milk to infant formula and add in some iron-rich foods such as meats and leafy greens.
- **E.** Switch the soy milk to half cow's milk and half infant formula, slowly increasing the amount of cow's milk.

**1-10.** A 1-month-old baby presents with his mother for a well-child check. At the last visit, the mother was breastfeeding exclusively. However, when you ask how the feeding is going today, she states she has stopped breastfeeding because she was diagnosed with mastitis and put on the antibiotic cephalexin. She was worried the antibiotics would get into the breast milk and affect the baby. The baby has been taking infant formula since yesterday, and the mother has not been pumping. The grandmother, who is also at the visit, states she is happy the baby is finally getting proper nutrition with infant formula. The mother asks you if she did the right thing. What do you recommend?

- **A.** The mother should continue the antibiotics but also continue to avoid breastfeeding until she finishes the antibiotic course. She should pump and discard the breast milk during the antibiotic course.
- **B.** The mother should continue her current course of antibiotics and restart breastfeeding as soon as possible.
- **C.** The mother should continue her antibiotics, avoid direct feeding for 24 to 48 hours, and pump and discard, but then can resume breastfeeding.
- **D.** The mother should stop the antibiotics and continue to breastfeed.
- **E.** The mother should contact her obstetrician and be placed on an alternative antibiotic so that she can continue to breastfeed.

**1-11.** A 2-month-old infant presents with his mother for a well-child check. The mother states the baby was very gassy and fussy and that they have switched him to a soy formula. She believes that there is possibly some improvement with the infant's symptoms. Which of the following statements is true about soy formula?

**A.** This baby is probably lactose intolerant; soy formula may help symptoms of gas and constipation.

**B.** Soy formula is recommended for babies who have cow milk protein–induced enterocolitis or enteropathy.

**C.** Soy formula is an acceptable alternative to milk-based formula for infants whose families want to maintain a vegan diet or cannot have human or cow's milk due to lactase deficiency or galactosemia.

**D.** Soy formula can be beneficial to treat colic and atopic dermatitis.

**E.** Soy formula is particularly beneficial for preterm infants for whom breast milk is not available.

**1-12.** A new patient arrives for an initial well-child check at 6 months of age. The baby was born at 30 weeks' gestation due to premature labor and weighed 1700 g at birth. She was discharged from the neonatal intensive care unit at corrected gestational age (CGA) of 37 weeks. The baby's mother states she has always had good milk supply and the baby was directly breastfeeding since CGA of 34 weeks, with 2 supplemental feeds with a preterm and transitional formula per day. The baby had been gaining weight well and has been in the 50% corrected for gestational age for height, weight, and head circumference. Her supplemental feeds were stopped at her 2-month well-child check by her previous pediatrician, and they have not seen a pediatrician since. Currently, the baby is chronologically 8 months old, but corrected to approximately 6 months old, and is directly breastfeeding only. What do you recommend for this baby's ideal nutrition?

**A.** The baby should be taking iron supplementation, 2 mg/kg, and vitamin D 400 IU daily, in addition to iron-rich solid foods.

**B.** The baby should restart supplemental feeds with preterm formula 2 times per day. This should be continued until 1 year of life.

**C.** The baby should restart supplementation with preterm formula, and iron-rich solid foods should be added.

**D.** The baby should continue breastfeeding and now start a variety of solid foods.

**E.** The baby should transition to exclusive formula feeding to ensure adequate calcium, phosphorus, and iron intake.

**1-13.** A 15-year-old girl presents for a well-child check. She has a normal body mass index (BMI), and experienced menarche at age 12. While obtaining a diet history, you find she has followed a strict vegan diet since she was 13 years old. In addition, she is a picky eater and does not like leafy greens or legumes. She is otherwise healthy, with no past medical history. She asks you if she is eating the correct foods. Which statement is the most accurate?

**A.** Her current diet meets all her nutritional needs.

**B.** She should increase her intake of leafy greens and iron-rich vegan foods but needs no other supplementation.

**C.** She needs vitamin $B_{12}$ supplementation, but otherwise, her diet is adequate.

**D.** She should add in more leafy greens and ensure she is eating nuts and legumes. She should also take a vitamin $B_{12}$ supplement and consider iron supplementation.

**E.** A vegan diet is not advisable for a teenager because it is not possible to meet an adolescent's nutritional needs.

**1-14.** You are seeing a 1-year-old boy with his grandmother. He was removed from his mother and father's care after witnessing intimate partner violence and suffering physical abuse in the form of shaking. During this visit, you note that he is growing well and developing normally in his grandmother's care. Which statement is correct about early childhood adversity?

**A.** All stressful events are detrimental to a child's health and well-being.

**B.** Children with a history of adverse childhood experiences (ACEs) may have symptoms such as poor concentration and impulsivity, which are easily distinguished from ADHD.

**C.** The more childhood adversity experienced, the less likely one will have medical and psychosocial problems as an adult.

**D.** Early childhood trauma is not associated with early death.

**E.** In the first 3 years of life, children are particularly vulnerable to traumatic exposures given the brain's plasticity in infancy and early childhood.

**1-15.** Which statement about childhood poverty is true?

**A.** Research shows increased hunger and malnutrition in the summer compared to the winter.

**B.** Few state and federal programs exist to address the food insecurity that is common in poor families.

**C.** Poor children of school age are more likely to participate in extracurricular activities because their parents need childcare while they are working.

**D.** Five percent of children in the United States will experience poverty at some point during their childhood.

**E.** The stress associated with childhood poverty may cause prolonged activation of the hypothalamic–pituitary–adrenal (HPA) axis.

**1-16.** You are seeing a 5-year-old boy for a routine well-child visit. You have known the family for 2 years, and at each visit, the mother and father argue about how to care for the child. Today, they report that the boy has been acting out during class. In addition, yesterday, he threw a chair against the wall. The mother reports that she does the majority of the childcare at home and attends to the child constantly. The father thinks that the mother does not allow the boy enough independence. They are talking to lawyers about separating and having joint custody. Throughout the visit, the child is silent. What should you do?

**A.** Advise that the mother should have full custody since she does the majority of the care.

**B.** Advise that the parents should have joint custody over the child since they have both been at every visit.

**C.** Contact the teacher and assess the child for attention-deficit hyperactivity disorder (ADHD).

**D.** Focus on the child's well-being, ensuring adequate growth, development, and mental health. Provide resources for effective co-parenting strategies.

**E.** Agree that the parents should separate since the child now has selective mutism.

**1-17.** Which statement about youth in the juvenile justice system is false?

**A.** Over the past decade, there has been a steady increase in crimes committed by juveniles.

**B.** Black boys and youths die from legal intervention at the same rate as white boys and youths.

**C.** Girls have represented the majority of incarcerated youth since the turn of the century.

**D.** Girls in the juvenile justice system tend to have a higher prevalence of reported traumatic exposures and psychiatric disorders.

**E.** Less than 5% of incarcerated youth have substance-use disorders.

**1-18.** You are seeing a 12-year-old boy for follow-up of anxiety and depression. Unfortunately, his symptoms have worsened, and he has been avoiding school due to bullying. He spends most of his time at home. He decided to stop going to therapy because he did not think it helped. You find out that the boy's father has a gun at home that he keeps for his personal safety. The gun is kept locked and separate from the ammunition. What do you tell the family?

**A.** The presence of a gun in the home only marginally increases the child's risk for suicide.

**B.** Few adolescent suicides involve the use of firearms.

**C.** The safest home for a child is one without guns.

**D.** The family should obtain more firearms to keep the child safe.

**E.** Few suicide attempts involving guns are lethal.

**1-19.** You are seeing a 15-year-old girl for a well-child examination. You have not seen her in a few years. She is presenting with her mother, who is worried about her daughter's relationship with her boyfriend. The mother reports that the boyfriend seems to text "all the time" and keep track of the patient's whereabouts through her mobile phone. He has strong opinions about the kinds of things she posts on social media, and he once slapped the patient after she posted a picture of herself with another male friend. When you speak with the patient separately from the mother, you learn from the patient that she and her boyfriend have been dating for a year. She states that he loves her so much and that is why he keeps close track of her. Her last menstrual period was 5 weeks ago. What is your next step?

**A.** Talk to the boyfriend to learn his side of the story.

**B.** Ask the patient specific questions about her relationship, assessing for physical safety, sexual health, and mental health.

**C.** Advise the mother to take the patient's mobile phone away for an extended time.

**D.** Perform a pregnancy test, and if it is negative, discharge her with close follow-up.

**E.** Refer the mother and patient to family therapy.

**1-20.** You are seeing a 15-year-old girl in urgent care with her boyfriend. Her chief complaint is nausea and vomiting. She seems hesitant to answer some basic questions including where she lives and where she goes to school. She makes little eye contact with you. She refuses to be interviewed without her boyfriend, and he answers many questions for her. When examining her abdomen, you notice a healing bruise on her rib. A urine pregnancy test is positive. You are suspicious that the patient is being coerced and may be a victim of human trafficking. Which statement about human trafficking is true?

**A.** Children with a history of family violence, sexual or physical abuse, or neglect are at higher risk for being victims of human trafficking.

**B.** Federal laws outline how clinicians can obtain consent from minors.

**C.** Mental health diagnoses such as anxiety and depression are uncommon among trafficked victims.

**D.** Trafficked victims rarely interface with healthcare professionals.

**E.** Currently, there are no screening tools to help providers identify victims of human trafficking.

**1-21.** You are evaluating a full-term, 6-week-old boy who presents with his 2 mothers for excessive crying. They report that he cries up to 2 hours per day, with the most crying occurring at 7:00 PM. Both parents appear tired and frustrated and are worried that "something is wrong with him." He is both breastfed and formula-fed. His growth chart, vital signs, and physical exam are normal. What is the most appropriate next step?

**A.** Tell the nursing mother to remove dairy from her diet.

**B.** Refer to pediatric neurology for electroencephalogram (EEG).

**C.** Initiate a histamine $H_2$ antagonist or proton pump inhibitor.

**D.** Change to a soy-based formula.

**E.** Reassure the parents that his behavior is normal.

**1-22.** Which statement about childhood maltreatment is true?

**A.** There has been an increase in substantiated physical abuse cases in the past 30 years.

**B.** Most children who die of abuse or neglect are between 5 and 10 years old.

**C.** Most maltreatment occurs outside the home.

**D.** The most common type of maltreatment is neglect, compared to physical abuse, sexual abuse, and psychological maltreatment.

**E.** Most perpetrators of child maltreatment are not parents, but other people known to the family, such as uncles or family friends.

**1-23.** You are seeing a 4-year-old boy for follow-up after a hospitalization. He presents with his mother, who appears to be very attentive to the boy. This is the third time the boy has been admitted to the hospital for abdominal complaints and vomiting. His mother recounts his hospital stay with numerous details, explaining that during this recent admission, he was made NPO and placed on total parenteral nutrition. His central line became contaminated with an unusual organism and he had a brief stay in the pediatric intensive care unit. His line infection resolved, but his mother reports that his abdominal pain and vomiting remain, even after multiple medications and an unrevealing endoscopy. What is the most likely diagnosis?

**A.** Factitious disorder by proxy

**B.** Immunodeficiency

**C.** Inflammatory bowel disease

**D.** Constipation

**E.** Mitochondrial illness

**1-24.** You are seeing a 2-year-old boy in the emergency department for excessive bleeding. The child had severe nosebleeds, to the point that the hematocrit is low and he has some vital sign instability. This episode is the boy's third visit to the emergency department for similar issues. Testing for bleeding disorders has been negative in the past.

He was also admitted once for failure to thrive as a baby, and during that time, he underwent several tests and procedures including a magnetic resonance imaging (MRI) scan and endoscopy, all of which were unrevealing. He gained weight in the hospital and was discharged home. On family history, there is no hemophilia or known bleeding disorders, but the grandfather has a history of stroke and takes warfarin. On social history, you find that the mother is a lab technician in the hospital. In discussing the case with the mother, she seems unusually calm when you tell her that the child needs to be admitted to the intensive care unit (ICU) for his vital sign instability. She comments that she knows all the personnel in the ICU and starts to gossip about one of the other doctors. Blood tests for warfarin and aspirin level come back negative. What is the most likely diagnosis?

**A.** Hemophilia A

**B.** Hemophilia B

**C.** Factitious disorder by proxy

**D.** Liver disease

**E.** Aspirin ingestion

**1-25.** A 17-year-old boy is presenting to you with his foster mother. He has been in foster care for 2 years and is about to age out of the foster care system. Which statement is true about children living in foster care?

**A.** The majority of children in foster care remain in the child welfare system for a number of years.

**B.** Children with behavioral problems are more likely to have multiple foster care placements.

**C.** On average, adolescents stay in the foster care system just as long as school-aged children.

**D.** Once children are placed in foster care, they have worsened conduct disorder behavior and hyperactivity.

**E.** The majority of children in foster care are eventually adopted.

**1-26.** You are seeing a new 6-year-old boy in your practice with his foster mother. He has a history of behavioral problems and learning difficulties at school. You take an appropriate history and perform a physical examination, with the plan to encourage the foster mother to seek educational testing and an individualized learning plan from the school. Of the following, which is true about children in foster care?

**A.** Rates of mood disorders such as depression and anxiety are similar in children in foster care compared to their peers.

**B.** Children in foster care are more likely to have been exposed to alcohol prenatally.

**C.** Most children sleep and eat well after placement in foster care because they feel safe compared to their previous home environment.

**D.** Most children are placed in foster care because of illness or death of parents or extreme poverty.

**E.** Infants in foster care frequently move from one foster care placement to another, compared to older children.

**1-27.** You are admitting a child for multiple bruises and an expedited workup for child abuse. The grandmother notes that there is a lot of stress and turmoil in the child's home. Which of the following is a risk factor for childhood maltreatment?

**A.** Parental depression

**B.** Single-parent household

**C.** Parent in the medical profession

**D.** Presence of > 4 children in the home

**E.** Presence of > 5 pets in the home

**1-28.** A 2-month-old infant comes to you for a routine healthcare visit. On physical exam, you notice multiple bruises over the abdomen and back. A fundoscopic examination reveals retinal hemorrhages. You suspect maltreatment in the home. What is the most likely stressor at home?

**A.** One parent works the night shift.

**B.** There are 4 older siblings.

**C.** The parent is a single parent.

**D.** Both parents have returned to work.

**E.** The mother has depression.

**1-29.** You are seeing a couple for a first prenatal pediatric visit in clinic. The woman is 36 years old and is 15 weeks pregnant with her first child but has declined all fetal testing and monitoring. She states that she was worried invasive tests would make her lose the pregnancy. She says she is willing to consider testing, if you feel the baby needs it. What would be the best advice for monitoring the health of the fetus?

**A.** Given the gestational age, she should complete blood testing with quad screen.

**B.** She should complete the 20-week anatomy ultrasound because it is not invasive and will provide information about the health of the baby.

**C.** She should continue with her current plan because the baby appears to be healthy and growing well, per the obstetrician.

**D.** Complete an ultrasound now and again at 20 weeks for the anatomy scan, as well as blood testing, such as the quad screen or cell-free DNA.

**E.** Given her age, she should proceed straight to amniocentesis.

**1-30.** You are seeing a new patient in clinic. He is a former 26-week premature infant and is now a 20-month-old boy. His mother states he had some complications in the neonatal intensive care unit (ICU); however, he has been growing and developing well since then. She asks if they are "out of the woods" now or if there is anything else they have to worry about. What is the best answer to this question?

**A.** Once he is 2 years corrected gestational age, we will know if he is free of neurologic sequelae from his prematurity.

**B.** He appears to be doing well now, but babies born earlier than 27 weeks' gestational age and with low birth weight are at high risk of developing comorbid intellectual and learning disabilities, which may not be diagnosed until later in life.

**C.** Now that he is past his first year and growing and developing normally, there are no longer any concerns of complications related to his prematurity.

**D.** Now with advancements in neonatal care, many babies born at less than 26 weeks have no long-term health problems.

**E.** He is still at great risk of growth abnormalities.

**1-31.** You are called urgently from the emergency department to see a woman who arrived and delivered a baby. The provider states the baby is 3 minutes old, appears well, and has a 1-minute Apgar score of 8. They are calling you because an oxygen saturation was noted to be 75%, and they would like you to assess the baby for urgent workup. When you arrive, the room is cold and the baby is unbundled on the bed. The baby appears to be full term, is pink, is crying loudly, and has good tone. What is the best first step?

**A.** Clamp the umbilical cord.

**B.** Put 100% oxygen on the baby via nasal cannula.

**C.** Provide positive-pressure ventilation via bag and mask.

**D.** Start cardiac compressions.

**E.** Warm and dry the infant.

**1-32.** You are called to the nursery to check on a 20-minute-old infant born at 39 5/7 weeks' gestation via cesarean section for breech presentation. Maternal prenatal history is unremarkable. You notice the infant has rapid breathing, with intercostal retractions. The delivery was uneventful, with rupture of membranes at the time of uterine incision, no maternal fever, and clear fluids. Mother was group B *Streptococcus* (GBS) culture negative. On exam, the baby looks pink and has normal tone and normal cardiac exam. Which of the following is the most likely cause of this baby's respiratory distress?

**A.** Transient tachypnea of the newborn

**B.** Surfactant deficiency

**C.** Neonatal pneumonia

**D.** Meconium aspiration

**E.** Improper suctioning of the oropharynx during delivery

**1-33.** During an initial admission exam, you are examining a term breech baby born via vaginal delivery. Mother was group B *Streptococcus* (GBS) negative, rupture of membranes was 4 hours, and there was no reported maternal fever. The baby is well appearing, is appropriate size for gestational age, and has normal newborn reflexes, except an absent grasp reflex on the left hand. The baby has a normal grasp reflex on the right. What is the most likely cause of the absent grasp reflex?

**A.** Central nervous system lesion

**B.** Congenital absence of the digital flexor muscles

**C.** Breech vaginal delivery

**D.** Early meningitis

**E.** Compression of nerves in utero

**1-34.** You are examining a healthy, term newborn shortly after birth and notice palpable ridges along the suture lines of the skull. The infant has normal tone with symmetric movement. Primitive reflexes are also symmetric. The infant responds to noxious stimuli appropriately. What is the next best step?

**A.** Order head ultrasound to further categorize the findings.

**B.** Obtain brain magnetic resonance imaging (MRI).

**C.** Monitor mental status closely.

**D.** Repeat exam of head and measure head circumference at discharge.

**E.** Refer for genetics consult.

**1-35.** A newborn is born in the emergency department, and you are called to assess the baby. The mother had no prenatal care and did not know she was pregnant. The baby weighs 3.6 kg. You conduct a Ballard assessment to determine the baby's gestational age and find the baby's score suggests a 39-week gestational age infant. On neurologic exam, you notice fully extended arms; the baby is able to bring his arms past midline and is able to lift part of his body weight with finger grasp. He has minimal head lag, his knees and hips are flexed, and he has a strong and sustained suck. He has a normal Moro and automatic walking reflex. What is your assessment of this baby?

**A.** He is a healthy 39-week infant with a normal neurologic exam.

**B.** He is a healthy 36-week infant with a normal neurologic exam.

**C.** He has low tone in the upper extremities and an abnormal neurologic exam and needs further evaluation.

**D.** It is too early to assign a proper gestational age.

**E.** His neurologic exam is grossly abnormal, and he needs emergent imaging.

**1-36.** You attend the delivery of a full-term baby girl with no known medical issues. Her mother had a normal pregnancy, with normal prenatal labs, including negative screen for gestational diabetes and negative group B *Streptococcus* (GBS) culture. You are examining the baby immediately after birth. She initially had poor respiratory effort, which quickly resolved with further stimulation. Her color is normal. On cardiac exam, you notice a heart rate of 180 bpm, with normal brachial and femoral pulses. You hear an irregular heartbeat, with approximately 4 ectopic beats per minute, and a harsh continuous 2/6 murmur, best heard at the upper left sternal border, that radiates to the left axilla. What is the next best step?

**A.** Obtain thyroid function tests on the infant.

**B.** Obtain an electrocardiogram (ECG).

**C.** Consult cardiology.

**D.** Initiate a septic workup with complete blood count (CBC) and blood culture.

**E.** Examine the infant again between 24 and 48 hours later and monitor vital signs.

**1-37.** You are conducting an admission history and physical on a term newborn boy born 20 hours ago via normal spontaneous vaginal delivery. His prenatal course and delivery were uneventful, and he has been going to the breast to feed every 2 to 3 hours. This is his mother's second child, and she has a large amount of colostrum. She states he has been latching well and feeding vigorously; he has been spitting up after every feed and occasionally coughs during feeds. On physical exam, he has normal color and tone, with no dysmorphic features, a normal cardiac and lung exam, and a slightly distended belly, which is nontender and soft. What is the next best step in the care of this child?

**A.** Obtain a chest x-ray assessing for lung and cardiac abnormalities.

**B.** Place an orogastric tube and obtain a radiograph to assess position.

**C.** Obtain a lactation consultation to assess positioning of child during feeds.

**D.** Send genetic testing looking for trisomies 13, 18, and 21.

**E.** Continue to observe the baby and assess weight loss at 24 hours of life.

**1-38.** You are caring for a term male infant. Maternal prenatal labs were normal. The 20-week anatomy scan noted right kidney pelviectasis of 8 mm, normal left kidney, and mild oligohydramnios. Third-trimester fetal ultrasound was unchanged. He is now 8 hours old and has voided once. Physical exam is normal. What is the best next step in the care of this child?

**A.** Obtain renal bladder ultrasound prior to discharge.

**B.** Begin prophylactic antibiotics and consult pediatric urology.

**C.** Obtain a same-day renal/bladder ultrasound and consult pediatric urology.

**D.** No further follow-up needed.

**E.** Obtain a bladder ultrasound at 1 month of age.

**1-39.** You are called by the lab about a critical white blood cell (WBC) count of $23 \times 10^3/\mu L$ in an infant born 2 hours ago that was found on a complete blood count (CBC) ordered by the delivery team. The differential shows very few immature WBCs. The infant is full term and was born via vaginal delivery after a short labor. Maternal history was significant for group B *Streptococcus* (GBS)-positive culture, for which the mother was treated with appropriate antibiotics 4 hours prior to delivery. Apgar scores were 9 at 1 minute after birth and 9 at 5 minutes after birth. No maternal fever was noted. On examination of the infant, you notice normal vital signs, normal tone and color, normal brachial and femoral pulses, and mild caput succedaneum. What would be the appropriate next step?

**A.** Obtain blood culture and C-reactive protein (CRP).

**B.** Administer antibiotics to the infant.

**C.** Repeat the CBC.

**D.** Observe the infant for 48 hours.

**E.** Observe the infant for 24 hours.

**1-40.** You are seeing a newborn baby for a first well visit after leaving the neonatal intensive care nursery. The family states she was a twin (dichorionic, diamniotic) but that her twin did not survive and the mother was induced at 33 weeks' gestation. They state this baby was growing well, with no known issues, and that her hospital stay was uneventful. They would like to know whether any further follow-up is necessary. What is the best answer?

**A.** She should have close neurodevelopmental assessments, in addition to monitoring for issues related to prematurity.

**B.** She should have routine well-child care.

**C.** She should have continued monitoring for her issues related to prematurity.

**D.** She should have genetic testing.

**E.** She should have a full cardiac workup, including electrocardiogram (ECG) and an echocardiogram.

**1-41.** You are called to the delivery of a newborn girl, born at 40 3/7 weeks. The mother initially went to a few prenatal visits, and all initial screening labs, ultrasound, and anatomy scan were normal. She was then lost to follow-up. The baby is well appearing, with Apgar scores of 8 and 9. Her birth weight is at the second percentile, her length is at the 45th percentile, and her head circumference is at the 55th percentile for gestational age. The mother states she is generally healthy, and she denies drug and tobacco use. A maternal hemoglobin A1c (HbA1c) upon admission was normal. What is the most likely cause of this baby's size?

**A.** Chromosomal abnormalities

**B.** Cytomegalovirus infection

**C.** Gestational diabetes

**D.** Inborn error of metabolism

**E.** Placental insufficiency

**1-42.** You speak with the mother of a newborn baby, telling her that the baby is well appearing but small for gestational age (SGA). The mother wants to know if there will be any complications related to the baby's diagnosis of SGA. What is the best answer?

**A.** Poor feeding

**B.** Learning disabilities

**C.** Increased risk of neonatal sepsis

**D.** Respiratory distress

**E.** Anemia

**1-43.** You are seeing a 55-hour-old infant in clinic for follow-up after initial birth hospitalization. He is a term baby who was born vaginally at 40 2/7 weeks' gestation to a mother with gestational diabetes requiring insulin. The rest of the prenatal labs were normal. His birth weight was 4.2 kg. He has a normal newborn exam. He had one initial low blood glucose level, which improved to normal with frequent feeds. Mother feels the feeding is going well. On exam, you notice a 20-g weight gain from discharge weight; the infant appears sweaty and is irritable but otherwise has a normal exam. What would be the best next step in his management?

**A.** Check a blood glucose level.

**B.** Check a serum bilirubin level.

**C.** Check a serum calcium level.

**D.** Admit him to the neonatal intensive care unit (ICU) for respiratory distress syndrome (RDS).

**E.** Check a magnesium level.

**1-44.** The American Academy of Pediatrics (AAP) recommends developmental screening with an evidence-based tool at 9, 18, and 30 months of age. You decide that the most efficient way to screen your patients at these times is with a general screening questionnaire that evaluates most developmental domains. Which screening tests best meets these objectives?

**A.** Modified Checklist for Autism in Toddlers (M-CHAT)

**B.** Ages and Stages Questionnaire (ASQ)

**C.** Strengths and Difficulties Questionnaire (SDQ)

**D.** Pediatric Symptom Checklist (PSC)

**E.** Social Communication Questionnaire (SCQ)

**1-45.** Temperament refers to the inborn, biologically based behavioral style with which an individual interacts with his or her environment. When children are assessed for 9 behavioral characteristics, temperament is classified as slow-to-warm-up, easy, difficult, or mixed. What percentage of infants are classified as slow-to-warm-up, easy, and difficult?

**A.** 25%, 60%, 20%

**B.** 15%, 40%, 10%

**C.** 5%, 40%, 20%

**D.** 10%, 50%, 5%

**E.** 20%, 20%, 20%

**1-46.** You have been concerned about the development of an infant in your practice since 6 months of age. At the 18-month health supervision visit, the child will sit without support and pull himself up to stand while holding onto a chair, but he will not cruise, stand unsupported, or walk without assistance. He has a crude pincer grasp, and his language is limited to consonants. He engages with you only briefly with minimal interest in a toy. There is no evidence of developmental regression, seizures, or dysmorphic facial features. The American Academy of Pediatrics (AAP) recommends which laboratory study?

**A.** Plasma amino acids

**B.** Liver functions tests

**C.** Urine organic acids

**D.** Chromosome microarray

**E.** DNA test for fragile X on all siblings

**1-47.** A sleep association is a common cause for night awakening in children. Which statement about sleep associations is true?

**A.** Sleep association usually refers to the theme of a screen time activity that a child experienced in the evening prior to sleep.

**B.** A sleep association is not associated with a transition from deep sleep to light sleep.

**C.** A sleep association occurs during a partial arousal when a child may awaken and find that the sleep-time environment is not the same as when he or she fell asleep. Falling back to sleep may be difficult.

**D.** An electroencephalogram (EEG) recording shows a specific pattern diagnostic of a sleep association.

**E.** Behavioral management is not effective when a child awakens due to a sleep association.

**1-48.** You are seeing a patient for his well-child visit. He babbles with consonants, recognizes his caregivers, reaches for objects, and transfers objects from one hand to another. He is rolling well and beginning to sit without support. What is the most likely developmental age of this child?

**A.** 4 months old

**B.** 6 months old

**C.** 9 months old

**D.** 12 months old

**E.** 15 months old

**1-49.** You are seeing a 9-month-old girl for her well-child visit. Her mother is worried that she is not developing appropriately. Which of the following would raise concern for developmental delay?

**A.** Mary is able to pull herself to stand but does not take independent steps.

**B.** Mary turns toward sounds and follows a point but does not point at objects to express interest.

**C.** Mary bangs 2 objects together but does not throw the objects.

**D.** Mary laughs and coos but does not babble with consonants and does not say "Mama" or "Dada."

**E.** Mary turns to her name but does not follow 1-step commands.

**1-50.** Your patient is able to make 3-word sentences and identifies her own name, gender, and age. She copies a circle, plays with her peers, and jumps on one foot, and her speech is 75% understandable. Her developmental age is consistent with which age?

**A.** 2 years

**B.** 2.5 years

**C.** 3 years

**D.** 4 years

**E.** 5 years

**1-51.** You are seeing a 14-year-old girl for a well-child check. Her weight, body mass index (BMI), height, vital signs, and exam are all within normal limits. Her breast development and pubic hair are both consistent with a sexual maturity rating (SMR) stage of 4, and she had menarche 6 months prior to your visit. She asks you, "How much more will I grow?" Which of the following is true regarding pubertal development in adolescents?

**A.** Peak height velocity in females increases after menarche.

**B.** Height velocity in females peaks at SMR 3 for breast development.

**C.** Height velocity in males peaks at SMR 3 for gonadal development.

**D.** Weight and height velocity peak around the same time in females.

**E.** Peak weight velocity occurs later than peak height velocity in males.

**1-52.** You are seeing an 11-year-old girl for "vaginal discharge." Her weight, height, and body mass index (BMI) are at the 50th percentile for age. She first noticed breast budding about 18 months ago, as well as development of pubic hair. She has noticed intermittent "discharge" on her underwear that can vary from watery to sticky. She has never been sexually active, denies douching or inserting anything into her vagina, and is otherwise not bothered by her symptoms. You educate her on physiologic discharge, and she asks you when she can expect to get her menstrual period. Which of the following is true?

**A.** The preovulatory phase of the menstrual cycle is predominately mediated by progesterone.

**B.** Approximately 12% body fat is required to achieve menarche.

**C.** Menarche typically occurs before females reach peak height velocity.

**D.** Menarche typically occurs between sexual maturity rating (SMR) stages 3 and 4.

**E.** Height increases an average of 9 cm in females after menarche.

**1-53.** A 13-year-old girl presents to your office with a chief complaint of "vaginal discharge." Her mother reports that she has complained of white, sticky discharge as well as more watery discharge for several weeks. On history, the patient has had breast development for 2 years but has not yet started menses. She denies any sexual activity or putting anything in her vagina and denies any other complaints but does note that the discharge is "weird." Mom is requesting treatment for "yeast infection." What is the best next step in management?

**A.** Reassurance

**B.** Prescribe oral antibiotics for bacterial infection

**C.** Prescribe topical antibiotics for bacterial infection

**D.** Prescribe oral antifungal for fungal infection

**E.** Prescribe topical antifungal for fungal infection

**1-54.** You are seeing an 18-year-old woman for her annual physical. Based on your chart review, she is up to date on immunizations, including human papillomavirus (HPV), and her past medical history is notable only for asthma. She is a high school senior, identifies as female, and is interested in males. She has been sexually active with one partner and has had oral and vaginal sex. She uses oral contraceptive pills for contraception and reports that she is inconsistent with condom use. You discuss screening for sexually transmitted infections (STIs), and she asks if she should also have a Pap smear at this visit. You discuss current screening guidelines. Which of the following is true regarding cervical development in adolescents?

**A.** During puberty, columnar epithelial cells replace squamous cells at the squamocolumnar junction.

**B.** During puberty, the squamocolumnar junction moves distally.

**C.** A major trigger for epithelial change during puberty is the alteration in the vaginal pH from alkaline (> 4.7) prior to puberty to acidic (< 4.5).

**D.** Squamous epithelial cells of the cervix are more susceptible to *Neisseria gonorrhoeae* and *Chlamydia trachomatis* infections than columnar epithelium.

**E.** Cervical cancers most frequently arise outside the transformation zone.

**1-55.** You are preparing a lecture for medical students on puberty. While preparing your slides, you review the hormonal changes that occur during male puberty. Which of the following is true regarding male puberty?

**A.** Sertoli cells, under the influence of luteinizing hormone (LH), mediate spermatogenesis.

**B.** Leydig cells, under the influence of follicle-stimulating hormone (FSH), mediate spermatogenesis.

**C.** Pulsatile gonadotropin-releasing hormone (GnRH) secretion occurs first during the day and leads to pituitary release of LH and FSH.

**D.** Sertoli cells, under the influence of FSH, mediate testosterone secretion.

**E.** Leydig cells, under the influence of LH, mediate testosterone secretion.

**1-56.** An 11-year-old boy presents to your office for a sports physical. His exam and history are within normal limits, and his weight, height, and body mass index (BMI) are at the 60th percentile for age. During the genitourinary exam, you note that his gonadal development is consistent with sexual maturity rating (SMR) stage 2. Which of the following is true?

**A.** Testicular length in SMR 2 is > 2.5 cm.

**B.** Testicular volume in SMR 2 is 3 mL.

**C.** Testicular volume in SMR 3 is 10 mL.

**D.** The first sign of puberty in males is an increase in penile length.

**E.** The first sign of puberty in males is an increase in penile width.

**1-57.** The mother of one of your patients asks to speak with you privately during a well visit. She reports that her 15-year-old daughter seems to be increasingly preoccupied with her friend group and has distanced herself from her parents and younger siblings, preferring to spend her time with friends. She has also started dating. Her mom states, "It's like all she wants to do is be with her friends, and we were such a close family!" She asks you whether this is normal for her age. Which of the following is true regarding adolescent development?

**A.** Adolescents do not develop sexual drive until late adolescence.

**B.** Late adolescents are typically most self-centered, leading to increased conflicts with parents.

**C.** Middle adolescence is marked by concrete thinking.

**D.** Middle adolescents are typically most concerned with peer relationships, with peer influence decreasing over time.

**E.** Cognitive development is complete by middle adolescence.

**1-58.** A 17-year-old girl presents to your office for a new patient visit. You gather the initial history with the patient and her mother together. Her mother provides most of the history, reporting that the family recently moved and is looking to establish care with a new primary care physician. She reports that her daughter has a history of asthma, allergic rhinitis, scoliosis, and irregular menstrual periods, as well as depression and anxiety. They have brought a copy of her previous medical and immunization records and medication list. You ask her mother to step out to gather more history from the patient privately, to which the mother expresses surprise. The mother notes that she has never been asked to leave the room during her daughter's medical visits in the past and asks what you plan on discussing "since we tell each other everything and I will want to know what she tells you." The best response to her concerns would be which of the following?

**A.** Adolescents have the right to confidentiality in all areas of their mental and physical health.

**B.** Parents have the right to access all of their children's medical and mental health records.

**C.** Adolescents have the right to confidentiality around sensitive topics, including sexual behavior, substance use, and mental health concerns, except in cases when the patient's or someone else's safety or life is at risk.

**D.** Discussing confidentiality and sensitive health topics is not a critical part of the adolescent health visit and may be waived if the parent does not think it is necessary.

**E.** Discussing confidential health topics with an adolescent is not necessary until the age of 18.

**1-59.** You are seeing an 18-year-old woman for a precollege physical. Her last well adolescent exam was 1 year ago, and she has had no health changes since that time. She currently lives with her parents but will be moving out of state to attend college. She denies drug or alcohol use. She is sexually active with one male partner and has had oral and vaginal sex; she uses condoms and the hormonal intrauterine device (IUD) for contraception. Her exam is unremarkable, and she is up to date on immunizations. She asks you if there are any other labs or tests she should be getting annually. Which of following screening tests is indicated annually for this patient?

**A.** Pelvic exam

**B.** Pap smear

**C.** Human immunodeficiency virus (HIV) testing

**D.** *Chlamydia trachomatis* testing

**E.** *Treponema pallidum* testing

**1-60.** You are asked to join a team of multidisciplinary providers to start a clinic aimed at helping transition children with chronic health issues to adult care. At the first clinic meeting, you are asked when the transition process should begin, in order to adequately prepare patients to move on to the adult healthcare system. Your best response would be which of the following?

**A.** The adult model of health care is similar to the pediatric model; therefore, conversations about transition may wait until the patient turns 18 years of age.

**B.** Providers should follow the patient's lead on when to transition to adult care.

**C.** Transition conversations should happen in early adolescence and at least 2 years prior to the projected transition date.

**D.** Transition conversations need not include detailed plans about patient expectations.

**E.** Transition conversations are best had with patients alone, as patients will be responsible for their own health care in the adult system.

**1-61.** A 16-year-old boy presents to your primary care office for "sleep issues." He reports that he is very stressed with school and is often up late at night doing homework, which he attributes to the fact that he often returns home from work late. When you interview him privately, he reports that his mood has been "down" and he has wondered if life is worth living. He denies having a plan to hurt or kill himself.

He admits that he smokes marijuana several times a week to help him go to sleep, as well as recreationally when out with friends. He reports that he has driven under the influence of marijuana but does not feel it alters his ability to drive safely. He reports that marijuana seems to be the only thing that he has tried that helps him fall asleep and is reluctant to discuss changing his use. When counseling him about his behavior, you mention that which of the following is true in the United States?

**A.** Nighttime restrictions and extended learners' permits have not been shown to reduce traffic mortality.

**B.** Suicide is the leading cause of death among teens and young adults.

**C.** Motor vehicle accidents are the leading cause of death among teens and young adults.

**D.** Males and females have similar rates of death by suicide and homicide.

**E.** The majority of teen deaths are due to chronic illnesses.

**1-62.** You are giving a presentation to medical students on morbidity and mortality in the pediatric population. At the end of the presentation, a student asks you how adverse childhood experiences (ACEs) affect morbidity specifically in the adolescent population. Which of the following is the best answer?

**A.** ACEs include abuse and neglect but do not include bullying, neighborhood violence, or family stressors.

**B.** Childhood and adolescent ACEs are associated with increased risk behaviors in adolescence, but not increased morbidity.

**C.** ACEs appear to have a limited effect on teens and do not appear to affect youth beyond adolescence.

**D.** In the United States, about half of 14-year-olds have experienced one ACE.

**E.** ACEs appear to have a cumulative effect on morbidity.

**1-63.** You are asked to give a presentation on adolescent health to a group of medical students. While discussing common causes of mortality in adolescents worldwide, you discuss the fact that complications from pregnancy or delivery are the second leading cause of death in adolescent females. In the United States, which of the following is true regarding teen pregnancy?

**A.** Adolescent pregnancy rates have decreased in the past 20 years, whereas abortion rates have increased.

**B.** Adolescent pregnancy rates have decreased in all racial and ethnic groups, except for African American females.

**C.** Increased adolescent access to contraception has not altered adolescent pregnancy rates.

**D.** Decreased adolescent access to comprehensive sexual health education is associated with higher teen pregnancy rates.

**E.** Less than half of teens report using some form of contraception at last intercourse.

**1-64.** You are seeing a 14-year-old boy brought in by his father, who has concerns today about his son's marijuana use. The patient has a history of attention-deficit hyperactivity disorder (ADHD), for which he takes methylphenidate, and acne, for which he takes doxycycline. Dad asks to speak with you prior to the visit and states that he is concerned that his son may be using marijuana with friends. He reports that, lately, his son has been spending more time with friends after school and on weekends. His son sometimes comes home smelling like marijuana. He has not noticed any other significant changes in behavior or school performance; however, he does think that the patient has been more irritable, particularly when questioned about his friends or drug use. The father is requesting that his son be drug tested today. What is the best response to this request?

**A.** A drug test should be obtained with the parent's consent.

**B.** A drug test should be obtained with the adolescent's consent.

**C.** Urine drug tests for marijuana may be positive up to 24 hours after last use.

**D.** Urine drug tests will not detect ADHD medications.

**E.** Doxycycline use will not affect the results of a urine drug test.

**1-65.** A 17-year-old girl presents to your office with complaints of a "breast mass." She reports that she has felt "bumps" in her breasts on both sides, most prominent at the upper outer quadrants, for several months. She notices that the bumps seem to come and go, but they can be very tender and painful during the week before her menstrual period. She has a maternal aunt who has a history of breast cancer, diagnosed in her 50s. The patient is very distressed and worried that she may have breast cancer as well. On exam, you note several < 1 cm mobile, firm lesions in the upper outer quadrants of her bilateral breasts that are nontender to palpation, with no overlying skin changes or nipple discharge. What is the best response to her concerns?

**A.** Fibrocystic breast changes are the most common cause of breast masses in adolescents.

**B.** Fibroadenomas are rarely noted on biopsy in adolescents.

**C.** The majority of breast cancers in adolescents are associated with *BRCA* positivity.

**D.** Later menarche is associated with higher risk of breast cancer.

**E.** Breast masses in adolescents are usually due to malignant tumors.

**1-66.** A 12-year-old boy presents with his mother for a "sensitive issue." You speak with the adolescent alone, who appears very uncomfortable. He finally tells you that he is worried he may have breast cancer. His grandmother was recently diagnosed with breast cancer, and when changing for physical education class a week ago, he noticed a "lump" on his right breast. He reports no other symptoms other than feeling very worried about having cancer.

On examination, he appears anxious but otherwise well. You note a firm, mildly tender lump under the right areola, measuring 3 cm. There are no overlying skin changes, and you note no axillary, cervical, or subclavian lymphadenopathy. His testes measure 3 cm in length. What is the best next step in management of this patient?

**A.** Obtain *BRCA* gene testing.

**B.** Obtain ultrasound.

**C.** Obtain urine drug testing.

**D.** Refer for surgical evaluation.

**E.** Offer reassurance.

**1-67.** A 13-year-old boy presents to your office for a sports physical. He has been healthy since his last well check and takes no medications. His only complaint is a feeling of "heaviness" or "achiness" in his scrotum after long periods of standing. He denies any history of sexual activity or trauma. On physical exam, you note a "bag of worms" on inspection and palpation of the right testis. Which of the following is the next best step in management?

**A.** Referral for surgical evaluation

**B.** Scrotal elevation

**C.** Nonsteroidal anti-inflammatory drugs (NSAIDs) and rest

**D.** A 3-day course of cefoxitin

**E.** Doppler ultrasound

**1-68.** A 16-year-old girl presents to your office for a new patient evaluation. She reports that she is generally healthy and has a past medical history notable for allergic rhinitis and an appendectomy at age 9. When asked if she has any health topics she would like to discuss today, she mentions that she has not yet had her first menstrual period and wonders if this is normal. She reports having breast budding around age 12 and believes that her mother had her first menstrual period at age 13. Which of the following is the best response to her concerns?

**A.** Primary amenorrhea is defined as lack of menses by age 12 in the absence of secondary sex characteristics.

**B.** Primary amenorrhea is defined as lack of menses by age 15, or within 3 years of thelarche.

**C.** Primary amenorrhea cannot be diagnosed at this time, and you would recommend watchful waiting for menarche.

**D.** Secondary amenorrhea is defined as cessation of menses for 6 months.

**E.** She likely has constitutional pubertal delay and does not need further workup at this time.

**1-69.** A 14-year-old girl presents to your office for evaluation of irregular periods. She reports that she had her first menstrual period about 9 months ago. She first noticed breast development 2 years ago and then notes that her height "shot up." After her first menstrual period, she started tracking her menses and noted that, although sometimes her cycles last around 30 days, they can be as short as 18 to 20 days and sometimes she skips months completely. Her menses usually last 4 to 5 days, and she uses 3 to 4 pads or tampons per day and denies soaking through pads or tampons. She finds not knowing when her period will occur frustrating. She and her mother are requesting a workup to "figure out what's wrong," especially as her mother has a history of uterine polyps. Which of the following is the best response?

**A.** Uterine polyps are a common cause of abnormal uterine bleeding in adolescents.

**B.** Once adolescents achieve menarche, the hypothalamic–pituitary–gonadal (HPG) axis has matured sufficiently to maintain regular, monthly menses.

**C.** About three-fourths of females begin to have regular, monthly menses by 1 year after menarche.

**D.** Anovulatory cycles are a common cause of irregular menses for 3 years after menarche.

**E.** She likely has von Willebrand disease and should have confirmatory lab testing.

**1-70.** A 13-year-old girl presents to your office for an annual physical. Since your last visit with her a year ago, she has been well, and she reports that she had her first menstrual period about 6 months ago. She notes that some of her friends complain of menstrual cramps with their periods and sometimes even miss school. She reports that she likes school and is worried that she may also develop cramps in the future. The best response to her concerns would be which of the following?

**A.** Menstrual cramps are rare, and she will likely not be affected by them in the future.

**B.** Menstrual cramps are not a common cause of school absenteeism or decreased quality of life.

**C.** The prevalence of menstrual cramps peaks 1 to 2 years after menarche.

**D.** Of those females who experience menstrual cramps, the majority have moderate to severe cramping.

**E.** There are few effective treatments available for menstrual cramps.

**1-71.** You are seeing a 15-year-old girl who presents to urgent care for abdominal pain. She is accompanied by her boyfriend. She reports a 4-week history of nausea and vomiting as well as abdominal discomfort. She further notes that she has not yet had her menstrual period this month. You obtain a urine pregnancy test, which is positive, and discuss the results with your patient privately. She expresses happiness, and after a discussion of options, she reports that she intends to continue the pregnancy. Which of the following screening tests is not indicated in the first trimester for a pregnant adolescent?

**A.** Human immunodeficiency virus (HIV)

**B.** Herpes simplex virus

**C.** Syphilis

**D.** *Chlamydia trachomatis*

**E.** *Neisseria gonorrhoeae*

**1-72.** A 16-year-old girl presents to your office for contraception. Her past medical history is notable for asthma, chronic abdominal pain, depression, and migraines. She reports that she gets "weird vision things" when she has a headache and that her migraines often prevent her from going to school.

She identifies as female and is interested in both males and females. She has had oral and vaginal sex with males and females in the past. She is currently sexually active with one male partner and uses condoms "sometimes." She reports she last had vaginal sex yesterday and did not use a condom. Her last menstrual period started 7 days ago. You review contraceptive options with her, and she expresses interest in an intrauterine device (IUD). What is the best next step in management of this patient?

**A.** Give her information about contraceptive options and ask her to return in 1 week for initiation of method.

**B.** Given her risk of unintended pregnancy, give Depo-Provera (depot medroxyprogesterone acetate [DMPA]) injection today and ask her to return for IUD placement.

**C.** Obtain a pregnancy test and place a hormonal IUD if negative.

**D.** Give oral emergency contraception today and ask her to return in 2 weeks for a follow-up pregnancy test before placing an IUD.

**E.** Obtain a pregnancy test and place a copper IUD today if negative.

**1-73.** A former 28-week-gestation premature infant, who is now 2 months of age, is brought to the emergency department with poor feeding and lethargy. On exam, the infant has a rectal temperature of 38.4°C, a heart rate of 189 bpm, and a respiratory rate of 55 breaths/min. The infant is barely responsive, and her skin is flushed and warm. You feel bounding pulses, and her capillary refill is immediate. Her lungs are clear, and cardiac exam is hyperdynamic and tachycardic, with no murmurs. What best describes the type of shock that this patient is experiencing?

**A.** Warm shock

**B.** Cold shock

**C.** Compensated shock

**D.** Cardiogenic shock

**E.** Hypovolemic shock

**1-74.** A 6-year-old child is brought in 1 hour after slipping in the shower and hitting the back of her head. She was initially alert after the injury but has become progressively somnolent. On your examination, there is a large hematoma over the left occiput. When you yell her name, she does not respond. When you firmly rub her sternum, she opens her eyes briefly and moans and extends both of her arms. What is her Glasgow Coma Scale (GCS) score according to the Pediatric GCS?

**A.** 3 (1 for eye opening, 1 for verbal response, 1 for motor response)

**B.** 6 (2 for eye opening, 2 for verbal response, 2 for motor response)

**C.** 8 (2 for eye opening, 3 for verbal response, 3 for motor response)

**D.** 10 (3 for eye opening, 4 for verbal response, 3 for motor response)

**E.** 12 (4 for eye opening, 4 for verbal response, 4 for motor response)

**1-75.** You are getting ready to renew your pediatric advanced life support (PALS) certification and are reviewing recommendations for infant and child cardiopulmonary resuscitation (CPR). You note that recommendations for chest compressions are to allow for complete chest recoil between compressions. What is the reason for allowing complete recoil?

**A.** To allow the lungs to fill with air

**B.** To ensure adequate cardiac venous return

**C.** To prevent injury to the ribs

**D.** To prevent injury to the heart

**E.** To prevent rescuer fatigue

**1-76.** A 3-month-old infant presents to your clinic with difficulty breathing. Her vital signs are notable for a temperature of 38.5°C, respiratory rate of 63 breaths/min, heart rate of 170 bpm, and oxygen saturation of 92% on room air. She is alert but in moderate respiratory distress, with nasal congestion; moderate suprasternal, intercostal, and supraclavicular retractions; and diffuse low-pitched wheezes, rhonchi, and rales on auscultation. What is the most likely diagnosis based on this clinical picture?

**A.** Asthma

**B.** Bronchiolitis

**C.** Croup

**D.** Foreign body aspiration

**E.** Pneumonia

**1-77.** You are asked to see a 14-hour-old neonate who was delivered at 36 weeks' gestation due to maternal rupture of membranes and fever. The infant appears lethargic and has a respiratory rate of 65 breaths/min, heart rate of 190 bpm, and blood pressure of 75/50 mm Hg. As you are beginning to stabilize the infant, the results of an arterial blood gas come back with a pH of 7.3, a $PCO_2$ of 30 torr, and a $HCO_3^-$ of 15 mEq/L. What is the best interpretation of this blood gas?

**A.** A primary metabolic acidosis with respiratory compensation

**B.** A primary metabolic alkalosis with respiratory compensation

**C.** A primary respiratory acidosis with metabolic compensation

**D.** A primary respiratory alkalosis with metabolic compensation

**E.** A mixed acid-based disorder

**1-78.** A previously healthy, 10-kg, 11-month-old infant is being seen in urgent care for vomiting from gastroenteritis. She is responsive, not ill appearing, and mildly tachycardic with strong pulses. Her capillary refill time is 3 to 4 seconds, and she has dry mucous membranes. She last urinated 8 hours ago. Despite oral ondansetron, she refuses to take oral fluids. You decide to give her an intravenous bolus. The best initial fluid and amount is which of the following?

**A.** Dextrose 5% (D5) in ½ normal saline (NS), 20 mL/kg

**B.** D5 ½ NS, 4 mL/kg/h

**C.** D5 ¼ NS, 20 mL/kg

**D.** NS, 20 mL/kg

**E.** NS, 4 mL/kg/h

**1-79.** You are seeing a 20-kg, 5-year-old child in urgent care clinic. The child has a fever and rash. The patient is ill appearing, with an oral temperature of 39°C, heart rate of 130 bpm, respiratory rate of 50 breaths/min, blood pressure of 90/50 mm Hg, and oxygen saturation on room air of 99%. He has cool extremities and poor perfusion, a nonblanching erythematous rash on the lower extremities, and clear lungs. After assuring airway patency and providing inhaled oxygen, what is the first step in stabilization of his hemodynamic status?

**A.** Epinephrine infusion

**B.** Dopamine infusion

**C.** Rapid administration of bolus isotonic fluids

**D.** Slow infusion of isotonic fluids

**E.** Administration of broad-spectrum antibiotics

**1-80.** A 6-month-old, former 37-week-gestation, previously well infant is described by her parents as having "stopped breathing." On further history, they describe that the infant had just fallen asleep when she suddenly gasped, turned "blue" around the mouth, appeared to be unable to breathe, and then after 30 seconds began to cry and returned to her normal color and tone. She has been in her usual state of health, with no recent fever or focal symptoms, and there are no sick contacts. Her exam is currently within normal limits. Appropriate diagnostic management, based on the American Academy of Pediatrics (AAP) clinical practice guideline for a brief resolved unexplained event (BRUE), should include which of the following?

**A.** Complete blood count (CBC), electrolytes, and electrocardiogram (ECG)

**B.** Head imaging

**C.** No further diagnostic testing

**D.** pH probe for gastroesophageal reflux (GER)

**E.** Nasopharyngeal swab for respiratory viruses

**1-81.** An 18-month-old child is brought in by ambulance after being found unresponsive at a relative's house. According to the relative, the child was playing in the living room during a party and then laid down to sleep on the floor. An hour later, they were unable to arouse the child, so they called an ambulance. On arrival, the child is minimally responsive to painful stimuli, with a heart rate of 80 bpm, a respiratory rate of 12 breaths/min, and a blood pressure of 80/50 mm Hg. Pupils are pinpoint. In addition to supportive care, what is the most important specific intervention at this time?

**A.** Sodium bicarbonate

**B.** Activated charcoal

**C.** Glucagon

**D.** *N*-Acetylcysteine

**E.** Naloxone

**1-82.** A 3-year-old child is brought in by a babysitter after she found him confused and vomiting. He was playing in his room alone on a cold day, and she had left the space heater on to keep the room warm. On exam, he appears confused and disoriented, is unable to stand on his own, and is dyspneic. His respiratory rate is 35 breaths/min, heart rate is 130 bpm, blood pressure is 100/75 mm Hg, and oxygen saturation on room air is 98%. Pupils are reactive bilaterally. The rest of the exam is unremarkable. What is the best test to confirm your suspected diagnosis?

**A.** Routine blood gas analysis

**B.** Serum toxicology screen

**C.** Carboxyhemoglobin (COHb) level via co-oximetry

**D.** Calculation of the anion gap

**E.** Methemoglobin level

**1-83.** A 3-year-old child is pulled unconscious from a body of water. He receives cardiopulmonary resuscitation (CPR) at the site by bystanders. On arrival, the paramedics detect a perfusing rhythm. He is stabilized and brought to the emergency department. What is the strongest predictor of outcome in this patient?

**A.** Whether the water was fresh or saltwater

**B.** The duration of submersion

**C.** The temperature of the water

**D.** The arrival time of paramedics

**E.** The child's ability to swim

**1-84.** You are talking to a family that has a 6-month-old child and a 3-year-old child. The family has just purchased a new house with a pool. They are interested in how best to keep their children safe from drowning. What should you tell them?

**A.** A pool cover is the best way to keep their children safe.

**B.** Teaching both children to swim is the best way to keep them safe.

**C.** Installing a self-latching fence around the pool is the most effective safety measure.

**D.** The children should only be allowed near the pool when an adult is outside.

**E.** Children can be taught to swim at an early age, including as young as 6 months.

**1-85.** What is the number one cause of death in the United States of children outside of the newborn period (1 month to 18 years of age)?

**A.** Infection

**B.** Trauma

**C.** Congenital abnormalities

**D.** Cancer

**E.** Poisoning

**1-86.** An 18-month-old child grabbed his grandmother's curling iron and sustained a burn on the palm of his hand. When you see him 2 hours later, the skin of his palm is erythematous, with areas of weeping and blistering, and is exquisitely painful to touch and to cold air. What is the most accurate description of the category of burn and approximate body surface area (BSA) affected?

**A.** Deep partial-thickness burn, 1% BSA

**B.** Deep partial-thickness burn, 5% BSA

**C.** Superficial partial-thickness burn, 1% BSA

**D.** Superficial partial-thickness burn, 5% BSA

**E.** Full-thickness burn, 5% BSA

**1-87.** A previously healthy 6-year-old boy is brought to medical attention several hours after being bitten by a neighbor's dog. He was trying to grab a toy out of the dog's mouth when the dog bit him on the hand. There are several puncture wounds and one jagged laceration that goes to the subcutaneous tissue. The patient's immunizations are up to date, and the dog is a family pet who is in good health. The patient is able to move all of his fingers normally, and there is faint erythema around the puncture wounds and the laceration. In addition to copious irrigation of the wounds, the most clearly indicated next step in management is which of the following?

**A.** Rabies immune globulin

**B.** Rabies vaccine

**C.** Tetanus booster

**D.** Suturing of the wounds

**E.** Systemic antibiotics (amoxicillin-clavulanate)

**1-88.** A family who is planning a camping trip with their 5-year-old twins calls the advice line asking for instructions on what to do in the event of a snakebite. They are traveling to an area of the United States that is home to rattlesnakes. In addition to reviewing prevention and rapid provision of medical care, what should you tell them to do in the event that one of the children is bitten on a limb?

**A.** Make a small incision near the bite and suck or squeeze out the venom.

**B.** Elevate the limb that is bitten above the heart.

**C.** Apply a tourniquet distal to the bite to prevent spread of the venom.

**D.** Immobilize and lower the bitten limb.

**E.** Do nothing, and seek professional care immediately.

**1-89.** A 30-month-old girl arrives in the emergency department with acute onset of fever of 40.1°C and severe stridor at rest. She is sitting in her parent's lap, appears ill and uncomfortable, and is drooling. Parents deny recent cough or upper respiratory infection symptoms. What is the first priority in this patient?

**A.** Perform a physical exam of the oropharynx.

**B.** Obtain intravenous access.

**C.** Obtain radiographs of chest and neck.

**D.** Obtain an arterial blood gas.

**E.** Perform airway management under controlled conditions.

**1-90.** A 3-year-old boy is being seen in the clinic for the second time with a "cold" and sore throat. On this visit, he has developed difficulty swallowing and is drooling. He has no cough and no stridor at rest, but his voice is "hoarse." He has a low-grade fever. His oxygen saturation is 99% on room air. He is tired but alert and well appearing. The left side of his neck is swollen and tender, but not erythematous, and he will not turn his head to that side or extend his neck. What is the most likely diagnosis?

**A.** Croup

**B.** Epiglottitis

**C.** Tracheitis

**D.** Retropharyngeal abscess

**E.** Peritonsillar abscess

**1-91.** An 18-month-old child is brought in with recurrent, severe coughing episodes. The episodes started when she was running around eating popcorn at a picnic earlier in the day; she suddenly began to cough, her face turned red, and she continued coughing for several minutes before being able to catch her breath. After this episode, she has had recurrent episodes of paroxysmal cough, with redness of the face and occasional posttussive vomiting over the remainder of the day. Her exam shows a normal respiratory rate and oxygen saturation. Her lung examination is notable for scattered wheezing on the right side. What is the best next step?

**A.** Pertussis polymerase chain reaction

**B.** Posteroanterior and lateral chest x-ray

**C.** Bilateral decubitus chest x-ray

**D.** Rigid bronchoscopy

**E.** Back blows or abdominal thrusts

**1-92.** There are anatomic and physiologic differences between the adult and pediatric airway and lungs. Which of the following anatomic factors places infants and young children at *higher* risk for decompensation from an upper airway obstruction?

**A.** Lower functional residual capacity

**B.** A relatively smaller tongue

**C.** A relatively smaller occiput

**D.** Relatively smaller adenoids and tonsils

**E.** Lower oxygen consumption

**1-93.** An 18-month-old child with a 2-day history of coryza now presents to the pediatric clinic with a cough. The mother describes the cough as "harsh" and "barking." Tonight, she noticed that the child is making a high pitched inspiratory noise when asleep. A neck radiograph is shown (Figure 118-2).

What is the diagnosis?

**A.** Pertussis

**B.** Croup

**C.** Epiglottitis

**D.** Retropharyngeal abscess

**E.** Foreign body

**1-94.** A 14-year-old soccer player is brought in by her parents after passing out during a soccer game on a hot summer day. The adolescent had come to the sidelines saying she felt overheated and dizzy, briefly lost consciousness, and then recovered within a few seconds. She continues to feel ill, complaining of muscle cramps, nausea, dizziness, and headache. Her core temperature is 38.6°C. Heart rate is 115 bpm. Respiratory rate is 20 breaths/min. She is alert and oriented, and her skin feels cool and moist. The best classification of her heat-related condition is which of the following?

**A.** Heat cramps

**B.** Heat edema

**C.** Heat syncope

**D.** Heat exhaustion

**E.** Heatstroke

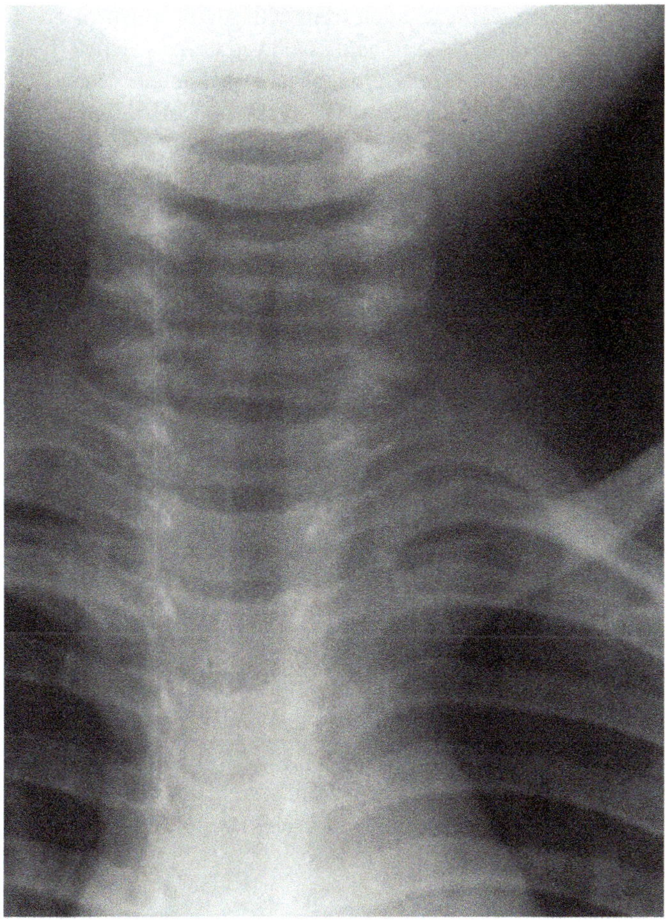

**FIGURE 118-2.** (Mark W. Kline, *Rudolph's Pediatrics*, 23rd Edition. Copyright © McGraw-Hill Education. All rights reserved.)

**1-95.** You are seeing a 3-year-old boy with trisomy 21 who has undergone cardiac surgery for complex congenital heart disease. He is oxygen dependent at night because of obstructive sleep apnea. He is taking levothyroxine for hypothyroidism and has just started to stand up with support. The medical student who is with you during the clinic visit asks about the current state of care for children with medical complexity in the United States. What is the best response?

**A.** Families are always included in healthcare decision-making for their children.

**B.** Parents of children with medical complexity may need to take time off from work and have fewer job opportunities.

**C.** Health care is often interdisciplinary with adequate communication among the different healthcare providers.

**D.** There are fewer medical errors that occur with this patient population.

**E.** Most health insurers have prioritized cost containment for this patient population.

**1-96.** What is the prevalence of children with medical complexity (CMC) in the United States?

**A.** 5% to 10% of all children in the United States

**B.** 1% to 5% of US children insured by Medicaid

**C.** 5% to 10% of US children insured by Medicaid

**D.** 15% to 20% of US children insured by Medicaid

**E.** 33% to 50% of US children insured by Medicaid

**1-97.** Your hospital has decided to develop a program to improve care for children with medical complexity (CMCs) and has identified both a hospitalist and a generalist to co-manage CMCs by assembling inpatient and outpatient teams to communicate and collaborate with each other and to provide seamless transition between inpatient and outpatient arenas. This approach is an example of which of the following models for care coordination?

**A.** Disease- or condition-specific care coordination program

**B.** Outpatient-based complex care service

**C.** Inpatient hospitalist-based complex care service

**D.** Integrated inpatient and outpatient services

**E.** Nurse visitation programs

**1-98.** You are seeing a 3-month-old infant with micrognathia, upper airway obstruction, and dysphagia. He has been fed through a nasogastric tube and has just been seen by a gastroenterologist, who recommends conversion of the nasogastric tube to a gastrostomy tube. What is the single most important consideration for this decision?

**A.** Reliance on the gastroenterologist on decision for gastrostomy tube conversion

**B.** Reliance on the pediatric surgeon on readiness for gastrostomy tube conversion

**C.** Reliance on the feeding therapist to indicate when therapy is not progressing

**D.** Shared decision-making between the primary care and subspecialist clinicians

**E.** Shared decision-making between the family and the care team

**1-99.** The parents of a 6-month-old infant with bronchopulmonary dysplasia and oxygen dependence at nighttime are exhausted because of the number of times they are wakened by the pulse oximetry alarm at night. The child is gaining weight well and beginning to achieve developmental milestones. According to her parents, every time they respond to the alarm, she appears well; she is sometimes woken up by the alarm and starts to cry. This makes it difficult for the parents to put her back to sleep. Oxygen saturation usually dips momentarily to 85% to 88% on room air and then returns to above 92%. The monitor is set to sound an alarm at 90%. The parents never have to intervene (ie, increase oxygen flow rate) because the saturation level returns to the normal range without intervention. What is the best next step?

**A.** Decrease the alarm setting to 85% and monitor how the patient does.

**B.** Refer the family to their pulmonologist; first available appointment is in 2 months.

**C.** Increase oxygen flow from 1 L/min to 2 L/min to prevent nighttime oxygen desaturation.

**D.** Direct the family to provide the patient with albuterol nebulization treatment 1 hour before sleep.

**E.** Recommend that the family bring their pulse oximeter to the vendor to get it fixed since that may be the reason why it is alarming so often.

**1-100.** You are seeing a 4-month-old infant for a hospital discharge follow-up visit for the first time. He was born preterm at 26 weeks of gestational age. During his hospitalization, he developed respiratory distress syndrome (RDS) and subsequent bronchopulmonary dysplasia. After a prolonged hospital stay for intensive respiratory support, he has just been discharged. He requires 2 L/min of oxygen by nasal cannula. His parents are negotiating with the vendor about his oxygen supply. You remind them about which of the following?

**A.** Liquid oxygen lasts longer than compressed oxygen.

**B.** Compressed oxygen can be cold and burn if it comes into contact with the skin.

**C.** The oxygen concentrator can deliver up to 2 L/min of 50% oxygen.

**D.** Backup compressed oxygen is recommended when using an oxygen concentrator.

**E.** Smoking is safe when oxygen is delivered with an oxygen concentrator.

**1-101.** You are seeing an adolescent with spastic quadriplegic cerebral palsy, neurogenic scoliosis, and restrictive lung disease for his annual health maintenance visit. Given recurrent aspiration pneumonias resulting in prolonged hospitalizations, he has recently undergone a tracheostomy. He does require nighttime oxygen but is not dependent on mechanical ventilation. A home visiting nurse accompanies him to the visit. The nurse is new at her position and asks about tips for tracheostomy care, especially on suctioning. Which of the following responses is correct?

**A.** Children with tracheostomies generally require suctioning once or twice daily.

**B.** Signs that a child needs suctioning include rattling mucus sounds, tachypnea, secretion pooling at the opening of the tracheotomy tube, and signs of respiratory distress.

**C.** Normal saline drops should not be instilled prior to suctioning because this can increase the risk of aspiration.

**D.** Suctioning until the catheter tip meets resistance from the carina is recommended to allow for complete clearance.

**E.** Suction pressure should only be applied on withdrawal of the suction catheter to avoid damaging the lining of the airway.

**1-102.** You are the primary care clinician for an infant with lissencephaly and seizure disorder. Her seizures are under relatively good control on antiepileptic medication, but she is quite developmentally delayed. She is 6 months old but is unable to hold her head up on her own. She has begun to move her extremities, but her lower extremities appear to have increased tone, and she has decreased truncal tone. You have just started a discussion with her family about her feedings and agree that learning to eat on her own without reliance on her nasogastric tube would be a desired goal. She has just started small amounts of pureed food for tasting purposes. Who would you refer this patient to for assessment and assistance in feeding?

**A.** Gastroenterologist

**B.** Physical therapist

**C.** Occupational therapist

**D.** Respiratory therapist

**E.** Speech and language pathologist

**1-103.** You are discussing wheeled mobility and seating with a 14-year-old patient with Duchenne muscular dystrophy and his parents. His neuromuscular dysfunction has been progressing. He is nonambulating, is now dependent on gastrostomy tube feeding because of difficulty with swallowing, and requires neck support when sitting up. He is no longer able to lift his shoulders; however, he can move his hands to use a keyboard and mouse. You agree with him and his family that maintenance of autonomy is a key goal in assuring his quality of life. What type of wheelchair would be most appropriate given his circumstances?

**A.** Stroller

**B.** Manual upright wheelchair

**C.** Manual tilt-in-space wheelchair

**D.** Power wheelchair

**E.** Scooter

**1-104.** You are following an 11-year-old child with trisomy 21 and mild to moderate intellectual disability. He has speech delay, mild conductive hearing loss, hypothyroidism, and elevated body mass index (BMI). He has recently undergone a tonsillectomy and adenoidectomy procedure for obstructive sleep apnea. Although he continues to have snoring attributable to postoperative upper airway inflammation, his parents are looking forward to resolution of his sleep problems. You remind them about which of the following?

**A.** Sleep disturbances are just as likely in children with intellectual disabilities as children without intellectual disabilities.

**B.** Attention to good sleep hygiene is not important in children with intellectual disabilities.

**C.** Poor sleep may be present in up to 25% of children with intellectual disability.

**D.** Symptoms of poor sleep include hyperactivity and aggressive behavior.

**E.** Melatonin should be considered if there is concern for obstructive sleep apnea.

**1-105.** Which of the following best exemplifies palliative care?

**A.** Nitrous oxide for acute respiratory distress in a 10-year-old child with moderate persistent asthma.

**B.** Human papillomavirus (HPV) immunization for a 14-year-old child with cerebral palsy and intellectual disability.

**C.** Anticipatory guidance to address recurrent elopement in an 8-year-old child with moderate autistic disorder and minimal verbal language.

**D.** Gastrostomy tube for failure to thrive in a 4-year-old child with developmental delay, hypotonia, and dysphagia.

**E.** Opioid treatment for moderate to severe pain in a 12-year-old child with metastatic osteosarcoma.

**1-106.** You are helping to guide decision-making by assessing interventions that meet identified goals rather than treat isolated medical problems. You remark during a meeting with parents of a child for whom you are providing palliative care, "Your child continues to receive exceptional care at home. My observation is that we are seeing fewer benefits from the treatment that we have available. What have you observed?" This communication is most consistent with which of the following objectives of palliative care?

**A.** Getting to know child and family

**B.** Determining goals of care as a guide to decision-making

**C.** Focusing on parent expertise

**D.** Acknowledging the limits of intervention

**E.** Offering continuity with a safety net

**1-107.** An interprofessional team provides expertise and collaboration in providing palliative care. Which of the following team members can best provide psychosocial assessment and supportive counseling for children and families adjusting to changes, skill in exploring hopes and worries of a patient and family, and expertise in identifying community resources?

**A.** Physicians

**B.** Nurses

**C.** Social workers

**D.** Chaplains

**E.** Child life specialists

**1-108.** You are providing palliative care to an 8-year-old child with muscular dystrophy who is dependent on gastrostomy tube feeding for dysphagia and failure to thrive. Medical interventions have not helped to decrease episodes of choking and coughing related to decreased ability to mobilize secretions. He has been hospitalized with increasing frequency for recurrent aspiration pneumonia. In the process of decision-making and defining a care plan, which of the following is an example of a step that can help determine how to proceed if the benefit hoped for from an intervention does not occur?

**A.** Define with the family the goals that you intend to meet.

**B.** Discuss with the patient what he would want family and friends to know.

**C.** Discuss with the patient and his family his resuscitation status.

**D.** Appoint a healthcare proxy.

**E.** Determine location of health care for acute illnesses.

**1-109.** You are about to have a discussion on pain control with a 7-year-old child, who has just been discharged from hospital after surgery for scoliosis, and his parents. The medical student who is with you during the clinic visit asks the patient to use a 0 to 10 scale to rate his pain. What rating tool would you suggest?

**A.** Poker chips

**B.** Oucher

**C.** Wong-Baker faces pain rating scale

**D.** 0 to 10 scale

**E.** FLACC scale

**1-110.** As the primary care pediatrician for a 12-year-old patient with moderate-to-severe cerebral palsy, spasticity and contractures of her extremities, scoliosis, restrictive lung disease, and dependence on gastrostomy tube feeding for nutrition, you are attempting to determine the cause of repetitive crying episodes. In the process of conducting a workup, you have excluded common etiologies such as otitis media, cholecystitis, urinary tract infection, pressure sores, and decubitus ulcers. In children with severe neurologic impairment who exhibit persistent pain-related behaviors, if extensive diagnostic workup does not yield a definitive source of pain, which of the following terms can be used to describe this scenario?

**A.** Nociceptive pain

**B.** Neuropathic pain

**C.** Constipation

**D.** Gastroesophageal reflux

**E.** Neuro-irritability

**1-111.** You are providing hospital discharge follow-up for your patient who underwent an osteotomy procedure for hip dysplasia. Which of the following statements is accurate with regard to management of pain?

**A.** Codeine has been demonstrated to be the most effective analgesic agent with the fewest side effects.

**B.** Ibuprofen has been demonstrated to achieve equivalent analgesia with fewer side effects than codeine.

**C.** Genetic variability in the metabolism of codeine places some individuals at higher risk for serious side effects, such as respiratory depression, at routine doses.

**D.** Integrative medicine, using approaches such as guided imagery, medication, and hypnosis, has been demonstrated not to be useful.

**E.** Acupuncture, hypnosis, and mind–body therapies have not been shown to be efficacious for pain and anxiety in children.

**1-112.** What is the most accurate statement about the use of opioids in pain treatment?

**A.** Opioids are the most effective agents for management of pain and dyspnea.

**B.** Opioid-induced respiratory depression is likely even when dosed appropriately.

**C.** Opioid use hastens death.

**D.** For optimal treatment of persistent, moderate-to-severe pain, opioid administration should be only as needed.

**E.** A reasonable trial dose of opioid for breakthrough pain is 25% of the 24-hour opioid requirement.

**1-113.** You are the primary care pediatrician for a 7-year-old child with acute lymphoblastic leukemia who has completed 3 cycles of chemotherapy. So far, she has not had any unusual or unexpected side effects of the chemotherapy, and her parents inform you that treatment is proceeding according to plan. However, the parents have noticed that she has become more quiet than usual. She does brighten up with play dates and has also expressed a desire to go back to school. She continues to eat well except during the few days following chemotherapy; her weight has remained stable, and she is able to fall asleep easily. Which of the following would you recommend to the family?

**A.** Social support systems to ameliorate distress

**B.** Targeted interventions and close monitoring

**C.** Consultation with behavioral health specialists, such as social workers or psychologists

**D.** Pharmacologic treatment with a medication such as melatonin

**E.** Psychopharmacologic treatment with medications such as selective serotonin reuptake inhibitors (SSRIs)

**1-114.** You are seeing a 14-year-old girl whom you have followed since she was an infant. She has moderate to severe cerebral palsy, intellectual disability, seizure disorder, scoliosis, and restrictive lung disease. She was recently hospitalized for recurrent aspiration pneumonia. You have been reminded by the hospitalist team that this would be an important time to begin discussions about advance care planning. Which of the following statements is most accurate about factors related to advance care planning?

**A.** Personal beliefs and experiences do not influence the definition of quality of life.

**B.** Many families routinely have discussions about advance care planning with their physicians.

**C.** Physicians are good prognosticators and can accurately predict survival.

**D.** Use of graphics can be helpful in communicating to families that planning is a flexible process.

**E.** Hope is similar to denial and can confuse end-of-life decisions.

**1-115.** The discussion of resuscitation plans may be more efficacious and effective when held in the context of a family's broader goals of care. You are facilitating such a discussion with the family of a 14-year-old child with severe cerebral palsy, intellectual disability, seizure disorder, scoliosis, and restrictive lung disease, who has been hospitalized several times recently for worsening respiratory symptoms. Which of the following communication recommendations is most helpful when discussing resuscitation plans?

**A.** Simplify decision-making and avoid confusion by presenting clear dichotomies, such as "doing everything" or "do nothing."

**B.** Discuss every single item that is included in a do not resuscitate (DNR) order.

**C.** Remind families that once they make a decision, they cannot change their mind.

**D.** Do not use the word "die" in discussions because family members can become upset.

**E.** Give legitimacy to both sides of a decision.

**1-116.** You are conducting rounds on the hospital ward and are about to enter the room of a 9-year-old patient with progressive muscular dystrophy who is wheelchair bound. The child recently lost his ability to swallow and is receiving palliative care. The medical student on your care team asks what the patient is able to understand about death and dying. What is the best response?

**A.** The patient has no intellectual concept of death.

**B.** The patient may believe that death is temporary and sleep-like and that people can return from death.

**C.** The patient understands death as universal and inevitable and may ask about details of the dying experience.

**D.** The patient understands death as universal and inevitable and may be concerned about physical appearance, such as hair loss and weakness.

**E.** The patient likely does not want to discuss death; therefore, healthcare providers should not raise the topic since it will be upsetting to do so.

**1-117.** During a routine well-child visit, you are informed by the parent of a 7-year-old child that her grandmother, who had been a close member of the family, had recently died. The 7-year-old patient has been experiencing episodes of sadness and difficulties with sleep. Which of the following is a helpful approach to support your patient who is grieving?

**A.** Try to "cheer up" the patient.

**B.** Encourage her to be strong and to minimize expressions of distress.

**C.** Do not tell her how she should feel; rather, ask her about her own feelings.

**D.** Do not offer to speak with children and adolescents by themselves.

**E.** Do not initiate such discussions because that may further upset her.

**1-118.** For a young child, which of the following factors may lead to guilt related to the death of a close family member?

**A.** Adults withhold information

**B.** Magical thinking and egocentrism

**C.** Narrow religious explanations

**D.** Exclusion from memorial activities, such as funerals

**E.** Underestimating the impact on children

**1-119.** You are the primary care hospitalist for a 16-year-old boy with metastatic osteosarcoma. Conventional chemotherapy has not resulted in anticipated improvements. Although your patient has confidentially revealed to you that he would like to stop further treatment and focus on palliative care, his parents are intent on pursuing experimental therapies. What is the most accurate statement about decision-making at the end of life?

**A.** Since your patient, when healthy, held a part-time job while living at home, he should be able to make medical decisions on his own.

**B.** Since your patient has lived with his condition for a long time and understands treatment choices, he should be able to make medical decisions on his own.

**C.** Given that you agree with your patient, you should question the parents' capacity to make medical decisions.

**D.** When there are disagreements between patients and families, healthcare providers can play an important role by engaging them in open dialogue to ensure that everyone's perspectives are heard.

**E.** Since parents have ultimate decision-making authority, if they wish to pursue experimental therapies, patient preference should not be considered in any decision-making discussions.

## ANSWERS

**Answer 1-1.** B

Carbon monoxide (CO) is an odorless gas produced by incomplete combustion of carbon fuels. Common sources include house fires and automobile exhaust. Other sources include improperly ventilated water heaters, stoves, or fireplaces. One should suspect CO poisoning if a patient is found unconscious in a house fire or a running automobile. The patient in the clinical vignette likely had his car running while he was listening to music from the car radio. Mild symptoms can include malaise, nausea/vomiting, headache, dizziness, or confusion. Severe symptoms include syncope, seizures, coma, respiratory depression, and death. CO detectors are available and are often used in conjunction with smoke detectors.

Influenza and meningitis are unlikely because there are no signs of infection or fever. Recreational drug use is also less likely given the negative drug screen.

(p. 32, Section 1: Foundations in Pediatric Practice and Child Health, Chapter 10: Environmental Pediatrics)

**Answer 1-2.** C

Lead is a metal that serves no physiologic function. In small amounts, even below the acceptable value of 5 μg/dL, lead can affect the developing brain.

Lead exposure most commonly comes from lead-based paint or lead-contaminated dust or dirt. Young children spend much of their time with their hands on the floor, and normal hand-to-mouth activity may contribute to exposure. Lead-based paint was banned in 1978, but exposures may continue if the home is older and chipping paint exists. Other sources include lead inhalation if there is a lead smelting or automobile battery plant near a child's home or the adults caring for the child work in those industries. Other sources can include fishing weights, ceramics, and contaminated herbal remedies, cosmetics, or spices.

Lead exposure can be associated with anorexia, constipation, abdominal pain, and vomiting. More serious lead exposure can cause seizures, high blood pressure, coma, and encephalopathy. The treatment is based on the child's symptoms and the blood lead level. Chelation therapy is usually reserved for children with a blood lead level > 45 μg/dL.

(pp. 32–33, Section 1: Foundations in Pediatric Practice and Child Health, Chapter 10: Environmental Pediatrics)

**Answer 1-3.** D

Early childhood caries are one of the most common pediatric health problems. It is estimated that 37% of children aged 2 to 8 years have some evidence of caries in their primary teeth. Children at high risk for development of caries include children of color, those in low- to moderate-income households, and those with special healthcare needs. Other risk factors include dry mouth or any condition that impairs salivary production, history of cavities in a sibling or parent, and frequent exposure to sugary foods such as cookies, juices, and candy.

Prolonged bottle use can certainly result in development of childhood caries, especially if a child is taking the bottle in sips on demand, between meals, and after infancy. Bottle use during infancy, however, is not considered to be a risk factor in future development of caries. Living in a high-altitude area does not increase the risk of caries. The presence of a high-arched palate, by itself, is not a risk factor for the development of caries.

(pp. 45–46, Section 1: Foundations in Pediatric Practice and Child Health, Chapter 12: Oral Health Supervision)

**Answer 1-4.** E

Vertical and horizontal transmission of *Streptococcus mutans* is known to cause caries in children. Horizontal transmission refers to the transmission of bacteria among members of a group, such as between siblings or among children at a daycare. Vertical transmission refers to the transmission of bacteria from a caregiver to a child. An example is a mother who wets a pacifier with her saliva before giving it to the child. Infants without teeth can still be colonized with *S mutans,* which can be a risk factor for developing early childhood caries and adult caries as well. It is important to review good dental hygiene practices at each pediatrics visit. These practices include brushing twice daily and flossing, using fluoridated toothpaste, and avoiding prolonged bottle use and high consumption of sugary foods.

The other bacteria, including *Streptococcus pyogenes, Streptococcus viridans, Staphylococcus epidermidis,* and *Staphylococcus aureus,* are not known to cause dental caries.

(pp. 46–48, Section 1: Foundations in Pediatric Practice and Child Health, Chapter 12: Oral Health Supervision)

**Answer 1-5.** A

Fluoride is effective in helping prevent dental caries. Therefore, fluoridated toothpaste is recommended for infants and children after tooth eruption. Infants and children younger than 3 years old can use a tiny smear approximately the size of a grain of rice when they brush their teeth. Children older than 3 years can use a pea-sized amount of fluoridated toothpaste. Older children may use a little more if they can spit it out after brushing. Excess fluoride can sometimes cause fluorosis, so it is important for children to use the appropriate amount.

Fluoride is found in toothpaste, tap water, and bottled water. However, some toothpastes are fluoride-free, and patients may live in areas without a fluoridated water supply. Bottled water may contain fluoride, but the amount varies between brands, and some have none. Fluoride can also be prescribed as a tablet or applied as a varnish on the teeth. Pediatricians should prescribe fluoride tablets if the child's water supply contains a fluoride level $< 0.6$ ppm. Fluoride varnish can be applied at the dentist's office or at the pediatrician's office.

(p. 48, Section 1: Foundations in Pediatric Practice and Child Health, Chapter 12: Oral Health Supervision)

**Answer 1-6.** B

Complementary and integrative medicine practices are common. It is important for pediatricians to be somewhat familiar with these practices so that they can meet the needs of their patients and families. There are many forms of complementary and alternative medicine, including meditation, yoga, hypnosis, homeopathy, music therapy, art therapy, and many others. Some mind-body practices, including meditation, yoga, and hypnosis, can have a calming effect and may be helpful for patients with impulsivity, including those with ADHD. This is one example of a nonpharmacologic approach to treating ADHD. Mind-body practices have shown to be helpful in a variety of conditions including chronic pain, mood disorders, and procedural anxiety.

This case does not warrant involvement of the court, and it is the parent's right to refuse to use medication for the child's ADHD. Fluoxetine is a selective serotonin reuptake inhibitor (SSRI) and is not the first-line treatment for ADHD. There is no indication for a sleep study at this time because the case does not mention any sleep difficulties. Multivitamins are good for children who may have dietary vitamin deficiencies but are not the first-line treatment for ADHD.

(pp. 51–52, Section 1: Foundations in Pediatric Practice and Child Health, Chapter 13: Complementary and Integrative Pediatrics)

**Answer 1-7.** C

Homeopathy is a whole medical system that was founded by a German physician, Samuel Hahnemann (1755–1843). Homeopathy is based on the idea that if a remedy would cause a set of symptoms in a healthy person, a dilution of this remedy would cure the same set of symptoms in a sick person. Homeopathic medicines are made from plants, animals, and minerals. They can be obtained without a prescription. In 2012, it was estimated that 5 million adults and 1 million children in the United States used homeopathy in the past year.

(pp. 53–54, Section 1: Foundations in Pediatric Practice and Child Health, Chapter 13: Complementary and Integrative Pediatrics)

**Answer 1-8.** D

Dietary supplements may include herbs, vitamins, and minerals and are among the most commonly used complementary and alternative medicine therapies. Fish oils, probiotics, and echinacea are common examples of dietary supplements. These supplements may be recommended by integrative pediatricians or conventional pediatricians and do not require a prescription but are readily available online or in most drugstores. The Dietary Supplement Health and Education Act (DSHEA) of 1994 defined herbal medicines and supplements as neither food nor drugs. Dietary supplements are regulated by the US Food and Drug Administration (FDA) but have less rigorous standards for safety and efficacy compared to prescription and over-the-counter drugs. Under the DSHEA, dietary supplements cannot claim to cure or treat disease.

Melatonin is a hormone that is involved in sleep–wake cycles and, as a supplement, may be effective for many patients with sleep problems. It is easily obtained over the counter.

(p. 55, Section 1: Foundations in Pediatric Practice and Child Health, Chapter 13: Complementary and Integrative Pediatrics)

**Answer 1-9.** D

Ideal infant nutrition consists of breastmilk and/or infant formula until 1 year of life, with the introduction of complementary foods from age 4 to 6 months. (The American Academy of Pediatrics [AAP] recommendation is starting solids at 6 months for exclusively breastfed infants.) An emphasis should be placed on additional sources of iron for both breastfed and formula-fed infants at 6 months of age. This can be accomplished by offering iron-rich foods (meats, fortified cereals, or leafy greens) or an iron vitamin. Recommended iron intake from 7 to 12 months of age is 11 to 40 mg/d. Breast milk contains adequate iron and zinc for the first 4 to 6 months. In addition, iron from breast milk has been shown to be better absorbed than iron from formula. Breast milk and infant formula also provide ideal calcium and phosphorus in the ratio of 2:1 for adequate bone mineralization. In addition to iron needs changing with age, so do protein needs.

There is an increased need for protein in the second year of life, which can be provided for with complementary foods and by switching to cow's milk, which has an increased protein per milliliter ratio compared to breast milk or infant formula. Cow's milk would not be appropriate for this infant under 1 year of age given the poor digestibility of fats; inadequate levels of vitamin C, zinc, iron, and essential fatty acids; and the high amounts of protein, sodium, chloride, and phosphorus. Soy milk is also not recommended at this age because it is not regulated by the FDA and so often is not consistent between brands. Neither soy milk nor cow's milk would provide the adequate amount of other nutrients and in the right concentrations for ideal growth, development, and bone mineralization.

(pp. 67–69, Section 2: Nutrition, Chapter 15: Normal Nutritional Requirements)

**Answer 1-10.** B

There are very few antibiotics and other medications without acceptable alternatives that are contraindicated in breastfeeding. This mother should continue the cephalexin because it is safe in breastfeeding.

Mastitis itself is not a contraindication to breastfeeding, and mothers should be encouraged to continue breastfeeding, especially on the affected side. Breastfeeding should be suspended for 24 to 48 hours only if a mother were to have mastitis complicated by a breast abscess or cellulitis. It is also important to counsel this mother about frequent emptying to maintain supply. She has gone 24 hours without emptying, which puts her at risk for clogged ducts, recurrent mastitis, and diminished milk supply.

The early postpartum period is a critical time for both establishing a healthy milk supply and supporting, educating, and counseling mothers through the difficulties of breastfeeding. There are large racial, ethnic, and socioeconomic disparities in initiation and continuation of breastfeeding. It is important to identify barriers to continued breastfeeding for each mother and attempt to support her efforts. For this mother, it would also be beneficial to address the familial pressure she may feel to formula feed and provide education about the superior nutritional and immunologic benefits of breast milk in comparison to formula.

(p. 76, Section 2: Nutrition, Chapter 16: Breastfeeding)

**Answer 1-11.** C

Infant formula is the only acceptable nutrition alternative for infants when breast milk is not available. Families have many options when it comes to choosing an infant formula, and for the most part, they are nutritionally very similar. However, the American Academy of Pediatrics (AAP) Committee on Nutrition recommends against the use of soy formula except for those infants whose families want to maintain a vegan diet, infants with hereditary lactase deficiency, or infants with galactosemia.

Soy-based infant formulas are specifically *not* recommended for preterm infants; to manage colic, allergies, or atopic disease; or as an alternative nutrition source for infants with cow milk protein–induced enterocolitis or enteropathy. The infant in this case is exhibiting fussiness and gas, which are both age appropriate and unlikely to be related to lactose intolerance because this is exceedingly rare in this age group. In addition, if this child were showing signs of cow milk protein–induced gastrointestinal disease, soy formula would not be recommended because there is often reaction to soy as well. There is no evidence to support the use of soy formula to manage colic or atopic dermatitis because there is no significant improvement in symptoms with its use.

(p. 77, Section 2: Nutrition, Chapter 17: Infant Formula and Complementary Foods)

**Answer 1-12.** A

Premature infants, especially those born at 31 weeks or earlier and < 1800 g, are at greatest risk of poor growth, protein deficiency, and poor bone mineralization after discharge. They have increased needs for calories, calcium, magnesium, phosphorus, vitamin D, and iron, and need supplementation of these with either a preterm infant formula or human milk fortifier in the breast milk.

Both preterm infant formula and human milk fortifier provide increased levels of protein, sodium, calcium, phosphorus, and other vitamins. In addition, preterm infants (born at 36 6/7 weeks and under) need iron supplementation sooner and at higher doses than for a term infant. Iron can be started at 2 weeks of age, with a dose of 2 to 3 mg/kg daily and continued through 1 year of life. It can be obtained from a multivitamin with iron, iron supplements, iron-fortified formula, and iron-containing complementary foods. If iron is provided by complementary foods alone, very close consideration should be paid to amounts of iron in those foods and how much the child is actually taking in because often these preterm infants will need iron supplementation as well to prevent anemia.

Given that this child has had good catch-up growth and is now at 50% for height, weight, and head circumference, there is no need for preterm/transitional formula or supplemental feeds. The American Academy of Pediatrics (AAP) recommends continuing transitional formula or supplementary feeds until weight for length is maintained at > 25th percentile or the infant reaches 6 months' CGA. It is common practice to continue the supplemented feeding plan until at least 48 weeks' CGA, as long as the child is growing well, to ensure good brain growth and bone mineralization during a critical period. This child has reached both milestones.

(pp. 84–85, Section 2: Nutrition, Chapter 18: Postdischarge Nutrition for the Premature Infant)

**Answer 1-13.** D

Adolescents, in general, are at risk of deficiencies in iron and calcium. Girls, given lower calorie intake, are more susceptible to vitamin and mineral deficiencies. In addition, menstruating girls are at further risk of iron deficiency due to blood loss. This girl is also vegan, which puts her at risk for further nutrient deficiencies. Vegan patients should be recommended to eat nuts, seeds, and grains combined with legumes (ideally at the same meal) so that adequate amounts of essential amino acids are available for protein synthesis. Iron, calcium, and zinc are also more difficult to get in vegetarian and vegan diets. Plant foods contain only nonheme iron and so are more susceptible to inhibitors of iron absorption than heme iron. Given she is also a menstruating female, this patient should increase her iron-rich foods and consider taking an iron supplement. She should also pay particular attention to eating calcium-rich foods, such as calcium-fortified soy milk, or take a calcium supplement. Vitamin $B_{12}$ is found only in products of animal origin, and so it is required for her to take a supplement. With careful attention to these factors, a vegan diet can provide adequate nutrition.

(pp. 86–88, Section 2: Nutrition, Chapter 19: Nutritional Issues: Toddler to Adolescent)

**Answer 1-14.** E

There has been an increasing focus on early childhood adversity and the relationship to adult medical and psychosocial problems. The landmark study was the Adverse Childhood Experiences (ACE) Study, which enrolled > 17,000 people and screened them for exposure to ACEs, including abuse, neglect, and household dysfunction, such as a parent with substance abuse or a parent who was incarcerated. One main finding was the shocking number of participants who experienced ACEs, including 25% who were physically abused and 20% who were sexually abused. The second main finding was the dose–response relationship between ACEs and adult medical and psychosocial problems and even early death.

Although adverse events can affect people at any age, children in the first 3 years of life seem particularly vulnerable to toxic stresses given the plasticity of the brain in infancy and early childhood. Symptoms in older children can be varied and can affect their functioning in school and in their social lives, with symptoms of impulsivity and poor concentration.

It is important to note that not all stressful events are detrimental to a child's life. Positive stress occurs when a child faces challenges and finds a positive outcome, which can build resilience and self-confidence.

(pp. 125–126, Section 3: Social-Environmental Factors, Chapter 28: Childhood Adversity and Toxic Stress)

**Answer 1-15.** E

Families living in poverty present with unique and complex challenges related to their health, mental well-being, development, and education. Poverty is defined based on the federal poverty level (FPL), which is derived from an estimation of how much food costs. The FPL for a family of 4 in 2015 was $24,036. Poverty can be brief, chronic, or cyclical, and about 37% of children in the United States will experience poverty during their childhood. Families often need to make difficult budget decisions, such as whether to pay for food or heating their home. As a result, hunger and malnutrition tend to be more common in the winter compared to the summer. Food insecurity is important to diagnose in the pediatrician's office, and there exist state and federal programs to assist with this, including the Women, Infants, and Children (WIC) program, the Supplemental Nutrition Assistance Program (SNAP), and the National School Lunch Program. Besides food insecurity, many families have struggles maintaining routines, and therefore, children are less likely to participate in extracurricular activities, which may lead to additional social isolation. Poverty can be associated with toxic stress, and research shows that there is a chemical basis for this chronic stress with prolonged activation of the HPA axis.

It is important to note that many families with poverty, associated food insecurity, or housing instability may go undiagnosed at the pediatrician's office. Therefore, it is important for pediatricians to screen regularly for social determinants of health.

(pp. 131–132, Section 3: Social-Environmental Factors, Chapter 30: Poverty, Homelessness, and Social Disorganization)

**Answer 1-16.** D

Parental discord, separation, and divorce can have lasting impacts on children. Children may feel insecure, have low self-esteem, and have difficulty with trust. Family discord and divorce are common, and many divorces happen during childbearing years. There can be varied symptoms depending on the age of the child. Infants and young children are influenced by the emotional state of their caregivers. Young school-aged children such as the boy in the vignette may have behavioral problems that can impact learning or socialization. Older children or adolescents may present with emotional disturbance, mood disorders, or psychosomatic complaints.

Both parents care for the child and have been present at each visit, but it is not the job of the pediatrician to determine custody arrangements. This decision will be determined by the court. The child may have a component of ADHD given impulsivity, but the overlying marital discord is likely impacting his behavior at school. It would be important to talk to the teacher about this behavior, but most important would be to assess the child's well-being in general. The child is silent during the visit, but this does not necessarily diagnose selective mutism. Given the family circumstances, it may reflect a developing emotional disturbance or mood disorder.

(p. 134, Section 3: Social-Environmental Factors, Chapter 31: Family Discord and Divorce)

**Answer 1-17.** D

There has been a decline over the past decade in crimes committed by juveniles. In 2014, the rate of violent crimes committed by juveniles was half the rate in 1980. The rate for girls, however, is unchanged. Girls account for approximately 19% of all juvenile arrests for violent crime. Mental health issues differ by sex, with girls reporting more traumatic exposures and psychiatric disorders. Unfortunately, nearly half of incarcerated youth have substance abuse issues. There has recently been more focus on deaths of African American boys and young men at the hands of law enforcement. Although the pediatric death rate is low overall (0.05 deaths per 100,000 in 2014), the majority of deaths occur in boys, and black boys and youth die at a rate 3 times that of whites. Pediatricians should be aware of this racial disparity when discussing safety and prevention with their patients.

(p. 140, Section 3: Social-Environmental Factors, Chapter 32: Family and Community Violence)

**Answer 1-18.** C

The child in the vignette has a diagnosed mood disorder and school avoidance. His history of depression combined with the normal impulsivity of adolescence make him at risk for suicide. Firearms are among the leading causes of death for children aged 10 to 19 years. The majority of suicides in adolescents involve firearms, and > 90% of those are completed suicides. The presence of guns in the home is associated with a 5-fold increase in risk of adolescent suicide. The pediatrician should counsel the family that the safest home for a child is one without guns.

(pp. 140–141, Section 3: Social-Environmental Factors, Chapter 32: Family and Community Violence)

**Answer 1-19.** B

Teen dating violence (TDV) encompasses physical, sexual, and mental abuse in adolescent relationships. With the advances in technology and social media, new and complex issues are emerging in this topic, as adolescent patients are navigating their relationships online as well as in person. Pediatricians should be aware of the risk factors for TDV, including a history of exposure to relationship violence or other adverse childhood events, involvement in the juvenile justice system, or a history of early or risky sexual behavior or alcohol or drug abuse. Patients may also have symptoms of mood disorders such as anxiety or depression or have irregular or fragmented medical care. It should not be reassuring that the patient is dismissive of the mother's concerns. Many victims of TDV accept the violent acts of their partners and may misinterpret controlling behavior for love and affection.

The pediatrician's first step should be to confirm the suspicion of TDV and assess for safety. Patients may be physically abused, including biting, hair-pulling, slapping, punching, kicking, or using a weapon. Sexual abuse may also be present in the form of unwanted or nonconsensual kissing or touching or even rape. Reproductive coercion may also be present when partners wish to control the patient's reproductive health. Psychological abuse is usually present if physical or sexual abuse is present and can be overt, such as ridiculing or yelling or threatening, especially in the presence of others, or can be very subtle, with intrusive or harassing behaviors such as excessive texting or surveillance that causes the patient mental distress. The other answers, including a pregnancy test, a break from screen time and use of the phone, and family therapy, may indeed be part of a therapeutic plan, but the immediate responsibility of the pediatrician is to identify TDV and assess for safety and associated medical and mental health problems. Discussing the relationship with the boyfriend could also be helpful, although this is not the immediate concern of the pediatrician.

(pp. 142–145, Section 3: Social-Environmental Factors, Chapter 33: Teen Dating Violence)

**Answer 1-20.** A

Child trafficking is a form of slavery. According to the social-ecological model, there are societal, community, relationship, and individual risk factors that place children at a higher risk for coercion and trafficking. One such risk factor is a history of maltreatment, although there are many more risk factors related to immigration, global health, politics, and human rights. Pediatricians should be aware of how to identify victims of human trafficking in order to treat their unique medical and mental health needs. Not surprisingly, trafficked victims suffer emotional trauma and are at risk for mental health diagnoses such as depression and anxiety. The patient in the vignette is a pregnant minor who presents with a companion who stays with her at all times, and she refuses to be interviewed without him. Patients may also have a poor or inconsistent history, a hesitation to answer basic questions like living or work situations, and may avoid eye contact or alternatively have hostile behavior or disorientation. Repeated sexually transmitted infections (STIs) or pregnancy may also be present. Signs of physical abuse such as abnormal bruises are also important to note. More subtle presentations such as repeated somatic complaints may also be present.

Trafficked victims report interfacing with medical professionals, with some estimates indicating that up to 88% of victims see a provider during their time of captivity. If a clinician suspects coercion, it is important to try to obtain consent to talk with the patient. State laws govern consent, and so providers should be aware of their state's laws around consent for contraception, STI evaluation and treatment, and other sensitive issues.

(pp. 146–148, Section 3: Social-Environmental Factors, Chapter 34: Child Trafficking)

**Answer 1-21.** E

Infant crying is a normal behavior with great variability between individuals. Colic is generally understood as excessive crying. Normal crying patterns include increased crying from birth to 6 weeks of life and decreased crying thereafter. One study showed an average duration of crying to be up to 110 to 118 minutes per day in the first 6 weeks, decreasing to 70 minutes per day by the 12th week. Crying also appears to cluster in the evening hours. Babies in the same family may have considerable variability, and an individual baby may also vary in the amount of crying from one day to the next.

The differential diagnosis for infant crying is wide, ranging from normal behavior to life-threatening illness. Crying may result from neurologic disease such as seizures, gastrointestinal disease such as reflux or food allergy, or cardiac disease such as congenital heart defects. These are just some of the possible explanations for infant crying. Red flags that may suggest a diagnosis other than colic are listed in Table 35-1.

The vignette describes a child with a typical pattern of crying behavior, at a classic age, with normal growth and a normal physical exam. With other causes ruled out, colic is an appropriate diagnosis of exclusion. Reassurance and continued observation are appropriate next steps.

Eliminating dairy would be appropriate if you were concerned about a milk protein allergy, which typically presents as bloody stools. Infants with severe reflux symptoms requiring treatment often present with poor weight gain. Lactose intolerance is rare in this age.

(p. 149, Section 3: Social-Environmental Factors, Chapter 35: Infant Colic)

**Answer 1-22.** D

Childhood maltreatment includes physical abuse, neglect, sexual abuse, exploitation, and emotional or psychosocial maltreatment. Neglect occurs when caregivers do not meet the child's needs including nutrition, shelter, clothing, or supervision. It may also mean failing to bring the child to necessary healthcare appointments or to provide the child with an education. The most common type of maltreatment is neglect, not physical abuse, sexual abuse, or emotional maltreatment.

Although the cases of reported childhood maltreatment have increased, the cases of substantiated claims based on the National Child Abuse and Neglect Data System have decreased between 1990 and 2013. Most children who die of abuse or neglect are younger than 3 years of age. Most maltreatment occurs in the home by parents.

(p. 152, Section 3: Social-Environmental Factors, Chapter 36: Child Maltreatment: Neglect to Abuse)

**Answer 1-23.** A

Factitious disorder by proxy (FDP), commonly known as Munchausen by proxy or medical child abuse, is a diagnostic description for abuse through fabrication. The abusive caretaker is most commonly the mother. The history may reveal chronic illness and ongoing physical ailments despite extensive workup, including numerous medications, procedures, and hospital stays. Caregivers can deceive physicians for years because they can convince others of their caring and may be unusually adept in medical knowledge and very supportive of the physician and the plans for diagnostic management and treatment. Abuse in cases of FDP persists for an average of 14 to 22 months before diagnosis. Characteristics of FDP are listed in Table 37-1.

The other answers, including immunodeficiency, inflammatory bowel disease, constipation, and mitochondrial illness, are possible but less likely. A child with immunodeficiency would likely have a history of multiple serious infections. A child with inflammatory bowel disease would have other physical exam findings and laboratory abnormalities. There is no history of constipation in the child. Although mitochondrial illness would present with a constellation of symptoms, FDP is a better fit for the clinical vignette.

(p. 159, Section 3: Social-Environmental Factors, Chapter 37: Factitious Disorder by Proxy)

**Answer 1-24.** C

Factitious disorder by proxy (FDP) is a form of abuse when a child's disease is falsified by the primary caregiver. This is most commonly the mother. This form of child abuse often goes undiagnosed for years before identification, as caregivers are often skilled in manipulating the medical team. The child has often had multiple procedures, hospitalizations, and medications without improvement in reported symptoms. Symptoms may also not be present when hospital personnel are present. Caregivers may be unusually calm or happy when their child needs a serious procedure or treatment. This patient was likely given the grandfather's warfarin, and the mother, who works in the lab, likely fabricated the negative warfarin results. A child with liver disease would likely have other symptoms including vomiting or jaundice.

(p. 159, Section 3: Social-Environmental Factors, Chapter 37: Factitious Disorder by Proxy)

**Answer 1-25.** B

Children in foster care face unique challenges. Pediatricians have a responsibility to address the mental health, medical, and developmental problems for children in foster care. Approximately 10% of children in foster care stay in the child welfare system for years, and about half return to their biological families within 6 months after placement. In 2014, 21% of children in foster care were adopted. Adolescents and children with behavioral problems tend to stay in the child welfare system for longer and may have multiple foster care placements.

Despite the challenges that foster children face, studies show that after foster care placement, children have improvements in their levels of conduct disorder behaviors, hyperactivity, and emotional stability, as well as better school attendance and performance.

**TABLE 35-1.** Physical Exam Findings Implying Pathologic Causes of Crying

| Exam | Concerning Findings for Underlying Pathology |
|---|---|
| Anthropomorphic parameters and vital signs | **Failure to thrive** (broad differential)<br>**Macrocephaly or microcephaly** (hydrocephalus, number of underlying genetic syndromes)<br>**Fever, tachycardia** (sepsis, urinary tract infection [UTI], congestive heart failure) |
| General appearance | **Decreased activity** (sepsis, abusive head trauma, metabolic derangements)<br>**High-pitched cry, excess sweating** (neonatal abstinence syndrome) |
| Head, eyes, ears, nose, and throat (HEENT) | **Photophobia, conjunctival erythema** (corneal abrasion)<br>**Mouth breathing** (choanal stenosis, nasal mass)<br>**Sneezing and congestion** (upper respiratory infection, neonatal abstinence)<br>**Oral ulcers** (herpangina)<br>**Bulging tympanic membrane** (acute otitis media)<br>**Decreased neck range of motion** (retropharyngeal abscess) |
| Cardiac | **Irregular rate** (supraventricular tachycardia)<br>**Gallop** (congestive heart failure, myocarditis) |
| Respiratory | **Asymmetric breath sounds** (foreign body aspiration)<br>**Wheezing, crackles** (bronchiolitis)<br>**Stridor** (croup or foreign body) |
| Neurologic | **Full fontanelle** (hydrocephalus, meningitis, encephalitis)<br>**Delayed motor skills or altered tone** (neurologic disease) |
| Gastrointestinal | **Distended abdomen** (malrotation, obstruction)<br>**Tender to palpation** (appendicitis, volvulus, gastroenteritis)<br>**Presence of mass** (pyloric stenosis, malignancy)<br>**Rectal tone increased** (Hirschsprung disease)<br>**Inguinal hernia** (incarcerated hernia) |
| Musculoskeletal | **Full range of motion of joints** (septic joint, dislocation)<br>**Deformity or palpable mass on long bones** (fracture, malignancy)<br>**Crying elicited by palpation of extremities** (osteomyelitis)<br>**Mucus or bloody stool in diaper** (cow's milk protein allergy, intussusception) |
| Skin | **Pallor** (anemia, malignancy)<br>**Jaundice** (hyperbilirubinemia, sepsis, urinary tract infection [UTI])<br>**Bruises or burn marks** (abuse)<br>**Eczema** (food allergy)<br>**Hair tourniquet** |
| Genitourinary | **Testicular mass or swelling** (torsion) |

Mark W. Kline, *Rudolph's Pediatrics*, 23rd Edition. Copyright © McGraw-Hill Education. All rights reserved.

(p. 163, Section 3: Social-Environmental Factors, Chapter 38: Foster Care and Adoption)

**Answer 1-26.** B

Pediatricians can provide needed medical treatment and appropriate referrals for children who are in foster care to help meet their unique physical, neurodevelopmental, and emotional needs. Children in foster care may present with different psychosocial, mental health, and physical ailments compared to other children. Children in foster care are 10 to 15 times more likely to have been exposed to alcohol prenatally and may have subsequent fetal alcohol spectrum disorder. Unfortunately, most cases of this disorder go undiagnosed.

**TABLE 37-1.** Clinical Profiles Suspicious for Factitious Disorder by Proxy

| **Child Presentations** |
|---|
| A child who presents with medical problems that do not respond to treatment or that follow an unusual course |
| Signs and symptoms of a child's illness fail to occur in the parent's absence |
| **Parent Presentations** |
| A parent who is medically knowledgeable and/or fascinated with medical details and hospital gossip |
| A parent who appears unusually calm or even giddy in the face of serious difficulties in the course of her child's illness and may at the same time be very supportive of the physician; some parents may become demanding and angry when further investigations and procedures are resisted by staff |
| Discrepancies in the medical history or presentation as reported by the parent |
| A parent who makes self-serving efforts at public acknowledgment |

Mark W. Kline, *Rudolph's Pediatrics*, 23rd Edition. Copyright © McGraw-Hill Education. All rights reserved.

Mental health problems, including depression and anxiety, are more common in children in foster care, with more use of prescription psychotropic medications as well. After placement, there is sometimes a "honeymoon period" in the initial months, but some significant problems may emerge thereafter, including sleep disturbances and poor appetite or overeating. Most children placed in foster care are placed because of parental abuse or neglect, rather than illness or death of the parent or extreme poverty. Compared to younger children, adolescents have the greatest placement instability, sometimes being placed directly from the juvenile justice system or having grown up in long-term foster care.

(pp. 161–162, Section 3: Social-Environmental Factors, Chapter 38: Foster Care and Adoption)

**Answer 1-27.** A

It is important for pediatricians to identify childhood maltreatment and provide appropriate referrals to ensure the child's safety. Several things make a child at higher risk for maltreatment, including parental depression, intimate partner violence, and drug or alcohol abuse. These topics are often difficult for families to discuss freely, so pediatricians may use screening tools to start the conversation. One such screening tool is from the primary care model called Safe Environment for Every Kid (SEEK). It starts with general safety questions regarding smoke detectors and other topics and then screens for things such as food insecurity, intimate partner violence, and drug or alcohol abuse.

Parents may have increased stress with more children in the home, but this is not necessarily associated with childhood maltreatment.

(pp. 166–167, Section 3: Social-Environmental Factors, Chapter 39: Preventing Child Abuse and Neglect: What Pediatricians Can Do)

**Answer 1-28.** E

This child likely has had an abusive head injury, or so-called "shaken baby syndrome." Pediatricians are responsible for identifying maltreatment, providing medical care, appropriate reporting to child abuse agencies, and helping to refer patients and families for treatment. Risk factors for childhood maltreatment include stressors in the home. One identified risk factor for child maltreatment is maternal depression.

Other risk factors for child maltreatment include paternal substance abuse and intimate partner violence (IPV). Some studies estimate that 33% to 77% of children living in homes with IPV are physically maltreated. For any case of child maltreatment, the pediatrician should try to identify and ameliorate these risk factors and provide support and appropriate referrals for parents and families. Other stressors that may increase risk of child maltreatment include poverty, unemployment, negative life events, poor social supports, and geographic moves.

The other options, including parents working the night shift, single parenting, multiple children, and both parents working, may increase stress at home, but maternal depression is the only risk factor shown to be associated with child abuse.

(p. 166, Section 3: Social-Environmental Factors, Chapter 39: Preventing Child Abuse and Neglect: What Pediatricians Can Do)

**Answer 1-29.** D

Proper prenatal care and monitoring are associated with improved outcomes for infants as well as better health for a population in general. Accurate assessment of gestational age and fetal growth is essential because that information may indicate when potential interventions are necessary or warranted. The assignment of gestational age is more accurate in early gestation and decreases with advancing gestation. This goal is most commonly accomplished with a first-trimester ultrasound in combination with a history of the last menstrual period. At this time, it is also helpful to establish how many fetuses are present. Maternal serum screening has been available since the late 1980s. Quad screening measures maternal serum α-fetoprotein, human chorionic gonadotropin, unconjugated estradiol, and inhibin A and can assess for risk of trisomy 21 and neural tube defects. More recently, cell-free DNA in the maternal serum has become an alternative method to screen for aneuploidy as well as identify sex.

Invasive testing, such as chorionic villus sampling, amniocentesis, and cordocentesis, does carry risk of rupture of membranes or preterm birth but is diagnostic for chromosomal/genetic disease and congenital infections. It would be most beneficial for both maternal and fetal health to proceed with maternal blood testing and both an early dating ultrasound and an anatomy ultrasound, reserving invasive testing as needed for further diagnosis.

(pp. 177–178, Section 4: Newborn, Chapter 41: Care of the Fetus)

**Answer 1-30.** B

Infant mortality rate is generally regarded as a good indicator of the overall health of a population. In the United States, currently, the rate is approximately 6/1000, with approximately one-third of those deaths being due to preterm birth. Of note, neonatal mortality rates are higher in infants who are non-Hispanic black, preterm, or products of multifetal pregnancy. Advances in perinatal care have led to increased survival of extremely preterm children, as well as decreased neurodevelopmental impairment. Long-term outcomes are variable and related to medical complications of prematurity and social risk factors.

Factors associated with risk of impaired neurodevelopmental outcomes include low birth weight, male gender, the presence of cerebral ultrasound abnormalities, bronchopulmonary dysplasia, and growth failure. Being born at a gestational age of < 27 weeks puts this patient at risk for impairment in early childhood. He is at risk for intellectual and learning disabilities. Extremely preterm children are also at increased risk for attention-deficit hyperactivity disorder (ADHD), particularly inattentive type, and are up to 5 times more likely to be diagnosed with autism. This child was at risk for poor growth early on but now appears to have normal growth and development. However, learning disabilities and ADHD may not be recognized until he is in school, and so his neurodevelopment should be closely monitored.

(pp. 188–189, Section 4: Newborn, Chapter 43: Neonatal Mortality and Morbidity)

**Answer 1-31.** E

There is little history provided for this baby, which makes it difficult to adequately prepare for its resuscitation. However, warming and drying a vigorous newborn are essential (Figure 44-1). Hypothermia of the newborn is associated with hypoglycemia, metabolic acidosis, and increased mortality. To minimize heat loss of the newborn, the delivery area temperature should be maintained at 74°F to 77°F, the baby should be dried, and warming aids such as hats, blankets, and radiant warmers can be used. You can also place the baby skin to skin.

The baby's oxygen saturation is within the normal range for this minute of life (3 minutes: 70%–75%), and so supplemental oxygen is not needed at this time. Furthermore, the baby is crying vigorously with no signs of respiratory distress and thus does not need further respiratory support. Cardiac compressions are not needed either as the baby has good circulation and respiratory effort, with a heart rate that is likely > 100 bpm. Clamping the umbilical cord should occur eventually; however, warming the infant takes priority, as there is evidence of benefits to delayed cord clamping for the infant.

(pp. 190, 192–194, Section 4: Newborn, Chapter 44: Delivery Room Resuscitation of the Newborn Infant)

**Answer 1-32.** A

Given the limited history and an otherwise well-appearing newborn, with little concern for neonatal infection or other abnormality, the most likely cause of the child's respiratory distress is transient tachypnea of the newborn. There are many organ systems that undergo transition immediately after birth. One of the most crucial is the respiratory system. Common factors that influence transition after birth are delayed cord clamping, cesarean section, and prematurity. It is not completely known what triggers transition to a regular postnatal breathing pattern, but it is likely loss of the umbilical circulation and the increase in systemic oxygen content.

Surfactant release, stimulated by lung inflation and an increase in circulating catecholamine concentration, is crucial to lowering surface tension in the alveoli and thus facilitating gas exchange. Surfactant production increases in the later stages of gestation. This child was full term and thus at less risk of surfactant deficiency. Meconium aspiration is another common cause of early respiratory distress; however, there was no history of meconium-stained fluid in this case. Although proper suctioning and clearing of oral secretions is important to facilitate breathing and stimulate the infant, it likely is not the cause of the child's distress. Clearance of fetal lung liquid at the time of birth occurs mostly via reabsorption across the respiratory epithelium and not out through the trachea.

(p. 197, Section 4: Newborn, Chapter 45: Transitional Changes in the Newborn)

**Answer 1-33.** C

This baby most likely suffered damage to the lower root of the brachial plexus (C8 or T1 vertebra), which affects nerves leading to the small muscles of the hand, resulting in the absence of or diminished grasp on the side of injury. This is a particular risk in breech vaginal deliveries.

Given this was observed in only the left hand and the baby was otherwise well appearing, meningitis and any other central nervous system lesion are less likely. Although you can have paralysis of muscles and nerve injury from compression in utero, typically that is observed in facial muscles. This injury is specifically an injury of the brachial plexus. Finally, congenital absence of the digital flexor muscles is exceedingly rare, especially without any other observed anatomic abnormalities.

(p. 208, Section 4: Newborn, Chapter 46: Examination of the Newborn Infant)

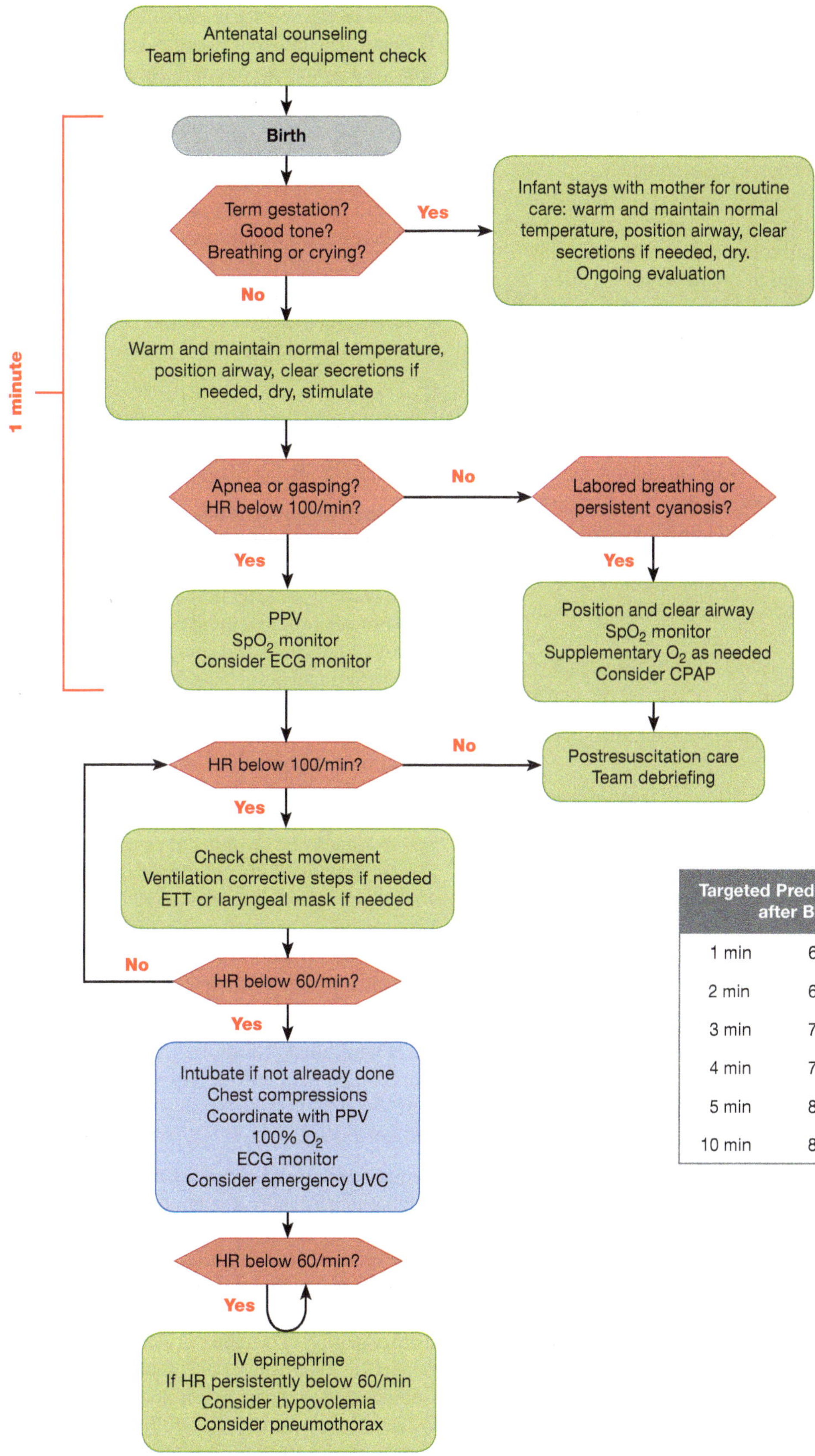


| Targeted Preductal $SpO_2$ after Birth | |
|---|---|
| 1 min | 60%–65% |
| 2 min | 65%–70% |
| 3 min | 70%–75% |
| 4 min | 75%–80% |
| 5 min | 80%–85% |
| 10 min | 85%–95% |

**FIGURE 44-1.** American Academy of Pediatrics/American Heart Association Neonatal Resuscitation Program Algorithm. CPAP, continuous positive airway pressure; ECG, electrocardiogram; ETT, endotracheal tube; HR, heart rate; IV, intravenous; PPV, positive-pressure ventilation; $SpO_2$, oxygen saturation level; UVC, umbilical venous catheter. (Reproduced with permission from Wyckoff MH, Aziz K, Escobedo MB, et al. Part 13: Neonatal resuscitation: 2015 American Heart Association guidelines update for cardiopulmonary resuscitation and emergency cardiovascular care. *Circulation*. 2015;132(18 Suppl 2):S543-S560.)

**Answer 1-34.** D

This newborn most likely has overriding sutures, which is a temporary overlap of the bony plates of the skull due to molding. This should be distinguished from craniosynostosis, or premature closure of 1 or more sutures. Craniosynostosis is much less common, occurring in approximately 1 in 2500 live births. Premature closing of the sutures prevents growth of the skull perpendicular to the fused suture line and will result in a sustained abnormal skull configuration. Occasionally, this abnormal skull configuration can be noticed at birth. If molding and overriding sutures are the cause of the palpable ridge, the bones should return to their normal position in a few days, and a small decrease in head circumference may be noticed. It is important to follow for resolution and/or abnormalities of the head shape. If craniosynostosis is suspected, a referral to a specialist who manages this condition is important. Head ultrasound or brain MRI is not commonly used to diagnose craniosynostosis and should not be ordered. Anticipatory guidance of insignificant molding is important, but the craniosynostosis should be considered and the baby's exam should be monitored. Mental status should not be altered in a baby with craniosynostosis or molding. Finally, a referral to genetics should only be considered if a diagnosis of craniosynostosis is made because it can be associated with certain genetic mutations.

(p. 207, Section 4: Newborn, Chapter 46: Examination of the Newborn Infant)

**Answer 1-35.** C

There are various tools that can be used to assess gestational age in an infant who is lacking consistent prenatal ultrasound gestational age measurements. Gestational age assessment can be done right from birth and is often done in the first 24 hours of life. In this case, the Ballard exam was used, and with those results and the infant's weight, it can be concluded that this baby is likely approximately 39 weeks of gestational age. However, his neurologic exam is not normal for a full-term infant. Namely, his upper extremity tone is low, with fully extended arms, ability to bring arms past midline, and inability to maintain his weight fully with finger grasp. The rest of his neurologic exam is normal for a term infant, which makes it less likely that his gestational age is actually younger than predicted. Given the focal neurologic abnormalities, further evaluation is warranted. However, urgent imaging is likely not required at this time because the infant is unlikely to require immediate intervention.

(pp. 209–210, Section 4: Newborn, Chapter 46: Examination of the Newborn Infant)

**Answer 1-36.** E

The cardiac exam described for this infant is within the normal limits for an infant in the first 10 minutes of life, and thus, the infant does not currently need further workup. In the first 10 minutes after birth, heart rate can vary from 120 to 180 bpm. Thereafter, the average is 120 to 130 bpm, with a range of 90 to 175 bpm. The murmur described is typical of a patent ductus arteriosus, which is commonly heard before full closure of the ductus by about 48 hours of life. An irregular heartbeat with ectopic beats is also occasionally encountered and often due to premature atrial contractions. They are usually inconsequential and resolve by 48 hours. If > 6 ectopic beats per minute are heard, an ECG should be obtained and a referral to cardiology considered. This infant was otherwise well, with normal color and pulses, making a cardiac abnormality less likely. At this point, this child has no risk factors or other signs of infection or thyroid dysfunction. A workup for these issues could be considered if her heart rate continued to be high.

(p. 213, Section 4: Newborn, Chapter 47: Postnatal Care and Observation of Low-Risk Newborns)

**Answer 1-37.** B

The concerning part of this infant's history is that he has vomited after every feed and is coughing during feeds. Although spitting up swallowed amniotic fluid or maternal blood is common early in the first day, it often subsides and does not occur only around feeds. Given this infant is now almost 24 hours old and coughs with feeds, esophageal atresia (EA) with tracheoesophageal fistula must be considered. Abdominal distension is often also seen with EA. The best first step in evaluating for EA is placing an orogastric tube and obtaining a radiograph to assess the position of the tube and esophageal patency. Not all forms of EA can be ruled out this way, and other imaging may be needed. A chest radiograph may eventually be helpful, but currently, there is no concern for cardiac or pulmonary abnormality. Genetic testing for trisomy 13, 18, or 21 should be considered only after a diagnosis of EA is made, given they are commonly associated. Although a lactation consultation could be beneficial, this infant appears to be latching and feeding well. The coughing during feeds and vomiting are not likely related to positioning.

(p. 213, Section 4: Newborn, Chapter 47: Postnatal Care and Observation of Low-Risk Newborns)

**Answer 1-38.** C

Urinary dilatation (eg, pelviectasis or hydronephrosis) diagnosed prenatally is common and occurs in approximately 1% of births. The extent of the dilatation can vary, and more severe cases carry more risk of significant uropathy. The general consensus is that mild unilateral pelviectasis or hydronephrosis (< 7 mm of dilatation) does not require further workup. Dilatation of > 7 mm or bilateral dilatation requires a renal/bladder ultrasound prior to discharge. If the findings persist, further consultation or imaging is required. Often, repeat imaging and an appointment with urology at about a month of age are recommended. Starting prophylactic antibiotics could be considered prior to discharge. In more severe cases, such as severe bilateral hydronephrosis, bilateral hydroureteronephrosis, multicystic dysplastic kidney, or male fetal hydronephrosis with prenatal history of oligohydramnios, such as in the infant in the case described in this question, urgent renal/bladder ultrasound and pediatric urology consult, as well as a chemistry panel at 12 hours of life, are recommended. In those cases, a voiding cystourethrogram is often obtained and prophylactic antibiotics started once pediatric urology has been consulted and prior to discharge.

(pp. 216–217, Section 4: Newborn, Chapter 47: Postnatal Care and Observation of Low-Risk Newborns)

**Answer 1-39.** D

This infant is at low risk for neonatal sepsis given the infant's well appearance and because the mother was adequately treated, 4 hours prior to delivery, with antibiotics for the GBS-positive culture. Risk factors for sepsis are prolonged rupture of membranes > 18 hours, fetal tachycardia, maternal fever, premature delivery, maternal chorioamnionitis, and birth depression. This infant has none of those risk factors. WBC counts are often elevated due to the demargination that occurs during the stress of delivery, and it is reassuring this child does not have elevated immature WBCs, which could indicate infection. If the infant had vital sign abnormality or appeared ill, the CBC may be interpreted differently and a repeat CBC, blood culture, CRP, and antibiotics could be considered. Given this infant's well appearance but GBS-positive mother, it is appropriate to observe the infant for 48 hours, not 24 hours.

(p. 217, Section 4: Newborn, Chapter 47: Postnatal Care and Observation of Low-Risk Newborns)

**Answer 1-40.** A

Multiple pregnancies are at higher risk of morbidity and mortality for the infants compared to singleton pregnancies. Those at most risk for demise of a twin and small for gestational age are monoamniotic, monochorionic twins due to the placental architecture. A single fetal demise, especially in monochorionic pregnancies, predisposes the surviving twin to cerebral lesions and subsequent neurodevelopmental delay. Absences of such lesions on magnetic resonance imaging (MRI) was associated with normal neurodevelopmental outcome. Given the twin demise in this case, the twin should be monitored for neurodevelopmental delay, with consideration for obtaining an MRI. This twin is at lower risk because the twins were dichorionic, diamniotic. She should also be monitored for complications related to prematurity; however, she is not at increased risk based on her twin gestation. Genetic testing would not be indicated for demise of the twin alone, especially given they are likely not monozygotic. There are no exam findings or symptoms concerning for cardiac disease, and she has otherwise been stable, and so cardiac workup is not indicated either. However, there is an increase in anomalies in multiple pregnancies, likely due to the higher incidence of abnormalities in monozygotic twins.

(p. 221, Section 4: Newborn, Chapter 48: Multiple Births)

**Answer 1-41.** E

This baby is small for gestational age (SGA), which is commonly defined as having a birth weight less than the 10th percentile of a population-specific birth weight versus gestational age relationship. SGA infants can also be thinner than normal when evaluating weight-to-length ratio. Intrinsic abnormalities that limit fetal growth usually begin early in gestation. Examples of intrinsic abnormalities are chromosomal abnormalities, cytomegalovirus infection early in gestation, inborn error of metabolism, and some early and sustained drug, alcohol, and/or tobacco use. This baby had normal growth up until mid-gestation, when the mother was lost to follow-up. The most common cause of late-gestation fetal growth restriction is placental insufficiency, which limits oxygen and nutrient transport to the fetus. Gestational diabetes mellitus (GDM) commonly causes large-for-gestational-age infants; however, if severe or with early onset, intrauterine growth restriction can ensue. Although this mother did not complete a glucose tolerance test, her HbA1c was normal, making severe GDM less likely.

(p. 222, Section 4: Newborn, Chapter 49: The Small-for-Gestational-Age Infant)

**Answer 1-42.** B

There are many short- and long-term complications associated with intrauterine growth restriction and the SGA infant. In the immediate neonatal period, hypoglycemia, hyperglycemia, increased energy expenditures, and altered lipid and protein metabolism are common. However, most term infants who are SGA do not exhibit poor feeding or respiratory distress at higher rates than appropriate-size-for-gestational-age (AGA) infants. SGA infants have an increased risk of polycythemia, not anemia, probably due to chronic intrauterine hypoxia. Although immune function in SGA infants can be impaired at birth, rates of sepsis are similar for SGA and AGA infants. Such infants often have deficiencies in lymphocyte numbers and function, low immunoglobulin levels during infancy, and attenuated antibody response to vaccines. Other long-term complications include continued short stature, low weight, and neurologic disorders.

SGA infants are 5 to 10 times more likely to suffer from neurologic disorders such as hyperactivity, inattention, learning disabilities, speech problems, fine motor incoordination, hyperreflexia, and other subtle behavioral problems.

(pp. 223–224, Section 4: Newborn, Chapter 49: The Small-for-Gestational-Age Infant)

**Answer 1-43.** C

Diabetes during pregnancy occurs in up to 10% of pregnancies and has serious consequences for the developing fetus that may last into adulthood. Most fetal complications are related to maternal glycemic control; however, even with strict glycemic control, fetal and infant complications persist. Some of the complications include intrauterine fetal demise, macrosomia or intrauterine growth restriction, birth trauma, perinatal depression, congenital anomalies, RDS, neonatal hypoglycemia, electrolyte abnormalities, polycythemia and hyperviscosity syndrome, hyperbilirubinemia, and cardiomyopathy. This baby did have macrosomia and one low blood glucose level during his hospitalization. Hypoglycemia usually develops during the first 24 hours and can present with symptoms of jitteriness, irritability, tachypnea, apnea, lethargy, hypotonia, poor feeding, or frank seizure. However, once good glycemic control is established and feeding is progressing, there is much less risk.

Hypocalcemia is also a risk and occurs in 20% to 50% of infants of diabetic mothers (IDMs), usually between 48 and 72 hours of life. Clinical signs of hypocalcemia include tremors, twitching, sweating, irritability, arrhythmia, seizures, and decreased myocardial contractility. This child showed some symptoms of hypocalcemia and so a serum calcium level should be checked in order to intervene if necessary. Hypomagnesemia is also a risk and occurs in one-third of IDMs; however, it is rarely of clinical significance. As a result, magnesium levels do not need to be specifically monitored. IDMs are also at risk for hyperbilirubinemia due to a combination of factors including risk of polycythemia and birth trauma related to macrosomia. In IDMs, bilirubin levels usually rise more rapidly and peak later; thus, they should be monitored early and frequently for development of hyperbilirubinemia. In this case, the baby did not appear jaundiced, and there was no report of jaundice in the hospital. This baby did not show signs of RDS, which would have presented soon after birth.

(pp. 225–226, Section 4: Newborn, Chapter 50: Infant of a Diabetic Mother)

**Answer 1-44.** B

The ASQ is an evidence-based tool that asks a parent to respond to questions that monitor gross motor, fine motor, social, and language skills. The M-CHAT is an evidence-based set of questions to assess risk for autism spectrum disorder. The SDQ and the PSC are behavioral screening tools for children age 3 to 4 years to adolescence. The SCQ screens for communication and social functioning beginning at age 4; it is primarily used for autism spectrum disorder screening.

(p. 369, Table 84-1, Section 6: Developmental and Behavioral Pediatrics, Chapter 84: Developmental and Behavioral Screening and Evaluation)

**Answer 1-45.** B

Studies of infant temperamental behavioral characteristics (Table 85-1) from parent questionnaires and direct clinical observation show that about 15% of children are slow to warm up, 40% have a behavioral pattern that is easy, and 10% are considered difficult to manage. About 35% have a mixed pattern of temperament behaviors.

Children with an easy temperament have regular patterns of eating, sleeping, and toileting. They comfortably change to a new environment. They are pleasant most of the time and do not become extremely agitated when their expectations are not met.

Children with a slow-to-warm-up temperament are typically shy and adapt slowly to new people and environments. They may hesitate to play with other children and take time to feel comfortable.

Children with difficult temperaments may be challenging for their parents to manage. They may not sleep, eat, or toilet at desired times. Children with difficult temperaments are more likely to have an irritable mood and react very negatively to unexpected changes in their routines or when their expectations are not met.

(p. 370, Section 6: Developmental and Behavioral Pediatrics, Chapter 85: Basics of Management of Common Behavior Problems)

**TABLE 85-1.** Temperamental Behavior Characteristics

| Behavior Characteristic | Description |
|---|---|
| Activity | The level and extent of motor activity |
| Rhythmicity | The degree of regularity of functions such as eating, elimination, and the cycle of sleeping and wakefulness |
| Approach or withdrawal | The response to a new object or person, in terms of whether the child accepts the new experience or withdraws from it |
| Adaptability | The adaptability of behavior to changes in the environment |
| Threshold of responsiveness | Sensitivity to a stimulus |
| Intensity of reaction | The energy level of responses |
| Quality of mood | The child's general mood or "disposition," whether cheerful or given to crying, pleasant or cranky, friendly or unfriendly |
| Distractibility | The degree of the child's distractibility from what he is doing |
| Attention span or persistence | The span of the child's attention and his persistence in an activity |

Mark W. Kline, *Rudolph's Pediatrics*, 23rd Edition. Copyright © McGraw-Hill Education. All rights reserved.

**Answer 1-46.** D

The developmental assessment is consistent with global development delay. The child does not meet milestones in gross motor, fine motor, language, or social skills. All children with global developmental delay or intellectual disability should be evaluated with chromosome microarray to assess for a specific genetic disorder.

A DNA test for fragile X should also be performed on the child with delayed global development even though there are no facial features seen in many patients with fragile X syndrome (the most common cause of inherited intellectual disability). It is not necessary to test all of this patient's siblings based on the information in the vignette. Plasma amino acids and urine organic acids are indicated if global developmental delay is associated with developmental regression, episodic encephalopathy, seizures, ataxia, involuntary movements, organomegaly, or episodic vomiting.

(pp. 378–379, Section 6: Developmental and Behavioral Pediatrics, Chapter 87: Global Developmental Delay and Intellectual Disability)

**Answer 1-47.** C

A sleep association refers to a child awaking in an environment that is different from where he or she fell asleep and the child struggles to fall asleep without the same environmental triggers. During the sleep cycle, the brain transitions from deep sleep to light sleep. At the time of this transition, the brain experiences a partial arousal, which is a break in the sleep cycle. The eyes may open, and as long as the environment remains consistent, the child will return to sleep. If the environment is different, the child will awaken to re-create the environment that occurred at bedtime. Although screen time in the bedroom before sleep may be the source of a sleep association, in young children, it is more typically a parent who reads or sings the child to sleep on a regular basis. Although an EEG may show a partial arousal pattern at the time of awakening, it is not diagnostic. An effective approach to a sleep association problem is to gradually reduce the associations (eg, singing, reading, rubbing). In this way, the child learns to fall asleep without an external prompt.

(p. 373, Section 6: Developmental and Behavioral Pediatrics, Chapter 85: Basics of Management of Common Behavior Problems)

**Answer 1-48.** B

The developmental milestones described in this vignette are most consistent with a 6-month-old child (Table 82-1). His ability to make consonants, transfer objects, and sit with support are all appropriate for a 6-month-old child. At 4 months, infants are still cooing and not able to sit. At 9 months, the child would be starting to pull to stand, and at 12 months, the child would be beginning to walk and ascribe meaning to sounds.

(p. 358, Table 82-1, Section 6: Developmental and Behavioral Pediatrics, Chapter 82: Introduction to Developmental-Behavioral Pediatrics: Pediatric Developmental Assessment)

**Answer 1-49.** D

At 9 months, a child who is not babbling with consonants likely has an expressive language delay (Table 82-1). Typically, children will begin to babble at 5 months with vowels and add consonants by 6 to 7 months. By 8 months, children use "Dada" nonspecifically for both of their parents, and by 9 months, they also begin to use "Mama" nonspecifically.

The child's gross motor and fine skills seem developmentally appropriate; children pull to stand or "bear walk" by crawling with their limbs straight at 9 months. Typically, children will be able to take independent steps at 12 months. She is banging blocks together, but would not be expected to throw objects until 10 to 11 months. Socially, the child is able to follow gestures at this age, but the ability to point to express interest is more typical at 12 months old. Her receptive language is normal as she orients to her name, but she does not follow commands, which again would be more typical for 12-month-olds.

(p. 358, Table 82-1, Section 6: Developmental and Behavioral Pediatrics, Chapter 82: Introduction to Developmental-Behavioral Pediatrics: Pediatric Developmental Assessment)

**Answer 1-50.** C

This child meets the developmental milestones for a typically developing 3-year-old. At 2 years old, a child is able to make 2-word sentences and exhibits parallel play (playing next to peers rather than interacting with peers). At 30 months, pronoun (I/you) confusion begins to dissipate. At 4 years old, 100% of speech should be understandable. A 5-year-old child should be able to recite their address and phone number.

(p. 358, Table 82-1, Section 6: Developmental and Behavioral Pediatrics, Chapter 82: Introduction to Developmental-Behavioral Pediatrics: Pediatric Developmental Assessment)

**Answer 1-51.** B

Height velocity peaks earlier for females than males, at SMR stage 3 for breast development for females. Height velocity peaks at SMR stage 4 for gonadal development in males. Because menarche usually occurs between SMR stages 3 and 4 for females, peak height velocity typically occurs before menarche. Weight velocity typically peaks after height velocity for females, whereas for males, height and weight velocity peak around the same time.

(p. 307, Section 5: Principles of Adolescent Care, Chapter 65: Somatic Growth and Development in Adolescence)

**Answer 1-52.** D

Menarche typically occurs between SMR stages 3 and 4; this is associated with increased, darker pubic hair and breast and areola enlargement. Menarche occurs after peak height velocity, and after menarche, linear growth slows and height typically increases an average of 7 cm in females. Although body fat percentage increases in females during puberty in order to initiate menarche and support regular menses, approximately 17% body fat is required for menarche and 22% for maintenance of normal ovulatory cycles. Therefore, assessing growth and development is critical during adolescent well checks to ensure adequate weight gain to support normal pubertal progression. The preovulatory phase of

**TABLE 82-1.** Sample Developmental Milestones to Consider When Eliciting Developmental Histories from Parents at Well-Child Visit Ages

| | Neurocognitive | | | | Neuromotor | | | Neurobehavior |
|---|---|---|---|---|---|---|---|---|
| **Age** | **Language** | **Social** | **Adaptive** | **Nonverbal/ Visual-Motor Problem Solving** | **Fine Motor** | **Gross Motor** | **Oral Motor/ Speech** | **Neurobehavioral Red Flags** |
| 1 month | | Visually focuses on face | | | | Lifts head up in prone | | Extreme irritability or docility in infancy |
| 2 months | | Social smile | | Visually tracks in horizontal and vertical planes | | Lifts chest up in prone | | Poor eye contact<br>Repetitive play (lining, sorting, spinning) |
| 4 months | Coos (3 months); laughs (4 months) | | | Visually tracks through 360 degrees (3 months) | Hands unfisted | Supports weight with arms straight in prone; head steady in supported sitting | | Visual or verbal perseveration<br>Restricted interests |
| 6 months | Babbles consonant sounds | Recognizes caregivers; exhibits stranger anxiety | | Reaches directly for objects; transfers objects from one hand to the other | | Rolls over both ways (5 months); sits without support | | Need for routine (picky eater who eats same food every day; upset with changes in usual car routes); upset with changes or transitions |
| 9 months | Uses nonspecific "Mama/Dada" (at 8 months); uses specific "Mama/Dada" (at 10 months); uses gestured language (waves "bye-bye") | Plays imitative games ("peek-a-boo," "pat-a-cake"); follows a point; looks preferentially when name is called; exhibits separation anxiety | Finger feeds; holds own bottle | Looks after fallen toy (9 months); uncovers hidden toy (10 months) | Inferior pincer grasp | At 8 months: crawls, pulls to stand, comes to sit<br>At 9 months: cruises around furniture | | Motor stereotypies (hand flapping, toe walking)<br>Sensory hypo- or hyperresponsiveness<br>Low frustration tolerance<br>Emotional lability |
| 12 months | 2-word vocabulary; follows single-step gestured command ("give me") | Points to request; shares objects of interest with others; social referencing | Helps with dressing; drinks from a cup | Shows intentional release of objects | | Walks independently | | Poor impulse control/ disinhibition<br>Hyperactivity<br>Inattention/easy distractibility |
| 15 months | Uses immature jargon (inflection); follows single-step ungestured command (16 months) | Points to show/ share interest; shows affection | Feeds self with spoon | Scribbles in imitation | | Rarely falls with walking; walks up stairs with one hand held | | |

| | | | | | | | |
|---|---|---|---|---|---|---|---|
| 18 months | 10-word vocabulary; uses mature jargon (single words mixed with jargon); points to body parts | Pretend play; imitates household chores | | Scribbles spontaneously; stacks 3 blocks | | Runs; walks down stairs with one hand held | |
| 24 months | At least 50-word vocabulary; uses 2-word sentences (noun/verb); follows 2-step ungestured command | Parallel play | Unzips | Builds horizontal train of blocks | | Walks up and down stairs independently marking time (21 months); jumps up, getting both feet off the ground (24 months) | |
| 30 months | Differentiates just one item from a greater number; differentiates "on" from "under"; pronoun ("I/you") confusion ceases; echolalia ceases | | | Copies horizontal and vertical stroke in the appropriate orientation; copies circle as a circular motion | | Alternates feet up stairs; pedals tricycle | |
| 3 years | 3-word sentences; identifies own name, gender, age | Interactive play; takes turns | Unbuttons | Copies a circle; recognizes colors | | Broad jumps; hops on one foot; alternates feet down stairs | Speech 75% understandable |
| 4 years | Verbally relates experiences/tells stories | | Buttons | Copies a cross (3½ years) and square (4 years) | Handedness established; uses scissors | Gallops | Speech 100% understandable |
| 5 years | Follows 3-step commands; tells address, phone number; identifies coins | | Ties shoes | Copies a triangle; differentiates right and left; recognizes all letters of the alphabet (5½ years) | | Skips rhythmically | |
| Red Flags | No gestured communication by 12 months; persistent echolalia beyond 30 months; pronoun ("I/you") confusion beyond 30 months | Flat facial expression/ no social smile; no pointing by 12 months; no response to name by 12 months | | Mouthing as primary means of exploration after 6 months | Fisting after 4 months; handedness before 1 year | Asymmetric movements; persistent primitive reflexes beyond 6 months; ↑ or ↓ muscle tone | Atypical/ monotonic speech prosody; stuttering after 5 years |

Mark W. Kline, *Rudolph's Pediatrics*, 23rd Edition. Copyright © McGraw-Hill Education. All rights reserved.

the menstrual cycle is predominately mediated by estrogen, whereas the postovulatory phase is predominately mediated by progesterone; the luteinizing hormone (LH) and follicle-stimulating hormone (FSH) surge are the primary drivers of ovulation mid-cycle.

(pp. 309–310, Section 5: Principles of Adolescent Care, Chapter 66: Reproductive Growth and Development in the Female Adolescent)

**Answer 1-53.** A

This patient is presenting with physiologic leukorrhea, often noticed in the months preceding menarche. Physiologic leukorrhea is caused by the shedding of desquamating squamous epithelial cells and can vary in appearance and consistency according to fluctuating hormone levels. Normal variants include copious thin, watery discharge during ovulation and thicker and cloudy or sticky discharge during the estrogenic and progesterone-dominant phases of the cycle. Although any patient presenting with the complaint of vaginal discharge should warrant a thorough history and physical exam, in a premenarchal female who has not had sexual contact or anything in the vagina, bacterial and fungal causes of vaginal discharge are less likely than physiologic leukorrhea with no other complaints.

Bacterial infections such as bacterial vaginosis (which presents with fishy smelling, watery or thin gray-white discharge, vaginal discomfort, or dyspareunia) are typically seen in sexually active adolescents and may be treated with either topical or systemic antibiotics. Chlamydia and gonorrhea often present with symptomatic cloudy or yellow vaginal discharge and are treated with systemic antibiotics, but they are unlikely in this patient, who is not sexually active. Oral or topical antifungals would only be indicated for treatment of vaginal candidiasis, which presents with thick, white, cottage cheese–like vaginal discharge and vaginal itching or burning.

(p. 309, Section 5: Principles of Adolescent Care, Chapter 66: Reproductive Growth and Development in the Female Adolescent)

**Answer 1-54.** C

During puberty, the change in vaginal pH from alkaline (> 4.7) to acidic (< 4.5) triggers a change in columnar epithelial cells to squamous epithelial cells through a process called squamous metaplasia. The squamocolumnar junction, termed the transformation zone, moves proximal on the cervix during puberty. The transformation zone is where most cervical cancers arise due to increased susceptibility to HPV due to increased replication. In contrast, columnar epithelial cells are more susceptible to *N gonorrhoeae* and *C trachomatis*.

(pp. 309–310, Section 5: Principles of Adolescent Care, Chapter 66: Reproductive Growth and Development in the Female Adolescent)

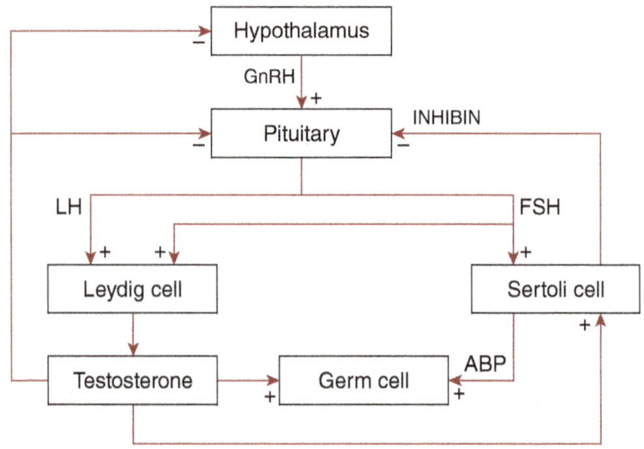


**FIGURE 67-2.** The hypothalamic–pituitary–testicular axis. ABP, androgen-binding protein; FSH, follicle-stimulating hormone; GnRH, gonadotrophin-releasing hormone; LH, luteinizing hormone. (Adapted with permission from Fitzgerald PA. *Handbook of Clinical Endocrinology*, 2nd ed. Norwalk, CT: Appleton & Lange; 1992.)

**Answer 1-55.** E

When puberty begins, pulsatile GnRH secretion occurs in the hypothalamus, first at night and then throughout the day. This leads to pituitary release of LH and FSH. LH influences the Leydig cells of the testes to secrete testosterone, which promotes Sertoli cell maturation. FSH influences the Sertoli cells to promote spermatogenesis (Figure 67-2).

(pp. 311–312, Section 5: Principles of Adolescent Care, Chapter 67: Reproductive Growth and Development in the Male Adolescent)

**Answer 1-56.** A

The first sign of puberty in males is testicular lengthening. SMR stage 2 gonadal development is defined by testicular length of > 2.5 cm or volume of at least 4 mL. SMR stage 3 testicular volume is at least 12 mL. Testicular size can be measured easily in the physician's office by using an orchidometer to estimate testicular size and volume and should be done routinely at well-child checks to ensure appropriate development. Although not the first signs of puberty, penile width and length increases occur after initial testicular growth, with length increasing before width. A rapid increase in penile growth occurs during SMR stage 3.

(p. 311, Section 5: Principles of Adolescent Care, Chapter 67: Reproductive Growth and Development in the Male Adolescent)

**Answer 1-57.** D

Middle adolescents are most concerned with their peer relationships as their sphere of influence shifts from the family unit to their social environment (Table 68-1). Middle adolescents are typically the most self-centered and focused

**TABLE 68-1.** Normal Development of the Stages of Adolescence and their Associated Impact on the Adolescent and on Delivery of Health Services

| Characteristics | Impact on Adolescents | Impact on Health Service Delivery |
|---|---|---|
| **Early Adolescence (Ages 10–13 Years)** | | |
| Onset of puberty; becomes concerned with developing body | Major questions concerning normality of physical maturation; often concerned about the stages of sexual development and how the process relates to peers of same gender; occasional masturbation | Important to normalize differences and explain range of normal development |
| Begins to expand social relationships beyond family | Adolescents concentrate on relationships with peers; begin to become more interdependent with parents | Encourage teens to begin to take responsibility for their own health and contact with health professionals, in consultation with parents (eg, part of visit time alone with health provider) |
| Beginning of transition from concrete to abstract thinking; new attractions and desires; socioemotional competencies of self-regulation still developing | Risky attitudes and health behaviors may emerge; opportunity for excitement and motivation | Shift in health provider's focus from anticipatory guidance to parents to risk reduction and prevention education to adolescent; still address most health situations with adolescents in a concrete manner with simple language |
| **Middle Adolescence (Ages 14–16 Years)** | | |
| Pubertal development usually complete, and sexual drives emerge | Explores ability to attract others; sexual experimentation (same and opposite sex) begins; masturbation increases | Provide sexual health screening; establish clinician's office as safe place to ask questions and discuss sexuality |
| Peer group sets behavioral standards, although family values usually persist | Peer group influences engagement in positive and negative health behaviors; peers rather than parents may also offer key support | Important to emphasize role of teen in making good choices and taking responsibility; focus on navigating social relationships and peer pressure |
| Conflicts over independence | Increased assumption of independent action, together with continued need for parental support and guidance; able to discuss and negotiate changes in rules | Increased involvement of teen in setting health-related goals and being clear on how to handle health situations (eg, time to take medication); reinforce adolescents' growing competencies |
| Emergence of abstract thinking with new cognitive competencies | Increased ability to process information, see other perspectives, and reflect; often leads to questioning adult behavior; while adolescent may consider broader range of possibilities/options, may not yet be able to integrate into real life | Important to be clear that individual understands and knows what he or she needs to do regarding health concerns |
| **Late Adolescence/Emerging Adulthood (Ages 17–21 Years)** | | |
| Physical maturation complete; body image and gender role definition clearer | Begins to feel comfortable with relationships and decisions regarding sexuality and preference; individual relationships become more important than peer group | Affirm decisions regarding sexuality and gender |
| Individuals less egocentric and self-centered; better at understanding others' points of view; greater ability to self-reflect and be insightful | More open to questioning regarding their behavior; interdependence with shared power and responsibility and greater reciprocity | Adolescent more able to work with clinician on setting goals and changing behavior; clinicians can help adolescents make better health decisions by involving them in their own health management |
| Idealistic | Idealism may lead to conflict with family or authority figures | May have own/alternative ideas of how to take responsibility for their health; clinicians can help adolescents see that they have a range of options |

*(Continued)*

**TABLE 68-1.** Normal Development of the Stages of Adolescence and their Associated Impact on the Adolescent and on Delivery of Health Services *(Continued)*

| Characteristics | Impact on Adolescents | Impact on Health Service Delivery |
|---|---|---|
| Identity exploration/life roles begin to be defined | People most likely to be exploring options in their lives | Often interested in discussion of life goals; depending on health status (eg, chronic illness), may influence life goals |
| Cognitive development nearing completion | Most are capable of understanding a full range of options for health issues | Important to help adolescents/emerging adults become competent in negotiating the healthcare system; encourage parents, when appropriate, to decrease their monitoring of clinical management issues, yet remain engaged and available to their son or daughter |

Mark W. Kline, *Rudolph's Pediatrics*, 23rd Edition. Copyright © McGraw-Hill Education. All rights reserved.

on peer relationships; these changes often lead to increases in conflicts with parents, and by late adolescence, youth are typically less self-centered. Dating and sexual relationships are often part of middle adolescent development; therefore, education about sexual health and contraception is particularly important, ideally before middle adolescents begin to have intimate relationships. Although early adolescence is characterized by concrete thinking, middle adolescents are typically able to demonstrate abstract thinking, characterized by an increased ability to reflect on multiple perspectives. Cognitive development continues throughout late adolescence and early adulthood, leading to increased ability to self-reflect and be insightful.

(pp. 313–315, Section 5: Principles of Adolescent Care, Chapter 68: Psychological Development)

**Answer 1-58. C**

In most states, adolescents have the right to confidentiality for certain sensitive health topics, including gender identity, sexual and reproductive health, substance use, and mental health counseling (medications for depression, anxiety, and other psychiatric disorders require parental consent until the age of 18 years). The limits of confidentiality should be discussed with patients and families at well visits starting in late childhood and early adolescence, ideally by age 10 to 12 years, to normalize the confidential interview and allow the patients to begin practicing relaying their history themselves and taking an active role in their medical care. The limits of confidentiality include if a patient or someone else's safety or life is at risk, such as if a patient has active suicidal or homicidal thoughts or behavior or is being or has been physically or sexually abused.

Discussion of confidential health topics should not wait until a child turns 18 years of age. Parents may access their minor children's medical records except for information regarding confidential health topics; many electronic medical records have the ability to mark certain documentation as sensitive or confidential to protect patient privacy. Discussing confidential health topics is a critical part of the adolescent health visit, and if parents are concerned about the need for confidentiality, this is best addressed by the clinician with the patient to empower the patient to decide how they would like to proceed. In some cases, it may be prudent to ask the patient to return on another day without their parent in order to adequately address any confidential health concerns. Although clinicians should strive to establish trusting relationships with adolescent patients, adolescents do not have the right to confidentiality in all areas of their health, only regarding certain sensitive topics, as mentioned.

(pp. 315–319, Section 5: Principles of Adolescent Care, Chapter 69: The Adolescent and Young Adult Visit)

**Answer 1-59. D**

The US Preventative Services Task Force (USPSTF), the Centers for Disease Control and Prevention (CDC), and the American Academy of Pediatrics (AAP) recommend annual screening of sexually active adolescents for *C trachomatis* and *Neisseria gonorrhoeae*.

While consideration of HIV testing for sexually active adolescents is important at every visit, particularly for those who are high risk (intravenous drug users, adolescents with a history of sex trafficking, adolescents with multiple partners, or adolescents who have a history of positive sexually transmitted infection [STI] testing), HIV testing is not recommended annually for low-risk adolescents. Syphilis testing is indicated for high-risk adolescents but not annually for low-risk adolescents. For adolescents with no pelvic complaints, annual screening pelvic exams are not recommended. The age to initiate screening Pap smears for cervical cancer has been changed to 21 years.

(pp. 318–319, Section 5: Principles of Adolescent Care, Chapter 69: The Adolescent and Young Adult Visit)

**Answer 1-60. C**

Transition to adult care for children with chronic diseases is an important part of adolescent health care. One in 5 families in the United States has a child with a chronic illness, and the majority of youth with special healthcare needs will enter adulthood and require adult medical providers. Increased morbidity and mortality have been reported in the posttransition period when transition is not adequately managed. The American Academy of Pediatrics (AAP) recommends beginning discussions about healthcare transition at age 14 and at least 2 years before projected transfer out of pediatric care to give youth and their family time to plan and prepare. The adult model of health care differs from the pediatric model; therefore, conversations about transition must begin before patients "age out" of pediatric specialties. Many patients and families may not be ready to think about transition early in adolescence when conversations and planning for transition should begin; furthermore, youth and their families may be reluctant to leave pediatric providers they have established care with and may need structure and encouragement to begin the transition process. Transition planning should include specific plans regarding who (the patient, parent, or providers) is responsible for which healthcare tasks (eg, making appointments, requesting refills) and when. One of the goals of transition is to have the adolescent (if cognitively appropriate) assume responsibility for his or her own health care. Even when adolescents assume more responsibility for their own health, transition conversations should include their parents or other responsible family members to discuss shifting responsibility away from parents toward the adolescent, as well as timing of transition.

(pp. 319–323, Section 5: Principles of Adolescent Care, Chapter 70: Healthcare Transition from Pediatric to Adult-Based Care for Youth and Young Adults with Special Healthcare Needs)

**Answer 1-61.** C

Motor vehicle accidents (MVAs) are the leading cause of unintentional injury in the United States and account for 54.9% of fatal accidents and 21.8% of all deaths among adolescents and young adults. It is estimated that 70.8% of adolescent and young adult deaths are due to preventable causes (in order of frequency: unintentional injury [including MVAs], suicide, and homicide). Contributors to MVA mortality include substance use, inexperience, fatigue, and lack of seatbelt use.

Restrictions on teen driving such as extended learners' permits and nighttime restrictions have been shown to be effective in reducing traffic mortality, leading to reductions in MVA mortality. Males have higher rates of suicide and homicide than females, with minority teens at highest risk. Chronic illnesses, including malignancy and heart disease, are responsible for 5.9% and 3.2% of deaths, respectively and, therefore, are not the leading cause of mortality in US teens.

(p. 324, Section 5: Principles of Adolescent Care, Chapter 71: Mortality)

**Answer 1-62.** E

ACEs are now recognized as a significant contributor to adolescent morbidity, which in turn affects youth into adulthood. ACEs include abuse, neglect, death of family or friends, incarceration or incarceration of family members, household dysfunction (eg, witnessing domestic violence, living with family members with mental illness, separated/divorced parents), and bullying and neighborhood violence. Experiencing any of these stressors can affect health throughout the life course.

Youth who have experienced ACEs are at higher risk for chronic toxic stress, which alters brain structure and increases lifetime incidence of chronic illnesses such as cerebrovascular disease, myocardial infarction, stroke, and asthma. ACEs appear to be cumulative; adolescents who have experienced more ACEs and more recent ACEs have poorer health outcomes than youth with fewer/more remote ACEs. In the United States, 90% of 14-year-olds have experienced at least one ACE, highlighting the importance of discussing ACEs with children and families; youth from poorer socioeconomic and minority backgrounds are at higher risk of experiencing ACEs.

(p. 325, Section 5: Principles of Adolescent Care, Chapter 72: Morbidity)

**Answer 1-63.** D

Increased adolescent access to comprehensive sexual health education and increased access to contraception are associated with lower teen pregnancy rates. Encouragingly, adolescent pregnancy rates have decreased in all racial and ethnic groups, including in African American females; however, African American and Hispanic females continue to have higher teen pregnancy rates than white females. Both teen pregnancy and abortion rates have declined over the past 20 years, according to recent statistics. According to the Youth Risk Behavior Survey, 86% of teens reported using some form of contraception at last intercourse.

(p. 326, Section 5: Principles of Adolescent Care, Chapter 73: Sexual Behavior)

**Answer 1-64.** B

The American Academy of Pediatrics (AAP) is opposed to drug testing without the adolescent's consent. Prior to obtaining a drug test, with the adolescent's consent, the provider should discuss what, if any, results the adolescent consents to be released to parents. When a parent requests that their child be drug tested, providers should have a discussion with the parent and patient about the need for consent for drug testing and facilitate an open conversation about the concerns around this request.

Most available drug screens include marijuana, cocaine, amphetamines, and opioids. Urine drug screens for marijuana may be positive for up to 48 hours if a patient uses 1 dose of marijuana but may remain positive for longer in more frequent users (up to 21–30 days in chronic users). Some prescribed medications, such as amphetamines for ADHD, may result in false-positive results on urine drug tests. Doxycycline may also cause false-positive opiate screen on urine drug tests. As a result, providers ordering and interpreting urine drug tests should be familiar with these limitations of testing.

(pp. 327–330, Section 5: Principles of Adolescent Care, Chapter 74: Substance Use and Abuse)

**Answer 1-65.** A

The majority of breast masses in adolescents are due to benign causes, with fibrocystic changes, fibroadenomas, and simple cysts being the most common causes. Fibrocystic changes, as in this patient's case, frequently present with diffuse, cord-like masses that change with the menstrual cycle and are often tender the week before the patient's menses.

Fibroadenomas are the most common breast masses on biopsy in adolescents and usually present as painless, well-demarcated, rubbery, mobile masses, between 1 and 3 cm in diameter, at the upper outer quadrants of the breast. Very few breast cancers (5%–9%) are associated with breast cancer–associated genes such as *BRCA*. Early menarche (prior to age 12 years) is associated with a higher risk of breast cancer. Adolescents who present with breast masses are often worried about malignant causes, and therefore, reassurance and anticipatory guidance are important parts of the visit.

(pp. 341–342; Section 5: Principles of Adolescent Care, Chapter 77: Breast Masses)

**Answer 1-66.** E

This patient's clinical presentation is most consistent with gynecomastia. Gynecomastia is a common condition in adolescent males, with peak incidence from sexual maturity rating (SMR) stages 2 to 4, affecting approximately one-third of males. This patient is SMR stage 2 based on his testicular length. Gynecomastia is typically transient and unilateral, and self-resolves without intervention in 90% of males within 2 years of presentation. Causes include decreased ratio of androgen to estrogen and a change in end-organ receptor sensitivity. Certain medical conditions and medications can contribute to gynecomastia and should be ruled out with history and physical exam.

Although the patient has a family history of breast cancer, his presentation is consistent with typical adolescent gynecomastia (eg, < 4 cm in size, lack of lymphadenopathy or other systemic symptoms), and therefore, *BRCA* gene testing is not indicated at this time. While marijuana can cause gynecomastia, history should be obtained first, and urine drug testing should only be obtained with the adolescent's permission. Given the size of his gynecomastia (< 4 cm), it is likely to self-resolve within 2 years; therefore, additional imaging and surgical evaluation are not indicated. Surgical evaluation would be warranted if his gynecomastia progresses to > SMR stage 3 breast development or > 4 cm in diameter, persists for > 2 years, or causes significant psychosocial impairment.

(p. 342, Section 5: Principles of Adolescent Care, Chapter 77: Breast Masses)

**Answer 1-67.** E

This patient is presenting with a symptomatic varicocele; 85% to 95% of varicoceles are left-sided, due to increased pressure transmitted to the left testicular vein through its right-angle insertion into the left renal vein. Right-sided varicoceles are associated with tumors and should prompt further evaluation with Doppler ultrasound to evaluate for inferior vena cava obstruction.

Scrotal elevation is an appropriate treatment for torsion of the appendix testis, along with NSAIDs. NSAIDs and rest are also appropriate treatments in cases of viral orchitis, such as in mumps. Antibiotic therapy would be indicated for treatment of bacterial epididymitis or orchitis (usually caused by spread of bacteria from the epididymis); the most common organisms in prepubertal children are enteric bacteria (such as *Escherichia coli*), whereas in sexually active adolescents, *Chlamydia trachomatis* and *Neisseria gonorrhoeae* are the most common causative organisms. Surgical evaluation would be indicated after evaluation for possible tumors given the right-sided and symptomatic nature of this patient's varicocele; surgical evaluation is also indicated in cases of bilateral varicoceles or testicular growth arrest or in cases where testicular torsion is suspected.

(pp. 343–345, Section 5: Principles of Adolescent Care, Chapter 78: Scrotal Masses)

**Answer 1-68.** B

This patient is presenting with primary amenorrhea, defined as a lack of initiation of menses by age 15, in the presence of breast development or within 3 years of thelarche, or by age 13 in the absence of secondary sex characteristics. Secondary amenorrhea refers to the cessation of menses for at least 3 months or 90 days in patients who have previously menstruated. Constitutional pubertal delay is a diagnosis of exclusion; therefore, additional workup, including further history, family history, and a physical exam including sexual maturity rating (SMR) staging should be obtained prior to diagnosing a patient with constitutional delay. While pregnancy is the most common cause of amenorrhea, the differential diagnosis for amenorrhea is broad and requires careful history, physical exam, and lab workup to assess for hypogonadotropic hypogonadism (eg, malnutrition, chronic diseases, eating disorders, and pituitary lesions), hypergonadotropic hypogonadism (eg, primary ovarian insufficiency, Turner syndrome, and androgen insensitivity syndrome), and eugonadotropic eugonadism (eg, polycystic ovarian syndrome or Mullerian duct defects). Initial labs typically include a pregnancy test, luteinizing hormone (LH), follicle-stimulating hormone (FSH), estradiol, thyroid-stimulating hormone, and prolactin, and possibly a karyotype and testosterone, 17-hydroxyprogesterone, and dehydroepiandrosterone sulfate levels depending on exam findings.

(pp. 345–349, Section 5: Principles of Adolescent Care, Chapter 79: Menstrual Problems)

**Answer 1-69. C**

Abnormal uterine bleeding, defined as vaginal bleeding that occurs in cycles shorter than 21 days or longer than 45 days, is common in the first 2 years after menarche, due to the immature HPG axis. Due to this immaturity, menstrual cycles are frequently anovulatory, characterized by oscillating estrogen levels and low progesterone levels, which lead to a thickened, fragile endometrium that sheds unpredictably, causing irregular vaginal bleeding. Even when females achieve menarche, the HPG axis is still maturing. By the end of the first year after menarche, three-fourths of females have regular, ovulatory menstrual cycles; 95% of women achieve regular menstrual cycles by 5 years.

While anovulatory cycles are a diagnosis of exclusion, requiring careful history and physical exam, other causes of abnormal uterine bleeding are relatively rare. Anatomic uterine abnormalities such as polyps are rare in adolescents. Although von Willebrand disease is the most common cause of heavy menstrual bleeding requiring hospitalization, with a prevalence of 1%, this patient is not presenting with heavy menstrual bleeding (bleeding lasting longer than 8 days, > 80 mL of blood loss in a menstrual cycle, or using > 8 full pads or tampons per day) and has no other complaints consistent with coagulopathy such as easy bruising or bleeding.

(pp. 349–350, Section 5: Principles of Adolescent Care, Chapter 79: Menstrual Problems)

**Answer 1-70. C**

The prevalence of menstrual cramps peaks at 1 to 2 years after menarche, coinciding with the establishment of ovulatory menstrual cycles. Primary dysmenorrhea is mediated by prostaglandins, leukotrienes, prostacyclin, and vasopressin. Increased levels of prostaglandin and leukotrienes stimulate uterine vasoconstriction, pain sensitization, and myometrium contractions. Decreased levels of prostacyclin, a vasodilator and muscle relaxant, occur in women with dysmenorrhea, and overproduction of vasopressin further increases uterine contractions. These 4 alterations lead to intense uterine contractions, vasoconstriction, and ischemic pain. Dysmenorrhea, or painful menstrual cramping, is common in adolescents, affecting 50% to 93% of menstruating adolescents, and is a leading cause of school and work absenteeism and decreased quality of life. The majority of adolescents who have dysmenorrhea experience mild to moderate pain; up to 10% to 20% of adolescents with dysmenorrhea experience more severe symptoms that can lead to incapacitation. There are good, evidence-based treatments for dysmenorrhea, including nonsteroidal anti-inflammatory drugs (NSAIDs), combined oral contraceptive pills, and supplements such as magnesium, omega-3 fatty acids, vitamin E, and vitamin $B_1$.

(p. 350, Section 5: Principles of Adolescent Care, Chapter 79: Menstrual Problems)

**Answer 1-71. B**

The Centers for Disease Control and Prevention (CDC) recommends screening all pregnant adolescents for HIV, syphilis, chlamydia, and gonorrhea at the first prenatal visit. The CDC also recommends screening all pregnant adolescents for hepatitis B early in pregnancy. Routine screening is not recommended for herpes simplex virus.

(pp. 351–352; Section 5: Principles of Adolescent Care, Chapter 80: Intrauterine and Ectopic Pregnancy)

**Answer 1-72. E**

This patient is at risk for unintended pregnancy given her inconsistent condom use and lack of a consistent contraceptive method. Answer choice E is the best choice; given that she has had unprotected sex in the past 5 days, she is a candidate for emergency contraception; the copper IUD is an ideal choice for this patient, as it functions both as emergency contraception as well as long-acting reversible contraception if placed within 5 days of unprotected sex. Given this patient has had inconsistent condom use beyond her sexual intercourse yesterday, she is at risk for pregnancy; therefore, it is important to rule out pregnancy before placing an IUD.

If she prefers the hormonal IUD, you could give oral emergency contraception and then place a hormonal IUD with strict counseling about the risks of unintended pregnancy if she has unprotected sex within 7 days of placement. A copper IUD functions as both emergency contraception and long-term contraception, unlike DMPA or a hormonal IUD. All patients initiating a hormonal form of contraception should be counseled on the need to use a backup method or abstain for 7 days. Asking this patient to return later for initiation of a contraceptive method increases her risk of pregnancy; therefore, it is advisable to initiate a method today if she is willing, rather than have her come back for another appointment.

(pp. 353–356, Section 5: Principles of Adolescent Care, Chapter 81: Contraception)

**Answer 1-73. A**

This patient has classic features of warm septic shock (also called distributive shock). Shock is defined as a state of cellular and tissue hypoxia due to reduced oxygen delivery and/or increased oxygen consumption or inadequate oxygen utilization. Septic shock is a clinical diagnosis based on evidence of abnormal temperature (hyper- or hypothermia), altered mental status, and altered vascular tone (increased or decreased). This patient shows signs of warm shock: a state of vasomotor paralysis with vasodilation, manifested by warm hands and feet, bounding peripheral pulses, and flash capillary refill. It is far less common in children than in adults, comprising only 20% of septic children. Warm shock usually responds to volume resuscitation and vasoconstrictors. Most children with warm septic shock will progress to cold shock. Cold shock is characterized by delayed capillary refill, diminished peripheral pulses, and mottled cool extremities. Compensated shock occurs when a patient experiences vasoconstriction and increased heart rate in attempt to keep perfusion and blood pressure adequate. Cardiogenic shock refers to a state of shock that is due to heart failure. Hypovolemic shock is defined by the origin due to low blood volume.

(p. 425, Section 8: Acute and Critical Illness, Chapter 97: Pathophysiology of Sepsis)

**Answer 1-74. B**

The GCS is the most well-known scale used to quantify arousal to stimuli, and in pediatrics, it is clinically most often used for patients who present with altered consciousness due to trauma, ingestion, or an unclear mechanism. The motor portion alone is most predictive of neurologic injury. The pediatric version of the score contains modifications of the verbal response to account for preverbal children. According to the scale (Table 98-3), this patient would get a score of 6—she is opening her eyes to pain (2), her best verbal response is a moan (2), and she extends her arms in response to pain (2).

(p. 431, Section 8: Acute and Critical Illness, Chapter 98: Acute Neurological Dysfunction)

**Answer 1-75. B**

Recommendations for chest compressions in both infants and children include compressing at a rate of 100 to 120/min, compressing to at least one-third of the chest depth, and allowing for complete chest recoil between compressions. Failing to allow chest recoil between compressions can impair venous return (ventricular filling) and thus impair adequate systemic blood flow with each compression.

As rescuers fatigue, they tend to lean into their compressions and become less likely to allow for adequate chest recoil, which is one reason to rotate rescuers about every 2 minutes during continuous CPR.

(p. 449, Section 8: Acute and Critical Illness, Chapter 102: Cardiopulmonary Resuscitation)

**TABLE 98-3.** Glasgow Coma Score

| Adult Glasgow Coma Score | | Pediatric Glasgow Coma Score | Nonverbal Glasgow Coma Score |
|---|---|---|---|
| **Best Eye-Opening Response** | | | |
| 1 | No eye opening | | |
| 2 | Eye opening to pain | | |
| 3 | Eye opening to speech | | |
| 4 | Spontaneous eye opening | | |
| **Best Verbal Response** | | | |
| 1 | No verbal response | No vocal response | No response to pain |
| 2 | Incomprehensible sounds | Occasional whimpers or moans | Mild grimace to pain |
| 3 | Inappropriate words | Cries inconsolably | Vigorous grimace to pain |
| 4 | Confused | Inappropriate interactions, cries but consolable | Less than usual ability or response to touch only |
| 5 | Oriented | Age-appropriate verbalization, smiles, orients to sound, tracks, interacts | Spontaneous facial and oromotor activity |
| **Best Motor Response** | | | |
| 1 | No motor response | | |
| 2 | Abnormal extension to pain | | |
| 3 | Abnormal flexion to pain | | |
| 4 | Withdraws from pain | | |
| 5 | Localizes pain or withdraws from touch | | |
| 6 | Obeys commands or performs spontaneous appropriate movement | | |

Mark W. Kline, *Rudolph's Pediatrics*, 23rd Edition. Copyright © McGraw-Hill Education. All rights reserved.

**Answer 1-76.** B

This infant's age, clinical appearance, and exam are all consistent with bronchiolitis. Bronchiolitis is a viral infection of the lower airways, most common prior to 2 years of age, resulting in lower airway obstruction characterized by hypoxia, increased work of breathing, and diffuse wheezes, rhonchi, and rales on exam.

Asthma usually presents later in infancy and would be characterized by reversible wheezing, often in the setting of an upper respiratory infection, but without the other lung sounds and with minimal hypoxia. Croup is a viral inflammation of the upper airways and usually presents with a hoarse voice, cough, and often inspiratory stridor. Foreign body aspiration would not explain the fever, low oxygen saturation, and diffuse lung findings. Although this infant may develop pneumonia as a complication of her bronchiolitis, there are no focal findings to suggest pneumonia at this point.

(p. 422, Section 8: Acute and Critical Illness, Chapter 96: Acute Respiratory Dysfunction)

**Answer 1-77.** A

This blood gas shows a primary metabolic acidosis with respiratory compensation. The first step in interpreting the blood gas is to look at the pH. Because the pH is < 7.4, this is an acidosis. The next question is whether this is primary metabolic or primary respiratory. Because the $HCO_3^-$ goes in the same direction as the pH, this makes this a primary metabolic acidosis (if it were a respiratory acidosis, the $PCO_2$ would be elevated, but it is decreased). Finally, respiratory compensation is demonstrated by the fact that the pH would be even lower if due entirely to the low $HCO_3^-$. The formula for this is as follows: for every 10 mM decrease in $HCO_3^-$, pH decreases by 0.15. Since the pH is only 0.1 below normal (7.4), this indicates some respiratory compensation. Overall, this blood gas is consistent with sepsis, which is the likely diagnosis in this case.

(pp. 436–437, Section 8: Acute and Critical Illness, Chapter 99: Physiologic Monitoring)

**Answer 1-78.** D

This child is moderately dehydrated and should be volume resuscitated with an initial bolus of 20 mL/kg of isotonic fluid, such as 0.45% NaCl (NS). Bolus fluids are typically dosed at 20 mL/kg/dose and should be repeated until the child is showing signs of restored intravascular volume or can take adequate oral fluids.

Either D5 ½ NS or D5NS would be an appropriate maintenance fluid in this age group, but D5 ½ NS should not be used for volume resuscitation. For maintenance fluids (once the child has been volume resuscitated), 4 mL/kg/h would be an appropriate rate for this 10-kg child.

(pp. 443–445, Section 8: Acute and Critical Illness, Chapter 101: Fluid Management of the Acutely Ill or Injured Child)

**Answer 1-79.** C

Rapid bolus administration of isotonic fluids is the first step in the acute resuscitation of hemodynamic compromise in presumed septic shock. Each bolus should be 20 mL/kg and should be followed by clinical assessment for both improvement and signs of fluid overload. Inotropes should only be given after adequate fluid resuscitation (60 mL/kg).

Recent studies performed in developing countries have highlighted the potential dangers of rapid fluid resuscitation in malnourished patients and without availability of high-level respiratory support, so slow administration of fluids should be considered in resource-poor settings where these conditions are common. Early administration of antibiotics (within 60 minutes) is recommended as well, but should not be prioritized over the immediate restoration of adequate intravascular volume.

(p. 106, Section 8: Acute and Critical Illness, Chapter 106: Early Management of Sepsis and Septic Shock)

**Answer 1-80.** C

This child meets criteria for a BRUE that is low risk. The low-risk features are as follows: age > 60 days, at least 32 weeks' gestation and corrected gestational age of at least 45 weeks, no cardiopulmonary resuscitation (CPR) by medical provider, event < 1 minute in duration, and first-time event.

According to the AAP guidelines, no routine laboratory or other diagnostic studies should be obtained for infants with a low-risk BRUE. If the history suggests pertussis or a cardiac dysrhythmia (which this one does not), then specific testing for these conditions may be obtained. If the infant did not meet low-risk criteria, then a targeted investigation guided by the infant's signs and symptoms could be undertaken (Table 113-1). Specifically, common causes to consider might include a respiratory virus, a central nervous system cause (seizures or unrecognized trauma), apnea or prematurity, an inborn error of metabolism, or GER.

(p. 498, Section 8: Acute and Critical Illness, Chapter 113: Caregiver-Reported Acute Infant Events)

**Answer 1-81.** E

This child demonstrates the classic toxidrome (clinical presentation) for opiate exposure. This toxidrome includes decreased responsiveness, respiratory and circulatory depression, and miosis. While opiates are not the only cause of this presentation (other causes might include carbon monoxide exposure or organophosphate poisoning), the history is highly suggestive of possible opioid exposure. In addition to supportive care of the respiratory and circulatory system, administration of naloxone would be the most important next step.

Sodium bicarbonate is used in cases of suspected or proven aspirin ingestion. Activated charcoal should not be used in patients with decreased consciousness such as this one, but in

**TABLE 113-1.** Diagnostic Testing for Infants Meeting Higher-Risk Brue Criteria

**Initial Assessment Appropriate in Most Infants Requiring Evaluation**

- Complete blood count with differential (evidence of infection)
- Plasma concentrations of glucose, electrolytes, blood urea nitrogen (BUN), calcium, and magnesium (evidence of $CO_2$ retention or bicarbonate loss, hyponatremia, hypoglycemia)
- Cardiorespiratory monitoring (evidence of dysrhythmia or irregular breathing)

**Tests Occasionally Indicated Based on Other Findings**

- Neurologic testing (EEG, brain imaging)
- Cardiac evaluation (chest radiograph, ECG, echocardiogram, Holter monitoring)
- Infectious disease evaluation (bacterial and viral screening, lumbar puncture, chest radiograph)
- Metabolic analyses (arterial blood gases, lactate, pyruvate, $NH_4$, urine amino and organic acids, aminotransferases)
- Polysomnography (simultaneous recordings of multiple physiologic signals, usually for at least 8 hours, with channels selected based on nature of symptoms)
- Esophageal pH and impedance monitoring with simultaneous polysomnography (pH probe alone is not useful for evaluation of ALTE)
- Child abuse investigation (skeletal survey, video surveillance)

ALTE, apparent life-threatening event; BRUE, brief resolved unexplained event; BUN, blood urea nitrogen; ECG, electrocardiogram; EEG, electroencephalogram.

Mark W. Kline, *Rudolph's Pediatrics*, 23rd Edition. Copyright © McGraw-Hill Education. All rights reserved.

an alert patient, it could be used for most suspected ingestions. It is most effective shortly after the ingestion and does not work for all ingestions, most notably iron and alcohols. Glucagon is specifically indicated for β-blocker poisoning, and *N*-acetylcysteine is used for acetaminophen toxicity.

(p. 507, Section 8: Acute and Critical Illness, Chapter 114: Toxic Ingestions and Exposures)

**Answer 1-82.** C

This clinical scenario is highly suggesting of carbon monoxide (CO) poisoning, which is the leading cause of poisoning death in the United States. Common sources of CO include house fires, automobile exhaust, and indoor sources of heat such as space heaters and furnaces. CO binds to hemoglobin with greater affinity than oxygen, displacing oxygen and, thus, depriving tissues of oxygen. Mild exposure may result in nonspecific symptoms such as malaise, nausea, headache, or dizziness. More significant exposure results in altered mental status that may progress to seizures and coma. Children are generally more sensitive than adults and may become symptomatic at lower exposure levels.

The diagnosis of CO poisoning is confirmed by determination of COHb level via co-oximetry of an arterial blood sample. A routine blood gas will typically be normal in CO poisoning due to dissolved oxygen. Methemoglobinemia does not fit this clinical picture as those patients appear cyanotic. A toxicology screen and anion gap would be reasonable but would not confirm the suspected diagnosis in this case.

(p. 509, Section 8: Acute and Critical Illness, Chapter 114: Toxic Ingestions and Exposures)

**Answer 1-83.** B

The strongest predictor of survival and long-term morbidity in drowning is the duration of submersion. Shorter arrival time of paramedics and saltwater are favorable factors in survival, but less significant than submersion duration. Hypothermia should be taken into account when deciding whether to terminate CPR in a drowning victim, as there have been case reports of victims surviving prolonged submersion in extremely cold water (< 5°C). Ability to swim may help to prevent drowning but is not associated with prognosis in a drowning victim.

(p. 516, Section 8: Acute and Critical Illness, Chapter 115: Submersion Injuries)

**Answer 1-84.** C

Fencing around home pools is the most effective prevention method for submersion injury. The fencing should be at least 4 feet high, narrow enough that a child cannot slip through, and include self-latching gates that a child cannot unlock.

Pool covers can give a false sense of security and do not prevent children from falling into a pool or drowning. Children should be taught to swim when old enough, but research has been equivocal on the efficacy of this measure, particularly at young ages, and it is not a substitute for physical preventive measures. Children this age should only be allowed in a pool with 1-to-1 supervision by an adult who is close enough to touch them.

(p. 516, Section 8: Acute and Critical Illness, Chapter 115: Submersion Injuries)

**Answer 1-85.** B

Trauma is the number one cause of pediatric death in children aged 1 month to 18 years. Trauma accounts for half of all pediatric deaths in this age group and occurs more frequently than infection, cancer, and heart disease combined. Motor vehicle crashes are the most common cause of traumatic death in children of all ages.

(p. 517, Section 8: Acute and Critical Illness, Chapter 116: Trauma, Burns, and Bites)

## Answer 1-86. A

Burn depth is categorized as either partial thickness (epidermis +/– portions of the dermis) or full thickness (involving all skin layers). The description of this burn is typical of a partial-thickness burn, which is characterized by erythema and exquisite tenderness and pain. A full-thickness burn would be dry, either pale or charred in color, and insensate.

The presence of weeping and blistering further characterizes this as a deep partial-thickness burn (formerly known as "second degree"). Multiple references can help estimate the BSA of a burn in a young child (Figure 116-2). However, a useful rule of thumb is that the palm of a young child represents about 1% of her entire BSA. So, in this case, this burn is approximately 1% BSA.

(p. 522, Section 8: Acute and Critical Illness, Chapter 116: Trauma, Burns, and Bites)

## Answer 1-87. E

Dog bites are the most common bite injury in children, and the upper extremity is the most commonly bitten area. Cat bites are less common but may carry a higher risk of infection. All bite wounds should be thoroughly irrigated and debrided of dead tissue, and antibiotics (amoxicillin-clavulanate to cover skin bacteria and oral anaerobes) should be routinely administered for all hand and face bites.

Closure of dog bite wounds is controversial, and the risks and benefits should be weighed by an experienced clinician. Due to the delay in care in this case and the depth of the wounds and difficulty in adequately cleaning them, delayed closure might be indicated. Postexposure rabies immunoglobulin G and vaccine are rarely indicated for dog bites in the United States, the majority of which occur from home pets. Rabies is far more likely in a bat or rodent bite. The local department of public health can aid in decisions about rabies prophylaxis. Tetanus toxoid is indicated only if vaccine status is unknown or incomplete.

(pp. 524–525, Section 8: Acute and Critical Illness, Chapter 116: Trauma, Burns, and Bites)

## Answer 1-88. D

First aid is important in the prehospital and in-hospital settings, and all snakebites should be preemptively managed as potentially serious envenomations from the moment of first suspicion. First aid for most venomous snakebites includes immobilizing the affected limb and ideally lowering it below heart level. This helps reduce the spread of the venom until medical care can be reached. For elapid bites (found only in Australia), pressure-immobilization can be used (wrapping the affected limb in a continuous elasticized bandage and applying a splint for immobilization). Tourniquets and sucking or squeezing out the venom should not be performed. The limb should be lowered, not elevated, to reduce spread of the venom.

(p. 526, Section 8: Acute and Critical Illness, Chapter 117: Envenomation)

## Answer 1-89. E

This child has symptoms that are concerning for a life-threatening infection of the upper airway, such as epiglottitis (supraglottitis). The first priority in this situation is to secure

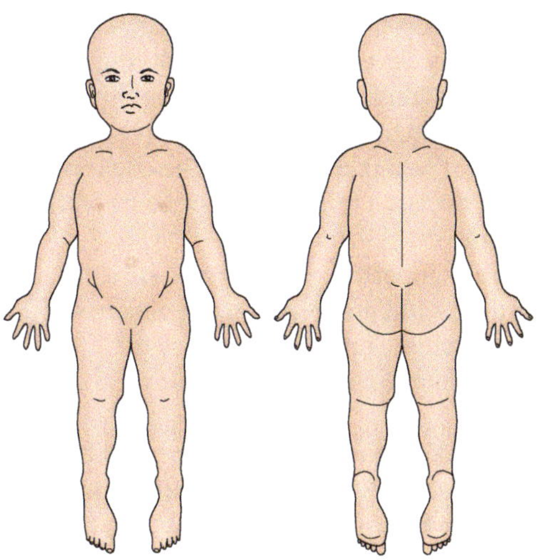

| Area | Age–Years | | | | | % 2° | % 3° | % Total |
|---|---|---|---|---|---|---|---|---|
| | 0–1 | 1–4 | 5–9 | 10–15 | Adult | | | |
| Head | 19 | 17 | 13 | 10 | 7 | | | |
| Neck | 2 | 2 | 2 | 2 | 2 | | | |
| Ant. Trunk | 13 | 13 | 13 | 13 | 13 | | | |
| Post. Trunk | 13 | 13 | 13 | 13 | 13 | | | |
| R. Buttock | 2–1/2 | 2–1/2 | 2–1/2 | 2–1/2 | 2–1/2 | | | |
| L. Buttock | 2–1/2 | 2–1/2 | 2–1/2 | 2–1/2 | 2–1/2 | | | |
| Genitalia | 1 | 1 | 1 | 1 | 1 | | | |
| R. U. Arm | 4 | 4 | 4 | 4 | 4 | | | |
| L. U. Arm | 4 | 4 | 4 | 4 | 4 | | | |
| R. L. Arm | 3 | 3 | 3 | 3 | 3 | | | |
| L. L. Arm | 3 | 3 | 3 | 3 | 3 | | | |
| R. Hand | 2–1/2 | 2–1/2 | 2–1/2 | 2–1/2 | 2–1/2 | | | |
| L. Hand | 2–1/2 | 2–1/2 | 2–1/2 | 2–1/2 | 2–1/2 | | | |
| R. Thigh | 5–1/2 | 6–1/2 | 8–1/2 | 8–1/2 | 9–1/2 | | | |
| L. Thigh | 5–1/2 | 6–1/2 | 8–1/2 | 8–1/2 | 9–1/2 | | | |
| R. Leg | 5 | 5 | 5–1/2 | 6 | 7 | | | |
| L. Leg | 5 | 5 | 5–1/2 | 6 | 7 | | | |
| R. Foot | 3–1/2 | 3–1/2 | 3–1/2 | 3–1/2 | 3–1/2 | | | |
| L. Foot | 3–1/2 | 3–1/2 | 3–1/2 | 3–1/2 | 3–1/2 | | | |
| | | | | Total BSA Burn | | | | |

Modified from Lund and Browder

• Hand Method for nonuniform burns—palm of child's hand approximates 1 percent of child's total BSA burn.

**FIGURE 116-2.** Modified Lund and Browder body surface area chart. (Mark W. Kline, *Rudolph's Pediatrics*, 23rd Edition. Copyright © McGraw-Hill Education. All rights reserved.)

the airway under controlled conditions. Anything that will upset the child or cause increased respiratory distress, such as labs, intravenous access, examining the oropharynx, or positioning supine, should be avoided. Radiographs of the neck can be helpful in visualizing the airway soft tissues, including the epiglottis, but should only be done in a stable patient, not one who is acutely ill with a tenuous airway.

(p. 537, Section 8: Acute and Critical Illness, Chapter 118: Acute Upper Airway Obstruction)

**Answer 1-90.** D

This child has a presentation that is most suggestive of a retropharyngeal abscess. The typical presentation is a preschool child with a preceding upper respiratory viral illness, followed by throat pain and unilateral neck swelling and pain, with or without stridor.

Croup would be accompanied by a harsh cough. Croup does not cause neck swelling or pain. Epiglottitis and tracheitis would result in a more ill-appearing child and do not cause neck swelling. A peritonsillar abscess would be very unusual in this age group, as it is most common in adolescents. A lateral neck radiograph would be helpful in establishing the diagnosis, as it would show widening of the retropharyngeal space. Treatment consists of intravenous antibiotics targeting *Streptococcus* species, *Staphylococcus aureus*, and oral anaerobes.

(p. 538, Section 8: Acute and Critical Illness, Chapter 118: Acute Upper Airway Obstruction)

**Answer 1-91.** D

This child is presenting with a history and physical examination that is strongly suggestive of a lower airway inhaled foreign body. The definitive diagnostic and therapeutic study is a rigid bronchoscopy. The acute onset after a choking episode, with no infectious symptoms, makes pertussis unlikely. Diagnostic radiography, such as a chest radiograph, may be normal in many cases of nonradiopaque inhaled foreign body. Furthermore, in a high-suspicion case, a chest radiograph is unlikely to change management. Back blows or abdominal thrusts are unlikely to dislodge the foreign body at this point and may increase the likelihood of the foreign body moving further distal.

(p. 539, Section 8: Acute and Critical Illness, Chapter 118: Acute Upper Airway Obstruction)

**Answer 1-92.** A

Compared to adults, pediatric patients have a larger occiput, larger tongue, shorter mandible, and prominent adenoids and tonsils (Figure 118-1). These differences combine with a relatively smaller airway, lower functional residual capacity, higher peripheral airway resistance, and higher oxygen to put infants and young children at higher risk for decompensation from an upper airway obstruction.

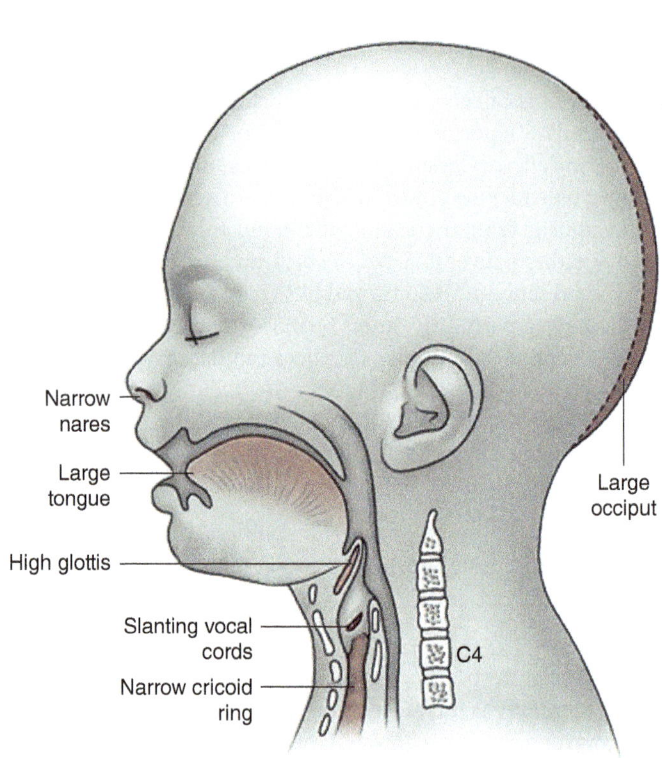


**FIGURE 118-1.** Anatomic differences in pediatric airways. (Mark W. Kline, *Rudolph's Pediatrics*, 23rd Edition. Copyright © McGraw-Hill Education. All rights reserved.)

(p. 539, Section 8: Acute and Critical Illness, Chapter 118: Acute Upper Airway Obstruction)

**Answer 1-93.** B

This child has croup, which begins with a prodrome of nasal congestion and rhinorrhea, similar to other viral upper respiratory infections. Fever usually occurs during the first 24 hours of illness. Within 12 to 48 hours, signs and symptoms of upper airway obstruction such as inspiratory stridor and the classic "barking seal" cough develop, with hoarseness appearing later. The illness may last 3 to 14 days, depending on the severity of the case.

In croup, the anteroposterior radiograph will show both subglottic narrowing and progressive tracheal narrowing as it reaches the subglottis. This is referred to as the "steeple sign" and is due to mucosal edema below the vocal cords (Figure 118-2).

Pertussis is less likely given the radiograph and the description of the cough. A cough with pertussis is usually described as paroxysmal and severe. The cough can be followed by a high-pitched "whoop" as the child inhales. Posttussive emesis is also not uncommon. Epiglottitis, retropharyngeal abscess, and foreign body are also unlikely given the presentation and the radiographic findings.

(p. 539, Section 8: Acute and Critical Illness, Chapter 118: Upper Airway Obstruction)

**Answer 1-94.** D

This patient has symptoms consistent with heat exhaustion, a moderately severe heat-related condition. While she did have syncope as part of her illness, her continued symptoms and abnormal vital signs put her in the category of heat exhaustion, rather than simply heat syncope. Heat exhaustion may progress to heatstroke, a life-threatening condition characterized by core body temperature of 40°C, accompanied by tachycardia, headache, and signs of central nervous system dysfunction. Sweating is usually absent in heatstroke.

(p. 541, Section 8: Acute and Critical Illness, Chapter 119: Temperature Dysregulation)

**Answer 1-95.** B

Children with medical complexity (CMCs) require multiple medical services and frequent hospital admissions. Care is often partitioned with limited communication among healthcare providers, contributing to duplicate or unnecessary investigations and therapies, the potential for costly medical errors, and frustration for families. Families complain that they are often excluded from decision-making and lack the information needed to care for their children at home. Society is impacted by the disproportionately high healthcare costs of CMC and by the loss of productivity because of parents taking time off from work and siblings missing school.

(p. 547, Section 9: Children with Medical Complexity, Chapter 120: Complex Care)

**Answer 1-96.** C

The prevalence of children with special healthcare needs (CSHCN), defined as children who have or are at risk of having a chronic physical, developmental, behavioral, or emotional condition that requires health and related services of a type or amount beyond that generally required by children, ranges from 12% to 19%. A small but growing subset of CSHCN can be described as CMCs, who have medical fragility and intensive care needs that are not easily met by existing healthcare models.

Common characteristics of CMCs include chronic conditions requiring multiple hospital and office-based medical and nonmedical services; a reliance on medical equipment and technology, multiple medications, specialized surgeries, and other therapies; and the need for effective care coordination. While there is not yet one commonly accepted definition of CMCs, they likely compose 5.8% of all US children insured by Medicaid and account for 34% of Medicaid spending for all children. Common frameworks for definitions include diagnostic condition, degree of impairment and disability, and risk for high healthcare costs.

(p. 547, Section 9: Children with Medical Complexity, Chapter 120: Complex Care)

**Answer 1-97.** D

In response to the complex management needs of CMCs, many tertiary centers in the United States have developed disease- or condition-specific programs that provide care coordination for CMCs (eg, diabetes programs, tracheostomy/ventilator programs). More recently, disease- or condition-independent care coordination programs have been developed to address the needs of CMCs whose conditions cross multiple specialty areas. Some offer a predominantly outpatient or hospital-based inpatient complex care service, in which direct primary and/or consultative care is provided by physician-led teams, some of whom also provide co-management with community primary care clinicians. Finally, a few programs offer integrated inpatient and outpatient services. Many of these models have shown a decrease in hospital days, increase in family satisfaction, and decrease in costs after enrollment in their program, but the lack of standardized definitions of the populations served makes comparisons among these models difficult.

(pp. 547–548, Section 9: Children with Medical Complexity, Chapter 120: Complex Care)

**Answer 1-98.** E

The rapid growth of medical knowledge and technology has led to an increase in the number of children with medical complexity (CMCs) who, through the use of technologic assistance, live longer and at home. If assistive technology is desired, the choice of support or device requires input from the family and multiple members of the healthcare coordination team. The primary care physician and subspecialists (eg, gastroenterologist, pediatric surgeon), along with providers with specialized expertise (eg, feeding therapist) must be able to advise the family on the potential benefits and possible limitations of a certain technology support.

Shared decision-making is the process between the family and the care team about whether to pursue the use of certain medical technologies. Although the gastroenterologist, pediatric surgeon, and feeding therapist may be able to provide advice on whether and when to consider conversion of the nasogastric tube to a gastrostomy tube in this case, the child's family is integral to deciding whether a particular technology support is consistent with their overall goals for their child.

(pp. 549–550, Section 9: Children with Medical Complexity, Chapter 121: Managing Technology in Children with Medical Complexity)

**Answer 1-99.** A

Children with medical complexity (CMCs) who receive supplemental oxygen may benefit from pulse oximetry to maintain safety and provide guidance in adjusting the level of support. The pulse oximeter alarms should be set at levels that alert the caregiver to assess the child and potentially intervene.

Setting limits too close to the child's baseline range will result in multiple alarms and decrease use of the monitor. Instructions for the caregivers should include specific parameters for when supplemental oxygen should be initiated and when the physician should be called.

Given that the child in this case does not exhibit any respiratory symptoms when the pulse oximetry alarm sounds and the oxygen saturation dips only momentarily, it would be reasonable to reset the alarm to a lower level to minimize multiple alarms. When making such an adjustment, it would be helpful to let the pulmonologist know. Because there is no indication that this child's respiratory status is worsening, there is no need at this time to refer her to the pulmonologist. While increasing oxygen flow and providing more frequent respiratory therapy, including medications, may be helpful when she has an upper respiratory infection and has more respiratory support needs, she currently is not exhibiting symptoms suggestive of an upper respiratory infection or respiratory support needs. All technology may malfunction and benefits from regular maintenance. While the multiple alarms appear to be related to the current alarm setting, if the alarms continue even after the alarm setting is reset or if there are other signs of malfunction, it would be important to notify the vendor for assessment and potential replacement.

(p. 550, Section 9: Children with Medical Complexity, Chapter 121: Managing Technology in Children with Medical Complexity)

**Answer 1-100.** D

Supplemental oxygen is commonly prescribed for home use in children with medical complexity (CMCs) who have chronic lung disease. While hospital case managers and pediatric pulmonologists often assist in the ordering of oxygen supplies, including mask, nasal cannula, tubing, and oxygen supply, the primary care clinician may be asked to refill such orders and discuss modifications as the specific needs of children and families change over time.

Oxygen is supplied in liquid form, as a compressed gas, or from an oxygen concentrator. Liquid oxygen is more portable; lightweight liquid oxygen tanks can be refilled from a large reservoir tank kept at home. Liquid oxygen, however, may cost more and may not last as long as compressed oxygen because it evaporates. Liquid oxygen is also cold and can burn if it comes into contact with the skin. Compressed oxygen is available in cylinders, ranging in size from small portable tanks to large stationary tanks for home use. An oxygen concentrator is an electric machine that can deliver approximately 4 L/min of 100% oxygen. The percentage decreases at higher flow rates. When an oxygen concentrator is used, a backup cylinder of compressed oxygen is recommended in case of power failure. All families should be reminded never to smoke or allow others to smoke when oxygen is used.

(p. 551, Section 9: Children with Medical Complexity, Chapter 121: Managing Technology in Children with Medical Complexity)

**Answer 1-101.** B

Children require tracheostomy tubes for a variety of indications including upper airway obstruction, airway protection, and long-term ventilation. Pediatric tracheostomy tubes are generally composed of silicone, which is quite flexible, or polyvinyl chloride, which may be either flexible or rigid. The tube is placed surgically, and children are often monitored in an intensive care unit (ICU) for about 1 week to address any complications.

Children with tracheostomies generally require suctioning at least 3 to 4 times per day and more frequently during times of respiratory illness. Signs that a child needs suctioning include rattling mucus sounds, tachypnea, secretion pooling at the opening of the tracheotomy tube, and signs of respiratory distress. Normal saline drops prior to suctioning help loosen the thick secretions or elicit a cough. Shallow suctioning removes secretions at the opening of the tracheostomy. Suctioning just past the tip of the tracheostomy tube allows complete clearance. Suctioning until the catheter tip meets resistance from the carina should generally be avoided because this may injure the lining of the airway. Applying suction pressure both on insertion and on withdrawal of the suction catheter facilitates removal of the secretions. Following suctioning, many children with tracheostomy tubes may benefit from a few manual ventilation breaths to recruit the lung.

(p. 551, Section 9: Children with Medical Complexity, Chapter 121: Managing Technology in Children with Medical Complexity)

**Answer 1-102.** E

In addition to pediatric subspecialists, physical and occupational therapists, speech and language pathologists, nutritionists, respiratory therapists, pharmacists, child life specialists, and nurse case managers can play a critical role in planning and delivering care to children with medical complexity (CMCs). Primary care pediatricians can play a crucial role in involving these specialized therapists when providing care for the most complex CMCs and encouraging communication among all members of the care team to ensure coordinated care.

Speech and language pathologists have expertise in human communication, including normal development and communication disorders. They are also trained to recognize neurologic and upper aerodigestive disorders that affect speech and swallowing. Thus, speech and language pathologists can address not only speech, language, and cognitive communication, but also the swallowing skills of children with disabilities. They can determine specific deficits, the severity of disorder, and possible etiologic and contributing factors. Recommended therapy based on comprehensive assessment may include exercises to improve oral-motor skills.

While the gastroenterologist and often accompanying nutritionist can address feeding difficulties that result in poor weight gain and growth and consult on decisions related to the consideration of feeding tubes, they are not the primary experts on the neuromotor aspects of feeding and swallowing. Physical therapists address problems associated with neuromuscular dysfunction and gross motor delay as they influence the child's ability to be mobile within the environment. Occupational therapists address problems associated with neuromuscular dysfunction, sensory perception, psychosocial competence, and fine motor delay as they influence the child's ability to participate in self-care, play, and school activities. In practice, there is often considerable overlap in the methods and techniques used by physical and occupational therapists. Respiratory therapists are often more active in the hospital setting and provide invaluable perspectives and services related to the care of a child's respiratory function. Although most respiratory therapists are involved in the care of children requiring respiratory support, such as oxygen, tracheostomy, and mechanical ventilation, they can also help recommend exercises to build more respiratory capacity as well as medications and equipment to assure patency of airways so that children can minimize the impairment and maximize activity to assure participation in age-appropriate activities.

(p. 552, Section 9: Children with Medical Complexity, Chapter 121: Managing Technology in Children with Medical Complexity)

**Answer 1-103.** D

A child's inability to master the environment independently may lead to decreased socialization, learned helplessness, and delayed development. Therefore, wheeled mobility should be considered as early as necessary to facilitate developmentally appropriate independence and functional activity. Because poor positioning and restriction of movement can result in pressure areas and musculoskeletal deformity, mobility devices are often combined with customized positioning or seating systems when the child needs assistance in maintaining appropriate position and use of the trunk, head, or limbs. The type of wheeled mobility should be based on the child's immediate and anticipated needs and goals (eg, duration of need, ability to self-propel, ability to partially ambulate), family issues (eg, transportation access, lifting restrictions), and the proposed environment in which the device will be used.

A power wheelchair is the most appropriate wheeled mobility equipment for the patient given his progressive neuromuscular disorder along with his current ability to operate computerized input devices with his hands. The direction and speed of movement for such wheelchairs can be specified by use of a hand-operated toggle device. Power wheelchairs have multiple seating and positioning options that are ideal to prevent pressure-related discomfort and injuries in an adolescent who is unable to move his body. The drawbacks of power wheelchairs are that they are heavy and generally require a vehicle lift for transportation. Additionally, repairs may be costly.

Strollers are appropriate for younger children with mild to moderate impairment. They are lightweight and easy to maneuver; however, they may not provide optimal body support and can become uncomfortable for children if used for long distances. A stroller would not be appropriate for a teenager and would not allow for independence. Manual upright wheelchairs can allow custom seating and encourage learning self-propulsion. When a child's endurance is low, however, maneuvering on a nonlevel surface may be challenging. A variety of types of wheelchairs, including those for sports, are available. Manual tilt-in-space wheelchairs, while heavier than the upright wheelchairs, can accommodate position changes and assistive technology. Scooters are specifically geared for older children and youth with impaired lower extremity strength; they are less expensive and lighter than power wheelchairs. However, there are minimal seating options, and they are inappropriate for those with progressive neuromuscular disorders.

(pp. 552–553, Section 9: Children with Medical Complexity, Chapter 121: Managing Technology in Children with Medical Complexity)

**Answer 1-104.** D

Children with intellectual disabilities are more likely to suffer from sleep disturbances. Poor sleep may be present in up to 85% of children with intellectual disabilities. Symptoms of poor sleep include excessive daytime sleepiness, hyperactivity, and aggressive behavior, all of which can lead to a decline in overall functioning. A sleep study should be considered if there is concern for obstructive sleep apnea or other sleep disorders. Melatonin is not a treatment for obstructive sleep apnea. Attention to good sleep hygiene is important but may be complicated by behavior disturbances and altered sleep–wake cycles.

(p. 556, Section 9: Children with Medical Complexity, Chapter 122: Managing Children with Intellectual and Developmental Disabilities)

**Answer 1-105.** E

Palliative care is a model of care to improve the quality of life of patients with serious illnesses and their families and includes the prevention and relief of suffering by promptly identifying and treating pain and other sources of distress, whether they are physical, psychosocial, or spiritual. Opioid treatment for moderate to severe pain in a 12-year-old child with metastatic osteosarcoma is an example of palliative care because it focuses on improving quality of life by effectively addressing pain.

The other responses do not exemplify palliative care because they are curative or disease-directed therapies. Treatment for acute asthma exacerbation, immunizations, and anticipatory guidance to address elopement, while important, are all disease-directed therapies. Gastrostomy tube placement for failure to thrive is also considered disease-directed. Foregoing such treatment, on the other hand, considers the impact of an intervention on quality of life and is often considered part of advance care planning in palliative care.

(p. 563, Section 10: Palliative Care, Chapter 125: Palliative and Hospice Care for Children)

**Answer 1-106.** D

Defining goals of care is a critical part of guiding decision-making by identifying interventions that meet identified goals rather than treat a medical problem in isolation. Communication tools useful for this purpose are reviewed in Table 125-1.

(p. 564, Table 125-1, Section 10: Palliative Care, Chapter 125: Palliative and Hospice Care for Children)

**Answer 1-107.** C

In palliative care, an effective interprofessional team approach enables collaboration among disciplines and enhances the holistic care for children and families. Among hospital-based pediatric palliative care programs and community-based hospice programs, the most common disciplines on staff are physicians, nurses, social workers, and chaplains. Social workers provide psychosocial assessment and supportive counseling for the child and family adjusting to changes, skill in exploring hopes and worries of a patient and family, and expertise in identifying community resources.

Physicians and nurses bring expertise in symptom management, treatment planning, and bedside care. Chaplains support faith traditions and spiritual values that promote hope and support families as they face change, loss, or grief. Child life specialists facilitate communication with children through activities that assist with emotional distress, can also explore a deeper understanding of patients' fears and wishes, and enhance psychosocial supports for siblings.

(pp. 564–565, Section 10: Palliative Care, Chapter 125: Palliative and Hospice Care for Children)

**Answer 1-108.** A

In the process of decision-making and defining a care plan, certain steps can help determine how to proceed if the benefit hoped for from an intervention does not occur:

- Define with the family the goals that you intend to meet.
- Identify the likelihood of an intervention meeting these goals.
- Know the evidence for the possible benefit and harm for the interventions available.
- Define a time period in which the intervention would be expected to meet the goal.
- Discuss a plan if the hoped-for benefit does not occur in this time period.

Advance care planning can help patients and families think through aspects of their care as they live with serious illness and approach the end of life. Advance care planning tools specific for children and adolescents, using developmentally appropriate language and medical terms, can be useful for clinicians in facilitating discussions about care preferences to cover the following themes:

- How I want people to treat me
- How I want to be comforted
- What I want my family and friends to know
- What I want my doctors and nurses to know

The discussion of resuscitation status requires an honest assessment of the likelihood of benefit and possible harm. Resuscitation status is a shared medical decision that incorporates both the medical assessment of benefit and the goals of care of the patient and family. Understanding the broader goals of care allows the clinician to discuss resuscitation in the context of what is most important to the patient and family. Clinicians should make recommendations based on the goals of care.

Appointment of a healthcare proxy allows a patient over 18 years of age to designate another person to make medical decisions if he is unable to make or communicate those decisions. A social worker or other trusted team member involved with the patient can assist with the process of identifying someone. This process is not relevant for your patient since he has not reached the age of maturity.

Great care is only possible when critical information is determined, documented, and communicated to those involved in the child's care. Areas of need discussed that are important in this process include the following:

- Location of care
- Individuals involved in care
- Information to include in documentation

(pp. 565–566, Section 10: Palliative Care, Chapter 125: Palliative and Hospice Care for Children)

**Answer 1-109.** C

Pain assessment tools are based on the concept of placing and understanding things in order of magnitude. Children from age 5 or 6 are developing the ability to create a series in order of size but only through trial and error. Pain rating tools appropriate for this functional age include poker chips and Oucher. Children from age 7 to 10 can more reliably use tools to quantify pain, such as the Wong-Baker faces pain rating scale. Adolescents develop the ability to use a numerical rating scale, such as a 0 to 10 scale, to rate their pain without the use of a tool. The FLACC (ie, face, legs, activity, crying, and consolability) pain scale was developed to help medical observers assess the level of pain in children who are too young to cooperate verbally. It can also be used in adults who are unable to communicate.

(p. 566, Section 10: Palliative Care, Chapter 125: Palliative and Hospice Care for Children)

**TABLE 125-1.** Communication Tools Used in Palliative Care

| Objectives | Suggested Language |
|---|---|
| Getting to know child and family | Tell us about your child before he or she became ill. |
| | What makes your child happy? Sad? |
| | What is your understanding of your child's illness/condition and its likely course? |
| | In light of your understanding of your child's illness, what is most important to you and your family? |
| | What are your hopes? What are your worries? |
| Determine goals of care as a guide to decision-making | We will always review how the interventions available meet the goals you've identified. |
| | Goals commonly include comfort and quality of life along with hope for life extension, although they may shift to providing care at home when less benefit or greater burden is seen from care in the hospital, may shift to comfort only when limited benefit is identified from the treatment available, and can be focused on a specific activity such as maintaining current health status for a family trip. |
| Focus on parental expertise | Although I will honestly reflect on changes in your daughter's health and functional status, you are the expert in how these changes look and affect her quality of life. |
| | Although we bring expertise in evaluating and managing health problems in children, you are the expert in how such problems look in your daughter. |
| Anticipate worries | We know that worries of parents at such times often include: Is my child suffering? Will my child get better? Is there more we can do? We will talk through these worries. |
| | We can talk through some of the "what ifs" so as to address any worries you may have, so you know what to expect, to assure that we have a care plan in place, and to allow you to focus on spending time with your daughter. |
| Reflect on the past as a guide to the future | I wonder if we are seeing less recovery and less time between each illness. |
| | Do you think we are seeing fewer good days now compared to 6 and 12 months ago? |
| | Your child's story will guide us along the way. Our job as parents and care providers is to watch, listen, and reflect honestly on what the story is telling us. |
| Acknowledge the limits of interventions | I cannot imagine how hard it is to be seeing fewer good days. I wish we had interventions that could reverse this. |
| | Your child continues to receive exceptional care at home. My observation is that we are seeing fewer benefits from the treatment we have available. What have you observed? |
| Limiting treatment does not mean limiting care | I worry that your child's body is getting tired despite the best treatment available. |
| | It might make sense to identify what we won't do if her body becomes too tired to sustain adequate breathing. We won't limit treatments that have reasonable benefit but will protect her from interventions that may harm or prolong suffering. |
| | We will always provide care that maximizes comfort throughout her life. |
| Hope for the best; prepare for the rest | We know families often hold simultaneously their hope for the best possible outcome with their realistic understanding of the severity of the problem. |
| Offer continuity with a safety net | We might not know when your child will have more problems, but you will always have a team available to help guide and support you on this journey. |
| Identify decision-making as a dynamic process | What might seem like the "right" decision today could change. Your decisions can change as the clinical course changes. |
| | Stopping a medical intervention is ethically and legally the same as not starting an intervention but can feel very different emotionally. |

Mark W. Kline, *Rudolph's Pediatrics*, 23rd Edition. Copyright © McGraw-Hill Education. All rights reserved.

**Answer 1-110.** E

Pain is usually classified as either nociceptive or neuropathic. Nociceptive somatic pain is caused by stimulation of nociceptors in skin, soft tissue, skeletal muscle, and bone. It is well localized and usually described as sharp, aching, squeezing, stabbing, or throbbing. Nociceptive visceral pain is caused by stimulation of nociceptors and stretch receptors in the viscera, and it is poorly localized and often described as dull, crampy, or achy. Neuropathic pain is caused by stimulation or abnormal functioning of damaged sensory nerves and is usually described as burning, shooting, or tingling.

Children with neurologic impairment experience pain more frequently than the general pediatric population. Identifying a source of pain in a nonverbal child with a developmental disability poses a unique and significant challenge. Commonly recognized pain sources in these children include acute etiologies, such as fracture, urinary tract infection, or pancreatitis; and chronic etiologies, such as gastroesophageal reflux, constipation, feeding difficulties, positioning, spasticity, hip pain, or dental pain.

Underlying central nervous system dysfunction poses the potential for altered pain modulation pathways in the brain, which may in turn alter the response to both noxious and nonpainful stimuli. In children with severe neurologic impairment who exhibit persistent pain-related behavior, extensive diagnostic workup may not yield a definitive nociceptor source of pain. As a diagnosis of exclusion, the term *neuro-irritability* can be used to describe this scenario.

Nociceptive pain and neuropathic pain are classifications of pain, and constipation and gastroesophageal reflux are commonly recognized chronic etiologies of pain.

(p. 566, Section 10: Palliative Care, Chapter 125: Palliative and Hospice Care for Children)

**Answer 1-111.** B

The World Health Organization revised its recommendation for medication selection for pain treatment in 2012 for children with chronic illness from a 3-step ladder to a 2-step approach, eliminating the category of moderate pain and the recommendation for weak opioids. Evidence has shown that codeine is not as effective or safe as was once thought, and it is no longer recommended for routine use. Codeine is ineffective in over one-third of individuals due to variability in conversion of codeine into its active metabolite, and ibuprofen has been demonstrated to achieve equivalent analgesia with fewer side effects than codeine, such as respiratory depression, at routine doses.

The first step of the 2-step approach is used for mild pain and includes the use of nonopioid analgesics, including acetaminophen, ibuprofen, and ketorolac. The second step is used for moderate to severe pain and includes the use of opioid analgesics, starting with a lower dose for moderate pain and a higher dose for severe pain. Adjuvant medication can be used at either step, especially for neuropathic pain. Integrative medicine offers approaches such as guided imagery, meditation, hypnosis, storytelling, music, art therapy, and acupuncture that may be useful. Acupuncture, hypnosis, and mind–body therapies have proven to be efficacious interventions for pain and anxiety in children. Hypnosis specifically has been effective in lessening procedural distress, reducing procedural time, and reducing procedural pain and anxiety for children.

(p. 568, Section 10: Palliative Care, Chapter 125: Palliative and Hospice Care for Children)

**Answer 1-112.** A

Opioids are the most effective agents for management of pain and dyspnea. However, fear of respiratory depression or addiction remains a barrier to the effective use of opioids, even at the end of life. This is unwarranted as opioid-induced respiratory depression is unlikely when dosed appropriately, adjusted for renal or hepatic impairment, and titrated in a standardized manner. The association of opioid use with end-of-life care can result in the misconception that opioid use either hastens death or indicates that someone is dying. When used effectively, opioids do not hasten death and are the mainstay of management for pain and dyspnea throughout the course of illness.

For optimal treatment of persistent, moderate-to-severe pain, opioid administration should be scheduled around the clock based on the duration of analgesic effect of the specific opioid. Once the opioid requirement is determined, it can be converted to a sustained-release formulation given 2 or 3 times daily, with immediate-release doses as needed for breakthrough pain. A reasonable trial dose for breakthrough pain is 10% of the 24-hour opioid requirement. It can be given as often as every 1 to 2 hours to achieve pain relief. Based on the patient's response and the requirement for breakthrough analgesia, the daily dose of analgesics may be increased by 25% to 50% per day until adequate analgesia is achieved or until there are intolerable or unmanageable side effects.

Opioid side effects are common, and management of these is important to assure continued use of necessary analgesics. Stimulant laxatives, such as senna or bisacodyl, should be initiated when opioids are prescribed to prevent constipation. For many other side effects, such as sedation and nausea, symptom improvement may occur without dose adjustment after several days.

(p. 568, Section 10: Palliative Care, Chapter 125: Palliative and Hospice Care for Children)

**Answer 1-113.** A

Pain, anxiety, distress, and suffering in children are best thought of as interrelated symptoms; addressing each is important to the relief of others. Children with cancer commonly encounter symptoms of worrying, sadness, nervousness, and irritability. Levels of distress in children and families can be stratified into 3 levels: a universal level that applies to all families, a targeted level that presents with acute needs, and a clinical level that is persistent and/or escalating. At the universal level, children and families often experience resilience and engage family and social support systems to ameliorate distress. At the targeted level, acute distress requires more targeted interventions and close monitoring. At clinical levels of distress, consultation with behavioral health specialists can inform the development of a plan of care that more fully addresses their risk factors.

Children with serious illness who experience psychological distress can benefit from a multidimensional approach to treatment. Psychotherapeutic and psychopharmacologic treatment options should be considered. Supportive interventions for depression and anxiety for the child include normalization of their experiences, supportive counseling, introduction to support groups or other children, and provision of psychoeducational resources. Clinical interventions include psychotherapeutic counseling, mindfulness-based interventions, support groups, art therapy, and bibliotherapy.

Sleep disturbances are common in children with serious illness, and consequences include fatigue, impaired daytime functioning, mood disturbances, reduced social/emotional well-being, reduced ability to cope, and impaired perception of illness severity. Sleep impairment may worsen symptoms of depression, anxiety, and pain. Pharmacologic treatment approaches include melatonin, antidepressants such as tricyclic antidepressants, trazodone, clonidine, and neuroleptics. Psychological and behavioral interventions include stimulus control, sleep education, and relaxation training.

Psychopharmacologic treatment can be considered for symptoms of depression and anxiety that persist despite nonpharmacologic interventions. Medications should always be used in conjunction with ongoing supportive counseling and psychosocial interventions. SSRIs have some safety data in medically ill children, although efficacy has been difficult to demonstrate. Therapeutic benefit may not be seen until 2 to 4 weeks after initiation. Side effects can occur within a few days of initiation and include dry mouth, constipation, urinary retention, sedation, anxiety, agitation, insomnia, irritability, impulsivity, akathisia, and hypomania. Suicidal thoughts may develop, making it important to recognize that worsening symptoms such as agitation and irritability may be precursor signs.

(pp. 571–572, Section 10: Palliative Care, Chapter 125: Palliative and Hospice Care for Children)

**Answer 1-114.** D

Discussing advance care planning topics with families of children with medical complexity (CMCs) presents unique challenges. The concept of "quality of life" is paramount to these discussions. Families and healthcare providers have personal beliefs and experiences that influence their definition of quality of life; thus, it can be difficult to agree on what is in the patient's best interest.

High-quality advance care planning provides benefits to patients, families, and healthcare providers. When parents have the opportunity to discuss their child's end-of-life care plan, they can increase the likelihood that their child will die in the family's preferred location and decrease levels of complicated grief after death. Many families are having these discussions privately; however, they do not feel able to have them with their physicians or other members of the healthcare team. Barriers cited by families include their fear of death or of losing hope, and those cited by providers include lack of training and of a dedicated palliative care team.

It is well established that physicians are poor prognosticators and typically overestimate survival. The length of the physician's relationship with the patient has been suggested to be inversely proportional to the physician's prognostic accuracy. This is important in CMCs because healthcare teams often care for patients from birth through adolescence and even into adulthood and thus may be less accurate in their ability to provide meaningful and precise prognostic information.

When communicating an uncertain prognosis, one helpful strategy is to use graphics to articulate the patient's waxing and waning to emphasize the overall downward trajectory. It is important to emphasize to families that planning for alterations in care is a flexible process that can and should change with the patient's clinical status (Figure 125-1).

Hope has an integral role in palliative and end-of-life care and should not be confused with denial. Although many hope for a miracle, most possess other hopes for themselves or

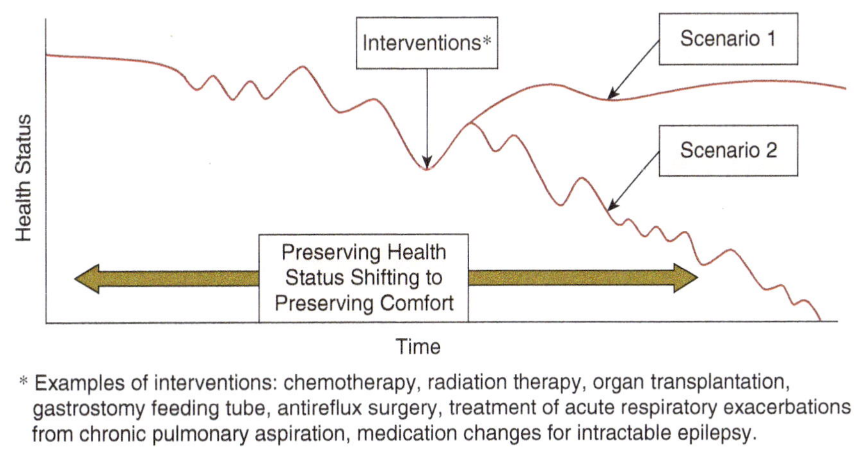


**FIGURE 125-1.** Health trajectories for children with serious illness. (Mark W. Kline, *Rudolph's Pediatrics*, 23rd Edition. Copyright © McGraw-Hill Education. All rights reserved.)

their child such as hope for time, hope for comfort, hope for companionship, hope to die at home, or a hope that loved ones do not suffer. Palliative care seeks to foster hope through open dialogue regarding prognosis, interventions, and goals of care. Studies support that such tasks increase caregiver hope and expressed goals of care when end of life approaches.

(pp. 574–576, Section 10: Palliative Care, Chapter 126: Palliative Care for Children with Chronic Diseases)

**Answer 1-115.** E

Some key communication tactics for discussing resuscitation plans include the following:

- Avoid dichotomies such as "doing everything" or "doing nothing." ("Do you want us to do everything for your child if her heart stops?") This implies that interventions could be helpful and can make parents feel as though they are "refusing" care for their child.
- Discuss a DNR order as a tool to protect a child from interventions that will not be helpful and may harm the child. Do not overemphasize the harm.
- It is not necessary to discuss every single item that is included in a DNR order. This can be overwhelming for parents and may lead to decisions that are inconsistent.
- Use the word "die": "If your child's heart stops, that would mean your child has died. The team could attempt to restart your child's heart ..."
- Give legitimacy to both sides of a decision: "Some loving parents choose to allow cardiac resuscitation, in the hopes that it would lead to more good time for the child down the road, while other loving parents choose to protect their child from cardiac resuscitation, valuing the opportunity to hold their child at the end of his or her life."
- Remind families that they can change their mind at any time and that, in an out-of-hospital setting, it is always up to them when, where, and with whom they choose to share a completed out-of-hospital DNR form.

(p. 576, Section 10: Palliative Care, Chapter 126: Palliative Care for Children with Chronic Diseases)

**Answer 1-116.** C

For typically developing children, prior to age 2 years, all interactions with the outside world are sensory and motor, and there is likely no intellectual concept of death. Starting in early childhood, at ages 2 to 7 years, orientation is self-centered, and the outside world is considered only from the child's personal and subjective view. To children, imaginary and magical things are important determinants of occurrences. At this stage, dead things should be able to eat and feel and breathe. Parents can be immortal, and dying animals should be able to return. From ages 7 to 11, thinking is less egocentric and more concrete. Reasoning is based on direct observation, and concepts of death are in the present tense. After age 12 years, full intellectual capacities develop and, with them, the ability to deal in abstractions. Since your patient is 9 years old, he understands that animals and people do not die because of a magical spell they or others cast, but perceives reality as he grasps universality and inevitability. Patients this age often ask repetitive questions secondary to their need to know the details of the dying experience. Adolescents, while capable with dealing with abstractions, become more concerned with changes in physical appearances and capacities. Like adults, children with full death conceptualizations worry not only about whether they will die, but also how they will die.

Children seldom ask for information for fear of causing the eruption of difficult emotions for all. However, the consequence of this reticence is a child's imagination running rampant and painting a picture worse than reality. It is therefore incumbent upon healthcare providers to encourage and support conversations between patients and their caregivers to ensure correct information and support of those difficult emotions. Such discussions can also identify hopes that a child or caregiver has, and consequently, a more robust healthcare plan can be devised.

(p. 577, Section 10: Palliative Care, Chapter 126: Palliative Care for Children with Chronic Diseases)

**Answer 1-117.** C

Virtually all children experience the death of a family member or friend. Bereavement is a normal and universal experience; however, it can cause significant adjustment difficulties. Pediatricians can play a vital role by building on their preexisting relationship to ensure that the child understands accurately what has occurred, provide advice to families on how to help promote adjustment and coping, and assist the child and family in identifying supportive resources within the community.

Pediatricians can begin by creating an environment where children and adolescents feel it is safe and where they are welcome to discuss their thoughts and feelings. Physicians often worry, however, that they do not know what to say that will be helpful and do not wish to make matters worse by raising the topic. Approaches that may be less helpful include (1) trying to "cheer up" those who are actively grieving, (2) encouraging people to be strong or to hide or minimize their expressions of distress, and (3) telling people how they should or do feel, rather than asking them about their own feelings.

It is helpful to offer to speak with children and adolescents alone so that they can talk freely and share their reactions without concern about upsetting their parents. Many healthcare providers are reluctant to initiate conversations with children out of concern that such discussions may upset them.

(pp. 578–579, Section 10: Palliative Care, Chapter 127: Supporting the Grieving Child and Family)

**Answer 1-118.** B

Young children's limited conceptual understanding, coupled with a tendency for adults to withhold information, often results in misconceptions and misunderstandings. The magical thinking and egocentrism of children prompt them to assume guilt related to the death for some thought, action, or failure to act. Often, this guilt is illogical (eg, "My father had a heart attack because I upset him that morning" or "If only I had stayed home from school that day, I would have been able to get help for my mother earlier") and too often remains fully unknown to others but may cause much distress for children; similar guilt feelings are common among adolescents and adults as well.

While religious explanations can be shared with children at any age, they are generally abstract and prone to literal misinterpretations and, especially for young children, should be accompanied by explanations about the physical realities of death (eg, "When people die, their body is no longer working; the person doesn't move, breathe, see, or feel pain"). Simply stating that the person "went to heaven" or "was chosen by God to be at His side" may lead to questions about how to get to or from heaven or worries that others close to the child (or the child himself or herself) may be chosen next.

Children who have been excluded from memorial events, such as funerals, miss an opportunity to benefit from the support of family members and friends, may have more difficulty understanding or accepting what has occurred, and often wonder what could have been done to their family member or friend that is so horrifying that they are not permitted to view. In general, it is helpful instead to explain to the child in clear and direct terms what is expected to occur at the funeral and to invite the child to participate to the level of his or her comfort, without any attempt to force or coerce participation. In addition, an adult who is not personally grieving but is well known to the child can accompany the child and monitor and address his or her needs and reactions, allowing the child to titrate the level of involvement.

Pediatricians can play an important role in helping adults identify and attend to their children's needs around the time of the death as well as during the period of readjustment, which often lasts months to years. Referral to support or counseling should be considered, especially when the death involves a close family member or friend, when risk factors for complicated mourning are anticipated, when the initial reactions are intense or unusual, or when intensive grieving is prolonged and associated with impairments in daily function. Children who are grieving should be expected to have at least some transient difficulties with schoolwork secondary to problems with attention, sleeping, and sadness. Ongoing communication and offers to meet for follow-up can be very helpful to the family in this setting.

(pp. 578–579, Section 10: Palliative Care, Chapter 127: Supporting the Grieving Child and Family)

**Answer 1-119.** D

Disagreements between patients and families can be traumatic to patients and ethically troubling to the medical team. One common scenario involves an adolescent patient who expresses fatigue and wishes to stop aggressive treatment and to focus on comfort, in conflict with parents who want to "do everything." Providers in these circumstances are challenged to engage the patient and his parents in open dialogue, ensuring that each party's message is heard by the other. Providers must be careful to ensure that the patient's preferences are taken into consideration, even though parents have ultimate decision-making authority.

As a general rule, parents have the rights to make medical decisions on behalf of minors in their care. In many states, however, emancipated minors are granted full medical decision-making capacity. Although your patient has held a part-time job in the past, since he continued to live at home during that time, he has not achieved emancipated minor status. Since he has lived with his condition for a long time, he is likely to have attained a greater maturity level and capacity of understanding the impact of treatment choices. Although minors generally cannot consent, even if parents wish to protect them from upsetting or painful information, they should be included in conversations about wishes at the end of life. The determination of capacity to make medical decisions should follow a standard protocol that reveals the parents' abilities to come to a complete understanding of risks, benefits, and alternatives to the medical decision being requested. Some parents' or legal guardians' capacity may be enhanced with the use of decision aids, written materials, or, if the parent or guardian has limited English proficiency, additional language services. Capacity should not be judged based on agreement or disagreement with medical advice.

(pp. 578–579, Section 10: Palliative Care, Chapter 128: Ethics, Law, and Medical Care Near the End of Life)

# CHAPTER 2 Fetal and Neonatal Care

W. Christopher Golden, Colleen A. Hughes Driscoll, Bernadette Crowder Johnson, Amaris M. Keiser, and Brittany L. Schwarz

**2-1.** A medical student from the United States is discussing infant mortality with a medical student from another country. Which of the following is the most important factor to consider when comparing infant mortality between the 2 countries?

**A.** The method by which gestational age is estimated in each country

**B.** The prevalence of multiple gestations in each country

**C.** The precise formula each country uses to describe infant mortality

**D.** The etiologies of infant death in each country

**E.** The differences in population size

**2-2.** A pregnant woman experiencing preterm labor at 23 weeks' gestation arrives at a small community hospital with special care neonatal services but no subspecialty care services. What is the most compelling rationale for transferring this woman to a regional subspecialty center prior to delivery?

**A.** Regional subspecialty centers have more support for establishing successful breastfeeding.

**B.** Regional subspecialty centers have more social work support for mothers of preterm babies.

**C.** Delivering the baby at a special care center would be more costly.

**D.** Delivering the baby at a regional subspecialty center reduces the risk of neonatal mortality.

**E.** Regional subspecialty centers provide parents support groups for preterm infants.

**2-3.** The on-call neonatologist is asked to counsel a pregnant woman who has just been diagnosed with a twin gestation. Which of the following statements about multiple pregnancies is true?

**A.** Pregnancy evaluation and management for monochorionic twins are the same as for dichorionic twins.

**B.** Twins have a decreased risk of chromosomal anomalies.

**C.** Multiple pregnancies account for approximately 10% of all preterm births.

**D.** The risk of neonatal morbidity is the same for singleton and twin pregnancies.

**E.** Growth of fetuses of a twin gestation is similar to that of a fetus of a singleton gestation.

**2-4.** A 5-hour-old male neonate born at 39 1/7 weeks' gestation was born through meconium-stained amniotic fluid. He was intubated in the delivery room. In the neonatal intensive care unit (NICU), he was placed on mechanical ventilation and supplemental oxygen, with a fraction of inspired oxygen ($FiO_2$) of 0.95. The baby's postductal oxygen saturation has been consistently 15% lower than the preductal oxygen saturation for the last 2 hours, although he is well ventilated. A chest radiograph shows patchy bilateral infiltrates, predominantly on the right side, with slight hyperinflation (Figure 52-3). The baby has appropriate blood pressure measurements. What is the appropriate next step in the management of this baby?

**A.** Hyperventilation

**B.** Maintenance of $PaO_2$ levels > 300 mm Hg

**C.** Maintenance of an arterial pH of 7.5

**D.** Treatment with inhaled nitric oxide

**E.** Initiation of extracorporeal membrane oxygenation

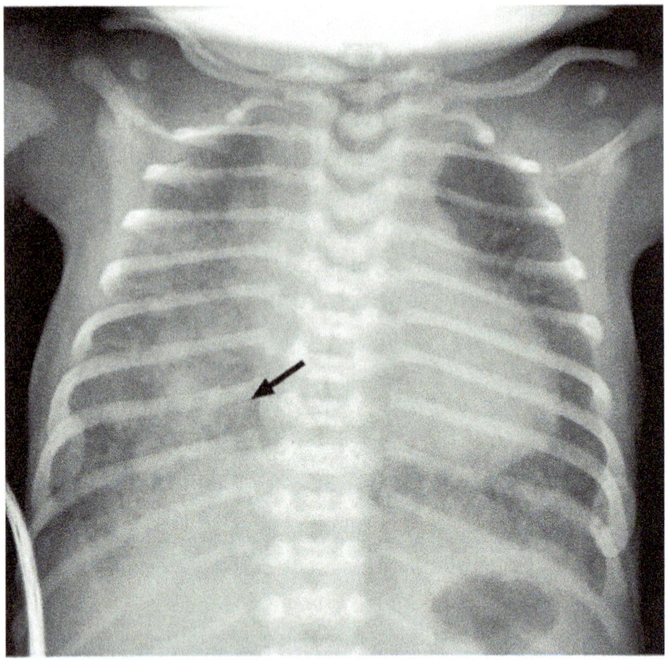

**FIGURE 52-3.** (Mark W. Kline, *Rudolph's Pediatrics*, 23rd Edition. Copyright © McGraw-Hill Education. All rights reserved.)

**2-5.** A 4-day-old baby born at 24 1/7 weeks' gestation is mechanically ventilated via an endotracheal tube and is being treated with indomethacin for a large patent ductus arteriosus. Abruptly, the baby develops increased respiratory distress, pallor, oxygen desaturation, and hypotension. A small amount of blood is seen in the endotracheal tube. Which of the following statements is true about this acute event?

**A.** This event occurs most commonly in term infants.

**B.** Chest radiography will demonstrate a focal lung finding.

**C.** Increasing the peak end-expiratory pressure on the ventilator may be useful in management.

**D.** Less than 5% of survivors develop chronic lung disease.

**E.** Neonatal hyperthermia is associated with this event.

**2-6.** A term newborn baby is born by vaginal delivery following prolonged rupture of membranes. The amniotic fluid is noted to be foul smelling. Shortly after birth, the baby is noted to have tachypnea, subcostal retractions, and grunting. The baby requires 0.5 $FiO_2$ to maintain normal newborn hemoglobin saturation levels. A chest radiograph demonstrates a diffuse, relatively homogenous, ground-glass appearance and a small left pleural effusion. A blood culture is obtained, and the baby is started on antibiotics. After several days of treatment, the baby no longer has a supplemental oxygen requirement, and symptoms of respiratory distress have resolved. The blood culture is sterile. Which of the following explains the low incidence of this baby's respiratory disease in the neonatal population?

**A.** Universal screening for group B *Streptococcus* (GBS) and intrapartum antibiotic treatment in pregnant women

**B.** Maternal administration of betamethasone and broad-spectrum antibiotics

**C.** Recommendations to avoid elective cesarean delivery before 39 weeks' gestation

**D.** Use of prenatal vitamins and fetal monitoring during labor

**E.** Frequent chest radiography and multiple blood culture samples

**2-7.** The neonatal resuscitation team is called to the delivery of a term baby whose mother received limited prenatal care. After birth, the baby develops cyanosis and severe respiratory distress, which becomes worse with positive-pressure ventilation administered through a face mask. On physical exam, bowel sounds can be auscultated prominently over the left chest, heart sounds are most apparent on the right chest, and the abdominal wall is flat. Which of the following steps should be performed next in management of this patient?

**A.** Increasing positive inspiratory pressure delivered through a face mask

**B.** Performing a needle thoracotomy

**C.** Administering surfactant administration

**D.** Placing a gastric drainage tube

**E.** Inserting a low-lying umbilical venous catheter

**2-8.** A 1-hour-old male newborn was born at 39 4/7 weeks via emergent cesarean section delivery. The delivery course was remarkable for fetal decelerations and suspicion of maternal placental abruption. The baby's Apgar scores were 2 and 7 at 1 and 5 minutes of age, respectively. Immediately after birth, the baby was limp and apneic. After several minutes of positive-pressure ventilation, the baby recovered. The umbilical venous cord blood gas showed a pH of 6.98. The pediatric neurology consultant describes the baby as having Sarnat 2 encephalopathy. Which of the following physical exam findings is consistent with this classification?

**A.** Periodic breathing

**B.** Irritability

**C.** Tachycardia

**D.** Absent Moro reflex

**E.** Flaccid muscle tone

**2-9.** Thirty minutes following birth, a term baby is noted to be lethargic with decreased activity, hypotonia, weak suck, incomplete Moro, bradycardia, and miosis. The baby's history is remarkable for fetal decelerations and suspicion of maternal placental abruption. The umbilical arterial cord pH was 6.91. The 5-minute Apgar score was 3. The baby was limp and apneic immediately after birth and required intubation with assisted ventilation. Which of the following therapies should be implemented standardly and immediately after birth to reduce the risk of disability for this baby?

**A.** Anticonvulsant therapy
**B.** Therapeutic hypothermia
**C.** Erythropoietin
**D.** Stem cell therapy
**E.** Permissive hyperthermia

**2-10.** Which of the following statements is true about perinatal stroke?

**A.** Newborns with perinatal stroke present with seizures at about 3 weeks of age.
**B.** Perinatal strokes most often occur in the distribution of the anterior cerebral artery.
**C.** Venous infarctions are more common than arterial infarctions.
**D.** Babies with intrauterine growth restriction are at risk for perinatal strokes.
**E.** Neuroimaging will clearly delineate vessel occlusion in a venous infarction.

**2-11.** A 1-day-old male infant, born at 23 6/7 weeks' gestation, acutely develops apnea, bradycardia, and increased ventilator support. His laboratory studies are notable for a significant anemia and acidosis. He appears pale, and his sutures are more widely spaced than at neonatal intensive care unit (NICU) admission. Which of the following studies would be most helpful in immediately diagnosing the infant's condition?

**A.** Cranial ultrasound
**B.** Echocardiogram
**C.** Cerebrospinal fluid analysis
**D.** Electroencephalogram
**E.** Complete blood count

**2-12.** Which of the following statements is true about strategies to reduce intraventricular hemorrhage (IVH) in preterm infants?

**A.** Completion of a course of antenatal steroids decreases the odds of a preterm infant developing an IVH.
**B.** Postnatal phenobarbital administration has been shown to reduce the incidence of IVH.
**C.** Rapid administration of intravascular volume replacement is indicated to reduce the risk of IVH.
**D.** Indomethacin prophylaxis is recommended to reduce the incidence of IVH in preterm infants.
**E.** Liberal use of inotropic agents decreases the likelihood of IVH in preterm infants.

**2-13.** The on-call neonatologist is asked to counsel a mother in preterm labor with a fetus at 24 3/7 weeks' gestation. Which of the following statements is most accurate regarding the risks of intraventricular hemorrhage (IVH)?

**A.** The incidence of IVH increases as birth weight increases.
**B.** Severe hemorrhages occur in 90% of babies born between 22 and 26 weeks' gestation.
**C.** Gestational age is the only factor that impacts the risk of IVH.
**D.** Ninety percent of IVHs will occur within the first hour of age.
**E.** The incidence of IVH since the mid-1990s for very-low-birth-weight infants has not changed.

**2-14.** A pediatrician attends the delivery of an estimated term newborn whose mother did not receive prenatal care. The baby is vigorous with good respiratory effort and a heart rate of 130 bpm. On exam, the baby has a 4-cm vertical opening in the skin over the lumbosacral spine, with protrusion of a cystic mass. The feet are plantar flexed and limited in motion with mild acrocyanosis. What is the most appropriate next step in the management?

**A.** Decompress the mass via needle aspiration
**B.** Intubate the infant
**C.** Wrap the mass with dry gauze
**D.** Place the infant prone
**E.** Provide supplemental oxygen via nasal cannula

**2-15.** The postpartum nurse is doing a routine assessment of an 18-hour-old newborn. The mother reports that the baby had 3 episodes of emesis in the past 6 hours and is not interested in breastfeeding. He has not yet stooled. The nurse finds that the baby has an estimated 5 mL of bright green emesis on his blanket. Physical exam reveals an irritable baby with intercostal retractions and a diffusely distended and tender abdomen. Which of the following diagnostic tests is urgently needed in this scenario?

**A.** Rectal biopsy
**B.** Esophageal manometry
**C.** Gastrointestinal contrast study
**D.** Chest radiograph
**E.** Left lateral decubitus abdominal radiograph

**2-16.** A 4-day-old male baby born at 39 3/7 weeks' gestation presents to a community hospital emergency department with decreased oral intake, lethargy, and mild tachypnea. The baby is jaundiced, tachycardic, and mottled. Rectal temperature is 36.9°C. He has a 15 mm Hg systolic blood pressure gradient between his upper and lower extremities and diminished femoral pulses. An arterial blood gas shows pH of 7.17, $PCO_2$ of 45 mm Hg, and base deficit of –10 mmol/L. The serum lactate is 10 mmol/L. You place an intravenous line, order a normal saline bolus, and arrange to have the baby transferred to an intensive care unit. Which of the following medications should be initiated first while awaiting arrival of the regional transport team?

**A.** Ibuprofen

**B.** Gentamycin

**C.** Acetaminophen

**D.** Prostaglandin E

**E.** Vitamin K

**2-17.** A 3800-g male infant is born at 42 0/7 weeks' gestation by cesarean section due to failed induction of labor. Rupture of membranes occurs 1 hour before birth and is notable for particulate meconium. The infant is limp and apneic upon arrival to the radiant warmer. What is the initial step in his resuscitation?

**A.** Begin positive-pressure ventilation with a T-piece resuscitator

**B.** Suction the hypopharynx with a meconium aspirator

**C.** Deliver blow-by oxygen with a self-inflating bag

**D.** Provide tactile stimulation, positioning, and warming

**E.** Initiate chest compressions coordinated with 100% oxygen delivery

**2-18.** A 3700-g female is born by emergent cesarean section at 37 1/7 weeks' gestation due to a placental abruption. The infant initially has no respiratory effort, a heart rate of 50 bpm, and hypotonia and cyanosis. She is dried, warmed, positioned, and stimulated. She then receives positive-pressure ventilation at 30 seconds of life (due to weak respiratory effort). At 90 seconds of age, she demonstrates a heart rate of 120 bpm and a strong cry; however, mild acrocyanosis is still noted. What is the next step in resuscitation?

**A.** Wrapping the infant in warm blankets

**B.** Placing an emergent umbilical line

**C.** Continuing positive-pressure ventilation

**D.** Providing supplemental oxygen

**E.** Initiating chest compressions

**2-19.** A woman presents at 32 1/7 weeks' gestation for a routine visit. During the visit, her fundal height measures only 28 cm. Due to concerns for low amniotic fluid levels or poor fetal growth, a uterine ultrasound is performed, which shows the fetus is at the 10th percentile for gestational age. An earlier scan at 25 2/7 weeks' gestation showed the fetus at the 50th percentile for gestational age, which raises concerns for intrauterine growth restriction (IUGR). Which of the following statements is true about IUGR?

**A.** IUGR is defined only by fetal growth less than normal for the population.

**B.** Fetuses with IUGR have symmetric growth restriction.

**C.** Adverse effects of IUGR are related to the size of the infant at birth.

**D.** IUGR results in normal brain development.

**E.** Very preterm infants with IUGR are particularly at risk for developmental complications.

**2-20.** You are discussing neonatal care with a student, who asks you about how to properly classify a newborn infant in terms of weight. Newborn infants can be classified according to birth weight, as well as by weight in relation to gestational age. Which of the following statements is correct?

**A.** A newborn infant who weighs 2000 g is always considered small for gestational age.

**B.** A newborn infant who weighs 2000 g could never be considered large for gestational age.

**C.** A newborn infant who weighs 2000 g is considered low birth weight.

**D.** A newborn infant who weighs 2000 g is considered very low birth weight.

**E.** A newborn infant who weighs 2000 g is considered extremely low birth weight.

**2-21.** Which of the following maternal risk factors most directly correlates with risk of congenital anomalies in the infant of a diabetic mother?

**A.** Age at onset of diabetes (maternal onset at age < 20 years)

**B.** Type 1 versus type 2 diabetes

**C.** Glycemic control (HbA1c)

**D.** History of a prior macrosomic child (> 4500 g at birth)

**E.** Use of oral hypoglycemics

**2-22.** A 28-year-old woman with gestational diabetes presents at 38 1/7 weeks' gestation in active labor. The estimated fetal weight is 4400 g. The male infant is born by vaginal delivery, with shoulder dystocia noted by the obstetricians. The neonate's resuscitation was unremarkable, and his physical exam at 2 hours of age is normal aside from occipital molding. What is the most appropriate initial step in management of this infant?

**A.** Serum glucose

**B.** Chest radiograph

**C.** Cranial sonogram

**D.** Abdominal sonogram

**E.** Serum bilirubin level

**2-23.** The pediatric resident is called to the nursery to evaluate a newborn who is "blue." The now 6-hour-old baby is a 39 6/7-week male infant born to a 28-year-old woman with sporadic prenatal care. The mother delivered the baby vaginally after 20 hours of ruptured amniotic membranes. Her group B *Streptococcus* (GBS) colonization status is unknown. She developed a temperature of 38.1°C in labor and received 1 dose of penicillin 2 hours before delivery. The infant cried after delivery and required only routine resuscitation in the delivery room. The mother noted increased work in breathing while feeding, and the baby was brought to the nursery. Physical exam reveals a tachypneic baby with intercostal retractions and audible grunting. Auscultation reveals coarse bilateral breath sounds but no stridor. Pulse oximetry is 81% (on the foot) in room air, but the pulse oximetry level improves to 98% when he is placed on a 2 L/min nasal cannula ($FiO_2$ 1.0). Chest radiograph reveals diffuse hazy lung fields and small, bilateral pleural effusions. What condition should be most suspected in this infant?

**A.** Respiratory distress syndrome

**B.** Tracheomalacia

**C.** Pneumonia

**D.** Bilateral choanal atresia

**E.** Congenital diaphragmatic hernia

**2-24.** Which of the following interventions has been shown to decrease the incidence of meconium aspiration syndrome?

**A.** Oropharyngeal suction at delivery of the head by the obstetrician

**B.** Labor induction at 41 weeks' gestation

**C.** Endotracheal intubation and suctioning by the pediatrician on the radiant warmer

**D.** Injection of hypotonic fluid into the amniotic sac prior to delivery

**E.** Elective cesarean section with detection of meconium-stained amniotic fluids

**2-25.** Which of the following statements is true about pulmonary surfactant?

**A.** Surfactant proteins A and D play an innate role in pulmonary immune defense.

**B.** Surfactant synthesis begins at about 20 weeks' gestation.

**C.** Surfactant is produced by type I alveolar cells.

**D.** Surfactant secretion begins at about 34 weeks' gestation.

**E.** Surfactant reduces alveolar surface tension primarily due to phosphatidylglycerol.

**2-26.** A 30 6/7-week male newborn is born via emergency cesarean section due to placental abruption after a motor vehicle accident. The infant received drying, warming, and continuous positive airway pressure (CPAP) in the delivery room. The infant is admitted to the neonatal intensive care unit (NICU) for respiratory distress. At 2 hours of age, physical exam reveals a well-perfused newborn with increased work in breathing, audible grunting, and coarse bilateral breath sounds. Chest radiograph shows hypoinflation and bilateral ground-glass lung opacities. He is intubated and administered surfactant. At 36 hours of age, the patient is extubated to CPAP. Which of the following most likely contributed to his clinical presentation?

**A.** Pulmonary infiltrates due to meconium aspiration

**B.** Pulmonary surfactant deficiency due to prematurity

**C.** Pneumonia due to group B *Streptococcus* (GBS) infection

**D.** Pulmonary edema due to delay in activation of alveolar sodium channels

**E.** Pulmonary surfactant dysfunction due to an *ABCA3* mutation

**2-27.** A 5-day-old, former 24 2/7-week female infant develops progressive hypotension and respiratory distress. Physical exam reveals bounding palmar pulses, 4- to 5-second capillary refill, and a machinery-like murmur heard best at the left sternal border between the second and third intercostal spaces. This baby's clinical presentation is most consistent with failure of closure of a fetal conduit between what structures after birth?

**A.** Right atrium and left atrium

**B.** Main pulmonary artery and descending aorta

**C.** Main pulmonary artery and superior vena cava

**D.** Left umbilical vein and inferior vena cava

**E.** Superior vena cava and brachiocephalic artery

**2-28.** A 36-hour-old former 26 4/7-week female newborn develops a new-onset murmur. Echocardiogram demonstrates a patent ductus arteriosus (PDA) measuring 1.8 mm in diameter. Clinically, the infant is ventilated with a mean airway pressure of 12 cm $H_2O$ and receiving supplemental oxygen with an $FiO_2$ of 0.5. The clinical team elects to treat her with intravenous indomethacin to close the PDA. Which of the following statements regarding indomethacin therapy is true?

**A.** Early indomethacin therapy increases the risk of necrotizing enterocolitis.

**B.** Isolated gastric perforation is associated with concomitant use of indomethacin and dexamethasone.

**C.** Indomethacin levels correlate with degree of ductal patency.

**D.** Indomethacin use is contraindicated in patients with serum creatinine levels > 1 mg/dL.

**E.** Prolonged indomethacin use is part of the routine management of PDA in the neonate.

**2-29.** Which of the following statements about patent ductus arteriosus (PDA) closure is true?

**A.** Functional closure of the PDA happens within hours of birth.

**B.** Anatomic closure of the PDA occurs after 2 months of life.

**C.** Surgical closure of the PDA is associated with lower risks of neurodevelopmental impairment.

**D.** Acetaminophen has been well studied in multiple, large, randomized controlled trials for PDA closure in preterm infants.

**E.** Catheter-based PDA closure is recommended over surgical ligation in infants who present prior to 1 month of age.

**2-30.** A 10-week-old infant was born at 26 3/7 weeks' gestation. He remains on supplemental oxygen via a high-flow nasal cannula. He is being treated with diuretics for bronchopulmonary dysplasia (BPD). His grandfather was born in 1968 at 32 weeks' gestation and was also treated for BPD in another neonatal intensive care unit (NICU). What lung pathology is most likely present in the current neonate (but not in the grandfather during his infancy)?

**A.** Smooth muscle hypertrophy

**B.** Alveolar hypoplasia

**C.** Epithelial metaplasia

**D.** Pulmonary fibrosis

**E.** Parenchymal emphysema

**2-31.** A male infant born at 28 weeks' gestation was intubated at birth and received mechanical ventilation and supplemental oxygen for 1 month after birth. He was extubated to continuous positive airway pressure (CPAP) at 33 weeks postmenstrual age and then transitioned to nasal cannula oxygen at 35 weeks postmenstrual age. Due to serial radiographic findings of pulmonary edema and chronic lung changes, he was treated with diuretics and an inhaled steroid beginning at 34 weeks postmenstrual age. He is currently 38 weeks postmenstrual age and remains on 0.5 L/min oxygen via nasal cannula with an $FiO_2$ of 0.33. The infant meets criteria for the diagnosis for BPD based on which of the following?

**A.** Need for mechanical ventilation in the first month of life

**B.** Use of chronic diuretics during hospitalization

**C.** Oxygen requirement at 36 weeks postmenstrual age

**D.** Use of steroid therapy at 36 weeks postmenstrual age

**E.** Radiographic evidence of chronic lung changes

**2-32.** A male infant is born at 25 1/7 weeks due to premature rupture of membranes and maternal chorioamnionitis. He is intubated in the delivery room due to respiratory distress and receives exogenous surfactant. He is treated with antibiotics for 7 days for *Klebsiella* bacteremia and with ibuprofen at 5 days of age for a patent ductus arteriosus (PDA). Which of the following is his greatest risk factor for developing bronchopulmonary dysplasia (BPD)?

**A.** Prematurity

**B.** Chorioamnionitis

**C.** Mechanical ventilation

**D.** PDA

**E.** Sepsis

**2-33.** A 6-week-old former 26 4/7-week female infant remains intubated on conventional mechanical ventilation with an $FiO_2$ of 0.6. She was delivered by urgent cesarean section due to maternal placental abruption. She was intubated in the delivery room and given surfactant. The residents and fellow discuss pharmacotherapy in the neonatal intensive care unit (NICU) and bronchopulmonary dysplasia (BPD). Which of the following medications used in neonatal care has been demonstrated as beneficial in the prevention and/or treatment of BPD?

**A.** Inhaled levalbuterol

**B.** Oral vitamin A

**C.** Inhaled budesonide

**D.** Oral caffeine

**E.** Oral furosemide

**2-34.** A 7-hour-old female infant is being examined by the pediatric intern after the postpartum nurse noted that the infant looked "pale." The infant was born vaginally with vacuum extraction at 38 5/7 weeks after 24 hours of ruptured amniotic membranes. Her mother is a 31-year-old woman whose pregnancy was complicated by gestational diabetes. On exam, the 4200-g infant has a large, tense fluid collection over her right occiput with a palpable fluid wave. Her right ear is displaced anteriorly. She has increased work in breathing and cool extremities, with a 4- to 5-second capillary refill. Which of the following is the next appropriate step in management of this baby?

**A.** Echocardiogram
**B.** Blood culture
**C.** Chest radiograph
**D.** Complete blood count
**E.** Urinalysis

**2-35.** Which of the following treatments in neonates has been suggested to reduce the risk of necrotizing enterocolitis (NEC)?

**A.** Delayed cord clamping
**B.** Preterm cow's milk formula
**C.** Extended indomethacin therapy (4 or more doses)
**D.** Oral immunoglobulin therapy
**E.** Delayed enteral feeds

**2-36.** A 65-hour-old former 36 1/7-week male infant is undergoing his daily newborn exam in the mother–baby unit. He was born after repeat cesarean section to a 27-year-old woman with a history of diabetes and a prior myomectomy. He is breastfeeding every 2 hours and has only lost 7% of his birthweight. The maternal blood type is O positive; the baby's blood type is B positive with a negative direct Coombs test. Physical exam reveals a well-hydrated, alert male infant with a strong suck and jaundice to the umbilicus. A total serum bilirubin (sent at 60 hours of age) is 13.5 mg/dL. The mother is planning a 96-hour hospitalization to recover from her cesarean section and work on breastfeeding further. A nomogram with the potential risk designation of term and near-term well newborns based on their hour-specific serum bilirubin levels (Figure 56-3) is shown below.

In addition, the nomogram for phototherapy is shown below (Figure 56-2).

What is the most appropriate next step in management of this infant?

**A.** Change the infant to a soy-based formula.
**B.** Space the infant's breastfeeding to every 4 hours.
**C.** Repeat the serum bilirubin now.
**D.** Continue routine newborn care.
**E.** Commence phototherapy.

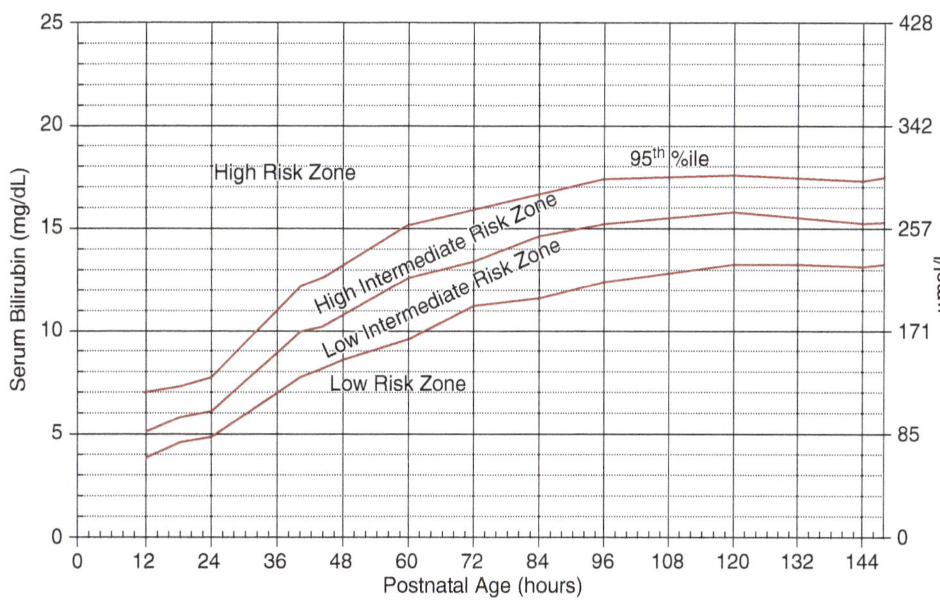


**FIGURE 56-3.** Risk designation of term and near-term well newborns based on their hour-specific serum bilirubin values. The high-risk zone is designated by the 95th percentile track. The intermediate-risk zone is subdivided to upper- and lower-risk zones by the 75th percentile track. The low-risk zone has been electively and statistically defined by the 40th percentile track. (Reproduced with permission from American Academy of Pediatrics Subcommittee on Hyperbilirubinemia. Management of hyperbilirubinemia in the newborn infant 35 or more weeks of gestation. *Pediatrics*. 2004;114(1):297-316.)

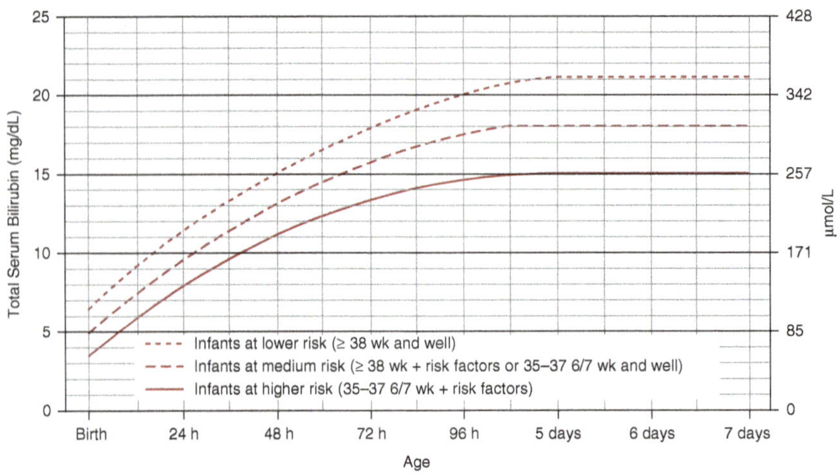


- Use total bilirubin. Do not subtract direct reacting or conjugated bilirubin.
- Risk factors = isoimmune hemolytic disease, G6PD deficiency, asphyxia, significant lethargy, temperature instability, sepsis, acidosis, or albumin < 3.0 g/dL (if measured).
- For well infants 35–37 6/7 wk can adjust TSB levels for intervention around the medium risk line. It is an option to intervene at lower TSB levels for infants closer to 35 wks and at higher TSB levels for those closer to 37 6/7 wk.
- It is an option to provide conventional phototherapy in hospital or at home at TSB levels 2–3 mg/dL (35–50 mmol/L) below those shown but home phototherapy should not be used in any infant with risk factors.

**FIGURE 56-2.** Guidelines for phototherapy in hospitalized infants of 35 or more weeks' gestation. TSB, total serum bilirubin. (Reproduced with permission from American Academy of Pediatrics Subcommittee on Hyperbilirubinemia. Management of hyperbilirubinemia in the newborn infant 35 or more weeks of gestation. *Pediatrics.* 2004;114(1):297-316.)

**2-37.** A 20-hour-old male infant is being examined by the nursery medical student. He was born vaginally at 39 6/7 weeks to a 24-year-old mother. Physical exam of the neonate reveals a large tuft of hair over the lumbosacral spine and a palpable mass over the symphysis pubis. Per the postpartum nurse, the baby has never voided. What is the next appropriate step in management of this newborn?

**A.** Ordering a urine culture

**B.** Performing a spinal sonogram

**C.** Performing an abdominal radiograph

**D.** Consulting a general pediatric surgeon

**E.** Ordering serum electrolytes

**2-38.** A 4-hour-old male infant is being examined by the pediatric intern after the mother noted the baby was "vomiting." He was born at 37 5/7 weeks' gestation to a 25-year-old primiparous woman with an unremarkable pregnancy. Examination of the patient reveals a vigorous, active newborn with normal tone. The cardiorespiratory exam is unremarkable. His abdominal exam reveals a soft abdomen with a periumbilical mass (that easily reduces when palpated) and active bowel sounds. The diaper contains a moderate-sized meconium stool. The vomitus, present on the mother's shoulder towel, is nickel-sized and contains curdled milk without bile or blood. Which of the following is the next appropriate step in management of this baby?

**A.** Complete blood count (CBC)

**B.** Reassurance to the mother

**C.** Pediatric surgical consultation

**D.** Upper gastrointestinal series

**E.** Blood culture

**2-39.** A 4-hour-old male infant is being examined by the pediatric intern after birth. He was born vaginally at 37 4/7 weeks to a 34-year-old mother. He had routine prenatal care and normal fetal sonograms throughout the pregnancy. Which of the following physical exam findings is normal for this baby?

**A.** A small gap in the midline abdominal wall musculature

**B.** A liver edge 3 cm before the right costal margin

**C.** A right kidney 5 cm in width

**D.** An umbilical stump with a small amount of clear drainage

**E.** A spleen tip 4 cm below the left costal margin

**2-40.** A 15-day-old former 28 2/7-week male infant develops abdominal distention, apnea, and bradycardia. Physical exam reveals an intubated, lethargic infant with no respiratory effort over the mechanical ventilator. His abdomen is tense with abdominal wall erythema (Figure 60-2). Arterial blood gas shows a pH of 7.10, $PCO_2$ of 49 mm Hg, $PaO_2$ of 70 mm Hg, and base deficit of −11 mmol/L. Abdominal radiograph demonstrates diffuse abdominal distention and gas within the wall of the small bowel.

Which of the following is the next appropriate step in management of this infant?

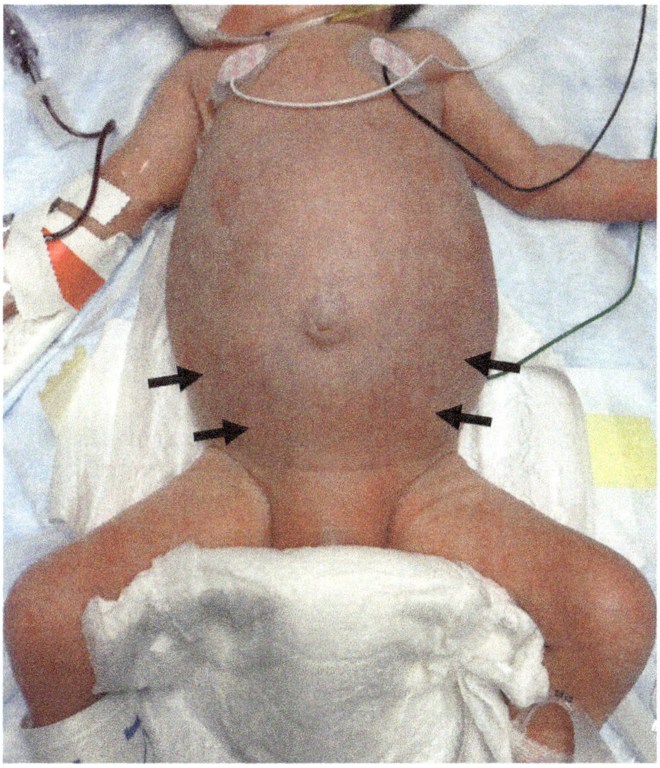

FIGURE 60-2. (Mark W. Kline, *Rudolph's Pediatrics*, 23rd Edition. Copyright © McGraw-Hill Education. All rights reserved.)

A. Placement of a large-bore nasogastric tube to low, intermittent wall suction
B. Administration of intravenous piperacillin-tazobactam
C. Initiation of continuous morphine infusion
D. Transfusion of platelets
E. Lumbar puncture

**2-41.** A 5-day-old male infant, born at 38 2/7 weeks' gestation, has completed 72 hours of therapeutic hypothermia for neonatal encephalopathy. His birth course was notable for perinatal depression after complete placental abruption, with a cord pH of 6.96 and base deficit of −17 mmol/L. He will undergo brain magnetic resonance imaging (MRI) today. His parents have questions about interpreting the results of the exam. Which of the following statements is correct regarding brain MRI in these patients?

A. Parasagittal lesions involving the vascular boundary zones are due to the hypothermia.
B. Brain imaging changes are static during the first 2 weeks of age.
C. White matter changes in these infants often are associated with visual defects.
D. Basal ganglia and thalamic injury may be associated with different forms of cerebral palsy.
E. MRI findings do not correlate with poor long-term neurodevelopmental outcomes.

**2-42.** Which of the following processes occurs during the primary phase of energy failure in hypoxic-ischemic brain injury?

A. Reduced high-energy phosphorylated compounds
B. Diminished neurotransmitter receptor activity
C. Decreased intracellular calcium
D. Accumulated excitatory neurotransmitters
E. Increased tissue pH

**2-43.** Which of the following statements is correct regarding neonatal circumcision?

A. Circumcision is associated with an increased risk of penile cancer.
B. The complication rate of circumcision is about 5%.
C. The American Academy of Pediatrics recommends circumcision as a routine procedure.
D. Circumcision may be performed in newborns with a chordee.
E. Circumcision is performed frequently to prevent balanoposthitis.

**2-44.** A 3-day-old former 39 2/7-week male infant is being seen by his pediatrician for a post-newborn visit. He was born vaginally to a 27-year-old woman with an uncomplicated pregnancy and delivery. He is breastfeeding every 2 hours and has only lost 8% of his birthweight. The parents are both African American. He and his mother both have A negative blood types. A total serum bilirubin at hospital discharge (48 hours of age) was 10 mg/dL. Physical exam reveals a sleepy male infant with normal skin turgor but jaundice to the elbows and knees. A total serum bilirubin measured in the office is 25 mg/dL, with a direct fraction of 0.4 mg/dL. What is the test most likely to confirm the etiology of this baby's hyperbilirubinemia?

A. Osmotic fragility test
B. Hemoglobin electrophoresis
C. Right upper quadrant abdominal sonogram
D. Serum electrolytes
E. Serum glucose-6-phosphate dehydrogenase level

**2-45.** Which of the following statements regarding fetal and perinatal thyroid hormone activity is correct?

**A.** The role of thyroid hormone in perinatal transition is clear.

**B.** The increase in thyroid-stimulating hormone at birth is related to increases in glucose.

**C.** Thyroid hormone levels increase 7-fold at the time of delivery.

**D.** Fetal thyroid hormone levels begin to increase at around 9 weeks of gestation.

**E.** Thyroid hormone activity is not associated with shivering thermogenesis.

**2-46.** Which of the following statements is true about the fetal circulation?

**A.** Inferior vena cava blood flow preferentially streams into the right ventricle.

**B.** Right and left ventricular blood flow contributes to systemic circulation.

**C.** Blood from the right ventricle perfuses the pulmonary circulation via the ductus arteriosus.

**D.** The fractional distribution of systemic blood flow to regional vascular beds is the same as in extrauterine life.

**E.** Approximately 20% of the ventricular output perfuses the placenta.

**2-47.** A 2-day-old female infant is being prepared for discharge. She was born vaginally at 38 5/7 weeks to a 19-year-old mother with limited prenatal care. Physical exam of the neonate reveals a cluster of vesicles on an erythematous base under a large left parietal cephalohematoma. Which of the following is the next appropriate step in management of this newborn?

**A.** Applying topical timolol to the lesions

**B.** Ordering a cranial sonogram

**C.** Performing a lumbar puncture

**D.** Aspirating the cephalohematoma

**E.** Ordering a complete blood count (CBC)

**2-48.** A 2-day-old female infant born at 23 5/7 weeks' gestation is being managed for respiratory distress syndrome (RDS) and hypotension. She has remained *nil per os* (nothing by mouth) since admission and is receiving total parenteral nutrition via an umbilical venous catheter. Her morning laboratories are remarkable for a serum calcium of 14 mg/dL and a serum phosphate of 2.7 mg/dL. The next appropriate step in management of this infant is administration of which of the following?

**A.** Intravenous sodium phosphate

**B.** Oral magnesium chloride

**C.** Intravenous normal saline

**D.** Intramuscular magnesium sulfate

**E.** Intravenous calcium gluconate

**2-49.** A 2-day-old former 26 2/7-week male infant is being treated for respiratory distress syndrome (RDS) and group B *Streptococcus* (GBS) bacteremia (documented by a positive blood culture at admission). The baby's mean arterial pressure, measured by an umbilical arterial catheter, is 23 mm Hg. The neonatal intensive care unit (NICU) resident asks you about improving the infant's blood pressure. Which of the following statements is true regarding therapeutics for circulatory support in preterm infants?

**A.** Delayed cord clamping at birth improves circulatory stability.

**B.** Intravenous hydrocortisone decreases left ventricular function in inotrope-resistant hypotension.

**C.** Intravenous albumin is superior to normal saline in terms of clinical outcomes.

**D.** Dobutamine decreases systemic blood flow relative to dopamine.

**E.** Dopamine therapy improves short-term outcomes in treated patients.

**2-50.** A 2-day-old former 38 2/7-week female infant is being prepared for hospital discharge. She was born vaginally to a 30-year-old woman with an uncomplicated pregnancy and delivery. She has been formula fed every 2 hours. The infant has only lost 6% of her birth weight. She and her mother both have O positive blood types. A total serum bilirubin at 46 hours of age is 13 mg/dL. Physical exam is remarkable for a well-perfused baby with jaundice to the abdomen. Her discharge weight is 3245 g. Which of the following is an appropriate component of the discharge plan for this infant?

**A.** Pediatric follow-up within a week of discharge

**B.** Agreement from the parents to send the name of the primary care provider after hospital discharge

**C.** Parental education about jaundice

**D.** Car seat observation test

**E.** Serum glucose-6-phosphate dehydrogenase (G6PD) level

**2-51.** Which of the following statements is correct regarding critical congenital heart disease (CCHD) screening in the newborn?

**A.** CCHD screening should be performed within 6 hours after delivery.

**B.** CCHD screening should be performed immediately in newborns with acrocyanosis.

**C.** Newborn physical exam and pulse oximetry are both components of CCHD screening.

**D.** CCHD screening is only useful for intracardiac lesions.

**E.** Ventricular septal defects are the primary lesion of concern in routine CCHD screening.

**2-52.** Which of the following statements is true about brown adipose tissue (BAT) in newborns?

**A.** The thermogenic response by BAT is regulated by neurogenic responses only.

**B.** BAT is less abundant in newborns relative to adults.

**C.** The perinephric region is a primary site for brown fat storage in newborns.

**D.** In BAT, uncoupling protein 1 (UCP1) inhibits heat generation.

**E.** The amount of heat generated by BAT in preterm newborns is well documented.

**2-53.** Which of the following statements regarding breast milk feedings in preterm infants is true?

**A.** Donor breast milk is ineffective in reducing necrotizing enterocolitis (NEC).

**B.** The risk of NEC is inversely related to breast milk exposure.

**C.** Relative to infants receiving formula, preterm infants receiving donor breast milk feedings were less likely to have cognitive scores < 85.

**D.** Exclusive breast milk feeding has been shown to be inferior to formula in reducing the risk of surgical NEC.

**E.** Donor breast milk decreases the likelihood of severe infections in preterm infants.

**2-54.** Which of the following are used during pregnancy to screen for the presence of fetal anomalies and neural tube defects?

**A.** Inhibin A, maternal α-fetoprotein, lecithin, sphingomyelin, and nuchal translucency

**B.** Nuchal translucency, lecithin, inhibin A, maternal α-fetoprotein, and estradiol

**C.** Inhibin A, maternal α-fetoprotein, human chorionic gonadotropin, estradiol, and nuchal translucency

**D.** Inhibin A, dipalmitoylphosphatidylcholine, maternal α-fetoprotein, estradiol, and nuchal translucency

**E.** Nuchal translucency, dipalmitoylphosphatidylcholine, lecithin, sphingomyelin, and estradiol

**2-55.** A newborn infant was born at 37 weeks' gestation after induction of labor due to development of intrauterine growth restriction (IUGR). Fetal ultrasound also demonstrated abnormal umbilical artery Dopplers with reversed end-diastolic flow. The newborn's birth parameters plot at the 30th percentile for head circumference, 8th percentile for weight, and 9th percentile for length. Which of the following conditions is the likely cause of this infant's IUGR?

**A.** Chromosomal anomaly

**B.** Intrauterine infection

**C.** Congenital malformation

**D.** Maternal ethnicity

**E.** Pregnancy-induced hypertension

**2-56.** Pregnant women who are at risk for delivering prematurely are administered glucocorticoid injections. For what purpose is this therapy indicated?

**A.** To accelerate fetal lung maturity

**B.** To stop preterm labor

**C.** To prevent postnatal hypoglycemia

**D.** To promote fetal weight gain

**E.** To prevent maternal hypoglycemia

**2-57.** A 39 5/7-week baby is born via emergency cesarean section for fetal bradycardia. The baby is brought to the warmer table and remains limp and apneic after you attempt drying and stimulating, so you initiate positive-pressure ventilation with bag and appropriate-sized face mask. However, the heart rate remains < 100 bpm. Which of the following is an initial corrective step to achieve chest rise and increase the baby's heart rate?

**A.** Increase the $FiO_2$

**B.** Lower the inflation pressure

**C.** Reposition the airway

**D.** Place a nasogastric tube

**E.** Use a larger face mask

**2-58.** A new mother is concerned about some of her newborn's movements. The baby was born at 39 2/7 weeks' gestation after an uncomplicated pregnancy and delivery. When she goes to pick up her daughter, the infant often extends her arms out to the side and opens her hands. On exam, you note that the infant is alert, is laying with upper and lower extremities flexed, and has an appropriate suck and root reflex. What is your next course of action?

**A.** Perform an electroencephalogram

**B.** Reassure the mother that this movement pattern is a normal reflex

**C.** Perform a cranial ultrasound

**D.** Arrange for outpatient neurodevelopmental follow-up

**E.** Consult a pediatric neurologist

**2-59.** A pediatric intern is examining a 2-day-old term infant in the newborn nursery. The mother had good prenatal care, with dating based on a first-trimester ultrasound and her last menstrual period. The pregnancy and delivery were uncomplicated. Which of the following would be an abnormal finding on neurologic exam for this term infant?

**A.** Laying with upper and lower extremities in flexion

**B.** Presence of the righting reaction

**C.** Spontaneous abduction of thumbs

**D.** Popliteal angle of > 120 degrees

**E.** Scarf sign in which the elbow does not reach midline.

**2-60.** The nursery team is caring for a male infant born at 38 3/7 weeks' gestation to a 16-year-old primigravida mother following induction of labor (due to preeclampsia and intrauterine growth restriction [IUGR]). The pregnancy was notable for poor maternal weight gain and multiple missed prenatal appointments in the third trimester. The baby was delivered vaginally with Apgar scores of 8 and 9. The birth weight is 2100 g (1st percentile for gestational age). Length was 45 cm (3rd percentile for gestational age). The head circumference was 33.5 cm (38th percentile for gestational age). Which of the following steps is most important in the care of this baby in the newborn nursery?

**A.** Urine cytomegalovirus assay

**B.** Daily serum electrolytes

**C.** Microarray assay

**D.** Preprandial plasma glucose checks

**E.** Blood culture

**2-61.** A 9-month-old male infant presents to the general pediatrics outpatient clinic for a routine health maintenance visit. The mother recalls being told shortly after delivery that her son was at increased risk for learning disabilities and behavioral problems and that he will likely be shorter than expected once he reaches adulthood. Which of the following clinical scenarios best correlates with the predicted outcomes explained to the mother?

**A.** 40-week gestation male with birth weight in 95th percentile born via cesarean section due to nonreassuring fetal heart tones

**B.** 37-week gestation male with birth weight in 7th percentile born vaginally following induction for severe intrauterine growth restriction (IUGR)

**C.** 38-week gestation male with birth weight in 15th percentile born via spontaneous vaginal delivery and required 24 hours of phototherapy in the newborn nursery

**D.** 37-week gestation male with birth weight in 65th percentile born via cesarean section to a mother with chorioamnionitis

**E.** 39-week gestation male with birth weight in 25th percentile born via vaginal delivery to a mother with hypothyroidism who was on levothyroxine during pregnancy

**2-62.** The neonatal intensive care unit (NICU) team is preparing to attend a cesarean section delivery of a woman at 28 4/7 weeks' gestation who received 2 doses of antenatal betamethasone. Prior to entering the operating room, the attending neonatologist discusses with the pediatric intern predisposing risk factors for development of respiratory distress syndrome (RDS) in premature infants. Which of the following factors would increase the risk of RDS for this newborn?

**A.** Female gender

**B.** Infant of a diabetic mother

**C.** Firstborn infant of a twin gestation

**D.** Maternal hypertension

**E.** Maternal narcotic abuse

**2-63.** A former 26 1/7-week male infant is now 37 0/7 weeks postmenstrual age. After intubation in the delivery room, surfactant administration, and conventional ventilation, he was extubated to continuous positive airway pressure (CPAP) by 3 weeks of age. He received caffeine and a short course of dexamethasone during his neonatal intensive care unit (NICU) course. Currently, he remains on 2 L/min nasal cannula, receiving 0.3 $FiO_2$. He has a history of bilateral grade II intraventricular hemorrhages (IVHs) and stage I retinopathy of prematurity. He was started on parenteral nutrition at birth but advanced to full enteral feeds (now fortified to 24 kcal/oz) by 6 weeks of age. He remains on vitamin A supplements. Which of the following interventions has been shown to reduce the rate of neurodevelopmental impairment?

**A.** Total parenteral nutrition

**B.** Postnatal dexamethasone

**C.** Caffeine

**D.** Vitamin A

**E.** Fortified enteral feeds

**2-64.** A former 27 1/7-week female child who spent 12 weeks in the neonatal intensive care unit (NICU) presents for neurodevelopmental follow-up at 24 months of corrected gestational age. Her physical exam reveals mildly increased lower extremity tone but normal upper extremity tone. She also can walk well on her own without support. Her mother is concerned about cerebral palsy because her daughter has been delayed in meeting her motor milestones compared to her 5-year-old sibling, who was born at 38 2/7 weeks. Which of the following statements is appropriate in addressing the mother's concern?

**A.** The child has cerebral palsy based on her history of delayed motor development and persistent hypertonia on exam.

**B.** The child has developmental coordination disorder based on physical exam findings.

**C.** The child's exam is normal, and she should not have any further delays or problems with her development.

**D.** The child has mild abnormalities on physical exam today, but she does not meet the criteria for the diagnosis of cerebral palsy.

**E.** The child will need brain magnetic resonance imaging (MRI) to make the diagnosis of cerebral palsy.

**2-65.** Former premature infants are at an increased risk for behavioral, socioemotional, and neuropsychiatric problems. Which of the following instruments can be used as a screening tool by pediatricians to assess for these concerns?

**A.** The Child Behavior Checklist (CBCL)

**B.** The Bayley Scales of Infant and Toddler Development

**C.** Modified Checklist for Autism in Toddlers (M-CHAT)

**D.** The General Movements Assessment

**E.** The Wechsler Individual Achievement Test (WIAT)

**2-66.** Cranial ultrasounds are commonly used to assess for brain injury in preterm infants. Which of the following cranial ultrasound results confers the greatest risk for future developmental delays?

**A.** Grade III intraventricular hemorrhage (IVH)

**B.** Grade I IVH

**C.** Cystic periventricular leukomalacia

**D.** Grade II IVH

**E.** Posthemorrhagic hydrocephalus with shunt placement

**2-67.** A woman with a history of cervical incompetence presents in preterm labor at 25 1/7 weeks' gestation. She had a prior 28 5/7-week male infant who had bilateral grade I intraventricular hemorrhages (IVHs), necrotizing enterocolitis (NEC), and *E coli* bacteremia during his neonatal intensive care unit (NICU) hospitalization and is "delayed." The woman is concerned about a similar outcome for her current baby if she delivers in the next 72 hours, since the baby will be more premature than her first child. In discussing outcomes with the mother, which of the following statements is correct regarding risks of neurodevelopmental abnormalities in preterm infants?

**A.** Surgical NEC is more strongly associated with adverse neurodevelopmental outcomes.

**B.** Among children with IVHs, infants with grade I IVH are at the highest risk of adverse neurodevelopmental outcomes.

**C.** Infection in preterm neonates is associated with increased risk of cognitive impairment at 12 months of age.

**D.** Babies developing NEC have decreased rates of cerebral palsy.

**E.** *Candida albicans* bacteremia poses a low risk of adverse neurodevelopmental outcomes.

**2-68.** A 26-year-old G2P1 woman at 23 1/7 weeks' gestation presents to the high-risk obstetrical clinic for further evaluation following a new diagnosis of fetal myelomeningocele. After thorough evaluation, she is deemed an appropriate candidate for fetal (in utero) myelomeningocele repair (Figure 42-4).

Which of the following statements about fetal myelomeningocele repair is accurate?

**A.** Compared to neonatal repair, fetal repair is associated with an increased probability of shunting at 12 months of age.

**B.** Compared to neonatal repair, fetal repair is associated with an increased probability of walking at 30 months of age.

**C.** This mother can expect a spontaneous vaginal delivery at term.

**D.** Compared to the open approach, the fetoscopic approach demonstrates improved outcomes.

**E.** After fetal repair, the risk of delivery prior to 30 weeks is about 50%.

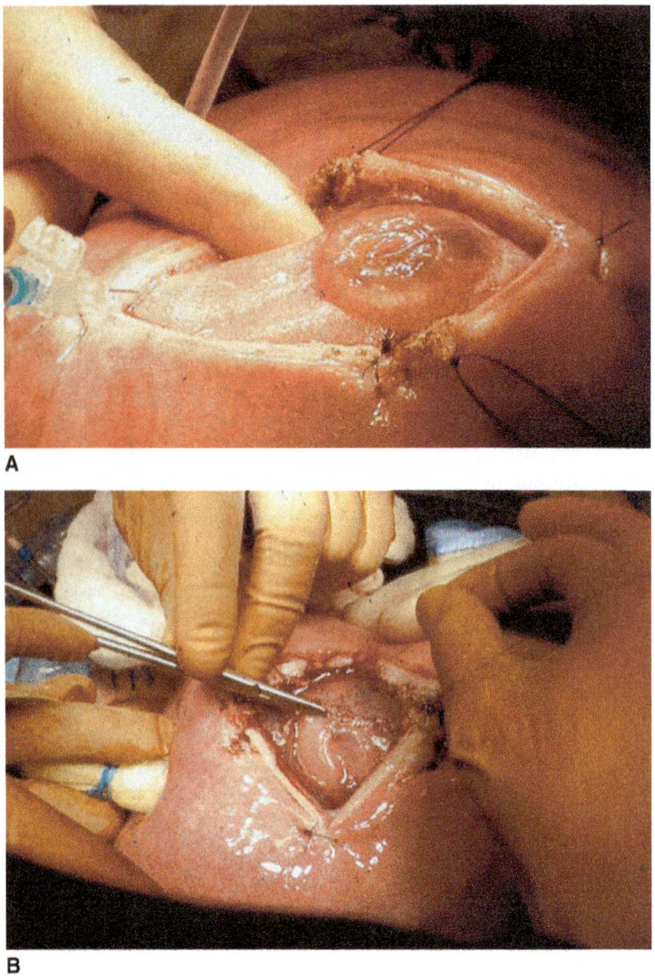


**FIGURE 42-4.** Fetal myelomeningocele. **A:** Surgical exposure of fetal myelomeningocele. **B:** Surgical closure of fetal myelomeningocele. (Mark W. Kline, *Rudolph's Pediatrics*, 23rd Edition. Copyright © McGraw-Hill Education. All rights reserved.)

**2-69.** A 34-year-old G4P0 woman is pregnant with monochorionic diamniotic twins conceived via in vitro fertilization. During a routine prenatal ultrasound at 23 1/7 weeks' gestation, there is a noted 45% size discordance between the twins and chorioangiopagus vascular connections between the twins. Given the ultrasonographic findings, she is diagnosed with twin–twin transfusion syndrome (TTTS). Which of the following interventions for TTTS is likely to result in the best outcome?

**A.** Selective amnioreduction for the "recipient" twin with polyhydramnios

**B.** Close clinical monitoring with elective delivery at 32 weeks gestational age

**C.** Ultrasound-guided radiofrequency umbilical cord ablation of the "donor" twin

**D.** Selective fetoscopic laser photocoagulation of the vascular connections between the twins

**E.** Termination of the pregnancy

**2-70.** A woman is referred to a pediatric cardiologist at 32 1/7 weeks' gestation after her most recent ultrasound revealed a fetal heart rate of 220 bpm. Fetal cardiac echocardiogram today demonstrates a structurally normal heart with trace pericardial effusion and a fetal heart rate that increased from 150 bpm to 200 bpm while the echocardiogram was being performed. You also note significant skin edema on the ultrasound images. There is no maternal or family history of cardiac arrhythmias. Which of the following is the most appropriate next step in management?

**A.** Arrange outpatient follow-up with obstetrics for nonstress tests every 2 weeks for the duration of the pregnancy

**B.** Call the referring obstetrician and recommend immediate delivery of the fetus

**C.** Obtain a baseline maternal electrocardiogram (ECG) and initiate therapy with digoxin to control the fetal arrhythmia

**D.** Obtain a baseline maternal ECG and initiate therapy with sotalol to control the fetal arrhythmia

**E.** Send testing for maternal anti-Ro and anti-La antibodies and, if positive, recommend administration of antenatal steroids

**2-71.** The pediatric residents are called to the mother–baby unit to evaluate a 1-hour-old male infant for "cyanosis." The baby was born at 39 weeks gestational age via precipitous vaginal delivery to a 21-year-old G2P1 mother with an unremarkable past medical history. The pregnancy was uncomplicated. The mother received 2 doses of penicillin prior to delivery of the infant due to group B *Streptococcus* colonization. Newborn exam reveals an appropriate-for-gestational-age male infant who is awake and alert in his bassinet. His oropharynx and tongue are pink. His respiratory exam is notable for mild periodic breathing and a soft I/VI systolic murmur. He is warm and well perfused with symmetric central and peripheral pulses, but he has a bluish discoloration to his feet. The bedside nurse asks what should be done to address the cyanosis. Which of the following interventions is recommended?

**A.** Continued routine care in the newborn nursery

**B.** Supplemental oxygen therapy

**C.** Echocardiogram

**D.** Chest radiograph

**E.** Hemoglobin electrophoresis

**2-72.** You are called to evaluate a 1-hour-old female infant in the mother–baby unit for difficulty feeding and respiratory distress. The mother reports no significant pregnancy history, although prenatal care was not initiated until late in the third trimester. Maternal group B *Streptococcus* status was negative. The baby was delivered vaginally 8 hours after spontaneous rupture of membranes. Physical exam reveals a term, pink, crying female infant with saturations of 98% on room air. She willingly accepts a pacifier, demonstrates a strong suck, and soothes easily. However, as the fellow listens to her heart and lungs, the oxygen saturations begin to drop, and she develops perioral cyanosis. The saturations then improve when she loses her pacifier and begins to cry. There is no stridor or wheezing. Which of the following is the most likely cause of this infant's intermittent hypoxia?

**A.** Transient tachypnea of the newborn

**B.** Phrenic nerve palsy

**C.** Laryngomalacia

**D.** Tracheoesophageal fistula

**E.** Choanal atresia

**2-73.** A 5-day-old infant is brought to the emergency department by her mother with concerns for increased sleepiness. Her mother reports an uncomplicated vaginal delivery at term. The infant was discharged home at 2 days of age. The baby was breastfeeding well. There is a history of voiding and stooling. There was a 7.5% weight loss noted at discharge. At home, however, the infant only nurses for 5 minutes at a time, sleeps almost all day, and has been more difficult to awaken for feeds. Exam reveals a cyanotic infant in moderate respiratory distress with 1+ symmetric distal pulses and cool hands and feet with sluggish capillary refill. You suspect congenital heart disease and start a prostaglandin infusion while awaiting cardiac echocardiogram. Within half an hour, the baby appears pinker with improved oxygen saturations and capillary refill. Which of the following is the most likely diagnosis?

**A.** Balanced atrioventricular canal defect

**B.** Tetralogy of Fallot without right ventricular outflow tract obstruction

**C.** Hypoplastic left heart syndrome

**D.** Muscular ventricular septal defect

**E.** Peripheral right pulmonary artery stenosis

**2-74.** A mother brings her 2-week-old female infant to the clinic for routine follow-up. The infant was born via spontaneous vaginal delivery following an uncomplicated pregnancy. The infant was discharged home at 24 hours of age. Over the past 24 hours, however, the mother notes the infant has been "sleepier," and she has to wake the baby to feed every 3 to 4 hours. The feeds are now lasting only 5 to 7 minutes as well. On physical exam, you note a female infant who barely rouses to exam, with mild generalized hypotonia, a large tongue, and normal female genitalia. Her right leg and arm appear larger than the left, which the mother confirms has been present since birth. The infant then exhibits nonsuppressible, rhythmic jerking of both upper extremities. A capillary glucose value is undetectable. Which of the following is the most likely etiology of this infant's seizure?

**A.** Hypoglycemia due to pancreatic hyperplasia and hyperinsulinism

**B.** Hypocalcemia due to absent parathyroid glands

**C.** Presence of a congenital brain malformation

**D.** Hyponatremia due to congenital adrenal hyperplasia

**E.** Intracranial hemorrhage due to vitamin K deficiency

**2-75.** A 3-day-old male infant with recurrent seizures is transferred to the neonatal intensive care unit (NICU) from an outside hospital. Fetal imaging was notable for a horseshoe kidney. Physical examination is remarkable for a submucosal cleft palate; hypertelorism; small, low-set ears; and a long narrow face. Which laboratory test and intervention are most likely to identify and treat the underlying cause of the child's seizure?

**A.** Electrolyte panel and 0.9% saline bolus administration intravenously

**B.** Coagulation studies and vitamin K administration intravenously

**C.** Serum glucose level and glucose administration intravenously

**D.** Serum ionized calcium level and calcium chloride administration intravenously

**E.** Emergent head computed tomography scan and phenobarbital administration intravenously

**2-76.** The neonatal intensive care unit (NICU) team is caring for a 40 1/7-week infant who completed 72 hours of therapeutic hypothermia for neonatal encephalopathy. Her neurologic exam has improved significantly, and she is slowly increasing her oral feeds while weaning her intravenous fluids. On reviewing her morning labs, you note that the serum potassium, which had previously been in the normal range, is elevated to 8.1 mEq/L. Her cardiac monitor demonstrates peaked T waves and widened QRS duration. Of the following, which is the most appropriate next step in the management of this patient?

**A.** Administer 200 mg/kg of intravenous calcium gluconate

**B.** Identify any potassium-containing fluids or medications and stop their administration

**C.** Resend her morning laboratories

**D.** Contact the nephrology service to perform renal replacement therapy

**E.** Administer 1 g/kg of an oral cation exchange resin

**2-77.** A 27 2/7-week very-low-birth-weight infant, now 3 weeks old, has not yet regained his birth weight. He has been tolerating full-volume gavage feeds of maternal breast milk, fortified to 24 kcal/oz with human milk fortifier, without issue. He does not require respiratory support and has occasional apneas and bradycardias on maintenance caffeine therapy. You order an electrolyte panel with the following results: $Na^+$ 136 mEq/L, $K^+$ 4.5 mEq/L, $Cl^-$ 106 mEq/L, $HCO_3^-$ 14 mEq/L, blood urea nitrogen (BUN) 22 mg/dL, and creatinine 0.6 mg/dL. Which of the following is the most likely cause of this infant's growth failure?

**A.** Chronic renal failure due to gentamicin exposure

**B.** An inborn error of metabolism causing chronic metabolic acidosis

**C.** Lactic acidosis secondary to sepsis

**D.** Proximal renal tubular acidosis with renal bicarbonate wasting

**E.** Hyponatremia due to aldosterone insensitivity

**2-78.** You are called to assess a 1-hour-old male infant born at 38 weeks gestational age via spontaneous vaginal delivery. The pregnancy was uncomplicated. The delivery was notable for a 25% placental abruption. Physical exam is notable for a pale but alert male infant. He is tachypneic (respiratory rate 70 breaths/min) and tachycardic (heart rate of 160 bpm), with mild subcostal retractions and soft, intermittent grunting. He has clear oral secretions. The remainder of his exam is normal.

Pulse oximetry reveals an oxygen saturation of 93% on room air. His complete blood count (CBC) shows a white blood cell (WBC) count of 10,000 cells/μL, hemoglobin of 11 mg/dL, hematocrit of 34%, and 250,000 platelets/μL. The mother and infant have O positive blood types. The maternal past medical and family histories are unremarkable for anemia.

Which of the following tests will reveal the most likely source of the anemia?

**A.** Peripheral smear

**B.** Apt test

**C.** Direct Coombs test

**D.** Kleihauer-Betke test

**E.** Osmotic fragility test

**2-79.** A 6-hour-old newborn delivered at 39 5/7 weeks' gestation is admitted to the neonatal intensive care unit (NICU) for hypoglycemia (capillary glucose, 20 mg/dL). The pregnancy was complicated by maternal type 2 diabetes requiring insulin therapy. The infant was delivered via cesarean section and weighed 4 kg at birth. In the NICU, he was started on continuous glucose-containing intravenous fluids. One hour later, the infant is noted by the bedside nurse to be "dusky." Physical exam reveals a lethargic, tachypneic male newborn with decreased peripheral pulses, perioral cyanosis, and 4- to 5-second capillary refill. Pulse oximetry reveals oxygen saturations of 82% on room air in both the upper and lower extremities. A STAT serum blood glucose is 35 mg/dL. A complete blood count (CBC) shows a hemoglobin of 25.2 mg/dL and a hematocrit of 75%. Which of the following is the next best step in the management of this infant?

**A.** Continue peripheral intravenous fluids at the current rate and recheck hematocrit in 8 hours

**B.** Place umbilical lines and prepare for double-volume exchange transfusion

**C.** Administer intravenous immune globulin (IVIG)

**D.** Send serum cortisol and growth hormone levels

**E.** Obtain central venous access and prepare for partial exchange transfusion with normal saline

**2-80.** A former 26 4/7-week gestational age intrauterine growth restriction (IUGR) infant, who is now 3 weeks old, has been demonstrating consistent weight gain on full-volume formula feeds fortified to 24 kcal/oz for the past week. Overnight, he was noted to have 3 episodes of small-volume emesis and abdominal distention. This morning, there were streaks of blood in his stool. He has also had increasing apnea, bradycardia, and desaturation episodes over the past 24 hours, requiring escalation of respiratory support. Abdominal radiograph demonstrates diffuse bubbly lucencies in the bowel wall and a fixed, dilated loop of bowel in the left lower quadrant. You diagnose the infant with necrotizing enterocolitis (NEC). Which of the following statements is true regarding management of this infant?

**A.** The antibiotic regimen of choice is vancomycin monotherapy.

**B.** Surgical intervention is only indicated when there is evidence of pneumoperitoneum on abdominal radiograph.

**C.** Antibiotic therapy should optimally be continued for 21 days.

**D.** As part of the initial workup, a complete blood count (CBC) should be obtained to assess for thrombocytosis, which is often associated with NEC.

**E.** Anaerobic antibiotic coverage will increase his risk of intestinal stricture.

**2-81.** During rounds in the neonatal intensive care unit (NICU), a medical student asks about methods to decrease the risk of developing necrotizing enterocolitis (NEC) in premature infants. You note that exclusive maternal breast milk feedings have been established as the most important strategy to prevent NEC. What is an additional method used to prevent NEC?

**A.** Use of a feeding protocol for all very-low-birth-weight infants in the NICU

**B.** Routine gastric aspiration to monitor gastric residuals

**C.** Use of acid-suppression medications

**D.** Prolonged (7–10 days) courses of antibiotic therapy for episodes of culture-negative sepsis

**E.** Use of acid-suppression medications during prolonged courses of antibiotic therapy

## ANSWERS

**Answer 2-1.** C

Comparison of infant mortality between entities (countries, regions) requires use of a common definition. The infant mortality ratio, the ratio of infant deaths to live births each year, is one way to standardize the reporting of infant mortality. This ratio relies on consistency in reporting of infant deaths and live births, which are very specifically defined. Although gestational age, causes of death, and multiple gestations impact the risk of infant mortality, they are not included in calculations for infant mortality. Differences in population size should not impact comparisons in infant mortality if infant mortality is being described by the infant mortality ratio.

(p. 185, Section 4: Newborn, Chapter 43)

**Answer 2-2.** D

Neonatal outcomes for very-low-birth-weight infants (including a reduction in neonatal mortality) are improved when delivery occurs at a regionalized, large subspecialty center. Notable differences in subspecialty centers, as compared to basic centers or special care centers, include 24-hour neonatologist coverage, availability of advanced respiratory support, availability of all medical and surgical specialists, and high-risk follow-up. Despite these additional services, delivery at a subspecialty center is not more costly when compared to delivery at a special care center. Therefore, transfer of this pregnant woman to a regional subspecialty center for potential delivery of a very-low-birth-weight baby should occur (if safe and feasible). Although regional subspecialty centers may or may not offer additional ancillary resources for parents of very-low-birth-weight infants, transfer of the mother is most justified by improved neonatal outcomes.

(p. 188, Section 4: Newborn, Chapter 43)

**Answer 2-3.** C

Whether due to preterm labor, fetal compromise, or obstetric concerns, there is a higher chance of preterm birth in a twin gestation. Preterm birth occurs in 50% of all twin pregnancies and accounts for 10% of preterm births, although only 10% of these births will occur before 32 weeks' gestation. Newborns of multiple gestations also are at increased risk of aneuploidy and structural abnormalities. Additionally, with higher order multiples, the risk of preterm birth increases to a greater extent. The mode of delivery for twin gestation is dependent on many factors, including the chorionicity of the fetuses. Generally, monochorionic twins should be delivered by cesarean section. However, vaginal delivery may be attempted for dichorionic twins based on the fetal lie and skill level of the obstetrician. Monochorionic twins face additional risks and complications of pregnancy compared to dichorionic twins, including growth retardation and twin–twin transfusion syndrome. Therefore, differences in pregnancy evaluation and management may exist. Overall, the risks of neonatal morbidity are higher for twin fetuses compared to singletons. One such morbidity includes poor fetal growth; twin fetuses have a higher risk of being small for gestational age or growth restricted compared to singletons.

(p. 219, Section 4: Newborn, Chapter 48)

**Answer 2-4.** D

This baby is showing signs of severe persistent pulmonary hypertension of the newborn (PPHN), which can occur in the setting of meconium aspiration syndrome (MAS). Principles in managing PPHN include lowering pulmonary vascular resistance, improving oxygenation and tissue perfusion, avoiding metabolic derangements (eg, acidosis, hypoglycemia, hypocalcemia), and using gentle mechanical ventilation. Inhaled nitric oxide, a pulmonary vasodilator that can be delivered directly to the lungs, would be the next intervention in treatment of this baby's PPHN.

Hyperventilation, hyperoxygenation, and pharmacologic alkalization are generally not helpful and can worsen outcomes for PPHN. Extracorporeal membrane oxygenation is a lifesaving treatment for newborns with PPHN; however, it is a high-risk therapy that should be implemented only when less invasive therapies have failed.

(pp. 236 and 239, Section 4: Newborn, Chapter 52)

**Answer 2-5.** C

This neonate has suffered a pulmonary hemorrhage, which occurs most commonly in preterm infants in the setting of a patent ductus arteriosus. Other etiologies, such as neonatal infection, maternal cocaine use, coagulopathy, surfactant administration, and hypothermia, have been implicated in this condition. Chest radiography findings are variable, with findings ranging from complete lung field opacification to patchy infiltrates. Although high-quality data are limited, strategies to treat pulmonary hemorrhage include increasing the peak end-expiratory pressure on the ventilator and administration of epinephrine (to cause pulmonary vasoconstriction). Approximately 60% of infants with pulmonary hemorrhage proceed to develop chronic lung disease, and the overall mortality from this condition ranges from 30% to 60% in premature infants.

(p. 236, Section 4: Newborn, Chapter 52)

**Answer 2-6.** A

The baby in the vignette has respiratory distress most likely associated with congenital pneumonia. Congenital pneumonia is most commonly caused by the same organisms that lead to early-onset neonatal sepsis: GBS, *Escherichia coli*, and *Listeria monocytogenes*. The incidence of congenital pneumonia has decreased to < 1% for term newborns due to universal screening of all pregnant women for GBS and recently instituted guidelines for maternal intrapartum antibiotic treatment. Betamethasone, given to mothers in early preterm labor, is used to promote lung maturity in preterm infants. Avoidance of elective cesarean delivery before 39 weeks has decreased morbidity from neonatal pulmonary disease but is not responsible for the lower rate of congenital pneumonia. Prenatal vitamins and fetal monitoring during labor, although important components of well-being, have not been shown to impact the incidence of congenital pneumonia. Judicious and timely use of chest radiography and blood cultures is an appropriate diagnostic strategy; however, chest radiography and blood cultures are not preventive strategies for congenital pneumonia.

(p. 235, Section 4: Newborn, Chapter 52)

**Answer 2-7.** D

The baby in this vignette has a congenital diaphragmatic hernia. Delivery room management in this case is focused on maximizing ventilation, which includes minimizing distention of the stomach and intestines herniated into the left chest. Of the choices listed, placement of a gastric drainage tube is the most appropriate next step in management. Endotracheal intubation (to provide positive pressure to the lungs) should also be performed.

Increasing the positive inspiratory pressure with a face mask may insufflate the gastrointestinal tract, making aeration of the lungs more challenging. A needle thoracotomy is an emergent intervention for a baby with a tension pneumothorax. However, the presence of a scaphoid abdomen is suggestive of a diaphragmatic hernia, rather than a tension pneumothorax. Surfactant administration has no demonstrated benefit in babies with congenital diaphragmatic hernia. Placement of a low-lying umbilical venous catheter (UVC) is indicated for volume and medication administration in the delivery room; however, a UVC is not the first step in management of this baby.

(p. 239, Section 4: Newborn, Chapter 52)

**Answer 2-8.** A

The baby in this vignette is suffering from neonatal encephalopathy. The low cord pH, fetal decelerations, placental abruption, and low Apgar score, while not diagnostic, are suggestive of an acute intrapartum hypoxic event. Diagnosis of neonatal encephalopathy should include serial neurologic examinations, and the degree of impairment should be classified based on the Sarnat criteria (Table 54-1).

Sarnat 1 (mild) encephalopathy is a hyperalert state characterized by irritability, tachycardia, regular respirations, and normal tone. Sarnat 2 (moderate) encephalopathy is characterized by several physical exam findings, including lethargy, a weak suck, an incomplete Moro response, and periodic breathing. Sarnat 3 (severe) encephalopathy is manifested by absent spontaneous activity and primitive reflexes (Moro, suck), flaccidity, and apnea.

(p. 253, Section 4: Newborn, Chapter 54)

**Answer 2-9.** B

The baby in the vignette has a history and physical exam findings suggestive of neonatal encephalopathy. In babies with neonatal encephalopathy, therapeutic hypothermia has been shown to reduce death or disability at 18 months of age in several randomized clinical trials, with a reasonable safety profile. Therefore, therapeutic hypothermia is endorsed by pediatric medical societies for the treatment of neonatal encephalopathy. Additionally, avoiding permissive hyperthermia may be beneficial as an immediate management strategy.

Although seizures may be a complication of neonatal encephalopathy, there are no data to support the use of prophylactic anticonvulsant therapy immediately after birth in preventing disability in infants. Stem cell therapy and erythropoietin treatment in humans with hypoxic-ischemic encephalopathy are in the early stages of investigation and are not routinely used in the immediate phase of neonatal encephalopathy.

(p. 255, Section 4: Newborn, Chapter 54)

**Answer 2-10.** D

Perinatal stroke (PS) is estimated to occur in approximately 1 in 4000 births. Risk factors include preeclampsia and intrauterine growth restriction. Clinical manifestations of PS may present at any time during infancy; however, seizures associated with PS occur within hours to days after the insult. Perinatal arterial strokes, the most common form of PS in newborns, present with wedge-shaped infarcts in the distribution of the middle cerebral artery. Venous infarcts, which occur in about one-third of cases of PS, may not always be demonstrable on magnetic resonance imaging (MRI)/magnetic resonance venogram imaging due to recanalization of the vessel or development of collateral circulation.

(pp. 254–255, Section 4: Newborn, Chapter 54)

**TABLE 54-1.** Stages of Encephalopathy According to the Sarnat Classification

| Variable | Stage 1 | Stage 2 | Stage 3 |
|---|---|---|---|
| Level of consciousness | Hyperalert, apparent awareness, responses to minimal stimuli | Lethargic | Stupor, coma |
| Spontaneous activity | Normal or decreased | Decreased | No activity |
| Posture | Mild flexion of distal joints (fingers, wrist usually) | Strong distal flexion, complete extension | Intermittent decerebration |
| Tone | Normal | Hypotonia, hypertonia | Flaccid, rigid |
| Reflexes | | | |
| Suck | Weak | Weak or absent bites | Absent |
| Moro | Intact, low threshold to illicit | Incomplete | Absent |
| Autonomic | | | |
| Pupils | Mydriasis | Miosis | Variable, often unequal, disconjugate eye movement, nonreactive |
| Heart rate | Tachycardia | Bradycardia (< 100 bpm) | Variable heart rate |
| Respirations | Regular respirations | Periodic breathing | Apnea, on ventilator |
| Seizures | None | Yes/no | Yes/no |

Mark W. Kline, *Rudolph's Pediatrics*, 23rd Edition. Copyright © McGraw-Hill Education. All rights reserved.

**Answer 2-11.** A

The infant in this vignette has most likely developed an intracranial hemorrhage. Given the infant's gestational age and clinical presentation, an intraventricular hemorrhage should be suspected. Infants may present with acute clinical changes (apnea, bradycardia) as well as laboratory findings (anemia, metabolic acidosis). The standard approach to diagnosing an intraventricular hemorrhage is with cranial sonography (Figure 61-3), which yields a high level of agreement among providers and is a feasible study to perform in this fragile population.

An echocardiogram would not be an appropriate diagnostic test for intraventricular hemorrhage. Cerebrospinal fluid analysis would be the test of choice to diagnose meningitis, but the presence of red blood cells in cerebrospinal fluid is not specific for intraventricular hemorrhage. An electroencephalogram may be able to diagnose seizures that are associated with intracranial hemorrhage in a newborn, but this study does not play a role in the diagnosis of intraventricular hemorrhage. A complete blood count may confirm neonatal blood loss following an intraventricular hemorrhage, but there are a variety of other causes of anemia in this preterm population.

(p. 290, Section 4: Newborn, Chapter 61)

**Answer 2-12.** A

Multiple studies have evaluated antenatal and postnatal interventions to reduce the incidence of IVH. As reported by the Neonatal Research Network, the odds ratio for the development of a severe IVH is 0.39 (95% confidence interval, 0.27–0.57) in preterm infants who complete a full course of antenatal steroids.

Due to the pressure-passive cerebral circulation of preterm infants (due to impaired cerebral autoregulation), slow administration of fluid replacement and judicious use of inotropic agents are recommended to prevent IVH. Indomethacin prophylaxis reduces the likelihood of severe IVH. However, the drug's immediate and long-term side effects (renal insufficiency, chronic lung disease, and ileal perforation) and lack of efficacy in improving long-term neurodevelopmental outcomes have limited its use in routine IVH prophylaxis. Other pharmacologic agents, such as phenobarbital, pancuronium, and vitamin E, have not demonstrated a clear protective effect.

(p. 294, Section 4: Newborn, Chapter 61)

**Answer 2-13.** E

IVH occurs most frequently in preterm infants, with the risk increasing as both birth weight and gestational age decrease. However, there are numerous intravascular, vascular, and extravascular factors that influence the pathogenesis of IVH and that complicate the prevention and management of this morbidity in the preterm population.

Over many decades, the incidence of IVH had decreased; however, since the mid-1990s, the incidence has been relatively

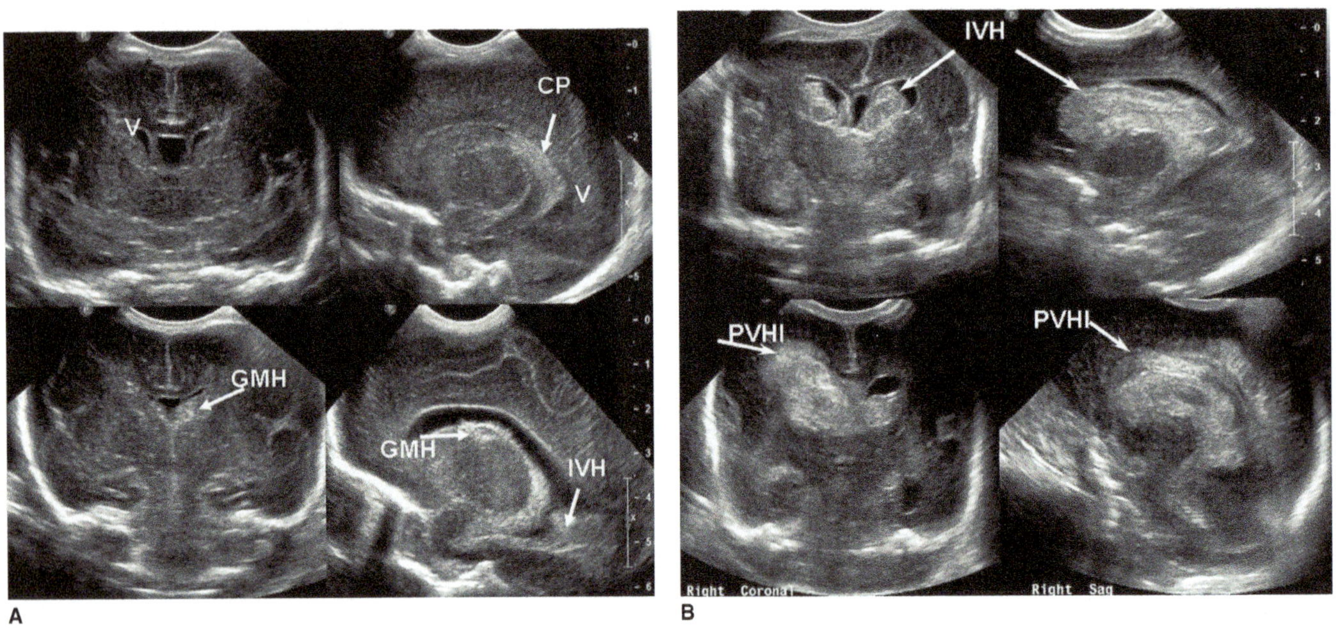


**FIGURE 61-3.** **A:** The top panel shows coronal (*left*) and sagittal (*right*) views from a normal preterm brain. The bottom left panel shows a coronal view with a left germinal matrix hemorrhage (GMH), or grade I. The bottom right panel shows a sagittal section showing blood in the lateral ventricle (intraventricular hemorrhage [IVH]) filling < 50% of the ventricular space; it is therefore a grade II germinal matrix hemorrhage/intraventricular hemorrhage. **B:** The top left panel shows a coronal view of bilateral hemorrhage (IVH) in the anterior ventricles, almost filling the ventricles. The top right panel shows a sagittal view of the hemorrhage or blood cast (IVH) filling and distending the lateral ventricle. This is a grade III hemorrhage. The bottom left panel shows a coronal view of hemorrhage with parenchymal involvement (*arrows*) representing periventricular hemorrhagic infarction (PVHI). The area of infarction is also noted in the sagittal view (*arrow*) in the bottom right panel. By Volpe criteria, the hemorrhage will be classified as a grade III with periventricular hemorrhagic infarction. CP, choroid plexus; V, ventricle. (Mark W. Kline, *Rudolph's Pediatrics*, 23rd Edition. Copyright © McGraw-Hill Education. All rights reserved.)

static despite advancements in intensive care for newborns. The most severe hemorrhages, grade III and IV, occur in as many as 20% of newborns with a birth weight of ≤ 750 g and in 17% to 28% of babies born between 22 and 26 weeks' gestation. Approximately 40% to 50% of IVHs will occur in the first day of life, and up to 90% will occur within the first 72 hours of age.

(p. 289, Section 4: Newborn, Chapter 61)

**Answer 2-14. D**

The baby in this vignette has an open neural tube defect (most likely a myelomeningocele). Prompt neurosurgical evaluation and treatment are necessary to optimize neurologic and developmental prognosis. In the delivery room, the pediatrician should keep the area over the lesion moist and clean and avoid manipulation of, or pressure on, the sac. Placing the baby prone or in the side-lying position can reduce the risk of pressure on the lesion.

Attempts to decompress or wrap the myelomeningocele can result in infection or neural trauma and should be avoided. The baby does have acrocyanosis, a normal finding in a newborn infant. His normal respiratory and heart rates suggest that he does not need respiratory support (intubation or supplemental oxygen) currently.

(p. 302, Section 4: Newborn, Chapter 63)

**Answer 2-15. C**

Bilious emesis in the newborn may occur due to a number of functional and anatomic causes. Malrotation with midgut volvulus is a surgical emergency that presents with bilious emesis, feeding disinterest, lethargy, and abdominal distention, as seen in this vignette. If not recognized and managed immediately, babies with midgut volvulus develop severe metabolic acidosis (due to gut ischemia) and hypovolemic shock, leading to death. An upper gastrointestinal contrast study can help diagnose midgut volvulus and is the study of choice in this case.

A left lateral decubitus radiograph can help to define free intraperitoneal air associated with a gastrointestinal perforation but cannot rule out a volvulus. A rectal biopsy, used to diagnose Hirschsprung disease (a cause of distal intestinal obstruction), is not the first-line test needed for this child with a likely small bowel obstruction. The child's increased work in breathing likely is a manifestation of pain and increased respiratory drive (secondary to metabolic acidosis) rather than a pulmonary process. Hence, a chest radiograph is not the first imaging test to order in this child. Esophageal manometry is indicated for motility disorders and is not indicated in this child.

(p. 301, Section 4: Newborn, Chapter 63)

**Answer 2-16. D**

The infant in this vignette has features of shock, which can result from a variety of conditions including newborn sepsis, dehydration, and congenital heart disease. Often, the exact etiology is unclear on presentation, but steps should be taken to restore circulation as quickly as possible. This infant has decreased perfusion in the lower extremities and lactic acidosis, suggesting coarctation of the aorta. Initiation of prostaglandin $E_1$ ($PGE_1$) is essential to maintain patency of the ductus arteriosus and maintain systemic blood flow in this infant. Intravenous prostaglandin should be initiated immediately whenever a ductal-dependent lesion is suspected.

The infant is afebrile; hence, administration of antipyretics (ibuprofen and acetaminophen) is not indicated in this child. Although septic shock must be considered in this infant, antibiotic administration should not precede prostaglandin administration in this case. In the absence of hemorrhage, vitamin K is not indicated as a first-line therapy in this baby.

(p. 301, Section 4: Newborn, Chapter 63)

**Answer 2-17. D**

Until recently, nonvigorous infants born through meconium-stained amniotic fluid were intubated and suctioned via an endotracheal tube to prevent meconium aspiration syndrome. However, a lack of evidence supporting this strategy led to a change in the Neonatal Resuscitation Program guidelines for depressed, meconium-stained newborns. The current recommendation is to perform routine steps (Figure 44-1) that would be performed for an infant born with clear fluid, with initial management including warming, positioning (opening the airway), and stimulation.

If an infant does not respond to the initial steps and there is a visual obstruction of the airway, airway suctioning may be indicated. If the airway is clear but the infant demonstrates bradycardia (heart rate < 100 bpm) or has poor respiratory effort, positive-pressure ventilation should be initiated. Chest compressions should be reserved for infants with a low heart rate (< 60 bpm) despite adequate positive-pressure ventilation. Supplemental oxygen may be administered to babies with heart rates > 100 bpm with labored breathing or persistent cyanosis.

(pp. 192–193, Section 4: Newborn, Chapter 44)

**Answer 2-18. A**

The baby described in this vignette demonstrated an appropriate response to resuscitative efforts, and the next step in her management involves postresuscitative care, which includes thermoregulation (wrapping in warm blankets). Acrocyanosis is common in newborn infants.

If the infant does not show central cyanosis and has good respiratory effort, other respiratory support (supplying supplemental oxygen and continuing positive-pressure ventilation) is not indicated. Placement of an umbilical line (for epinephrine administration) or initiation of chest compressions is indicated when initial respiratory steps have not improved the baby's heart rate.

(p. 192, Section 4: Newborn, Chapter 44)

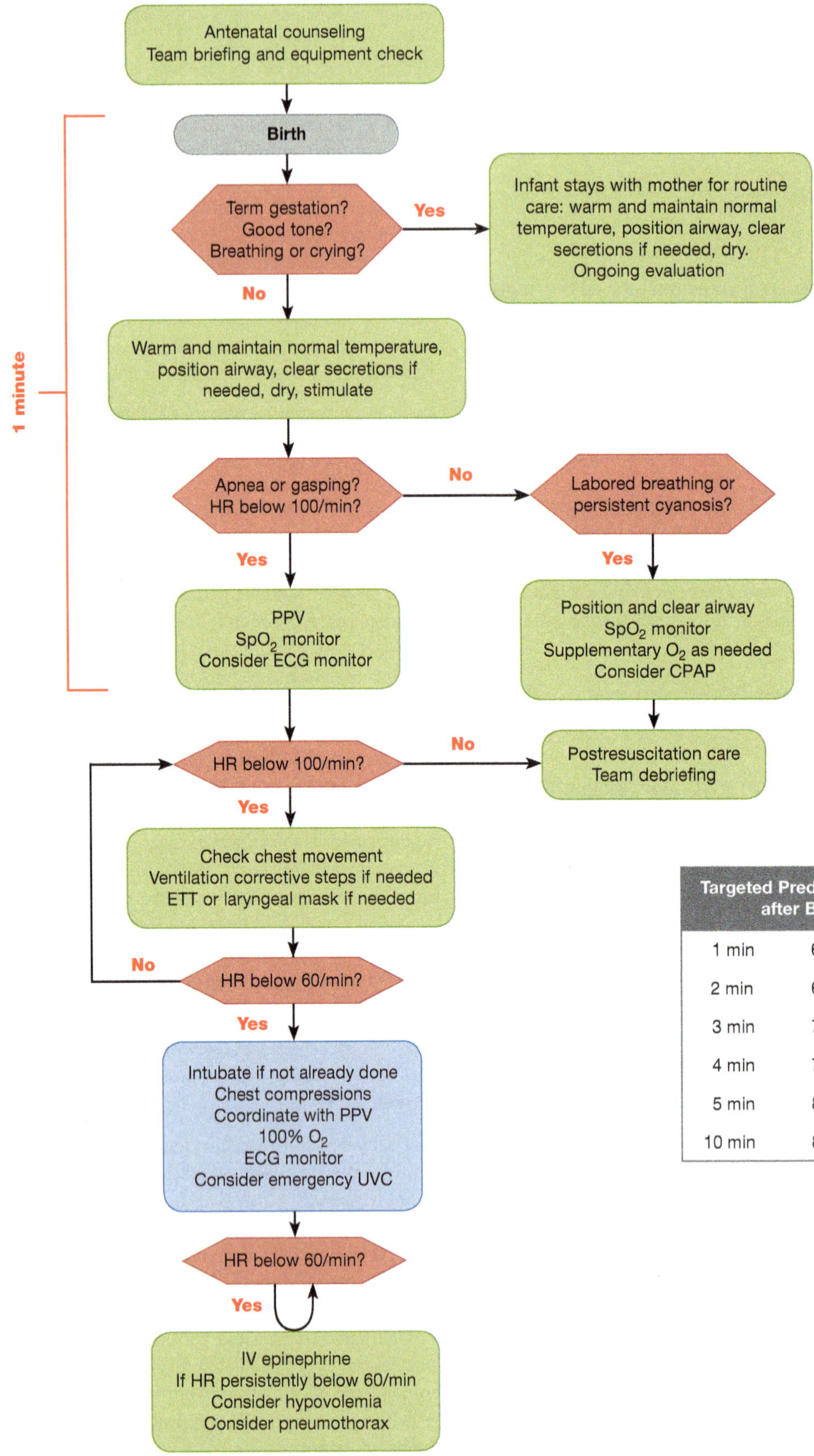


| Targeted Preductal $SpO_2$ after Birth | |
|---|---|
| 1 min | 60%–65% |
| 2 min | 65%–70% |
| 3 min | 70%–75% |
| 4 min | 75%–80% |
| 5 min | 80%–85% |
| 10 min | 85%–95% |

**FIGURE 44-1.** American Academy of Pediatrics/American Heart Association Neonatal Resuscitation Program Algorithm. CPAP, continuous positive airway pressure; ECG, electrocardiogram; ETT, endotracheal tube; HR, heart rate; IV, intravenous; PPV, positive-pressure ventilation; $SpO_2$, oxygen saturation level; UVC, umbilical venous catheter. (Reproduced with permission from Wyckoff MH, Aziz K, Escobedo MB, et al. Part 13: Neonatal resuscitation: 2015 American Heart Association guidelines update for cardiopulmonary resuscitation and emergency cardiovascular care. *Circulation*. 2015;132(18 Suppl 2):S543-S560.)

**Answer 2-19.** E

IUGR is defined as a rate of fetal growth that is less than normal for the population and for the growth potential of a specific infant. The adverse complications of IUGR are due to the processes that lead to growth restriction and the concomitant fetal adaptations rather than the actual anthropometric measurements. Fetuses with IUGR often have asymmetric ("head sparing") effects, with more restriction in organ, muscle, and fat growth than in the brain and long bones. However, neurologic complications are higher in IUGR infants due to impaired central nervous system (CNS) development (fewer neurons, shorter axons, fewer dendrites, and less arborization and synaptic formation). Notably very preterm infants with IUGR are at risk for developmental complications.

(p. 222, Section 4: Newborn, Chapter 49)

**Answer 2-20.** C

Newborn infants can be classified according to birth weight, as well as by weight in relation to gestational age (Table 49-1). Infants who weigh < 2500 g are considered low birth weight. The weight cutoffs for low birth weight and very low birth weight are 1500 g and 1000 g, respectively.

It is not possible to determine whether a 2000-g infant is large for gestational age, appropriate for gestational age, or small for gestational age without information about the gestational age.

Weight in relation to gestational age in conjunction with other anthropometric measurements (eg, length, head circumference, ponderal index) can be helpful in determining the etiology of the size difference, as well as potential adverse outcomes.

(Section 4: Newborn, Chapter 49)

**TABLE 49-1.** Classification of Fetal Growth[a]

| | | |
|---|---|---|
| SGA | Small for gestational age | Birth weight < 10th percentile for gestational age |
| AGA | Average for gestational age | Birth weight between 10th and 90th percentile for gestational age |
| LGA | Large for gestational age | Birth weight > 90th percentile for gestational age |
| IUGR | Intrauterine growth restriction | Slower than normal rate of fetal growth |
| LBW | Low birth weight | < 2500 g |
| VLBW | Very low birth weight | < 1500 g |
| ELBW | Extremely low birth weight | < 1000 g |

[a]Normal birth weight is > 2500 g at term gestation.

Mark W. Kline, *Rudolph's Pediatrics*, 23rd Edition. Copyright © McGraw-Hill Education. All rights reserved.

**Answer 2-21.** C

Major congenital anomalies occur in 6% to 12% of infants of diabetic mothers, in contrast to the incidence of 2% to 3% in infants in the general population. Many studies suggest that the risk of these anomalies is directly correlated with glycemic control early in pregnancy (during organogenesis) and may even be affected by glycemic control immediately prior to conception. Age of onset of diabetes, use of oral hypoglycemics, diabetes type, and a history of a prior macrosomic infant do not increase the risk of congenital anomalies.

(pp. 224–225, Section 4: Newborn, Chapter 50)

**Answer 2-22.** A

Macrosomic infants of diabetic mothers have increased risks of many morbidities, including neurologic injury (eg, subdural hemorrhage, brachial plexus injury), clavicular fractures, abdominal organ injury, and hypocalcemia. In the absence of any significant physical exam findings, however, the first step in management of this infant should be measurement of a serum glucose. All infants of diabetic mothers are at risk of hypoglycemia due to the abrupt cessation of maternal glucose upon severing of the umbilical cord.

Occipital molding is seen in many infants after vaginal delivery, and a clinically significant subdural hematoma would not be suspected in this infant with a normal physical exam. In the absence of clavicular trauma, abdominal distention, or jaundice, the remaining interventions are not indicated immediately.

(pp. 224–226, Section 4: Newborn, Chapter 50)

**Answer 2-23.** C

The infant presents with cyanosis and respiratory distress as well as with maternal risk factors for infection (prolonged [> 18 hours] rupture of amniotic membranes, intrapartum fever, unknown GBS colonization status, and antibiotic administration < 4 hours prior to delivery). Coupled with the radiographic findings, the presentation is most consistent with pneumonia, likely due to GBS or gram-negative bacteria (eg, *E coli*).

Respiratory distress syndrome can present with similar findings on exam and imaging but is less likely in an infant born at term gestation. The increase in saturations with placement of a nasal cannula makes bilateral choanal atresia unlikely. Laryngomalacia presents with audible stridor at birth, which is not noted on exam. Finally, the absence of peritoneal contents (stomach, bowel, liver) in the thorax on chest radiograph makes congenital diaphragmatic hernia unlikely.

(p. 230, Section 4: Newborn, Chapter 51)

**Answer 2-24.** B

Meconium aspiration syndrome (MAS) occurs in approximately 4% to 5% of babies exposed to meconium-stained amniotic fluid. Advanced gestation (> 42 weeks) increases the risk of fetal meconium passage, putting post-dates infants at higher risk of MAS relative to term or preterm infants.

Of the strategies noted, induction of labor (to prevent post-dates delivery) is the only approach demonstrated to reduce the incidence of MAS. The antenatal (elective cesarean section, amnioinfusion) and postnatal (oropharyngeal suctioning by the obstetrician, endotracheal suctioning by the pediatrician) strategies listed have not been demonstrated to reduce the risk of MAS.

(pp. 236–237, Section 4: Newborn, Chapter 52)

**Answer 2-25. A**

The cardinal feature of respiratory distress syndrome in preterm newborns is a deficiency in pulmonary surfactant. Produced and stored by type II alveolar cells beginning at about 16 weeks' gestation, surfactant consists of 90% phospholipids and 10% protein. The components of surfactant primarily involved in reduction of alveolar surface tension are the phospholipid dipalmitoylphosphatidylcholine (DPPC) and surfactant proteins B and C. Surfactant proteins A and D are responsible for modulation of immune function in the lung. Surfactant secretion can be detected in amniotic fluid as early as 28 weeks' gestation.

(pp. 198 and 265, Section 4: Newborn, Chapters 45 and 57)

**Answer 2-26. B**

This infant was born by emergent cesarean section after a motor vehicle accident and developed progressive respiratory symptoms after birth. Due to his gestational age, gender, and lack of antenatal maternal steroid administration, this infant is at highest risk for surfactant deficiency and respiratory distress syndrome (RDS). Neonates with RDS present with respiratory distress and hazy ("ground-glass") infiltrates on chest radiograph.

Pulmonary disease due to an *ABCA3* mutation (which causes surfactant dysfunction) would have presented with a more protracted and severe disease course not resolving in the first 48 hours of age despite exogenous surfactant administration. GBS pneumonia may present with ground-glass lung opacification but is less likely than RDS in this case. Fetuses typically do not pass meconium prior to 32 weeks' gestation; hence, meconium aspiration is unlikely the cause of this neonate's lung disease. Transient tachypnea of the newborn, resulting from failure of alveolar sodium channel activation and subsequent fluid absorption, occurs more commonly in male infants born via cesarean section. Additionally, transient tachypnea of the newborn occurs more commonly in term and late preterm infants, with streaky bilateral infiltrates on chest radiograph.

(pp. 234–236 and 265–268, Section 4: Newborn, Chapters 52 and 57)

**Answer 2-27. B**

During fetal life, most of the cardiac output from the right ventricle bypasses the lungs due to high resistance in the pulmonary vascular bed (Figure 45-2). Blood is therefore shunted via the main pulmonary artery through the ductus arteriosus to the descending aorta. With lung inflation after birth, pulmonary vascular resistance and ductus arteriosus flow both decrease. Ductal closure occurs within hours in about 95% of infants born at > 28 weeks' gestation. However, patent ductus arteriosus persists in about 70% of infants born before 28 weeks' gestation.

(pp. 228 and 270, Section 4: Newborn, Chapters 51 and 58)

**Answer 2-28. B**

This baby has evidence of a hemodynamically significant PDA based on size (diameter > 1.5 mm) and clinical status. Indomethacin, a cyclooxygenase (COX) inhibitor, is more effective than placebo in closing a PDA. Controversies remain regarding use in neonates. Indomethacin use initiated prior to 2 days of age (early therapy) increases the likelihood of PDA closure and decreases the risk of other preterm comorbidities (eg, bronchopulmonary dysplasia and necrotizing enterocolitis).

However, relative to indomethacin treatment at 3 to 6 days of age or > 7 days of age, early therapy did not reduce the incidence of PDA surgical closure or death. Additionally, indomethacin use is contraindicated (Table 58-3) in neonates with a variety of renal conditions (including oliguria and elevation of serum creatinine > 1.8–2 mg/dL). Indomethacin use increases the risk of gastric perforation when used concomitantly with postnatal dexamethasone. A multicenter randomized controlled trial also showed that high serum indomethacin concentrations were not associated with lower rates of PDA. Finally, use of indomethacin (including multiple courses and prolonged use) is not recommended in routine PDA management.

(p. 275, Section 4: Newborn, Chapter 58)

**Answer 2-29. A**

At birth, increases in the partial pressure of oxygen after birth trigger a cascade of cellular and molecular events, including inhibition of voltage-gated potassium channels, activation of the endothelin-1 pathway, and reduction in prostaglandin $E_2$ ($PGE_2$). These mechanisms lead to ductal smooth muscle constriction and functional closure of the ductus arteriosus within hours of birth.

Anatomic closure of the ductus arteriosus follows in the next few days of age due to vascular remodeling and permanent ductal closure. Surgical closure results in permanent closure of the ductus arteriosus but has significant associated morbidities, including earlier complications (eg, pneumothorax, bleeding, vocal cord paralysis) and long-term complications (increased risk of chronic lung disease, retinopathy of prematurity, and neurodevelopmental

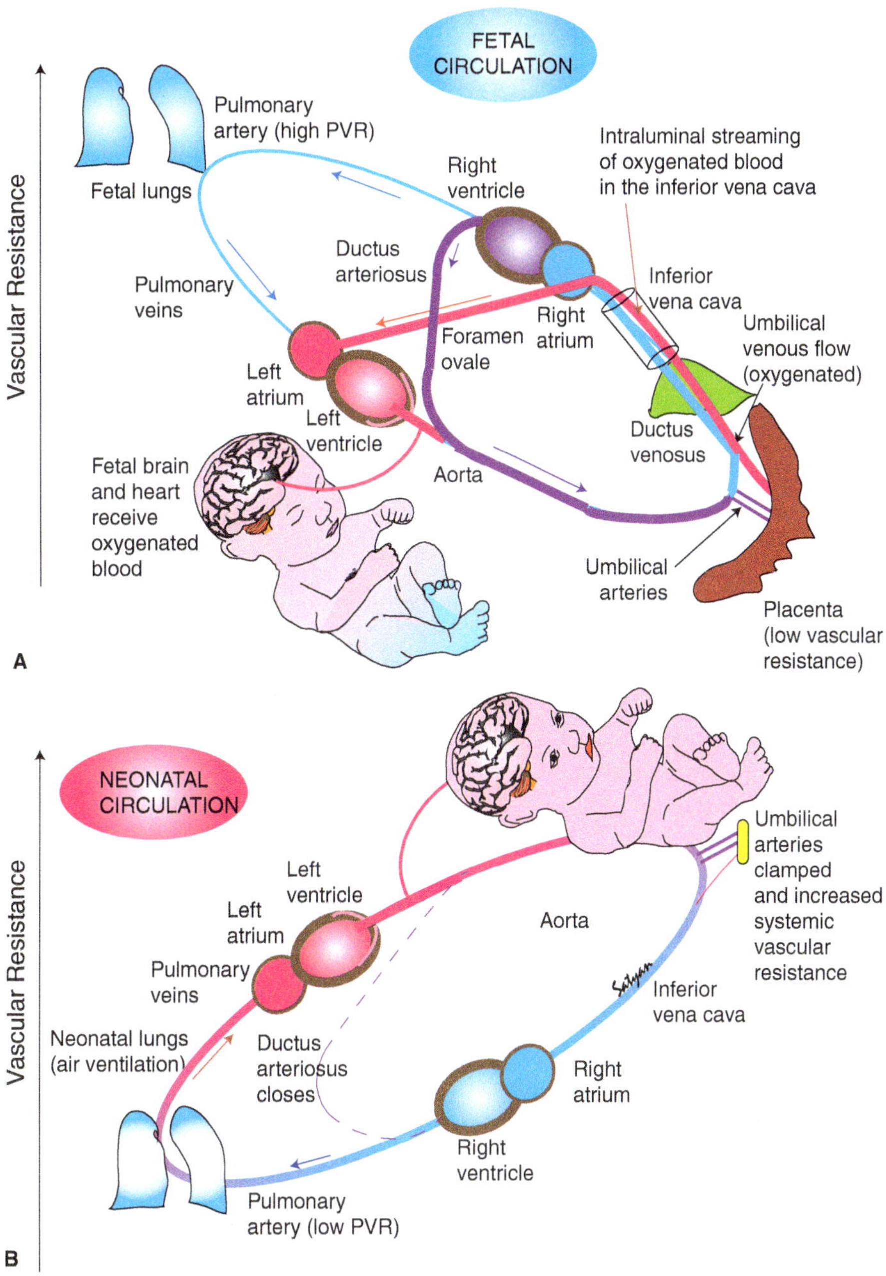


**FIGURE 45-2.** Cardiovascular transition at birth. (**A**) Fetal circulation and (**B**) neonatal circulation are shown, demonstrating flow from areas of high resistance to low resistance. During fetal life, pulmonary vascular resistance (PVR) is high and placental vascular resistance is low. Therefore, right ventricular output flows away from the lungs through the ductus arteriosus and perfuses the placenta to pick up oxygen from the maternal blood. Oxygenated blood flows through the umbilical vein and ductus venosus and streams along the inferior vena cava and enters the left atrium through the foramen ovale to perfuse the heart and brain. Following birth, the onset of ventilation and clamping of the umbilical cord lead to a decrease in pulmonary vascular resistance and an increase in systemic vascular resistance, respectively. Right ventricular output perfuses the lung, and the left ventricle pumps blood to the systemic circulation. Increased oxygenation leads to closure of the ductus arteriosus. (Mark W. Kline, *Rudolph's Pediatrics*, 23rd Edition. Copyright © McGraw-Hill Education. All rights reserved.)

impairment). Indomethacin is known to decrease intestinal blood flow. Acetaminophen has been demonstrated in observational studies to serve as an effective treatment for PDA closure; however, the risk–benefit profile among preterm infants remains unknown. Catheter-based PDA closure is the procedure of choice for PDA closure beyond the neonatal period. This procedure may present with technical challenges in low-weight infants.

(pp. 270–276, Section 4: Newborn, Chapter 58)

**Answer 2-30.** B

The introduction of mechanical ventilation and supplemental oxygen in the 1960s improved survival of infants with respiratory distress syndrome (RDS). However, prolonged use of these therapies to sustain these infants resulted in chronic lung changes first described by Northway in 1967 as BPD. Pathologically, lungs from these infants (with "old" BPD) demonstrated airway smooth muscle hypertrophy and epithelial

**TABLE 58-3.** Contraindications to Use of Indomethacin

- Active gastrointestinal bleeding
- Necrotizing enterocolitis, active or suspected
- Creatinine ≥ 1.8–2.0 mg/dL
- Urine output < 1 mL/kg/h
- Platelet count < 50,000/μL
- Active infection
- Suspected congenital heart disease
- Known gastrointestinal or renal anomaly

Mark W. Kline, *Rudolph's Pediatrics*, 23rd Edition. Copyright © McGraw-Hill Education. All rights reserved.

cell hyperplasia as well as alternating parenchymal fibrosis and emphysema. With the advent of antenatal corticosteroids, exogenous surfactant, and noninvasive ventilatory strategies, the architecture of BPD has changed. Infants with the "new" BPD now demonstrate reduced numbers of alveoli and pulmonary capillaries, with minimal areas of hyperinflation and focal collapse.

(p. 295, Section 4: Newborn, Chapter 62)

**Answer 2-31.** C

The diagnostic criteria for BPD have evolved over time (Table 62-1). The initial definition of BPD required an infant to be on supplemental oxygen for at least 28 days and demonstrate radiographic evidence of lung injury. A 2000 National Institutes of Health (NIH) workshop created a stratified BPD definition for infants born at < 32 weeks gestational age, which included supplemental oxygen for a minimum of 28 days and different degrees of oxygen support at the earlier of hospital discharge or 36 weeks of postmenstrual age. This definition does not consider radiographic changes in making the diagnosis. Pharmacologic therapies (eg, corticosteroids, diuretics) are not considered in making the diagnosis of BPD. Recent studies on infants born at < 32 weeks, however, have suggested that the mode of respiratory support at 36 weeks postmenstrual age, not the amount of oxygen delivered, is best in defining bronchopulmonary dysplasia (BPD).

(p. 295, Section 4: Newborn, Chapter 62)

**TABLE 62-1.** Current Definitions of Bronchopulmonary Dysplasia

| Definition | Criteria |
|---|---|
| **Shennan** | |
| (Originally defined for infants with BWs < 1500 g) | Treatment with supplemental oxygen at 36 weeks PMA |
| **2000 Workshop** | |
| (Originally defined for infants with GAs < 32 weeks) | Treatment with supplemental oxygen for at least 28 days plus the following criteria to distinguish BPD severity: |
| Mild | Breathing in room air at 36 weeks PMA or discharge, whichever comes first |
| Moderate | Treatment with < 30% $O_2$ at 36 weeks PMA or discharge, whichever comes first |
| Severe | Treatment with ≥ 30% $O_2$ and/or positive airway pressure at 36 weeks PMA or discharge (whichever comes first) |
| **Physiologic** | |
| (Originally defined for infants with BWs 501–1500 g) | Infants treated with mechanical ventilation, continuous positive airway pressure, or $O_2$ ≥ 30% at 36 weeks PMA diagnosed with BPD<br>Infants treated with $O_2$ < 30% at 36 weeks PMA diagnosed with BPD if they failed a timed stepwise reduction to room air |

BW, birth weight; GA, gestational age; PMA, postmenstrual age.

Mark W. Kline, *Rudolph's Pediatrics*, 23rd Edition. Copyright © McGraw-Hill Education. All rights reserved.

**Answer 2-32.** A

Although likely due to a combination of prenatal and postnatal effects, multiple risk factors have been identified as causative in BPD. Prematurity is the most important risk factor for BPD, as evidenced by data showing that > 50% of infants born at 24 to 25 weeks' gestation will develop BPD. BPD is inversely proportional to gestational age and birth weight.

Chorioamnionitis has not been independently or conclusively attributed to BPD in human subjects but does predispose babies to preterm birth. Mechanical ventilation and supplemental oxygen are well described as postnatal risk factors for BPD development. However, clinical trials have shown minimal to no effect on BPD incidence of avoiding supplemental oxygen or mechanical ventilation or minimizing supplemental oxygen. Although the presence of a PDA beyond the first days of life is another well-established risk factor for BPD, a causal relationship is unclear based on lack of efficacy of treatment on BPD outcomes. Finally, neonatal sepsis appears to be an independent risk factor for BPD, but its direct effect remains unclear.

(pp. 296–297, Section 4: Newborn, Chapter 62)

**Answer 2-33.** D

The Caffeine for Apnea of Prematurity trial demonstrated that caffeine reduces the risk for BPD and neurodevelopmental impairment. Caffeine is one of the most prescribed medications in the NICU.

Bronchodilators (eg, albuterol and levalbuterol) aid in mucociliary airway clearance and dynamic compliance, but limited data exist on the safety and efficacy in newborn infants.

Vitamin A plasma levels have been found to be lower in infants with BPD, but recent observational studies of supplemental vitamin A in preterm infants showed no differences in development of BPD. Inhaled corticosteroids (eg, budesonide) have been implemented as an alternative to systemic corticosteroids for BPD treatment, but efficacy has not been established, and early use has been associated with increased mortality. Diuretics are a mainstay in the treatment of BPD, but their long-term safety and efficacy have not been demonstrated in large, randomized controlled trials.

(pp. 298–299, Section 4: Newborn, Chapter 62)

**Answer 2-34.** D

This newborn has evidence of hypovolemic shock in the setting of a large, tense scalp mass. Subgaleal hemorrhages, seen in infants born after instrumented delivery, present in the first 24 hours after delivery with a large scalp fluid collection that crosses the cranial suture lines (see figure below). Affected newborns also may have anterior displacement of the ears and subcutaneous fluid tracking in the neck. Of the choices listed, a complete blood count (CBC) would be appropriate to determine the patient's hematocrit and platelet count, both of which are decreased in the setting of a subgaleal hemorrhage.

This patient is less likely to have congenital heart disease, pulmonary disease (eg, pneumonia, transient tachypnea of the newborn), or neonatal sepsis; hence, the other choices are less appropriate as initial management steps.

(p. 206, Section 4: Newborn, Chapter 46)

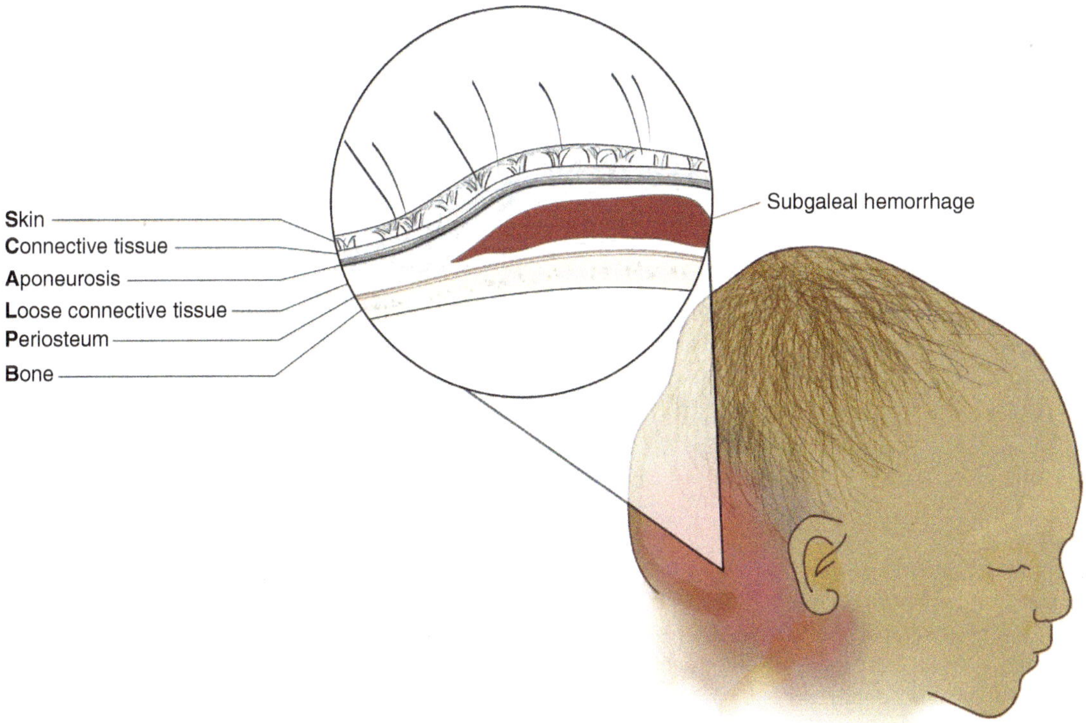


Subgaleal hemorrhage: Perinatal and postnatal hemorrhage can occur into the subgaleal space. Sheering forces caused by traumatic delivery or vacuum extraction can cause tearing of veins within the loose connective tissue space (the *L* in the acronym SCALP), resulting in significant and sometimes lethal overwhelming hemorrhage as the space can expand to hold the entire neonatal blood volume. (Reproduced from Stevenson DK, Cohen RS, Sunshine P, eds. *Neonatology: Clinical Practice and Procedures*. New York, NY: McGraw-Hill; 2015.)

**Answer 2-35.** A

A number of systematic reviews and meta-analyses of randomized studies of therapies with NEC as a primary or secondary outcome have been reported. Of the 5 therapies listed, delayed cord clamping is the only treatment demonstrated to reduce the risk of NEC. However, the results are based on small studies, making reliable conclusions difficult to ascertain. Preterm formula (relative to breast milk) and extended indomethacin therapy have been associated with an increased risk of NEC, whereas oral immunoglobulin (Ig) G and/or IgA therapy and delayed enteral feeds have shown no effect in reducing the risk of NEC.

(pp. 281 and 288, Section 4: Newborn, Chapters 59 and 60)

**Answer 2-36.** E

This newborn has several risk factors for hyperbilirubinemia, including being the infant of a diabetic mother (increased red blood cell volume), having ABO blood group incompatibility, and being born prematurely. Based on the risk designation for infants > 35 0/7 weeks' gestation (Figure 56-3), his bilirubin level at 60 hours of age places him in the high-intermediate-risk zone if a neonatal discharge was being considered. However, given that the mother is planning to stay (and, by default, the baby) to work on breastfeeding, the appropriate next step is to begin phototherapy and continue breast milk feeding every 2 hours.

A repeat bilirubin should be obtained after 2 to 4 hours of phototherapy. Spacing the enteral feeds to every 4 hours would impair the baby's hydration and stooling pattern, increasing the risk of worsening hyperbilirubinemia. Changing the infant to feeding with a soy-based formula will not decrease the child's risk of worsening hyperbilirubinemia.

(pp. 261–264, Section 4: Newborn, Chapter 56)

**Answer 2-37.** B

The newborn in this case has examination findings concerning for an occult spinal dysraphism (eg, a tethered cord). An associated neurologic finding in neonates with this condition is urinary retention, which results in bladder distention (and the midline mass seen in this case). The appropriate next steps in management include spinal and urinary tract sonography, consultation with pediatric neurosurgery and pediatric urology, and decompression of the bladder by urethral catheterization or suprapubic aspiration.

(p. 209, Section 4: Newborn, Chapter 46)

**Answer 2-38.** B

This patient has an unremarkable physical exam, save for a reducible umbilical hernia (a normal finding in a newborn). The vomitus in this 4-hour-old patient is normal newborn regurgitation given the absence of bloody or bilious contents or abdominal distention. Additionally, the baby has passed a meconium stool, making a distal bowel obstruction less likely. At this time, the mother should be reassured that the baby is clinically well and that newborns usually regurgitate a small amount of milk with most feeds. Additional laboratory and imaging tests and surgical consultation should be performed only if the infant develops persistent vomiting, abdominal distention, or a change in the color or content of the vomitus, which could reflect an acute abdominal process (malrotation with midgut volvulus) or neonatal sepsis.

(pp. 208 and 213, Section 4: Newborn, Chapters 46 and 47)

**Answer 2-39.** A

The newborn may have a fuller than normal abdomen at birth but should be generally soft and minimally distended. Diastasis recti, a small gap in the midline abdominal wall musculature, is a normal finding in neonates and most pronounced when the child is crying. Organomegaly is never normal in a newborn. Generally accepted normal findings for abdominal organs on neonatal physical exam include a spleen tip palpated ≤ 1 cm below the left costal margin, a liver edge felt 1 to 2 cm below the right costal margin, and kidneys approximately 2 cm in width. The umbilical cord should contain 2 arteries and 1 vein. The cord should be clear of drainage. Clear fluid noted at the umbilicus raises the suspicion for urine egress due to a patent urachus.

(p. 208, Section 4: The Newborn, Chapter 46)

**Answer 2-40.** A

Necrotizing enterocolitis (NEC) is the most common gastrointestinal complication of prematurity, causing significant short-term and long-term gastrointestinal and extragastrointestinal complications. Babies with NEC need aggressive management of their acute illness, including respiratory support and correction of other complications of the disease. Of the choices listed, decompression of the gastrointestinal tract via nasogastric suctioning is an appropriate next step.

Workup and management of a possible infection (eg, blood, urine, and cerebrospinal fluid cultures, antibiotic administration) and hematologic abnormalities (platelet transfusion for thrombocytopenia) and pain control (morphine infusion) should occur after addressing the acute abdominal distention.

(pp. 284–286, Section 4: Newborn, Chapter 60)

**Answer 2-41.** D

Brain MRI findings are useful in identifying potential long-term outcomes after neonatal encephalopathy. The major areas affected in term and near-term newborns with neonatal encephalopathy include those in a watershed-related pattern (white matter and, in severe cases, cortical gray matter), as well as deep gray nuclei, the perirolandic complex, and the posterior limb of the internal capsule. With mild to moderate hypotension (which occurs in neonatal encephalopathy), parasagittal lesions occur and are unrelated to therapeutic hypothermia. Importantly, MRI changes are dynamic during the first 2 weeks of age, with abnormal areas on initial exam normalizing over time and normal areas worsening on repeat imaging. Based on the degree of basal ganglia and thalamic involvement, patients may develop dyskinetic, spastic, or both spastic and dyskinetic cerebral palsy. White matter lesions in these children often present with cognitive defects.

(pp. 253–254, Section 4: Newborn, Chapter 54)

**Answer 2-42.** A

The pathophysiology of hypoxic-ischemic encephalopathy is based in 2 phases of energy failure that lead to brain injury. The primary phase involves multiple biochemical processes, including decreased high-energy compounds (eg, adenosine triphosphate [ATP] and phosphocreatine) and tissue acidosis, which precipitate a variety of neuronal derangements (loss of membrane homeostasis, increases in neurotransmitter activity and intracellular calcium, and osmotic deregulation). A secondary phase of energy failure occurs later in the process and involves accumulation of excitatory neurotransmitters, oxidative stress, inflammation, and apoptosis (programmed cell death). Resolution of hypoxia-ischemia reverses the loss of high-energy compounds and tissue acidosis and promotes neurotransmitter recycling, providing a period to prevent secondary energy failure. This therapeutic window forms the basis of initiating therapeutic hypothermia to prevent neuronal injury after hypoxic-ischemic encephalopathy.

(pp. 252–253, Section 4: Newborn, Chapter 54)

**Answer 2-43.** E

Neonatal circumcision, often performed for personal, religious, or cultural reasons, prevents balanoposthitis and foreskin constriction problems (eg, paraphimosis). Circumcision also has been shown to decrease the risk of penile cancer, urinary tract infections, and sexually transmitted infections. However, despite these benefits, a policy statement by the American Academy of Pediatrics indicates that the procedure is not recommended as a routine procedure. Contraindications to circumcision include a family history of bleeding disorders (eg, hemophilia), structural abnormalities of the penis (eg, chordee, epispadias, hypospadias), prematurity, small penis size, and clinical illness of the patient. The complication rate of circumcision is about 1%, and complications typically include hemorrhage and infection at the surgical site.

(p. 217, Section 4: Newborn, Chapter 47)

**Answer 2-44.** E

This newborn has an unexplained spike in his bilirubin at 3 days of age in the absence of dehydration or red blood cell group incompatibility. Glucose-6-phosphate dehydrogenase (G6PD) deficiency occurs in approximately 10% of male infants born to parents of African descent and presents with acute hyperbilirubinemia with or without anemia. Of the choices listed, a serum G6PD level is the most appropriate test to order, although the results must be interpreted in setting of acute hemolysis (where results may be normal). An abnormal osmotic fragility test is diagnostic of hereditary spherocytosis, which is less likely in this neonate. Hemoglobin electrophoresis is useful in diagnosis of hemoglobinopathies common in African Americans (eg, sickle cell anemia); however, neonatal jaundice is not a manifestation of sickle cell disease or thalassemias. A right upper quadrant ultrasound is useful in the diagnosis of cholestatic jaundice due to obstructive liver disease; however, the baby's direct bilirubin level is normal for age. A neonate with < 10% weight loss and normal skin turgor is unlikely to be dehydrated, making serum electrolytes less useful in this case.

(pp. 261–264, Section 4: Newborn, Chapter 56)

**Answer 2-45.** C

Fetal thyroid hormone concentrations rise in mid-gestation, increasing significantly during the last weeks of a term gestation to approximately 7-fold at the time of birth. This increase is related to an increase in thermal stress at delivery, which likely relates to the thyroid hormone's role in nonshivering thermogenesis and postnatal cardiac function. However, the overall role of thyroid hormone in the transition to extrauterine life is unclear, because children with congenital hypothyroidism rarely have clinical abnormalities that require medical attention immediately after birth.

(p. 202, Section 4: Newborn, Chapter 45)

**Answer 2-46.** B

In utero circulation is adapted to the unique circumstances of the fetus. To provide well-oxygenated blood from the placenta to the systemic circulation, inferior vena cava blood preferentially streams into the right atrium and across the foramen ovale into the left atrium. Pulmonary vascular resistance is higher in the fetus than in the newborn, and as a result, only 10% to 15% of right ventricular output reaches the pulmonary circulation, all through the pulmonary artery. Systemic circulation results from combined ventricular output, with right ventricular blood shunted through the ductus arteriosus to the descending aorta. About 50% of this ventricular output perfuses the placenta, the organ of intrauterine gas and nutrient exchange.

(pp. 197–198, Section 4: Newborn, Chapter 45)

**Answer 2-47.** C

The newborn in this case has cutaneous findings consistent with herpes simplex virus (HSV) infection. The "classic" rash of neonatal HSV is isolated or clustered vesicles on an erythematous base, although other skin findings may be seen. The baby should undergo a full evaluation for neonatal HSV disease, which includes culture and/or polymerase chain reaction assay (PCR) of swabs of the skin lesions, lumbar puncture, and serum chemistries (including transaminases).

A CBC may identify abnormalities consistent with disseminated HSV disease (eg, neutropenia, lymphocytosis) but is not the next step in management of this infant. Topical timolol is used in infants with cutaneous hemangiomas, not with cutaneous HSV disease. Aside from exaggerated hyperbilirubinemia in the neonatal period, the cephalohematoma should resolve on its own, and cranial imaging and direct aspiration are not indicated.

(p. 206, Section 4: Newborn, Chapter 46)

**Answer 2-48.** C

This preterm neonate has concomitant hypercalcemia and hypophosphatemia, which in preterm infants occurs in the setting of total parenteral nutrition with insufficient phosphate content. Short-term treatment of hypercalcemia in this case involves removal of the improper intravenous nutrition, volume expansion (administering normal saline, 10–20 mg/kg intravenously), and loop diuretic therapy (intravenous furosemide).

Hypophosphatemia should not be corrected with intravenous phosphate (unless the serum phosphate is < 1.5 mg/dL) due to the risk of extraskeletal calcification. Hypomagnesemia is associated with hypocalcemia; hence, supplemental magnesium therapy is not indicated. In a patient with hypercalcemia, supplemental calcium likely will aggravate the hypophosphatemia and is not indicated in this child.

(pp. 247–248, Section 4: Newborn, Chapter 53)

**Answer 2-49.** A

Trials in the use of therapies to improve circulation in the preterm infant have been designed to evaluate changes in a clinical parameter instead of clinical outcomes. However, data on delayed cord clamping, a natural means of volume resuscitation at birth, have demonstrated better circulatory stability as well as a decreased incidence of intraventricular hemorrhage (IVH) and a decreased risk of nectrotizing enterocolitis (NEC).

Albumin and normal saline are not superior to dopamine in improving blood pressure in preterm infants, and neither improves clinical outcomes in this population. Dopamine, a naturally occurring precursor to epinephrine and norepinephrine, is superior to dobutamine, a β-adrenergic catecholamine, in terms of increasing blood pressure, but this effect does not translate into better short-term outcomes. Dobutamine, which causes systemic vasodilatation, produces increased, not decreased, systemic blood flow relative to dopamine. Hydrocortisone has been demonstrated in one small study to increase left ventricular function, but its effects on cerebral blood flow are unclear.

(pp. 280–281, Section 4: Newborn, Chapter 59)

**Answer 2-50.** C

This term newborn has experienced a relatively uncomplicated newborn course. Discharge planning for this infant should include a scheduled follow-up visit with a primary care provider within 48 to 72 hours of discharge, with particular attention at that visit to feeding, weight gain, elimination, and jaundice. This provider should be established by the family prior to hospital discharge and documented in the hospital medical record. Given this infant's gestational age and bilirubin level (which places her in the high-intermediate–risk zone for bilirubin complications), she should be seen ideally within 48 hours of discharge. Discharge instructions to this baby's parents should include education about jaundice, including signs of bilirubin encephalopathy (lethargy, progressive jaundice, poor feeding).

The infant does not require a car seat observation test given her gestational age (> 37 weeks' gestation). G6PD deficiency is an X-linked disorder that occurs primarily in male infants. Furthermore, G6PD testing is not required prior to hospital discharge due to a lack of availability in all hospitals and timeliness for use in decision-making.

(pp. 218 and 264, Section 4: Newborn, Chapters 47 and 56)

**Answer 2-51.** C

CCHD screening is a relatively new addition to testing during the newborn hospitalization. CCHD screening is designed to identify both cyanotic and acyanotic heart lesions in babies. The screen consists of physical examination (including auscultation of heart sounds and palpation of peripheral pulses) and pulse oximetry done at 24 hours of age (or at the time of discharge for babies discharged within 24 hours of birth). CCHD screening is delayed until this time to allow for functional closure of the ductus arteriosus, which may induce cyanosis, pallor, hypoperfusion, or a murmur in ductal-dependent lesions. CCHD screening is useful in detecting both intracardiac lesions (eg, tetralogy of Fallot) and extracardiac lesions (eg, total anomalous pulmonary venous return). Abnormal CCHD screens result in neonatal echocardiography and referral to a pediatric cardiologist. Owing to mild persistence of elevated right ventricular pressures in the immediate newborn, ventricular septal defects may not be detected by CCHD screening. Acrocyanosis is a common finding in newborns and, in the absence of other abnormal physical exam findings, does not indicate congenital heart disease.

(pp. 205 and 215, Section 4: Newborn, Chapters 46 and 47)

**Answer 2-52.** C

BAT is the source of heat during nonshivering thermogenesis, although its role in thermogenesis in preterm infants is not clearly known. Primary areas of BAT storage include the upper back and neck, mediastinum, and perinephric region. Although it increases in postnatal life for some time, BAT is more abundant in newborns than adults. BAT is regulated both by neurogenic (hypothalamic and thermoreceptive afferents) and biochemical (cyclic adenosine monophosphate and intracellular lipases) processes. Within BAT, UCP1 facilitates proton entry into the mitochondria in the absence of normal adenosine 5′-disphosphate/adenosine 5′-triphosphate synthase pathway, producing heat instead of adenosine triphosphate (ATP).

(p. 201, Section 4: Newborn, Chapter 45)

**Answer 2-53.** B

Breast milk exposure has been demonstrated to reduce NEC; donor breast milk has also been shown to be effective in reducing NEC (and, in particular, surgical NEC). Donor breast milk in premature babies has been associated with decreased cognitive scores < 85, but with no difference in mean cognitive score or anthropometrics at 18 months of age (relative to babies receiving preterm formula). In addition, despite the presence of immunoprotective proteins in breast milk (eg, lactoferrin, lysozyme, and immunoglobulins), a study in the Netherlands demonstrated no effect on the likelihood of severe infections.

(p. 287, Section 4: Newborn, Chapter 60)

**Answer 2-54.** C

Inhibin A, maternal α-fetoprotein, human chorionic gonadotropin, and estradiol are the 4 biomarkers that make up the quad screen, which is used prenatally to identify fetuses at increased risk for fetal anomalies such as Down syndrome and neural tube defects. This screen is used in conjunction with the nuchal translucency measurement to assess risk.

Lecithin and sphingomyelin are 2 phospholipids that are present in amniotic fluid. The ratio of these molecules was historically used to assess for fetal lung maturity, not risk of anomalies. Dipalmitoylphosphatidylcholine is a surfactant phospholipid synthesized by type II alveolar epithelial cells.

(pp. 178 and 265, Scction 4: Newborn, Chapters 41 and 57)

**Answer 2-55.** E

This infant's growth parameters are consistent with asymmetric growth restriction, with preservation of head size despite a decrease in weight and length. This pattern of growth is typically seen in the setting of placental insufficiency, evidenced by reversed end-diastolic flow seen on the umbilical artery Dopplers. Pregnancy-induced hypertension is one of the most common causes of placental insufficiency.

Chromosomal anomalies, congenital malformations, constitutionally small size (due to factors such as maternal ethnicity, parity, and body mass), and intrauterine infections are common causes of symmetric IUGR.

(p. 178, Section 4: Newborn, Chapter 41)

**Answer 2-56.** A

Neonatal respiratory distress syndrome (RDS) is a major complication of premature birth and is associated with significant morbidity and mortality. Glucocorticoids administered to the mother prior to delivery have been shown to accelerate fetal lung maturity and therefore decrease morbidity and mortality. Other benefits of antenatal corticosteroid administration include decreased rates of necrotizing enterocolitis (NEC) and improved developmental outcomes.

(p. 178, Section 4: Newborn, Chapter 41)

**Answer 2-57.** C

MRSOPA is an acronym to remember strategies that can be used to improve chest rise and ultimately improve the newborn's heart rate when using bag-mask ventilation in newborn resuscitation. The acronym stands for *m*ask adjustment, *r*eposition airway, *s*uction mouth and nose, *o*pen the mouth, (inflation) *p*ressure increase, and *a*lternate airway. A change in oxygen is not part of ventilation corrective measures. Using a larger face mask may prevent formation of an adequate seal, hampering delivery of positive pressure. Nasogastric tube placement may be indicated for children with gastric distention after extended resuscitation or with congenital diaphragmatic hernias but is not an initial corrective step.

(p. 194, Section 4: Newborn, Chapter 44)

**Answer 2-58.** B

The baby is demonstrating a normal physical exam for a term infant. She has appropriately flexed upper and lower extremities and demonstrates normal Moro (abduction of the arms and opening of the hands upon lifting of the head), root, and suck reflexes. Based on these findings, the neonate does not need additional testing or consultation.

(pp. 209 and 212, Section 4: Newborn, Chapter 46)

**Answer 2-59.** D

All the answer choices describe part of a normal neurologic exam for a term newborn except for the popliteal angle (Figure 46-3). Assessed at the knee with the infant's thigh flexed and the knee extended, the popliteal angle should measure 90 degrees or less in a term infant. A popliteal angle of > 120 degrees in a term infant would indicate decreased passive tone.

(pp. 209–211, Section 4: Newborn, Chapter 46)

**Answer 2-60.** D

This infant is small for gestational age based on birth weight less than the 10th percentile. Additionally, the newborn described here demonstrates asymmetric growth restriction, commonly seen with extrinsic factors leading to placental insufficiency, for which there are multiple risk factors listed in the case (Table 49-2).

This baby is at increased risk for hypoglycemia after delivery, compared to appropriate-for-gestational-age newborns of the same gestation. Small-for-gestational-age infants require early and frequent blood glucose checks in the first 48 hours after birth. Early enteral feedings are helpful in limiting hypoglycemia. Although chromosomal abnormalities and congenital infections may lead to small-for-gestational-age status in the newborn, these are typically associated with symmetric growth restriction. In the absence of risk factors or clinical evidence of bacteremia or dehydration, blood culture and serum electrolytes are not indicated.

(pp. 222 and 223, Section 4: Newborn, Chapter 49)

**Answer 2-61.** B

Newborns who are born small for gestational age are at increased risk for a variety of long-term sequelae following delivery. Compared to appropriate-for-gestational-age infants, small-for-gestational-age infants are 5 to 10 times more likely to have neurologic disorders such as learning disabilities,

| | Weeks Gestation | Below 32 | 32–33 | 34–35 | 36–37 | 38–39 | 40–41 |
|---|---|---|---|---|---|---|---|
| PASSIVE TONE | Popliteal angle | 130° or more | 120°–110° | 110°–100° | 100°–90° | 90° | 90° or less |
| | Scarf-sign | No resistance | Very weak resistance | Largely passes midline | Slightly passes midline | Does not reach midline | Very tight |
| | Return to flexion of forearms | Posture in extension most of the time | | Weak or absent | Present, less than 4 times | 4 Times or more brisk but inhibited | 4 Times or more very strong & not inhibited |
| | Foot-dorsiflexion angle | ≥50° | 40°–30° | | 20°–10° | | Null |
| ACTIVE TONE | Righting reaction lower limbs and trunk | No support | Brief support lower limbs only | Begins to maintain trunk | Trunk more firm | Begins to raise head | Complete righting for a few seconds |
| | Raise-to-sit (neck flexor muscles) | No movement of the head forward | | Face View<br>Head rolls on the shoulder | Passes briskly in the axis | More powerful | Perfect, minimal lag |
| | | | | Better Backward | Progressive Equalization | | Symmetrical |
| | Back-to-lying (neck extensor muscles) | No movement of the head backward | Head begins to lift but cannot pass backward | Passes briskly in the axis | Powerful movement backward | | Perfect, minimal lag |
| PRIMARY REFLEX | Finger grasp and response to traction | Absent | | Very weak or absent | Able to lift part of the body weight | Able to lift all body weight for 1 second | Maintains 2 to 3 second with head passing forward |
| | Crossed extension | | Good extension but no adduction | | Tendency to adduction | Reaches the simulated foot | Crosses immediately |
| | Sucking | Sucks/burst<br>Rate of sucks<br>Negative pressure<br>interburst time | 3 or less<br>1/second<br>Weak or none<br>15–20 second | 4–7<br>1.5/second<br>intermediate<br>5–10 second | 8 or more<br>2/second<br>high<br>5–10 second | Idem | Idem |

**FIGURE 46-3.** Neurologic criteria described at 2-week intervals, from 32 to 40 weeks' gestation. Periods of rapid modifications are enclosed by heavy borders, indicating the most discriminative period for each observation. Idem = refers to same response as 36–37 weeks; null = no flexion. (Adapted with permission from Levene MI, Bennett MJ, Puni J. *Fetal and Neonatal Neurology and Neurosurgery*, 2nd ed. London: Churchill Livingstone; 1995.)

**TABLE 49-2.** Maternal Conditions Associated with Intrauterine Growth Restriction

| |
|---|
| Both very young and advanced maternal age |
| Maternal prepregnancy short stature and thinness |
| Poor maternal weight gain during the third trimester of pregnancy |
| Maternal illness during pregnancy |
| Failure to obtain normal medical care during pregnancy |
| Lower socioeconomic status |
| Black race (in the United States) |
| Multiple gestation |
| Uterine and placental anomalies |
| Polyhydramnios |
| Preeclampsia |
| Hypertension, both chronic and pregnancy induced |
| Chronic, severe diabetes |
| Intrauterine infections |
| Cigarette smoking, cocaine use, and other substance abuse |

Mark W. Kline, *Rudolph's Pediatrics*, 23rd Edition. Copyright © McGraw-Hill Education. All rights reserved.

behavioral problems, and fine motor dyscoordination. In addition, infants with severe IUGR may have short stature that persists into adulthood, ultimately not reaching their predicted mid-parental height. These infants are also at increased risk for impaired immunologic function at birth and in early childhood, as well as for cardiovascular disease as adults.

(p. 224, Section 4: Newborn, Chapter 49)

**Answer 2-62.** B

Infants of diabetic mothers are 5 times more likely to have RDS compared to infants born to mothers without diabetes. RDS is less common in female infants and in firstborn twins compared to male infants and second-born twins, respectively. Maternal hypertension and maternal narcotic abuse have also been shown to decrease the incidence of RDS.

(p. 265, Section 4: Newborn, Chapter 57)

**Answer 2-63.** C

This patient has multiple risk factors for neurodevelopmental impairment, including his degree of prematurity, development of bronchopulmonary dysplasia (BPD), IVH, and retinopathy of prematurity. Caffeine is the only treatment that has been shown to decrease the incidence of neurodevelopmental impairment (as well as BPD and death in preterm infants).

Vitamin A may reduce the composite outcome of BPD or death, but it has not been shown to affect developmental outcomes. Although antenatal steroids have been shown to reduce rates of neurodevelopmental impairment, postnatal steroids increase the risk of cerebral palsy. Advances in nutrition (including fortification of enteral feeds and aggressive parenteral nutrition) have not been shown to improve developmental outcomes.

(pp. 304–305, Section 4: Newborn, Chapter 64)

**Answer 2-64.** D

Despite the patient's physical exam findings, she does not meet criteria for diagnosis of cerebral palsy. Specifically, her mild lower extremity hypertonia does not have a corresponding functional limitation (based on her ability to walk well). Cerebral palsy is a clinical diagnosis and is not dependent on imaging studies (eg, brain MRI). The patient remains at risk for developmental coordination disorder, a problem of motor coordination that may interfere with activities of daily living or academic achievement. However, developmental coordination disorder is not diagnosed with confidence until a child is 5 years old.

(p. 303, Section 4: Newborn, Chapter 64)

**Answer 2-65.** A

The CBCL and the Brief Infant and Toddler Social and Emotional Assessment (BITSEA) are commonly used to screen for behavioral or socioemotional problems during childhood. The Bayley Scales of Infant and Toddler Development are used to assess developmental outcomes, including motor, cognitive, and language development. The M-CHAT is a validated tool used in children aged 16 to 30 months to screen for signs of autism. The General Movements Assessment is a motor evaluation used in preterm infants to assess for the risk of cerebral palsy. The WIAT measures academic skills in school-age children.

(p. 303, Section 4: Newborn, Chapter 64)

**Answer 2-66.** E

Cranial ultrasounds, although not diagnostic, are commonly used in preterm infants to predict the risk of future developmental delays. Controversy exists regarding the impact of grade I and grade II IVH on long-term neurodevelopmental complications. However, grade III IVH and intraparenchymal hemorrhage are known to be associated with adverse developmental outcomes. Infants with grade III IVH and intraparenchymal hemorrhage are also at risk for posthemorrhagic hydrocephalus, which further increases the risk for developmental delays, especially when shunt placement is required. It is important to remember that a normal head ultrasound in a preterm infant does not exclude the possibility of later developmental impairment, and these infants still require close monitoring of their neurodevelopment.

(p. 304, Section 4: Newborn, Chapter 64)

**Answer 2-67.** A

Premature infants are at risk for abnormal neurodevelopmental outcomes due to a variety of morbidities. Infants with NEC are at increased risk of cerebral palsy, cognitive delay, developmental impairment, and death at 18 months of age. In one observational study, surgical NEC, not medical NEC, was most strongly associated with this increased risk for impairment. Infection is also associated with abnormal neurodevelopmental outcomes (cerebral palsy, cognitive delay, and visual impairment) at 18 to 22 months of age, with fungal infections and meningitis posing higher risks. However, data on outcomes after grade I and grade II IVHs are still unclear, with some studies showing no impact on developmental delay and others showing a small increase in risk.

(pp. 304–305, Section 4: Newborn, Chapter 64)

**Answer 2-68.** B

The National Institutes of Health (NIH)-funded Management of Myelomeningocele Study (MOMS) demonstrated that open fetal myelomeningocele repair led to a decreased rate of shunting for hydrocephalus at 12 months of age, reversal of hindbrain herniation (from the associated Chiari II malformation), and increased probability of walking at 30 months of age. Deliveries are by scheduled cesarean section near term or at 34 weeks in the event of premature rupture of membranes. Preterm labor is one of the risks associated with fetal myelomeningocele repair, and approximately 10% of cases deliver before 30 weeks. Minimally invasive (fetoscopic) techniques are currently under investigation, but the available evidence at this time demonstrates results inferior to those seen with open repair.

(p. 183, Section 4: Newborn, Chapter 42)

**Answer 2-69.** D

TTTS affects 10% to 15% of monochorionic twin pregnancies. In TTTS, abnormal placental vascular connections result in increased blood flow to the "recipient" twin at the expense of the "donor" twin. Depending on the severity, this can progress to macrosomia, polycythemia, polyhydramnios, hydrops, and fetal death in the recipient, or intrauterine growth restriction (IUGR), anemia, anhydramnios, and fetal death in the donor. Left untreated, TTTS is almost uniformly fatal. In the past, selective amnioreduction was the treatment of choice for this condition, but newer treatment modalities, such as selective fetoscopic laser photocoagulation, have become first-line therapy due to the ability to prevent progression of the condition. Umbilical cord ablation is performed as salvage therapy to protect the surviving twin in cases of fetal demise of the co-twin. Survival rates of 64% to 92% have been reported in cases of TTTS treated with laser photocoagulation.

(pp. 181–182, Section 4: Newborn, Chapter 42)

**Answer 2-70.** D

The fetus in this scenario has supraventricular tachycardia (SVT) with associated hydrops fetalis. SVT is the most common fetal arrhythmia. It can be successfully treated in utero through maternal administration of antiarrhythmic medications. Of the choices listed, initiation of maternal sotalol is the best management strategy.

Digoxin is the first-line antiarrhythmic unless hydrops is present, which limits transplacental transfer of the medication. Because successful therapeutic medical interventions exist, it would be inappropriate to send the mother home with monitoring alone or recommend immediate delivery of the fetus. Maternal corticosteroid administration is indicated in the management of complete heart block, which manifests with bradycardia (not tachycardia) and is most often associated with maternal lupus and transplacental transfer of anti-Ro/SSA antibodies.

(p. 180, Section 4: Newborn, Chapter 42)

**Answer 2-71.** A

The infant in this vignette has acrocyanosis, or dark blue discoloration of the hands and/or feet, which is considered a normal finding in healthy newborns. This condition is due to relatively slow blood flow through the capillary beds and increased time for oxygen extraction by the tissues, resulting in the accumulation of 3 to 5 g/dL of deoxyhemoglobin in the peripheral tissues. Isolated acrocyanosis does not require further intervention and will resolve on its own within days after birth. In the absence of other abnormal findings, additional testing (eg, chest radiograph, echocardiogram, hemoglobin electrophoresis) and supplemental oxygen in the neonatal intensive care unit (NICU) are not warranted.

Central cyanosis, characterized by bluish discoloration of the skin (trunk, face, and lips) and mucous membranes, is always abnormal, and intervention and further workup are indicated. Of note, extremities can appear pale or blue and cool in the context of poor perfusion with peripheral vasoconstriction; however, other aspects of the clinical exam will also be abnormal, an indication that further evaluation is warranted.

(pp. 227, 230–231, Section 4: Newborn, Chapter 51)

**Answer 2-72.** E

The infant in this vignette demonstrates the classical clinical findings associated with bilateral choanal atresia. Because air exchange can only occur via the mouth in babies with this condition, oral occlusion (via a pacifier, bottle, or breast) compromises air exchange, leading to desaturations.

Transient tachypnea of the newborn is less likely in this full-term infant born vaginally with an uncomplicated delivery course. Phrenic nerve palsy could cause respiratory distress and desaturations, but the desaturations would not preferentially occur when calm. Laryngomalacia may be present at birth but more commonly presents at several weeks of age and is associated with inspiratory stridor and respiratory distress that worsens with crying, feeding, and respiratory infections. Tracheoesophageal fistulae, with or without esophageal atresia, may present as choking and gagging with feeds and respiratory distress and desaturations at rest due to aspiration of saliva;

however, respiratory symptoms are not reliably alleviated by crying.

(pp. 228–230, Section 4: Newborn, Chapter 51)

**Answer 2-73. C**

Cyanosis is associated with congenital heart disease in which there is obstruction to pulmonary blood flow, obstruction to systemic blood flow, or parallel circulations with inadequate mixing. Mixing of oxygenated and deoxygenated blood occurs through the ductus arteriosus, which is patent during fetal life but closes in the days following birth.

The infant in this vignette exhibits the classic presentation of a ductal-dependent cardiac lesion; that is, well-appearing immediately after birth and at discharge from the birth hospitalization, but with progressive hypoxemia and cyanosis during the following days as the ductus arteriosus closes and the pathway enabling adequate blood flow to the lungs or body is removed. Of the lesions listed, only hypoplastic left heart syndrome is ductal dependent.

A balanced atrioventricular canal defect is usually associated with intracardiac mixing of oxygenated and deoxygenated blood, but babies with this condition most often present at 3 to 8 months of age with overcirculation and pulmonary edema as the pulmonary vascular resistance decreases. Tetralogy of Fallot *without* right ventricular outflow tract obstruction is also associated with intracardiac mixing through a ventricular septal defect, but because there is adequate pulmonary blood flow, the infants are not typically cyanotic. Muscular ventricular septal defects are infrequently associated with clinical symptomatology during infancy and often close spontaneously during childhood. Peripheral pulmonic stenosis is more often seen in preterm infants; when unilateral in presentation, this condition rarely presents with cyanosis.

(p. 233, Section 4: Newborn, Chapter 51)

**Answer 2-74. A**

Seizures in the newborn can have many different etiologies, including electrolyte and glucose abnormalities, central nervous system (CNS) malformations, and intracranial hemorrhage. This infant demonstrates multiple symptoms of hypoglycemia, including lethargy, hypotonia, and poor feeding. The findings of hemihypertrophy (large right arm and leg) and macroglossia (large tongue), coupled with the hypoglycemia, are most consistent with Beckwith-Wiedemann syndrome. Beckwith-Wiedemann syndrome is associated with hyperplasia of multiple organs, including the pancreas, which can lead to hyperinsulinism and hypoglycemia. If severe and prolonged, the hypoglycemia can cause seizures.

Hypocalcemia due to absent parathyroid glands is associated with 22q11.2 deletion syndrome (also known as DiGeorge syndrome or the velocardiofacial syndrome), which presents with cardiac defects and distinct facial features (ie, small ears, hooded eyelids, cleft lip and/or palate, bulbous nose) in infancy. Congenital adrenal hyperplasia can cause ambiguous genitalia in female infants (not seen in this case) and result in electrolyte abnormalities (eg, hyponatremia, hyperkalemia) and adrenal crisis due to low levels of aldosterone and cortisol.

(pp. 242–243, Section 4: Newborn, Chapter 53)

**Answer 2-75. D**

The patient described in this vignette has DiGeorge syndrome (22q11.2 deletion syndrome), which is associated with craniofacial, cardiac, renal, and immunologic abnormalities. Hypocalcemia (due to parathyroid gland hypoplasia) is seen in children with DiGeorge syndrome. Although hypoglycemia, hyponatremia, intracranial hemorrhage, and other structural central nervous system (CNS) abnormalities may be etiologies of neonatal seizures, the baby in this vignette most likely has hypocalcemia, which will respond to administration of intravenous calcium.

(pp. 243 and 247, Section 4: Newborn, Chapter 53)

**Answer 2-76. A**

Hyperkalemia is a life-threatening emergency because it can precipitate cardiac arrhythmias and dysfunction, as noted by the abnormal electrocardiogram (ECG) findings in this case. Of the options listed, the most appropriate next step is to administer calcium gluconate to lower the cell membrane threshold. Although transient, this intervention can be lifesaving and should be the first step in treating symptomatic hyperkalemia.

Potassium-containing fluid should be discontinued completely until serum levels have returned to normal; however, this step should not delay immediate administration of calcium gluconate. In the setting of ECG changes, the laboratory value is unlikely to be spurious. As a result, repeat laboratories are not an appropriate next step. Dialysis is an option for removing the excess potassium; however, this process takes time to coordinate and is not an immediate solution for hyperkalemia in this case. Oral cation exchange resins will not immediately correct hyperkalemia.

(p. 250, Section 4: Newborn, Chapter 53)

**Answer 2-77. D**

Chronic metabolic acidosis produces reversible growth failure. In this otherwise well-appearing preterm infant, the most likely cause of his growth failure is a mild, developmentally regulated, proximal renal tubular acidosis with renal bicarbonate wasting. This renal tubular acidosis of prematurity represents the most common cause of normal anion gap metabolic acidosis in the preterm newborn.

There is no evidence of chronic renal failure because the BUN and creatinine are within normal limits for age. An undiagnosed inborn error of metabolism in a 3-week-old, clinically well-appearing infant tolerating full-volume, fortified feeds would be unlikely. The infant does not demonstrate signs or symptoms of sepsis, such as an increase in the frequency of apnea/bradycardia, temperature instability, or hypoperfusion. The serum sodium concentration is within acceptable limits for a preterm infant and is less likely a result of aldosterone insensitivity.

(p. 251, Section 4: Newborn, Chapter 53)

**Answer 2-78.** D

The infant in this vignette has congenital anemia and exhibits clinical signs and symptoms including pallor, tachycardia, tachypnea, hypoxia, and respiratory distress. The absence of concerns during the pregnancy (ie, elevated middle cerebral artery Doppler flow, intrauterine growth restriction [IUGR], hydrops fetalis) makes the congenital anemia more likely due to an acute condition (eg, maternal–fetal hemorrhage) as opposed to a chronic condition (eg, fetal hemolysis or red cell aplasia). The Kleihauer-Betke test looks for the presence of fetal hemoglobin in the maternal blood and is indicative of maternal–fetal hemorrhage (as can be seen in the setting of a placental abruption).

Hemolytic disease of the newborn, an immune-mediated hemolytic anemia, is diagnosed using the direct Coombs test, which looks for the presence of maternal antibody bound to the surface of infant red blood cells. When mother and infant have the same blood type, this test is unlikely to be positive. Both the peripheral smear and the osmotic fragility test can aid in diagnosing red cell membrane defects, such as hereditary spherocytosis or pyropoikilocytosis. However, the diagnosis is less likely in the absence of a family history of red cell disorders or anemia. Furthermore, the findings on a peripheral smear associated with mild anemia due to blood loss are nonspecific. The Apt test, which looks for the presence of maternal blood in newborn specimens (stool or vomit), is helpful in determining the maternal or fetal origin of blood in newborn emesis. In the absence of bloody oral secretions, an Apt test is not indicated in this case.

(pp. 257–258, Section 4: Newborn, Chapter 55)

**Answer 2-79.** E

The infant in this vignette demonstrates symptomatic polycythemia, defined as a central venous hematocrit of > 65% with clinical signs and symptoms, which can include plethora or rubeosis ("ruddiness"), lethargy, tachypnea, and delayed capillary refill. In addition to supporting the infant's respiratory status and titrating intravenous fluids to prevent hypoglycemia, partial exchange transfusion should be initiated, especially if there is further deterioration in the clinical status.

Maintenance of current intravenous fluids will not reverse symptomatic polycythemia (via a dilutional effect) in this case. Hypoglycemia in this case likely is a transient phenomenon mediated by the large red cell mass and elevated neonatal insulin levels (in this infant of a diabetic mother). Thus, investigation for other endocrine causes of hypoglycemia is not indicated at this time. A double-volume exchange transfusion is generally indicated for severe hyperbilirubinemia to prevent bilirubin encephalopathy and kernicterus, not for polycythemia, which is not noted in this case. IVIG is used to treat hyperbilirubinemia due to alloantibody-mediated hemolytic disease of the newborn, but not for polycythemia.

(pp. 242–243 and 258–259, Section 4: Newborn, Chapters 53 and 55)

**Answer 2-80.** E

The infant in this vignette exhibits classic signs and symptoms of medical (stage II) NEC, including the sudden onset of abdominal distention, bloody stool, apnea and bradycardia, and radiographic evidence of pneumatosis intestinalis. The diagnostic evaluation for this infant includes blood and urine cultures and serial monitoring of the CBC and serum chemistries for thrombocytopenia, neutropenia or neutrophilia, anemia, coagulopathy, and electrolyte abnormalities.

Most NEC-associated bloodstream infections are caused by gram-negative bacteria such as *E coli* and *Klebsiella* and are treated for 7 to 10 days, although there is a paucity of data to guide the optimal duration of therapy. Although variability exists in the initial choice of antibiotic treatment, the most common regimen is vancomycin plus gentamicin. Infants receiving anaerobic antimicrobials at the onset of NEC therapy have a higher risk of post-NEC stricture formation but also have a lower mortality risk. Although pneumoperitoneum (free intra-abdominal air) is the primary indication for surgical intervention, additional criteria may also be considered, including portal venous gas, a "fixed" intestinal loop on abdominal radiograph, or abdominal wall erythema.

(pp. 284–286, Section 4: Newborn, Chapter 60)

**Answer 2-81.** A

The risk of NEC is related inversely to the amount of breast milk exposure, which likely relates to important components of human milk (lactoferrin, long-chain polyunsaturated fatty acids, immunoglobulins). Of the choices listed, standardized feeding protocols are the only strategy demonstrated to decrease NEC. Although limited evidence exists to support any specific single feeding plan to reduce the risk of NEC, observational studies have demonstrated that the implementation of a standardized feeding protocol is associated with a decrease in the incidence of NEC. Acid-suppression medications, such as $H_2$ antagonists, increase the risk of NEC by decreasing gastrointestinal bacterial diversity and selectively increasing the abundance of pathogenic bacteria due to the reduced bactericidal effect of stomach acid. Antibiotic duration for > 3 days is associated with higher risk of colonization with gram-negative bacteria and development of NEC; thus, prompt discontinuation of empiric antibiotic therapy helps to decrease the chance of infection with gram-negative species. Routine monitoring of gastric aspirates remains controversial; this practice has not been shown to decrease the incidence of NEC or adverse outcomes.

(pp. 287–289, Section 4: Newborn, Chapter 60)

# CHAPTER 3 Principles of Adolescent Care

Adam W. Dell and Nicole L. Mihalopoulos

**3-1.** A 17-year-old boy presents to your office for an acute care visit. He has come without his parents' knowledge or consent. He recently started having sexual intercourse and has not always been using a condom. He would really prefer that his parents not know that he has started having sex. He states that he has had some yellow discharge from his penis and is concerned he may have a sexually transmitted infection (STI). What is your next step?

**A.** Call his parents and explain the situation without telling him that you are calling.

**B.** Call his partner and explain the situation without telling him that you are calling.

**C.** Tell him that you cannot see him without notifying his parents.

**D.** Explain the rules of confidentiality in the state where you practice and offer confidential STI testing and treatment as able.

**E.** Explain to him that under federal law, you cannot treat him for an STI without notifying his parents.

**3-2.** A 14-year-old African American boy presents to your office for an urgent care visit. He presents with sudden onset of severe left-sided hip and thigh pain and is unable to bear weight. His body mass index (BMI) is 35 $kg/m^2$. You are concerned he might have a slipped capital femoral epiphysis (SCFE). If he does in fact have an SCFE, which sexual maturity rating (SMR) would you expect on physical examination?

**A.** SMR 1

**B.** SMR 3

**C.** SMR 4

**D.** SMR 5

**E.** SMR 6

**3-3.** Which hormone is the most influential in promoting glandular development of the breast during puberty?

**A.** Progesterone

**B.** Thyroxine

**C.** Luteinizing hormone

**D.** Insulin

**E.** Estrogen

**3-4.** At what mean age and mean sexual maturity rating (SMR) does spermarche occur?

**A.** 12 years; SMR 2

**B.** 13 years; SMR 3

**C.** 13.5 years; SMR 2.5

**D.** 14.5 years; SMR 3.5

**E.** 15 years; SMR 4

**3-5.** A patient presents for a physical examination for school. Overall, he reports that things are going well. On your Home, Education/Employment, Eating, Activities, Drugs, Sex, Suicidality, Safety (HEEADSSS) assessment, he reports that he lives with his parents. While they get along well generally, they have been fighting more because he has been staying out later than they would like. He states he is attracted to females and just recently began dating for the first time. He reports that he and the girl broke up, and his friends were his main support. He reports he has used alcohol, as all of his friends drink as well. As a result, he is unclear if he really wants to stop drinking at this time. You note that he has never driven in a car with someone who is drinking. When thinking about his biopsychosocial development, what stage would you estimate him to be?

**A.** Early adolescence (age 10–13)

**B.** Middle adolescence (age 14–16)

**C.** Late adolescence (age 17–21)

**D.** Young adulthood (age 21–24)

**E.** Adulthood (age 25+)

**3-6.** A 14-year-old girl, who is a new patient, presents for a physical examination. You obtain a medical history and want to do a social history. You decide to complete a Home, Education/Employment, Eating, Activities, Drugs, Sex, Suicidality, Safety (HEEADSSS) assessment. You ask the parent to leave the room so you can ask the patient about these sensitive topics. After mom has left, you begin. Which of the following is true about the HEEADSSS assessment model?

**A.** It is a good model to assess the health and well-being of the adolescent in a number of different domains.

**B.** You must report all the information obtained back to her parent.

**C.** If you complete a HEEADSSS assessment, you do not need to complete a physical examination.

**D.** You should not ask the patient about suicidal ideations because that might lead the patient to have thoughts about suicide.

**E.** HEEADSSS is a series of questions used to definitively diagnose specific conditions.

**3-7.** A 16-year-old boy presents for a physical examination. Overall, he seems to be healthy and doing well. His last physical examination was so long ago that he cannot remember the date of the visit. His mother wants to make sure he is caught up in his immunizations, but she did not bring his immunization records. What will you advise the patient and his mother about immunizations?

**A.** Adolescence is a crucial time for catching up on vaccines that were started and not finished, and there may be new vaccines specific to adolescents.

**B.** If it has been <5 years since he received any vaccines, he should receive a tetanus, diphtheria, and pertussis (TdAP), given recent concern about pertussis outbreaks.

**C.** Adolescents typically do not require any vaccinations, even though he has not had any in at least 5 years.

**D.** He needs his third measles-mumps-rubella (MMR) immunization at 16 years of age.

**E.** He needs to repeat all of his vaccines since his mother did not bring his vaccination records.

**3-8.** You are asked to give a presentation to a local group of high school students. The school has asked that you present information related to adolescent health. A teacher reports that they recently had a student in the school who died, and the students have been quite upset about this. The teachers would like to be sure that you mention the major causes of adolescent mortality. Which of the following should you report to them as the leading cause of death in teens?

**A.** Suicide

**B.** Homicide

**C.** Late effects from the treatment of childhood neoplasms

**D.** Malignant neoplasms

**E.** Unintentional injuries, including motor vehicle accidents

**3-9.** A 13-year-old boy presents for a physical examination. You notice on review of his chart that he is overweight and has been overweight since he was about 3 years old. You want to discuss your concerns about the health consequences of being overweight with him. What will be your next step in managing this patient about his weight?

**A.** Say nothing, since he is so young that there are no health consequences to his current weight.

**B.** Document the body mass index (BMI) for now and track over time. Most overweight adolescents do not become overweight or obese adults.

**C.** Discuss with him some of the health consequences that are associated with overweight and obesity such as diabetes, hypertension, and high cholesterol.

**D.** Counsel him that he should not worry, given that only 25% of overweight adolescents become overweight or obese adults.

**E.** Offer to start a stimulant medication to help promote weight loss.

**3-10.** What percentage of adolescents use contraception at their first intercourse?

**A.** 10%

**B.** 25%

**C.** 50%

**D.** 75%

**E.** 95%

**3-11.** A 14-year-old boy is brought into the emergency department (ED) by his friends. His friends explain that the patient had been with them at a party earlier that night when he suddenly lost consciousness. They are not exactly sure what he had ingested. After his airway is secured and intravenous fluids are administered, his labs return and you learn that his blood alcohol level is 250 mg/dL. With severe alcohol intoxication, what other laboratory abnormalities can you expect to find?

**A.** Hyperkalemia

**B.** Hyperglycemia

**C.** Elevated osmolar gap

**D.** Metabolic alkalosis

**E.** Hyponatremia

**3-12.** A mother presents to clinic with her 15-year-old daughter. The mother is concerned because her daughter used to be very close with the rest of the family, an excellent student, and captain of the soccer team. However, over the past few months, she has been refusing to join the family at dinner, her grades are deteriorating, and she has been missing soccer practice. You meet with the patient alone. On examination, she is tachycardic and appears anxious. Her pupils are dilated, she has injected conjunctiva, and she has poor coordination and balance. What is the patient's diagnosis?

**A.** Panic disorder

**B.** Schizophrenia, paranoid type

**C.** Opiate intoxication

**D.** Ethanol intoxication

**E.** Cannabis intoxication

**3-13.** Which of the following statements correctly describes the American Academy of Pediatrics (AAP) position on drug testing of adolescents?

**A.** Adolescents can be tested for drugs of abuse involuntarily with their parent's consent.

**B.** With few exceptions, involuntary testing of adolescents for drugs of abuse should not be done.

**C.** Adolescents can be tested for drugs of abuse if their parent, teacher, or doctor suspects that they are using drugs.

**D.** Involuntary testing of adolescents for drugs of abuse can be done if the results are kept confidential.

**E.** Involuntary testing of adolescents for drugs of abuse can be done on a case-by-case basis.

**3-14.** A 16-year-old girl presents complaining of symptoms of depressed mood and worthlessness. She states, "Nothing matters." Her parents report that her performance in school has declined over the course of this year, and she no longer seems interested in her school clubs, which she used to enjoy. Both the patient and parents are interested in starting a treatment that may help her. What is your next step in the management of this patient?

**A.** You ask them to follow up with you in 3 months.

**B.** Medications are not recommended for the management of depression in adolescents, so you refer them for therapy.

**C.** You discuss options for medications, including potential risks and benefits, and reach a decision with the patient and family.

**D.** You ask her specific questions in order to assess her risk of suicide in order to determine the acuity of her depressive symptoms.

**E.** You order a hemoglobin level and thyroid-stimulating hormone (TSH) levels to screen for anemia and hypothyroidism.

**3-15.** A 15-year-old girl presents to the emergency department (ED) for chest pain. She reports that she was at school and she began to feel dizzy and light-headed and then noticed that her heart felt like it was beating so hard it was going to pop out of her chest. She reports that she felt like she was going to die of a heart attack. She has a family history positive for asthma, but she herself has no other significant medical history, and her physical examination is within normal limits. What is your next step in the management of this patient?

**A.** Order echocardiography and an electrocardiogram in order to rule out a myocardial infarction.

**B.** Discharge home with an albuterol inhaler.

**C.** Recommend and prescribe lorazepam for her to use regularly.

**D.** Refer her for a psychological assessment for cognitive-behavioral therapy and psychiatric evaluation for medication.

**E.** Review the results of your examination with the parents and patient. Reassure them that nothing is wrong. No further treatment is needed.

**3-16.** The mother of a 17-year-old patient of yours calls you to express her concerns about her son. She is crying when she speaks to you. She reports that he was caught shoplifting and seems to have no understanding of the potential consequences. His mom reports that she feels like he has been out of control for the last week, staying up all night playing music. He has started talking about being a rock star. She feels like she can't get a word in when she speaks to him as he speaks so quickly. You are reviewing the chart when you speak with her. You notice last year when you saw him for his annual physical examination, you were concerned that he was depressed. Currently, in speaking with mom, you are most concerned about which of the following?

**A.** He is having a manic episode, which untreated may put his safety at risk.

**B.** He is abusing alcohol, which untreated may put his safety at risk.

**C.** He has symptoms of barbiturate abuse, which may put his safety at risk.

**D.** He has symptoms of post-traumatic stress disorder (PTSD), which will be difficult to treat.

**E.** This episode of shoplifting may put his chances of being accepted into a competitive university at risk.

**3-17.** A 12-year-old girl is brought in by her parents because they are worried about her. About a month ago, the house was burglarized at night while the family was home asleep. Your patient woke up to get a drink of water and saw the burglars who threatened her and her family if she told anyone what she had seen prior to their fleeing the home. Since then, she has had nightmares and hasn't wanted to sleep in her room by herself. She is jumpy and hypervigilant. Her parents are looking to you for what they should do next for their daughter. What is your next step in management of the patient?

**A.** Prescribe a sleeping pill such as zolpidem.

**B.** Criticize the parents for involving the police given the threat to their safety.

**C.** Refer the patient and her family for a psychological assessment for appropriate therapy.

**D.** Inform the parents that this condition is transient and will improve with time, especially if the police catch the burglars.

**E.** Inform the parents that this condition is less common among females than among males.

**3-18.** A 15-year-old girl presents for her annual physical examination. You review her growth chart prior to seeing her and notice that both her weight and body mass index have dropped significantly since you saw her last year (from the 50th percentile to the 10th percentile). On history, she reports that she is on the cross-country team and running many miles weekly. Additionally, she reports that while onset of menarche was at age 12, she has not had a period in the past 6 months. She denies sexual activity, substance use, and any other physical complaints and is doing very well in school. Her mother reports that she has been worried about her daughter's recent weight loss and social isolation, particularly around meal times. What is your next step?

**A.** Obtain vital signs, including a resting heart rate, blood pressure, and body temperature, because you are concerned she may require hospitalization.

**B.** Order lab tests, including a complete blood count (CBC) and serum electrolyte levels.

**C.** Reassure mom that dieting is normal adolescent behavior.

**D.** Call her coach to see if the coach has any concerns.

**E.** Hospitalize the patient.

**3-19.** A 19-year-old woman presents to your office for a physical examination. Her weight and body mass index (BMI) are at the 60th percentile. Her heart rate and blood pressure are within normal limits. She reports that overall things are going well at home and at school. She does endorse that she is experimenting with alcohol and marijuana. She also states that she wishes that she were thinner, and that she has been dieting. You proceed to your physical examination. Which of the following physical examination findings would make you more concerned that the patient is engaging in disordered eating behaviors?

**A.** Acanthosis nigricans on her neck and axillae

**B.** Russell's sign on her hands

**C.** Dilated pupils

**D.** Hyperthermia

**E.** Kayser-Fleischer rings

**3-20.** A 16-year-old girl presents to your office having recently been hospitalized for medical complications due to anorexia nervosa. She was hospitalized for 2 weeks and was able to gain weight in the hospital. Since hospital discharge, she has been eating better, including 3 meals and 3 snacks, and has limited her physical activity. Her parents would like her to start mental health treatment and would like some next steps in finding appropriate treatment for her. You make which of the following recommendations, thinking it has the strongest evidence base in the treatment of anorexia nervosa?

**A.** You refer her to a psychiatrist to begin psychotropic medication, such as an antidepressant.

**B.** You refer her to a nutritionist, as studies show she has the best chance to do well if she can reach a higher weight.

**C.** You refer her to an individual therapist, as research demonstrates she will do better if the parents play a minimal role in treatment.

**D.** You refer her to a family-based therapist, as this psychotherapeutic modality has the strongest evidence base.

**E.** None of the above.

**3-21.** A 14-year-old girl presents for her annual physical examination. During the review of systems, she says that she has bilateral breast pain in the upper outer quadrants of her breasts. On physical examination, you find diffuse cordlike thickening as well as discrete mobile lesions throughout her breasts. Which additional piece of history or examination finding would aid in confirming the diagnosis?

**A.** The pain begins in the premenstrual phase of the menstrual cycle.

**B.** The pain begins in the ovulatory phase of the menstrual cycle.

**C.** She has a positive family history for *BRCA1* genes.

**D.** She is having fevers.

**E.** She was recently in a car accident and was wearing a seat belt that laid over her breasts.

**3-22.** A 14-year-old boy presents to your clinic with the chief complaint of breast development. He and his mother explain that they first noticed the enlargement of his breasts 1 year ago. You obtain a detailed history and physical examination and determine that he has pubertal gynecomastia. Which of the following about pubertal gynecomastia is a true statement?

**A.** It is common and occurs in 90% of boys.

**B.** It peaks in incidence during Tanner stage (or sexual maturity rating [SMR]) 5.

**C.** It is a permanent condition.

**D.** Spontaneous resolution occurs in 90% of boys.

**E.** Starting an aromatase inhibitor or a selective estrogen receptor modulator is appropriate at this time.

**3-23.** A 14-year-old previously healthy boy presents with severe left-sided scrotal pain. In addition, he complains of nausea and fever. On physical examination, the left scrotum is erythematous with moderate swelling. His cremasteric reflex is absent. What is the best treatment for this patient?

**A.** Empiric treatment with antibiotics.

**B.** Supportive treatment including analgesics, anti-inflammatory agents, and scrotal elevation.

**C.** Surgical exploration and detorsion.

**D.** Surgical exploration and detorsion, as well as scrotal orchiopexy.

**E.** Additional testing is required prior to treating this patient.

**3-24.** A 16-year-old boy presents with fever, abdominal pain, and pain in his right scrotum. In reviewing his history, you learn that he has no other significant past medical history, but that 1 week ago he had parotitis. What is the most common cause of this patient's diagnosis in adolescent males?

**A.** *Chlamydia trachomatis*

**B.** *Staphylococcus aureus*

**C.** Coxsackievirus

**D.** Adenovirus

**E.** Mumps virus

**3-25.** An 18-year-old man presents for his annual physical examination. He is otherwise healthy but does report that over the past few months, his right scrotum has been swollen. He denies any pain. On his testicular examination, you note a firm irregular mass that does not transilluminate. The examination is also significant for gynecomastia. Which of the following is a risk factor for this patient's diagnosis?

**A.** Cryptorchidism

**B.** An uncircumcised penis

**C.** Anabolic steroid use

**D.** Obesity

**E.** Unprotected intercourse

**3-26.** Which of the following choices best describes a spermatocele?

**A.** It is an inflammatory disease of the epididymis.

**B.** It is the result of fluid tracking down into the tunica vaginalis.

**C.** It is a dilation of the pampiniform venous plexus within the scrotum.

**D.** It is a cystic accumulation of sperm within the epididymis.

**E.** It is a dilation of the pampiniform venous plexus within the epididymis.

**3-27.** A 16-year-old girl presents to your clinic for her annual physical examination. During the history, you learn that despite having a history of regular periods, she has not had a period in 3 months. After you complete the history and physical examination, what test would you order next?

**A.** A dual-energy x-ray absorptiometry (DEXA) scan to evaluate her bone density

**B.** A qualitative urine human chorionic gonadotropin (HCG) test

**C.** Follicle-stimulating hormone (FSH) and luteinizing hormone (LH)

**D.** A karyotype

**E.** A urine drug screen

**3-28.** A 15-year-old girl with cystic fibrosis (CF) presents to your clinic complaining, "I have never had a period." You do a pregnancy test, which is negative. You suspect that the patient has amenorrhea from nutritional deficiencies secondary to having a chronic disease. What labs would confirm your suspicion?

**A.** High luteinizing hormone (LH), high follicle-stimulating hormone (FSH), and low estrogen

**B.** High LH, high FSH, and high estrogen

**C.** Low LH, low FSH, and low estrogen

**D.** High gonadotropin-releasing hormone (GnRH), high LH, and high FSH

**E.** Low GnRH, high LH, and high FSH

**3-29.** A 15-year-old girl presents to your clinic with 6 months of painful menstrual periods. She is otherwise healthy and had menarche at age 13. Unfortunately, the painful periods have led to missing a significant amount of school. You begin to counsel your patient about managing dysmenorrhea. Which of the following would not help your patient in managing her symptoms?

**A.** Avoid dietary omega-3 polyunsaturated fatty acids

**B.** Take ibuprofen 1 to 2 days before the onset of menses

**C.** Take combination oral contraceptive pills

**D.** Avoid smoking

**E.** Take mefenamic acid 1 to 2 days before the onset of menses

**3-30.** You receive a phone call from your colleague informing you that one of your patients has been admitted to the hospital. You learn that the patient is a 14-year-old girl with menorrhagia who requires hospitalization for excessive menstrual bleeding. Your patient is undergoing an evaluation to determine the etiology of the bleeding. What is the most common cause of excessive menstrual bleeding requiring hospitalization?

**A.** Polycystic ovarian syndrome

**B.** Spontaneous abortion

**C.** Hemangioma

**D.** Bleeding disorder

**E.** Cervical polyps

**3-31.** A 15-year-old girl presents to your clinic with concern that she may be pregnant. She explains that she had unprotected intercourse with her boyfriend 2 weeks ago. You perform a urine pregnancy test, which confirms that she is pregnant. Which of the following statements about teenage pregnancy is correct?

**A.** Only 50% of adolescents who maintain a pregnancy to term decide to parent the child themselves.

**B.** Confidentiality does not apply to adolescents who become pregnant.

**C.** A pelvic examination is not part of the evaluation of a possible pregnancy for an adolescent.

**D.** Urine β-human chorionic gonadotropin (β-hCG) testing at 1 week after implantation is unlikely to be positive.

**E.** Unusual vaginal bleeding is a sign of a possible pregnancy.

**3-32.** A 17-year-old girl presents to the emergency department (ED) with the chief complaint of severe lower abdominal pain. You begin interviewing the patient and learn that she has not had a period in 2 months. On physical examination, she has abdominal tenderness and adnexal tenderness. You send some labs; her β-human chorionic gonadotropin is positive, and you are concerned that your patient may have an ectopic pregnancy. Which of the following is *not* a risk factor for developing an ectopic pregnancy?

**A.** Urinary tract infection

**B.** Previous pelvic surgery

**C.** Early sexual debut

**D.** Multiple sexual partners

**E.** Cigarette smoking

**3-33.** A 16-year-old healthy girl presents for routine primary care. While talking alone with the patient, she discloses to you that she is sexually active with her boyfriend. She has been using condoms but wants to start taking oral contraceptive pills. You discuss her history and side effects of the medication and determine that she is a good candidate for this method. Her last menstrual period was 2 days ago. When should the patient begin taking the pill?

**A.** At the time of her next menses

**B.** After you have discussed the plan with the patient's parents

**C.** Immediately

**D.** After she has a negative pregnancy test

**E.** After she has a normal pelvic examination

**3-34.** A 15-year-old girl presents for follow-up after being treated for a deep venous thrombosis in her left calf. In reviewing her history, you learn that the patient is sexually active with her boyfriend and is taking oral contraceptive pills. What is an appropriate management step for you to take?

**A.** Discontinue her current oral contraceptive pills and start the patient on a lower-dose pill

**B.** Continue her current oral contraceptive pill and encourage condom use

**C.** Discontinue her current oral contraceptive pill and advise her to abstain from having sex

**D.** Do not change her medication regimen while the patient is sexually active

**E.** Discontinue her current oral contraceptive pill and place the etonogestrel 68-mg implantable rod

**3-35.** A 17-year-old girl presents to your clinic. She appears anxious as she explains to you that she had unprotected intercourse 3 days ago with her boyfriend. You perform a urine pregnancy test, which is negative. You explain the results to the patient, and she is relieved. Which of the following management steps would be most indicated at this time?

**A.** Progestin-only emergency contraception (EC)

**B.** Reassurance and counseling to the patient

**C.** Estrogen–progestin EC

**D.** Place a levonorgestrel intrauterine device

**E.** Providing condoms and asking the patient to follow up in 1 week

**3-36.** A 16-year-old girl presents for her annual physical examination. While discussing her social history, you learn that she is sexually active with her boyfriend. She is interested in starting contraception. You discuss the different options and together decide that depot medroxyprogesterone acetate (DMPA) would be an appropriate method for the patient. Before starting the method, you discuss the side effects. Which of the following is a side effect of DMPA?

**A.** Nausea

**B.** Breast tenderness

**C.** Weight loss

**D.** Amenorrhea

**E.** Increased bone mineral density

**3-37.** Which of the following common sexually transmitted infections (STIs) is a reportable bacterial infection in the United States?

**A.** *Chlamydia trachomatis*

**B.** Human papillomavirus (HPV)

**C.** *Candida albicans*

**D.** *Trichomonas vaginalis*

**E.** Bacterial vaginosis

**3-38.** A 17-year-old sexually active girl presents with 1 week of abnormal vaginal discharge. She describes the discharge as being thin in consistency and white in color. You sample the discharge and note a pH of 8 and an amine odor. No additional findings are seen on the wet prep. What is the best treatment for this patient?

**A.** Azithromycin 1 g orally for 1 dose

**B.** Ceftriaxone 250 mg intramuscularly for 1 dose and doxycycline 100 mg orally twice daily for 7 days

**C.** Metronidazole 500 mg orally twice daily for 7 days

**D.** Fluconazole 150 mg orally for 1 dose

**E.** Additional workup is necessary prior to determining treatment.

**3-39.** A sexually active 15-year-old boy presents with a 3-hour history of left-sided testicular pain. He reports no history of trauma. In addition, he is complaining of dysuria. On examination, the scrotum is painful and red. The patient does report pain relief when you elevate the testis. Which of the following diagnostic tests can help confirm your diagnosis?

**A.** A Doppler ultrasound

**B.** Nucleic acid amplification tests for *Chlamydia trachomatis*

**C.** A complete blood count (CBC)

**D.** Dark field microscopy

**E.** Radionuclide imaging

**3-40.** A 15-year-old boy presents to your clinic with the concern that he has acquired a sexually transmitted infection (STI). He reports painful sores on his penis. On examination, he has multiple grouped vesicles with an erythematous base on the shaft of his penis. He also has tender inguinal adenopathy. You suspect that he has genital herpes. Which of the following statements can you tell your patient about genital herpes?

**A.** Most genital herpes infections are symptomatic.

**B.** Herpes simplex virus type 1 (HSV-1) is now the most common cause of genital herpes in the United States.

**C.** Stress and sexual intercourse can precipitate recurrences.

**D.** Close to 90% of genital herpes infections occur in people younger than 19 years old.

**E.** Seroepidemiologic studies show that 75% of adults in the United States are seropositive for herpes simplex virus type 2 (HSV-2).

**3-41.** A 17-year-old girl presents to the emergency department (ED) with fever and lower abdominal pain. She is sexually active and occasionally uses condoms. On physical examination, you note a temperature of 38.4°C and lower abdominal and pelvic tenderness. She has mucopurulent vaginal discharge as well as cervical motion tenderness. You suspect pelvic inflammatory disease (PID). Which of the following is true regarding this patient?

**A.** Inpatient treatment with intravenous (IV) antibiotics is necessary.

**B.** Outpatient treatment with combination empiric broad-spectrum intramuscular and oral antibiotics is appropriate.

**C.** She should come in for follow-up 1 week after completion of antibiotic therapy.

**D.** She can have sex with her partner after she takes the first dose of antibiotic.

**E.** Her partner only needs to be treated if he is symptomatic.

**3-42.** You answer a call for your clinic and speak with a 16-year-old girl who is concerned about a vaginal infection. She explains her symptoms to you over the phone, and you suspect that she has vaginal candidiasis. You ask that she come to clinic to be examined prior to initiating any treatment. Which of the following is *not* consistent with vaginal candidiasis?

**A.** Pruritus

**B.** Vaginal pH > 5.0

**C.** Pseudohyphae in potassium hydroxide (KOH) preparation

**D.** White lesions on vaginal mucosa

**E.** Erythematous vaginal mucosa

**3-43.** A 15-year-old girl presents for her annual physical examination. The patient's mother would like to make sure she is screened for scoliosis. The patient denies any concerns including back pain. You complete a Home, Education/Employment, Eating, Activities, Drugs, Sex, Suicidality, Safety (HEEADSSS) psychosocial screening, which demonstrates that she is making a number of healthy choices and avoiding risky behaviors. On her physical examination, her vital signs are stable, and both her weight and height are at the 60th percentile for age. In order to screen her for scoliosis, what is your next step?

**A.** Order a magnetic resonance imaging (MRI) scan of the entire spine

**B.** Obtain standing posteroanterior and lateral x-ray views of the spine

**C.** Perform an Adams forward bend test during your examination

**D.** Given the patient has no back pain, she is unlikely to have scoliosis and does not require screening

**E.** None of the above

**3-44.** A 19-year-old man presents for an acute care visit for back pain. He states that he just got a new job and is doing a lot of lifting. Previously, he was in fairly good physical shape and has not previously had any back pain. On further history, which complaint would prompt you to obtain a radiograph?

**A.** He reports that his pain is the worst at the end of the work day.

**B.** He reports that his pain radiates to the lower extremities.

**C.** He reports that his pain improves with rest.

**D.** He reports that his pain is localized to his lower back.

**E.** Radiographs are not indicated for back pain.

**3-45.** A 14-year-old male athlete comes to your office 2 days after a championship soccer game. He explains that during the game, while running, he twisted his leg. He immediately felt pain in his left ankle. On examination, he has swelling and pain along the ligament. You suspect a grade I or II ankle sprain. Which of the following does *not* describe appropriate management for a grade I or II sprain?

**A.** Treat your patient with the rest, ice, compression, elevation (RICE) protocol.

**B.** During the initial 72 hours after the injury, begin range of motion exercises.

**C.** During the initial 72 hours after the injury, begin weight bearing.

**D.** Slowly return to activity as pain and swelling resolve.

**E.** Refer your patient to a musculoskeletal specialist for further evaluation.

**3-46.** A 17-year-old boy presents to your office because of concerns about his acne. He has never been treated previously but would like to start. On physical examination, he has mild comedonal acne centralized on his face, particularly his nose and forehead. He has no lesions on his chest or back. He has no cysts and no evidence of scarring. What is the first line of treatment for this patient?

**A.** Topical benzoyl peroxide

**B.** Oral minocycline

**C.** Oral isotretinoin

**D.** Topical adapalene

**E.** Referral to a dermatologist

**3-47.** A 17-year-old girl presents with moderate acne over her forehead and cheeks and with several lesions on her back with no evidence of scarring. For the past 6 months, she has been using topical tretinoin and benzoyl peroxide with minimal improvement. As a result, she is very interested in additional treatment. She is still quite embarrassed by her acne and really would like her skin to look better. Which is the next best step in management of her acne?

**A.** Instruct her to make changes to her diet, such as removing chocolate and pizza.

**B.** Recommend she continue her topical treatment, as she has not given it enough time to work.

**C.** Insist at this point that she should start oral isotretinoin as nothing else will help.

**D.** Discuss adding a combined estrogen–progesterone oral contraceptive pill to her current treatment regimen.

**E.** Referral to a dermatologist.

**3-48.** A 15-year-old boy presents to your office concerned about a rash. He said it started with a single, large, well-circumscribed lesion on his trunk (back), and about a week later, he has developed a number of oval salmon-colored flat patches. He says it has been itchy. On physical examination, you notice a number of lesions on his back that resemble the branches of a Christmas tree. He also has lesions in his axillae. He has no lesions on the palms of his hands. He has no past medical history of any skin conditions and is on no medications. Which of the following is the next best step to manage his rash?

- **A.** You prescribe a 5-day course of an oral corticosteroid.
- **B.** You prescribe topical clotrimazole.
- **C.** You prescribe oral doxycycline.
- **D.** You recommend oatmeal baths to help with the itching and reassure him that it should self-resolve.
- **E.** You administer an intramuscular injection of penicillin in the office.

**3-49.** A 14-year-old boy presents to clinic for his physical examination. You complete a Home, Education/Employment, Eating, Activities, Drugs, Sex, Suicidality, Safety (HEEADSSS) interview and find that he is making very healthy choices. On his physical examination, his vital signs are stable, and both his height and weight are at the 50th percentile. On your physical examination, you notice that he has a rash on his chest. He has noticed it but is unsure how long it has been there. The rash includes sharply demarcated and hypopigmented macules and papules with some scaling. He says that sometimes it might be a little itchy, and he thought it got worse this summer following his job as a lifeguard. What is your next step in diagnosing this rash?

- **A.** A potassium hydroxide (KOH) examination of scrapings from the lesions
- **B.** A bacterial culture of scrapings from the lesions
- **C.** A rapid plasma reagin (RPR)
- **D.** A scabies preparation of scrapings from the lesions
- **E.** A skin biopsy

**3-50.** A 17-year-old girl presents for an acute care visit. She is concerned that she has "lumps in her armpits." She is afebrile, her vital signs are stable, and she is overweight. On physical examination, you notice she has several large and tender cysts in both axillae. She reports that she has had these before, but they were milder and resolved on their own. You perform a culture, which is negative for growth. What is your next step in managing these lesions?

- **A.** Oral isotretinoin
- **B.** Oral diphenhydramine
- **C.** Topical clindamycin
- **D.** Immediate surgical excision
- **E.** Skin biopsy with potential surgical excision

**3-51.** You are caring for a 12-year-old girl who is brought to your office by her mother. The patient's parents are divorced, and she just spent the weekend at her father's house. Her mother is concerned because she noticed a white stain in her daughter's underwear. Examination shows sexual maturity rating (SMR) 3 breast and SMR 3 pubic hair. On genitourinary exam, there is white mucus at the vaginal opening. You obtain a wet prep of vaginal secretions, which shows lactobacilli, squamous epithelial cells, and a few polymorphonuclear leukocytes. Which of the following findings would also be present on the wet prep?

- **A.** Vaginal squamous epithelial cells coated with the anaerobic gram-variable coccobacilli
- **B.** Budding yeast
- **C.** Vaginal pH $< 4.5$
- **D.** Vaginal pH $> 4.5$
- **E.** Mobile pear-shaped flagellated organisms

**3-52.** A 16-year-old girl presents to the emergency department (ED). She was found unresponsive in the bathroom by her mother. Her mother tells you that the patient has a history of bulimia nervosa. On physical examination, you note a normal weight, lethargic young woman. There is vomitus on her clothing. Which of the following laboratory findings would you expect to find on further evaluation?

- **A.** Peaked T waves on electrocardiogram (ECG)
- **B.** U waves on ECG
- **C.** Serum potassium of 6.2 mmol/L
- **D.** Serum creatinine of 2.8 mg/dL
- **E.** Serum sodium of 138 mmol/L

**3-53.** A 13-year-old girl presents to your clinic. She is a new patient and has been struggling with irregular and heavy periods for the past 6 months. She endorses vaginal bleeding for the past 10 days. Her heart rate is 92 bpm, and blood pressure is 96/72 mm Hg. She does not have any orthostatic changes. Physical examination demonstrates pallor. Abdominal and pelvic exams are unremarkable. Initial laboratory findings show a hemoglobin of 10.1 g/dL and a negative urine pregnancy test. What is the next best step in management for this patient?

**A.** Hospitalize the patient for intravenous (IV) fluids and IV estrogen

**B.** Type and cross and transfuse 1 unit of packed red blood cells

**C.** Start iron therapy and perform iron studies in 2 months

**D.** Begin a monophasic estrogen–progestin oral contraceptive and administer at set intervals until the bleeding stops

**E.** Refer to a gynecology specialist

**3-54.** You are caring for a 15-year-old girl who is hospitalized for nutritional rehabilitation in the setting of anorexia nervosa. You initiate a caloric goal of 30 to 40 kcal/kg/d. In addition, you plan to monitor the patient closely for refeeding syndrome. Which of the following clinical measures is not typically present with refeeding syndrome?

**A.** Hypophosphatemia

**B.** Bradycardia on electrocardiogram (ECG)

**C.** Hypomagnesemia

**D.** Thiamine deficiency

**E.** U waves on ECG

**3-55.** A 17-year-old girl presents to your clinic with the chief complaint of irregular and less frequent periods over the past 18 months. Her last period was over 6 months ago. Menarche occurred at the age of 13. Previously, she had monthly periods lasting 5 days. Physical examination is unremarkable. She takes no medication. Lab studies include negative urine pregnancy test, normal prolactin, normal thyroid-stimulating hormone (TSH), normal follicle-stimulating hormone (FSH), and normal estradiol levels. Her body mass index (BMI) is in the 33rd percentile (22.4 kg/m$^2$). What would be the next best step in evaluating the patient's irregular and less frequent bleeding?

**A.** Order a pelvic ultrasound

**B.** Refer to gynecology

**C.** Encourage diet and exercise to promote weight loss

**D.** Prescribe a 10-day course of medroxyprogesterone acetate 10 mg once daily

**E.** Order a brain magnetic resonance imaging (MRI)

**3-56.** A 20-year-old man is presenting to your clinic for a wellness appointment. He is a new patient to your clinic. The patient discloses to you that he identifies as bisexual and has had sex with 3 partners in the past year. He is interested in the human papillomavirus (HPV) vaccination. Which of the following statements regarding the HPV vaccine is true?

**A.** HPV vaccine is only effective when given to girls aged 9 to 26 years.

**B.** HPV vaccine increases risk of developing autism.

**C.** HPV vaccine is most effective when given as a 3-dose series.

**D.** HPV vaccine is only effective in preventing genital warts.

**E.** HPV vaccine is recommended as a 2-dose series.

**3-57.** A 14-year-old African American boy presents for a well-adolescent visit. Physical exam and laboratory values are significant for moderate pustular acne on the face and back; genital exam is sexual maturity rating (SMR) 4; alkaline phosphatase is 221 IU/L, alanine aminotransferase (ALT) is 20 IU/L, aspartate aminotransferase (AST) is 18 IU/L, hemoglobin is 14.6 g/dL, and hematocrit is 41.2%. Which of the following is the most appropriate next step for this boy?

**A.** Evaluate for hemochromatosis

**B.** Evaluate for bone tumor

**C.** Reassure the patient and family that he is developing normally

**D.** Evaluate for liver disease

**E.** Prescribe isotretinoin oral therapy for acne

**3-58.** The period of middle adolescent psychological development includes all but which of the following characteristics?

**A.** Concrete thought processes

**B.** Experimentation with social role

**C.** Experimentation with substances (eg, tobacco, alcohol, marijuana)

**D.** Experimentation with sexual experiences

**E.** Impulsive behaviors and "it won't happen to me"

**3-59.** The period of late adolescence includes all but which of the following characteristics?

**A.** Completion of physical maturation

**B.** Relationships with parents become more important

**C.** Personal identity begins to be defined

**D.** Capable of understanding a full range of options for health issues

**E.** Sense of idealism

**3-60.** A 19-year-old female patient with moderate congenital heart disease tells her pediatrician she is engaged to be married and would like to transition her health care to an adult provider. She has limited knowledge of the extent of her heart disease. Her mother has always taken care of medication management, including organizing the pillbox each week. Which of the following is the best option for a successful healthcare transition?

**A.** Ask the patient if her family is going to be able to continue to assist with her healthcare needs.

**B.** Counsel the patient to find an adult provider who is knowledgeable about her condition.

**C.** Develop a transition roadmap and provide the patient with a list of questions to prepare for transition.

**D.** Encourage her to postpone her wedding until she has transitioned to a new healthcare team.

**E.** Discuss the importance of behaving like an adult in all aspects of her life.

**3-61.** Although the mortality rate for adolescents and young adults has decreased over the past decades, this time of life remains high risk. Which of the following scenarios presents the highest risk for death?

**A.** A 13-year-old Hispanic boy wearing a helmet while mountain biking with friends

**B.** A 17-year-old American Indian girl who is the designated driver at a Saturday night party

**C.** A 19-year-old black man who struggles with depression, who lives at home, and whose father is a police officer

**D.** A 21-year-old black woman who is pregnant

**E.** A 24-year-old white woman who works a swing shift at a local convenience store

**3-62.** A 15-year-old boy presents for a well-adolescent exam. He completed the Home, Education/Employment, Eating, Activities, Drugs, Sex, Suicidality, Safety (HEEADSSS) assessment, and there were no red flags. Physical exam was unremarkable, and sexual maturity rating (SMR) is 4. Just as you are about to walk out of the room, the boy states he had sex with a friend. You sit down and thank him for being honest with you and ask him about his concerns. He tells you that he had oral and anal sex about 2 days ago. Which of the following is the most appropriate next step?

**A.** Swab anus and obtain a urine specimen to test for gonorrhea and chlamydia

**B.** Counsel him to stop having sex and remain abstinent until marriage

**C.** Obtain a urine specimen to test for gonorrhea and chlamydia

**D.** Empirically treat for gonorrhea and chlamydia

**E.** Tell him his partner needs to be tested and treated for gonorrhea and chlamydia

**3-63.** A 16-year-old girl with a body mass index (BMI) of 36.4 presents complaining of heavy periods. Her last menstrual period was 38 days ago. Menarche was at age 14. She states that she gags when she tries to swallow a pill and often forgets to take medication when prescribed. She gets straight As and plans to graduate from high school 1 year early to start college and pursue a career in medicine. She has never been sexually active but is getting very serious with her boyfriend. On physical exam, she has obesity, and breasts and external genital exam are sexual maturity rating (SMR) 5. She became extremely anxious prior to and during genital examination. Which of the following is the most appropriate for her?

**A.** Combined oral contraceptive pills; dissolve under tongue each day

**B.** Transdermal combined contraceptive patch (6 mg norelgestromin/75 mg ethinyl estradiol)

**C.** Depot medroxyprogesterone acetate (DMPA) 150 mg intramuscular injection every 3 months

**D.** Etonogestrel 68-mg implantable rod

**E.** Copper intrauterine device

**3-64.** A 16-year-old gay young man comes for a well-adolescent visit. On Home, Education/Employment, Eating, Activities, Drugs, Sex, Suicidality, Safety (HEEADSSS) assessment, he reports that he enjoys using several different dating apps on his smart phone. Upon further questioning, he tells you that he "hooks up" with a new partner at least once a day. He denies sore throat, dysuria, and hematochezia. He states that sex is fun for him and he enjoys "giving and receiving." He often has partners who he is certain are older than 21 years. On physical exam, you note a faint rash on his palms and soles; otherwise, exam is normal, and sexual maturity rating (SMR) is 4. What is the most appropriate next step?

**A.** Order serum rapid plasma reagin (RPR)

**B.** Recommend treatment with topical terbinafine twice daily for 14 days

**C.** Perform swab of oropharynx for rapid strep test

**D.** Obtain urine for urine culture

**E.** Administer ceftriaxone 250 mg intramuscular 1 time

**3-65.** A 10-year-old girl presents for a well-child check and to establish care. She and her parents tell you that since the age of 3 she has identified as a boy. As a young child, she threw tantrums when wearing a dress. She has always engaged in stereotypical boy activities (eg, playing with cars and trains, sports). More recently, she has become anxious and withdrawn. On physical exam, she has breast development stage of sexual maturity rating (SMR) 3. Her parents are very concerned and want to know what the options are. How should you proceed?

**A.** Begin fluoxetine 10 mg by mouth once daily
**B.** Refer to a mental health provider
**C.** Reassure that she is experiencing normal puberty
**D.** Begin treatment with testosterone cypionate 25 mg intramuscular every 2 weeks
**E.** Measure serum estradiol concentration

## ANSWERS

### Answer 3-1. D

In the 1960s, in order to prevent foregone treatment of adolescent STIs, all state legislatures enacted statutes allowing minors to receive treatment for STIs without parental involvement. These laws vary in specifics state to state and are not mandated by federal law. You should be able to see an adolescent and discuss their concerns confidentially without parental involvement, and thus do not need to call the parent to discuss these issues. Billing for these services, however, may not be confidential depending on the insurance carrier and state regulations.

(Pages 16–17, Section 1: Foundations in Pediatric Practice and Child Health, Part 1, Chapter 5: Law, Ethics, and Clinical Judgment)

### Answer 3-2. B

The musculoskeletal system is affected significantly by the biological changes of puberty. The growth spurt typically occurs at SMR 2 to 3 for girls and SMR 4 for boys. SCFE typically occurs during the period of maximal skeletal growth, such as occurs concurrently with puberty at SMR 3. SMR 1 is prepubescent (prior to growth spurt or developmental changes), and SMR 5 is complete adult development (postpubertal).

(Pages 307–308, Section 5: Principles of Adolescent Care, Part 1, Chapter 65: Somatic Growth and Development in Adolescence)

### Answer 3-3. E

Estrogen is the most influential hormone affecting glandular breast development during puberty. It binds to the breast tissue resulting in stimulation of the glandular ductal system, whereas progesterone is linked to alveolar growth. Other hormones, such as insulin, prolactin, thyroxine, and cortisol, do play an important role in breast development, particularly in their interactions with estrogen. Luteinizing hormone and follicle-stimulating hormone are released by the ovaries and stimulate ovarian growth, not breast development.

(Page 309, Section 5: Principles of Adolescent Care, Part 1, Chapter 66: Reproductive Growth and Development in the Female Adolescent)

### Answer 3-4. C

"Spermarche," or the onset of spermatogenesis, occurs relatively early in puberty. It typically corresponds with a time of rapid increase in testicular weight, as well as in seminiferous tubular diameter, length, and relative volume. Testosterone initiates and maintains the process of spermatogenesis in humans.

(Pages 311–312, Section 5: Principles of Adolescent Care, Part 1, Chapter 67: Reproductive Growth and Development in the Male Adolescent)

### Answer 3-5. B

In middle adolescence, teenagers are now able to understand complex concepts and have begun to question the thinking and behavior of adults. They begin to think in more abstract terms, which allows for shifts from same-sex relationships/friendships to romantic dating. Risky health behaviors are of critical importance in middle adolescence, as peer norms include engaging in risky behaviors as individuals make more independent choices.

Early adolescents typically focus on their developing bodies and on their peer group, and their concerns are often around acceptance and conformity.

During late adolescence, individuals are less egocentric and self-centered, are better at understanding others' points of view, and have greater ability to self-reflect and be insightful. Identity exploration/life roles begin to be defined. At this point, physical maturation is complete, and body image and gender role definition clearer. A description of the different stages of adolescence is listed in Table 68-1.

(Pages 313–315, Section 5: Principles of Adolescent Care, Part 1, Chapter 68: Psychological Development)

### Answer 3-6. A

The HEEADSSS (Home, Education/Employment, Eating, Activities, Drugs, Sex, Suicidality, Safety) assessment tool is based on the biopsychosocial model of adolescent development (Table 69-1). HEEADSSS is a screening tool, not a diagnostic tool. It allows clinicians to assess a variety of domains; however, a positive HEEADSSS assessment is not diagnostic. More

**TABLE 68-1.** Normal Development of the Stages of Adolescence and their Associated Impact on the Adolescent and on Delivery of Health Services

| Characteristics | Impact on Adolescents | Impact on Health Service Delivery |
|---|---|---|
| **Early Adolescence (Ages 10–13 Years)** | | |
| Onset of puberty; becomes concerned with developing body | Major questions concerning normality of physical maturation; often concerned about the stages of sexual development and how the process relates to peers of same gender; occasional masturbation | Important to normalize differences and explain range of normal development |
| Begins to expand social relationships beyond family | Adolescents concentrate on relationships with peers; begin to become more interdependent with parents | Encourage teens to begin to take responsibility for their own health and contact with health professionals, in consultation with parents (eg, part of visit time alone with health provider) |
| Beginning of transition from concrete to abstract thinking; new attractions and desires; socioemotional competencies of self-regulation still developing | Risky attitudes and health behaviors may emerge; opportunity for excitement and motivation | Shift in health provider's focus from anticipatory guidance to parents to risk reduction and prevention education to adolescent; still address most health situations with adolescents in a concrete manner with simple language |
| **Middle Adolescence (Ages 14–16 Years)** | | |
| Pubertal development usually complete, and sexual drives emerge | Explores ability to attract others; sexual experimentation (same and opposite sex) begins; masturbation increases | Provide sexual health screening; establish clinician's office as safe place to ask questions and discuss sexuality |
| Peer group sets behavioral standards, although family values usually persist | Peer group influences engagement in positive and negative health behaviors; peers rather than parents may also offer key support | Important to emphasize role of teen in making good choices and taking responsibility; focus on navigating social relationships and peer pressure |
| Conflicts over independence | Increased assumption of independent action, together with continued need for parental support and guidance; able to discuss and negotiate changes in rules | Increased involvement of teen in setting health-related goals and being clear on how to handle health situations (eg, time to take medication); reinforce adolescents' growing competencies |
| Emergence of abstract thinking with new cognitive competencies | Increased ability to process information, see other perspectives, and reflect; often leads to questioning adult behavior; while adolescent may consider broader range of possibilities/options, may not yet be able to integrate into real life | Important to be clear that individual understands and knows what he or she needs to do regarding health concerns |
| **Late Adolescence/Emerging Adulthood (Ages 17–21 Years)** | | |
| Physical maturation complete; body image and gender role definition clearer | Begins to feel comfortable with relationships and decisions regarding sexuality and preference; individual relationships become more important than peer group | Affirm decisions regarding sexuality and gender |
| Individuals less egocentric and self-centered; better at understanding others' points of view; greater ability to self-reflect and be insightful | More open to questioning regarding their behavior; interdependence with shared power and responsibility and greater reciprocity | Adolescent more able to work with clinician on setting goals and changing behavior; clinicians can help adolescents make better health decisions by involving them in their own health management |
| Idealistic | Idealism may lead to conflict with family or authority figures | May have own/alternative ideas of how to take responsibility for their health; clinicians can help adolescents see that they have a range of options |

*(Continued)*

**TABLE 68-1.** Normal Development of the Stages of Adolescence and their Associated Impact on the Adolescent and on Delivery of Health Services (*Continued*)

| Characteristics | Impact on Adolescents | Impact on Health Service Delivery |
|---|---|---|
| Identity exploration/life roles begin to be defined | People most likely to be exploring options in their lives | Often interested in discussion of life goals; health status (eg, chronic illness) may influence life goals |
| Cognitive development nearing completion | Most are capable of understanding a full range of options for health issues | Important to help adolescents/emerging adults become competent in negotiating the health care system; encourage parents, when appropriate, to decrease their monitoring of clinical management issues, yet remain engaged and available to their son or daughter |

Mark W. Kline, *Rudolph's Pediatrics*, 23rd Edition. Copyright © McGraw-Hill Education. All rights reserved.

**TABLE 69-1.** Heeadsss Assessment for Psychosocial Concerns: Screening History

| Assessment Area | Questions |
|---|---|
| Home | How is the adolescent's home life? How are his/her relationships with family members? Where and with whom does the patient live? Is his/her living situation stable? |
| Education (or employment) | How is the adolescent's school performance? How is she/he doing in school? If adolescent is working, is he/ she working full time or part time and what are his/her plans for the future? |
| Eating (incorporates body image) | Does the patient have a balanced diet? Is the adolescent trying to lose weight, and if so, is it in a healthy manner? How does the patient feel about his/her body? Has there been significant weight gain or loss recently? |
| Activities | How does the patient spend her/his time? Is he/she engaged in sports or other extracurricular activities? Is he/ she engaging in dangerous or risky behaviors? Is the adolescent supervised during free time? With whom does the adolescent spend most of his/her time? Does he/she have a supportive peer group? |
| Drugs (including alcohol and tobacco) | Does the patient drink caffeinated beverages (including energy drinks)? Does the patient smoke or use electronic nicotine devices? Does the patient drink alcohol? If so, explore amount including frequency and context. Has the patient used other substances, including marijuana, over-the-counter drugs, or opioids? If there is any substance use, to what degree, and for how long? Consider using a screening tool (eg, CRAFFT) if the patient endorses substance use to establish the severity. |
| Sexuality | What is the patient's current gender identity? Is the patient attracted to males, females, or both? What is the patient's sexual orientation (heterosexual, homosexual, bisexual, or other)? Has the patient ever been sexually active and if so, with males, females, or both? Has the patient ever been tested for sexually transmitted infections? Is the patient using any contraception? Has the patient ever been pregnant or gotten someone pregnant? Has the patient ever been forced into having sex? Does the patient's family know about the patient's gender identity and sexual behavior? |
| Suicidality (including general mood assessment) | What is the patient's mood from day to day? Has he/she thought about or attempted suicide? Consider using the Patient Health Questionnaire-2 (PHQ-2) as a screening tool and advance to the Patient Health Questionnaire-9 (PHQ-9) for further assessment. |
| Safety | Does the patient feel safe at home, school, in the neighborhood? Has the patient been bullied or felt he/she had to carry a weapon to protect himself/herself? Has the patient been in physical fights in school or the neighborhood? Does the patient wear a seatbelt in the car and safety equipment for sports/physical activities? Has the patient ever ridden with a driver that was drunk or high? Does the patient send text messages while driving? |

Mark W. Kline, *Rudolph's Pediatrics*, 23rd Edition. Copyright © McGraw-Hill Education. All rights reserved.

specific questions and investigation are necessary for a specific diagnosis.

Certain topic areas are confidential, and confidentiality and its limits should be explained to both parent and adolescent at the start of the visit. The HEEADSSS is part of the history but does not take the place of a physical examination. There is no evidence to support that asking an adolescent about suicidal thoughts will lead to suicidality.

(Pages 315–316, Section 5: Principles of Adolescent Care, Part 1, Chapter 69: The Adolescent and Young Adult Visit)

**Answer 3-7.** A

The adolescent visit is an important time to make certain that teens have received all their necessary vaccines. Clinicians should be familiar with the Centers for Disease Control and Prevention (CDC) Advisory Committee for Immunization Practices (ACIP) and check for recent updates to vaccine recommendations. More recent vaccines are adolescent- and young adult–specific and include vaccines for meningococcal disease, varicella, hepatitis A, human papillomavirus (HPV), and influenza. For an adolescent female, it is important to determine possibility of pregnancy prior to giving vaccines because some are contraindicated. In general, adolescents do not need an MMR if they have received 2 MMR immunizations earlier during childhood.

(Page 318, Section 5: Principles of Adolescent Care, Part 1, Chapter 69: The Adolescent and Young Adult Visit)

**Answer 3-8.** E

Unintentional injuries account for about 70.6% of adolescent deaths. The majority of these are motor vehicle accidents. Other etiologies of unintentional injuries include drowning, fires, burns, falls, and poisoning. Alcohol is a cofactor in injuries associated with boating, swimming, bicycles, and skateboards. Additionally, male adolescents and young adults have a higher unintentional injury rate than females, and this disparity increases with age. Homicide is the second leading cause of death in adolescents and young adults, and suicide is third. Malignant neoplasms lead to almost 6% of adolescent mortality.

(Page 324, Section 5: Principles of Adolescent Care, Part 2, Chapter 71: Mortality)

**Answer 3-9.** C

The percentage of adolescents who are overweight and obese has more than tripled over the past 25 years. With this major increase, associated health consequences of obesity such as diabetes, hypertension, and high cholesterol have begun occurring at much younger ages and at much higher rates. It is important that teens understand the associated health consequences as this knowledge may help to motivate some behavior change. Overweight adolescents have a 70% chance of becoming overweight or obese adults. Young people with obesity may be targeted by bullying due to their weight, and advising him about dating may be damaging to an already potentially low self-esteem. Using stimulant medications is not an appropriate management option for obesity.

(Page 325, Section 5: Principles of Adolescent Care, Part 2, Chapter 72: Morbidity)

**Answer 3-10.** D

Over the past 15 years, fewer adolescents have initiated sexual intercourse and more adolescents are using effective contraception when they initiate sexual activity. Approximately 75% of adolescents report using some form of contraception at first intercourse. Given rates of younger (middle-school) adolescents' sexual activity are low, with a major increase at the start of high school (ninth grade), this may be an important time to counsel teens about available contraceptive methods so that they are prepared at the time of onset of sexual behavior.

(Page 326, Section 5: Principles of Adolescent Care, Part 2, Chapter 73: Sexual Behavior)

**Answer 3-11.** C

The patient in the vignette has moderate-to-severe alcohol intoxication. Laboratory findings that you may find include an elevated osmolar gap, hypoglycemia, hypokalemia, and metabolic (lactic) acidosis. You would not expect to see hyponatremia with alcohol intoxication.

(Pages 327–328, Section 5: Principles of Adolescent Care, Part 2, Chapter 74: Substance Use and Abuse)

**Answer 3-12.** E

The patient in the vignette has intoxication effects from cannabis/marijuana. Patients typically experience euphoria, tachycardia, postural hypotension, anxiety, psychosis, time-space distortion, impaired balance and coordination, confusion, panic, and increased appetite. Eye findings include dilated pupils and injected conjunctiva.

Although patients with panic disorder and schizophrenia may become more socially isolated, you would not expect to see dilated pupils, injected conjunctiva, or impaired balance and coordination with these diseases. Patients with opiate intoxication typically have constricted pupils, not dilated. Although patients with ethanol/alcohol intoxication may present with impaired coordination, you would not expect patients to be anxious or have dilated pupils. Instead, patients with ethanol intoxication present with altered cognition, disinhibition, and euphoria. Typical eye findings with severe ethanol intoxication include nystagmus, but normal pupil size.

(Pages 327–328, Section 5: Principles of Adolescent Care, Part 2, Chapter 74: Substance Use and Abuse)

**Answer 3-13.** B

The AAP opposes involuntary testing of adolescents for drugs of abuse. "Testing adolescents requires their consent, unless (1) a patient lacks decision-making capacity; or (2) there are strong medical indications or legal requirements to do so" (AAP, 1996). Laboratory testing for drugs under any circumstances is improper unless the patient and clinician can be assured that the test procedure is valid and reliable and that patient confidentiality is ensured.

(Pages 327–328, Section 5: Principles of Adolescent Care, Part 2, Chapter 74: Substance Use and Abuse)

**Reference**

American Academy of Pediatrics, Committee on Substance Abuse. Testing for drugs of abuse in children and adolescents. *Pediatrics*. 1996;98:305–307 [the statement was reaffirmed by the AAP in 2006].

### Answer 3-14. D

Based on the history given here, the patient most likely suffers from symptoms of depression and may have major depressive disorder. In an adolescent suffering from major depressive disorder, it is critical to assess potential risk for suicide, including obtaining a history about suicidal ideation, a potential suicide plan (if they have thought about any mechanism by which they would commit suicide), history of suicide in family or friends, and prior suicide attempts. This approach will assist in determining level of acuity and if the patient is safe to go home or potentially requires an acute psychiatric hospitalization. If it has been determined that the patient is safe to go home, discussing options for treatment including medications and therapy (in particular cognitive-behavioral therapy) is appropriate. Close monitoring and follow-up are important with children and adolescents with depression in order to ensure they are receiving appropriate treatment and tolerating medications if prescribed.

(Pages 331–332, Section 5: Principles of Adolescent Care, Part 3, Chapter 75: Depression, Anxiety, and Other Disorders in Adolescence)

### Answer 3-15. D

This patient most likely had a panic disorder. Panic disorder presents with episodes of increasing anxiety typically lasting for about 10 minutes. Patients typically feel a sense of doom and often believe they are about to die. Patients often present to the ED due to these symptoms. Panic disorder is best treated with cognitive-behavioral therapy to educate patients about how to respond to possible triggers and strategies for self-soothing. Medications also have a role in treatment of panic disorder both as prophylaxes against panic episodes (selective serotonin reuptake inhibitors) and to immediately relieve a panic episode (benzodiazepines). Benzodiazepines should be closely monitored due to their potential for dependency and abuse; therefore, they should not be prescribed for regular use in an ED that cannot provide regular follow-up care.

(Page 333, Section 5: Principles of Adolescent Care, Part 3, Chapter 75: Depression, Anxiety, and Other Disorders in Adolescence)

### Answer 3-16. A

Bipolar disorders can begin at any age, but most often between the ages of 15 and 19 years. This teen's sensation-seeking behavior (shoplifting), rapid speech, and prolonged period of excitation (staying up all night) are all potential symptoms of a manic episode. Other symptoms include grandiosity, euphoria, and racing thoughts. Depressive symptoms in adolescents with bipolar disorder include hypersomnia, psychosis, and very low energy. Adolescents with bipolar disorder are more likely than adults to present with rapid cycling (moods shifting rapidly between depression and mania), sometimes presenting with symptoms of both in the same day. Diagnosis of bipolar disorder is based on careful history and mental status examination. The goal of treatment is mood stabilization and typically includes medication, such as lithium. Alcohol is a central nervous system depressant, and abuse would typically not present with the symptoms of rapid speech and grandiosity the mother describes. PTSD typically presents with patients being hypervigilant, easily startled, depersonalization, and derealization. Barbiturate use is unlikely in this case, as it is associated with sedation, pinpoint pupils, bradycardia, hypothermia, as well as central nervous system and respiratory depression.

(Page 332, Section 5: Principles of Adolescent Care, Part 3, Chapter 75: Depression, Anxiety, and Other Disorders in Adolescence)

### Answer 3-17. C

The patient has had a significant stressor and may be experiencing post-traumatic stress disorder (PTSD). PTSD occurs after experiencing or witnessing a terrifying physical or emotional event in which life is lost, injured, or threatened (as in this case). The symptoms of PTSD include frequent and persistent thoughts, memories, nightmares, and flashbacks. People with PTSD are hypervigilant and easily aroused. PTSD is twice as common among women compared with men. Combat is reported to be the most common source of PTSD among men, versus sexual assault for women.

The diagnosis of PTSD is established by a thorough and careful assessment by a skilled clinical professional, as the interview itself may be traumatic. Therapy, particularly cognitive-behavioral therapy and other therapeutic modalities such as exposure therapy, is effective. Certain medications (eg, selective serotonin reuptake inhibitors) may have a role with associated symptoms such as anxiety and depression, and other medications may help reduce the hyperarousal symptoms. A sleeping medication, such as zolpidem, has little role on its own in the treatment of PTSD.

(Page 335, Section 5: Principles of Adolescent Care, Part 3, Chapter 75: Depression, Anxiety, and Other Disorders in Adolescence)

### Answer 3-18. A

You are concerned that this patient has anorexia nervosa, given her severe weight loss, amenorrhea, and her mother's concerns.

The majority of patients with anorexia nervosa may express denial of the seriousness of being at such a low weight or the degree of weight loss. The first step in your management is to determine if the patient is medically stable, so obtaining vital signs is the next step. In the setting of severe weight loss, you may see bradycardia, orthostatic changes by pulse or blood pressure, hypotension, and hypothermia. Depending on the severity of vital sign changes, the patient may require hospitalization. Assuming the patient is medically stable, you may then consider ordering lab tests, including a CBC, serum electrolyte levels, a pregnancy test, thyroid hormones, liver function tests, and an electrocardiogram. Reassuring the patient's mother and calling the coach are not appropriate steps at this time given your concerns.

(Pages 337–340, Section 5: Principles of Adolescent Care, Part 3, Chapter 76: Disordered Eating)

**Answer 3-19.** B

The patient is expressing body dissatisfaction by her desire for thinness and dieting behaviors, despite having a weight and BMI in the healthy range. Given this, it is important to evaluate for signs or symptoms of disordered eating/eating disorder. Russell's sign is callusing on the back of the hand due to abrasions from self-induced vomiting. Other symptoms and findings that may be seen with disordered eating include hypothermia (not hyperthermia), bradycardia, hypotension, fatigue, growth stunting, delayed puberty, irregular periods (oligomenorrhea and amenorrhea), lanugo and hair loss, brittle nails and hair, tooth decay and gingivitis, and salivary gland enlargement. Acanthosis nigricans is seen in patients with insulin resistance. Dilated pupils may be seen with certain substance use such as marijuana but are not classically seen in eating disorders. A Kayser-Fleischer ring is a brown-green ring at the edge of the cornea. Kayser-Fleischer rings are associated with disorders of copper accumulation, such as Wilson disease.

(Pages 337–340, Section 5: Principles of Adolescent Care, Part 3, Chapter 76: Disordered Eating)

**Answer 3-20.** D

Family-based treatment/family therapy has the strongest evidence base as a psychotherapeutic modality in the treatment of adolescents with anorexia nervosa. Malnutrition alone can worsen anxiety and depression symptoms, so restoring nutrition is critically important. A nutritionist may assist with this, and it may be important to have a nutritionist as a part of an interdisciplinary treatment team; however, there is no evidence that a nutritionist alone can provide the necessary support needed for an optimal outcome. Antidepressant medications, particularly selective serotonin reuptake inhibitors, may be beneficial in treating coexisting symptoms of depression or anxiety, but have little evidence in treating the anorexia nervosa itself and thus are not first-line management without a patient also being in therapy.

(Page 340, Section 5: Principles of Adolescent Care, Part 3, Chapter 76: Disordered Eating)

**Answer 3-21.** A

The patient described in the vignette has fibrocystic breast change (benign proliferative breast change), which is a physiologic response of breast tissue to cyclic hormonal activity. The pain begins in the premenstrual phase of the menstrual cycle and subsides thereafter. Supportive care, including nonsteroidal anti-inflammatory agents for pain and a well-fitting supportive bra, is the primary treatment modality. In addition, oral contraceptives reduce symptoms in 70% to 90% of cases.

The pain from fibrocystic breast changes begins in the premenstrual phase, not the ovulatory phase of the menstrual cycle. A positive family history of *BRCA1* and *BRCA2* genes is associated with the development of breast cancer, not fibrocystic breast change. Fevers would aid in the diagnosis of infection. However, fibrocystic breast changes are not associated with fevers. Obtaining a history of a recent car accident would aid in the diagnosis of fat necrosis.

(Pages 341–342, Section 5: Principles of Adolescent Care, Part 4, Chapter 77: Breast Masses)

**Answer 3-22.** D

Pubertal gynecomastia does spontaneously resolve in 90% of boys within 3 years. This is usually not a permanent condition. Pubertal gynecomastia is a common condition, seen in 40% to 60% of 10- to 16 year olds. It peaks in incidence at SMR 2 to SMR 4 (age 14 years), not SMR 5. The medications listed in answer choice E are generally not recommended because of their side effect profiles, lack of documented efficacy, and frequent return of breast tissue after the drug is discontinued.

(Page 342, Section 5: Principles of Adolescent Care, Part 4, Chapter 77: Breast Masses)

**Answer 3-23.** D

The patient in the vignette has testicular torsion. Common presentation includes abrupt onset of severe scrotal pain, with associated nausea, vomiting, fever, and abdominal pain. On examination, if the adolescent presents early, the testicle may have a horizontal lie with minimal swelling. Typically, the adolescent presents later, and the scrotum is swollen, tender, erythematous, and difficult to examine. The cremasteric reflex is usually absent. Testicular torsion is a surgical emergency and is a clinical diagnosis. Time is of the essence with treatment because testicular viability declines to zero after 24 hours. An ultrasound with Doppler should not hinder a surgical evaluation. Treatment involves prompt surgical exploration and detorsion. Given the high incidence of retorsion, as well as torsion of the contralateral testis, once detorsed, the affected testis and the contralateral testis are fixed to the scrotum in a procedure called scrotal orchiopexy.

Empiric antibiotics are not necessary for this patient because he does not have epididymitis. Patients with epididymitis often present with scrotal pain and swelling but not with an absent cremasteric reflex as described in this patient. Supportive treatment including analgesics, anti-inflammatory agents, and scrotal elevation is the appropriate management for torsion of testicular or epididymal appendage but not for torsion of the testis. Diagnosis of testicular torsion can be made by physical examination alone. A Doppler ultrasound can assist in the diagnosis but should not delay treatment and is not necessary if there is a high index of suspicion.

(Page 343, Section 5: Principles of Adolescent Care, Part 4, Chapter 78: Scrotal Masses)

**Answer 3-24.** E

The patient in this vignette has orchitis. The mumps virus is the most common cause of orchitis. Mumps orchitis usually follows parotitis by about 4 to 8 days, but presentation up to 6 weeks later has been reported. The typical presentation includes edema, erythema, and tenderness of testicles. In addition, you may see constitutional symptoms (eg, fever, nausea, and lower abdominal pain). Other viruses (coxsackievirus, echovirus, adenovirus, varicella) or bacteria may cause orchitis but not as commonly as mumps. Bacterial orchitis is usually associated with an epididymal infection.

(Pages 344–345, Section 5: Principles of Adolescent Care, Part 4, Chapter 78: Scrotal Masses)

**Answer 3-25.** A

The patient in the vignette has a testicular tumor, the most common solid tumor seen in males aged 15 to 34 years. Patients present with painless scrotal swelling of gradual onset. On physical examination, you see a firm irregular mass that is opaque to transillumination. Gynecomastia can be present because stromal tumors tend to produce androgens and/or estrogen, which can cause feminization in a pubertal male. Cryptorchidism is the absence of 1 or both testes from the scrotum. About 1 in 500 males born with 1 or both testes undescended develop testicular cancer, roughly a 4- to 40-fold increased risk.

An uncircumcised penis does not increase a patient's risk for cancer. Anabolic steroids can cause gynecomastia in males but do not increase their risk for testicular cancer. Obesity increases the risk of developing many medical conditions, including but not limited to hypertension, diabetes, and hyperlipidemia. It does not, however, increase the risk of developing testicular cancer. Unprotected intercourse puts patients at risk of developing sexually transmitted infections (STIs). Human papillomavirus (HPV), a STI, is associated with cancer of the anus and penis, but not with testicular cancer.

(Page 345, Section 5: Principles of Adolescent Care, Part 4, Chapter 78: Scrotal Masses)

**Answer 3-26.** D

Spermatocele refers to the accumulation of sperm within the head of the epididymis. Spermatoceles are benign cysts that do not require intervention unless symptomatic. On palpation, they are predominantly smooth, soft, well circumscribed, and found on the superior aspect of the testicle.

Epididymitis is an inflammatory disease of the epididymis. A communicating hydrocele is an abnormality that develops when fluid tracks down the inguinal canal into the tunica vaginalis. A varicocele is a dilation of the pampiniform venous plexus within the scrotum, not within the epididymis.

(Pages 343–345, Section 5: Principles of Adolescent Care, Part 4, Chapter 78: Scrotal Masses)

**Answer 3-27.** B

Pregnancy is the most common cause of secondary amenorrhea. Therefore, the most important test to order next is the urine human chorionic gonadotropin test to check for pregnancy. Patients with amenorrhea secondary to nutritional deficiencies, such as anorexia nervosa, can develop osteopenia and osteoporosis and be at an increased fracture risk. Obtaining DEXA scans in these patients can be useful to evaluate their bone density. FSH and LH levels are useful in evaluating amenorrhea. Low levels of these hormones indicate inadequate hypothalamic–pituitary stimulation, as occurs with hypogonadotropic hypogonadism. High levels of these hormones can result from ovarian failure (hypergonadotropic hypogonadism). Normal levels of FSH and LH (eugonadotropic eugonadism) are seen with conditions that cause an increase in circulating androgens (polycystic ovarian syndrome, virilizing ovarian tumors, and adrenal tumors), as well as with some medications. Although these hormone levels are useful in diagnosing the etiology of amenorrhea, a pregnancy test is still the next best test to order. A karyotype is also a useful test in the workup of amenorrhea and can help diagnose Turner syndrome (45,XO) or androgen insensitivity (46,XY), but is not more important than a pregnancy test in the workup of amenorrhea. Certain medications and illicit drugs, such as phenothiazine derivatives, methadone, and heroin, can result in amenorrhea by producing dysregulation at the hypothalamus and pituitary (hypogonadotropic hypogonadism). If any of these drugs are suspected, a drug screen can be useful.

(Pages 345–349, Section 5: Principles of Adolescent Care, Part 4, Chapter 79: Menstrual Problems)

**Answer 3-28.** C

Hypogonadotropic hypogonadism indicates inadequate hypothalamic–pituitary stimulation of the ovary and is characterized by low levels of FSH, LH, and estrogen. Hypothalamic amenorrhea results from partial or complete inhibition of GnRH release. This may be associated with constitutional delay of puberty; nutritional deficiencies secondary to chronic diseases such as regional enteritis, CF, diabetes, or poorly controlled anorexia nervosa; excessive exercise resulting in malnutrition; stress; isolated GnRH deficiency; endocrinopathies such as hypothyroidism, congenital adrenal hyperplasia, and Cushing disease; and specific drugs.

Answer choice A correlates with hypergonadotropic hypogonadism, which is characterized by high levels of LH and FSH and low estrogen. Hypergonadotropic hypogonadism would result from ovarian failure, not from a chronic disease. Answer choices B, D, and E, all with high levels of hormones, would not be expected in a patient with amenorrhea from a chronic disease.

(Pages 346–349, Section 5: Principles of Adolescent Care, Part 4, Chapter 79: Menstrual Problems)

**Answer 3-29.** A

Your patient should be counseled to increase, not decrease, her dietary omega-3 polyunsaturated fatty acids because omega-3 polyunsaturated fatty acids have been found to have a beneficial effect on adolescents with dysmenorrhea. In addition, treating dysmenorrhea focuses on inhibiting the synthesis or action of prostaglandins. Standard therapy includes nonsteroidal anti-inflammatory drugs (NSAIDs) such as ibuprofen, naproxen sodium, or mefenamic acid starting 1 to 2 days before the onset of expected menses. Combination oral contraceptive pills also improve symptoms in 90% of young women with dysmenorrhea but may take 3 cycles to achieve maximum therapeutic benefit. Patients should be told to avoid smoking, as it is a risk factor leading to dysmenorrhea.

(Page 350, Section 5: Principles of Adolescent Care, Part 4, Chapter 79: Menstrual Problems)

**Answer 3-30.** D

The most common cause of heavy menstrual bleeding requiring hospitalization is a bleeding disorder. Excessive bleeding at the time of menarche might be the initial manifestation of a bleeding disorder. The most common bleeding disorder is von Willebrand disease, which has a prevalence of 1%.

The remainder of the choices—polycystic ovarian syndrome, a spontaneous abortion, a hemangioma, and cervical polyps—are all causes of abnormal vaginal bleeding. However, bleeding disorders are more likely to require hospitalization.

(Page 349, Section 5: Principles of Adolescent Care, Part 4, Chapter 79: Menstrual Problems)

**Answer 3-31.** E

Unusual vaginal bleeding or amenorrhea should alert the physician to the possibility of pregnancy. In addition to menstrual changes, other symptoms of pregnancy include nausea, vomiting, breast tenderness, unexplained weight gain, urinary frequency, and fatigue.

Close to 800,000 adolescents between 15 and 19 years old in the United States experience a pregnancy each year, with 30% of pregnancies terminated by therapeutic abortion, 14% resulting in spontaneous abortion, and the balance resulting in a live birth. Of those who maintain the pregnancy to term, about 95% of adolescents decide to parent the child. Confidentiality should be offered to the adolescent and maintained at the request of the adolescent, based on state minor consent laws, as appropriate.

During the evaluation for a possible pregnancy, a physical assessment, including a pelvic examination, should be done. In addition, a pregnancy test should be done. Urine testing using monoclonal antibodies to β-human chorionic gonadotropin provides an accurate, sensitive, easy, and inexpensive screening tool to detect early pregnancy. In fact, testing performed as early as 1 week after implantation will be positive for 98% of pregnant women.

(Page 351, Section 5: Principles of Adolescent Care, Part 4, Chapter 80: Intrauterine and Ectopic Pregnancy)

**Answer 3-32.** A

Ectopic pregnancy is an expanding problem for young, sexually active women. The most common factor that predisposes the young woman to tubal damage and therefore ectopic pregnancy is acute salpingitis, especially chlamydial infection, not a urinary tract infection.

Other predisposing factors include previous pelvic or abdominal surgery and prior ectopic pregnancies. Other factors linked to ectopic pregnancy include multiple sexual partners and early sexual debut, as well as cigarette smoking and vaginal douching. Endometriosis is also a risk factor for ectopic pregnancy.

(Pages 351–352, Section 5: Principles of Adolescent Care, Part 4, Chapter 80: Intrauterine and Ectopic Pregnancy)

**Answer 3-33.** C

Effective use of a hormonal method is enhanced if the adolescent can initiate her contraceptive method right away rather than waiting for her next menses. This is termed the "quick start" approach and means starting the patient on their method immediately. Waiting for the patient's next menses is not necessary and delays the patient's use of an effective contraceptive method. With the quick start method, a pregnancy test is only necessary if it has been greater than 5 days since the last menstrual period. Since the patient in the vignette had a period 2 days ago, a pregnancy test is unnecessary.

The primary reason adolescents hesitate or delay obtaining family planning or contraceptive services is concern about confidentiality. Without confidentiality, adolescents may forego necessary health care, especially those teens at greatest risk. As a result, professional health organizations recommend that clinicians provide confidential contraceptive care. Therefore, the provider does not need to discuss the plan for prescribing oral contraceptive pills prior to initiating the method. A pelvic examination is not necessary prior to initiating oral contraceptive pills.

(Pages 353–355, Section 5: Principles of Adolescent Care, Part 4, Chapter 81: Contraception)

**Answer 3-34.** E

Absolute contraindications for use of estrogen–progestin combination contraception include abnormal vaginal bleeding of unknown cause, estrogen-dependent tumor, liver disease, thromboembolic disease, and cerebrovascular disorders. The patient's history of having a deep venous thrombosis constitutes thromboembolic disease and should prompt the clinician to discontinue this medication. An appropriate method is one that does not contain any estrogen.

The most effective progestin-only option for this patient is the etonogestrel implant, which is a long-acting reversible contraceptive that is effective for 3 years. Depot medroxyprogesterone acetate is an appropriate progestin-only method that would be safe for this patient if she does not want the implantable rod. Starting the patient on a lower-dose combination oral contraceptive pill would not be appropriate, as all estrogen-containing methods may increase the patient's risk for another clot. The hormonal patch and vaginal ring also contain estrogen and are therefore inappropriate methods for the patient. Advising the patient to abstain from sex is not an appropriate next step and an instruction that the patient may not be able to follow. Instead, providing a safe contraceptive method will ensure that the patient is protected from pregnancy.

(Page 355, Section 5: Principles of Adolescent Care, Part 4, Chapter 81: Contraception)

**Answer 3-35.** A

Progestin-only EC products are more efficacious and easier to dose and have fewer side effects than combined (estrogen–progestin) oral contraceptive pills. They are indicated for use after unprotected or underprotected intercourse. EC is extremely time sensitive with an increased risk of pregnancy as the time from unprotected intercourse to EC use increases. Although you may provide reassurance and offer counseling to the patient if you determine it is indicated, it should not delay the use of EC. US Food and Drug Administration (FDA) approval of EC is to provide it within a 72-hour window, but clinical practice is to use it up to 5 days. Placement of a copper intrauterine device, not a levonorgestrel intrauterine device, is the most effective form of EC. A pelvic examination is not indicated unless the patient is complaining of vaginal or pelvic symptoms.

(Page 355, Section 5: Principles of Adolescent Care, Part 4, Chapter 81: Contraception)

**Answer 3-36.** D

DMPA appeals to adolescents because it is comparably long lasting, easy to use, and invisible to parents and partners. However, there are some significant side effects associated with the method. The 3 main side effects are weight gain, irregular bleeding/amenorrhea, and a reduction in bone mineral density. Nausea and breast tenderness are common side effects with combined hormonal contraceptives.

(Page 355, Section 5: Principles of Adolescent Care, Part 4, Chapter 81: Contraception)

**Answer 3-37.** A

*C trachomatis* is the most commonly reported bacterial STI in the United States, and the rates of *Chlamydia* are highest in adolescent women. An estimated 2.8 million infections occur annually in the United States. Underreporting is substantial because most people with *Chlamydia* are not aware of their infections and do not seek testing.

HPV is common in the United States with an annual incidence of 5.5 million. However, HPV is a virus and therefore an incorrect answer to this question. *C albicans* is a fungal infection, not bacterial, so this is incorrect. *T vaginalis* is a protozoan infection, not bacterial. Bacterial vaginosis is the most common cause of abnormal vaginal discharge, but the transmission is not clearly from a direct sexual route. It is therefore not the correct answer to this question asking about STIs.

(Pages 1089–1097, Section 17: Infectious Diseases, Part 2, Chapter 228: Sexually Transmitted Infections)

**Answer 3-38.** C

Bacterial vaginosis (BV) results from replacement of normal vaginal flora with a number of anaerobic bacteria in high concentrations, including *Bacteroides* species, *Mobiluncus* species, and other bacteria such as *Gardnerella vaginalis* and *Mycoplasma hominis*. Symptoms include pruritus, irritation, and a thin white vaginal discharge with a "fishy" odor. With BV, vaginal pH is > 4.5, and when potassium hydroxide (KOH) is added, there is a fishy amine odor noted. Treatment with metronidazole 500 mg orally twice a day for 7 days yields a 95% cure rate.

Azithromycin and ceftriaxone plus doxycycline is the treatment for *Chlamydia trachomatis* and *Neisseria gonorrhoeae*, respectively. Neither of these infections would present with a basic vaginal discharge with a fishy amine odor. Additionally, you would expect to see polymorphonuclear leukocytes on the wet prep with these infections. Fluconazole is appropriate treatment for candidal vaginitis. With candidal vaginitis, vulvar pruritus is the dominant feature. There is often little or no discharge; that which is present is typically white and clumpy, not thin in consistency as described in the question stem. The vaginal pH is typically 4 to 4.5, which also distinguishes it from BV. In addition, with candidal vaginitis, you would expect to see pseudohyphae on the wet prep.

(Page 1097, Section 17: Infectious Diseases, Part 2, Chapter 228: Sexually Transmitted Infections)

**Answer 3-39.** B

The patient in the vignette has epididymitis. Key findings of epididymitis include scrotal pain and edema, as well as abdominal or flank pain, urethral discharge, or dysuria. On physical exam, the lessening of pain with scrotal elevation (ie, a positive Prehn sign) may help to distinguish epididymitis from testicular torsion. Epididymitis is a clinical syndrome of inflammation of the epididymis caused by infection or trauma. *C trachomatis* and *Neisseria gonorrhoeae* are the most common organisms causing epididymitis in sexually active adolescents. Evidence of urethritis, with a positive test for *C trachomatis* or *N gonorrhoeae*, can help confirm the diagnosis.

Diagnosis of testicular torsion may be confirmed by Doppler ultrasound demonstrating decreased testicular perfusion. Dysuria is not a symptom of testicular torsion. Dysuria is expected with urethritis, as seen with this patient. Although the white blood count may be elevated in a patient with epididymitis, a CBC would not confirm the diagnosis. Dark field microscopy is a helpful test to see treponemes if a diagnosis of syphilis was suspected. However, the patient in the vignette does not have signs or symptoms of syphilis. Radionuclide imaging can reveal a "hot dot" sign to help diagnose torsion of the appendix testis. This would not help in the diagnosis of epididymitis.

(Page: 1099, Section 17: Infectious Diseases, Part 2, Chapter 228: Sexually Transmitted Infections)

**Answer 3-40.** C

Factors implicated in precipitating recurrences of herpes simplex virus lesions include emotional stress, menses (in females), and sexual intercourse. Most genital herpes infections are actually asymptomatic. In fact, only 10% to 25% of people with HSV-2 antibodies have a history of genital herpes. There is an increasing prevalence of HSV-1, and it has become the predominant cause of genital herpes in some countries. However, in the United States, HSV-2 remains the most common cause of genital herpes. At least 30%, not 90%, of genital herpes infections occur in people aged 19 years old or younger. Seroepidemiologic studies show that 17% of adults, not 75%, in the United States are seropositive for HSV-2.

(Page 1366, Section 17: Infectious Diseases, Part 7, Chapter 304: Herpes Simplex Virus Infections)

**Answer 3-41.** B

Based on history and physical examination, this patient most likely has PID. There is not a single definitive diagnostic test for PID, which can make the diagnosis challenging and necessitates a low threshold for suspicion. Diagnostic criteria for PID are shown in Table 228-2. The Centers for Disease Control and Prevention sexually transmitted infection treatment guidelines recommend presumptive treatment for PID for young women who are sexually active, are experiencing pelvic or lower abdominal pain (without other identifiable cause for illness), and who have one or more minimum clinical criteria.

The majority of cases of PID are polymicrobial, usually *Neisseria gonorrhoeae* and/or *Chlamydia trachomatis*, although increased screening and treatment of *N gonorrhoeae* and *C trachomatis* have decreased the incidence of PID due to these pathogens. There are multiple different antibiotic regimens

**TABLE 228-2.** Diagnostic Criteria for Pelvic Inflammatory Disease (PID)

| **Diagnostic Criteria** |
|---|
| *Treat empirically if any are present and no other illness can be identified as causal:* |
| Cervical motion tenderness |
| OR uterine tenderness |
| OR adnexal tenderness |
| **Additional Criteria to Enhance and Support Diagnosis** |
| Oral temperature > 38.3°C |
| Abnormal cervical mucopurulent discharge or cervical friability |
| Elevated erythrocyte sedimentation rate or C-reactive protein |
| Laboratory-documented *Neisseria gonorrhoeae* or *Chlamydia trachomatis* cervical infection |
| Abundant white blood cells on saline wet prep |
| **Definitive Criteria (Selected Cases)** |
| Evidence of endometritis on biopsy |
| Thickened or fluid-filled tubes with or without free pelvic fluid or tubo-ovarian mass on transvaginal ultrasound |
| Laparoscopic findings of PID |

Data from Workowski KA, Bolan GA. Sexually transmitted diseases treatment guidelines, 2015, *MMWR Recomm Rep*. 2015;64(RR-03):1-137. Check https://www.cdc.gov/std/tg2015/ for the most current updates to the treatment guidelines.

recommended for the treatment of PID, for both inpatient and outpatient treatment (Table 228-3). All regimens used to treat PID must provide empiric, broad-spectrum coverage and should be effective against *N gonorrhoeae* and *C trachomatis* because even negative endocervical screening for these organisms does not rule out upper reproductive tract infection. Ceftriaxone 250 mg intramuscular 1 time plus doxycycline 100 mg by mouth twice daily plus metronidazole 500 mg by mouth twice daily for 14 days would effectively treat both *N gonorrhoeae* and *C trachomatis*, as well as anaerobic organisms.

Hospitalization is not necessary unless the woman is pregnant, is immunocompromised, or cannot tolerate oral administration of antibiotics. Follow-up should occur 72 hours after initiation of antibiotics to ensure clinical improvement. She should be counseled to abstain from all sexual encounters during treatment with antibiotics. Her partner(s) should be presumptively treated for *N gonorrhoeae* and *C trachomatis*.

(Pages 1097–1098, Section 17: Infectious Diseases, Part 2, Chapter 228: Sexually Transmitted Infections)

**Answer 3-42.** B

Patients with vaginal discharge that is seen with candidiasis have a pH < 4.5. This helps to distinguish it from the basic discharge seen in bacterial vaginosis and *Trichomonas* vaginitis.

**TABLE 228-3.** Treatment Regimens for Acute Pelvic Inflammatory Disease (PID)

| **Recommended Inpatient Regimens** |
|---|
| Parenteral regimen A |
| Cefotetan 2 g IV q12h or cefoxitin 2 g IV q6h, plus doxycycline 100 mg IV q12h. Use IV for minimum of 24 hours after patient improves. After hospital discharge, continue doxycycline 100 mg PO twice daily to complete 14-day course. |
| or |
| Parenteral regimen B |
| Clindamycin 900 mg IV q8h, plus gentamicin 2 mg/kg IV or IM in 1 loading dose followed by a maintenance dose of 1.5 mg/kg IV q8h in patients with normal renal function. |
| Transition to oral outpatient therapy can be initiated 24–48 hours after clinical improvement. For those on cefotetan or cefoxitin, continue doxycycline 100 mg orally twice daily to complete 14-day total; for those on clindamycin/gentamicin regimen, continue clindamycin 450 mg orally 4 times daily or doxycycline 100 mg twice daily to complete 14-day course therapy. If tubo-ovarian abscess is present, clindamycin or metronidazole, 500 mg twice daily, should be used to complete the 14 days of therapy with doxycycline. Alternative regimens can be found at CDC website. |
| **Recommended Outpatient Regimens** |
| Ceftriaxone 250 mg IM |
| or |
| Cefoxitin 2 g IM and probenecid 1 g PO given concurrently in a single dose |
| or |
| Other third-generation cephalosporin (ceftizoxime or cefotaxime) |
| PLUS |
| Doxycycline 100 mg PO twice daily for 14 days |
| with or without |
| Metronidazole 500 mg PO twice daily for 14 days |
| Patients should demonstrate substantial clinical improvement within 3 days of start of treatment. For a diagnosis of chlamydial or gonococcal PID, patients should be retested 3 months after treatment. |
| **Management of Sex Partners** |
| Partners with sexual contact within 60 days prior should be evaluated and treated empirically for *Neisseria gonorrhoeae* and *Chlamydia trachomatis* infection. If a woman's last intercourse was > 60 days ago, then her most recent sexual partner should be evaluated and treated. |

CDC, Centers for Disease Control and Prevention; IM, intramuscular; IV, intravenous; PO, orally; q, every.

Data from Workowski KA, Bolan GA. Sexually transmitted diseases treatment guidelines, 2015, *MMWR Recomm Rep.* 2015;64(RR-03):1-137.

The remainder of the answer choices correctly describe vaginal candidiasis, which is characterized by pruritus and a thick, white, cottage cheese–like discharge. The vaginal mucosa is erythematous with white lesions like those seen in thrush.

(Pages 1095–1096, Section 17: Infectious Diseases, Part 2, Chapter 228: Sexually Transmitted Infections)

### Answer 3-43. C

Idiopathic scoliosis is the most common type of scoliosis and is often seen in adolescent girls. Patients do not typically present with pain but with an observed deformity noticed by family members or school nurses. The Adams forward bend test is performed by having the patient bend forward at the waist with the arms dangling in front, which allows rotational deformity of the spine to be easily visualized (Figure 213-4). Significant curves require referral to an orthopedist and x-rays of the spine. An MRI may be required in infantile and juvenile scoliosis when there more likely is concern regarding a potential underlying diagnosis.

(Pages 1011–1015, Section 16: The Musculoskeletal System, Chapter 213: Disorders of the Neck and Spine)

### Answer 3-44. B

Back pain in adolescents is common. Mechanical back pain results from muscle spasm as the paraspinal muscles fatigue during or following activities. Treatment for mechanical back pain includes core strengthening and physical therapy. Common features of mechanical back pain include worsened pain at the end of an active day, localized pain to the lower back without radiation to lower extremities, improvement

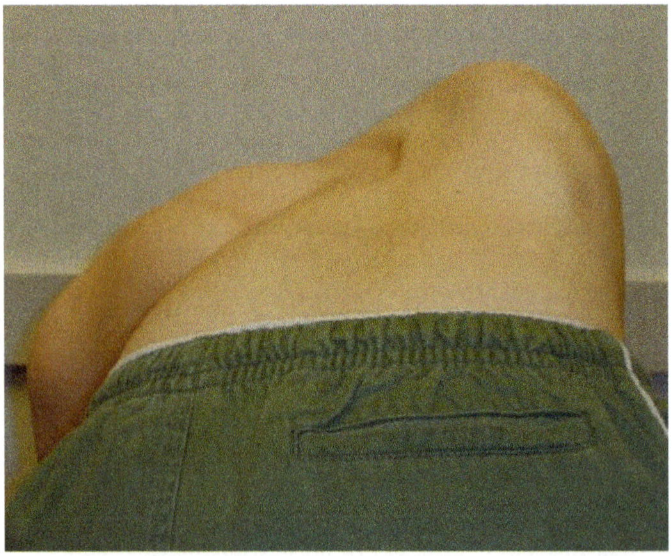

**FIGURE 213-4.** The Adams forward bend test is used to visualize the axial plane deformity seen in idiopathic scoliosis. (Mark W. Kline, *Rudolph's Pediatrics*, 23rd Edition. Copyright © McGraw-Hill Education. All rights reserved.)

with rest, and no association with bowel or bladder symptoms. Concerning symptoms for another etiology of back pain that may warrant a radiograph include radiation to the lower extremities, night pain that awakens the patient from sleep, constitutional symptoms such as fever, and pain with palpation of the bone.

(Pages 1015–1017, Section 16: The Musculoskeletal System, Chapter 213: Disorders of the Neck and Spine)

**Answer 3-45.** E

Sprains are classified into 3 clinical grades. Grade I sprains involve pain along a ligament but no laxity in comparison to the contralateral joint. Grade II sprains involve some detectable degree of asymmetry in laxity testing. Grade III sprains describe injuries to a ligament that result in > 10 mm of laxity in comparison to the contralateral joint. Most sprains are grade I or grade II injuries with minimal fiber injury and are appropriately treated by the RICE protocol. The RICE protocol consists of rest, ice, compression, and elevation and is appropriate for most nonbony injuries.

In addition to the RICE protocol during the initial 72 hours, low-grade sprains benefit from early range of motion and weight bearing as tolerated. Slow return to activity is allowed as pain and swelling resolve over 3 to 4 weeks. However, only suspected grade III sprains and lower-grade sprains that fail to improve following the initial 3 weeks should be referred to a musculoskeletal specialist for further evaluation. Therefore, answer choice E does not describe appropriate management.

(Pages 1024–1026, Section 16: The Musculoskeletal System, Chapter 215: Injuries)

**Answer 3-46.** A

Benzoyl peroxide is a suitable first-line choice for the treatment of mild inflammatory acne. It is particularly effective given its bactericidal nature, and daily use inhibits the development of bacterial resistance. Side effects include irritation and erythema and bleaching of clothing or towels. Other topical options may also be beneficial in this case including topical retinoids (eg, tretinoin, adapalene, and tazarotene). Topical antibiotics may also be first-line therapy and may be used together in combination with topical benzoyl peroxide for maximal effect. Oral antibiotics, including doxycycline and tetracycline, may be tried if a patient does not respond to topical therapy, presents with moderate to severe acne, or presents with acne on the back or chest that may be more difficult to reach or is too large of an area for use of topical medications. Minocycline may be more efficacious but is more expensive and has more serious associated side effects. Oral isotretinoin is highly effective but is typically only used for very severe acne with concerns for significant scarring given its side effect profile.

(Pages 1572–1575, Section 18: Disorders of the Skin, Chapter 360: Acne and Other Disorders of the Pilosebaceous Unit)

**Answer 3-47.** D

Typically, patients with acne who begin topical treatment should begin to see some results after 4 to 6 weeks of therapy. Since she has been using the medications consistently by her report for 6 months without improvement, it makes sense to consider another agent. Starting either an oral contraceptive pill or an oral antibiotic would make sense in this case. Oral contraceptives have been shown to be efficacious in adolescent females with moderate to severe or persistent inflammatory acne. Oral antibiotics such as doxycycline and tetracycline may also be of benefit in the management of her acne. Oral isotretinoin is highly effective, but given its significant side effects, including teratogenicity, its use is typically limited to patients with severe scarring acne or who have failed adequate trials of conventional therapy.

(Pages 1572–1575, Section 18: Disorders of the Skin, Chapter 360: Acne and Other Disorders of the Pilosebaceous Unit)

**Answer 3-48.** D

The patient in the scenario most likely has pityriasis rosea, a common, generalized, and self-limited dermatosis. The etiology of the rash is unclear. Typically, it presents with a single patch, as described in the case, known as a herald patch, which may be mistaken for nummular eczema (which may require treatment with topical steroids) or tinea corporis (which you would treat with an antifungal, such as clotrimazole). Days to weeks following the development of the herald patch, patients with pityriasis rosea develop a progressive eruption of numerous lesions as described in the question stem. Pityriasis rosea typically spares the face, hands, and feet, differentiating it from secondary syphilis, which typically affects the palms and soles. Treatment of pityriasis rosea is typically not necessary, as it will self-resolve in 4 to 6 weeks. Treatment of syphilis would include an intramuscular injection of penicillin.

(Pages 1529–1530, Section 18: Disorders of the Skin, Chapter 353: Disorders of the Epidermis)

**Answer 3-49.** A

This patient's most likely diagnosis is tinea versicolor, a superficial skin infection caused by the fungus *Malassezia furfur*. This infection typically occurs on the chest, back, and face. It is diagnosed by KOH examination of the scrapings, demonstrating short stubby hyphae that appear like "spaghetti and meatballs." Culture is not useful because *Malassezia furfur* is a normal skin inhabitant. An RPR would be the test for secondary syphilis, which presents differently from the rash in this patient. Scabies is extremely pruritic and typically is located at the wrists, finger web spaces, and waistline. Often scabies burrows appearing like a threadlike trail of scale on the skin are present.

(Pages 1592–1593, Section 18: Disorders of the Skin, Chapter 362: Skin Infections and Exanthems)

**Answer 3-50.** C

Based on the case, this patient likely has hidradenitis suppurativa. This condition is a chronic inflammatory disease of the apocrine gland–bearing areas of the body. It can be mild or more severe and can cause formation of sinus tracts and fistulas. Typically, first-line treatment may include topical antibacterials, such as topical clindamycin and/or benzoyl peroxide, incision and drainage, or intralesional steroids. Other treatment options may include systemic steroids or, in severe cases that are recalcitrant to other treatments, surgical excision. The fact that she is afebrile and the culture was negative makes an abscess much less likely. The treatment of choice for an abscess would be incision and drainage. Oral isotretinoin is used for severe scarring acne but has not been described as a treatment for hidradenitis suppurativa.

(Pages 1575–1576, Section 18: Disorders of the Skin, Chapter 360: Acne and Other Disorders of the Pilosebaceous Unit)

**Answer 3-51.** C

Normal-appearing epithelial cells, lactobacilli, and polymorphonuclear cells are typical findings of physiologic leukorrhea. Physiologic leukorrhea is a normal increase in vaginal secretions that often occurs 6 to 12 months prior to the onset of menses. The production of the vaginal secretions is stimulated by estrogen. Typically, secretions are clear to grayish-white and without odor.

A vaginal pH of > 4.5 and clue cells are typical findings of bacterial vaginosis (BV). In BV, normal lactobacilli are most commonly replaced by *Gardnerella vaginalis* and other anaerobic bacteria that promote a basic pH environment.

Budding yeast on a wet prep is seen with candidiasis. Mobile pear-shaped organisms with flagella (trichomonads) are seen with trichomoniasis.

(Page 309, Section 5: Principles of Adolescent Care, Part 1, Chapter 66: Reproductive Growth and Development in the Female Adolescent)

**Answer 3-52.** B

Individuals with extremely severe bulimia nervosa engage in inappropriate compensatory weight loss behaviors > 14 times per week. Self-induced vomiting and laxative abuse can lead to hypokalemia and hypochloremia with a metabolic alkalosis. Typical ECG findings of hypokalemia include depression of ST segments, flattened T waves, and U waves.

Peaked T waves on ECG are often seen in patients with hyperkalemia. Elevated serum creatinine is seen in patients with acute renal injury.

(Page 339, Section 5: Principles of Adolescent Care, Part 1, Chapter 76: Disordered Eating; Page 2311, Section 26: Disorders of the Cardiovascular System, Part 4, Chapter 487: Electrocardiography)

**Answer 3-53.** D

Prolonged abnormal uterine bleeding is classified as mild, moderate, or severe based on the duration of vaginal bleeding or frequency of menses and the severity of anemia. This patient has moderately prolonged abnormal uterine bleeding, defined as > 7 days and/or frequent menses every 1 to 3 weeks, with moderate to heavy menstrual flow and hemoglobin ≥ 10 g/dL. Abnormal uterine bleeding in this age group is often caused by anovulatory cycles secondary to an immature hypothalamic-pituitary-ovarian axis. Anovulatory cycles are common during the first 1 to 2 years after the onset of menses. **Mild** anovulatory bleeding is defined as menses lasting > 7 days and/or shortened cycles (< 24 days) for ≥ 2 months, with slightly to moderately increased menstrual flow and a normal or mildly decreased (10–12 g/dL) hemoglobin. **Severe** anovulatory bleeding is defined by irregular menses and a hemoglobin < 10 g/dL, which may or may not be associated with hemodynamic instability.

The patient does not have orthostatic changes on examination and appears to be hemodynamically stable. The next best step in caring for the patient is to begin a combined monophasic estrogen–progestin oral contraceptive and administer at set intervals until the bleeding stops.

The following regimen is recommended: 1 pill every 8 hours until the bleeding stops; then 1 pill every 12 hours for 5 days; then 1 pill once daily for a total of at least 21 days.

Iron therapy will be helpful to correct the anemia but will not stop active bleeding. The patient requires acute intervention, and referral to a specialist will delay treatment.

(Pages 349–350, Section 5: Principles of Adolescent Care, Part 1, Chapter 79: Menstrual Problems)

**Answer 3-54.** B

Refeeding syndrome is a potentially life-threatening complication caused by fluid and electrolyte shifts during nutritional rehabilitation of malnourished patients. Hypophosphatemia, hypomagnesemia, and hypokalemia are the electrolyte disturbances most commonly seen in refeeding syndrome. With the initiation of nutritional rehabilitation, glucose causes a release of insulin that triggers intracellular uptake of phosphate, magnesium, and potassium.

U waves on ECG are often seen with hypokalemia, a common electrolyte disturbance seen with refeeding syndrome.

Individuals with anorexia nervosa also experience deficiency in vitamins and trace minerals. Thiamine is often low in these patients.

Bradycardia is common in this patient population and is not a typical finding of refeeding syndrome. A normal sinus rhythm or sinus tachycardia may suggest heart failure and refeeding syndrome.

(Pages 338–340, Section 5: Principles of Adolescent Care, Part 1, Chapter 76: Disordered Eating)

**Answer 3-55.** D

The patient presents with secondary amenorrhea defined as the absence of menses for 3 cycles or 6 months. Common causes of secondary amenorrhea include pregnancy, endocrinopathies such as thyroid disorders, polycystic ovarian syndrome, and ovarian failure. Often there is a disruption of the pulsatile release of gonadotropin-releasing hormone. This affects downstream production of luteinizing hormone and FSH, promoting anovulation. In the setting of anovulation, there is a lack of a progesterone surge, which is responsible for menstrual bleeding.

The progesterone challenge is helpful to assess whether there is an adequate estrogen effect on the uterine lining. Daily progesterone is given for 10 days. This exogenous progesterone should promote the change to the secretory uterine lining often seen during the second half of the menstrual cycle. Stopping the progesterone on day 10 promotes a withdrawal bleed similar to that of a normal menstrual cycle.

A pelvic ultrasound would be of utility to determine if there are any anatomic abnormalities promoting amenorrhea. However, the patient has had normal menstrual cycles in the past, indicating that anatomy is intact.

The patient is at a healthy weight based on her BMI. She does not have clinical manifestations of hirsutism or acne due to hyperandrogenism that is seen in polycystic ovarian syndrome.

An MRI would be helpful in the setting of elevated serum prolactin levels to determine the presence of a prolactinoma.

(Pages 346–349, Section 5: Principles of Adolescent Care, Part 1, Chapter 79: Menstrual Problems)

**Answer 3-56.** E

The US Food and Drug Administration (FDA) licensed 3 HPV vaccines: bivalent, quadrivalent, and 9-valent. Since late 2016, only the 9-valent HPV vaccine is available for distribution in the United States. The 9-valent vaccine protects against 9 types of HPV, including 7 that can cause cancer. The other 2 can cause genital warts. The CDC recommends routine HPV vaccination for adolescents (boys and girls) at 11 or 12 years, but can be started as early as age 9 years. The vaccine is also recommended for males aged 13 through 21 years, females aged 13 through 26 years, and high-risk groups (men who have sex with men, transgender people, and those with immunocompromising conditions). Ideally the vaccine is given before exposure to HPV occurs (see https://www.cdc.gov/hpv/index.html).

(Page 1098, Section 17: Infectious Diseases, Part 1, Chapter 228: Sexually Transmitted Infections)

**Answer 3-57.** C

Puberty in boys begins between ages 9 and 14 years. Boys experience peak height velocity later in puberty, usually around SMR 4 and 5. During this period of rapid growth, bones are growing rapidly; therefore, alkaline phosphatase is elevated.

The increasing production of testosterone causes increased production of red blood cells. Normal range for hemoglobin and hematocrit in adult males is 13.5 to 17.5 g/dL (Table 65-1). Oral isotretinoin is appropriate for severe cystic acne and is not first-line treatment for moderate pustular acne.

(Pages 307–308, Section 5: Principles of Adolescent Care, Part 1, Chapter 65: Somatic Growth and Development in Adolescence)

**Answer 3-58.** A

During middle adolescence, typically ages 14 to 16 years, there is an emergence of abstract thinking and the ability to take perspective and reflect. Rules often apply to others but not to self. The middle adolescence is characterized by intense feelings and importance of peer group, not often family values. Conflicts with parents become more frequent as the adolescent focuses on his or her peers. Concern over appearance and body image continues. Heterosexual relationships, in addition to same-sex peer relationships, begin to become important, often associated with initiation of sexual experimentation with the opposite sex. Involvement with groups may be both beneficial (eg, sports, school clubs) and harmful (eg, gangs). Idealism is often replaced, at least in part, with more realistic vocational and academic goals. However, rapidly maturing limbic structures in imbalance with a still immature prefrontal cortex often leads to overactive, emotionally driven responses with underactive executive controls, which can place adolescents at risk of harm from accidents, substance abuse, and sexual experimentation.

(Page 314, Section 5: Principles of Adolescent Care, Part 1, Chapter 68: Psychological Development)

**Answer 3-59.** B

During the period of late adolescence, typically age 17 to 21 years, but as old as 25 years, there is continued exploration of identity and social role. There is increased self-reflection and insight. Individual relationships become more important than those with peer groups and parents. Most adolescents in this age group are described as restless and anxious to separate from family. No longer concerned and self-absorbed over pubertal changes, they become more comfortable with themselves, their values, and identity. The physical body is in adult form. A strong sense of idealism and altruism may lead to conflict with family and society. In the healthcare setting, clinicians can support the developmental process by engaging the adolescent in shared decision-making and encouraging them to make better health decisions.

(Pages 314–315, Section 5: Principles of Adolescent Care, Part 1, Chapter 68: Psychological Development)

**Answer 3-60.** C

Healthcare transition for youth with complex chronic health conditions is a process. The most successful transitions

**TABLE 65-1.** Clinical Correlates of Pubertal Maturation

| | SMR 1 | SMR 2 | SMR 3 | SMR 4 | SMR 5 |
|---|---|---|---|---|---|
| **Girls** | | | | | |
| *Hematocrit (%)* | | | | | |
| White (mean) | 39.1 | 39.2 | 39.6 | 39.2 | 39.2 |
| (range) | 36.1–42.1 | 37.1–41.3 | 37.0–42.2 | 36.9–41.6 | 36.2–42.2 |
| Black (mean) | 37.3 | 38.9 | 39.0 | 38.4 | 38.7 |
| (range) | 34.6–39.9 | 35.7–42.1 | 35.2–42.6 | 34.9–42.8 | 35.9–41.5 |
| *Alkaline phosphatase (IU/L) (serum)* | | | | | |
| White (mean) | 70 | 89 | 76 | 33 | 38 |
| (range) | 51–90 | 49–134 | 36–108 | 16–60 | 23–76 |
| Black (mean) | 84 | 95 | 86 | 44 | 31 |
| (range) | 69–108 | 65–138 | 26–148 | 18–144 | 13–70 |
| Peak height velocity | | + | ++ | + | |
| Menarche | | + | ++ | ++ | |
| Slipped capital femoral epiphysis | | + | ++ | | |
| Acute worsening of scoliosis | | + | ++ | + | |
| Osgood-Schlatter disease | | + | ++ | | |
| Acne vulgaris | | + | ++ | ++ | |
| Physiological leucorrhea | | + | ++ | | |
| **Boys** | | | | | |
| *Hematocrit (%)* | | | | | |
| White (mean) | 39.5 | 39.8 | 40.9 | 42.3 | 43.8 |
| (range) | 37.1–41.8 | 36.7–42.8 | 38.2–43.5 | 39.7–44.8 | 41.1–46.4 |
| Black (mean) | 37.7 | 38.4 | 39.7 | 41.1 | 42.7 |
| (range) | 35.2–40.2 | 36.0–40.9 | 37.3–42.0 | 38.3–43.8 | 39.6–45.9 |
| *Alkaline phosphatase (IU/L) (serum)* | | | | | |
| White (mean) | 72 | 77 | 101 | 75 | 58 |
| (range) | 54–110 | 42–106 | 53–141 | 41–158 | 21–120 |
| Black (mean) | 77 | 94 | 122 | 116 | 75 |
| (range) | 43–130 | 53–204 | 46–240 | 32–228 | 23–228 |
| Peak height velocity | | | + | ++ | + |
| Ejaculation onset | | + | ++ | ++ | + |
| Ejaculation with fertility | | | + | ++ | ++ |
| Slipped capital femoral epiphysis | | + | ++ | + | |
| Acute worsening of scoliosis | | + | ++ | ++ | + |
| Osgood-Schlatter disease | | + | ++ | ++ | |
| Acne vulgaris | | + | ++ | ++ | + |
| Gynecomastia | | + | ++ | + | |

+ = May occur during this stage but is less likely than ++.

++ = Occurs most often during this sexual maturity rating.

SMR, sexual maturity rating.

Adapted with permission from Joffe A, Blythe MJ. Adolescent medicine: state of the art reviews. Handbook of adolescent medicine, *Adolesc Med State Art Rev* 2009 Aug;20(2):261-859.

begin at least 2 years in advance of when the patient will transition from a pediatric to an adult-based healthcare team. In preparation for transition, the pediatric provider can use one of several assessment tools to determine where in the process the patient is. These tools assess knowledge, skills, confidence, and experience of the patient to be able to navigate the adult healthcare system. Direct communication between pediatric and adult providers, in addition to having a formalized transition roadmap that summarizes past medical history, medications, list of providers, and so on, improves the likelihood that a young adult will make and keep a first appointment with an adult provider. Transition to adulthood includes new relationships, roles, and responsibilities. In the case of this patient, she will need a provider who is skilled at family planning.

(Pages 319–323, Section 5: Principles of Adolescent Care, Part 1, Chapter 70: Healthcare Transition from Pediatric to Adult-Based Care for Youth and Young Adults with Special Healthcare Needs)

**Answer 3-61.** C

The mortality rate for adolescents and young adults increases with each age group: 10 to 14 years (14.0 deaths per 100,000), 15 to 19 years (45.5 deaths per 100,000), and 20 to 24 years (83.8 deaths per 100,000). The top 3 causes of death are unintentional injury (typically due to motor vehicles), suicide, and homicide. Black males have the highest suicide and homicide rates (67.7 deaths per 100,000). Hispanic, compared to non-Hispanic, adolescents have the lowest mortality rates.

(Page 324, Section 5: Principles of Adolescent Care, Part 2, Chapter 71: Mortality)

**Answer 3-62.** A

An estimated 3 million adolescents are diagnosed with a sexually transmitted infection (STI) annually. Chlamydia and gonorrhea are the most common STIs in the United States. The Centers for Disease Control and Prevention (CDC) recommends annual screening for gonorrhea and chlamydia for all sexually active women younger than 25, and men who have sex with men who have had insertive intercourse should be screened for urethral chlamydial infection and rectal infection at least annually; screening for pharyngeal infection is not recommended. In someone who presents with specific symptoms, nucleic acid amplification test (NAAT) swabs of the symptomatic regions (pharyngeal, rectal) and urine specimen should be obtained.

National data on adolescent sexual behavior are the most robust for vaginal intercourse, for which incidence has decreased in the past 20 years. Most adolescents use some form of contraception at first intercourse (79%) and last intercourse (86%). About 41% of high school males and females have experienced coitus at least 1 time. The National Survey on Family Growth showed that 49% of males and 45% of females aged 15 to 19 years reported they had received oral sex. Slightly smaller percentages (38% of males, 39% of females) reported having given oral sex. Reports of anal sex are similar among males (10.2%) and females (10.5%). These data are limited because not all states include questions about sexual identity and sexual behavior in the CDC's Youth Risk Behavior Survey.

(Page 318, Section 5: Principles of Adolescent Care, Part 1, Chapter 69: The Adolescent and Young Adult Visit; Page 345, Section 5: Principles of Adolescent Care, Part 4, Chapter 78: Scrotal Masses)

**Answer 3-63.** D

This patient has several concerning health problems. Her BMI places her in the class II obesity status. She has irregular periods, which may be an indication of anovulatory cycles or polycystic ovarian syndrome. She is unable to swallow pills or remember to take them daily. She is in a serious relationship and at high risk for having vaginal intercourse and an unplanned pregnancy and needs a reliable form of contraception. Combined oral contraceptive pills may decrease menstrual volume but are not an appropriate option if she cannot remember to take them every day, as intermittent use of oral contraceptives increases risk for pregnancy. The transdermal patch is not an appropriate option because it has decreased effectiveness in women who weigh more than 200 lb or have a BMI > 35 kg/m$^2$. The DMPA injection, while effective, is associated with increased weight gain. The copper intrauterine device is more appropriate in a woman who is already sexually active and can tolerate unexpected, irregular bleeding. Most adolescents do not tolerate this option very well. The best choice is the etonogestrel implantable rod, which will be an effective form of contraception for 3 years but may cause unexpected intermittent vaginal bleeding.

(Pages 353–354, Section 5: Principles of Adolescent Care, Part 1, Chapter 81: Contraception)

**Answer 3-64.** A

This patient engages in high-risk sexual behaviors with multiple male partners. He most likely has secondary syphilis, which commonly presents about 2 to 8 weeks after the nonpainful chancre lesion of primary syphilis. Symptoms of secondary syphilis include skin rash on the palms and soles, swollen lymph nodes, and fever. The signs and symptoms of secondary syphilis can be mild and may not be noticed. Presumptive diagnosis of syphilis begins with a nontreponemal serum test such as the RPR. A positive nontreponemal test should be followed by a serum treponemal test such as the fluorescent treponemal antibody absorption (FTA-ABS) or treponema pallidum particle agglutination (TP-PA) assay to confirm the diagnosis of syphilis. Topical terbinafine is used to treat fungal infection. A rapid strep test will not assist with diagnosing syphilis. Urine culture is not appropriate to diagnose syphilis but may be useful in a patient with dysuria in whom *Neisseria gonorrhoeae* is suspected. Ceftriaxone 250 mg intramuscularly is used to treat infection with *N gonorrhoeae*. Penicillin is the treatment for syphilis.

(Pages 1299–1300, Section 17: Infectious Diseases, Part 5, Chapter 283: Syphilis)

**Answer 3-65. B**

The prevalence of gender dysphoria (GD)/gender incongruence is estimated at 0.7% among adolescents aged 13 to 17 years. Children with GD/gender incongruence that is extreme in early childhood, similar to the child in this scenario, are more likely to have persistence of GD/gender incongruence into adolescence. GD/gender incongruence may be accompanied with psychological problems. At this time, it is most appropriate to refer this patient to a mental health provider with expertise in GD/gender incongruence. Treatment with fluoxetine is not recommended before establishing care with a mental health therapist. This child is experiencing normal female puberty; however, the child's gender identity as male makes assessment by a clinician who can discuss gender-affirming treatment important. Treatment with testosterone cypionate is not recommended at this early age. The most appropriate treatment option is a gonadotropin-releasing hormone agonist ("puberty blocker") to allow this child to further explore gender identity without continuing through a feminizing puberty. Measuring serum estradiol concentration is not helpful because there are not differences in circulating levels of sex steroids between transgender and nontransgender (cisgender) individuals.

(Pages 333–334, Section 5: Principles of Adolescent Care, Part 1, Chapter 75: Depression, Anxiety, and Other Disorders in Adolescence)

**References**

American Academy of Pediatrics. Ensuring comprehensive care and support for transgender and gender-diverse children and adolescents. 2018. http://pediatrics.aappublications.org/content/142/4/e20182162. Accessed November 12, 2020.)

The Endocrine Society. Endocrine treatment of gender-dysphoric/gender-incongruent persons: An Endocrine Society Clinical Practice Guideline, 2017. https://academic.oup.com/jcem/article/102/11/3869/4157558. Accessed November 12, 2020.

World Professional Association for Transgender Health. www.wpath.org. Accessed November 12, 2020.

# CHAPTER 4 Clinical Genetics and Dysmorphology

Julia Shelburne, Charu J. Sehgal, Jennifer Benjamin, Heather Moore, and Angelo Giardino

**4-1.** A previously healthy, Hispanic, 3-month-old male infant comes in to clinic with a complaint of a possible seizure. His mother was attempting to feed him his formula via a bottle, which he used to eat well but lately has been having trouble taking in, when she noticed a twitching of his extremities and eye rolling. The episode lasted about 1 minute. The mother is scared because there is a history of males in her family with seizures and developmental delay.

Upon exam, you note an alert infant who has truncal hypotonia with poor head control as compared to your exam a month earlier. He has a full head of hair, but it is coarse in texture and shorter and paler than his mother's and sibling's hair. He has a pectus excavatum and umbilical hernia, and his face has developed more than before with saggy cheeks and large ears. He has a high-arched palate. He seems to have loose skin on his neck and axilla. What is the most likely diagnosis?

A. Hemochromatosis
B. Acrodermatitis enteropathica
C. Menkes disease
D. Wilson disease
E. Lead toxicity

**4-2.** You are seeing 1-month-old baby girl, a new patient in your clinic who was just discharged from the neonatal intensive care unit (NICU). She was born at 33 weeks' gestation, has a history of supravalvular artery stenosis, and is being followed by cardiology. The infant also presented with seizures while in the NICU, so she is on antiepileptic medication. She also had an abnormal brain magnetic resonance imaging (MRI) scan. Her discharge summary notes that genetics was consulted while she was inpatient and the patient was found to have a chromosomal deletion of the short arm of chromosome 7. The child also had some issues with hyponatremia and hypercalcemia. Your exam is significant for large bulging eyes with stellate pattern of the irides, long philtrum with upturned nose, flat nasal bridge, full cheeks, full lips, and elfin facies. What is her most likely diagnosis?

A. CHARGE syndrome
B. DiGeorge syndrome
C. Cri-du-chat syndrome
D. Williams-Beuren syndrome
E. Turner syndrome

**4-3.** You are evaluating a 6-hour-old male infant in the well-baby nursery. Upon exam, you notice a missing fourth digit on the left hand, and his left forearm seems curved. His anus seems more anterior than it should be and smaller in circumference. He has not passed meconium yet. You order a left arm and hand x-ray and surgery consult for a possible imperforate anus. Which of the following should you *not* order or perform at this time?

A. Pass a nasogastric tube to determine whether it goes into the stomach
B. Echocardiogram
C. Renal ultrasound
D. Skeletal survey
E. Head ultrasound

**4-4.** You are called to the delivery of a newborn via cesarean section for fetal distress. A male infant weighing 7 lb is born with good Apgar scores of 8 and 9 at 1 and 5 minutes, respectively. On examination you notice a tuft of white hair and depigmented patches of skin on his torso. Investigations for the infant should include which of the following?

A. Abdominal ultrasound
B. Audiology evaluation
C. Echocardiography for cardiac defects
D. Electrolytes including glucose
E. Skeletal survey

**4-5.** You are managing a 12-month-old boy with DiGeorge syndrome in clinic. He is known to be immune deficient and is on antibiotic prophylaxis to prevent infection. He had a tetralogy of Fallot defect that was previously repaired, and he is gastrostomy tube dependent for feeds, with no signs of cardiac failure. Which of the following statements is *true* regarding the management of this patient?

**A.** He needs regular immunizations of DTaP (diphtheria, tetanus, and pertussis), hepatitis A, *Haemophilus influenzae* B, pneumococcal conjugate vaccine, MMR (measles, mumps, and rubella), and varicella.

**B.** The incidence of autism is the same as in the normal population.

**C.** Velopharyngeal incompetencies are usually corrected with surgery and therapies in the neonatal period.

**D.** Hypercalcemia is commonly seen in patients with DiGeorge syndrome.

**E.** Seventy-five percent of patients with DiGeorge syndrome have cardiac defects.

**4-6.** A 10-month-old male infant presents with history of chronic rhinorrhea and acute-onset ear pain. On examination, he is noted to have erythematous bulging tympanic membranes and is diagnosed with acute otitis media. His history is remarkable for 2 previous episodes of ear infections requiring antibiotics and a hospitalization with pneumonia. His mother reports that he is on oral antihistamines and nasal spray, but he always has a runny nose. On examination, he has coarse breath sounds that are better heard on the left than the right hemithorax. His height and weight are tracking along the 50th percentile. Which of the following statements regarding his underlying condition is true?

**A.** A triad of situs inversus, bronchiectasis, and recurrent pneumonia is suggestive of Kartagener syndrome.

**B.** Chest x-ray (CXR) findings are most likely to show chronic airway changes in his upper lobes.

**C.** Fifty percent of patients with primary ciliary dyskinesia (PCD) have situs inversus totalis.

**D.** He has a mutation of the *CFTR* gene.

**E.** Fertility in adulthood is not affected if treatment is started early.

**4-7.** You are seeing a 3-month-old male infant in the emergency department. He has been transferred from an outside facility with lethargy and new onset seizures. He was born after an uneventful pregnancy. He was treated for sepsis soon after birth and was noted to have marked acidosis. He was discharged home at 2 weeks and noted to have poor weight gain and delayed development. He has recently been ill with diarrhea and vomiting, and he has developed seizures in the last 2 hours. The parents report recent viral illness, although he does not have any fever. On examination, he has marked central hypotonia, with poor head control, and appears to be drowsy. What is the next best step in management?

**A.** Obtain blood gas and metabolic screen including cultures and administer broad-spectrum antibiotics.

**B.** Perform a full septic screen including lumber puncture before starting on broad-spectrum antibiotics.

**C.** Perform a computed tomography (CT) scan to rule out intracranial bleed.

**D.** Secure airway, obtain blood gas, perform fluid resuscitation if needed, and obtain labs for a metabolic screen.

**E.** Call for the genetics service to consult on the patient while in the emergency department.

**4-8.** You are following up a 7-year-old boy with developmental delay. He has been lost to follow-up for the past 2 years. On examination, he has macrocephaly and freckling around his mouth and neck. You notice that he has 5 café-au-lait spots measuring around 7 mm, and he has reduced vision when checking visual fields. His blood pressure is 99/56 mm Hg. Which of the following statements is true about his genetic condition?

**A.** An affected person has a 50% chance of transmitting the disease to the child.

**B.** If the parents are examined and neither has clinical signs, the child has incomplete penetrance.

**C.** Long bone dysplasia is a clinical manifestation in adults.

**D.** Most optic gliomas need surgery.

**E.** Plexiform neurofibromas are only seen in adolescence.

**4-9.** A 3-hour-old infant girl is vomiting. The mother received scant prenatal care but otherwise had an uneventful pregnancy. This is her first infant. On exam, the child is not ill appearing but is noted to be diffusely hypotonic. She has a short neck with loose folds on the back of the neck, a protruding tongue, and upslanting palpebral fissures. She is noted to have short fifth fingers that curve inward and a gap between the first and second toes. Her pediatrician will need to follow her closely for common associated problems, including which of the following?

**A.** Bicuspid aortic valve

**B.** Gonadoblastoma

**C.** Celiac disease

**D.** Abnormal pubertal development with absence of secondary sexual characteristics

**E.** Optic nerve defects

**4-10.** An infant is born at 36 weeks after induction of delivery for severe oligohydramnios. The infant is noted to have respiratory distress with hypoxemia. He exhibits large, folded ears; a flattened appearance to the facial features; wrinkled skin; and clubbed feet. What is true about this condition?

**A.** It results from a developmental field defect.

**B.** It results from a disruption.

**C.** It is caused by a single-gene disorder.

**D.** It is caused by dysplastic connective tissue.

**E.** It usually results from a renal or urogenital malformation in the fetus.

**4-11.** A newborn infant is noted to have microcephaly along with other dysmorphisms. The pediatrician evaluating the infant is highly suspicious of a specific genetic disorder. Which of the following conditions could be confirmed by routine chromosomal analysis?

**A.** Williams syndrome

**B.** Cri-du-chat syndrome

**C.** 16p11.2 deletion syndrome

**D.** Patau syndrome

**E.** Smith-Lemli-Opitz syndrome

**4-12.** A pediatrician is seeing a 5-year-old boy in clinic for evaluation of developmental delays, for which he has been receiving therapies through his public school system. He has recently moved to the area, and the new therapists would like him to have a medical evaluation prior to resuming his therapies.

He had a history of hypotonia and poor feeding as an infant, for which he needed supplemental feeds by gastrostomy tube for 2 years to ensure sufficient intake. However, for the past 2 years, he has gained weight very rapidly despite the removal of the gastrostomy tube and efforts by the family to restrict his eating. Testing shows that he has moderate to severe intellectual disability.

On exam, he is friendly, although his social skills are delayed. It is difficult to examine him because he is fixated on his mother's purse, where he has seen a snack. He is noted to be obese with a body mass index of 22 (which is well above the 99% for age), whereas his height is 5% for age. His facial features do not strike the physician as being dysmorphic. He has small hands and feet and small testes as well. What genetic condition would best explain this patient's history and findings?

**A.** Fragile X syndrome

**B.** Klinefelter syndrome

**C.** Prader-Willi syndrome (PWS)

**D.** Rett syndrome

**E.** Spinal muscular atrophy

**4-13.** You are seeing a 47-year-old woman for a prenatal visit. She is expecting her first child and is concerned about whether her infant will be at risk for any genetic conditions. Which common aneuploidy is *not* associated with increasing maternal age?

**A.** Down syndrome

**B.** Edwards syndrome

**C.** Patau syndrome

**D.** Turner syndrome

**E.** All of the above

**4-14.** A 2-month-old female infant is diagnosed with phenylketonuria (PKU), which is caused by a deficiency in phenylalanine hydroxylase (PAH). She has a 10-year-old brother who is clinically normal. Assuming that the brother is not affected with PKU, what is his risk of carrying a mutation affecting PAH activity?

**A.** 1 in 4

**B.** 1 in 3

**C.** 1 in 2

**D.** 2 in 3

**E.** 3 in 4

**4-15.** You are attending in the nursery and suspect that the child pictured in the figure has Down syndrome. Which of the following statements is correct?

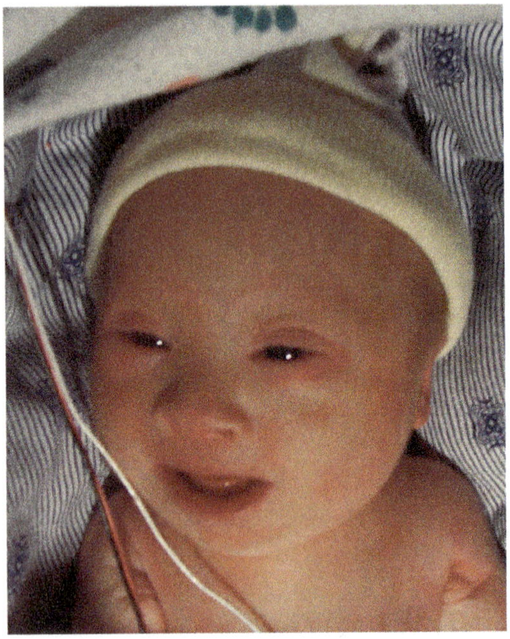

(Reproduced, with permission, from Rudolph CD, Rudolph AM, Lister GE, First LR, Gershon AA, *Rudolph's Pediatrics*, 22nd Edition New York: McGraw-Hill, 2011.)

**A.** Down syndrome is relatively rare and occurs in 1 in 8000 infants.

**B.** All individuals with Down syndrome have 3 copies of the entire chromosome 21.

**C.** The presence of a single transverse crease is pathognomonic for Down syndrome.

**D.** Physical examination is likely to reveal hypertonia and exaggerated primitive reflexes.

**E.** Referral for echocardiogram is not necessary for routine health supervision for children with Down syndrome.

**4-16.** A newborn female infant weighs 4.6 kg. She has a large tongue and an umbilical hernia. She is noted to have facial hemangiomata, pits on the backs of her ear helices, and double creases in her earlobes. Abdominal ultrasound reveals enlarged, lobulated kidneys. Her likelihood of having cognitive impairments is most related to the presence of which of the following?

**A.** Hemihyperplasia

**B.** Hypoglycemia

**C.** Jaundice

**D.** Obstructive apnea

**E.** Wilms tumor

**4-17.** A newborn has a round, flattened face; accessory fontanelle; small ears and mouth; upslanted palpebral fissures; a short rib cage; short fingers; bilateral transverse palmar creases; widely spaced first and second toes; and generalized hypotonia. Echocardiogram reveals an ostium primum atrial septal defect. Radiographic examination of the chest and abdomen reveals a "double bubble" sign. What is the most appropriate genetic test to provide the parents with complete diagnostic and recurrence risk counseling?

**A.** Chromosome breakage study

**B.** Cytogenomic microarray analysis

**C.** Fluorescence in situ hybridization

**D.** Routine karyotype

**E.** Whole-exome sequencing

**4-18.** Abnormality of chromosome number (ie, aneuploidy) is the leading known cause of which of the following conditions?

**A.** Cognitive impairment

**B.** Growth aberration

**C.** Heritable disorders

**D.** Major malformations

**E.** Spontaneous abortion

**4-19.** With regard to the inheritance of genetic conditions, the concept of *penetrance* refers to which of the following?

**A.** Clinical diagnosis assigned when more than one condition is caused by mutations in the relevant gene (ie, allelic conditions)

**B.** Degree of variation or severity among people who express the phenotype

**C.** Incidence of familial cases as compared to cases caused by de novo genetic mutation

**D.** Percentage of affected individuals within a given generation of a family

**E.** Proportion of individuals with the genotype who manifest any part of the phenotype

**4-20.** With regard to inheritance of genetic conditions, the concept of *expressivity* refers to which of the following?

**A.** Clinical diagnosis assigned when more than one condition is caused by mutations in the relevant gene (ie, allelic conditions)

**B.** Degree of variation or severity among people who express the phenotype

**C.** Incidence of familial cases as compared to cases caused by de novo genetic mutation

**D.** Percentage of affected individuals within a given generation of a family

**E.** Proportion of individuals with the genotype who manifest any part of the phenotype

**4-21.** Collagen protein is comprised of 3 intertwining strands. Most commonly, there are 2 identical strands ("A" strands) and 1 nonidentical strand ("B" strand). A and B strands are coded by separate genes. A mutation in the gene for the B strand will interfere with the structure of that polypeptide so that the final collagen protein will be abnormal. This is an example of which mechanism of mutation?

**A.** Dominant negative

**B.** Gain of function

**C.** Haploinsufficiency

**D.** Imprinting

**E.** Pleiotropy

**4-22.** A 3-year-old girl with a history of autism presents for a second opinion. She has delayed language development. You note paroxysmal laughter and tongue thrusting. On examination, you note prognathism and an abnormal gait. Examination is negative for any rash. What is the most likely diagnosis?

**A.** Angelman syndrome

**B.** Prader-Willi syndrome

**C.** Rett syndrome

**D.** Tuberous sclerosis

**E.** Fragile X syndrome

**4-23.** A 3-year-old child is diagnosed with Angelman syndrome. When taking the family history, you learn that his first cousin—his mother's sister's child—also has been diagnosed with Angelman syndrome. Both mothers are normal, and there is no other history of the condition in the family. What is the most likely explanation for this familial occurrence of Angelman syndrome?

**A.** Coincidence

**B.** Deletion of the Prader-Willi/Angelman region on the maternal chromosome 15

**C.** Maternally inherited *UBE3A* mutation

**D.** Nonpaternity

**E.** Uniparental disomy of chromosome 15

**4-24.** A 3-year-old boy presents to your clinic for the first time. He is a former full-term infant who was originally noted to have hypotonia and a poor swallow. He has since recovered; however, he is now noted to have a body mass index approaching the 90th percentile. He learned how to walk at 15 months of age. His language development is delayed. On examination, he has almond-shaped eyes, as well as small hands and feet (see figure). The remainder of the examination is unremarkable. What is the most likely diagnosis?

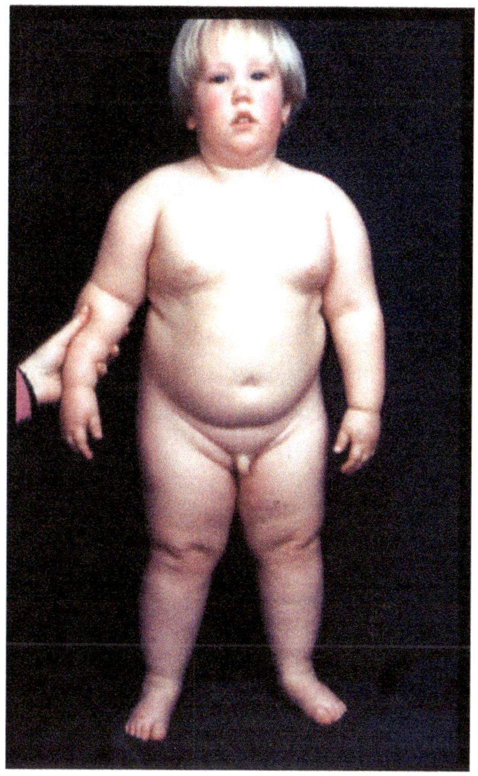

(Reproduced, with permission, from Kappy MS, Allen DB, Geffner ME. *Pediatric Practice: Endocrinology*. New York, NY: McGraw-Hill; 2010.)

**A.** Angelman syndrome

**B.** Prader-Willi syndrome (PWS)

**C.** Rett syndrome

**D.** Tuberous sclerosis

**E.** Fragile X syndrome

**4-25.** Tay-Sachs disease is an autosomal recessive degenerative neurologic disease. It is relatively common in the Cajun population of Louisiana. Cajuns descended from a group of French-speaking immigrants (Acadians) from eastern Canada in the 18th century. It is postulated that one of them was a man who was a carrier for the Tay-Sachs mutation. His descendants carry the mutation, and intermarriage has led to appearance of the disease. This phenomenon of a mutation originating with a single individual is known as which of the following?

**A.** Consanguinity

**B.** Endogamy

**C.** Decreased fitness

**D.** Founder effect

**E.** Genetic drift

**4-26.** By studying monozygotic versus dizygotic twins, it is possible to estimate the relative contribution of genetics to a given trait or birth defect. The best type of study design to indicate the difference between environmental and genetic influences involves which of the following?

**A.** Children born to mothers who are themselves monozygotic twins

**B.** Dizygotic twins discordant for structural birth defects

**C.** Dizygotic twins of the same sex

**D.** Monozygotic twins who are raised apart

**E.** Triplets composed of one set of monozygotic twins and an independent triplet

**4-27.** A child is born with bilateral microtia, colobomata of the lower eyelids, absent zygomata, micrognathia, and a high but intact palate. What is the most likely diagnosis?

**A.** Pierre Robin sequence

**B.** Smith-Lemli-Opitz syndrome

**C.** Goldenhar syndrome

**D.** Treacher Collins syndrome

**E.** CHARGE syndrome

**4-28.** A child is born with bilateral microtia, colobomata of the lower eyelids, absent zygomata, micrognathia, and a high but intact palate. A diagnosis of Treacher Collins syndrome is made. What is the most important intervention that should be done to maximize speech development?

**A.** Hearing aid placement

**B.** Mandibular distraction

**C.** Pharyngeal flap surgery

**D.** Sign language training

**E.** Speech therapy

**4-29.** Osteogenesis imperfecta is caused by mutations in the genes for type I collagen (*COL1A1* and *COL1A2*). Mutations that decrease polypeptide synthesis typically result in less severe disease than point mutations that change a single amino acid. Why?

**A.** Amino acid changes almost always involve *COL1A2*.

**B.** Epigenetic factors are more important in the context of missense mutations.

**C.** Mutations deleting a gene are less likely to be inherited.

**D.** Null mutations are more likely to result in spontaneous abortion.

**E.** Point mutations interfere with tertiary protein structure.

**4-30.** A child is born with micrognathia, glossoptosis, and a U-shaped cleft palate. This combination of findings is most appropriately classified as which of the following?

**A.** Association

**B.** Disruption

**C.** Field defect

**D.** Sequence

**E.** Syndrome

**4-31.** A 12-year-old girl presents as a new patient to your clinic. She has a diagnosis of intellectual disability with autism spectrum disorder. Her general physical health is good. Her mother requests referral to dermatology because the patient has facial acne that has been resistant to therapy (Figure 355-4), including dermabrasion; a bumpy rash over the left scapula; and "fungus" of the toenails. On physical exam, you also note 3 areas of hypopigmentation on the abdomen. What is the most appropriate next step in patient management?

**A.** Biopsy of the facial lesions

**B.** Brain magnetic resonance imaging (MRI)

**C.** Prescription of isotretinoin

**D.** Referral to dermatology

**E.** Technetium nuclear medicine evaluation

**4-32.** Hutchinson-Gilford syndrome (short stature, sparse hair, osteopenia), Hallermann-Streiff syndrome (short stature, sparse hair, premature cataracts), and cutis laxa (loose, inelastic skin) are all what type of condition?

**A.** Collagenopathies

**B.** Disorders of accelerated aging

**C.** Ectodermal dysplasias

**D.** Laminopathies

**E.** Nucleotide excision repair disorders

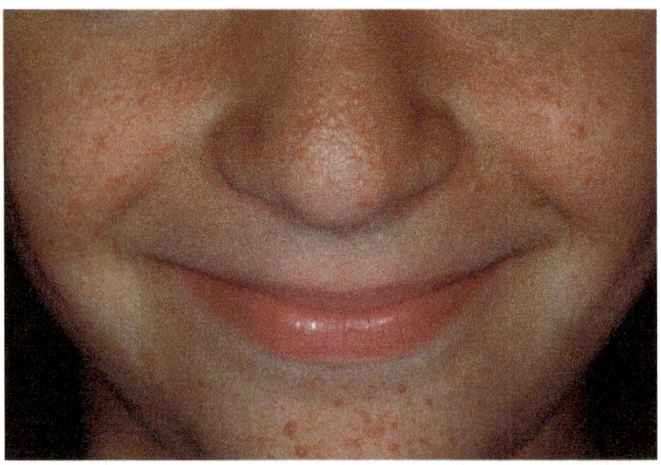

**FIGURE 355-4.** Facial acne. (Mark W. Kline, *Rudolph's Pediatrics*, 23rd Edition. Copyright © McGraw-Hill Education. All rights reserved.)

**4-33.** To determine whether a child's head size is inappropriately large or small, it is best measured and compared against what other growth parameter?

**A.** Arm length

**B.** Chest circumference

**C.** Height or length

**D.** Inner canthal distance

**E.** Weight

**4-34.** A healthy 2-week-old baby presents for routine newborn pediatric evaluation. Her mother reports that the baby has been diagnosed with a balanced chromosomal translocation involving chromosomes 2 and 13. The mother also has this translocation, having been diagnosed after her third miscarriage. The birth weight was 3450 g, and the Apgar scores were 7 and 9. She went home with her mother at 36 hours and has had no subsequent hospitalizations. She is breastfeeding without problems and has good weight gain. There is a normal red reflex, and the child is not dysmorphic. There is no heart murmur or abdominal mass. The genitalia and extremities are normal. What is the most likely reason that the newborn was found to have the balanced translocation?

**A.** Amniocentesis because of the maternal diagnosis

**B.** Evaluation because of intrauterine growth restriction

**C.** Placental testing after complicated delivery

**D.** Prenatal diagnosis of a structural heart defect

**E.** Umbilical cord blood testing for stem cell banking

**4-35.** Congenital contractures are caused by which of the following?

**A.** Any factor that diminishes movement

**B.** Autosomal dominant mendelian mutations

**C.** Constricting maternal anatomy

**D.** Environment such as maternal nutritional state

**E.** Epigenetic factors

**4-36.** There are estimated to be 20,000 to 25,000 genes in the human genome. It is observed that some genes have variable splicing and that a single stretch of DNA may produce more than one gene depending on the direction of transcription. Additionally, there are polymorphisms that lead to hundreds of normal variant base pair differences between even closely related people. What is the ultimate source of person-to-person variation in the genome?

**A.** Epigenetic factors

**B.** Fertilization

**C.** Recombination

**D.** Meiotic crossover

**E.** Mutation

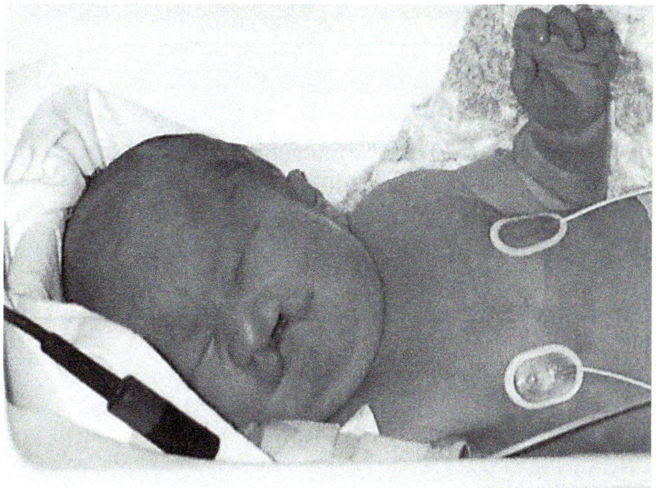

**FIGURE 166-5.** Infant with Trisomy 13. Newborn showing typical features of trisomy 13 (Patau syndrome), including bilateral cleft lip and broad nasal bridge and postaxial polydactyly of the left hand. (Reproduced with permission from Jorde LB, Carey JC, Bamshad MJ, White RL: *Medical Genetics*, St. Louis, Mosby, 2000.)

**4-37.** The baby in Figure 166-5 was diagnosed prenatally with intrauterine growth restriction, facial malformations, and structural abnormalities of the brain and heart. Based on the child's facial features, what is the most likely brain malformation affecting the child?

**A.** Dandy-Walker malformation

**B.** Holoprosencephaly

**C.** Hydrocephalus

**D.** Polymicrogyria

**E.** Schizencephaly

**4-38.** What genetic test is appropriate to confirm the diagnosis of the baby in Figure 166-5?

**A.** 7-Dehydrocholesterol level

**B.** Cytogenomic microarray analysis

**C.** Routine karyotype

**D.** Sequencing of the *SHH* gene

**E.** Whole-exome sequencing

**4-39.** You see a patient in an urgent care center and notice the presence of microbrachycephaly and micrognathia. The patient has a low hairline, synophrys, arched eyebrows, long eyelashes, a thin upper lip, and low-set ears. In examining the patient's extremities, you note spade-like hands and 2-3 syndactyly of toes. What is the most likely syndrome?

**A.** Moebius sequence

**B.** Sturge-Weber syndrome

**C.** Cornelia de Lange syndrome

**D.** Beckwith-Wiedemann syndrome

**E.** Cleidocranial dysplasia

## ANSWERS

**Answer 4-1. C**

Hemochromatosis is caused by mutations in proteins that govern iron homeostasis, hepcidin, and ferroportin. Iron overload caused by hemochromatosis can be managed with monthly phlebotomies to remove iron. Hemochromatosis presents with enlarged liver; cirrhosis of the liver, which causes increased bilirubin and jaundice; weakness; edema; and enlarged heart.

Acrodermatitis enteropathica is caused by low zinc levels and presents with acral skin lesions, alopecia, dermatitis, diarrhea, irritability, and failure to thrive. The diagnosis is made on the basis of a low serum zinc level (< 60 μg/dL), although symptomatic infants with normal or only slightly decreased serum zinc levels have been reported.

Menkes disease is an X-linked recessive disorder of copper transport caused by diverse mutations in a copper-transporting ATPase, *ATP7A* (OMIM no. 309400). Menkes disease typically presents in males at 2 to 3 months of age with loss of previously obtained developmental milestones and the onset of hypotonia, seizures, and failure to thrive. Characteristic physical changes of the hair and facies in conjunction with typical neurologic findings often suggest the diagnosis. Scalp hair in classically affected infants is short, sparse, coarse, and twisted. Light microscopy of the hair will illustrate pathognomonic pili torti (180-degree twisting of the hair shaft) and often other abnormalities, including trichoclasis (transverse fracture of the hair shaft) and trichoptilosis (longitudinal splitting of the shaft). The hair tends to be lightly pigmented and may show unusual colors such as white, silver, or gray, but in some cases, it is normally pigmented. The face is jowly with sagging cheeks and ears that often appear large. The palate tends to be high-arched and tooth eruption delayed. Pectus excavatum is a common thoracic finding. Umbilical and/or inguinal hernias may be present. The skin often appears loose and redundant, particularly at the nape of the neck, at the axillae, and on the trunk. Neurologically, profound truncal hypotonia with poor head control is invariably present. Appendicular tone may be increased with thumbs held in an adducted, cortical posture. Deep tendon reflexes are often hyperactive. The patient in the question has several of these symptoms, with the truncal hypotonia, activity reminiscent of seizures, and the physical findings of coarse and short hair that is lighter than that of family members, sagging cheeks, large ears, and high-arched palate. The patient in the question has several of these symptoms, with the truncal hypotonia, activity reminiscent of seizures, and the physical findings of coarse and short hair that is lighter than that of family members, sagging cheeks, large ears, high-arched palate, pectus excavatum, and umbilical hernia.

Wilson disease, or hepatolenticular degeneration, is due to mutations in the *ATP7B* gene (OMIM no. 277900) and is an autosomal recessive disorder of copper metabolism with an incidence of approximately 1 in 30,000 live births. Affected individuals accumulate abnormal levels of copper in the liver and (later) in the brain. Presenting clinical features of Wilson disease include nonspecific liver disease, neurologic abnormalities, psychiatric illness, hemolytic anemia, renal tubular Fanconi syndrome, and various skeletal abnormalities. In addition to the brain and liver, the eye is a primary site of copper deposition in Wilson disease, producing a pathognomonic sign, the Kayser-Fleischer ring. Laboratory findings that support the diagnosis of Wilson disease include low levels of serum copper and serum ceruloplasmin, elevated hepatic transaminase levels, aminoaciduria, and hemolytic anemia. Wilson disease also does not present as young as the patient in the clinical vignette.

Lead toxicity in the immature, developing brain, even moderate toxicity, is associated with neurobehavioral abnormalities and decreased intelligence quotients. Lead can cause neuronal demyelination, decreased numbers of neurons, decreased neuronal growth, interference with neuronal transmission, and sensorineural hearing loss that may result in significant delays in the acquisition of language and difficulty in auditory processing. At very high levels, lead can cause encephalopathy and cerebral edema, resulting in death or severe neurologic damage in survivors. The infant in the clinical question has no history of lead exposure mentioned. Lead toxicity causes mostly neurologic issues, as the patient's hypotonia and progressive encephalopathy would suggest, but his physical findings do not include a bulging fontanelle indicating cerebral edema.

(Section 11: Inherited Disorders of Metabolism, Chapter 164: Disorders of Metal Metabolism)

**Answer 4-2. D**

CHARGE is an acronym for ocular **c**oloboma, congenital **h**eart defects, choanal **a**tresia, **r**etardation of growth and development, **g**enital hypoplasia, and **e**ar anomalies associated with deafness. Cardiovascular malformations are found in 75% to 85% of patients. The most characteristic defects include conotruncal anomalies. Atrioventricular canal defects, vascular ring, and aberrant subclavian artery are also described frequently. The phenotype is highly variable. The patient in the question was not noted to have eye issues, respiratory distress due to choanal atresia, hearing issues, or underdevelopment of genitalia.

The most common genomic disorder linked to congenital heart defect (CHD) is DiGeorge syndrome/velocardiofacial syndrome due to 22q11.2 deletion, with a prevalence of 1 in 4000 live births. CHD is reported in almost 75% of affected individuals and is typically observed as conotruncal and aortic arch defects. The conotruncal defects include tetralogy of Fallot (TOF), truncus arteriosus, interrupted aortic arch type B, and double-outlet right ventricle. An aberrant subclavian artery may present with feeding difficulties or respiratory symptoms. About 15% of all TOF cases are attributed to this syndrome. Extracardiac problems include characteristic features (small palpebral fissures, small dysplastic ears, bulbous nose, long digits), velopharyngeal insufficiency with or without cleft palate, hypocalcemia due to hypoparathyroidism, immunodeficiency secondary to thymic hypoplasia, renal problems, and learning disabilities.

Cri-du-chat syndrome, also known as 5p minus syndrome, is characterized by a high-pitched, cat-like cry, growth retardation, and distinct craniofacial features including microcephaly, round facies, hypertelorism, epicanthal folds, down-slanting palpebral fissures, preauricular tags, and downturned corners of the mouth. About 30% of affected infants have CHDs including atrial septal defect, ventricular septal defect, and patent ductus arteriosus. Right ventricular outflow tract obstructive anomalies including TOF and pulmonary atresia have also been reported. The patient in the question has a chromosome 7 deletion, and patients with cri-du-chat have a discrepancy in chromosome 5.

The patient in this question has Williams-Beuren syndrome, which results from recurrent deletion of 7q11.23 and is frequently characterized by cardiac defects. The characteristic facial features include periorbital fullness, a stellate pattern of the irides, flattened nasal bridge, full cheeks, an upturned nose, long philtrum, wide mouth, and full lips. Hypercalcemia is reported in about half of all patients. The classic cardiac lesion observed in Williams-Beuren syndrome is supravalvular aortic stenosis, which is seen in approximately 75% of children. Peripheral pulmonary artery stenosis is also encountered at a higher frequency (~60%). Turner syndrome only affects females and results when one of the X chromosomes is missing or partially missing. Signs of Turner syndrome during infancy may include a wide or web-like neck; low-set ears; broad chest with widely spaced nipples; a high, narrow palate; fingernails and toenails that are narrow and turned upward; receding or small lower jaw; cardiac defects; and slowed growth. Short stature is universal in this condition due to loss of the *SHOX* gene on the distal short arm of the X chromosome. Girls with Turner syndrome are prone to recurrent otitis media as well as conductive and sensorineural hearing loss. They are also at risk for the development of autoimmune conditions, such as hypothyroidism and celiac disease.

(Section 12: Clinical Genetics and Dysmorphology, Chapter 181: Genetics of Congenital Heart Disease)

**Answer 4-3.** E

The baby in the vignette has some of the several findings in VACTERL syndrome, which stands for **v**ertebral anomalies, **a**nal atresia, **c**ardiac defects, **t**racheo**e**sophageal fistula, **r**enal anomalies, and **l**imb defects. VACTERL is an association, which is defined as 2 or more anomalies that are not pathogenetically related but occur together more frequently than expected by chance alone.

If when passing a nasogastric tube, it does not end up in the stomach but curled up in the esophagus, this indicates a possible tracheoesophageal fistula, which can be confirmed via magnetic resonance imaging (MRI). Even without a murmur, getting an echocardiogram in a patient with VACTERL is advisable in case there are cardiac defects that cannot be heard yet and may need immediate attention. It is warranted simply because of the association, as is the renal ultrasound. A skeletal survey is a way to look at all the bones to see whether there are further limb or vertebral anomalies to define the syndrome further and assess whether any need treatment.

A head ultrasound is not warranted at this time because the infant is not defined as premature and does not have seizures or focal neurologic defects. However, a head ultrasound may be ordered later if the newborn shows any signs of neurologic issues or decline or in the workup for possible genetic syndromes.

(Section 12: Clinical Genetics and Dysmorphology, Chapter 171: Birth Defects, Malformations, and Syndromes)

**Answer 4-4.** B

The infant has Waardenburg syndrome. Waardenburg syndrome is one of the most common types of autosomal dominant syndromic hearing loss. It is attributed to a mutation in the *PAX3* gene. Clinical findings include heterochromia iridis, white forelock, synophrys, and unilateral or bilateral sensorineural hearing loss (see table on next page).

(Section 12: Clinical Genetics and Dysmorphology, Chapter 174: Hearing Loss)

Major And Minor Criteria for Waardenburg Syndrome

| Major Criteria | Minor Criteria |
|---|---|
| Sensorineural hearing loss | Skin depigmentation |
| Pigmented changes of iris | Synophrys |
| Hair depigmentation | Broad high nasal root |
| Affected first-degree relative | Nostril hypoplasia |
| Dystopia canthorum (W index > 1.95) | Premature graying hair |
| Waardenburg Syndrome Consortium recommendations: criteria for diagnosis are two major criteria or one major and two minor criteria. | |

From Wong J. A male infant who has a white hair tuft and hypopigmented macules. *Pediatr Rev.* 2012;33(3):e18-e21.

**Answer 4-5.** E

The most common genomic disorder linked to congenital heart defect (CHD) is the DiGeorge/velocardiofacial syndrome due to 22q11.2 deletion, with a prevalence of 1 in 4000 live births. CHD is reported in almost 75% of affected individuals and typically involves conotruncal or aortic arch defects. Extracardiac problems include characteristic features

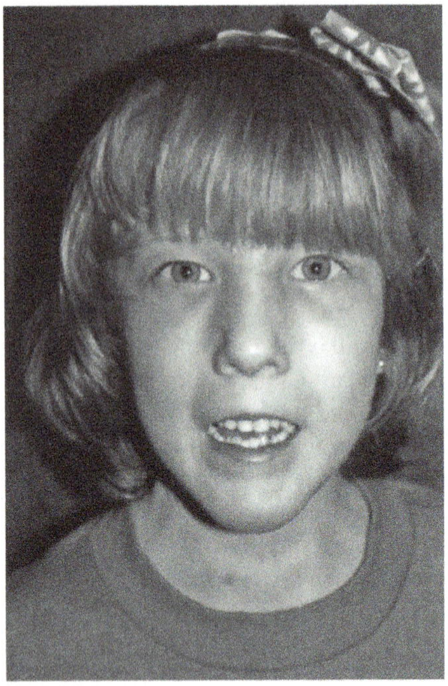

**FIGURE 166-6.** Child with DiGeorge syndrome. Note the tall nasal root and bridge with a bulbous nasal tip and small mouth. (Reproduced with permission from Jorde LB, Carey JC, Bamshad MJ, White RL. *Medical Genetics*. St. Louis, MO: Mosby; 2000.)

(small palpebral fissures, small dysplastic ears, bulbous nose, long digits), velopharyngeal insufficiency with or without cleft palate, hypocalcemia due to hypoparathyroidism, immunodeficiency secondary to thymic hypoplasia, renal problems, and learning disabilities (Figure 166-6). The diagnosis is confirmed either by fluorescence in situ hybridization (FISH) for 22q11.2 deletion or chromosomal microarray analysis. Most cases are from de novo mutations. Increased incidence of autism and behavioral problems are present. Patients need to be monitored for velocardiofacial abnormalities with hypernasal speech and swallowing dysfunction. Hypocalcemia is commonly seen in the neonatal period and during times of stress. Independent of the cardiac or palatal issues, one-third of patients have feeding difficulties related to dysphagia. Involvement of speech-language therapists and aggressive feeding protocols are essential. Nasogastric or gastrostomy tube feeding may be needed to assure proper energy intake, especially in infancy and childhood, when most corrective surgeries take place.

Live vaccines are avoided in those with T-cell deficiency. Immunologic abnormalities, usually involving T lymphocytes, are common in individuals with 22q11.2 deletion. Most patients have thymus hypoplasia, which can result in impaired T-cell function; at its most extreme, thymus aplasia can lead to life-threatening infections in early infancy. The parathyroid glands can also be affected. Some patients manifest severe hypocalcemia with tetany in the newborn period that can be intractable to treatment. However, most children have normal serum calcium concentrations, although hypocalcemic events, especially in neonates or during times of stress, can occur.

(Section 12: Clinical Genetics and Dysmorphology, Chapter 181: Genetics of Congenital Heart Disease)

**Answer 4-6.** C

Primary ciliary dyskinesia (PCD) is an autosomal recessive disorder secondary to absent or immotile cilia. Patients present with both upper and lower respiratory infections, and recurrent sinusitis, chronic rhinitis, and recurrent otitis media are the cardinal symptoms. It can present in the neonatal period as transient tachypnea or pneumonia. Almost all patients present with rhinosinusitis. The triad of situs inversus, chronic sinusitis, and bronchiectasis is referred to as Kartagener syndrome, a subgroup of PCD. Unlike findings in cystic fibrosis, PCD pulmonary findings are seen in the middle and lower lobes on CXR. Genetic testing is challenging due to heterogeneity. Treatment is supportive with aggressive airway clearance. Men with PCD are infertile due to immotile spermatozoa, and females have a 50% chance of infertility.

(Section 27: Disorders of the Respiratory System, Chapter 503: Disorders Causing Airway Obstruction)

**Answer 4-7.** D

This child has an underlying urea cycle disorder. Urea cycle disorders are a result of inherited deficiencies in the 6 enzymes or 2 transporters in the urea cycle pathway, leading to hyperammonemia. Children with complete defects normally present in the newborn period, due to immaturity of the neonatal liver accentuating the defects in the urea cycle. Neonates can appear normal at birth but rapidly develop cerebral edema with signs of lethargy, poor feeding, hyper- or hypoventilation, hypothermia, seizures, neurologic posturing, and coma. In the newborn period this can often be mistaken for sepsis or can present as acute worsening of mental status at 48 hours of life. In milder forms with partial enzyme deficiency, the symptoms are more subtle and the hyperammonemia can be triggered by illness or stress. Seizures are a common presentation of acute hyperammonemia. Ammonia concentration > 150 μmol/L or higher, with a normal anion gap and normal glucose is indicative of UCD. Once suspected, testing plasma amino acids will help identify specific deficiency in the urea cycle. Diagnosis is usually made with clinical, biochemical, and molecular genetic data. The main goal of treatment is to rapidly reduce ammonia levels in the blood in the critical care unit by addressing causes such as infections, catabolic states, reducing nitrogen load by eliminating protein intake, and preventing protein breakdown with dextrose infusion. Sodium benzoate can facilitate nitrogen disposal through alternate pathways. Patients resistant to intravenous therapy should be started on hemodialysis. Liver transplantation is considered in patients who do not respond to therapies.

ABP content specifications include:

1. Recognize clinical features associated with urea cycle defects
2. Plan appropriate immediate and long-term management of urea cycle defects while considering long-term prognosis

PREP pearls include:

- Urea cycle disorders clinically manifest with immediate decompensation in the first 24 to 72 hours of life with progressive respiratory alkalosis, obtundation, and hyperammonemia in the presence of a normal anion gap.
- Hyperammonemia is very toxic to the brain and can cause irreversible damage in the absence of immediate intervention. It is very important to check the serum ammonia level and quickly implement measures to decrease the ammonia level as soon as possible (dialysis, hemofiltration, nitrogen scavenger medications, and protein restriction).

(Section 11: Inherited Disorders of Metabolism, Chapter 141: Urea Cycle Disorders)

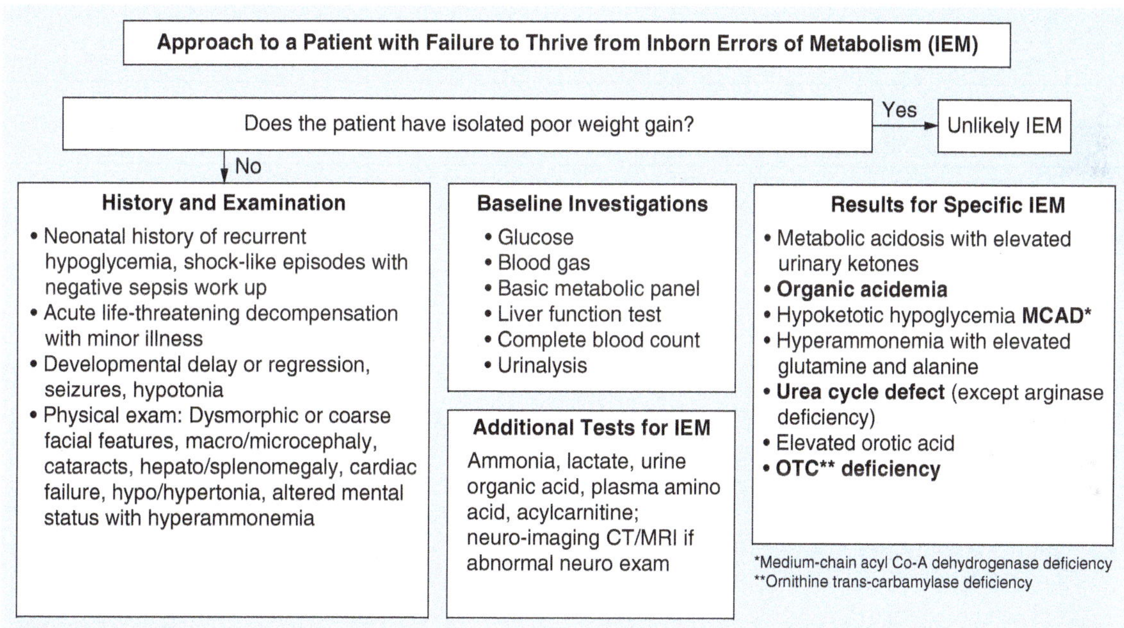


**Answer 4-8.** A

Neurofibromatosis (NF) type 1 is transmitted as an autosomal dominant trait with complete penetrance but variable expression. An affected person has a 50% chance of transmitting NF1 to a child. Fifty percent of cases occur sporadically due to a new mutation. If the parents of a child with NF1 are examined and neither has signs (eg, café-au-lait macules, neurofibromas), then the child is most likely affected due to new mutation and the parents face a low risk of recurrence. The most common pediatric-onset manifestations are café-au-lait macules and plexiform neurofibromas (see table on next page and Figure 176-1). Plexiform neurofibromas are commonly seen in children. NF1 presents with different clinical findings in different age groups; neurofibromas, long bone dysplasia, and macrocephaly can be seen soon after birth. Recognition of the possibility of NF1 in a child with any of these early signs can help make a diagnosis and guide management to avoid delay in recognizing potentially serious complications. Most optic gliomas are self-limiting in their growth and do not require surgical excision for treatment. If progression occurs, it usually does so by age 6 years. Current guidelines suggest annual ophthalmologic examination to detect optic pathway tumors, at least until about age 6 to 7 years.

(Section 12: Clinical Genetics and Dysmorphology, Chapter 176: Neurocutaneous Disorders)

**Manifestations of Neurofibromatosis Type 1 (NF1) by Age**

| | | |
|---|---|---|
| Birth to 2 years | Café-au-lait spots | > 6 spots larger than 5 mm are diagnostic |
| Birth | Plexiform neurofibromas | Arise in peripheral nerve sheath, occur at birth, and develop during infancy. Large lesions causing overgrowth and disfigurement |
| Birth | Macrocephaly | Benign |
| Birth | Bone dysplasia | Tibial dysplasia with or without pseudo-arthrosis |
| 2–6 years | Optic glioma | Usually asymptomatic; some may cause visual loss<br>Hypothalamic involvement if chiasm abnormal<br>Need yearly ophthalmology evaluation |
| 3–5 years | Skinfold freckles | Axillary, inguinal, submammary regions |
| Adolescence | Neurofibromas | Cutaneous lesions occur at birth and progress throughout life |
| Adults | Pheochromocytoma | Hypertension in children is often from renal artery stenosis |
| | Moyamoya disease | Can lead to stroke |
| | Cognitive deficit/attention-deficit/hyperactivity disorder | |
| | Scoliosis | |

From Korf BR, Bebin EM. Neurocutaneous disorders in children. *Pediatr Rev*. 2017;38:119.

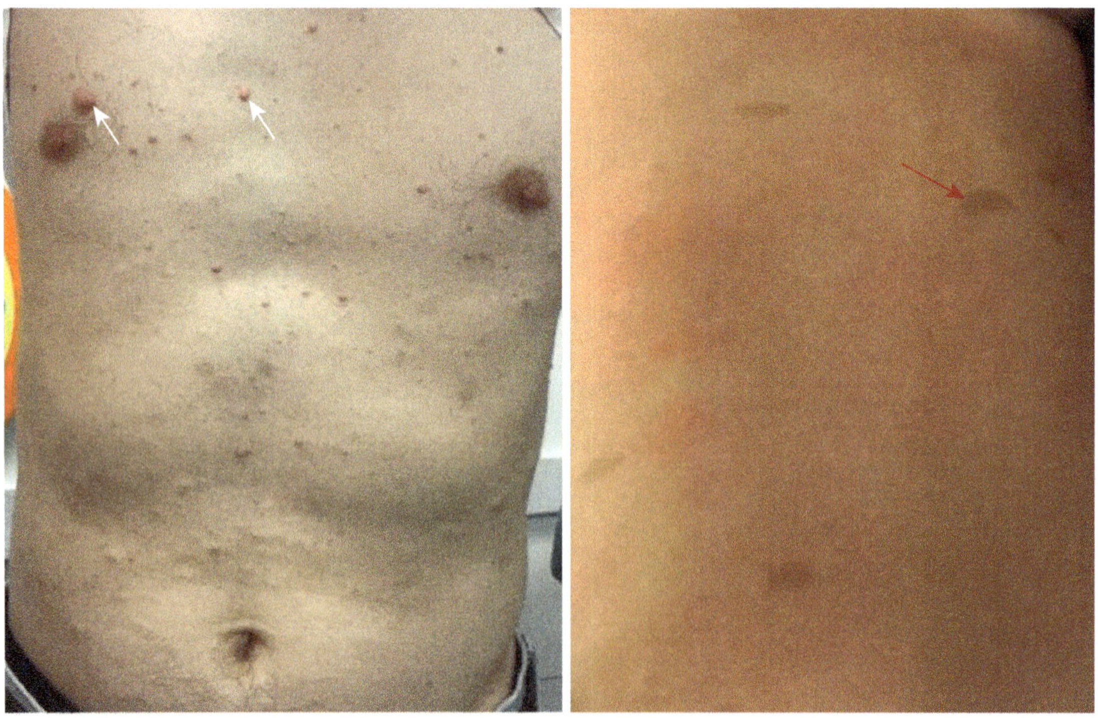

A B

**FIGURE 176-1.** **A:** Adult individual affected with neurofibromatosis type 1 (NF1) displaying neurofibromas (*white arrows*) and café-au-lait (CAL) macules affecting the torso. **B:** Child with NF1 with multiple CAL macules (*red solid arrow*) on the back.

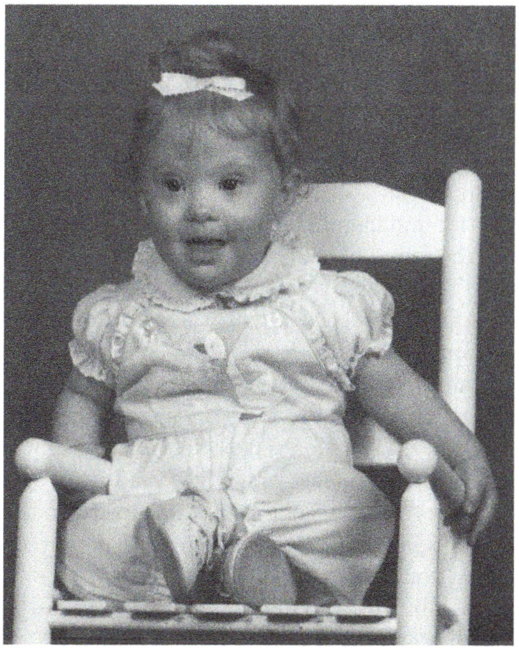

**FIGURE 166-3.** Child with Down syndrome. Note the upslanting palpebral fissures, epicanthal folds, and flat facial profile. (Reproduced with permission from Jorde LB, Carey JC, Bamshad MJ, White RL. *Medical Genetics*. St. Louis, MO: Mosby; 2000.)

**Answer 4-9.** C

This infant has features of Down syndrome. Down syndrome is caused by an extra copy of chromosome 21, usually due to trisomy 21 but sometimes due to mosaic trisomy 21 or Robertsonian translocations.

Clinical features include typical facial features (epicanthal folds, upslanting palpebral fissures, speckling of the iris, flat nasal bridge, protruding tongue, and small ears) and a short neck with redundant skin folds (Figure 166-3). The extremities often show short broad hands with clinodactyly of the fifth fingers and a single transverse palmar crease. The feet may show a "sandal gap," which is a large space between the first and second toes.

Short term, the child is at risk for congenital heart defect (CHD) (most commonly, an atrioventricular canal defect or ventricular septal defect), gastrointestinal malformations (duodenal atresia or Hirschsprung disease), cataracts, and hypothyroidism. Longer-term complications include intellectual disability, autoimmune disease (Graves disease, type 1 diabetes mellitus, and celiac disease), orthopedic problems (eg, atlantoaxial instability and hip dislocation), and hearing loss associated with recurrent otitis media.

Children with Down syndrome are at increased risk of blood disorders, including neonatal transient myeloproliferative disorder, acute lymphoblastic leukemia (20-fold increased risk), and acute megakaryoblastic leukemia (500-fold risk).

Children with Turner syndrome have a single X chromosome, and 6% are a mosaic of 45X and 46XY. Phenotypically female, but with a lack of development of secondary sexual characteristics at puberty, they also may have CHD (usually bicuspid aortic valve or coarctation of the aorta) and hand and foot abnormalities at birth (lymphedema causing typical swelling of the dorsum of the hands and feet). They, too, have a short neck, although their necks show webbing rather than redundant skin folds, and they have varying degrees of intellectual disability. Patients with mosaicism are at risk for gonadoblastoma in residual gonadal tissue. Optic nerve defects are not commonly seen in either disorder.

(Section 12: Clinical Genetics and Dysmorphology, Chapter 166: Chromosomal and Genetics Disorders)

**Answer 4-10.** E

This is Potter sequence, a constellation of physical findings due to oligohydramnios, usually resulting from a renal malformation or urogenital obstruction that causes decreased urine output by the fetus, although it can be due to other causes of oligohydramnios.

It is not a single-gene disorder, as it is the end point of several different potential causes of oligohydramnios.

A developmental field defect refers to a pattern of anomalies caused by a disturbance of a physical contiguous region of the embryo, such as in holoprosencephaly. Potter sequence, in contrast, affects the development of multiple regions.

A disruption is caused by external interference with development, resulting in destruction of irreplaceable normal developing tissues, such as in the loss of a limb due to an amniotic band.

A dysplasia occurs when the intrinsic architecture of a tissue is not maintained during development, as in achondroplasia.

(Section 12: Clinical Genetics and Dysmorphology, Chapter 171: Birth Defects, Malformations, and Syndromes)

**Answer 4-11.** D

Williams syndrome is caused by a 7q11.2 deletion. Cri-du-chat is caused by a 5p deletion, whereas the 16p11.2 deletion syndrome causes low body mass index, autism spectrum disorder, and other mental health issues. These diagnoses can be made using chromosomal microarray, which is a genome-wide approach for detecting copy number variants (deletions and duplications) at a high resolution.

Smith-Lemli-Opitz syndrome is diagnosed via elevated serum concentration of 7-dehydrocholesterol and low or low-normal plasma cholesterol.

Patau syndrome is caused by trisomy 13. Because this is trisomy of an entire chromosome rather than an isolated deletion or duplication, this diagnosis can be confirmed using routine chromosomal analysis.

(Section 12: Clinical Genetics and Dysmorphology, Chapter 167: Laboratory Analysis of Copy Number and Single Nucleotide Variants, Chapter 169: Diagnostic Algorithms)

**Answer 4-12.** C

Early feeding problems and hypotonia, followed by obesity due to extremely poor satiety, accompanied by intellectual disability (ID) is highly suggestive of PWS. The physical features of obesity, short stature, small hands and feet, and small testes would support the clinical suspicion of PWS. Facial dysmorphisms tend to be subtle in PWS.

Patients with Klinefelter syndrome can also have ID and hypogonadism but are generally tall and do not have the feeding issues associated with PWS.

Fragile X syndrome can also cause ID, although the facial features are generally more distinct and include a large head, long face, and protruding ears. They tend to have large testes after puberty but normal testes in childhood.

Rett syndrome is typified by normal development in infant girls, followed by rapid regression and development of ID and stereotypic hand movements.

Spinal muscular atrophy can cause hypotonia and poor feeding in infancy, but the weakness is progressive and intelligence is normal.

(Section 12: Clinical Genetics and Dysmorphology, Chapter 169: Diagnostic Algorithms)

**Answer 4-13.** D

Turner syndrome is most commonly related to abnormalities of the sperm (failure of the sperm to have a sex chromosome). This fact is important for genetic counseling. Down (trisomy 21), Patau (trisomy 13), and Edwards (trisomy 18) syndromes are all associated with advanced maternal age.

(Section 12: Clinical Genetics and Dysmorphology, Chapter 166: Chromosomal and Genomic Disorders)

**Answer 4-14.** D

All forms of PKU affecting PAH activity are inherited in an autosomal recessive manner.

If "R" represents a normal allele and "r" represents a recessively mutated allele, the parents are Rr and Rr. Offspring of these parents can be RR (normal), Rr (carriers), or rr (affected). The ratio of risk is 1 RR to 2 Rr to 1 rr for each pregnancy.

| | **R** | **r** |
|---|---|---|
| **R** | RR | Rr |
| **r** | Rr | rr |

The affected child is rr. The normal brother cannot be rr (because if he were, he would have the disease). So that possibility drops out, and there are 3 remaining possible combinations for him. Of these 3 possibilities, the likelihood that he is a carrier (Rr) is 2 in 3.

(Section 12: Clinical Genetics and Dysmorphology, Chapter 165: Principles for the Practice of Clinical Genetics: Monogenic Conditions)

**Answer 4-15.** C

Although the overall phenotypic pattern of Down syndrome is characteristic and identifiable, specific physical examination findings can be found in patients without Down syndrome. For example, the presence of a single transverse crease is a nonsensitive and nonspecific physical examination finding for Down syndrome.

Down syndrome is the most common autosomal chromosomal abnormality, with a frequency of 1 in 800 infants. Physical examination is likely to reveal hypotonia in approximately 90% of infants with Down syndrome. Congenital cardiac issues occur in 40% of infants with Down syndrome. As a result, an echocardiogram is commonly a part of routine health supervision for Down syndrome.

Over 90% of infants with Down syndrome have 3 separate copies of chromosome 21; however, approximately 10% have trisomy due to a translocation of only a part of the long arm of chromosome 21.

(Section 12: Clinical Genetics and Dysmorphology, Chapter 166: Chromosomal and Genomic Disorders)

**Answer 4-16.** B

The child has Beckwith-Wiedemann syndrome. These patients generally do quite well cognitively unless there are problems with untreated hypoglycemia in infancy. The other features on the list are possible complications of Beckwith-Wiedemann syndrome but have not been associated with the development of cognitive impairment.

(Section 12: Clinical Genetics and Dysmorphology, Chapter 171: Birth Defects, Malformations, and Syndromes)

**Answer 4-17.** D

The baby has Down syndrome, caused by trisomy of chromosome 21. It is a clinical diagnosis. A routine karyotype test is necessary to evaluate for a translocation trisomy as this has implications for higher recurrence and indicates a need to test the parents. Fluorescence in situ hybridization studies do not differentiate free from translocation trisomy and are not indicated in this situation. The other testing is inappropriate for the question being asked.

(Section 12: Clinical Genetics and Dysmorphology, Chapter 166: Chromosomal and Genomic Disorders and Chapter 167: Laboratory Analysis of Copy Number and Single Nucleotide Variants)

**Answer 4-18.** E

Chromosomal aneuploidy is thought to account for the majority of early-pregnancy losses. While important in all of the other signs and symptoms, most genetic disease is not chromosomally based and so chromosomal aneuploidy as a whole is not the single leading cause of any of the other conditions.

(Section 12: Clinical Genetics and Dysmorphology, Chapter 165: Principles for the Practice of Clinical Genetics, Chapter 166: Chromosomal and Genomic Disorders, Chapter 167: Laboratory Analysis of Copy Number and Single Nucleotide Variants)

**Answer 4-19.** E

Penetrance is defined as the proportion of individuals with the genotype who manifest any part of the phenotype. Answer choice B is the definition of expressivity. The other statements are not standard definitions of common terms.

(Section 12: Clinical Genetics and Dysmorphology, Chapter 165: Principles for the Practice of Clinical Genetics)

**Answer 4-20.** B

Expressivity is defined as the degree of variation or severity among people who express the phenotype. Answer choice E is the definition of penetrance. The other statements are not standard definitions of common terms.

(Section 12: Clinical Genetics and Dysmorphology, Chapter 165: Principles for the Practice of Clinical Genetics)

**Answer 4-21.** A

This situation describes a dominant negative mutation, which is, itself, a type of loss-of-function mutation. Haploinsufficiency results when 50% of the gene product is insufficient for normal development and/or function. The other 2 answers are not mechanisms of mutation.

(Section 12: Clinical Genetics and Dysmorphology, Chapter 166: Chromosomal and Genomic Disorders)

**Answer 4-22.** A

Although Angelman syndrome, Rett syndrome, tuberous sclerosis, and fragile X syndrome can be associated with autism, the phenotype of prognathism, paroxysmal laughter, and tongue thrusting make Angelman syndrome more likely. Angelman syndrome occurs when a mutated *UBE3A* is inherited through the mother. Prader-Willi syndrome results if the gene is inherited from the father. Methylation testing for UPD15 can help confirm the diagnosis.

(Section 12: Clinical Genetics and Dysmorphology, Chapter 173: Genetic Evaluation of Intellectual Disability and Autism)

**Answer 4-23.** C

Both mothers/sisters inherited a mutated *UBE3A* from their father. Because it is inactive when inherited from the father, the mutation is silent and the women are healthy. But when they conceived their own children, the mutated gene became active again. Inheritance by their children of the mutated gene will result in Angelman syndrome. The children will have no active or normal copy of the gene because the allele inherited from the father will be inactive. Coincidence and uniparental disomy of 15 are possible but much less likely. Deletion of the entire region would either have to have occurred separately in each pregnancy, which is highly unlikely, or be carried by both women as inherited from a parent.

If the women had inherited the deletion, they would have one of the conditions. Specifically, they would have Angelman syndrome if inherited from their mother and Prader-Willi syndrome if inherited from their father.

Nonpaternity is irrelevant to this condition because the paternal gene is inactive.

(Section 12: Clinical Genetics and Dysmorphology, Chapter 166: Chromosomal and Genomic Disorders)

**Answer 4-24.** B

PWS is caused by a deletion of 2 to 4 Mb of chromosome 15. When the deletion is inherited from the father, the child will have PWS. The phenotype includes severe neonatal hypotonia, obesity, small hands and feet, and intellectual disability. Although infants may be described as having a "failure to thrive" during infancy due to the initial hypotonia, the syndrome is also associated with polyphagia and subsequent obesity.

Angelman syndrome is also caused by a microdeletion on chromosome 15. When this microdeletion is inherited via the mother, Angelman syndrome results, which has a different phenotype.

(Section 12: Clinical Genetics and Dysmorphology, Chapter 173: Genetic Evaluation of Intellectual Disability and Autism)

**Answer 4-25.** D

This scenario is considered a standard example of the founder effect; however, other factors must come into play for the founder effect to manifest. Endogamy (marriage within the group) and consanguinity (mating between related individuals) are part of the process perpetuating the mutation. In addition, a population "bottleneck" occurred. Tay-Sachs does confer decreased fitness, but that is not what is driving the increased prevalence. Genetic drift is random fluctuation in gene frequencies and is essentially the opposite of this situation.

(Section 12: Clinical Genetics and Dysmorphology, Chapter 165: Principles for the Practice of Clinical Genetics)

**Answer 4-26.** D

Studies in monozygotic twins who are raised apart are the best twin studies because the children are presumed to be genetically identical (or near-identical) but they have been exposed to different postnatal environments. This works for behavioral and psychological studies but not, obviously, for studies of birth defects. For that, the studies compare monozygotic and dizygotic twins, but that is not one of the choices. The other choices are not relevant to this question.

(Section 12: Clinical Genetics and Dysmorphology, Chapter 165: Principles for the Practice of Clinical Genetics)

**Answer 4-27.** D

The description is most consistent with Treacher Collins syndrome. Persons with Treacher Collins syndrome are typically cognitively normal, but they often have conductive hearing loss (see figure below).

Goldenhar syndrome, or oculoauriculovertebral syndrome, is also associated with anomalies involving the head and neck. The phenotype includes hemifacial microsomia and anomalies of the pinna with associated deafness. Other findings include ear tags, vertebral anomalies, and Arnold-Chiari type I malformations (herniation of the cerebellum into the cervical spinal canal).

Pierre Robin sequence is characterized by a triad of cleft palate, micrognathia, and glossoptosis.

Smith-Lemli-Opitz syndrome is associated with cleft palate, micrognathia, short nose, ptosis, high square forehead, microcephaly, hypospadias, cryptorchidism, ventricular septal defect, tetralogy of Fallot, hypotonia, mental retardation, postaxial polydactyly, 2-3 toe syndactyly, and defect in cholesterol biosynthesis.

CHARGE syndrome consists of coloboma of the eye, heart malformations, atresia (choanal), retardation, genital anomalies, ear abnormalities and/or deafness, facial palsy, cleft palate, and dysphagia.

(Section 12: Clinical Genetics and Dysmorphology, Chapter 166: Chromosomal and Genomic Disorders)

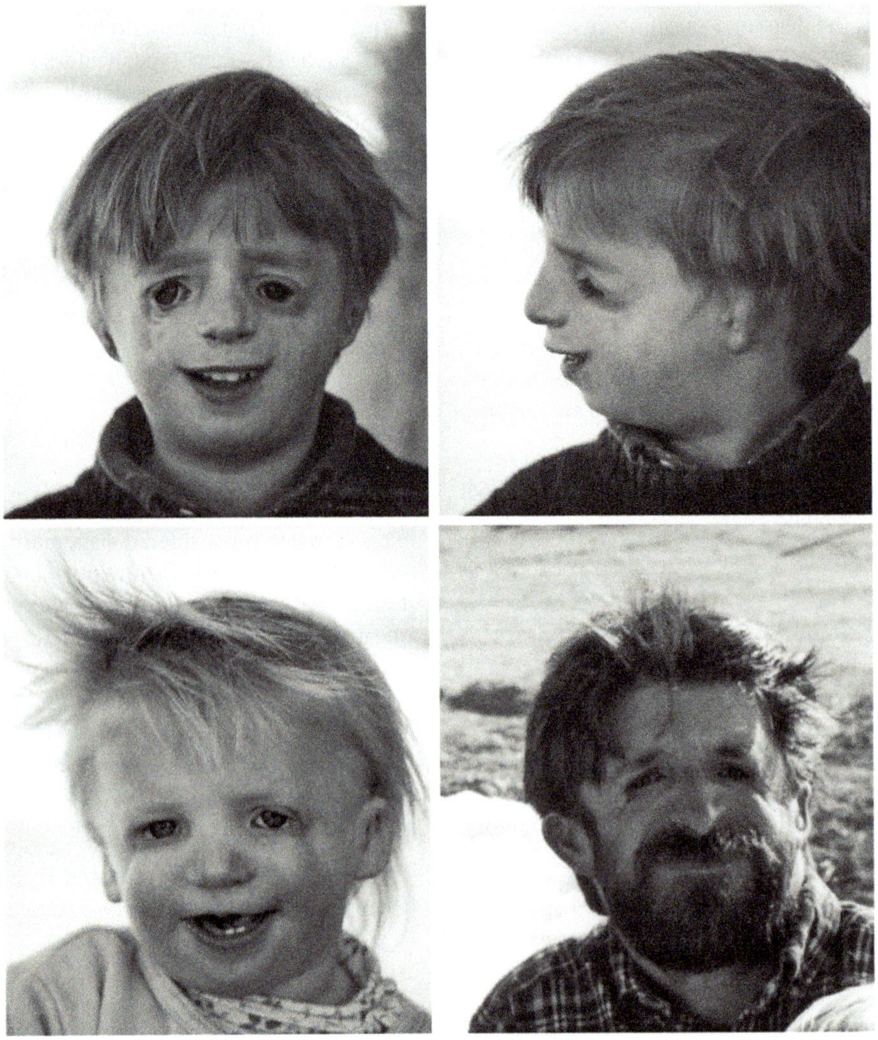

Treacher Collins syndrome. Two siblings (top and lower left) with variable manifestations of autosomal dominant Treacher Collins syndrome. The father (lower right panel) was the first individual in his family known to have Treacher Collins syndrome. Both children were born with cleft palate, but their father has an intact palate. (Reproduced, with permission, from Rudolph CD, Rudolph AM, Lister GE, First LR, Gershon AA. *Rudolph's Pediatrics*. 22nd ed. New York, NY: McGraw-Hill; 2011.)

**Answer 4-28.** A

People with Treacher Collins syndrome are typically cognitively normal, but they often have conductive hearing loss. The single most important intervention is placement of bone conduction hearing aids as young as possible. Other hearing assistive devices can be explored over time. Palate surgery is not indicated at this time in this child. The mandible may need to be distracted and the child may need speech therapy, but those are not of urgent importance. Sign language training may be useful depending on the situation, but it may slow rather than assist spoken language development.

(Section 12: Clinical Genetics and Dysmorphology, Chapter 166: Chromosomal and Genomic Disorders)

**Answer 4-29.** E

The collagen I protein is a triple helix consisting of 2 A1 polypeptides and 1 A2 polypeptide. As with twisted fibers of a rope, abnormality of 1 polypeptide—A1 or A2—will interfere with the structure of the final protein. Deletions or other mutations that lead to decreased polypeptide synthesis result in decreased but otherwise normal protein. Epigenetic factors are not relevant to this question. Gene deletions are more likely to be inherited because they are less likely to result in lethal disease or spontaneous abortion.

(Section 12: Clinical Genetics and Dysmorphology, Chapter 180: Connective Tissue Disorders)

**Answer 4-30.** D

The combination of findings describes the Pierre Robin sequence. It is not a syndrome because it does not have a single consistent etiology. It is a sequence of embryologic events starting with failure of the jaw to grow. The tongue then prevents the palatal folds from fusing. A disruption is a chemical or physical interference of a structure with normal primary embryogenesis. A field defect results from spatially related abnormalities. An association is a set of defects that occur more frequently together than expected by chance alone.

(Section 12: Clinical Genetics and Dysmorphology, Chapter 165: Principles for the Practice of Clinical Genetics)

**Answer 4-31.** B

This child presents with autism spectrum disorder and skin findings. Her clinical presentation is consistent with a diagnosis of tuberous sclerosis. The child has adenoma sebaceum, which is composed of numerous angiofibromas (skin-colored to red papules) over the central face. They continue to increase in size and number with age.

The 1- to 4-cm hypopigmented macules can be shaped like "ash leaves" (eg, "ash leaf spots"), but they can also be round, oval, irregular, or confetti-like in their appearance. The presence of 3 or more hypomelanotic macules at birth should raise suspicion for tuberous sclerosis and warrants further evaluation.

Connective tissue nevi, which include a fibrous forehead plaque and shagreen patches (collagenomas, a type of connective tissue nevus), may also aid in early diagnosis, especially when the fibrous forehead plaque is present at birth. Other cutaneous findings of tuberous sclerosis include periungal fibromas and gingival fibromas.

While dermatology referral may be useful, there is no directed treatment that will cure the skin and nail findings. Brain MRI or computed tomography is indicated because 75% or more of patients with tuberous sclerosis will have brain hamartomata. None of the other options is indicated.

(Section 12: Clinical Genetics and Dysmorphology, Chapter 173: Genetic Evaluation of Intellectual Disability and Autism, Chapter 176: Neurocutaneous Disorders)

**Answer 4-32.** B

These are all disorders of accelerated aging: they all have features that are generally associated with normal advanced age (eg, loss of hair, loose skin, osteopenia, cataracts). None of these is a disorder of collagen or a nucleotide excision repair disorder, although some of the diseases of accelerated aging fall in that group. They are not ectodermal dysplasias. Cutis laxa is not a laminopathy, and the causative gene for Hallermann-Streiff has not been identified.

(Section 12: Clinical Genetics and Dysmorphology, Chapter 165: Principles for the Practice of Clinical Genetics)

**Answer 4-33.** C

Height or length is the best comparator. Weight is too variable with environmental factors. The other parameters are not useful. Age is not a growth parameter either, although comparison of the child's head circumference against growth standards can be useful to determine whether the problem is an overall growth deficiency or just microcephaly.

(Section 12: Clinical Genetics and Dysmorphology, Chapter 165: Principles for the Practice of Clinical Genetics)

**Answer 4-34.** A

Balanced translocations are those in which there is no net gain or loss of genetic material. It is not unusual for otherwise healthy fetuses or newborns to be diagnosed by amniocentesis because of maternal issues such as advanced maternal age. In these instances, the finding is coincidental. Umbilical cord blood testing because of stem cell banking is a possible way to find the translocation but is much less likely than the amniocentesis diagnosis. The other choices are not indicated because the child did not have any of those findings.

(Section 12: Clinical Genetics and Dysmorphology, Chapter 166: Chromosomal and Genomic Disorders)

**Answer 4-35.** A

Any factor that decreases joint mobility—intrinsic genetic neuromuscular abnormality, teratogen, or mechanical construction—will lead to joint contractures.

(Section 12: Clinical Genetics and Dysmorphology, Chapter 171: Birth Defects, Malformations, and Syndromes)

**Answer 4-36.** E

It is true that no 2 people have exactly the same genome—identical twins coming the closest. However, for the vast majority of genes, there is a standard sequence, which varies little if at all from person to person. This level of variation is nonpathogenic. The way that this base pair variation happens is through the various mechanisms of mutation. The mutation stays in the population through failure of DNA repair mechanisms *and* the fact that the variation does not negatively impact the reproductive fitness of the individual. All of the other possible answers do create person-to-person variation but do not cause change in the primary base pair sequence of the genome.

(Section 12: Clinical Genetics and Dysmorphology, Chapter 165: Principles for the Practice of Clinical Genetics)

**Answer 4-37.** B

The child has a midline cleft lip: cleft with absence of the prolabium represents a primary midline craniofacial defect and is on the holoprosencephaly spectrum. When midline cleft lip is present, the child should be assumed to have holoprosencephaly until it is ruled out. While any of the other brain malformations can occur with facial abnormalities, holoprosencephaly is the most likely.

(Section 12: Clinical Genetics and Dysmorphology, Chapter 166: Chromosomal and Genomic Disorders)

**Answer 4-38.** C

The baby has trisomy 13. The infant has a midline cleft and postaxial polydactyly. In addition, intrauterine growth restriction and structural abnormalities of the heart and brain are present. The appropriate test to confirm trisomy 13 is a routine karyotype.

(Section 12: Clinical Genetics and Dysmorphology, Chapter 166: Chromosomal and Genomic Disorders)

**Answer 4-39.** C

This patient most likely has Cornelia de Lange syndrome.

Moebius sequence is associated with congenital facial palsy, cranial nerve VI and VII palsy, distal limb deficiencies, occasional arthrogryposis, and/or intellectual disability.

Sturge-Weber syndrome is associated with hemangiomata in the distribution of the trigeminal nerve, glaucoma, and seizures.

Beckwith-Wiedemann syndrome is associated with coarse facial features, macroglossia (often with secondary maxillary and mandibular deformity), earlobe creases, posterior auricular pits, mid-face hypoplasia, omphalocele, generalized overgrowth or hemihypertrophy, visceromegaly, Wilms tumor (and other malignancies), cryptorchidism, and cardiomyopathy.

Cleidocranial dysplasia is associated with brachycephaly, frontal and parietal bossing, wormian bones, persistent open anterior fontanelle, maxillary hypoplasia, delayed eruption of deciduous and permanent teeth, supernumerary and fused teeth, hypoplastic to absent clavicles, brachydactyly, and joint laxity.

(Section 12: Clinical Genetics and Dysmorphology, Chapter 171: Birth Defects, Malformations, and Syndromes)

# CHAPTER 5 Disorders of Metabolism

Ayesha Ahmad, Elizabeth G. Ames, and Kristen N. Lee

**5-1.** Most inborn errors of metabolism are inherited by an autosomal recessive mode of inheritance. Which of the following is an example of an inborn error of metabolism with X-linked recessive inheritance and significant variability in clinical phenotype?

- **A.** Ornithine transcarbamylase deficiency
- **B.** Propionic acidemia
- **C.** Methylmalonic acidemia
- **D.** Biotinidase deficiency
- **E.** Citrullinemia

**5-2.** A 3-day-old male neonate presents to the emergency department (ED) with a 1-day history of poor feeding. He was born to a 21-year-old primigravida after a normal pregnancy and delivery. In the ED, you note that he is lethargic. Vitals are notable for temperature of 36.7°C, heart rate of 185 bpm, respiratory rate of 46 breaths/min, and blood pressure of 65/35 mm Hg. During your evaluation, the patient becomes increasingly hypotonic and does not respond to sternal rub. Arterial blood gas reveals a respiratory alkalosis, normal glucose, and normal lactic acid level. Of the following, which is the most important next diagnostic test?

- **A.** Urine organic acids
- **B.** Plasma amino acids
- **C.** Urine-reducing substances
- **D.** Plasma ammonia level
- **E.** Plasma acylcarnitine profile

**5-3.** A 3-day-old male neonate presents to the emergency department (ED) with a 1-day history of poor feeding. He is lethargic, and vitals are notable for temperature of 36.7°C, heart rate of 185 bpm, respiratory rate of 46 breaths/min, and blood pressure of 65/35 mm Hg. During your evaluation, the patient becomes increasingly hypotonic and does not respond to sternal rub. Arterial blood gas reveals a respiratory alkalosis, normal glucose, and normal lactic acid level. A plasma ammonia level test shows the neonate has hyperammonemia. You complete a normal saline bolus of 20 mL/kg. His heart rate is now 162 bpm, and blood pressure is now 76/46 mm Hg. What type of fluids do you now order?

- **A.** Repeat normal saline bolus of 20 mL/kg
- **B.** 5% dextrose at maintenance rate
- **C.** 5% dextrose at 150% (1.5 times) maintenance
- **D.** 10% dextrose at maintenance rate
- **E.** 10% dextrose at 150% (1.5 times) maintenance

**5-4.** Which of the following scenarios should prompt you to evaluate further for a possible underlying metabolic disorder?

- **A.** A previously healthy 2-year-old child with increasing fever for 5 days, poor oral intake for 2 days, and metabolic acidosis
- **B.** A neurocognitively normal, healthy 3-year-old child in the care of his grandmother, with sudden onset of lethargy and anion gap metabolic acidosis
- **C.** A 3-week-old infant with emesis, somnolence, anion gap metabolic acidosis, and significant ketosis (urinary ketones 4+)
- **D.** A 5-year-old child with lethargy, anion gap metabolic acidosis, and blood glucose of 351 mg/dL
- **E.** A 7-month-old baby with a 3-day history of persistent diarrhea and hyperchloremic, non–anion gap metabolic acidosis

**5-5.** You are meeting with a pregnant couple for a prenatal visit. They request information on current newborn screening. Which statement are you *most* likely to include in your discussion?

**A.** A positive newborn screen is almost always diagnostic for a specific condition, and confirmatory testing is often not needed.

**B.** The advent of newer technology now allows for the detection of > 50 different metabolic disorders by newborn screening.

**C.** Only disorders that are fatal if left untreated are included in newborn screening.

**D.** Blood spot cards for newborn screening have to be collected immediately after birth, within the first 6 hours.

**E.** Only disorders that have an incidence of > 1 in 10,000 births are included in newborn screening.

**5-6.** You have just been informed by your state newborn screening laboratory that one of your patients has a positive newborn screen for phenylketonuria (PKU). This child is a healthy, term, 5-day-old male child. You have scheduled an appointment to see the patient and meet with the parents, who are white. Which of the following statements about PKU do you include in your discussion with the parents?

**A.** PKU is an extremely rare genetic disorder and is especially rare in whites.

**B.** If the newborn is feeding well and has a normal physical examination, he is unlikely to have PKU.

**C.** PKU can be treated by dietary manipulation and its effects prevented by timely intervention.

**D.** This is most likely a false-positive newborn screening result, and no further action is needed.

**E.** About 50% of individuals with untreated PKU develop severe mental disability.

**5-7.** A 2-year-old new patient presents to clinic for initial evaluation. Her mother reports 2 episodes in the past year of unsteady gait associated with viral illness with resolution of symptoms when well. She also reports an intermittent "sweet caramel-type" odor to her child's skin. Past medical history is otherwise normal. Neurodevelopmental parameters are age appropriate. Current growth parameters and physical examination are normal. What is your recommendation?

**A.** Further evaluation for a biotin-responsive disorder

**B.** Further evaluation for a branched-chain amino acid disorder

**C.** Plasma glucose and urinalysis to evaluate for type 1 diabetes mellitus

**D.** Referral and an evaluation by an infectious disease specialist

**E.** Magnetic resonance imaging (MRI) of the brain to ensure no intracranial abnormalities

**5-8.** A 5-day-old term neonate presents to the emergency department (ED). Her parents report a 2- to 3-day history of poor feeding and a 1-day history of increasing lethargy. She has an anion gap of 22, pH of 7.17, and a glucose level of 24 mg/dL. Urinalysis reveals the presence of large urinary ketones. Which of the following laboratory evaluations is *most* likely to lead to an underlying diagnosis?

**A.** Urine organic acids

**B.** Free and total carnitine levels

**C.** Very-long-chain fatty acids

**D.** Urine-reducing substances

**E.** Urine amino acids

**5-9.** An 18-year-old with a history of cognitive impairment is referred for evaluation from an ophthalmologist with a diagnosis of downward subluxation of the ocular lens (see following figure). Which of the following tests is most likely to be abnormal and lead to an underlying diagnosis?

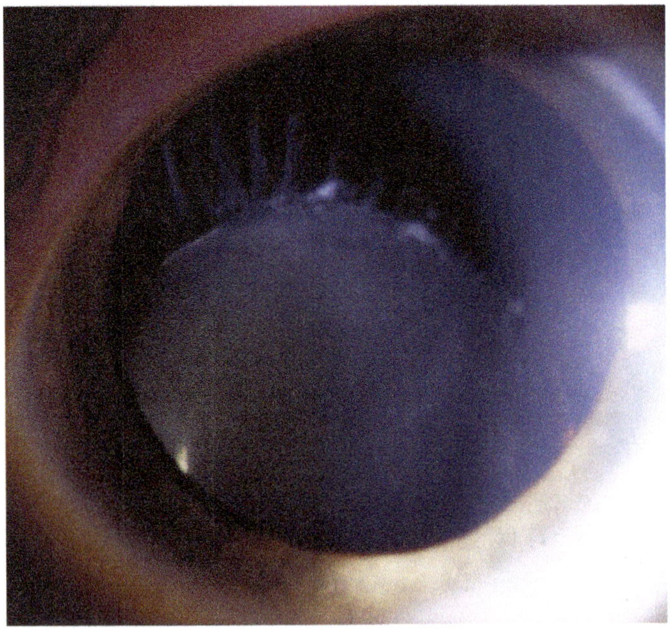

(Reproduced, with permission, from Lueder GT. *Pediatric Practice Ophthalmology*. New York, NY: McGraw-Hill; 2011.)

**A.** Chromosomal analysis

**B.** Free and total carnitine levels

**C.** Urine organic acids

**D.** Total homocysteine level

**E.** Acylcarnitine profile

**5-10.** A term neonate is transferred to the neonatal intensive care unit from the well-baby nursery secondary to new onset of seizures noted at 16 hours of age. He was born after a normal pregnancy with no complications during delivery. He appeared normal at birth. At 16 hours of age, he developed myoclonic seizures and recurrent hiccups. A sepsis evaluation was completed and intravenous antibiotics initiated. All cultures are negative at 24 hours. Over the next day, he develops apnea. He is unresponsive and has continued seizure activity despite use of antiepileptic medications. Electroencephalogram (EEG) reveals burst suppression. Laboratory evaluation reveals normal pH, glucose, ammonia, and lactic acid levels. There is no ketonuria. What is the most likely underlying inborn error of metabolism?

**A.** Homocystinuria

**B.** Glutathione synthase deficiency

**C.** Hyperprolinemia type 1

**D.** Hyperlysinemia

**E.** Nonketotic hyperglycinemia

**5-11.** A 5-month-old, previously healthy infant has sudden onset of hypotonia and dystonia after an intercurrent illness. She was born with macrocephaly and adopted from China at the age of 2 months. A brain magnetic resonance imaging (MRI) is completed and shows degeneration of the caudate and putamen with frontal atrophy. Which of the following diagnostic tests is most likely to reveal the underlying diagnosis?

**A.** Galactose-1-phosphate level

**B.** Urine organic acids

**C.** Ceruloplasmin level

**D.** Copper level

**E.** Urine mucopolysaccharides

**5-12.** A 10-year-old boy presents with recurrent episodes of lower back and abdominal pain. He has a history of passage of stones. He is on a regular diet. An ultrasound of the kidneys and bladder reveals stones in the urinary bladder. He is neurocognitively normal. Review of past medical history reveals no other medical problems. What is the most likely diagnosis?

**A.** Cystinuria

**B.** Cystinosis

**C.** Lysinuric protein intolerance

**D.** Hartnup disease

**E.** Creatine metabolism defect

**5-13.** A 3-day-old comatose male neonate is noted to have an ammonia level of 550 μmol/L. What is the next most critical treatment option that should be initiated emergently to provide the best neurocognitive outcome?

**A.** Administer a bolus of intravenous (IV) arginine

**B.** Make immediate arrangements to initiate hemodialysis

**C.** Administer lactulose for gut sterilization

**D.** Start a 20-mg/kg bolus of normal saline

**E.** Administer IV sodium benzoate

**5-14.** A 6-month-old male infant is brought in by his adoptive parents for evaluation of a skin rash. He has been exclusively formula fed with standard infant formulas. He was recently adopted from an orphanage overseas. He has history of recurrent diaper rashes and seizures. During evaluation for seizures, he was also found to have an increased anion gap metabolic acidosis. In your office, he is noted to have alopecia, an eczematous periorificial skin rash, and candidiasis, and he is hypotonic. This history should prompt you to evaluate for a deficiency of which compound?

**A.** Folate

**B.** Vitamin D

**C.** Zinc

**D.** Biotin

**E.** Vitamin $B_{12}$

**5-15.** A 4-month-old, previously healthy female infant is brought to the emergency department (ED) with a 2-day history of poor oral intake associated with diarrhea and vomiting. Mother reports decreased oral intake and decreased activity level over the past few days. The infant has not been febrile. Mother found the child in her crib this morning, limp and lethargic, and immediately came to the ED. A serum glucose level is collected and is noted to be 25 mg/dL. A dextrose bolus is initiated. No hepatomegaly is noted on physical examination. Electrolytes reveal a bicarbonate level of 18 mg/dL and glucose level of 25 mg/dL, without other significant abnormalities. A stat ammonia level is noted to be normal. A venous blood gas reveals a pH of 7.35, $CO_2$ of 38 mmHg, and $HCO_3$ of 18 mmol/L. Urinalysis reveals a specific gravity of 1.030, negative glucose, negative protein, and negative ketones. Rhythm strip in the ED shows an arrhythmia, and follow-up stat echocardiogram shows a mild to moderately dilated right atrium and ventricle. What is the most likely underlying class of diagnosis?

**A.** Organic acidemia

**B.** Fatty acid oxidation disorder

**C.** Glycogen storage disease

**D.** Urea cycle disorder

**E.** Type 1 diabetes mellitus

**5-16.** You are evaluating a 4-month-old male infant, who is currently hospitalized after his parents brought him to the emergency department (ED) after a generalized tonic-clonic seizure related to an episode of hypoglycemia, with a glucose level of 20 mg/dL on arrival to the hospital. He was in his normal state of health until 2 days prior to admission, when he was noted to have increased upper airway congestion associated with poor oral intake. He normally feeds every 4 to 5 hours. His mother states she skipped his overnight feeding the night before admission.

He was given a bolus of dextrose intravenously and was started on dextrose-containing intravenous (IV) fluids. On physical examination, you note a protuberant abdomen, and you feel the liver edge 6 to 7 cm below the right costal margin. The spleen tip is also palpable. Laboratory evaluation is remarkable for an elevated lactic acid level, elevated uric acid level, mildly elevated transaminases, and an elevated triglyceride level. What is the most likely diagnosis?

**A.** Glycogen storage disease type I
**B.** Phosphofructokinase deficiency
**C.** Fructose 1,6-bisphosphatase deficiency
**D.** Uridine diphosphate galactose-4-epimerase deficiency
**E.** Ribose-5-phosphate isomerase deficiency

**5-17.** A 4-month-old male infant is hospitalized after a generalized tonic-clonic seizure related to an episode of hypoglycemia. The infant also has an enlarged liver, elevated lactic acid level, elevated uric acid level, and an elevated triglyceride level, leading to a diagnosis of glycogen storage disease (GSD) type I. In your discussion with the parents of the infant, what is the most appropriate mechanism to prevent nighttime hypoglycemia?

**A.** Regularly administering glucagon
**B.** Adding cornstarch to all his feeds
**C.** Providing continuous nighttime nasogastric feeds
**D.** Feeding him *ad libitum* with a standard infant formula fortified to 24 kcal/oz
**E.** Ensuring he does not go longer than 6 hours between feeds

**5-18.** One of your 15-year-old patients presents to clinic with complaints of muscle cramps and muscle pain with exercise. He is not especially physically active; however, recently he decided to join his school's track team. He reports one incident of tea-colored urine after a 400-m sprint. He denies any other medical problems. He reports that if he rests at the first sign of pain, he can resume exercise at a slower pace after a short period of time. You check a creatine phosphokinase level, which is mildly elevated; electrolyte levels, renal function, and aspartate aminotransferase/alanine aminotransferase levels are normal. You suspect a diagnosis of McArdle disease. Which of the following diagnostic modalities would you recommend to establish the diagnosis?

**A.** Plasma acylcarnitine profile
**B.** Liver biopsy for enzymatic analysis
**C.** An ischemia exercise test
**D.** Urine organic acid analysis
**E.** Molecular sequencing

**5-19.** You are evaluating a 3-month-old infant in the emergency department (ED) with tachypnea and tachycardia. The family reports he has always "seemed a bit floppy." He was born at term gestation, after an unremarkable pregnancy and delivery. Birth weight and length were in the 50th percentile. Parents note they have had an increasingly difficult time with feeding, as he is taking longer to finish bottles. On examination, he is noted to be at the 3rd percentile for weight and 25th percentile for length and has macroglossia, hepatomegaly, and diffuse hypotonia. Deep tendon reflexes are present bilaterally. Chest x-ray reveals cardiomegaly. Stat electrocardiogram reveals high-voltage QRS complexes and shortened PR intervals. Echocardiogram reveals biventricular wall thickening. Complete blood count, blood gas, and lactate are within normal limits for age. Comprehensive metabolic panel is significant for elevated transaminases. Creatine phosphokinase level is 2500 IU/L. What is the most likely underlying diagnosis?

**A.** McArdle disease (muscle phosphorylase deficiency)
**B.** Pompe disease (acid glucosidase deficiency)
**C.** X-linked phosphorylase kinase deficiency
**D.** Glycogen synthase deficiency
**E.** Muscle phosphofructokinase deficiency

**5-20.** A 4-day-old breastfed female neonate presents with poor feeding, lethargy, jaundice, and hypotension. A concurrent septic and metabolic workup is initiated, the baby is pan-cultured, and appropriate intravenous (IV) fluids and antibiotics are started. Blood and urine cultures reveal sepsis due to *Escherichia coli*. On physical examination, she is lethargic, her skin appears icteric, and she has hepatomegaly. Testing on urine reveals presence of non–glucose-reducing substances. What is the most likely underlying diagnosis?

**A.** Glycogen storage disease (GSD)

**B.** Maple syrup urine disease (MSUD)

**C.** Organic acidemia

**D.** Galactosemia

**E.** Urea cycle defect

**5-21.** The respiratory chain is the terminal pathway of mitochondrial metabolism, where most energy is produced as adenosine triphosphate (ATP). Defects of the respiratory chain cause an extremely heterogeneous group of disorders that affect both children and adults and can affect single tissues as well as have multiorgan involvement. Which statement best describes mitochondrial respiratory chain genetics?

**A.** The rules of mitochondrial genetics are the same as the rules of Mendelian genetics.

**B.** Each cell contains 50 to 100 copies of mitochondrial DNA, which distribute randomly among daughter cells at cell division.

**C.** At cell division, the proportion of mutant mitochondrial DNA in daughter cells always remains constant.

**D.** All respiratory chain disorders, when inherited, always come from the maternal lineage.

**E.** At fertilization, all mitochondrial DNA is derived from the oocyte.

**5-22.** A 15-year-old girl presents with a 4- to 6-month history of recurrent vomiting and migraine-like headaches and 2 stroke-like episodes associated with hemiparesis. Early developmental milestones are normal. Magnetic resonance imaging (MRI) of the brain reveals basal ganglia calcifications and "infarcts" in the posterior cerebral hemispheres, not corresponding to the distribution of major vessels. Molecular analysis reveals a mitochondrial DNA pathogenic variant in the tRNA-Leu gene. Which of the following statements is correct?

**A.** This patient is likely to have an elevated lactic acid level.

**B.** Ophthalmoplegia is a characteristic finding in this disorder.

**C.** This condition is an autosomal recessive disorder.

**D.** This patient will most likely develop cataracts in the next 2 to 3 years.

**E.** Treatment for this condition with mitochondrial cofactors is well established.

**5-23.** A 1.5-year-old patient with mucopolysaccharidosis (MPS) type I (Hurler syndrome) is followed in your practice. Which of the following statements is important to review with her parents?

**A.** Anesthesia is particularly difficult, and surgery should only be performed in centers with experience in managing difficult pediatric airways.

**B.** Most patients with MPS type I syndrome do not survive beyond the age of 2 to 3 years.

**C.** This is an X-linked disorder; therefore, recurrence risks for the parents of this child may be as high as 50% if the subsequent child is a boy.

**D.** Patients with MPS type I are at high risk for seizures as the disorder progresses.

**E.** This is a progressive, lysosomal storage disorder with no effective treatment options.

**5-24.** A 9-year-old white girl presents with a history of recurrent bruising and nosebleeds. She also reports a longstanding history of nonprogressive bilateral leg pain that seems to be worse at night. No developmental or neurocognitive concerns are identified. Examination reveals painless hepatosplenomegaly. Neurologic examination is normal. Complete blood count reveals a low platelet level and mild anemia. You recommend a referral to hematology/oncology. Extensive evaluation by this service, including a bone marrow examination, does not reveal a malignancy or primary hematologic disorder. Which of the following conditions should be on your differential diagnosis?

**A.** Sandhoff disease

**B.** Krabbe disease

**C.** Farber disease

**D.** Gaucher disease

**E.** Tay-Sachs disease

**5-25.** A 13-year-old boy presents to clinic with onset of episodic, severe, burning pain in his hands and feet. He states this episode began during a family ski vacation after he was out on the mountain all day. He has had similar episodes at least twice over the past 5 years, triggered by activity or illness. Physical examination is significant for tenderness to palpation of the small joints in his hands, periumbilical tenderness of the abdomen, and significant allodynia in his distal extremities. Additionally, he is noted to have several reddish-black papular lesions around his umbilicus. He states that 2 of his maternal uncles have a similar rash and shares that one of these uncles is receiving dialysis; the other is currently recovering at home after suffering a stroke. What therapy would you recommend initiating now for the most effective treatment of the complications that result from the pathophysiology of this disorder?

**A.** There is no effective therapy for this disorder.

**B.** Surgical referral for abdominal pain

**C.** Bone marrow transplantation

**D.** Liver transplantation

**E.** Enzyme replacement therapy (ERT)

**5-26.** A 1-month-old female infant is hospitalized for evaluation of conjugated hyperbilirubinemia and failure to thrive. She is noted to have a large high forehead, large anterior fontanelle, epicanthal folds, a small nose, broad nasal bridge, and micrognathia. She is profoundly hypotonic. Ophthalmology evaluation reveals cataracts and a pigmentary retinopathy. Which of the following evaluations is most likely to provide a diagnosis?

**A.** Plasma very-long-chain fatty acids

**B.** Serum free and total carnitine levels

**C.** Plasma amino acids

**D.** Biotinidase enzyme assay

**E.** Urine organic acids

**5-27.** Glycosylation is an important posttranslational protein modification. A growing family of genetic disorders, called congenital disorders of glycosylation (CDGs), are caused by defects in protein glycosylation. Which of the following statements best describes the phenotype associated with CDGs?

**A.** Most CDGs are benign disorders with normal neurocognitive development.

**B.** The majority of CDGs can be easily treated with enzyme replacement therapy (ERT).

**C.** Most CDGs are severe multisystem disorders with neurologic involvement.

**D.** Most CDGs show an X-linked mode of inheritance.

**E.** Important tools in the diagnostic evaluation of suspected CDGs include very-long-chain fatty acid analysis.

**5-28.** A 25-year-old primigravida delivers a term male infant with growth restriction. Prenatal maternal screening revealed low estriol levels. On physical examination, the newborn is microcephalic, has a cleft palate, and has 2 to 3 toe syndactyly. What is the most likely underlying diagnosis?

**A.** Desmosterolosis

**B.** Mevalonic aciduria

**C.** Chondrodysplasia punctate

**D.** Smith-Lemli-Opitz syndrome

**E.** CHILD syndrome

**5-29.** Disorders affecting low-density lipoprotein (LDL) receptor (LDLR) activity lead to elevations in LDL cholesterol. Which of the following statements best describes familial hypercholesterolemia (FH), a disorder that results from mutations in the LDL receptor?

**A.** FH is an X-linked disorder that presents in adolescence.

**B.** Heterozygosity for FH affects about 1 in 5000 people.

**C.** Twenty-five to 50% of untreated adults with heterozygous FH will develop cardiovascular disease by age 50.

**D.** Patients who are homozygotes for FH have milder manifestations than patients with heterozygous FH.

**E.** About 1 in 50,000 individuals are homozygous for FH.

**5-30.** Which of the following statements best describes the porphyrias (disorders of heme biosynthesis)?

**A.** The enzyme deficiencies leading to the porphyrias are all inherited as autosomal recessive disorders.

**B.** These disorders are primarily classified as hepatic or erythropoietic, depending on the primary site of overproduction or accumulation of the porphyrin.

**C.** Manifestations of the erythropoietic porphyrias characteristically include abdominal pain, neuropathy, and mental disturbance.

**D.** Manifestations of the hepatic porphyrias characteristically include cutaneous photosensitivity.

**E.** There are currently no known environmental factors involved in the pathophysiology of these disorders.

**5-31.** A 1-year-old boy presents with a history of irritability and generalized muscle weakness. His mother reports a history of "brownish-red sand" in his diapers. She reports normal development in the first 4 months of life with concern for developmental delay and low muscle tone noted around 6 months of age. Your review of prior laboratory tests reveals an elevated uric acid level. What is the most likely diagnosis?

**A.** Purine nucleoside phosphorylase deficiency

**B.** Phosphoribosylpyrophosphate synthetase superactivity

**C.** Adenosine deaminase deficiency

**D.** Hypoxanthine-guanine phosphoribosyltransferase deficiency

**E.** Deoxyguanosine kinase deficiency

**5-32.** Metals are indispensable elements of cell biology. They function as cofactors in many specific proteins and are involved in all major metabolic pathways. Clinical presentations of disorders of metal metabolism are diverse and involve all major organs and systems. A 3-month-old infant presents with persistent diarrhea and severe periorificial dermatitis (see following figure). What is the most likely metal deficiency associated with these symptoms?

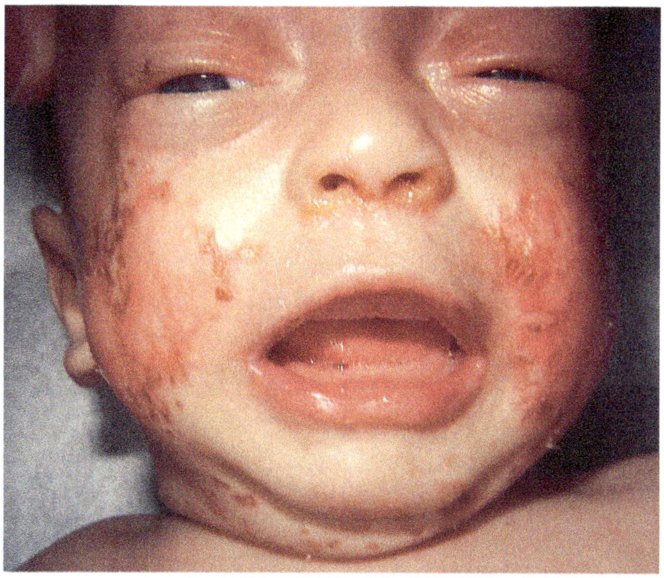

(Reproduced, with permission, from Weinberg S, Prose NS, Kristal L. *Color Atlas of Pediatric Dermatology.* 4th ed. New York, NY: McGraw-Hill; 2008.)

**A.** Copper

**B.** Iron

**C.** Zinc

**D.** Magnesium

**E.** Manganese

## ANSWERS

**Answer 5-1.** A

Most inborn errors of metabolism (IEMs) are inherited as autosomal recessive conditions. A significant minority are inherited as X-linked recessive disorders and a few as dominant disorders. However, in developed countries, where consanguinity is rare and the size of sibships small, many cases appear to be sporadic with a negative family history. It is important to remember that ornithine transcarbamylase deficiency, the most common urea cycle defect, is an X-linked disorder with a very variable phenotype in females that can lead to fatal hyperammonemia in both affected males and females. The other disorders listed are inherited in an autosomal recessive form.

(Section 11, p. 644: Ornithine Transcarbamylase Deficiency, and p. 643: Table 141-1)

**Answer 5-2.** D

The neonate has a limited repertoire of responses to severe illness, and inborn errors of metabolism (IEMs) may present with nonspecific symptoms (Table 129-1). Consider IEMs in parallel with other more common conditions such as sepsis. Rapid clinical deterioration is concerning for IEMs.

Isolated hyperammonemia can occur without acidosis or an elevated lactate. An elevated ammonia level alone can induce respiratory alkalosis. Respiratory alkalosis is rare in septic neonates who usually present with metabolic acidosis. A finding of respiratory alkalosis in a neonate who appears "septic" should prompt rapid evaluation for hyperammonemia with a stat ammonia level.

(Section 11, p. 588: Hypotonia, p. 644: Ornithine Transcarbamylase Deficiency, p. 588: Figure 129-2, p. 589: Table 129-1, and p. 591: Table 129-3)

**Answer 5-3.** E

First ensure adequate cardiorespiratory function (eg, ABCs [airway, breathing, and circulation]) and treat hypotension when noted. Adequate fluid status is essential to maintain urine output because many of the offending metabolites in inborn errors of metabolism (IEMs) are freely filtered at the glomerulus. Intravenous fluids should be judicious because cerebral edema can occur. During resuscitation of patients with suspected metabolic disease, it is also critical to reverse the catabolic state. Ten percent dextrose run intravenously at 150% maintenance will provide a glucose infusion rate of approximately 9 to 10 mg/kg/min of glucose to neonates and infants. The other fluids listed do not provide an adequate glucose infusion rate to reverse catabolism.

(Section 11, p. 592: Approach to Therapy)

**TABLE 129-1.** Neurologic Presentations in Neonates and in Early Infancy

| Predominant Clinical Symptom | Main Clinical Signs | Biological Signs | Best Diagnoses (Disorder/Enzyme Deficiency) |
|---|---|---|---|
| Neurologic deterioration: mostly metabolic and treatable | Lethargy, coma, hiccups<br>Poor sucking, hypothermia<br>Hypotonia, hypertonia<br>Abnormal movements<br>Large-amplitude tremor<br>Myoclonic jerks<br>Burst suppression<br>Abnormal odor | Ketosis, acidosis<br>Hyperlactacidemia<br>Hyperammonemia<br>Bone marrow suppression<br>Characteristic changes of AAC or OAC | MSUD (odor)<br>MMA, PA, IVA (odor)<br>MCD<br>Urea cycle defects<br>CAVA deficiency<br>GA type II (odor) |
| Seizures: sometimes metabolic, sometimes treatable | Isolated<br>Generalized | Metabolic ketoacidosis<br>Typical OAC profile | MCD |
| | | None | Pyridoxine responsive, folinic acid responsive<br>(antiquitin deficiency) |
| | | Hypocalcemia with hypomagnesemia | Congenital magnesium malabsorption |
| | | Severe hypoglycemia | PHHI |
| | Generalized hypsarrhythmia<br>Major microcephaly | Low serine (plasma/CSF) | 3-PGD |
| | Severe hypotonia<br>Myoclonic jerks<br>Burst suppression | Low HVA, 5-HIAA in CSF, vanillactic acid (urine)<br>Hyperglycinemia<br>None<br>S-Sulfocysteine | PNPO (pyridoxamine phosphate responsive)<br>NKH<br>Glutamate transporter<br>Sulfite oxidase |
| | Facial dysmorphia<br>Malformations<br>Severe hypotonia | VLCFA, phytanic, plasmalogen<br>Glycosylated transferrin<br>Sterols in plasma | Peroxisomal defects<br>CDG syndrome<br>Cholesterol biosynthesis |
| Severe hypotonia: rarely metabolic, many not treatable | Isolated | None | Prader-Willi syndrome |
| | | Massive cystinuria | Hypotonia cystinuria syndrome |
| | Predominant dysmorphia<br>Malformations | VLCFA, phytanic, plasmalogen<br>Sterols in plasma<br>Glycosylated transferrin<br>APO-B glycosylation | Peroxisomal defects<br>Cholesterol defects<br>Glycosylation defects<br>Polymalformation syndromes with muscular dystrophy (Walker-Warburg syndrome, with muscle, eye, brain, and other anomalies) |
| | Cataract | Lactic acidemia | Lowe syndrome |
| | Tubulopathy | Enzyme/DNA analyses | Respiratory chain |
| | Cardiomyopathy | Vacuolated lymphocytes | Pompe disease |

*(Continued)*

**TABLE 129-1.** Neurologic Presentations in Neonates and in Early Infancy *(Continued)*

| Predominant Clinical Symptom | Main Clinical Signs | Biological Signs | Best Diagnoses (Disorder/Enzyme Deficiency) |
|---|---|---|---|
| | Abnormal movements (dystonia-parkinsonism, oculogyric crises), feeding difficulties, temperature instability | Abnormal CSF<br>Biogenic amines/pterines, glycine | Neurotransmitter disorders |
| | Pyridostigmine-responsive congenital myasthenic syndrome | Serum transferrin IEF type 1 pattern in some<br>Normal CK | ALG2, ALG14, DPAGT1, GFPT1, and GMPPB CDGs |
| | Macroglossia | Lactic acidemia | Respiratory chain |
| | Hepatopathy | Acylcarnitine | Trifunctional enzyme (FAO)<br>Carnitine transporter<br>Riboflavin transporter |
| | | COQ10 fibroblasts, muscle | Primary COQ10 defects |

3-PGD, 3-phosphoglycerate dehydrogenase; 5-HIAA, 5-hydroxy indole acetic acid; AAC, amino acid chromatography; CDG, congenital disorders of glycosylation; CAVA, carbonic anhydrase VA isoform; CK, creatine kinase; COQ10, coenzyme Q10; CSF, cerebrospinal fluid; FAO, fatty acid oxidation; GA II, glutaric aciduria type II; HVA, homovanillic acid; IEF, isoelectric focusing; IVA, isovaleric acidemia; MCD, multiple carboxylase deficiency; MMA, methylmalonic aciduria; MSUD, maple syrup urine disease; NKH, nonketotic hyperglycinemia; OAC, organic acid chromatography; PA, propionic acidemia; PHHI, persistent hyperinsulinemic hypoglycemia of infancy; PNPO, pyridox(am)ine-5′-phosphate oxidase; VLCFA, very-long-chain fatty acids.

Mark W. Kline, *Rudolph's Pediatrics*, 23rd Edition. Copyright © McGraw-Hill Education. All rights reserved.

**Answer 5-4.** C

Metabolic acidosis can result from a large variety of acquired conditions, including infections (patient described in answer choice A), severe catabolic state, severe dehydration, and intoxication/ingestion (patient described in answer choice B). Evaluation of patients with metabolic acidosis includes calculating the anion gap. In patients with metabolic acidosis caused by loss of bicarbonate (gastrointestinal or renal loss), the plasma chloride is elevated and anion gap is normal (patient described in answer choice E). The patient described in answer choice D most likely has diabetic ketoacidosis.

Metabolic acidosis in inborn errors of metabolism (IEMs) often develops as a result of accumulation of a fixed anion, such as lactate, ketone bodies, organic acid, or a combination of these, leading to increased anion gap metabolic acidosis. Ketonuria should always be considered abnormal in a neonate and, when associated with metabolic acidosis, should prompt evaluation for metabolic disease (patient described in answer choice C).

(Section 11, p. 590: Initial Approach to the Investigation, p. 591: Table 129-3, p. 595: Metabolic Acidosis and Ketosis)

**Answer 5-5.** B

The application of tandem mass spectrometry to newborn screening has greatly changed both newborn screening and the diagnosis of many inborn errors of metabolism (IEMs). This technology allows for detection of many disorders at one time. A positive newborn screen is considered a screening test and must be confirmed (making answer choice A incorrect). False-positive results can occur. It is recommended the sample for newborn screening be collected after 24 hours of age to allow for oral intake of formula or breast milk that may be necessary to show characteristic elevations of metabolites (not in the first 6 hours as in answer choice D). Current newborn screening panels include several conditions with a much lower frequency than 1 in 10,000, and many of the disorders screened for are not fatal (making answer choices C and E incorrect).

(Section 11, p. 605: Newborn Screening)

**Answer 5-6.** C

PKU has a very distinct role in the field of metabolic disorders. It is the first genetic disease that can be treated exclusively by dietary manipulation and entirely prevented by universal newborn screening and presymptomatic dietary intervention.

PKU is one of the most common inherited metabolic diseases and has a higher incidence in whites than people of African, Hispanic, or Asian descent. Children with severe hyperphenylalaninemia do not show any symptoms at birth. If untreated, symptoms usually appear after 6 months of age. Newborn screening for PKU is fairly specific, and false positives are more often seen in premature or sick babies. All positive newborn screens must be promptly followed by confirmatory testing. For patients with PKU, initiation of treatment before the age of 2 weeks is recommended. Approximately 90% of individuals with untreated PKU have severe mental disability. The damage to the brain is believed to occur from direct toxicity of phenylalanine and depletion of tyrosine, tryptophan, and other large neutral amino acids that compete with phenylalanine for uptake into the brain.

(Section 11, pp. 607–610: Hyperphenylalaninemias and Phenylketonuria)

**Answer 5-7.** B

The 3 essential branched-chain amino acids (BCAAs)—leucine, isoleucine, and valine—encompass about 25% of human protein. The most frequent inborn errors affecting the BCAA catabolic pathway are maple syrup urine disease (MSUD) and isovaleric, propionic, and methylmalonic acidemias. In the typical patient with MSUD, symptoms appear at 3 to 5 days of age and can progress rapidly to death. Early manifestations include poor feeding, irregular respirations, lethargy, muscle rigidity, and opisthotonos.

The characteristic maple syrup odor can be detected in urine, skin, hair, or ear wax. Milder intermittent forms of the disease can occur and present with episodic ataxia or episodes of lethargy, which can progress to coma without mental retardation. These episodes are often precipitated by intercurrent illness, as descried in this vignette. Early diagnosis is essential because treatment with special diets with closely controlled intake of the BCAA leads to normal neurocognitive outcome.

Biotinidase deficiency usually presents in infancy with periorificial dermatitis resembling acrodermatitis enteropathica, patchy alopecia, neurologic abnormalities, and metabolic acidosis related to impaired activity of the carboxylases, which use biotin as a cofactor.

Type 1 diabetes mellitus is associated with a fruity odor due to acetone and ketosis, but symptoms would not be expected to be intermittent over the course of months. A referral to a geneticist is appropriate to evaluate for MSUD, not an infectious disease referral. An MRI of the brain will most likely be normal and will not add toward establishing the underlying diagnosis.

(Section 11, pp. 613–614, Chapter 132: Disorders of Branched Chain Amino and Organic Acid Metabolism)

**Answer 5-8.** A

Most organic acidemias present in the newborn period with lethargy, feeding intolerance, encephalopathy, metabolic acidosis (with an increased anion gap), hypoglycemia, and ketosis/ketonuria. Characteristic, diagnostic metabolites are noted on urine organic acids, especially if collected during an acute event. Free and total carnitine levels will indicate a carnitine deficiency and possible need for carnitine supplementation but are not diagnostic. Alternatively, an acylcarnitine profile (which is a different test from free and total carnitine levels and is not one of the choices listed) uses tandem mass spectrometry to quantitate specific acylcarnitines and is an extremely useful adjunct diagnostic test for organic acidemias.

Very-long-chain fatty acids are used in diagnosis of peroxisomal disorders, not organic acidemias. Testing for urine-reducing substances is a nonspecific test sometimes used to detect carbohydrates like galactose and would not lead to a diagnosis. Urine amino acid results are nondiagnostic in organic acidemias. Amino acids are best sampled in plasma, not urine, because they are effectively cleared by the kidneys.

(Section 11, pp. 614–617, Chapter 132: Disorders of Branched Chain Amino and Organic Acid Metabolism)

**Answer 5-9.** D

Classical homocystinuria (cystathionine β-synthase deficiency) presents as a multisystem disease with dysplasia of connective tissue, a predisposition to thromboembolism, and cognitive impairment. The most characteristic feature of this disorder is subluxation of the ocular lens, which occurs in almost all untreated individuals by adulthood. Severe hyperhomocysteinemia is identified by homocysteine levels in the range of 80 to 300 μmol/L. Plasma amino acids can be collected once hyperhomocysteinemia has been detected and generally reveal high methionine and low cysteine levels.

Subluxation of the ocular lens can also be seen in Marfan syndrome, but patients with Marfan syndrome do not have cognitive impairment. Presence of cognitive impairment in patients with marfanoid skeletal features and/or lens subluxation should prompt evaluation for homocystinuria. Chromosome analysis would be normal in both Marfan syndrome and homocystinuria.

The other tests listed would also be normal/nondiagnostic in patients with homocystinuria. Free and total carnitine levels are used to identify carnitine deficiency. Urine organic acids are often diagnostic in organic acidemias. An acylcarnitine profile is extremely useful in the diagnosis of fatty acid oxidation disorders and organic acidemias but would be normal in homocystinuria.

(Section 11, pp. 618–619, Chapter 133: Disorders of Sulfur-Containing Amino Acid Group Metabolism)

**Answer 5-10.** E

Glycine encephalopathy, or nonketotic hyperglycinemia, is an inherited metabolic disorder in which large amounts of glycine are found in body fluids, without further metabolic derangement. Glycine encephalopathy typically presents with severe neonatal epileptic encephalopathy, like the clinical picture described in the vignette, and recurrent hiccupping is common. EEG shows a typical burst suppression pattern. It is caused by defects in the mitochondrial glycine cleavage system.

Diagnosis is made by documentation of elevated cerebrospinal fluid (CSF) glycine levels and a characteristic CSF/plasma glycine ratio (by collecting CSF and plasma amino acids). There are limited effective treatments, and prognosis is generally poor in the severe form of this disorder.

The other disorders listed do not present with neonatal seizures. Patients with hyperprolinemia type 1 and hyperlysinemia are typically asymptomatic. Glutathione synthase deficiency presents with hemolytic anemia.

(Section 11, p. 622: Disorders of Glycine Metabolism, Nonketotic Hyperglycinemia (Glycine Encephalopathy))

**Answer 5-11.** B

Glutaric acidemia type 1 is caused by defects in glutaryl-CoA dehydrogenase. Many patients are born with macrocephaly and develop normally until they suddenly develop hypotonia and dystonia after an intercurrent illness. MRI scans show frontal and cortical atrophy, and after the onset of dystonia, degeneration of the caudate nucleus and putamen, often described as a "bat wing" in appearance. Urine organic acids are often diagnostic and show increased excretion of glutaric acid and 3-hydroxyglutaric acid. Diagnosis can also be made by collecting a plasma acylcarnitine profile, which shows elevation of glutarylcarnitine. Most patients are now diagnosed by newborn screening. Effective treatment is possible with early diagnosis.

Galactose-1-phosphate levels are used in diagnosis and follow-up of patients with galactosemia. Copper and ceruloplasmin levels are used in the diagnosis of Wilson disease. Assessment of urine mucopolysaccharides is done to diagnose the mucopolysaccharidoses.

(Section 11, p. 627: Glutaric Acidemia Type 1)

**Answer 5-12.** A

Inherited defects in amino acid transport at cell membranes (Figure 139-1) are expressed as selective renal aminoaciduria

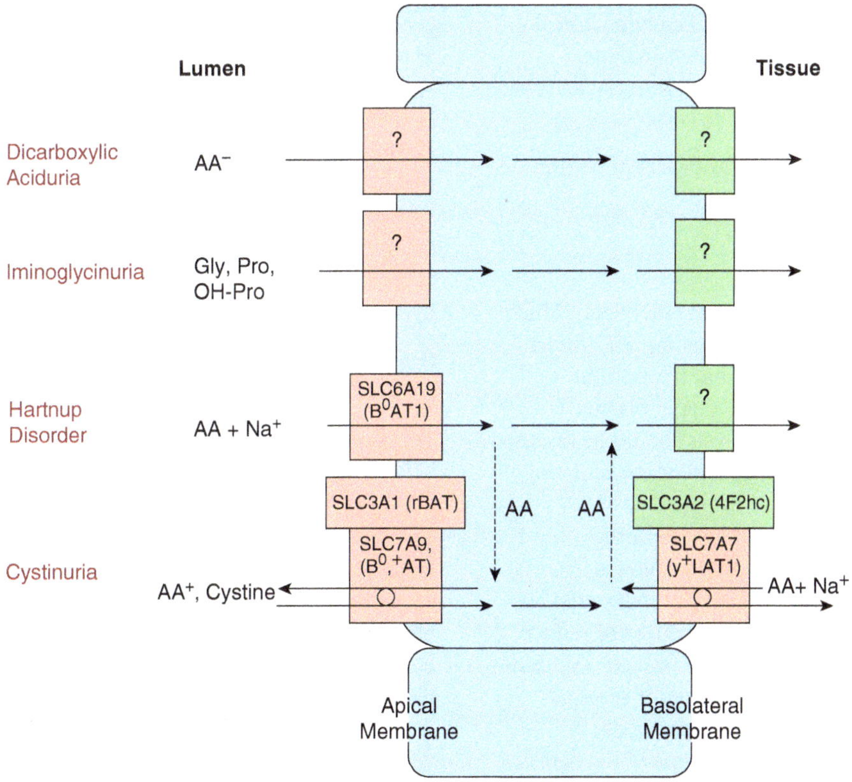


**FIGURE 139-1.** Simplified schematic representation of amino acid transport in proximal tubular epithelial cell including transport systems for negatively charged dicarboxylic amino acids ($AA^-$); imino acids (glycine, proline, and hydroxyproline); neutral amino acids (AA); and cystine and positively charged dibasic amino acids ($AA^+$). The sites of the presently known molecular transporter defects are indicated in red.

Cystine and the dibasic amino acids are transported into the epithelial cells by a luminal transporter (in exchange for neutral amino acids), and further from the epithelial cell into tissues by an antiluminal (basolateral) transporter (in exchange for neutral amino acids and sodium). Both these transporters are heteromers of a heavy subunit (*N*-glycosylated type 2 membrane glycoprotein) and a light subunit (nonglycosylated polytopic membrane protein) linked by a disulfide bridge. The light subunit $b^{0,+}$AT I and the heavy subunit rBAT of the luminal transporter are encoded by the genes *SLC7A9* and *SLC3A1*, and the light subunit $^+$LAT1 and the heavy subunit 4F2hc of the basolateral transporter by the genes *SLC7A7* and *SLC3A2*, respectively.

The neutral transporter system ($b^{0,+}$ATI encoded by the gene *SLC6A19*) is expressed only at the luminal border of the epithelial cells. It transports alanine, asparagine, citrulline, glutamine, histidine, isoleucine, leucine, phenylalanine, serine, threonine, tryptophan, tyrosine, and valine into the epithelial cells. Dicarboxylic amino acids are transported by *SCL1A1* and proline, hydroxyproline, and glycine by *SLC36A2*. (Mark W. Kline, *Rudolph's Pediatrics*, 23rd Edition. Copyright © McGraw-Hill Education. All rights reserved.)

and impaired intestinal absorption. Their symptoms result from excess of certain amino acids in the urine or lack of them in the tissues. Examples of disorders in this category include cystinuria (not cystinosis), lysinuric protein intolerance, and Hartnup disease.

Cystinuria leads to formation of cystine stones secondary to high urinary concentration of poorly soluble cystine and can be detected by checking urine amino acids. Nephropathic cystinosis is characterized by renal tubular Fanconi syndrome, poor growth, hypophosphatemic rickets, impaired glomerular function, and accumulation of cystine crystals in almost all cells, leading to tissue destruction. The typical untreated child has short stature, growth failure noted between 6 and 9 months, rickets, and photophobia. Prior to the use of renal transplantation and cystine-depleting therapy, the life span in nephropathic cystinosis was no longer than 10 years.

In lysinuric protein intolerance, the transport of dibasic amino acids is impaired, leading to lack of the urea cycle intermediates arginine and ornithine, with resultant hyperammonemia and protein intolerance. Deficiency of tryptophan, the precursor to niacin, leads to a pellagra-type dermatitis and ataxia in Hartnup disease. The main clinical symptoms seen in creatine metabolism defects include developmental delay, cognitive impairment, pronounced speech delay, autistic behavior, and seizures.

(Section 11, pp. 636–638: Chapter 139: Disorders of Amino Acid Transport Across Cell Membranes)

**Answer 5-13.** B

Acute hyperammonemia presents a medical emergency. Studies have shown that hyperammonemic coma lasting > 72 hours invariably leads to severe brain damage and intellectual disability. When newborns are comatose due to plasma ammonia levels > 200 μmol/L, hemodialysis should be initiated. This is the most rapid and effective mechanism for reducing ammonia levels.

IV arginine, IV sodium benzoate, and IV sodium phenylacetate (Ammonul) are used to provide alternate pathways for nitrogen excretion and should be initiated while preparing for hemodialysis, but this therapy does not reduce exceedingly high ammonia levels in a timely fashion. IV fluids should be used judiciously because of the risk for cerebral edema. Lactulose does not have a role in the emergency management of severe hyperammonemic coma in neonates.

(Section 11, pp. 645–646: Urea Cycle Disorders, Treatment)

**Answer 5-14.** D

Profound biotinidase deficiency usually presents in infancy with periorificial dermatitis resembling acrodermatitis enteropathica, patchy alopecia, neurologic abnormalities (eg, seizures, hypotonia, developmental delay), hearing loss, optic atrophy, recurrent viral or fungal infections caused by immunologic dysfunction, and metabolic acidosis related to impaired activity of the carboxylases, which use biotin as a cofactor. Patients respond dramatically to treatment with large doses of biotin, usually at 10 mg/d. Early recognition is critical because it can be so easily treated. Untreated biotinidase deficiency can lead to permanent neurologic sequelae; optic atrophy, hearing loss, and developmental delay may not be reversible, even with treatment. Based on these factors, most states in the United States perform newborn screening by enzymatic assay for this disorder.

(Section 11, p. 653, Chapter 143: Biotin Responsive Disorders)

**Answer 5-15.** B

Mitochondrial fatty acid oxidation provides the main source of energy when the supply of glucose is limited. Patients present with hypoketotic hypoglycemia during fasting or stress. Several untreated fatty acid oxidation disorders, especially long-chain fatty acid oxidation defects, can also present with severe rhythm or conduction abnormalities and cardiomyopathy during infancy.

Defects in fatty acid oxidation do not allow generation of adequate acetyl-coenzyme A (acetyl-CoA) for ketone body production; therefore, there is no ketosis. Hypoglycemia related to poor oral intake and increased loss from viral gastroenteritis should lead to an appropriate physiologic ketone body response in patients with a normal fatty acid oxidation pathway (note negative urinary ketones in the urinalysis). Organic acidemias would also lead to significant ketonuria and acidosis.

Glycogen storage diseases are most often associated with hepatomegaly. Ammonia level would be elevated in urea cycle defects. Type 1 diabetes mellitus usually presents with hyperglycemia.

(Section 11, p. 657, Chapter 145: Disorders of Fatty Acid Oxidation)

**Answer 5-16.** A

Type I glycogen storage disease (GSD) is due to a defect in glucose-6-phosphatase in liver, kidney, and intestine. Patients with GSD type I typically present with hypoglycemia and hepatomegaly at 3 to 4 months of age. The biochemical hallmarks of the disease are hypoglycemia, lactic acidosis, hyperuricemia, and hyperlipidemia. The other disorders listed are disorders of carbohydrate metabolism but do not lead to the classic biochemical abnormalities described in the vignette.

(Section 11, Chapter 149, p. 666: Type I Glycogen Storage Disease)

**Answer 5-17.** C

Treatment of glycogen storage disease (GSD) type I is designed to maintain normal blood glucose levels, which is achieved by continuous infusion of glucose or oral administration of uncooked cornstarch. Nasogastric feeds, especially at night, are used in infancy and may consist of an elemental formula or a glucose polymer to maintain normoglycemia during the night.

Frequent meals with a high-carbohydrate content are given during the day.

Uncooked cornstarch provides a slow-release form of glucose, but this supplementation can only be used after the age of 9 months, when pancreatic amylase activity is mature. Administration of glucagon causes little or no rise in glucose but can increase lactate levels significantly. *Ad libitum* feeding or feeds spaced out more than every 4 hours would most likely lead to further hypoglycemia in this disorder.

(Section 11, Chapter 149, p. 666: Type I Glycogen Storage Disease)

**Answer 5-18.** E

Symptoms of glycogen storage disease (GSD) type V (McArdle disease) are characterized by exercise intolerance and muscle cramps. Brief periods of intense activity or less intense but sustained activity lead to symptoms. Most patients report a "second wind" phenomenon, as described by the patient in the vignette. About half of patients report burgundy-colored urine after exercise, the consequence of myoglobinuria secondary to rhabdomyolysis. Intense myoglobinuria after vigorous exercise can cause renal failure. Serum creatine kinase is usually elevated at rest and increases more after exercise. This is an autosomal recessive disorder. One common pathogenic variant (R49X) accounts for 90% of North American patients with this disorder. Lack of an elevated blood lactate level and exaggerated ammonia elevations are noted after an ischemia exercise test.

The abnormal exercise test, however, is *not* limited to type V GSD and can be seen in other defects of glycogenolysis or glycolysis. Definitive diagnosis is made by enzymatic assay in muscle tissue (not liver) or by mutation analysis of the myophosphorylase gene. Mutation analysis offers the least invasive test to establish a diagnosis. Plasma acylcarnitine profile and urine organic acids are normal in patients with GSD. These tests are used in diagnosis of fatty acid oxidation disorders, some of which can also present with exercise intolerance.

(Section 11, p. 671, Type V Glycogen Storage Disease (Muscle Phosphorylase Deficiency, or McArdle Disease))

**Answer 5-19.** B

The vignette describes the typical infantile presentation of Pompe disease. This disease is also a lysosomal storage disease and is characterized by accumulation of glycogen in lysosomes as opposed to its accumulation in the cytoplasm in other glycogen storage diseases (GSDs). The disorder encompasses a range of phenotypes, with the severe infantile form as described in the vignette (which includes skeletal, cardiac, and smooth muscle involvement) and a late-onset form characterized by skeletal muscle manifestations. It is important to establish the correct diagnosis because enzyme replacement therapy (ERT) is currently available for Pompe disease and leads to improved cardiac and skeletal muscle function, although response to ERT is variable.

As of 2015, Pompe disease was added to the Recommended Universal Screening Panel in the United States, which makes recommendations on which disorders should be added to state newborn screening programs. Not all states have yet implemented newborn screening for Pompe disease. The other GSDs listed have a primary liver (hepatomegaly) or skeletal presentation (exercise intolerance), without cardiomegaly.

(Section 11, p. 672, Glycogen Storage Disease Type II (Acid α-1,4-Glucosidase Deficiency, Acid Maltase Deficiency, or Pompe Disease))

**Answer 5-20.** D

Classic galactosemia is due to deficiency of galactose-1-phosphate uridyl transferase. Incidence is approximately 1 in 60,000. Symptoms typically appear by the first to second week of life for newborns receiving breast milk or regular formulas (with lactose). Manifestations include jaundice, hepatomegaly, and feeding intolerance. Patients are at increased risk for *E coli* sepsis. A preliminary diagnosis of galactosemia is made by demonstrating reducing substances in urine (both glucose and galactose are reducing substances; it is easy to exclude glucosuria as contributing to the presence of reducing substances by completing a urinalysis to check for glucose in urine).

Only patients with galactosemia receiving lactose will have positive reducing substances. Enzymatic testing for galactose-1-phosphate uridyl transferase in erythrocytes or molecular analysis confirms the diagnosis. Treatment includes elimination of galactose from the diet with use of galactose-free formulas (lactose-free/soy-based formulas). Most patients with galactosemia are now diagnosed by newborn screening.

Patients with GSD, MSUD, organic acidemia, or urea cycle disorders have different clinical presentations to what is described in this vignette and are not prone to *E coli* sepsis. In addition, these disorders do not lead to presence of non–glucose-reducing substances.

(Section 11, pp. 674–675, Disorders of Galactose Metabolism, Galactosemia)

**Answer 5-21.** E

The rules of mitochondrial genetics differ from those of Mendelian genetics in the following ways. Each cell contains hundreds or thousands (not 50–100) of copies of mitochondrial DNA (mtDNA) which distribute randomly among daughter cells at cell division. In normal tissues, all mtDNA molecules are identical (homoplasmy). Most deleterious mtDNA mutations affect some, but not all, mtDNA within a cell, tissue, or individual (heteroplasmy). The clinical expression is determined by the relative proportion of normal and mutant mtDNA. A minimum critical number of mtDNA is required to cause mitochondrial dysfunction (threshold effect).

At cell division, the proportion of mutant mtDNA in daughter cells may shift and change the phenotype (mitotic segregation). At fertilization, all mtDNA derives from the oocyte.

A mother carrying a mitochondrial point mutation will transmit it to all her children, male and female. But only her daughters will transmit it to their progeny. Of the approximately 80 subunits of the respiratory chain, only 13 are encoded by mtDNA, with the rest encoded by nuclear DNA. Disorders due to mutations in nuclear DNA are inherited as Mendelian traits.

(Section 11, p. 684, Chapter 153: Respiratory Chain Disorders)

**Answer 5-22.** A

This vignette describes a patient with MELAS (mitochondrial encephalomyopathy, lactic acidosis, and stroke-like episodes). Lactic acidosis is a common finding in defects of the respiratory chain, and the lactate-to-pyruvate ratio is usually elevated. Ophthalmoplegia is not seen in MELAS; it is a feature of other mitochondrial disorders, such as Kearns-Sayre syndrome and progressive external ophthalmoplegia. Inheritance of MELAS is maternal because it is due to a pathogenic variant in the mitochondrial DNA. Ocular findings are *not* typically seen in patients with MELAS. Therapy for mitochondrial disorders, including MELAS, is still inadequate.

(Section 11, pp. 685–690, Table 158-1)

**Answer 5-23.** A

All MPS disorders are multisystem diseases, and effective management depends on a multidisciplinary approach. The pediatrician has a major role in orchestrating the various members of the therapeutic team. Anesthesia is particularly difficult in patients with Hurler syndrome (MPS type I), and surgery should only be performed in centers with access to anesthesiologists used to dealing with difficult pediatric airways. With the advent of newer therapeutic strategies, many patients now survive through adolescence and into adulthood, and careful planning of transition from pediatric to adult services is necessary.

MPS type I is an autosomal recessive disorder with a recurrence risk of 25% for parents of an affected child. Hurler syndrome is not associated with increased risk for seizures. There are several treatment options, including bone marrow or stem cell transplantation, for patients who are < 2 years of age. Enzyme replacement therapy (ERT) is also available and leads to improvement in endurance, respiratory status, hepatosplenomegaly, and cardiac status. ERT does not cross the blood–brain barrier, and the only option for a good neurologic outcome is stem cell/bone marrow transplantation, often in combination with ERT.

(Section 11, pp. 693–694, Chapter 160)

**Answer 5-24.** D

The most common of the sphingolipidoses, Gaucher disease is an example of how sphingolipid storage diseases may present at any age. Gaucher disease can present in the neonatal or early infantile period with severe central nervous system (CNS) impairment and hepatosplenomegaly. However, the most common presentation is in late childhood or adulthood (type 1 Gaucher disease) without CNS impairment. A typical presentation is described in the vignette. Although chronic bone pain is typically reported, acute bone pain may resemble that of a sickle cell crisis and may also be clinically indistinguishable from osteomyelitis.

All the other disorders listed are examples of sphingolipidoses; however, the presentation for these disorders includes CNS impairment.

(Section 11, pp. 706–708, Sphingolipidoses, Clinical Presentation)

**Answer 5-25.** E

The patient described in this vignette has classic features of Fabry disease, an X-linked lysosomal storage disorder. Fabry disease usually presents in the late first decade of life with acroparesthesia, which is episodic and precipitated by extreme temperature, exertion, or fever. Pain in the joints may be indistinguishable from pauciarticular arthritis, and abdominal pain can resemble an acute abdomen or inflammatory bowel disease. Angiokeratomas develop around the umbilicus and on the skin of the buttocks. Renal function deteriorates over time. Other complications include cardiac disease and strokes.

ERT has emerged as one of the most important advances in the treatment of sphingolipidoses. ERT with biweekly infusions of agalsidase-β is available for treatment of Fabry disease, although its effect in preventing cardiac disease, strokes, and renal failure is unproven. None of the other options listed are valid treatment options for Fabry disease. Hemodialysis and kidney transplantation may be offered to those with end-stage renal disease.

(Section 11, pp. 706-709, Fabry Disease, Sphingolipidoses, Clinical Presentation and Management)

**Answer 5-26.** A

Peroxisome disorders are divided into 2 main classes: peroxisome biogenesis disorders (PBD), which are characterized by a deficiency of multiple peroxisome functions due to mutations in the *PEX* genes, leading to dysfunctional organelle biogenesis; and single-enzyme disorders, in which only one peroxisome function is deficient. PBD-Zellweger spectrum disorders (ZSD) have severe, intermediate, and mild forms. Severe cases are recognized in the neonatal period and are characterized by the clinical phenotype described in this question. The *PEX* gene defects in these patients are null or strong hypomorphic alleles. The most frequently used laboratory diagnostic test for PBDs detects elevated levels of very-long-chain fatty acids, which are elevated about 10-fold in severe cases. The other tests listed are expected to be normal or nondiagnostic in patients with PBD-ZSD.

(Section 11, pp. 711–714, Figure 157-4A-B, Chapter 157: Peroxisome Disorders)

**Answer 5-27.** C

Glycosylation is an important posttranslational protein modification that occurs in cytoplasm, the endoplasmic reticulum, and Golgi apparatus. A rapidly growing group of genetic disorders, collectively called CDGs, is due to defects in *N*- or *O*-glycosylation. Most CDGs are severe multisystem disorders with neurologic involvement.

There is no effective treatment for the majority of patients with CDGs; ERT is not available for this group of disorders. CDG type 1b (which is much rarer than CDG type 1a) is the only known CDG that is efficiently treatable with oral mannose. Many CDGs show autosomal recessive inheritance, not X-linked inheritance. The most important initial diagnostic tool is transferrin isoelectric focusing, not very-long-chain fatty acid analysis (which is used in the diagnostic evaluation of patients with peroxisomal disorders).

(Section 11, pp. 717–722, Chapter 158: Congenital Disorders of Protein Glycosylation)

**Answer 5-28.** D

All the disorders listed are disorders of cholesterol synthesis; however, the phenotype described in the question is most consistent with Smith-Lemli-Opitz syndrome. Cholesterol is an important constituent of cell membranes and has important interactions with signaling proteins involved in embryogenesis and development. Disorders of this pathway lead to dysmorphic features and malformations of internal organs.

The signs and symptoms of Smith-Lemli-Opitz syndrome vary in severity. Typical features include intrauterine growth restriction with low maternal estriol levels. At birth, dysmorphic features include microcephaly, ptosis, anteverted nares, cleft palate, other midline defects such as congenital heart disease, genital abnormalities, and 2 to 3 toe syndactyly. Hypotonia, feeding problems, and failure to thrive are common. Patients with growth restriction, microcephaly, and 2 to 3 toe syndactyly warrant further evaluation for this disorder. This is an autosomal recessive disorder. Diagnosis requires analysis of plasma sterols and shows elevated concentration of 7-dehydrocholesterol.

(Section 11, pp. 723–728, Chapter 159: Disorders of Cholesterol Synthesis)

**Answer 5-29.** C

Heterozygous FH is an autosomal dominant disorder that presents at birth and early in life with 2- to 3-fold elevations in LDL cholesterol. Heterozygosity for FH affects about 1 in 500 people and is due to > 900 different mutations in LDLR. Fifty percent of male adults with untreated heterozygous FH and 25% of female adults with untreated heterozygous FH will develop cardiovascular disease by age 50.

Patients who are homozygotes for FH have significantly more severe manifestations than patients with heterozygous FH and can die from cardiovascular disease in the second decade. About 1 in a million individuals are homozygous for FH.

(Section 11, pp. 743–744: Familial Hypercholesterolemia)

**Answer 5-30.** B

The porphyrias are a group of inherited and acquired metabolic disorders, each resulting from the deficient activity of a specific enzyme in the heme biosynthetic pathway. These disorders are inherited as autosomal dominant, autosomal recessive, and sporadic (porphyria cutanea tarda) conditions. They are primarily classified as hepatic or erythropoietic, depending on the primary site of overproduction or accumulation of the porphyrin precursor or porphyrin.

Manifestations of the *hepatic* porphyrias characteristically include abdominal pain, neuropathy, and mental disturbance. Manifestations of the *erythropoietic* porphyrias characteristically include cutaneous photosensitivity.

The porphyrias are echogenic disorders in which environmental, physiologic, and genetic factors interact to cause disease. Steroid hormones, drugs, and nutrition influence the production of porphyrin precursors and porphyrins, thereby precipitating or increasing the severity of some porphyrias.

(Section 11, p. 749, Chapter 162: Disorders of Heme Biosynthesis: The Porphyrias, Table 162-1, p. 749)

**Answer 5-31.** D

Lesch-Nyhan syndrome (hypoxanthine-guanine phosphoribosyltransferase [HPRT] deficiency) is an incapacitating neurologic disorder that is typically limited to males based on X-linked inheritance. It is characterized by choreoathetosis, spasticity, compulsive self-mutilation, and 3- to 4-fold elevations in plasma and urine uric acid levels.

The first indication of the disease may be brownish to red "sand" (crystals of uric acid tinged with blood) in diapers, especially with dehydration. Infants show normal development in the first 4 to 6 months, followed by irritability (possibly related to renal colic) and hypotonia. These events are followed in the second year of life by choreiform movements, development of spasticity, and subsequent onset of self-mutilatory behavior. Severely affected children are never able to walk. The excessive production of uric acid in HPRT deficiency is explained by an enhanced purine synthesis rate. Milder and intermediate variants have been described.

(Section 11, p. 760, Chapter 163: Disorders of Purine and Pyrimidine Metabolism)

**Answer 5-32.** C

Zinc is the cofactor for > 100 enzymes and, as such, is involved in all major metabolic pathways. Patients with mutations in the intestinal zinc-specific transporter *SLC30A2* develop acrodermatitis enteropathica characterized by diarrhea and severe periorificial dermatitis. Diagnosis is established by a low serum zinc level followed by DNA testing. Treatment includes high doses of zinc sulfate.

(Section 11, pp. 766–772, Chapter 164: Disorders of Metal Metabolism, p. 770: Zinc Metabolism)

# CHAPTER 6 Mental and Behavioral Health

Eva C. Ihle and Megen Vo

**6-1.** An 8-year-old boy with moderate intellectual disability and suspected autism spectrum disorder arrives for a new patient appointment. He is reported to have had routine medical care up until this point, which included normal hearing screens. Which medical workup is expected for all such patients?

**A.** Sleep study

**B.** Genetic workup

**C.** Metabolic workup

**D.** Electroencephalography (EEG)

**E.** Audiology referral

**6-2.** A 14-year-old girl is brought into her pediatrician's office because her mother has become concerned about her increased "clinginess" for the past 2 months, ever since the mother had to be hospitalized after a car accident. The mother stated that the girl has recently started refusing to return to school, stating that she has a variety of physical complaints, such as headache, stomach ache, or fatigue. The mother also stated that the girl is having more trouble falling asleep at night. She will either come into her parents' room to sleep with them or demand that her mother stay with her until she is asleep. The girl is reported to have had similar behaviors when she was 3 years old, but these behaviors resolved by the time she was 5 years old. What is the most likely diagnosis?

**A.** Post-traumatic stress disorder (PTSD)

**B.** Generalized anxiety disorder

**C.** Social anxiety disorder

**D.** Major depressive disorder

**E.** Separation anxiety disorder

**6-3.** A 17-year-old boy with a history of intellectual disability diagnosed in high school is hospitalized for dehydration and hypotension. In the days leading up to the hospitalization, he spent several days alone in his room, refusing to come down for meals or to interact with his family. His family reports that he has been more reclusive for several months. One family member remembered the patient telling him that his favorite radio station was broadcasting specifically to him. In addition, the patient stated that he "received the message too fast." On exam, he appears to be staring blankly and is disheveled, malodorous, and mute. What is the most likely diagnosis underlying his catatonia?

**A.** Schizophrenia

**B.** Major depressive disorder

**C.** Bipolar I disorder

**D.** Autism spectrum disorder

**E.** Schizotypal personality disorder

**6-4.** A 12-year-old girl is brought in to clinic for a chief complaint of fatigue. On examination, she also reports decreased energy, decreased concentration, poor appetite, decreased interest in pleasurable activities, and increased sleep latency. She also reports low mood but no thoughts of self-harm. Prior to selecting an antidepressant to treat the neurovegetative symptoms associated with a major depressive episode, what needs to be the next step in the treatment plan?

**A.** Obtain parental consent to prescribe antidepressant medication

**B.** Obtain baseline laboratory testing

**C.** Review medication black box warning with patient and parents

**D.** Obtain a Patient Health Questionnaire-9 (PHQ-9) score

**E.** Provide information about crisis hotlines

**6-5.** For both inhibited and excited catatonia, what is the first-line treatment for the behavioral and motor symptoms?

**A.** Aripiprazole

**B.** Propranolol

**C.** Risperidone

**D.** Lorazepam

**E.** Electroconvulsive therapy (ECT)

**6-6.** A 9-year-old boy with mild autism spectrum disorder and intellectual disability has recently started scratching his arms and pushing on his eyes. Bilateral corneal abrasions are noted on physical exam. In addition, there are numerous linear abrasions on his bilateral upper extremities. When asked about this behavior, he says he is "upset." His mother reported that his special education teacher recently went out on maternity leave and the substitute teacher is having difficulty managing the classroom. She also noted that she has gone back to work part time. Which of the following is the first-line intervention for the patient's self-injurious behavior?

**A.** Dialectical behavioral therapy

**B.** Applied behavior analysis

**C.** Risperidone

**D.** Paroxetine

**E.** Quetiapine

**6-7.** A 13-year-old boy was recently diagnosed with attention-deficit/hyperactivity disorder (ADHD), combined subtype. He was started on methylphenidate immediate release 5 mg twice a day and had mild improvement in his behavioral control and focus. This medication was titrated to 20 mg twice a day, then converted to methylphenidate extended-release tablets 36 mg daily. Modest additional improvement was noted, but symptoms re-emerged in the last few hours of the school day. When the methylphenidate extended-release dose was increased further, the patient complained of agitation but also of feeling like a "zombie." Which medication would be the best option to switch to next?

**A.** Atomoxetine

**B.** Extended-release guanfacine

**C.** Mixed dextroamphetamine salts

**D.** Fish oil

**E.** Bupropion

**6-8.** A 16-year-old female cross-country runner is hospitalized for bradycardia and weight loss to < 75% of her ideal body weight. She endorsed a history of converting to veganism and switching to a gluten-free, casein-free diet. She also reported eating dinner with her family but standing up at the kitchen counter while she does so. She states that she snacks throughout the remainder of the day because if she eats another meal she feels nauseated and is likely to vomit. She acknowledged that she likes her current weight and is fearful that if she regains the weight she has lost she will no longer be a competitive athlete. What is the most likely diagnosis?

**A.** Avoidant/restrictive food intake disorder

**B.** Other specified feeding and eating disorder (OSFED)

**C.** Bulimia nervosa

**D.** Anorexia nervosa, restricting type

**E.** Binge eating disorder

**6-9.** Which of the following risk factors for suicide can a pediatrician most readily modify?

**A.** Previous suicide attempt

**B.** Family history of suicide

**C.** Chronic medical disorder

**D.** Self-injurious behavior

**E.** Access to means

**6-10.** A 10-year-old boy presents to clinic for attention-deficit/hyperactivity disorder (ADHD) medication. His father reports that his teacher has complained about the boy's impulsivity and other disruptive behaviors. These behaviors have worsened since the family has started to live out of their car after the patient's mother was incarcerated 6 weeks ago. Which of the following is the best medication to treat the underlying cause of the boy's symptoms?

**A.** α-Adrenergic agents

**B.** Stimulants

**C.** Antipsychotics

**D.** Antidepressants

**E.** Anxiolytics

**6-11.** A 6-year-old girl has started showering twice a day. She occasionally wakes up in the middle of the night to shower as well. When she comes in for her well-child check she has red, chapped skin on both hands, and she acknowledges that she washes her hands "a lot." Her mother reports that she spends a total of 2 hours each afternoon, after she comes home from school, washing her hands because she believes her desk at school is "covered in germs." Which medication is approved by the US Food and Drug Administration (FDA) to treat these symptoms for a 6-year-old patient?

**A.** Fluoxetine (Prozac)

**B.** Paroxetine (Paxil)

**C.** Fluvoxamine (Luvox)

**D.** Sertraline (Zoloft)

**E.** Clomipramine (Anafranil)

**6-12.** A 3-year-old girl is brought in to clinic because of her parents' concerns about her development. She has only 100 words, and her parents state that she "makes up" for not having language by having great nonverbal communication. They state that she is eager to share her experience with them and does so through gestures, facial expressions, and demonstrations of empathy/affection. However, they also note that at times she flaps her hands and toe-walks. Which therapeutic intervention is most appropriate for the likely diagnosis?

**A.** Applied behavior analysis

**B.** Speech therapy

**C.** Occupational therapy

**D.** Play therapy

**E.** Augmentative communication

**6-13.** A 15-year-old girl who was diagnosed with anorexia nervosa returns to her pediatrician's office after undergoing family-based therapy and having her weight restored to 94% of her ideal body weight. The anxiety symptoms that predated and exacerbated her anorexia nervosa persist. What is the appropriate intervention for the pediatrician to take in treating the patient's anxiety?

**A.** Prescribe sertraline (Zoloft)

**B.** Prescribe bupropion (Wellbutrin)

**C.** Refer to dialectical behavior therapy

**D.** Refer to exposure-and-response prevention therapy

**E.** Continue to monitor anxiety symptoms

**6-14.** After undergoing multiple surgeries for tetralogy of Fallot earlier in his life, an 11-year-old boy experienced the loss of his favorite caregiver following a protracted and painful cancer treatment, as well as the divorce of his parents. He and his mother, with whom he lives full time, were recently displaced from their home following a fire. What is the lifetime prevalence rate of post-traumatic stress disorder (PTSD) in adolescents with similar exposure to adversity?

**A.** 1%

**B.** 4%

**C.** 9%

**D.** 15%

**E.** 20%

**6-15.** Which of the following clinical scenarios is most consistent with the diagnosis of disruptive mood dysregulation disorder?

**A.** A 9-year-old girl who cries and hits her mother when it is time for her to go to bed

**B.** An 8-year-old boy who is irritable, distractible, and fidgets and squirms in his seat

**C.** A 10-year-old girl who is angry and vindictive toward her brother and also defies her parents and teachers

**D.** A 9-year-old girl who is persistently irritable and has frequent episodes of poorly modulated behavioral responses

**E.** An 8-year-old boy who is irritable, isolative, apathetic, and has poor sleep

**6-16.** Which of the following clinical scenarios is most consistent with a diagnosis of avoidant/restrictive food intake disorder?

**A.** A 12-year-old boy who is distressed by his waking up in the middle of the night to snack on junk food

**B.** An 11-year-old girl with dependence on enteral feeding after an episode of choking

**C.** A 9-year-old girl who eats only vegetables because she is afraid of looking "fat"

**D.** A 9-year-old girl who, twice a week, eats 3 servings of dinner and then forces herself to throw up

**E.** A 15-year-old boy who eats only 1 meal a day and exercises 3 hours each day because he thinks his abdomen is "flabby"

**6-17.** Pharmacotherapy for bipolar disorder includes lithium and atypical antipsychotic medications such as olanzapine and risperidone. At what point or interval in the course of treatment is lab monitoring similar for both classes of mood stabilizer?

**A.** With dosage changes

**B.** Every 5 days

**C.** Every 6 months

**D.** Daily

**E.** Baseline

**6-18.** In the treatment of attention-deficit/hyperactivity disorder (ADHD) with stimulant medications, abdominal pain is often cited as 1 of the 2 most common side effects. What is the other most common side effect of stimulants?

**A.** The "zombie effect"

**B.** Sleep disturbance

**C.** Appetite suppression

**D.** Jitteriness

**E.** Headache

**6-19.** There are a number of psychological factors that characterize the eating disorders of anorexia nervosa and bulimia nervosa. In addition to anxiety, what other psychological factor is common to these 2 disorders?

**A.** Perfectionism

**B.** Obsessive behavior

**C.** Depression

**D.** Substance use

**E.** Low self-esteem

**6-20.** In 2004, the US Food and Drug Administration (FDA) applied a black box warning to selective serotonin reuptake inhibitors (SSRIs) and, subsequently, to all antidepressants. The black box warning recommends that when pediatricians first prescribe antidepressants they do which of the following?

**A.** Monitor for hyponatremia

**B.** Ask parents to monitor changes in appetite

**C.** Check in with the patient on a weekly basis

**D.** Check in with the patient on a biweekly basis

**E.** Ask parents to monitor weight gain

**6-21.** A 9-year-old girl is brought in by her mother because of concern for auditory hallucinations. The mother reports that the girl is often found to be talking as though in a conversation but when no one else is around. The girl used to play animatedly with her teddy bear. Her mother reports that on 2 to 3 nights each week she is so engaged with the conversation, which seems to be positive and enjoyable, that she does not fall asleep until late at night. She is often irritable the day after but otherwise does not express distress. What is the most likely diagnosis?

**A.** Schizophreniform disorder

**B.** Age-appropriate imagination

**C.** Manic episode, bipolar disorder

**D.** Delusional disorder

**E.** Disruptive mood dysregulation disorder

**6-22.** What distinguishes cyclothymia from bipolar disorder?

**A.** Duration of symptoms

**B.** Lack of episodicity

**C.** Lack of elevated mood

**D.** Lack of depressed mood

**E.** Severity of symptoms

**6-23.** A 10-year-old boy returns to clinic for a refill on his stimulant medication, prescribed for attention-deficit/hyperactivity disorder (ADHD), hyperactive/impulsive subtype. What information can you provide his parents about what is known regarding the typical natural course of his hyperactive symptoms?

**A.** Hyperactivity will manifest as restlessness or impatience.

**B.** Hyperactivity will convert to inattention.

**C.** Hyperactivity will increase.

**D.** Hyperactivity will persist unabated.

**E.** Hyperactivity will completely resolve.

**6-24.** The parents of a 4-year-old boy express concern about his limited vocabulary. He said "mama" at 18 months and has acquired 25 additional words, mostly nouns. He participates in shared attention through nonverbal communication. He walked at 12 months and was toilet trained at 19 months. He can jump, throw a ball, hop, and take off his clothes. He cannot yet draw a circle, cannot identify > 3 colors, and cannot use pronouns appropriately. You refer for early intervention services. What is the most likely diagnosis?

**A.** Intellectual disability

**B.** Autism spectrum disorder

**C.** Expressive language disorder

**D.** Global developmental delay

**E.** Specific learning disability

**6-25.** A 12-year-old girl is asked by her pediatrician, "Do you have any thoughts about your body?" The girl responds, "I hate it! I'm so ugly and fat! My hips are so big! I'm dieting all the time and I'm supposed to be a size 0 like my friends! I can only get down to a size 4!" The patient has not yet achieved menarche, and she is in the 10th percentile for height and weight. What is the most appropriate intervention in the treatment of the described disorder?

**A.** Dialectical behavior therapy

**B.** Cognitive behavioral therapy (CBT)

**C.** Psychodynamic psychotherapy

**D.** Family-based therapy

**E.** Interpersonal therapy

**6-26.** A 7-year-old boy presents to the emergency department with a painful and swollen left arm. Radiographs indicate a spiral fracture in the left humerus. Information obtained from the parents reveals a several-month history of irritability, decreased sleep, increased self-stimulation, and attempts to touch women's breasts. There are also numerous occasions when the patient has declared himself to be a "superhero," with superpowers, including the ability to fly. He was demonstrating this ability to fly for his friends when he leapt from his treehouse to the ground. What is the patient's likely diagnosis?

**A.** Nonaccidental trauma

**B.** Bipolar disorder, manic episode

**C.** Childhood imagination

**D.** Victimization (sexual abuse)

**E.** Childhood-onset schizophrenia

**6-27.** A 5-year-old boy with delayed milestones (walking, talking, and toileting) is brought into clinic for concerns about his social development. He has difficulties interacting with other children and has a limited number of friends. Observations of the boy while he is in clinic reveal that he is able to follow a point and to use gestures to share his interests and convey his needs. He also demonstrated concern for his mother when she started to cry during the appointment, giving her a hug and saying, "No cry, mommy; okay mommy?" What diagnosis can be ruled out?

**A.** Intellectual disability

**B.** Expressive language disorder

**C.** Autism spectrum disorder

**D.** Attention-deficit/hyperactivity disorder (ADHD)

**E.** Social anxiety disorder

**6-28.** A 6-year-old girl comes into clinic for a well-child check. Her parents are concerned about the girl's ability to engage in conversation with her friends and her friends' parents. They describe her as "speaking like a little headmistress," lecturing anyone around her about her interests but not accommodating her conversational partners. Her interests are age appropriate. During your interaction with her, she demonstrates the ability to use gestures and eye contact. What is the most likely diagnosis?

**A.** Social (pragmatic) communication disorder

**B.** Nonverbal learning disability

**C.** Attention-deficit/hyperactivity disorder (ADHD)

**D.** Autism spectrum disorder

**E.** Expressive language disorder

**6-29.** The parents of a nonverbal 6-year-old boy with autism spectrum disorder bring their child into clinic for recent changes in behavior. They are specifically concerned about irritability, decreased appetite, and hitting his abdomen with his hands. The parents ask about "any treatments" that could be helpful in treating their child's change in behavior. Which treatment is the most appropriate intervention?

**A.** Exclusion diet

**B.** Antifungal medication

**C.** Laxative medications

**D.** Megadoses of vitamin C

**E.** Hyperbaric oxygen therapy

**6-30.** Which medication is approved by the US Food and Drug Administration (FDA) for the treatment of irritability in the setting of autism spectrum disorder?

**A.** Quetiapine

**B.** Citalopram

**C.** Ziprasidone

**D.** Olanzapine

**E.** Aripiprazole

**6-31.** A 17-year-old boy presents to the acute care clinic for treatment of an infected arm laceration. On exam, it becomes apparent that there are numerous linear lacerations on both forearms in various stages of healing. Upon interview, he acknowledges that he feels depressed. He engages in cutting to "feel something other than numb." Further interview reveals that he frequently feels hopeless and isolated from peers, in part because he doesn't drink alcohol and doesn't like going to parties. He reports that he has good grades and his teachers are encouraging him to join the debate team. His teachers are also willing to help him practice. What is a protective factor against suicide in this boy's history?

**A.** Age

**B.** Gender

**C.** Academic success

**D.** Teacher support

**E.** Abstinence from alcohol

**6-32.** What is the most common type of mental health disorder encountered in an adolescent primary care clinic?

**A.** Depressive disorders

**B.** Psychotic disorders

**C.** Bipolar disorder

**D.** Anxiety disorders

**E.** Disruptive mood dysregulation disorder

**6-33.** Anxiety disorders are characterized by several key features, among them being significant interference with social or academic functioning, avoidance or procrastination, and physiologic symptoms such as sweating or increased heart rate. What additional feature distinguishes anxiety disorders from other psychiatric disorders?

**A.** Excessive or extreme worries

**B.** Decreased interest in pleasurable activities

**C.** Impaired reality testing

**D.** Impaired concentration

**E.** Increased activity level

**6-34.** A 15-year-old girl with a history of living in poverty after her emotionally distant parents divorced now presents for treatment for her fear of "not being good enough." She reports having considerable worry about a number of different situations and difficulty controlling her worry. Her worry is now causing her to avoid completing assignments because her heart races and her chest tightens when she thinks about getting to work on them. She thinks she might not get a good grade and will disappoint her mother and her teachers. After obtaining consent from the girl's parents to prescribe medication, what is the first-line pharmacotherapy for the treatment of the patient's symptoms?

**A.** Paroxetine

**B.** Gabapentin

**C.** Duloxetine

**D.** Lorazepam

**E.** Hydroxyzine

**6-35.** A 16-year-old girl is brought to her pediatrician's office by her parents because of their concern about the recent changes in her behavior. For the past several months, they report that she has started spending time with new "goth" friends, has been dressing in black, and has been talking about getting a tongue piercing. She is reported to be spending less time on homework and in family activities, often complaining about how "boring" these activities are and that she no longer finds pleasure in them. They stated that she is often irritable and stays up most of the night and then doesn't get up for school the next day because she is so tired. She also is reported to have stated that she doesn't see the point of school because she is hopeless about improving her grades. What is the most likely diagnosis?

**A.** Persistent depressive disorder

**B.** Major depressive disorder

**C.** Bipolar disorder

**D.** Normal adolescence

**E.** Learning disability

**6-36.** A 12-year-old girl meets criteria for persistent depressive disorder. The parents ask for advice about pursuing treatment. What can you tell them is the most effective intervention, based on research evidence for treatment of depression?

**A.** Cognitive behavior therapy (CBT) alone

**B.** Selective serotonin reuptake inhibitors (SSRIs) alone

**C.** Interpersonal therapy alone

**D.** Interpersonal therapy and a mood stabilizer

**E.** CBT and SSRIs

**6-37.** A 17-year-old girl is found to meet criteria for bipolar disorder, after having experienced a manic episode in which she stayed up for 4 straight days, cheated on her boyfriend with boys she hardly knew, and stole her mother's credit cards and maxed them out on makeup and shoes. She is started on lithium both to treat the acute manic episode and to prevent recurrence. As an alternative to lithium for the prevention of recurrence, what atypical antipsychotic could be prescribed?

**A.** Asenapine (Saphris)

**B.** Quetiapine (Seroquel)

**C.** Olanzapine (Zyprexa)

**D.** Aripiprazole (Abilify)

**E.** Risperidone (Risperdal)

**6-38.** According to the 2015 Youth Risk Behavior Surveillance System, what percentage of high school students surveyed had carried out a suicide attempt?

**A.** 6.7%

**B.** 8.6%

**C.** 11.4%

**D.** 14.6%

**E.** 17.7%

**6-39.** A 4-year-old girl is in the waiting room of a pediatrician's office; the doctor has fallen behind in her schedule, and the little girl is hungry and irritable. She begins to demand candy. Her mother tries to soothe her verbally without success. She then hands her a lollipop, asking her, "If I give you this, will you please be quiet?" The little girl eagerly accepts the lollipop—and has an even louder tantrum once she finishes the lollipop. In terms of contingencies of reinforcement, which aspect of the clinical scenario is the problematic consequence?

**A.** The mother giving the lollipop

**B.** The mother's attempt to verbally soothe

**C.** The girl's irritability with having to wait

**D.** The girl's tantrum after finishing the lollipop

**E.** The girl's crying after becoming irritable

**6-40.** A temper tantrum can erupt in response to an unexpected change in plans. When such a temper tantrum becomes violent and a child displays aggression toward parents, what intervention can be implemented in the moment to minimize the likelihood that the tantrum will be reinforced?

**A.** Distract

**B.** Model using words

**C.** Time-out/remove from situation

**D.** Establish a routine

**E.** Engage in fun activities

**6-41.** A 4-year-old boy is brought to the emergency department by his father after falling from the top of the bookcase in their living room. His father suspects that the child climbed up to retrieve the television remote control. It had been hidden away so that he would stop watching cartoons and get ready for bed. The boy's father acknowledged that he has difficulty setting limits and disciplining his child because when the child's wishes are thwarted he will tantrum aggressively and will destroy property, including his father's eyeglasses. What is the most evidence-based treatment modality for the disruptive behaviors described?

**A.** Pharmacotherapy

**B.** Parent management training

**C.** Dialectical behavior therapy

**D.** Interpersonal therapy

**E.** Individualized education plan

**6-42.** A 13-year-old boy discloses during his well-child check that his grades have dropped this semester because he has not been doing the assigned oral reports. He skips school on the days when his assignments are due. He states that he feels "queasy," flushed, and sweaty when he gets in front of an audience. The pediatrician asks open-ended questions to facilitate further disclosure and normalizes the boy's experience, which encourages him to acknowledge that he also has been sitting alone at lunch. He refuses to attend school events that require him to mingle with peers. What is the most likely diagnosis?

**A.** Panic disorder

**B.** Generalized anxiety disorder

**C.** Separation anxiety disorder

**D.** Post-traumatic stress disorder (PTSD)

**E.** Social anxiety disorder

**6-43.** The parents of an 11-year-old girl express concerns about the behaviors she has been engaging in for "the past year or two." They report that she has been truant from school. She spends time with her friends setting fire to their siblings' toys. They state that they also know that she is getting into physical fights with her younger brother and then lying about it or blaming others when confronted about her behavior. Which of the features described predicts a *less* favorable prognosis?

**A.** Aggression

**B.** Destructive behaviors

**C.** Deceitfulness

**D.** Truancy

**E.** Preadolescent onset

**6-44.** To meet *Diagnostic and Statistical Manual of Mental Disorders, Fifth Edition* (DSM-5) diagnostic criteria for schizophrenia, a patient *must* exhibit which of the following symptoms?

**A.** Delusions

**B.** Disorganized behavior

**C.** Decreased emotional expressiveness

**D.** Reduced speech output

**E.** Avolition

**6-45.** A 16-year-old boy was recently diagnosed with a psychotic disorder. He was started on an atypical antipsychotic to address his symptoms of paranoia and auditory hallucinations of multiple voices telling him "to do bad things." In addition to monitoring for weight gain, waist circumference, and total cholesterol levels, what additional lab tests should be periodically performed?

**A.** Liver function tests

**B.** Thyroid function tests

**C.** Complete blood count (CBC)

**D.** Fasting blood glucose

**E.** Serum electrolyte levels

**6-46.** First-line pharmacotherapy for treating attention-deficit/hyperactivity disorder (ADHD) involves medications that increase synaptic dopamine and norepinephrine levels. Methylphenidate blocks reuptake of these neurotransmitters. Amphetamine causes release from synaptic storage sites. Both classes are approved by the US Food and Drug Administration (FDA) for use in young children, and both come in a wide variety of formulations. Which of the following formulations of stimulants is common to both the methylphenidate and the amphetamine classes?

**A.** Elixir

**B.** Patch

**C.** Pro-drug

**D.** Osmotic "pump"

**E.** Chewable tablets

**6-47.** The parents of a 14-year-old girl, who was recently diagnosed with attention-deficit/hyperactivity disorder (ADHD) and has no comorbidities, come to clinic requesting pharmacotherapy. They assert that they requested an individualized education plan and that the patient is involved in a social skills group at school. What additional nonpharmacologic intervention can be implemented before initiating a trial of pharmacotherapy?

**A.** Increasing omega-3 intake

**B.** Increasing zinc intake

**C.** Eliminating foods containing artificial ingredients

**D.** Prohibiting homework

**E.** Involvement in appropriate extracurricular activities

**6-48.** Adolescents with attention-deficit/hyperactivity disorder (ADHD) often have comorbid mood, conduct, and substance use disorders. This combination puts them at increased risk for what problem as young adults?

**A.** Oppositional behavior

**B.** Low self-esteem

**C.** Emotional dysregulation

**D.** Suicide attempt

**E.** Low frustration tolerance

**6-49.** Cognitive behavior therapy (CBT) is an effective psychotherapeutic intervention for a variety of anxiety disorders. It is a brief intervention (16–20 weeks) that features a number of components, including psychoeducation, cognitive restructuring, and exposure to feared situations. What additional component is also an important aspect of CBT?

**A.** Mindfulness

**B.** Self-hypnosis

**C.** Self-monitoring

**D.** Exclusively individual engagement

**E.** Interpersonal effectiveness

**6-50.** A 9-year-old boy is brought into clinic at the request of his school. The patient's parents state that his teacher expressed concern about his frequent, intense anger outbursts triggered by minimal provocation (eg, losing a turn in a game, a peer bumping in to him, or being asked to wait his turn when he tried to cut in line). The parents acknowledge that they have noticed similar behaviors occurring almost daily for the past 18 months, as well as persistent irritability; they state that there was 1 month during the summer when his mood seemed to "lighten" but then the irritability resumed again and has persisted. They report no change in appetite, energy, or interest levels. What is the most likely diagnosis?

**A.** Major depressive disorder

**B.** Disruptive mood dysregulation disorder

**C.** Bipolar disorder

**D.** Attention-deficit/hyperactivity disorder (ADHD)

**E.** Oppositional defiant disorder

**6-51.** The parents of a 7-year-old girl bring her in for evaluation. She was bitten on the hand by a dog at 4 years old. Ever since that event, she has been afraid of dogs. When she encounters a dog, she will shriek and run away, which has led to some additional negative encounters when the dogs have actually run after her. The situation is so problematic that the family cannot go to the park or anywhere outdoors. If she sees a dog, she screams, hyperventilates, and demands to go home, which the family accommodates. She also now refuses to walk to school because there is a dog in one of the yards along the way. What is the most likely diagnosis?

**A.** Normative fear

**B.** Specific phobia

**C.** Obsessive-compulsive disorder (OCD)

**D.** Post-traumatic stress disorder (PTSD)

**E.** Panic disorder

**6-52.** In addition to dopamine, imbalance in what other neurotransmitter is understood to be implicated in the pathogenesis of attention-deficit/hyperactivity disorder (ADHD)?

**A.** Norepinephrine

**B.** Glutamate

**C.** $\gamma$-Amino butyric acid (GABA)

**D.** Serotonin

**E.** Acetylcholine

**6-53.** In studies of the etiology of attention-deficit/hyperactivity disorder (ADHD), differences in the structure and function of the frontal lobe and cerebellar vermis have been implicated. Differences in what other structure are understood to contribute to the etiology of ADHD?

**A.** Thalamus

**B.** Basal ganglia

**C.** Raphe nucleus

**D.** Anterior cingulate cortex

**E.** Amygdala

**6-54.** The parents of a 9-year-old boy come to clinic requesting referral to a behavioral specialist. They report concerns about a number of social difficulties that their son demonstrates. These issues include problems playing with friends, being impatient, missing social cues, and blurting out inappropriate remarks. He is struggling academically because he forgets to turn in his homework. When the boy was younger, he would often run off from them without regard for his own safety. The parents note that he would express concern when his little brother would cry and would try to "kiss away the boo-boo" like he saw his father do. A specialty clinic for what diagnosis would be most helpful for this patient?

**A.** Depressive disorder
**B.** Learning disability
**C.** Intellectual disability
**D.** Attention-deficit/hyperactivity disorder (ADHD)
**E.** Autism spectrum disorder

**6-55.** In conceptualizing the clinical manifestations of attention-deficit/hyperactivity disorder (ADHD), what is the most appropriate framework for understanding this disorder?

**A.** Disorder of complete lack of attention
**B.** Disorder of lack of common sense
**C.** Disorder of boredom
**D.** Disorder of motivation
**E.** Disorder of attention allocation

**6-56.** The father of an 11-year-old girl brings her to clinic because of concern for her obesity. He reports that she often eats "voraciously" and quickly at mealtime. She eats multiple snacks each day. When redirected, she sneaks food into her room to eat during the night. He states that when he confronts her about her eating behavior, she acknowledges that she feels that her eating is "out of control." What is the most likely diagnosis?

**A.** Binge eating disorder
**B.** Night eating syndrome
**C.** Bulimia nervosa
**D.** Anorexia nervosa, binge-purge type
**E.** Overeating

**6-57.** A 16-year-old girl asks her pediatrician about how to address her low energy. She explains that she doesn't have any energy to do anything even though she seems to sleep all the time. She also reports that she has no appetite or interest in things that she used to enjoy. She can't concentrate at school and feels guilty about her resulting bad grades. She describes her mood as "sad all the time." Of the population of adolescents with this patient's diagnosis, 20% to 40% of them will develop what disorder in the next 5 years?

**A.** Panic disorder
**B.** Major depressive disorder
**C.** Attention-deficit/hyperactivity disorder (ADHD)
**D.** Bipolar I disorder
**E.** Schizophrenia

**6-58.** The parents of a 15-year-old boy are concerned about their son's worsening anxiety. They state that they recognized that he was struggling with social anxiety disorder and post-traumatic stress disorder (PTSD), related to a motor vehicle accident (MVA). The MVA was not his fault; however, it resulted in the death of one of the passengers riding in his car. They report that he now is describing episodes of intense anxiety associated with frightening physical sensations, such a difficulty breathing, chest tightening, and tunnel vision. They state that he is having trouble leaving the house out of concern that he will not be able to seek medical attention if one of these episodes occurs when he is alone. Research suggests that, in the setting of comorbid anxiety disorders, there is increased risk of this patient developing what disorder?

**A.** Panic disorder
**B.** Obsessive-compulsive disorder (OCD)
**C.** Schizophrenia
**D.** Bipolar disorder
**E.** Depressive disorder

**6-59.** An 8-year-old girl is brought in to clinic for her well-child check. Her mother recalls that when her daughter was in preschool, she was afraid of the dark for a short period. She got over this fear with the help of a nightlight and parental reassurance. The mother wonders, however, if the child will develop additional fears in elementary school. The pediatrician provides anticipatory guidance about the normative fears that occur at this age. What types of concerns tend to be associated with elementary school-aged children?

**A.** Separation from parents
**B.** Anticipatory worry
**C.** Harm and competence
**D.** Rejection by peers
**E.** Anxiety about performance

**6-60.** A 12-year-old girl presents to your office for an annual physical exam. She is transferring care to you after moving from another state. You review her growth chart and note that her weight and body mass index (BMI) from birth to the age of 10 years were consistently at the 75th percentile for age. Her weight and BMI today are the 1st percentile for age. Her vital signs are notable for a heart rate of 48 bpm. Her blood pressure is 88/48 mm Hg, with an orthostatic heart rate change of 36 bpm from lying to standing. On exam, she is pale. She has hypoactive bowel sounds and lanugo over her trunk and extremities. Her hands are cool and mottled. On history, which of the following would be most consistent with this presentation?

**A.** Recurrent episodes of eating large quantities of food in a short period of time, followed by compensatory vomiting

**B.** Life-long picky eating with long-standing issues with food textures leading to persistent food aversion

**C.** History of diarrhea and flatulence after consuming dairy products

**D.** Recent change to a gluten-free, vegetarian diet

**E.** History of marijuana use

**6-61.** You are asked to give a presentation on eating disorders to parents at a local school. You include a discussion of warning signs, as well as symptoms, diagnosis, and treatment. At the end of the presentation, a concerned mother asks what parents should know regarding the prognosis of adolescents with eating disorders. What would be the best response?

**A.** Younger age at diagnosis is associated with lower rates of clinical remission.

**B.** Early weight gain during treatment is not associated with a change in prognosis.

**C.** Longer duration of symptoms prior to diagnosis is associated with better response to treatment.

**D.** Rates of clinical remission at 1 year are > 50%.

**E.** Early recognition and entry into treatment are associated with better prognosis.

**6-62.** A 15-year-old boy is brought in by his parents for evaluation of depression. On history, he and his family note that he has had increased irritability, decreased interest in school and extracurricular activities he used to enjoy, and difficulty sleeping and early waking despite feeling tired. He also has had decreased appetite for the past month. You interview him privately, and he further reports that he has episodes of feeling "down" and hopeless. He has had thoughts that he would be better off dead; however, he denies a plan to hurt himself or end his life. You meet with his parents separately to gather additional history. They ask you if he is at risk for suicide. Which of the following is not associated with a higher risk of suicide in adolescents?

**A.** Female gender

**B.** History of nonsuicidal self-injury

**C.** Previous suicide attempt

**D.** History of substance abuse

**E.** Social isolation

## ANSWERS

**Answer 6-1.** B

It is recommended that all children with autism spectrum disorder undergo chromosomal microarray analysis and testing for fragile X syndrome in the effort to determine the etiology for their autism spectrum disorder.

The other medical studies included are indicated based on clinical findings. Audiology evaluations are important to perform if the child has never had his hearing tested; hearing impairment can result in symptoms similar to those of autism spectrum disorder. Many patients with autism have sleep disturbances. As a result, a sleep study can be helpful in ruling out conditions such as obstructive sleep apnea, which can result in behavioral dysregulation. Metabolic workup is usually reserved for situations in which physiologic symptoms are manifested. For children whose neurodevelopmental disorders are thought to be causing seizures, an EEG is indicated. However, in this vignette, there was no mention of concern for seizures.

(p. 398, Section 6: Developmental and Behavioral Pediatrics)

**Answer 6-2.** E

Although more often associated with younger children, separation anxiety disorder can occur in adolescents, especially those who had separation anxiety early in their development. Although the patient's mother did experience a trauma, the patient was not directly affected by the car accident. She is reacting to the separation from her mother that was a result of the hospitalization from the car accident. Also, the 2-month interval between trauma and symptoms does not meet the time criteria for PTSD.

The patient's symptoms are specifically related to being away from her mother. Generalized anxiety is more diffuse and is associated with worry about numerous issues, not just separation from a caregiver. Although the patient has somatic complaints, they are not consistent with neurovegetative symptoms associated with a depressive disorder. There is nothing in the vignette that suggests that the patient's anxious behaviors are related to social scrutiny or fear of being embarrassed or rejected.

(p. 402, Section 7: Pediatric Mental Health)

**Answer 6-3.** A

The patient is demonstrating the hallucinations, disorganized behaviors, and negative symptoms (withdrawal, poor attention to activities of daily living) that characterize schizophrenia. The relatively late diagnosis of intellectual disability could represent the cognitive decline that often precedes the psychotic break characteristic of first-episode schizophrenia.

The patient's sadness and withdrawal can be mistaken for a severe depressive disorder; however, the level of disorganization, the cognitive symptoms, and the hallucinations are more characteristic of a psychotic disorder. The patient's recent decline in function suggests that a neurodevelopmental disorder such as autism is less likely. Although catatonia is more often associated with mood disorders than psychotic disorders, there is little in the patient's presentation besides hallucinations to suggest that mania is responsible for his symptoms, thereby ruling out bipolar I disorder. Schizotypal personality disorder tends to have briefer episodes of less intense symptomatology, such that activities of daily living are not impacted.

(p. 416, Section 7: Pediatric Mental Health)

**Answer 6-4.** B

Because mood symptoms can be caused or exacerbated by other medical conditions, it is important to obtain baseline laboratory studies to rule out conditions such as anemia, hypothyroidism, and mononucleosis.

While it is good to know PHQ-9 scores to quantify the degree of depression and to be able to track changes in severity of symptoms, it is not necessarily the next step in the treatment course, as it is part of the evaluation. When the laboratory testing has ruled out other medical causes for neurovegetative symptoms, it is important to obtain (and document) parental consent for psychotropic medications. Although the studies that compelled the black box warning have now been called into question, it is still necessary to discuss the black box warning with the patient and caregivers because it has not been removed from the prescribing information and prescribers remain obligated to follow monitoring guidelines. Information about crisis hotlines can be offered as part of the counseling provided to patients and parents to prevent the potentially devastating outcome of major depressive disorder; however, this information does not treat the symptoms of this disorder.

(p. 409, Section 7: Pediatric Mental Health)

**Answer 6-5.** D

Catatonia is often associated with psychosis, although it is more commonly associated with mood disorders and neurodevelopmental disorders (NDDs). Pediatric catatonia often goes undiagnosed. A high index of suspicion is necessary to avoid missing this syndrome, particularly given the high morbidity and mortality associated with delayed diagnosis. Despite a low overall incidence, certain pediatric populations are at much greater risk for catatonia, including patients with NDDs such as autism and developmental delay. Although rating scales such as the Bush Francis Catatonia Rating Scale can be helpful in making the diagnosis, the approach needs to be modified in NDDs because many patients could meet criteria at baseline as a result of their NDD.

Unlike psychotic disorders, which are treated with antipsychotic medications like aripiprazole or risperidone, catatonia does not respond to these medications. Instead, the first-line intervention for catatonia is lorazepam. When this medication is not effective, ECT is indicated.

(p. 416, Section 7: Pediatric Mental Health)

**Answer 6-6.** C

Behavioral dysregulation can be mistaken for or misinterpreted as nonsuicidal self-injury (NSSI). Although dialectical behavioral therapy is an effective intervention in NSSI, it is unlikely to be effective in treating self-injurious behavior related to dysregulation. This condition is treated with either risperidone or aripiprazole, antipsychotics that have been approved by the US Food and Drug Administration (FDA) as first-line agents to treat agitation or aggression in autism spectrum disorder.

Other antipsychotics (eg, quetiapine) can be used; however, they are not considered first-line agents because they have not been approved by the FDA for this purpose. Applied behavior analysis would be a reasonable long-term intervention, once the severity of the patient's symptoms has been mitigated with pharmacotherapy. The patient's level of dysregulation is too severe to accommodate behavior shaping through applied behavior analysis.

(p. 398, Section 6: Developmental and Behavioral Pediatrics)

**Answer 6-7.** C

Stimulants are effective in 70% to 80% of patients. Because the mechanism of action of increasing synaptic dopamine and norepinephrine is different for methylphenidate and for the mixed amphetamine salts, a stimulant trial is not considered complete until both classes of stimulant are tried. Furthermore, patients can have different responses to the 2 classes of stimulants. Thus, if one class of stimulant is not effective or has prohibitive side effects, then the other class should be tried before switching to a nonstimulant agent.

Atomoxetine and extended-release guanfacine are good nonstimulant options that directly affect norepinephrine neurotransmission. These medications are second-line agents when stimulants are not effective, but can be used first if there are concerns about psychotic disorders or diversion or misuse of stimulants. Bupropion has weaker activity as a dopamine reuptake blocker but may have sufficient efficacy to adjust dopamine tone in the frontal cortex and basal ganglia, especially in the setting of affective symptoms. There is limited evidence regarding fish oil for psychotic and mood disorders, but the evidence is more mixed (and anecdotal) for ADHD.

(pp. 390–391, Section 6: Developmental and Behavioral Pediatrics)

**Answer 6-8.** D

The patient's thoughts (fear of regaining weight) and behaviors related to her weight and her efforts to decrease weight by limiting caloric intake meet diagnostic criteria for anorexia nervosa, not OSFED. Although she does avoid numerous foods, which is consistent with avoidant/restrictive food intake disorder, she has numerous symptoms beyond being very selective about her food choices. Because the patient does not report any episodes of increased food intake in the form of binges, she does not meet criteria for binge eating disorder or bulimia nervosa (even though she does engage in behaviors that compensate for caloric intake).

(p. 337, Section 5, Part 3: Mental Health Disorders in the Adolescent)

**Answer 6-9.** E

No one can change history, so prior attempt and family history are not modifiable. Medical disorders are the realm of pediatricians, but chronic conditions are not readily changed. Likewise, self-injurious behavior can be treated but this is not usually the role of the pediatrician.

The pediatrician does have the opportunity to intervene most directly by working with their patients' parents to remove means of suicide such as medications and firearms.

(p. 411, Section 7: Pediatric Mental Health)

**Answer 6-10.** A

The disruptive behaviors described in the scenario are likely secondary to the recent trauma that the family has experienced. The heightened stress response can lead to impulsive behaviors that appear similar to those seen in ADHD. Because the etiology of the patient's impulsivity is trauma rather than executive dysfunction, the most appropriate medication is an α-adrenergic agent like guanfacine or clonidine. Focus, attention, and impulsivity will improve with stimulants, but they do not target the stress response that is actually driving the behaviors. Stimulant medications also can result in agitation and insomnia, as well as appetite suppression.

Situational depression may be an etiology for the patient's symptoms; if more depressive symptoms were elaborated in the history, then antidepressants could be a possible intervention. Antipsychotics and anxiolytics will sedate the patient; however, they will not address his underlying symptoms.

(p. 415, Section 7: Pediatric Mental Health)

**Answer 6-11.** D

The symptoms described are those of obsessive-compulsive disorder. There a number of medications approved by the FDA for treatment of these symptoms; of those listed, only paroxetine is not approved for this use. The distinguishing characteristic (in addition to side effect profile) to consider when selecting a medication is the age for which FDA approval has been given (Table 93-4).

**TABLE 93-4.** Medications Approved for Anxiety Disorders in Children and Adolescents

| Generic Name (Brand Name) | Subclass | Dosing | FDA-Approved Uses | Ages | Additional Information |
|---|---|---|---|---|---|
| Fluoxetine (Prozac) | SSRI | 20–60 mg/d<br>Start 10 mg/d, increase to 20 mg/d on day 14 | OCD | 7 y and older | Long half-life (4–6 d)<br>Available in liquid form |
| Sertraline (Zoloft) | SSRI | 25–200 mg/d<br>Start at 25 mg/d and increase to 50 mg after 7 days; increase to 50 mg and then may increase every 4 weeks | OCD | 6 y and older | Available in liquid form |
| Fluvoxamine (Luvox) | SSRI | 50–200 mg/d<br>Oral daily dosing to twice/day<br>Start 25 mg at bedtime, increase by 25 mg/d q4–7 d; maximum dose is 200 mg/d up to 11 y, 300 mg/d for > 11 y | OCD | 8 y and older | |
| Duloxetine (Cymbalta) | SNRI | 30–60 mg/d<br>Start 30 mg/d; may increase by 30 mg/d after 2 weeks | GAD | 7 y and older | Used for treatment of neuropathic pain in adults |
| Clomipramine (Anafranil) | TCA | 100–200 mg at bedtime<br>Start 25 mg qd, increase by 25 mg/d q4–7 days; maximum 3 mg/kg/d up to 100 mg/d in first 2 wk and up to 200 mg/d maintenance | OCD | 10 y and older | |

GAD, generalized anxiety disorder; OCD, obsessive-compulsive disorder; q4–7, every 4 to 7; qd, once daily; SNRI, serotonin norepinephrine reuptake inhibitor; SSRI, selective serotonin reuptake inhibitor; TCA, tricyclic antidepressant.

Mark W. Kline, *Rudolph's Pediatrics*, 23rd Edition. Copyright © McGraw-Hill Education. All rights reserved.

Only sertraline has been approved to treat children as young as 6 years old.

(pp. 404 and 407, Section 7: Pediatric Mental Health)

**Answer 6-12.** B

The most likely diagnosis is expressive (receptive) language disorder. The fact that the child's nonverbal communication and relatedness are intact makes the diagnosis of autism spectrum disorder less likely. As a result, applied behavior analysis would not be as beneficial for the patient's symptoms. Some symptoms of motoric overflow (hand flapping and toe-walking) may be misinterpreted as representative of autism spectrum disorder but are often normal behaviors, often associated with excitement. Occupational therapy is less indicated for these behaviors and more suited for difficulties with fine motor control.

Speech therapy is the most targeted (and appropriate) intervention for a language disorder; it can be helpful in autism spectrum disorder as well, but it does not target the core symptoms of this disorder. Augmentative communication is helpful in the setting of providing support for nonverbal children or of plateauing of speech therapy gains. Play therapy is a type of psychotherapy that addresses psychological factors more so than language disorders.

(p. 397, Section 6: Developmental and Behavioral Pediatrics)

**Answer 6-13.** A

Eating disorders are often comorbid with other psychiatric disorders, such as anxiety or depressive disorders. The eating disorder is often treated first, and then the residual anxious or mood symptoms are addressed later. Regardless of whether anxiety disorders are or are not comorbid with eating disorders, the safest and most effective treatment is a selective serotonin reuptake inhibitor, such as sertraline.

Bupropion is contraindicated in eating disorders due to the increased risk of seizures that is associated with the electrolyte disturbances and elevated serum levels of medication that can occur if the eating disorder symptoms recur. Neither dialectical behavior therapy nor exposure-and-response prevention therapy is indicated for anxiety that is not associated with emotion dysregulation or compulsions, respectively. Additional monitoring will delay necessary treatment.

(p. 340, Section 5, Part 3: Mental Health Disorders in the Adolescent)

**Answer 6-14.** C

PTSD can result from a singular traumatic event in which there is the possibility of bodily harm or death (eg, accidents, natural disasters, and medical trauma) or a series of adverse childhood experiences, such as violence in the home, emotional abuse, or the loss of a caregiver to divorce, incarceration, or the like. The 12-month prevalence approaches 5%, but the lifetime prevalence is estimated to be 9%.

The risk factors that predispose individuals to PTSD are varied, especially because 50% of the population is estimated to be exposed to traumatic events during childhood and adolescence; they include (but are not limited to) female gender, a history of psychiatric illness, low levels of social support, and higher than expected release of catecholamines during a traumatic event.

(p. 335, Section 5, Part 3: Mental Health Disorders in the Adolescent)

**Answer 6-15.** D

Disruptive mood dysregulation disorder is a depressive disorder associated with persistently irritable or angry moods and outbursts of behavioral dysregulation that occur at least 3 times per week. Other disorders associated with irritability are major depressive disorders (answer choice E, where neurovegetative symptoms are prominent) and PTSD (answer choice B). The behaviors described in answer choice C are most consistent with oppositional-defiant disorder. The behaviors described in answer choice A are consistent with separation anxiety disorder.

(p. 408, Section 7, Chapter 94: Pediatric Depression and Bipolar Spectrum Disorders)

**Answer 6-16.** B

The scenario in answer choice B describes a situation in which the patient avoids oral intake because of a traumatic experience with food. There is no mention of fears of gaining weight or other concerns about body image, which is the key distinguishing feature of avoidant/restrictive food intake disorder compared to anorexia nervosa (answer choices C and E) and bulimia nervosa (answer choice D). Night eating syndrome (answer choice A) does not involve food avoidance or impaired social functioning.

(pp. 337–338, Section 5, Part 3: Mental Health Disorders in the Adolescent, Chapter 76)

**Answer 6-17.** E

Both classes of mood stabilizer should have laboratory tests performed at baseline (answer choice E); for lithium, these tests include pregnancy tests, thyroid function tests, serum blood urea nitrogen, and serum creatinine level, whereas for atypical antipsychotics, these tests include fasting blood glucose and lipid panel. Lithium blood levels should also be checked after dosage changes (answer choice A) but not every 5 days (answer choice B). Both lithium and antipsychotics should have follow-up labs drawn every 3 months initially, and then lithium-related labs should be checked every 6 to 12 months (answer choice C), whereas antipsychotic-related labs can be checked every 12 months. Neither class of medication requires daily labs (answer choice D).

(p. 411, Section 7: Pediatric Mental Health, Chapter 94)

**Answer 6-18.** C

Appetite suppression is one of the most frequent side effects of stimulant medications, especially the longer acting stimulants, which tend to interfere with appetite at lunchtime. By scheduling doses after breakfast and ensuring that patients have access to nutritious, high-calorie meals and snacks after the medication wears off, appetite suppression can be compensated for. Sleep disturbance (answer choice B), jitteriness (answer choice D), and headache (answer choice E) are also common side effects, but not as common as abdominal pain and appetite suppression. The "zombie effect" (answer choice A) is occasionally described by parents when they notice the patient being more subdued while taking the stimulant medication. This effect wears off as the stimulant is metabolized.

(p. 391, Section 6: Developmental and Behavioral Pediatrics, Chapter 90)

**Answer 6-19.** E

Perfectionism (answer choice A) and obsessive behavior (answer choice B) are associated with anorexia nervosa, whereas depression (answer choice C) and substance use (answer choice D) are more typically associated with bulimia nervosa. Low self-esteem (answer choice E) and anxiety are shared between anorexia nervosa and bulimia nervosa.

(p. 338, Section 5: Principles of Adolescent Care, Chapter 76)

**Answer 6-20.** C

The black box warning addresses the potential consequence of increased suicidal ideation associated with the use of antidepressants. The expectation established by the FDA in the warning is that prescribers check in weekly for the first 4 weeks after initiating or changing the dose of an antidepressant (answer choice C).

After the first month of monitoring, the check-ins can occur every 2 weeks (answer choice D). The black box warning does not address the metabolic consequences of antidepressant medications. The monitoring for hyponatremia (answer choice A) or weight gain (answer choice E) is established by pharmacologic guidelines. Monitoring for appetite change (answer choice B) is more often associated with counseling around stimulant medications and is a useful suggestion when any medication is prescribed; however, it is not a part of the black box warning.

(p. 410, Section 7: Pediatric Mental Health, Chapter 94)

**Answer 6-21.** B

Imaginary friends can be part of normal development for younger children, so enthusiastic conversations with beings (people or otherwise) who are not real can be part of age-appropriate imagination (answer choice B). This behavior tends to fade around 10 years of age. Auditory hallucinations may cause patients to appear as though they are having a conversation with a person whom only they hear, but the emotional tone tends to be more negative (ego-dystonic).

Because the patient's behaviors are play based and not psychotic, schizophreniform disorder (a *forme fruste* of schizophrenia; answer choice A), bipolar disorder (answer choice C), and delusional disorders (answer choice D) can be ruled out. Although irritability is described in the clinical scenario, it is limited in its scope and situational, unlike the irritability associated with disruptive mood dysregulation disorder (answer choice E).

(p. 416, Section 7: Pediatric Mental Health, Chapter 95)

**Answer 6-22.** E

In cyclothymia, the duration of hypomanic (but not manic) and depressive symptoms can endure for 1 year (longer than the 1- or 2-week criterion for mania or depression, respectively), but importantly, the severity of the symptoms never reaches criterion level (eg, remains subsyndromal). The frequency of symptom fluctuation can actually be increased in cyclothymia, and the impairment and distress caused by the subsyndromal symptoms are what brings the affected individual to clinical attention. Both disorders have episodic mood fluctuations.

(p. 332, Section 5: Principles of Adolescent Care, Chapter 75)

**Answer 6-23.** A

Hyperactive symptoms of ADHD are more common in boys than in girls and tend to manifest early as excessive motoric activity or talkativeness. Over time, the symptoms evolve (likely as a result of the maturation of the frontal lobe) and become attenuated, not increased (answer choice C); these attenuated symptoms are more likely to be described as restlessness or impatience (answer choice A). The hyperactivity is less likely to persist without change (answer choice D) or resolve completely (answer choice E), although the symptoms can decrease enough so that they are subclinical and not problematic for the patient. Hyperactivity and inattention are different symptom clusters, stemming from different brain functions; they can appear in tandem, but they are not interchangeable, nor does one symptom cluster convert to the other (answer choice B).

(p. 387, Section 6: Developmental and Behavioral Pediatrics, Chapter 90)

**Answer 6-24.** A

Although the patient is struggling with language development, appearing that perhaps he has an expressive language disorder (answer choice C), he is also struggling with other cognitive functions as well. As a result, this symptom constellation suggests that he has cognitive deficits that are best characterized as an intellectual disability (answer choice A).

Because he does not have deficits in the social or motor domains of development, he does not meet criteria for global developmental delay (answer choice D). Specific learning disabilities are usually diagnosed at later ages, when children are in elementary school, when difficulty with mastering the academic concepts of reading, writing, or arithmetic becomes apparent. At this time, the patient's symptoms are not consistent with specific learning disabilities (answer choice E). The diagnosis of autism (answer choice B) is unlikely because of the patient's intact theory of mind, as evidenced by joint attention.

(p. 397, Section 6: Developmental and Behavioral Pediatrics, Chapter 91)

**Answer 6-25.** D

Because the patient is articulating concerns about her weight and appearance and is already engaging in behaviors to counteract these concerns and these behaviors are having an impact on her physiology, she meets criteria for anorexia nervosa. Family-based therapy (answer choice D) is an evidence-based intervention that has demonstrated considerable efficacy in the treatment of anorexia nervosa.

CBT (answer choice B), interpersonal therapy (answer choice E), and even psychodynamic psychotherapy (answer choice C) in some situations can be helpful in addressing the affective symptoms that predate or are comorbid with anorexia nervosa. Dialectical behavior therapy (answer choice A) and CBT may have some efficacy in treating bulimia nervosa.

(p. 340, Section 5: Principles of Adolescent Care, Chapter 76)

**Answer 6-26.** B

Although many children use their imaginations and pretend that they are superheroes and pretend to fly (answer choice C), there are some children who have difficulty distinguishing their fantasies from reality, with unfortunate consequences. This impairment in reality testing, as described here, is less consistent with childhood-onset schizophrenia (answer choice E) and more consistent with a manic episode of bipolar disorder (answer choice B) because of the associated symptoms of irritability, decreased sleep, and increased sexualized behavior.

This last symptom might also be associated with sexual abuse (answer choice D), and this possibility should always be investigated and ruled out before establishing the diagnosis of mania. Nonaccidental trauma (answer choice A) is another diagnosis to be ruled out when a child presents with a humeral fracture. Given the overall clinical picture, bipolar disorder with a manic episode remains the most likely diagnosis.

(p. 408, Section 7: Pediatric Mental Health, Chapter 94)

**Answer 6-27.** C

Because the patient demonstrates intact nonverbal interactions, reciprocity, and empathy, his social communication and social interactions are relatively appropriate. As a result, the diagnosis of autism spectrum disorder can be ruled out. Autism spectrum disorder is characterized by deficits in the social communication/interaction domain as well as restricted interests and behaviors.

Given his delayed milestones and difficulty with expressive language, neither intellectual disability (answer choice A) nor expressive language disorder (answer choice B) can be ruled out. It remains possible that his social difficulties with peers relate to poor attention to social cues, suggestive of ADHD (answer choice D) inattentive subtype. His delays may make him feel self-conscious when interacting with peers, leading to social anxiety (answer choice E). These disorders remain plausible and need to be evaluated more extensively before ruling them out.

(p. 397, Section 6: Developmental and Behavioral Pediatrics, Chapter 91)

**Answer 6-28.** A

The patient is reported to have deficits in the realm of communication for social interaction with no impairments in the realm of restricted interests or behaviors. This dissociation of the symptom clusters distinguishes social (pragmatic) communication disorder (answer choice A) from autism spectrum disorder (answer choice D). Individuals with nonverbal learning disability (answer choice B) also have difficulty reading social situations (appreciating nuanced conversation and facial expressions) but recognize the relevance of others in the interaction. Conversational difficulties in ADHD (answer choice C) are related to not attending to the conversational partner's contribution to the conversation or to blurting out responses in an untimely fashion. The patient has little difficulty expressing herself through her vocabulary and complex sentence structure, deficits that are typical of expressive language disorder (answer choice E).

(pp. 395 and 397, Section 6: Developmental and Behavioral Pediatrics, Chapter 91)

**Answer 6-29.** C

The timing of the change in the patient's behavior and the symptoms described suggest that he is likely experiencing discomfort related to a gastrointestinal disorder. A very common gastrointestinal issue for children with autism is constipation, and the most straightforward intervention, which is both diagnostic and therapeutic, is providing a laxative (answer choice C) to relieve the child of his stool burden.

Unfortunately, interventions of questionable validity are directly marketed to parents who seek unconventional treatment for their child. Exclusion diets (answer choice A) such as the gluten-free, casein-free diets; antifungal medications (answer choice B), purported to treat fungal overgrowth of normal gut flora; and megadoses of vitamins (answer choice D) are popular interventions that are considered by the lay public to be relatively harmless. More complicated (and riskier) interventions, such as hyperbaric oxygen (answer choice E), may be sought by parents when over-the-counter remedies are ineffective.

(p. 398, Section 6: Developmental and Behavioral Pediatrics, Chapter 91)

**Answer 6-30.** E

Along with risperidone, aripiprazole (answer choice E) received FDA approval for treating the agitation and aggression (to self and to others) that can be associated with autism spectrum disorders.

Other atypical antipsychotic medications, such as quetiapine (answer choice A), ziprasidone (answer choice C), and olanzapine (answer choice D) are not FDA approved; when and if they are used, mostly for sedation, their use is "off label." Citalopram (answer choice B) was theorized to be a treatment for irritability, but controlled studies have not validated this hypothesis.

(p. 415, Section 7: Pediatric Mental Health, Chapter 95)

**Answer 6-31.** D

While the patient's age (older adolescent) and gender are known risk factors for suicide, his community support (in the form of teacher investment in his success) is a protective factor against suicide. Also important is the fact that he is presenting to clinical care and is disclosing his distress. Academic success and abstinence from alcohol are positive aspects of this patient's functioning; however, they are not shown to be as protective as the support of a caring adult.

(p. 332, Section 5, Part 3: Mental Health Disorders in the Adolescent, Chapter 75)

**Answer 6-32.** D

Although the stereotypical image of an adolescent is a gloomy, irritable, oppositional teenager, suggestive of depression, most adolescents suffer from anxiety disorders. The lifetime prevalence of anxiety disorders is estimated to be 30%. Approximately half of all anxiety disorders in adults are present by early adolescence. Psychotic disorders are uncommon and tend to manifest in later adolescence or young adulthood. Bipolar disorder has a lifetime prevalence of 3%, whereas disruptive mood dysregulation disorder is a subtype of depressive disorder, which has a lifetime prevalence of 12%.

(p. 333, Section 5, Part 3: Mental Health Disorders in the Adolescent, Chapter 75)

**Answer 6-33.** A

When anxiety is extreme, it can impact several different functions. In addition, anxiety indirectly can cause a loss of interest in activities that were once pleasurable, because they may now cause anxiety and are avoided. In these cases, the anxiety becomes so extreme as to border on the delusional and the patient can no longer rationally address the reality of his or her anxiety. Alternatively, the responses to anxiety become distracting and interfere with concentration or become activating and cause hyperkinetic activity to distract from the anxiety or to allow scanning of the environment.

Only answer choice A is directly associated with anxiety disorders. Answer choice B is associated with depressive disorders, answer choice C is associated with psychotic disorders, and answer choices D and E are associated with attention-deficit/hyperactivity disorder (ADHD).

(p. 333, Section 5, Part 3: Mental Health Disorders in the Adolescent, Chapter 75)

**Answer 6-34.** C

The patient has risk factors for and describes symptoms consistent with generalized anxiety disorder. Duloxetine is considered first-line treatment of generalized anxiety disorder, given its approval by the US Food and Drug Administration (FDA) for its use in adolescents with anxiety.

Although selective serotonin reuptake inhibitors (SSRIs), such as paroxetine, can be used to treat anxiety disorders, they do not have an indication for use in children and adolescents. Paroxetine is especially problematic given its short half-life and considerable withdrawal effects. Gabapentin, lorazepam, and hydroxyzine can briefly mitigate peaks of anxious symptoms but are not truly treatments for the disorder.

(pp. 333–334, Section 5, Part 3: Mental Health Disorders in the Adolescent, Chapter 75)

**Answer 6-35.** B

The scenario describes both mood (irritability) and neurovegetative (eg, sleep disruption and diminished energy) symptoms consistent with a major depressive disorder. Her withdrawal from family and descriptions of boredom and lack of pleasure and hopelessness are especially concerning. The symptoms are less consistent with persistent depressive disorder because there has not been 1 year of symptoms and the symptoms themselves are more severe than what is typically experienced in persistent depressive disorder.

Although the patient is described as irritable and her sleep pattern has changed, the symptoms are less likely to be associated with bipolar disorder because the sleep pattern has shifted but not decreased; likewise, there appears to be less goal-directed activity, not more of this activity. The symptoms reported are not consistent with normal adolescence because anhedonia, isolation, and hopelessness are not normative. Finally, the patient's academic dysfunction is less likely to be a learning disability because her poor grades are recent and more likely related to lack of engagement in schoolwork associated with her overall anhedonia.

(p. 331, Section 5, Part 3: Mental Health Disorders in the Adolescent, Chapter 75)

**Answer 6-36.** E

The Treatment for Adolescents with Depression Study (TADS) demonstrated that CBT and SSRIs when used alone are not as effective as the combination of CBT and SSRIs. The 12-week data in this study showed response rates of 61% with fluoxetine monotherapy, 43% with CBT only, and 71% with combination therapy. Although interpersonal therapy can be an effective intervention for adolescents struggling with role transitions, it does not have the same efficacy as CBT and SSRIs, either alone or in combination with a mood stabilizer.

(p. 410, Section 7: Pediatric Mental Health, Chapter 94: Pediatric Depression and Bipolar Spectrum Disorders)

**Answer 6-37.** D

There are a number of atypical antipsychotics that are US Food and Drug Administration (FDA) approved for the treatment of the acute manic episodes associated with bipolar disorder in individuals younger than 18 years old; these include asenapine, quetiapine, and risperidone. Olanzapine is unique in that it can be used to treat acute episodes of both mania and depression.

There are fewer medications that are indicated for the maintenance of remission (or prevention of recurrence) of bipolar disorder symptoms; one of them is aripiprazole.

(p. 411, Section 7: Pediatric Mental Health, Chapter 94: Pediatric Depression and Bipolar Spectrum Disorders)

**Answer 6-38.** B

Nearly 1 in 12 adolescents (8.6%) attempted suicide in the year prior to the survey; 14.6% of students made a plan for suicide, and 17.7% had suicidal ideation. The prevalence of major depressive disorder in adolescents is 11.4%, and the reported prevalence of bipolar spectrum disorder is 6.7%. Pediatricians are on the primary care front lines of individuals who can intervene to save the lives of adolescents who are suffering from affective disorders.

(pp. 408 and 411, Section 7: Pediatric Mental Health, Chapter 94: Pediatric Depression and Bipolar Spectrum Disorders)

**Answer 6-39.** A

The scenario describes a very common situation, where the behavior of tantrums or tears (answer choice E) serve as a means of self-expression in the setting or antecedent of frustration or irritability (answer choice C). This behavior is understandable, but it can ultimately become maladaptive, especially when a child develops alternative means (language) for communicating distress or displeasure. Tantrums and disruptive behavior often elicit consequences in the form of responses from parents. These consequences, such as an attempt to soothe (answer choice B), can be reassuring, but they can also be inadvertently reinforcing, and thus problematic, such as when a treat is offered as a bribe (answer choice A). In this case, the consequence of offering a lollipop can result in an escalation of behaviors, such as a louder tantrum after the lollipop is consumed (answer choice D).

(p. 412, Section 7: Pediatric Mental Health, Chapter 95: Disruptive Behavior Disorders and Psychotic Disorders)

**Answer 6-40.** C

Behavior shaping can occur at the level of antecedents of behaviors or responses to the behaviors. Establishing a routine (answer choice D) can be helpful in minimizing the precipitants of a tantrum that occurs when unexpected changes occur in a child's day. Distraction (answer choice A) or helping a child learn to use verbal (rather than physical) means of expression (answer choice B) can shape behaviors in the moment when the behaviors are mild in intensity. If the child continues (or is encouraged to continue) engaging in fun activities during the tantrum (answer choice E), then the tantrum will likely be reinforced. If a tantrum is violent, then the child can be disengaged from the situation (answer choice C) that caused the tantrum so that the behavior is not reinforced and instead is more likely to extinguish.

(pp. 413–414; Section 7: Pediatric Mental Health, Chapter 95: Disruptive Behavior Disorders and Psychotic Disorders)

**Answer 6-41.** B

Because the behavior of parents can so profoundly influence the behavior of their children, it is important for parents to develop the skills required to address potentially disruptive behaviors. Parent management training is an intervention to support parents in this effort through education about and practicing of behavior principles that reinforce adaptive behavior and model prosocial interactions.

Pharmacotherapy is second line or adjunctive to parent management training. Dialectical behavior therapy and interpersonal therapy may be helpful in addressing psychological comorbidities, such as depression, associated with disruptive behaviors engaged in by older (adolescent) patients. An individualized education plan could include goals related to aggression at school, but the father in the clinical scenario is having difficulty managing behavior at home and could benefit from an intervention targeting his responses to the patient's behaviors.

(p. 415; Section 7: Pediatric Mental Health, Chapter 95: Disruptive Behavior Disorders and Psychotic Disorders)

**Answer 6-42.** E

Social anxiety disorder (otherwise known as social phobia) is the culmination of an individual's fear of the scrutiny of peers and the worry about how the individual will be judged as a consequence of such scrutiny. Social anxiety disorder is associated with fears of embarrassment or rejection in social situations.

Separation anxiety disorder can occur in adolescents, especially those who had separation anxiety early in their development. It can be associated with school refusal; however, the patient in the scenario does not avoid school entirely. He only misses class when he is expected to speak in front of his peers. Generalized anxiety disorder is a more diffuse form of anxiety and is associated with worry about numerous issues, not social scrutiny alone. There is no evidence to suggest that the patient's avoidance of certain classes is related to a traumatic event that occurred at school, which decreases the likelihood of PTSD. The clinical scenario enumerates physiologic symptoms that can be associated with panic disorder but does not include reports of a sense of doom or of "going crazy," which are key symptoms of panic disorder.

(p. 333, Section 5: Principles of Adolescent Care, Chapter 75: Depression, Anxiety, and Other Disorders in Adolescence)

**Answer 6-43.** E

All of the behaviors described are concerning as potential symptoms of conduct disorder. Aggression against others, destruction of property, especially by fire, lying about the behavior, and truancy represent disregard for the rights of others and for societal norms. These are the cardinal features of conduct disorder. The fact that the age of onset for these behaviors was around or before 10 years of age is most concerning for an unfavorable prognosis. With earlier onset, there is a greater likelihood of delinquency or evolution into antisocial personality disorder.

(p. 414, Section 7: Pediatric Mental Health, Chapter 95: Disruptive Behavior Disorders and Psychotic Disorders)

**Answer 6-44.** A

Delusions, hallucinations, and disorganized speech or thoughts are cardinal symptoms of schizophrenia.

Decreased emotional expressiveness, reduced speech output, and avolition are all negative symptoms, which are characteristic of a schizophrenia diagnosis, but not 1 of the 3 cardinal symptoms. Disorganized (or catatonic) behavior, such as inability to attend to activities of daily living, is also a possible symptom, but not one of the key criteria for the diagnosis of schizophrenia. To confirm the diagnosis, the symptoms must endure for 6 months or more and cause significant impairment or disruption of developmental trajectories in academic and social functioning.

(p. 416, Section 7: Pediatric Mental Health, Chapter 95: Disruptive Behavior Disorders and Psychotic Disorders)

**Answer 6-45.** D

The lab tests that should be periodically performed in the setting of atypical antipsychotic use help monitor for metabolic syndrome and include (fasting) total cholesterol levels and fasting blood glucose.

Thyroid function tests and serum electrolytes are monitored when a patient is prescribed lithium to ensure that lithium is not having a deleterious effect on the thyroid or the kidneys. Liver function tests and CBC are monitored when certain mood stabilizers (valproic acid and carbamazepine) are prescribed. Mood stabilizers are not typically prescribed for psychotic disorders alone but may be used in the setting of comorbid mood disorders.

(p. 417, Section 7: Pediatric Mental Health, Chapter 95: Disruptive Behavior Disorders and Psychotic Disorders)

**Answer 6-46.** A

Only the elixir formulation is shared by both the methylphenidate and the amphetamine classes of stimulant (Quillivant XR and ProCentra, respectively). Only methylphenidate comes in a patch (Daytrana), which is helpful for patients who cannot or will not take oral medication. Likewise, only methylphenidate comes in an osmotic controlled-release delivery system (Concerta) and in a chewable form (Methylin). The only pro-drug formulation in the class of stimulants is lisdexamfetamine (Vyvanse).

(pp. 390–391, Section 6: Developmental and Behavioral Pediatrics, Chapter 90: Attention-Deficit/Hyperactivity Disorder)

**Answer 6-47.** E

Appropriate extracurricular activities are those that allow hyperkinetic children an outlet for their physical energy and that promote a sense of mastery and prosocial experiences. Dietary changes (increasing fatty acid or mineral intake or following elimination diets) are alternative approaches to treatment that have not been rigorously assessed. Although it is appropriate to adjust homework assignments or decrease the amount of homework, completely eliminating homework from a patient's academic expectations is not expected.

(pp. 389–390, Section 6: Developmental and Behavioral Pediatrics, Chapter 90: Attention-Deficit/Hyperactivity Disorder)

**Answer 6-48.** D

It is imperative for pediatricians to appreciate the serious consequences of ADHD beyond academic struggles. Suicide is likely the most serious. Low self-esteem and emotional dysregulation are often seen with mood disorders. Oppositional behavior and low frustration tolerance are associated with conduct disorders.

(p. 388, Section 6: Developmental and Behavioral Pediatrics, Chapter 90: Attention-Deficit/Hyperactivity Disorder)

**Answer 6-49.** C

Self-monitoring, or information gathering about triggers and responses (both physiologic and cognitive), is a key stage of the CBT process. Mindfulness and interpersonal effectiveness are components of dialectical behavior therapy. Self-hypnosis has no role in CBT. Importantly, family engagement is another key component in CBT.

(p. 406, Section 7: Pediatric Mental Health, Chapter 93: Anxiety)

**Answer 6-50.** B

The description of the patient's persistent irritability and frequent, intense anger outbursts are the hallmarks of disruptive mood dysregulation disorder, which is classified as a depressive disorder.

Because no neurovegetative symptoms (eg, change in appetite or sleep or interest levels) are reported and the patient's mood is irritable and not depressed, the diagnosis of major depressive disorder is unlikely. Likewise, although irritability can be the mood presentation of pediatric bipolar disorder, the irritability would be more episodic and there would likely be changes in sleep (as well as inflated self-esteem, flight of ideas, or distractibility), making bipolar disorder less likely. ADHD can manifest as aggressive impulsivity, but the patient only started manifesting symptoms 18 months ago, whereas impulsive symptoms of ADHD would have been apparent for even longer. Likewise, ADHD is not characterized by persistent irritability, although children can develop secondary mood symptoms because of poor academic performance or social interactions. Finally, oppositional defiant disorder is commonly comorbid with disruptive mood dysregulation disorder.

(pp. 408–409, Section 7: Pediatric Mental Health, Chapter 94: Pediatric Depression and Bipolar Spectrum Disorders)

**Answer 6-51. B**

The circumstances described are most consistent with specific phobia because the fear described is associated with a particular situation (proximity to dogs).

The reaction is considerably greater and more impairing than normative fears exhibited by other children the patient's age. Although she has been traumatized by her dog bite experience and she demonstrates avoidance, consistent with PTSD, there are no other obvious or described cardinal symptoms (eg, hyperarousal, re-experiencing, dissociation, or negative mood states). The clinical scenario does not describe physiologic symptoms or reports of a sense of doom or of "going crazy," which are associated with panic disorder. The child's reaction to dogs occurs in the moment but is not performed repeatedly. In addition, she is not described as having recurring thoughts about her fear of dogs, all of which suggest that OCD is unlikely to be the diagnosis.

(p. 402, Section 7: Pediatric Mental Health, Chapter 93: Anxiety)

**Answer 6-52. A**

In addition to delays in cortical maturation, imbalances in dopamine and norepinephrine neurotransmission are implicated in the pathophysiology of ADHD. Glutamate and GABA function in excitatory and inhibitory neurotransmission, which are key for overall brain function but not specifically related to ADHD pathogenesis. Serotonin is the neurotransmitter that plays a key role in affective (mood and anxiety) disorders. Cholinergic neurons are found in the basal ganglia/striatum and forebrain; acetylcholine neurotransmission underlies certain aspects of attention and motivation, but this neurotransmitter is not associated with ADHD.

(p. 387, Section 6: Developmental and Behavioral Pediatrics, Chapter 90: Attention-Deficit/Hyperactivity Disorder)

**Answer 6-53. B**

The basal ganglia, especially the ventral tegmentum and the caudate nucleus, plays a role in supporting motivation and attention. These are behaviors that are impaired in ADHD. The caudate is another target (in addition to the frontal lobe) of stimulant medications, such as methylphenidate and amphetamine preparations.

The raphe nucleus is the structure that innervates much of the brain with serotonin neurons and thus is implicated in depressive disorders. The anterior cingulate cortex is a part of the limbic circuitry responsible for empathy and emotion regulation, whereas the amygdala is understood to be an important structure in fear responses of certain anxiety and stress-related disorders, such as post-traumatic stress disorder (PTSD). The thalamus is a subcortical structure responsible for relaying signals between the cortex and brainstem but is not directly implicated in ADHD pathogenesis.

(p. 387, Section 6: Developmental and Behavioral Pediatrics, Chapter 90: Attention-Deficit/Hyperactivity Disorder)

**Answer 6-54. D**

Social deficits are often associated with ADHD because social cues are often missed due to inattention and social norms are often violated because of impulsivity (eg, not taking turns or engaging reciprocally in interactions) or hyperactivity (eg, excess motor activity causing accidental injury). These social deficits are often misinterpreted for the theory of mind deficits seen in autism spectrum disorders. A specialty clinic for ADHD will be able to provide social skills training designed to address the social deficits characteristic of this disorder.

Children with ADHD may have comorbid depressive disorders either as a result of poor emotion modulation or as a response to the consequences of their ADHD (eg, poor academic or social functioning). Therefore, treatment for their ADHD can have a direct, positive effect on mood, obviating the need for a specialty mood clinic. The scenario describes academic dysfunction, but it is related to executive dysfunction (eg, not turning in homework) rather than not being capable of doing homework, which might suggest a learning disability. Likewise, the patient is not described as having cognitive impairment separate from his inattention and impulsivity symptoms. This clinical observation makes intellectual disability a less likely diagnosis.

(pp. 387–388, Section 6: Developmental and Behavioral Pediatrics, Chapter 90: Attention-Deficit/Hyperactivity Disorder)

**Answer 6-55. E**

Individuals with ADHD do not completely lack attention. In fact, there are times when they are hyperfocused, especially on activities of interest, and they struggle to shift attention from preferred to nonpreferred activities. Children with ADHD may often appear bored; however, they are actually struggling with paying attention. Likewise, while intrinsic motivation, or the lack thereof, can play a role in the symptomatology of ADHD, extrinsic motivators such as rewards or token economies can play a role in helping individuals to internalize organizing principles that support improved executive functioning. Lack of common sense is a negative judgment of an individual's struggles with impulsivity. When ADHD is understood as a disorder of attention allocation, then interventions to help direct attention appropriately can be designed and implemented.

(p. 388, Section 6: Developmental and Behavioral Pediatrics, Chapter 90: Attention-Deficit/Hyperactivity Disorder)

**Answer 6-56.** A

Binge eating disorder is characterized by feeding behaviors that are in clear excess of what is considered typical, as well as the experience of eating being out of the individual's control. Night eating syndrome is characterized by eating behavior that occurs in the middle of the night and is distressing but that is not felt to be "out of control."

Bulimia nervosa involves similar feeding behaviors as those in binge eating disorder but also includes compensatory behaviors such as purging through self-induced vomiting or the use of laxatives; in the clinical scenario described, no such purging behavior is described. Likewise, the binge-purge subtype of anorexia nervosa has the hallmarks of distorted body image and the desire to achieve low weight, but includes episodes of binge eating or purging; the clinical scenario suggests that low weight is not a problem for the patient. Overeating that is not compulsive can have physiologic consequences that are similar to binge eating disorder (or compulsive overeating) but is not associated with feeling out of control.

(pp. 336–337, Section 5: Principles of Adolescent Care, Chapter 76: Disordered Eating)

**Answer 6-57.** D

Bipolar disorder tends to demonstrate the depressive "pole" first, before manic symptoms develop. As a result, it is important to monitor for symptoms of mania even in the setting of a major depressive disorder (eg, the symptoms of which are what the patient is reporting currently) by asking about episodes of irritability or euphoria, increased goal-directed activity, decreased need for sleep, or using poor judgment.

The patient is already describing symptoms consistent with a major depressive episode, so the likelihood of recurrence in 5 years (and thus a diagnosis of major depressive disorder, answer choice B) is estimated to be as high as 70%. ADHD (answer choice C) and anxiety disorders such as panic disorder (answer choice A) tend to be comorbid with depressive disorders, but depressive symptoms do not predict the development of ADHD or panic disorder. The negative symptoms of schizophrenia (answer choice E), such as social withdrawal and anhedonia, are similar in presentation to depressive symptoms. Severe depressive episodes can be associated with psychotic symptoms, such as paranoid delusions or auditory hallucinations; however, these associations do not predict the development of schizophrenia.

(p. 331, Section 5: Principles of Adolescent Care, Chapter 75: Depression, Anxiety, and Other Disorders in Adolescence)

**Answer 6-58.** E

The patient is described to already have 3 comorbid anxiety disorders: social anxiety disorder and PTSD, as well as the panic disorder (answer choice A) that was described in the vignette. A longitudinal study from New Zealand found that with increasing numbers of comorbid anxiety disorders, individuals are at increased risk of a depressive disorder (not necessarily major depressive disorder, but depression more generally; answer choice E). Although anxiety disorders do have increased likelihood of homotypic comorbidity, OCD (answer choice B) is not necessarily any more likely to develop than any other anxiety disorder. The study found that patients with comorbid anxiety disorders have increased risk of substance use and suicidal behavior but not schizophrenia (answer choice C) or bipolar disorder (answer choice D).

(p. 406, Section 7: Pediatric Mental Health, Chapter 93: Anxiety)

**Answer 6-59.** C

During elementary school ages (approximately 7–12 years old), children often have fears related to anticipation of dangerous events that can cause harm. In addition, they also worry about social scrutiny and competence (answer choice C).

Anticipatory worry (answer choice B) tends to occur during preschool ages, whereas concerns about separation from parents (answer choice A) tend to occur even earlier. Worries about rejection by peers (answer choice D) and performance (answer choice E) are fears that can be normative for adolescence. If these fears become impairing and interfere with functioning, then a social anxiety disorder may develop.

(p. 403, Section 7: Pediatric Mental Health, Chapter 93: Anxiety)

**Answer 6-60.** D

This patient's presentation is most consistent with anorexia nervosa, restricting subtype. The diagnostic criteria for anorexia nervosa are fear of weight gain or being fat, low weight for the patient's age and historical growth trajectory, disturbance in the way the patient experiences their own body weight/shape/size or an undue influence of weight on the patient's self-evaluation, and denial regarding the seriousness of the patient's low weight. It is common to find that such patients may use "socially acceptable" ways to restrict their intake. Examples include adopting vegetarian or gluten-free or other restrictive diets that have become more acceptable and mainstream recently. This behavior results in the patient not meeting their caloric needs with subsequent weight loss.

Bulimia nervosa (answer choice A) is incorrect as it is characterized by recurrent episodes of binge eating, accompanied by a feeling of loss of control or guilt. These actions are followed by a compensatory behavior such as vomiting, fasting, or excessive exercise. Unlike patients with anorexia nervosa, patients with bulimia nervosa are typically normal or high weight and therefore do not typically present with signs of malnutrition on exam. Avoidant restrictive food intake disorder (answer choice B) is characterized by pathologic picky eating and a failure to meet caloric needs without body image disturbance. Patients with avoidant restrictive food intake disorder often have significant issues with food intake due to texture, smell, taste, or other characteristics of food that do not disturb others. Lactose intolerance (as described in answer choice C) is characterized by gastrointestinal symptoms after consumption of dairy and would not be expected to cause weight loss and vital sign instability of this severity. Likewise, these symptoms are not consistent with marijuana use (answer choice E). Marijuana use alone would not be expected to cause such significant weight loss. Although substance abuse, infection, or other chronic diseases should be on the differential for weight loss, this patient's presentation is most consistent with inadequate intake due to anorexia nervosa.

(pp. 336–340, Section 5: Principles of Adolescent Care, Chapter 76: Disordered Eating)

**Answer 6-61.** E

Eating disorders have the highest mortality rates of any psychiatric disorders. Deaths are most commonly due to suicide, followed by medical complications of starvation and malnutrition. Therefore, early recognition and treatment are essential, as both are associated with better prognosis and higher rates of remission.

Answer choice D is incorrect. Despite increased research around eating disorder treatment, rates of clinical remission at 1 year remain < 50%. Answer choices A, B, and C are also incorrect. Better prognosis is associated with younger age at diagnosis (age < 14 years) and early weight gain during the first 4 weeks of treatment. The most frequently cited study associated a 1 pound a week weight gain over the first 4 weeks with higher rates of clinical recovery at 1 year. In addition, better prognosis is associated with a shorter duration of symptoms prior to diagnosis. The Society for Adolescent Health and Medicine recommends a multidisciplinary approach to diagnosis and treatment of eating disorders, and the best evidence supports a family-based treatment approach to therapy and re-nourishment.

(pp. 336–340, Section 5: Principles of Adolescent Care, Chapter 76: Disordered Eating)

**Answer 6-62.** A

Suicide is the second leading cause of death in adolescents in the United States. History of nonsuicidal self-injury, clinically diagnosed depression, previous suicide attempt or attempts, history of substance abuse or alcohol abuse, social isolation, male gender, and older age are associated with higher risk of suicide in adolescents. Protective factors include family, community, and mental health support. Suicide risk is highest during a major depressive episode. Therefore, assessing adolescents for symptoms of depression and recommending effective clinical care are critical during adolescent medical visits.

(p. 331, Section 5: Principles of Adolescent Care, Chapter 75: Depression, Anxiety, and Other Disorders in Adolescence)

# CHAPTER 7 Child Abuse and Neglect

Larissa Hines and Kristine Campbell

**7-1.** Which of the following statements is correct, based on epidemiologic data collected about child abuse?

**A.** Most child maltreatment occurs outside the home.

**B.** Females are as equally likely as males to be perpetrators of sexual abuse.

**C.** Of substantiated child abuse cases, neglect is the most common type.

**D.** If all types of child abuse are included, males are the most likely perpetrators of child abuse.

**E.** Females are more commonly perpetrators in child abuse death cases.

**7-2.** A single mother brings a developmentally normal 16-month-old child to the emergency department (ED) for not moving his left arm for the past 3 days. The mother reports that he stopped moving his arm 3 days ago when they were walking to the bus stop. Mother reports that she was holding his hand while they were walking and he tripped off a curb. She pulled him up by his left arm. He cried initially. He has seemed fine other than not moving his left arm. On exam, he has a nursemaid's elbow of the left arm. When asked by the nurse when alone whether somebody hurt him, the child replies "no." Which of the following factors makes this injury most suspicious for child abuse?

**A.** The mother is single and thus is at increased risk for abusing her child.

**B.** The history of tripping off a curb is not within a 16-month-old child's developmental abilities.

**C.** The mother delayed seeking care for the child soon after the injury.

**D.** The child's response when asked by the nurse when alone whether somebody hurt him.

**E.** The child appears very fearful and cries when even experienced pediatricians try to examine him.

**7-3.** A newborn is being evaluated by you in the newborn nursery. The mother is a 17-year-old girl living in her parents' basement with her 17-year-old boyfriend, the father of the baby. The maternal grandparents are very involved and plan to assist the new parents in raising this child. In reviewing the parents' background, which of the following factors that are identified is *not* associated with an increased risk of abusing their child?

**A.** The mother is a teenager.

**B.** The parents are supported by the maternal grandparents.

**C.** The father has a substance abuse problem.

**D.** There is a history of intimate partner violence in the family.

**E.** The mother was maltreated as a child.

**7-4.** A 2-year-old boy is brought to your clinic by child protective services for a clearance examination. The child is noted to have a bruise on the glans of his penis with some swelling. The child can urinate. Urinalysis reveals no blood. There are no other injuries to the child's genitals or anus noted. The child is also noted to have multiple bruises on the abdomen and buttocks and cheeks. This child's findings would be best classified as which of the following types of maltreatment?

**A.** Exploitation

**B.** Emotional abuse

**C.** Neglect

**D.** Physical abuse

**E.** Sexual abuse

**7-5.** A 19-month-old child comes into your clinic for hot water burns. There are scalding water burns on both the toddler's feet. The second-degree burns cover the feet and the lower part of the legs. On each leg, there are straight, well-demarcated burn lines approximately 2 cm above the ankles.

The child is developmentally normal and was born full term. He has no past medical history, and his immunizations are up to date. His parents have missed 2 appointments since birth that had to be rescheduled. The father reports that the bathtub was running with hot water as he prepared the bath for the child. He went into another room to clean up the child's soiled underwear. He also reports he has been trying to potty train the child. He reports that when he came back into the bathroom, the child had climbed into the bathtub and was found crying in the water. The father did not bring the child in for care until he noticed blistering of the burn site later in the evening.

Which factor makes this burn most suspicious for abuse?

**A.** The delay in bringing in the child for care
**B.** The unlikely ability of the 19-month-old child to climb into the bath
**C.** The fact that the child was potty training and soiled his underwear
**D.** The history of missed appointments
**E.** Sharply demarcated lines of the burn

**7-6.** A 2-year-old child is brought in for buttock bruising noticed by a daycare worker when changing the child's diaper. In clinic, the child is acting developmentally normally for the child's age, and the child does not seem fearful or in pain. After complete history and physical, the best workup for this patient would be which of the following?

**A.** Complete blood and platelet count, prothrombin, and partial thromboplastin time
**B.** Skeletal survey
**C.** Abdominal computed tomography (CT) scan
**D.** CT scan of the head and neck without contrast
**E.** Ophthalmology examination with dilated pupils

**7-7.** Which of the following is an accurate statement about violence exposure?

**A.** A child's exposure to intimate partner violence (IPV) is associated with a greater likelihood of being abused.
**B.** Sibling violence is more benign and less harmful than other forms of peer violence.
**C.** Over 95% of victims of IPV are women.
**D.** Dating violence is reported to occur in > 50% of relationships.
**E.** A child's exposure to violence affects mental, but not physical, health.

**7-8.** You are referred a 3-month-old nonambulatory child from daycare center staff who noticed bruising on the infant's buttocks during a diaper change. The parents and other caretakers deny any history of trauma. The child appears well on examination and is interactive and playful. Although you are concerned about abusive injuries given the location of the bruising, you create a differential diagnosis. Which of the following should *not* be included in your differential diagnosis?

**A.** Henoch-Schönlein purpura
**B.** Idiopathic thrombocytopenic purpura
**C.** Acute lymphocytic leukemia
**D.** Dermal melanocytosis
**E.** Vitamin A deficiency

**7-9.** You see a 3-year-old girl brought in for possible sexual abuse. The mother says the girl has made statements about being touched by her father's brother, who lives in the house with the family. The girl is well appearing. The mother denies any bleeding, itching, dysuria, or frequency. The girl has otherwise been acting her normal self per the mother's report. You perform a physical examination, including a genital examination. The finding most indicative of sexual abuse in this case would be which of the following?

**A.** A confirmed genital human papillomavirus (HPV) wart on the child's labia majora
**B.** A crescentic hymen through which the vaginal mucosa can be seen
**C.** A 1-cm circular bruise on the inner thigh
**D.** A finding of erythema of the labia majora and minora
**E.** The child's disclosure during a forensic interview of digital-vaginal contact

**7-10.** A 30-month-old developmentally normal boy presents to your clinic with a chief complaint of not walking and inability to bear weight on his right leg. The parents noted this yesterday and are bringing the child in today because the apparent pain with weight bearing has not resolved. The parents give no history of falls or trauma. The child has not had any other complaints. On contacting their primary pediatrician, you learn that there have been no previous fractures or other significant past medical history concerning for abuse.

On physical examination of the entire body, there is no evidence of bruising or other concerning findings, and neurologic and mental status examinations are normal. You are not able to obtain an adequate retinal examination. In examining the right leg, there are no obvious bruises. There is full range of motion, with a question of some point tenderness over the distal tibial plateau on the right side. The child is reluctant to walk and cries when prompted to do so, with a noticeable limp on the right leg. There are no other significant physical examination findings. A radiograph reveals a nondisplaced spiral fracture of the distal right tibia. What is the next best diagnostic procedure for this child?

**A.** Check levels of calcium, phosphorus, alkaline phosphatase, and 25-hydroxyvitamin D.

**B.** No further workup is indicated given the information at this point.

**C.** Obtain a computed tomography (CT) scan of the head looking for subdural hemorrhages.

**D.** Get an ophthalmology consult to look for retinal hemorrhages.

**E.** Perform a full skeletal survey, looking for occult abusive fractures.

**7-11.** A 6-month-old, typically developing infant is referred to the emergency department (ED) for radiographs after presenting to the primary pediatrician's office with a swollen left thigh. The physical exam reveals stable vital signs, normal growth parameters, and no cutaneous injuries. There was pain on examination when the left lower extremity was moved. There are no bruises, and the leg is distally neurovascularly intact. The radiograph shows an oblique/spiral fracture through the left femoral diaphysis with associated soft tissue swelling.

The day prior to presentation, the infant had been fussier than usual after spending the day in childcare. The mother decided to bring her infant in the next day when the fussiness continued and she noticed the left thigh swelling. Neither the childcare provider nor the mother recalls any falls or other traumatic injuries. A family history is reviewed and reveals no history of recurrent fracture, unexplained short stature, hearing loss, or dental concerns. Which of the following is the most accurate statement concerning the likelihood of abuse associated with this fracture?

**A.** Over 20% of oblique/spiral femur fractures in nonmobile infants are attributable to abuse.

**B.** Over 50% of fractures in children $< 3$ years of age are attributable to abuse.

**C.** Physical exam and family history are not reliable in excluding most cases of osteogenesis imperfecta.

**D.** The overnight delay in seeking care for a femur fracture is an indicator of probable abusive injury.

**E.** A skeletal survey is unnecessary as the child has no other findings of traumatic injury.

**7-12.** A 3-month-old girl is admitted for suspicion of abusive head trauma. The mother gives a history of the baby falling off a couch. The baby cried immediately but then became lethargic and unresponsive. The baby was rushed to a nearby hospital, where she was stabilized. A computed tomography (CT) scan of the head shows a thin-layer subdural hemorrhage over the right hemisphere. A chest radiograph reveals a number of posterior rib fractures with sharp fracture lines and no callous formation. On ophthalmology examination, retinal hemorrhages are noted. The most accurate statement regarding retinal hemorrhages would be which of the following?

**A.** Birth-associated retinal hemorrhages often persist to 4 months of age.

**B.** Only 1 type of retinal hemorrhage is associated with abusive head trauma.

**C.** Retinal hemorrhages usually cause irreversible blindness for the child.

**D.** Retinal hemorrhages only occur near the macula due to presence of retinal blood vessels.

**E.** Retinal hemorrhages can result from certain types of infections.

**7-13.** A 14-month-old typically developing boy is brought to the hospital with concerns for abuse by his mother. The mother states she has noticed marks on the child over the past several days when picking him up from daycare. At first, she thought these were normal bruises from the child playing, but she has been more concerned recently given the number and type. The child also seems to be crying and scared when dropped off at daycare, which is a new phenomenon. On physical examination, the child is noted to have a number of cutaneous findings. Which of the following findings would be most concerning for abusive injuries?

**A.** Bruising to the pretibial region of multiple colors, suggesting different ages

**B.** Large, palpable, painless bruises over soft tissues

**C.** Three perioral ulcerated lesions approximately 12 mm in diameter with yellow crusting

**D.** Four oval bruises in the submandibular region

**E.** A bruise on the right forehead, just above the eye

**7-14.** A 17-month-old boy is admitted for suspicion of abuse. The boy was noted to have multiple bruises on the buttocks, upper arms, trunk, and ears. On physical examination, the child is interactive and otherwise well appearing. A complete blood count reveals normal platelets, and coagulation factors are normal as well. A skeletal survey is done to evaluate for possible fractures. Which of the following statements about a skeletal survey is most accurate?

**A.** Is a series of x-rays of the long bones, chest, and spine, but not the skull

**B.** Usually shows evidence of any fractures within the last year

**C.** Should be obtained for every child < 7 years old with suspicious fractures

**D.** Is typically repeated in 2 weeks to look for additional fractures not observed on initial skeletal survey

**E.** Can rule out abuse if it is found to be negative

**7-15.** A 15-year-old girl is brought in for possible sexual assault by an adult man. She met the man on the Internet and eventually agreed to go to his apartment to meet him. She became intoxicated while drinking alcohol with him and eventually "blacked out." She does not recall anything else, except waking up in a park, where police officers found her and brought her into the hospital. Her blood alcohol level was 0.02 on arrival at the emergency department (ED). Examination was otherwise unremarkable, except for some abrasions over her knees and right shoulder, and several 1- to 2-cm circular bruises on her left arm. The girl complains of pain in the genital area. A sexual assault examination is performed. The examination is found to be normal. The girl tests positive for chlamydia on the urine test and culture performed on the day of the possible sexual assault. Which of the following statements is correct?

**A.** The normal genital examination does not rule out a sexual assault.

**B.** The positive chlamydia test is proof that the girl was raped.

**C.** The bruises suggest that the girl was assaulted.

**D.** The girl would not benefit from postexposure prophylaxis.

**E.** The blood alcohol level suggests the girl was raped.

**7-16.** A previously full-term 4-month-old girl presents to the emergency department with a brief resolved unexplained event (BRUE). The baby was sleeping with the mother and was noted to turn blue and stop breathing for > 1 minute. Mother reports starting cardiopulmonary resuscitation (CPR) before the baby responded. The baby was brought in by ambulance with the mother. Emergency medical technicians (EMTs) reported a well-appearing baby when they got to the house. In the ED, physical examination was normal, and a history and review of symptoms was unremarkable. The baby was observed in the hospital over the next several days. She had 6 more events of stopping breathing over the next several days and continues to be observed in the hospital. Workup for infections including blood and urine cultures, respiratory syncytial virus, and pertussis was negative. An electrocardiogram (ECG) was normal, as was a pH probe, and the events do not seem to be associated with feeding. There is no reported seizure activity, and an electroencephalogram (EEG) is normal. Head computed tomography (CT) scan is unremarkable. Before further workup is initiated, one of the members of your team points out that the only time the events occur are when mother is with the baby alone in her room. You begin to suspect pediatric condition falsification. Which statement about pediatric condition falsification is most accurate?

**A.** Pediatric condition falsification rarely results in truly life-threatening events.

**B.** Pediatric condition falsification is usually straightforward to diagnose based on a complete medical history and physical exam.

**C.** BRUEs are most likely to reflect pediatric condition falsification when infectious and neurologic causes have been excluded.

**D.** Caregivers involved in pediatric condition falsification are often nonparent caretakers.

**E.** A complete review of all medical records may help identify cases of pediatric condition falsification.

**7-17.** A boy who recently turned 3 years old is being evaluated for poor weight gain noted during your well-child check. The child has crossed 2 percentile lines for weight in the past 6 months, going from the 50th percentile at 32 lb to between the 5th and 10th percentiles at 27 lb. Height and head circumference have not crossed percentile lines. There are multiple family stressors, including a recent divorce, and the primary caregiver has been struggling with finances and employment. The child also has had multiple upper respiratory infections over the past several months, although he has never been hospitalized.

On physical examination, the child appears thin but not cachectic. He is quiet and does not engage with you or with his mother during the encounter. He has multiple bruises over his left and right shins, has 2 café-au-lait spots on his trunk, and is noted to have a faint 1/6 systolic ejection murmur at the left sternal border, which the mother says was noted in previous visits since the age of 18 months, and she was told it was a "Still's murmur." His examination is otherwise unremarkable. You are concerned about neglect but realize you must also evaluate the child for other possible causes of poor weight gain. The most appropriate next step is which of the following?

**A.** Obtain an electrocardiogram (ECG) and 4-limb blood pressures.

**B.** Get baseline electrolytes prior to feeding.

**C.** Obtain a skeletal survey.

**D.** Obtain a careful feeding history.

**E.** Obtain a head computed tomography (CT) scan.

**7-18.** A 2-month-old baby fell onto a hardwood floor from a 4-ft-high changing table when the mother's boyfriend was reaching to get the diapers. He reports instinctively grabbing the child by the left forearm to try to prevent him from hitting the floor but heard a hard thump before forcefully pulling the infant up. There was no reported loss of consciousness and no vomiting. The boyfriend decided to bring the baby to the emergency department (ED) out of concern. On exam, the baby is noted to have superficial soft tissue swelling with erythema over the right parietal area. A head computed tomography (CT) scan identifies a simple linear parietal skull fracture with a scalp hematoma and minimal extra-axial blood adjacent to the skull fracture. You advise the ED doctor to get a full history, a skeletal survey, and a complete metabolic panel, as a skull fracture in a nonmobile infant without independent witnesses may reflect an episode of physical abuse. Of the following known or possible findings on evaluation, which is the most specific for abuse?

**A.** The linear skull fracture of the right parietal bone

**B.** Hepatic transaminases > 80 IU

**C.** Linear bruising and petechiae below the left zygomatic arch

**D.** A classic metaphyseal lesion of the left distal radius

**E.** A healing mid-diaphyseal fracture of the right clavicle

**7-19.** A 3-month-old baby presents with apnea and unresponsiveness at home under the care of a babysitter. The sitter says she went to get a bottle for the baby, and when she returned, the baby was blue and not breathing. Cardiopulmonary resuscitation (CPR) was performed by the sitter while waiting for emergency medical technicians (EMTs) to arrive, and the baby responded and became alert. On arrival by EMTs, the baby appeared alert and responsive but began to have seizure activity in the ambulance on the way to the hospital. In the emergency department (ED), the baby was stabilized, and apparent seizures resolved with medication. On chest x-ray, several acute posterior rib fractures were noted. A head computed tomography (CT) scan showed a right subdural hemorrhage layering over the hemisphere and into the convexity. Otherwise, the baby appeared to have an unremarkable physical examination, with no bruising or other signs of head trauma. The next step that would be most helpful in supporting the diagnosis of abusive head trauma would be to obtain which of the following?

**A.** Liver function tests

**B.** Coagulation studies and a complete blood count (CBC)

**C.** A dilated retinal examination by ophthalmology

**D.** Serum $Ca^{2+}$, $PO_4^-$, and alkaline phosphatase

**E.** Serum amino acids

**7-20.** A 2-year-old girl is brought in when her divorced mother gets concerned after picking her up from a weekend visit with the girl's father. The mother noted blood in the girl's underwear and called the father to ask if he had noticed this as well. The father says the girl fell and hit her perineal area while playing on a tricycle. She reportedly cried when this occurred but settled down and was consoled easily. The father reports he did not notice any bleeding and did not think anything more of it, as the girl continued to play without problems. On genital examination of the girl, the most concerning finding for sexual abuse would be which of the following?

**A.** Bruise and shallow laceration of the labia majora

**B.** Transection of the hymen with active bleeding

**C.** Prolapsed urethra with bleeding

**D.** Thinning of the skin with subepidermal hemorrhages of the vulva

**E.** Perianal group A streptococcal infection with bleeding

**7-21.** Which of the following descriptions is concerning for a sentinel injury?

**A.** A bruise on the forehead of a 9-month-old child

**B.** A red mark on the back of the neck of a 1-month-old infant

**C.** A bruise on the arm of a 3-month-old infant

**D.** A subconjunctival hemorrhage in the eye of a 10-day-old infant

**E.** A bruise on the anterior lower leg of a 15-month-old child

**7-22.** A mother brings her 4-year-old daughter in for concerns for sexual abuse. The school reported that her child has been showing her genitals to her friends at preschool. The mother also noted that her daughter has been touching private parts while in the family room watching television. The mother asked her daughter if she had ever been touched "down there," and the child denied ever being touched. Which of the following behaviors is most concerning for potential sexual abuse?

**A.** Showing genitals to peers

**B.** Touching peer or new sibling genitals

**C.** Rubbing body against others

**D.** Insisting that other children touch their genitals

**E.** Touching or masturbating genitals in public

**7-23.** A 4-month-old male infant is brought to the emergency department (ED) for seizure activity. The mother reports that he was in his normal state of health until this evening when she noticed his eyes rolling back into his head and him going limp. He has been fussy for the past week, and his mother thinks he is teething. A head computed tomography (CT) scan demonstrates a high-attenuation subdural fluid collection. Which of the following is *not* indicated in the initial evaluation of this patient?

**A.** Skeletal survey

**B.** Ophthalmologic exam

**C.** Complete blood count (CBC), prothrombin time (PT), partial thromboplastin time (PTT)

**D.** Liver function tests (LFTs)

**E.** Magnetic resonance imaging (MRI) of the brain

**7-24.** A 16-year-old girl presents to the emergency department (ED) after acute sexual assault. She reports that she was at a party drinking heavily. An acquaintance took her into the bathroom and had penile-vaginal sex with her. She returned home later that night and disclosed what happened to her mother the next morning. What is the most appropriate next step in her evaluation?

**A.** A forensic interview

**B.** Evidence collection

**C.** Police interview

**D.** Testing for herpes simplex virus (HSV)

**E.** Testing for *Neisseria gonorrhoeae*

**7-25.** A 14-year-old girl presents to the emergency department (ED) after disclosure in a forensic interview of penile-anal intercourse with an unknown adult male 4 weeks ago. She reported that she met up with the man at a train station and went back to his apartment to do drugs. She woke up the next morning with pain and bleeding of her anus, which has resolved. She initially disclosed to a friend at school that she thought she was raped. The friend reported the incident to the school resource officer. What is the next step in evaluation?

**A.** Evidence collection

**B.** Postexposure human immunodeficiency virus (HIV) prophylaxis

**C.** Pregnancy prophylaxis

**D.** Chlamydia prophylaxis

**E.** Sexually transmitted infection (STI) testing

**7-26.** A 2-month-old infant presents to your office for a well-child examination. On exam, you note a torn upper labial frenulum. The mother does not report any history of blood from the mouth. The exam is otherwise normal. Complete evaluation for physical abuse, including skeletal survey, head computed tomography (CT) scan, and liver enzyme testing, did not reveal any occult injuries. What is the next step in the care of this patient?

**A.** Magnetic resonance imaging (MRI) of the brain

**B.** Report to child protective services

**C.** Routine follow-up at the 4-month well-child check

**D.** Follow-up in 2 weeks to evaluate for healing

**E.** Reassurance to the mother that this was likely accidental

**7-27.** Which of the following scenarios is most concerning for teen dating violence (TDV)?

**A.** A 12 years old in a serious dating relationship

**B.** A 17 years old who is dating multiple people at the same time

**C.** A 15 years old who is sexually active with her boyfriend

**D.** A 16 years old who has a history of risky behaviors

**E.** A 14 years old in a controlling relationship

**7-28.** Which of the following is true regarding adverse childhood experiences (ACEs)?

**A.** Tolerable stress is one of the ACEs.

**B.** Adverse effects are not seen until at least 4 ACEs have been documented.

**C.** Abuse and neglect have more of an effect than household dysfunction.

**D.** Intimate partner violence (IPV) is not an ACE.

**E.** ACEs have a dose-response relationship with adult outcomes.

**7-29.** A 6-month-old infant is evaluated in the hospital for abusive head trauma. A large subdural hematoma was found on head computed tomography (CT) scan and confirmed as an acute subdural hematoma on magnetic resonance imaging (MRI) of the brain. There were no other injuries on exam or skeletal survey. Which of the following explanations is most consistent with the injury?

**A.** Bleeding from scalp veins

**B.** Bleeding from the subarachnoid space

**C.** Bleeding from torn bridging veins

**D.** Bleeding from the dural sinuses

**E.** Bleeding from the brain parenchyma

**7-30.** A mother brings her 6-week-old infant to your clinic for evaluation of crying. She reports that the infant cries 4 hours a day, usually in the evenings, at least 5 days a week. She reports that nothing in particular incites the crying or improves it once it has started. She thinks that the infant is "gassy" and has been giving the infant simethicone drops at home, which she feels help somewhat. What is the most appropriate next step in evaluation for this infant?

**A.** Maternal education on normal infant crying

**B.** Abdominal radiograph

**C.** Complete metabolic profile

**D.** Computed tomography (CT) of the head

**E.** Skeletal survey

**7-31.** A 16-year-old girl presents to your urgent care for sexually transmitted infection (STI) testing. You want to screen the patient for sex trafficking. Which of the following questions is most specific for sex trafficking?

**A.** Is there a previous history of drug and/or alcohol use?

**B.** Has the youth ever had an STI?

**C.** Does the youth have a history of sexual activity with > 5 partners?

**D.** Has the youth ever traded sexual acts for a place to stay?

**E.** Has the youth ever run away from home?

**7-32.** A 6-year-old child is placed into foster care due to parental drug use. You are seeing the patient for an exam after placement. Which of the following should be included in your evaluation of this patient?

**A.** Skeletal survey

**B.** Hair follicle testing for drug exposure

**C.** Mental health screening

**D.** Complete metabolic panel

**E.** Computed tomography (CT) of the head

**7-33.** A 5-month-old male infant presents to the emergency department (ED) for concerns of a brief resolved unexplained event (BRUE). This is the third time this infant has been seen for these concerns. Which of the following reassures you that there is a medical cause for these events?

**A.** Blood in the nose and mouth

**B.** Multiple reported episodes of apnea

**C.** A sibling with a major illness

**D.** Multiple caregivers have witnessed the episodes

**E.** A sibling who has died of sudden infant death syndrome

**7-34.** A 3-month-old female infant presents to the emergency department for respiratory distress. You initiate an evaluation that includes a chest radiograph. On the radiograph, you note 6 healing posterior medial rib fractures. Which of the following mechanisms is consistent with the fractures?

**A.** Anterior posterior compression of the chest

**B.** Direct blow to the chest

**C.** Caregiver fingers pressing on the ribs

**D.** Cardiopulmonary resuscitation (CPR)

**E.** Forceful coughing

**7-35.** Which of the following bruises is *not* highly concerning for abuse?

**A.** A 2 years old with ear bruising

**B.** A 4 months old with shin bruising

**C.** A 3 years old with neck bruising

**D.** A 5 years old with abdominal bruising

**E.** A 16 months old with forehead bruising

**7-36.** A 2-month-old male infant is admitted to the hospital for failure to thrive (FTT). Which of the following is most consistent with an organic cause for the FTT?

**A.** Poor maternal bonding

**B.** Maternal postpartum depression

**C.** Low volumes reported on feeding history

**D.** Projectile vomiting

**E.** Dilution of the formula

**7-37.** A 5-month-old infant is brought to her primary care provider after her mother notes an unusual growth in the diaper area. In your clinic, the infant is growing along her trajectory, interactive with the examiner, rolling from front to back, and in good health. On exam, you note 2 dry, flesh-colored papules, each < 0.5 cm across, on the labia minora. The lesions have an irregular, rough surface without excoriation or erosion. There is no indication of pain with palpation. Her genital exam is significant for a normal Tanner I female phenotype without any other lesions. Her hymen is crescentic without transection or clefting. There is no vaginal discharge. Perianal exam is notable for an anal fissure at 11 o'clock. Her mother reports that no one else in the family has similar lesions, although her 5-year-old son has a history of molluscum contagiosum. She has no concern for sexual or physical abuse. Her daughter has been in a daycare 3 days a week for the past 2 months. What is the most appropriate next step in this case?

**A.** Contact child protective services to report suspected child sexual abuse.

**B.** Obtain bag urine to test for gonorrhea, chlamydia, and trichomoniasis.

**C.** Review the natural history of molluscum contagiosum with the mother.

**D.** Scrape lesions and send for darkfield microscopy.

**E.** Review maternal medical records for history of genital human papillomavirus (HPV).

**7-38.** A previously healthy 7-month-old boy is found unresponsive in his crib by his mother. She calls emergency medical services and provides cardiopulmonary resuscitation (CPR) while awaiting the ambulance. Paramedics arrive and continue resuscitation efforts. This infant is transported to your hospital where he is admitted to the pediatric intensive care unit, requiring mechanical ventilation and pressor support. Initial physical examination reveals a well-developed but unresponsive infant. His pupils are fixed and dilated, and you observe no independent respiratory effort. Labs demonstrate multiorgan failure and coagulopathy, whereas cardiac echocardiography reveals poor cardiac output. A head computed tomography (CT) scan identifies diffuse brain edema with the possibility of a thin subdural hemorrhage. A first brain death exam is ongoing, and he is not stable enough for a skeletal survey or ophthalmology examination. Which of the following should be obtained immediately to help determine the cause of this unexpected collapse?

**A.** A full-body CT with 3-dimensional reconstruction to identify any occult fractures or intra-abdominal trauma

**B.** Magnetic resonance imaging (MRI) of the brain to clarify the presence and age of possible subdural hemorrhage

**C.** A complete social history identifying recent caregivers and any past concerns for child maltreatment

**D.** Scene investigation by law enforcement to document sleep environment and secure physical evidence

**E.** Multidisciplinary consultation to evaluate for cardiac, hematologic, infectious, or genetic processes explaining the infant's condition

**7-39.** A 7-year-old boy is being discharged from your hospital to his maternal aunt and uncle, who will serve as foster parents while his biological mother receives treatment for disabling mental illness and substance use disorder. Your patient was initially hospitalized with severe failure to thrive (FTT) and has demonstrated significant developmental delay during his inpatient stay. He is beginning to gain weight and has started to engage with nurses and therapists on the floor. He becomes distraught when he learns that he will not be going back to his mother's home upon discharge. The medical team is upset and believes that the plan to discharge him to family members is inadequately protective of his safety and well-being. You are asked to participate in a team meeting to explore these concerns. What do you understand about foster care placement that should be reassuring to your medical team?

**A.** Placement in a kinship foster family setting has been found to reduce child traumatic stress, improve child well-being, and maintain connections with biological parents.

**B.** Your patient is at low risk for return to his biological mother given her history of substance use and mental illness.

**C.** You would expect rapid resolution of your patient's FTT and developmental delay once he is placed in a stable and nurturing home.

**D.** You would advise child welfare to limit contact between your patient and his mother in order to reduce disruption to his new household.

**E.** The new foster parents will receive highly specialized training on how to manage their nephew's feeding and behavioral problems.

**7-40.** A 15-year-old girl is brought to your clinic by her stepmother. Family and teachers have noted multiple large bruises on her arms in the past week. When asked by the school nurse about the source of the bruising, she shrugged and replied, "I guess I'm cursed or something." Her stepmother is worried that her boyfriend may have hurt her. The boyfriend is 17 years old, and the stepmother has heard that he is involved with a violent local gang. The stepmother reports that she has been parenting alone since the young woman's mother died 5 years ago and her father was sentenced to 10 years in prison last year. She worries about how this social history affects her decision-making. On physical exam, you observe a bright, engaged young woman with very large tender bruises on the back of the right arm, left bicep, and right forearm. She has additional bruising over her lower back and thighs. There is no clear pattern to the bruising and no overlying skin injury. When you ask her about the source of the bruises, she says, "I don't know—they just started popping out. I guess I'm cursed." When you ask her about dating violence, she denies this and reports that her family history taught her to stay away from violence, gangs, and drugs. What is the best next step?

**A.** Conduct a magnified genital examination to look for physical evidence of sexual assault or date rape.

**B.** Send bloodwork for a complete blood count (CBC), prothrombin time/international normalized ratio, partial thromboplastin time, and von Willebrand panel to look for evidence of a bleeding diathesis.

**C.** Notify law enforcement of your suspicion for dating violence and assault.

**D.** Provide the patient's stepmother with local resources for trauma-focused mental health services.

**E.** Reassure the patient's stepmother that the patient is making protective and healthy choices in her relationships.

**7-41.** You and your partners have become aware of several families in your practice in which unsuspected intimate partner violence (IPV) between parents has resulted in physical or emotional injury to children that you care for. In response to this recognition, you have proposed introduction of a standardized screening instrument for IPV at every visit. Clinic colleagues and staff raise concerns about whether universal IPV screening is a good idea. Which of the following statements about screening for IPV in the pediatric clinic is correct?

**A.** Studies find that most women are reluctant to be screened for risks such as IPV or postpartum depression in a pediatric clinic.

**B.** There is no mandated reporting associated with a report of IPV in the pediatric clinic.

**C.** Pediatricians should discuss IPV with parents and children together in order to support open family dialogue about this difficult topic.

**D.** Prior to implementing any standardized screening for IPV, pediatricians and clinic staff should be prepared to respond to positive screeners with community resources.

**E.** Although there are exceptions, most children living in homes with IPV do not demonstrate physical or emotional harm associated with IPV.

**7-42.** Six-month-old twins die after being left in a hot car while their parents spent the afternoon in a casino. Prior to this tragedy, there had been several child protective services (CPS) investigations for concerns of neglect that were closed without substantiation. The event gets significant news coverage, and the local community is shocked and outraged. A reporter from the local newspaper contacts you for background information on this story. Which of the following statements about the epidemiology of child abuse and neglect are true?

**A.** Rates of substantiated child neglect rose dramatically during the Great Recession.

**B.** CPS interventions have been effective in reducing recurrent episodes of child neglect.

**C.** CPS carefully investigates every report of suspected child maltreatment and substantiates those cases where maltreatment has happened.

**D.** On average, child maltreatment is evenly distributed between child neglect, physical abuse, and sexual abuse.

**E.** Almost 1600 children die of child maltreatment in the United States every year.

## ANSWERS

**Answer 7-1.** C

Among the types of maltreatment, neglect makes up almost two-thirds of substantiated cases. National data suggest that women make up more than half of the perpetrators of child abuse, although perpetrators of sexual abuse are overwhelmingly male. In addition, more than two-thirds of child abuse deaths are perpetrated by males. National survey data also suggest that most child abuse occurs in the child's home.

(pp. 152–153, Chapter 36: Child Maltreatment: Neglect to Abuse)

**Answer 7-2.** C

Five types of history should raise the suspicion of child abuse. These include (1) a child with a serious injury and no history of trauma offered; (2) a history that is not consistent with the mechanism, severity, or timing of an injury; (3) a delay in seeking care for a significant injury; (4) a history that changes during the course of evaluation; and (5) a history of recurrent injuries.

Although single parenting is a risk factor for child abuse, in this case, it is not the most concerning factor. In addition, the majority of single parents do not abuse their children. A 16-month-old child described as developmentally normal would be expected to be able to run and fall. As a result, from a developmental standpoint, the injury is not suspicious. A developmentally normal 16-month-old child's reply to a question of whether they were hit or not is probably not helpful in determining a cause of the injury. Sixteen-month-old children would also be considered developmentally normal if they were fearful and crying when strangers tried to examine them, regardless of abuse history.

(pp. 153–154, Chapter 36: Child Maltreatment: Neglect to Abuse)

**Answer 7-3.** B

There are a number of factors associated with abuse or neglect of children, including those associated with the child, the parents, the family unit, and the social setting. Parental risk factors for child abuse include young maternal age and abuse of alcohol or drugs. There is also a strong association between a history of abuse as a child and abusing one's own child (the intergenerational transmission of abuse), although the majority of parents who were abused as children do not abuse their own children. Intrafamilial violence such as intimate partner or domestic violence is an independent risk factor for child maltreatment. The family support offered by having the maternal grandparents present and involved is a protective factor for potential child abuse.

(p. 153, Chapter 36: Child Maltreatment: Neglect to Abuse)

**Answer 7-4.** D

Maltreatment includes physical abuse, neglect, sexual abuse, exploitation, and emotional maltreatment. Physical abuse is an act of commission toward the child by a parent or other caregiver that results in harm or intended harm to the child. Neglect is an act of omission, such as failure to provide adequate nutrition, shelter, or health care, among other needs. Sexual abuse is the involvement of children or adolescents in sexual activities that they do not fully understand, to which they cannot give informed consent because of their developmental understanding, and that break societal or family taboos. Exploitation is the use of a child in work or other activities for the benefit of others, such as child labor, commercial sexual exploitation of children, and child trafficking. Emotional maltreatment is the most difficult form of maltreatment to define and can include repeated verbal denigration.

In the case presented, the bruise is associated with other bruises that suggest physical abuse. Although one might argue the bruise to the penis is sexual in nature, bruising of the penis is commonly a result of punishment (eg, for potty training accidents when the penis is pinched or shut in the toilet seat). In addition, the lack of other suggestion of sexual abuse in this case and the associated bruising in areas concerning for physical abuse make physical abuse the most likely classification for this case.

(p. 152, Chapter 36: Child Maltreatment: Neglect to Abuse)

**Answer 7-5.** E

Demarcated lines are associated with abusive scald injuries, whereas nonabusive scalds tend to be asymmetric from one extremity to the other and have less sharply demarcated borders. Nonabusive scalding should reveal splash marks that indicate the child tried to avoid the injury. In this case, if the child climbed into a tub himself, one would expect splash marks as the child tried to avoid the pain of the hot water.

Delay in bringing a child into care is certainly a concerning factor in abuse. However, burns may not appear immediately concerning to a layperson. In addition, delay in seeking care is not as specific for abuse as the physical findings in this case. In this case, it may be part of an overall concern and suspicion, but not as clearly suspicious as the absence of splash marks and the sharply demarcated lines of the burn. Although it may seem implausible that 19-month-old children could get into a bathtub by themselves, a 2005 study in *Pediatrics* revealed that of 176 children between 10 and 18 months of age, 35% were able to climb into a standard bathtub on their own.

Providers need to be careful in their assumptions about the developmental abilities of young children. The fact that the child was potty training may indeed have been a trigger for frustration in a caregiver, but in itself, it is not as clearly suspicious as the physical examination in this case. The history of missed appointments, although potentially indicating a pattern of avoidance of medical care or neglect, is also quite nonspecific as a concern. The developmental ability of a child needs to be matched with the history offered for an injury; inconsistencies raise serious concerns and suspicion.

(p. 154, Chapter 36: Child Maltreatment: Neglect to Abuse)

**Answer 7-6.** A

In every case of suspected abuse, a complete history and physical examination are indicated. Often, healthcare providers neglect to perform a full examination of the skin, including the perigenital and anal areas. Providers should pay close attention to the ears and the mouth, as injuries are missed. With bruising, in general, a complete blood count, platelet count, prothrombin time, and partial thromboplastin time are indicated as a first set of laboratory tests to be sure there is not an obvious bleeding disorder (eg, idiopathic thrombocytopenic purpura, leukemia). Although any of the tests listed may be indicated with further history and physical examination, the initial labs should be obtained given the bruising noted, as unsuspected medical conditions could obviate the need for further testing.

A skeletal survey is generally indicated in a child < 2 years of age who presents with a history or physical examination suspicious for physical abuse. In children ≥ 2 years of age, there may be some yield to a skeletal survey, but this should usually be considered after the blood cell, platelet, and coagulation studies, and in consultation with a child abuse expert.

An abdominal CT scan may be indicated if there was abdominal bruising on exam or if screening liver transaminases were > 80 IU/L. A CT scan of the head may be indicated when there is suspected physical abuse in a young child with concern for head injury, particularly in a child younger than 1 year with history or physical examination suggesting physical abuse. In the absence of acute neurologic symptoms, a magnetic resonance imaging (MRI) scan of the head is a more revealing study, without the radiation exposure risks. An MRI is a more expensive study that often requires sedation. Similarly, ophthalmology examinations are useful in cases of suspected abusive head trauma to evaluate the presence of retinal hemorrhages.

(p. 157, Chapter 36: Child Maltreatment: Neglect to Abuse)

**Answer 7-7.** A

The risk of child maltreatment increases as the level of violence in the household increases. Children exposed to IPV are 6 to 15 times more likely to be abused. Overall, sibling violence tends to result in fewer serious injuries than peer violence and involves the use of fewer potentially injurious weapons; however, sibling violence is more likely to be chronic and therefore may hold greater potential for trauma symptoms. Although IPV is present in relationships across class, culture, race/ethnicity, and sexual orientation, this phenomenon is characterized by a gender disparity; in 2001, the US Bureau of Justice Statistics reported that 85% of victims of IPV are women. Dating violence is reported in up to 25% of relationships. An estimated 7% to 26% of adolescent females report violence during pregnancy inflicted by a partner or family member. There are overwhelming data that exposure to violence affects mental health and more and more data to support that long-term physical health is also affected.

(pp. 136–137, Chapter 32: Family and Community Violence)

**Answer 7-8.** E

Buttock bruises are concerning for child abuse in many cases. The differential diagnosis for bruises can include a number of acute or chronic medical conditions. Henoch-Schönlein purpura is a disease that can cause abdominal and joint pain, as well as purpura, often on the buttocks, which may be mistaken for bruising. Abnormalities affecting the coagulation process such as idiopathic thrombocytopenic purpura, an autoimmune disorder leading to platelet destruction resulting in decreased platelet counts, can increase the propensity to bruise easily. Similarly, a bone marrow infiltrative process such as acute lymphocytic leukemia can present with easy bruising. Birthmarks such as dermal melanocytosis (previously called Mongolian spots) are often located in the buttocks area and can easily be mistaken for bruises. Bruising may be associated with malnutrition, such as deficiencies of vitamins $B_{12}$, C, and K or folic acid. However, vitamin A is not likely to be a cause of easy bruising by itself.

(p. 157, Chapter 36: Child Maltreatment: Neglect to Abuse)

**Answer 7-9.** E

The child's statements about being touched by her uncle are concerning for sexual abuse. A forensic interview would be the appropriate next step in this case. A child's disclosure during a forensic interview of digital-vaginal contact by her uncle is consistent with sexual abuse, regardless of the exam findings.

HPV is not diagnostic of sexual abuse and can result from nonsexual autoinoculation. Like herpes simplex virus (HSV), genital warts in a prepubertal child should trigger an evaluation for possible sexual abuse. Normal prepubertal girls may have any of a variety of hymen shapes including crescentic, annular, and fimbriated or redundant. Vaginal mucosa can be seen through such a normal hymen. There is a myth that the hymen covers the vaginal opening and that it can be "popped" or broken. However, in normal prepubertal girls, there is generally a hymenal opening through which one may see the vaginal mucosa on routine examination. Lack of a hymenal opening is called hymenocolpos and can present at puberty when menstrual blood cannot exit the vagina. A small bruise on the inner thigh of a 3-year-old girl could raise concerns; however, it is not diagnostic of sexual abuse. Erythema of the genitals of a 3-year-old girl is nonspecific for sexual abuse and most commonly indicates poor hygiene.

(pp. 155–157, Chapter 36: Child Maltreatment: Neglect to Abuse)

**Answer 7-10.** B

Spiral fractures in themselves are not diagnostic of physical abuse. Careful consideration of the nature and severity of the injury, the proposed mechanism of injury, and the developmental abilities of the child should be undertaken when spiral fractures are diagnosed. In a nonambulatory child, spiral fractures certainly raise suspicion for abuse. In an ambulatory 2- or 3-year-old child, spiral fractures can occur accidentally. The term *toddler's fracture* refers to a nondisplaced spiral fracture, usually of the distal tibia. Although one cannot rule out abuse, such fractures can occur with a twisting or planting motion in an ambulatory child as they are running or walking. It would be expected that the parents may not witness or be aware of the actual injury.

Given the overall lack of other findings or other concerns, this would be a reasonable diagnosis to make for this child. When there are fractures that are not consistent with the developmental age of a child or mechanism or history provided, obtaining laboratory tests to rule out some underlying disease that could affect bone strength, such as rickets, may be helpful. Checking levels of calcium, phosphorus, alkaline phosphatase, and 25-hydroxyvitamin D would be a reasonable first step. Other labs might include a workup for osteogenesis imperfecta or other rare disorders that might affect bone fragility such as Menkes disease. If there is suspicion of head trauma in a young child, then a workup might include a retinal examination to evaluate for retinal hemorrhages and a CT or magnetic resonance imaging (MRI) scan of the head to evaluate for intracranial bleeding. In this case, with a normal mental status examination and no findings concerning for head trauma, these diagnostic studies would not be indicated. A skeletal survey is a series of radiographs examining all the long bones as well as the skull, chest, and spine. A skeletal survey is a helpful screening tool when suspicion of abuse is present in children < 2 years old. A skeletal survey can be helpful in children up to 5 years old in certain clinical situations.

(pp. 155 and 157, Chapter 36: Child Maltreatment: Neglect to Abuse)

**Answer 7-11.** A

Approximately 1 in 3 long bone fractures in hospitalized infants are attributed to abuse. About 25% of fractures in children < 3 years old are believed to be from abuse. Whereas an oblique/spiral femur fracture in an ambulatory child could be accidental from a planting and twisting motion during running or walking, a femur fracture in a nonambulatory infant without any history of trauma is very concerning for abuse.

Underlying bone diseases must be considered, but most of these are rare and can be excluded by a thorough physical examination, medical history, family history, laboratory testing, and careful review of the radiographs. Osteogenesis imperfecta (OI) is a constellation of diseases that affect collagen and bone strength. Severe forms of OI present at birth and would not be confused with inflicted injury in an older infant. Milder forms of OI are inherited in an autosomal dominant fashion and are frequently associated with clinical findings such as blue sclerae, dental abnormalities, hyperflexibility, and short stature. Radiographs may reveal wormian bones (extra sutures) in the skull. A careful family history and physical exam can reasonably exclude milder forms of OI that may be mistaken for abusive fractures, although genetic consultation and/or testing should be considered in select cases. Fractures of the femur may not be readily apparent, and a delay by a mother of 1 night to bring in her child in this case would not be overly concerning, although in general, delay in care for obvious injuries is a red flag. One study reported that femur fractures in newborns were not recognized by medical personnel often for days and sometimes weeks. In this case, as in all cases of children < 2 years old who have injuries suspicious for abuse, a skeletal survey would be indicated to look for non-clinically evident fractures.

(pp. 154–155, Chapter 36: Child Maltreatment: Neglect to Abuse)

**Answer 7-12.** E

Retinal hemorrhages can occur from a number of causes, including infections causing meningitis, sepsis, or coagulation disturbances; birth; and abusive head injury. Retinal hemorrhages from birth usually resolve within 2 weeks, although hemorrhages have been documented lasting almost 2 months. There are a number of types of retinal hemorrhages including preretinal and intraretinal hemorrhages, and hemorrhages may have descriptions such as "splinter" hemorrhages and "blot and dot" hemorrhages. All of these types of hemorrhages have been associated with abusive head trauma.

Retinal hemorrhages usually resolve without any effect on vision, although severe hemorrhages can affect vision. Retinal hemorrhages can occur anywhere in the retina and are not found only near the macula. Greater numbers of retinal hemorrhages distributed throughout the retina are more specific for abusive head trauma than a few scattered hemorrhages around the macula. In general, it is important for an ophthalmologist with pediatric experience to photodocument the number, type, and location of retinal hemorrhages when there is concern for abusive head trauma.

(pp. 155 and 157, Chapter 36: Child Maltreatment: Neglect to Abuse)

**Answer 7-13.** D

Any bruising in an infant < 4 months of age should raise questions regarding possible abuse. In children between 4 months and 4 years of age, bruising of the trunk, ears, and neck may raise concern for abuse. Accidental bruises on the front of the typical 1-year-old boy would not be unexpected. Bruises over bony prominences such as shins, elbows/forearms, and the face are not unusual, especially when children are learning to walk and might fall forward. Multiple bruises in these areas, especially the shins, are common. The color of bruises can vary, and dating bruises is inexact. Although inflicted or accidental injury is the most common cause of bruising, large, painless, palpable lesions may reflect purpura rather than bruising and warrant consideration of medical pathology such as coagulopathy or vasculitis. Round ulcerated lesions may raise concern for cigarette burns. Cigarette burns are typically 7 to 10 mm in diameter with a deep central scar and rolled edges. The perioral location and yellow crusting described here are more likely to represent impetigo.

(pp. 154 and 157, Chapter 36: Child Maltreatment: Neglect to Abuse)

**Answer 7-14.** D

The skeletal survey is a series of radiographs that includes frontal and lateral views of the skull, lateral views of the cervical spine and thoracolumbosacral spine, and single frontal views of the long bones, hands, feet, chest, and abdomen. Oblique views of the ribs may be added for improved accuracy of diagnosis of rib fractures. A skeletal survey is the primary screening tool for detecting occult skeletal injury when there is suspicion of abuse or neglect in children < 2 years old. In specific cases, skeletal surveys may be indicated for children up to 5 years of age. The skeletal survey can detect unsuspected recent or old fractures that may be clinically undetectable. Many fractures will heal within 6 months or less, and so the survey does not detect all previous fractures in a child. Due to callous formation over time, which makes fractures more apparent, repeating a limited skeletal survey in 10 to 14 days may reveal fractures that were not obvious initially.

(p. 157, Chapter 36: Child Maltreatment: Neglect to Abuse)

### Answer 7-15. A

A normal genital examination does not rule out sexual abuse or assault. A study of pregnant adolescents found that 2 of 36 had definitive findings of vaginal penetration. Only 5% of children referred for sexual abuse have positive findings on their genital examinations. Among those cases in which a perpetrator was convicted, only 23% of the genital examinations were considered suspicious. A chlamydia test being positive on the day of a sexual contact in a postpubertal girl would more likely be the result of a previously existing infection, particularly in a sexually active person. In this case, a positive chlamydia test would not be proof of rape. In cases of suspected or known sexual assault, postexposure prophylaxis for pregnancy, syphilis, chlamydia, gonorrhea, and human immunodeficiency virus (HIV) may be indicated, depending on the situation. State laws around age of consent and ability to provide these medications vary, but in this case, such prophylaxis may benefit the girl. In general, for HIV and pregnancy prophylaxis, the earlier the medications are taken, the more effective they are. Beyond 72 hours, the benefit is greatly diminished.

For syphilis, chlamydia, and gonorrhea, the decision is often made to treat before results of diagnostic tests are returned, especially due to poor follow-up rates. There is no treatment to prevent hepatitis C, although immunization against hepatitis B should be ensured. A blood alcohol level that is elevated only suggests alcohol ingestion and does not suggest rape in itself.

(p. 157, Chapter 36: Child Maltreatment: Neglect to Abuse)

### Answer 7-16. E

Pediatric condition falsification is a spectrum of abuse types (often referred to as Munchausen syndrome by proxy, factitious disorder by proxy, medical child abuse, and other names), in which a parent exaggerates or fabricates symptoms of an illness or causes a child to be ill. It has a fatality rate of 6% to 9% because it is often difficult to recognize or diagnose, because often the focus is on the child's symptoms rather than the possibility that they could be caused by a parent. The most common presentations of pediatric condition falsification are seizures, apnea, diarrhea, and fever. The etiology of BRUEs is unknown as often as half the time. Pediatric condition falsification should be considered as a possible etiology in cases of recurrent BRUEs that are reported only by a single caregiver. Diagnosis of pediatric condition falsification requires in-depth review of medical records, including clarification around established diagnoses, invasive interventions, and documentation of communication between a child's caregiver and medical providers.

(pp. 159–160, Chapter 37: Factitious Disorder by Proxy)

### Answer 7-17. D

Neglected children commonly present with poor growth due to inadequate nutrition. Weight usually is the first parameter affected, then height, and then head circumference. Often there is accompanying developmental delay, particularly in language and social interactions. Although there are a myriad of possible causes of poor weight gain (or failure to thrive), whether evaluating for organic or nonorganic causes, a careful feeding history is critical in order to estimate the caloric intake of the child as well as evaluate the potential social and environmental contributions to the weight loss. Evaluation might focus on questions such as how food is prepared and how the child responds to it, past feeding problems, and parental concerns.

Any feeding history for a child with poor weight gain should include evaluation of food insecurity. Family separation, unemployment, and poverty may be contributing to lower quantity or quality of food available in the household. Standardized questions, such as the 2 included on the Safe Environment for Every Kid (SEEK) Questionnaire, may be helpful in uncovering food insecurity in a household:

1. In the past 12 months, did you worry that your food would run out before you could buy more?
2. In the past 12 months, did the food you bought just not last and you did not have money to get more?

Prior to other medical tests, a complete developmental history is also an important next step. Standardized evaluation of the child's developmental milestones, temperament, and interactions with family and others may identify behavioral or developmental concerns that could be contributing to poor weight gain. Even in the setting of suspected physical neglect, in the absence of concerning signs of physical abuse, a skeletal survey in a 3-year-old child is not necessarily indicated, nor is a CT scan of the head. The murmur may require further workup but would not be as important as a feeding history in this situation. Assessment of serum electrolyte levels would not be useful given the child does not have other signs to suggest that he is severely malnourished at this point.

(p. 131, Chapter 30: Poverty, Homelessness, and Social Disorganization; pp. 155–157, Chapter 36: Child Maltreatment: Neglect to Abuse)

### Answer 7-18. C

Linear skull fractures are consistent with a simple fall onto a hard surface, and an underlying epidural (and even localized subdural) hematoma could be consistent with this mechanism of injury, assuming no other suspicious findings. Hepatic transaminase elevation is worrisome for occult intra-abdominal trauma in the setting of suspected child physical abuse, and an abdominal CT may be warranted in children with likely physical abuse and transaminase elevation > 80 IU. In the absence of findings supporting suspicion of abuse, however, transaminase elevation is not in and of itself worrisome for occult trauma. Two types of fractures that are commonly associated with abusive head trauma are classic metaphyseal fractures (also called bucket handle or corner fractures related to their appearance depending on the angle of the x-ray) and posterior (or posterior-lateral) rib fractures. There are almost no household accidents that would be commonly associated with a posterior rib fracture in a young infant. In this case, however, the boyfriend describes a scenario that may be a reasonable explanation of a classic metaphyseal fracture of the distal radius, which typically involves shearing forces at the joint. It is also worth noting that his history associated with the left radial injury was provided prior to the skeletal survey. A transverse clavicle fracture could be associated with birth trauma in an infant. Although birth fractures may be healed at 2 months of age, they may still be seen as healing fractures on a skeletal survey.

(pp. 154–155, Chapter 36: Child Maltreatment: Neglect to Abuse)

**Answer 7-19. C**

Head injuries are the most common cause of death and severe disability from child physical abuse. Abusive head trauma may present with a spectrum of external and internal head injuries, with or without spinal, skeletal, cutaneous, ophthalmologic, or abdominal injuries. In many cases, however, there are no external signs of head trauma such as bruises or swelling. Infants with abusive head trauma can be asymptomatic or present with severe findings and even coma or death. Seizures, apnea, and respiratory symptoms are not uncommon. A high index of suspicion is required as caregivers may not give a trauma history to healthcare providers. When trauma histories are provided, they may be inconsistent with the spectrum of injuries identified.

Abusive head trauma often is accompanied by retinal hemorrhages. Although there are multiple etiologies for retinal hemorrhages, those that are considered most specific for severe head trauma are numerous, involve multiple layers of the retina, and extend out to the periphery of the retina. Given the importance of precise documentation of the characteristics of retinal hemorrhages, a retinal examination with a full indirect examination through a dilated pupil by an ophthalmologist with pediatric experience is important to obtain when there is suspicion of abusive head trauma. Photodocumentation of retinal hemorrhages is also strongly advised. Important labs to rule out potential mimics of abusive head trauma would include coagulation studies with a CBC to evaluate for coagulation abnormalities. It should be noted that head trauma, particularly severe trauma, can cause coagulation disorders as a secondary response to injury. Some rare disorders, such as glutaric acidemia type 1, can present with retinal hemorrhages and subdural hemorrhages, and tests for these might include serum amino acids. Liver function tests can screen for occult abdominal injuries in young infants and children with suspicious injuries but would not directly support the diagnosis of abusive head trauma in the same manner as retinal hemorrhages. Serum calcium, phosphorus, and alkaline phosphatase would be labs to obtain to work up fractures.

(pp. 154–155, Chapter 36: Child Maltreatment: Neglect to Abuse)

**Answer 7-20. B**

Complete transection of the hymen is only associated with penetrating genital injury. A physical finding of genital injury is seen in < 3% of cases of sexual abuse in prepubertal children but would be concerning based on the available history. There are multiple case reports of penetrating genital injury from accidental falls onto protruding objects, but these are typically immediately recognized based on a child's symptoms. There is commonly a toy, post, or other object immediately recognized as the source of the injury, and law enforcement should be given information like this to guide scene investigation. In the absence of a likely accidental history, child sexual abuse must be carefully considered as a likely diagnosis.

A bruise and/or laceration to the external female genitalia such as the labia majora would be consistent with a straddle injury, as described by the father. Prolapsed urethra often presents with bleeding, occurs more often in obese African American girls, and is often mistaken for sexual abuse on examination by an inexperienced provider. Treatment is usually with topical steroids. Lichen sclerosus et atrophicus presents with hypopigmented thinning of the skin in the perianal or genital area and is often associated with subcutaneous or submucosal hemorrhages, lacerations, itching, and pain. The etiology of lichen sclerosus in children is unknown but is likely immune-mediated, and treatment with topical steroids is commonly recommended. Although lichen sclerosus in adult women may be a perineoplastic condition, this is not described in children with this condition. Perianal streptococcal dermatitis is a sharply demarcated bright red rash caused by group A β-hemolytic streptococci. It is not sexually transmitted, although this may be misunderstood by anxious caregivers. Symptoms can include blood-streaked stools in one-third of patients, and it primarily occurs in children between 6 months and 10 years of age. A rapid streptococcal test of the area can make the diagnosis, and treatment is similar to that for strep throat, with amoxicillin or penicillin being effective.

(pp. 156–157, Chapter 36: Child Maltreatment: Neglect to Abuse)

**Answer 7-21. C**

Sentinel injuries are mild injuries, such as bruising, intraoral injuries, or subconjunctival hemorrhages, in premobile infants that are visible by the caretakers and are poorly explained. Sentinel injuries indicate abusive actions by a caretaker, which could lead to escalating abuse. It is important for pediatric providers to recognize sentinel injuries and complete a full evaluation for physical abuse at the time they are discovered. A full evaluation of a sentinel injury includes a full physical exam, including intraoral exam, skeletal survey, laboratory evaluation for bleeding disorders (prothrombin time, partial thromboplastin time, complete blood count), screening abdominal labs (aspartate aminotransferase and alanine aminotransferase), and a head computed tomography (CT) scan. A study of infants being evaluated for abuse found that 27.5% of infants diagnosed with abuse had a previous sentinel injury and 42% of those were documented by the pediatric provider.

Bruising on the forehead of a 9-month-old child is consistent with the developmental abilities of cruising. A bruise on the shin of a 15-month-old child is consistent with the developmental capabilities and walking. A red mark on the posterior neck of a 1-month-old infant is most consistent with a congenital nevus simplex. Subconjunctival hemorrhage in a 10-day-old infant is consistent with residual birth trauma. A bruise on the arm of a 3-month-old infant is not consistent with the developmental abilities of a child that age and is concerning for inflicted injury, which should be further evaluated.

(p. 154, Chapter 36: Child Maltreatment: Neglect to Abuse)

**Answer 7-22.** D

Sexual behaviors in children are often brought to the attention of the pediatric provider due to parental concern for sexual abuse. It is important to recognize that a wide variety of sexual behaviors are considered normal in children. Showing genitals to peers, touching or masturbating genitals in public or private, and touching peer or new sibling genitals are normal and common behaviors in children age 2 to 6 years. A child rubbing their body against others is less common but still a normal behavior in a 4-year-old child. Sexual behaviors that involve coercion are rarely normal and should prompt further evaluation for abuse and a report to child protective services.

(p. 155, Chapter 36: Child Maltreatment: Neglect to Abuse; Kellogg N. Clinical report: the evaluation of sexual behaviors in children. *Pediatrics* 2009;124:992–998.)

**Answer 7-23.** E

This infant was found to have a subdural fluid collection, which is concerning for subdural hematoma and physical abuse. The initial evaluation for suspected physical abuse in an infant includes a skeletal survey to evaluate for occult fracture and LFTs to evaluate for occult abdominal trauma. The subdural hematoma should lead to evaluation by ophthalmology for retinal hemorrhages and bleeding labs, including a CBC, PT, and PTT. Although an MRI is recommended for further evaluation of the subdural fluid collection and the brain parenchyma, this is not recommended until 3 to 5 days after injury to allow for full evaluation. Therefore, this would not be indicated in the initial evaluation.

(p. 155, Chapter 36: Child Maltreatment: Neglect to Abuse)

**Answer 7-24.** B

The recommendations for evaluation of acute sexual assault that has occurred within the past 72 hours in a pubertal patient include forensic evidence collection, including body swabs and clothing collection. This should be the first step in evaluation after obtaining the history. A forensic interview is indicated, but due to the timing and need for evidence collection, this can be completed at a later time. The same is true for the police interview, which can be included in the forensic interview. Testing for HSV is not indicated in sexual assault unless there are concerning lesions on exam. Sexually transmitted infection testing that is indicated for acute sexual assault includes urine sample for β-human chorionic gonadotropin, chlamydia, and gonorrhea and serum testing for human immunodeficiency virus (HIV), syphilis, and hepatitis B and C. Although these are recommended at the initial assessment, they should not delay the forensic evidence collection and should be obtained afterward.

(p. 157, Chapter 36: Child Maltreatment: Neglect to Abuse)

**Answer 7-25.** E

The recommendations for evaluation of sexual abuse that involves penetration in a pubertal female include STI testing, no matter the timing of the abuse. However, due to the remote timing of the sexual contact, forensic evidence collection, postexposure HIV prophylaxis, pregnancy prophylaxis, and chlamydia prophylaxis are not indicated. Forensic evidence should be collected if the last contact was within 72 hours. Postexposure HIV prophylaxis must be initiated within 72 hours of exposure; however, the sooner it is initiated, the better. Pregnancy prophylaxis can be given within 72 hours and 120 hours depending on the specific medication given. Chlamydia prophylaxis should be given within 72 hours of exposure.

(p. 157, Chapter 36: Child Maltreatment: Neglect to Abuse)

**Answer 7-26.** B

A sentinel injury is defined as a minor injury, such as a bruise or intraoral injury (torn labial frenulum) in a premobile infant, that is visible to the caregiver and poorly explained. The torn frenulum in a 2-month-old infant is consistent with a sentinel injury. The evaluation for a sentinel injury includes full exam, skeletal survey, head CT, and screening liver function tests (LFTs), all evaluating for occult trauma. The evaluation in this patient revealed no further injuries. The next step in the evaluation would include a report to child protective services. A sentinel injury is an early indicator of escalating physical abuse and meets the mandate to report. A study showed that 27.5% of patients diagnosed with physical abuse had a previous sentinel injury and 42% of those were known by a medical provider.

This patient did not have any hemorrhage detected on head CT, and therefore, an MRI of the brain is not indicated. Routine follow-up at the 4-month well-child visit is appropriate, but not the next step due to the current diagnosis of physical abuse, which must be reported. Follow-up in 2 weeks to evaluate healing is not indicated. Reassurance that this was likely an accidental injury is not appropriate in this patient, because due to the premobile status and sentinel injury, this is not an accidental injury. In older children who are walking, a frenulum tear is most consistent with accidental injury.

(pp. 154–158, Chapter 36: Child Maltreatment: Neglect to Abuse)

**Answer 7-27.** E

TDV includes physical, sexual, and psychological maltreatment in a relationship and occurs in approximately 25% of teen relationships. Although a serious dating relationship at the age of 12 may be concerning, it does not necessarily include violence. A 17 years old dating multiple people may be risky but does not fit the definition of dating violence. A sexually active 15 years old may be having consensual sexual contact and not be sexually maltreated. A 16 years old with risky behaviors, such as alcohol or drug use, multiple sexual partners, or police involvement, is at higher risk of dating violence and trafficking. A 14 years old in a controlling relationship meets the definition of psychological dating violence and should be addressed.

(pp. 143–144, Chapter 33: Teen Dating Violence)

**Answer 7-28.** E

The ACEs study demonstrated the relationship between childhood adversity and adult health outcomes. ACEs demonstrate a dose-response relationship, in that the more ACEs a patient has, the higher are the rates of negative health behaviors and morbidities in adulthood. The rates of poor outcomes are higher in those with 4 or more ACEs, but those with less still experience an effect. The defined adverse experiences include abuse (physical, emotional, and sexual), neglect (physical and emotional), and household dysfunction (substance abuse, mental illness, violence against mother, parental separation or divorce, incarcerated household member, and criminal behavior). No one adverse experience is worse than another. Tolerable stress occurs when the degree of adversity is not overwhelming and the child can overcome, whereas toxic stress is severe and unremitting stress in childhood due to ACEs.

(pp. 125–126, Chapter 28: Childhood Adversity and Toxic Stress)

**Answer 7-29.** C

The mechanism of subdural hemorrhage in abusive head trauma is due to shearing forces on the bridging veins from repeated acceleration and deceleration. Scalp veins are not in an anatomic location that would cause subdural hematoma because they are outside the skull. Bleeding from these veins would result in a subgaleal hematoma or a cephalohematoma. Bleeding from the subarachnoid space can result in spread to the subdural space, but this is more isolated and not the most common mechanism of a subdural hemorrhage. Bleeding from the dural sinus is not the cause of a subdural hemorrhage, but bleeding into the dural sinus can occur with a subdural hemorrhage. Bleeding from the brain parenchymal would result in parenchymal hemorrhage or subpial hemorrhage, rather than subdural hemorrhage.

(p. 155, Chapter 36: Child Maltreatment: Neglect to Abuse)

**Answer 7-30.** A

Infantile colic is defined in multiple ways but, in general, is considered excessive crying, at least a few hours a day, multiple days a week, with no recognized cause of onset or resolution. Infantile colic is concerning because of the risk of physical abuse by the caregiver in response to the crying. There is no known cause of infantile colic at this point. Multiple theories exist regarding neurodevelopment and gastrointestinal causes. Without specific signs or symptoms other than crying, there is no indication for medical workup. Infantile colic resolves on its own as the infant grows and matures.

(pp. 149–151, Chapter 35: Infant Colic)

**Answer 7-31.** D

Sex trafficking of a minor is defined as trafficking a person under the age of 18 for commercial sex. This includes the exchange of sexual activities for money, drugs, food, clothing, or shelter and is defined as survival sex. In screening a patient for sex trafficking, the use of the questions regarding risky behaviors (drug or alcohol use, running away, law enforcement involvement, history of STIs, and multiple sexual partners) is important as these increase the risk of sex trafficking. However, these screening questions are not specific for sex trafficking. The use of survival sex is more specific for sex trafficking and should be included in screening for trafficking.

(pp. 146 and 148, Chapter 34: Child Trafficking)

**Answer 7-32.** C

The pediatric provider's role in the care of a patient in foster care includes routine well examination, providing a medical home, screening for mental health concerns, and providing support for the family. Given this child's age, skeletal survey, head CT, and complete metabolic panel to screen for occult trauma are not indicated. Routine hair follicle testing is not recommended for the evaluation of children who have been placed into foster care. Rather, serum or urine drug testing should be used if there are specific concerns for current intoxication.

(p. 164, Chapter 38: Foster Care and Adoption)

**Answer 7-33.** D

Multiple BRUEs or sudden infant death syndrome is concerning for intentional suffocation when the following are present: (1) multiple episodes of reported apnea, (2) a child

> 6 months, (3) a sibling with a major illness, (4) a sibling who has died, (5) index child or sibling with child abuse, (6) blood in the nose or mouth, and (7) a single witness present for all episodes. The most reassuring part of this case is having multiple caregivers witness the episodes, making intentional suffocation less likely.

(p. 160, Chapter 37: Factitious Disorder by Proxy)

**Answer 7-34.** A

The mechanism for posterior medial rib fractures is anterior posterior compression of the chest leading to the posterior medial rib fracturing against the transverse process of the spine. Direct blows to the chest or caregiver fingers can cause other types of rib fractures, but the posterior medial portion of the rib is highly protected by the spine. CPR is unlikely to cause rib fractures and would more commonly cause lateral or anterior rib fractures rather than posterior medial rib fractures. Coughing in an infant does not generate enough force to cause rib fractures and would not cause rib fractures in the posterior medial location.

(p. 155, Chapter 36: Child Maltreatment: Neglect to Abuse)

**Answer 7-35.** E

The TEN-4 rule for evaluating bruising indicates that bruising of the torso, ear, and neck of any child under the age of 4 years and any bruising at all in infants under 4 months of age should prompt clear concern for physical abuse. Bruising on the forehead of a mobile (walking) infant is consistent with their developmental capabilities and does not meet the TEN-4 rule.

(p. 154, Chapter 36: Child Maltreatment: Neglect to Abuse)

**Answer 7-36.** D

The most common manifestation of neglect in infants and young children is poor growth and developmental delay. FTT can be a result of organic (medical cause) or nonorganic (nonmedical cause or neglect) causes. Signs of FTT as a result of neglect include poor maternal bonding, maternal postpartum depression, dilution of the formula, and inadequate food volume provided, among others. A history of projectile vomiting in a patient with FTT should prompt further workup for a medical cause, such as pyloric stenosis for the poor weight gain.

(p. 155, Chapter 36: Child Maltreatment: Neglect to Abuse)

**Answer 7-37.** B

Genital warts as described in this case are caused by HPV. HPV can present in infancy as a result of vertical transmission, casual household contact, or sexual abuse. In the absence of additional history of abuse, physical findings of abuse, or additionally sexually transmitted infections (STIs), it may be difficult to distinguish the source of infection. Testing to rule out co-infection with other STIs is recommended unless a nonsexual source of transmission can be clearly identified. Reporting to child protective services without additional evidence of sexual abuse may create confusion and mistrust without a strong evidence for child sexual abuse. Although molluscum contagiosum can present in the genital region, these lesions are typically smooth and umbilicated in contrast to the rough, cauliflower-like surface of HPV. Condyloma lata, the wart-like lesions associated with secondary syphilis, are highly contagious, and scrapings of these lesions are typically positive for *Treponema pallidum* by darkfield microscopy. In comparison with HPV, however, these lesions are typically moist. In the setting of likely HPV, reactive plasma reagin and human immunodeficiency virus (HIV) testing should be considered. While we often gather medical histories for maternal HPV status, the prevalence of subclinical HPV infection may make such inquiries unhelpful in identifying the source of infection in an infant.

(pp. 156–157, Chapter 36: Child Maltreatment: Neglect to Abuse)

**Answer 7-38.** D

If this infant progresses to death, this case will be classified as a sudden unexplained infant death (SUID). In these cases, the medical teams face many complex and difficult decisions related to diagnosis and treatment alongside the need to provide social and emotional support for frightened or grieving caregivers. One aspect of these cases that may be easily forgotten within the high-intensity medical context is the importance of a timely scene investigation by outside agencies. Critical evidence to identify the cause of injury or death may be lost, including clear description of the sleep environment, collection of food or bottles for toxicology testing, and understanding of household risks. Standard skeletal survey or full-body CT is recommended for children < 2 years of age with suspected physical abuse or as part of a postmortem evaluation of infants and young children. This would not be appropriate for an infant who is too clinically unstable to tolerate this procedure. MRI would again be inappropriate for an infant this unstable. Additionally, optimal MRI timing is approximately 3 days from the most likely injury to improve the ability to characterize traumatic or hypoxic parenchymal injuries. A social history is always appropriate, but high-risk social circumstances are neither specific nor sensitive enough to support a diagnosis of child physical abuse. Finally, multidisciplinary consultation may be indicated in some cases where there is historical, physical, or laboratory evidence of underlying disease leading to the current presentation. It is important to recall, however, that coagulopathy and metabolic derangements are common in the setting of multiorgan system failure and may reflect the critical condition of the infant rather than underlying disease.

(pp. 154–155, Chapter 36: Child Maltreatment: Neglect to Abuse)

**Answer 7-39.** A

Foster care placement is typically a last resort in cases of child abuse or neglect in which a child cannot be safely returned to his or her own home. Kinship care placement has increased in the past decade due to evidence suggesting that such placements may improve placement stability, ties with the family of origin, and child behavioral outcomes. Half of all children entering foster care return to their biological families within 6 months of placement, and three-quarters return within 24 months. This should remind pediatricians and others of the importance of supporting engagement of biological families in the care of a child in foster care within the boundaries of child safety and legal mandates. While FTT and developmental delay in cases of extreme neglect may resolve with entry into a more stable household, these may persist. Pediatric evaluation for underlying and unrecognized chronic medical conditions should occur alongside trauma-informed behavioral health interventions to improve chances of recovery. Foster families, whether kin or unrelated, undergo standard background checks and training that varies by state. Standard foster care trainings may be basic. Health care may be able to identify additional supports needed to manage the medical and behavioral health needs of children placed into foster care.

(pp. 125–126, Chapter 28: Childhood Adversity and Toxic Stress; pp. 162–163, Chapter 38: Foster Care and Adoption)

**Answer 7-40.** B

The physical exam findings of large, nonpatterned bruises in locations that are common sites of minor trauma without any evidence of other injury or history of inflicted injury are most consistent with an acquired bleeding diathesis such as idiopathic thrombocytopenia or leukemia. Appropriate lab testing for mimics of inflicted injury should not be overlooked in the context of a complex or worrisome social history. There is no history provided by the patient to suggest sexual assault. Given the poor predictive value for genital findings to either confirm or exclude sexual assault, there is no indication to proceed with a genital examination in the absence of patient concerns. Similarly, notification of law enforcement of concerns for assault based on the evidence available at this point would be premature. It is possible that your patient is choosing not to disclose risky behaviors in your clinic, so a standardized screener for teen dating violence, substance abuse, self-injury, suicidal ideation, and/or trafficking may be very helpful in understanding the risks that her stepmother is reporting to you. Although it will not alter your diagnostic approach to the bruising, your patient's past history places her at high risk for post-traumatic stress disorder (PTSD). Regardless of the outcome of the evaluation in clinic, offering referrals to mental health resources capable of evaluation and treatment of childhood PTSD is warranted.

(p. 127, Chapter 28: Childhood Adversity and Toxic Stress; p. 144, Chapter 33: Teen Dating Violence; p. 157, Chapter 36: Child Maltreatment: Neglect to Abuse)

**Answer 7-41.** D

Although many pediatricians are uncomfortable with screening for IPV, research consistently demonstrates that parents are open to screening for these household risks in the pediatric clinic. Prior to implementing a universal IPV screening process, however, pediatricians must plan for safe and effective responses to positive screens including identification of potential for lethality (history of strangulation, access to household guns), counseling on creating safety plans, and knowing local IPV resources. State laws vary, and there are several states in the United States for which exposure to IPV is a reportable form of child abuse; other states may support a report of IPV exposure in cases where this exposure is causing emotional or physical injury to a child in the home. Pediatricians may be able to identify behavioral symptoms that reflect the toxic stress associated with exposure to IPV, including aggressive or disruptive behavior problems, sleep disruptions, or inattention that may be confused with attention-deficit/hyperactivity disorder. IPV screening should occur outside of the earshot of children, as parents may be uncomfortable disclosing or discussing IPV in front of their children. Pediatricians may help parents consider how to talk effectively with children about IPV if this is requested.

(pp. 137–138, Chapter 32: Family and Community Violence)

**Answer 7-42.** E

Physicians play an important role in child advocacy by providing reliable information to the media in these circumstances, and developing these relationships with reporters in the community can be valuable to protecting child health. The public should realize that the epidemiology of child maltreatment is challenging due to important variability in definitions of child maltreatment and identification of child maltreatment. Official counts of child maltreatment in the United States are typically reflected through the National Child Abuse and Neglect Data System (NCANDS), which collects and reports child maltreatment numbers from state child welfare systems on an annual basis. These numbers reflect state definitions of abuse or neglect, which vary from state to state. They also fail to capture child abuse or neglect not reported to a child welfare agency. Despite these limitations, the annual NCANDS report of child maltreatment represents a reliable resource to understand trends in child maltreatment across the United States over time. One trend that has been noted in recent years is that despite increasing numbers of reports of child maltreatment to child welfare agencies, the number of substantiated cases of child maltreatment has actually declined since 1990. These declines have been most notable in cases of physical and sexual abuse, although cases of neglect have also either declined or remained stable over time. Despite these declines, state child welfare agencies still receive > 3 million reports of suspected child maltreatment involving > 6 million children every year. CPS agencies must make difficult decisions with limited information in responding to these reports and typically open just over half of these reports for investigation. These investigations substantiate concerns of maltreatment in only about one-third of cases where sufficient evidence of maltreatment can be identified. Failure to substantiate a concern of maltreatment does not mean that maltreatment has not occurred or that household risks are not identified. Child neglect is the most common form of substantiated child maltreatment nationally, representing 75% of substantiated cases, followed by physical abuse (17%) and sexual abuse (8%). Unfortunately, child neglect is also the most common form of child maltreatment to result in repeated reports, and there are few evidence-based interventions to address child neglect. This may reflect the strong association between child neglect and poverty.

(p. 152, Chapter 36: Child Maltreatment: Neglect to Abuse)

# CHAPTER 8 Emergency and Critical Care

Katherine Ban, Dana Foradori, Heather Haq, and Brent Mothner

**8-1.** A 24-month-old girl is brought to the emergency department after an episode of choking and coughing. The child was playing alone in another room when her mother heard her choking and gagging. En route to the hospital, the coughing resolved. She now appears calm. Oropharyngeal examination is normal. Expiratory wheezes are present over the right lower lobe of the lung. What is the most likely cause of the child's symptoms?

A. Epiglottitis

B. Tracheal foreign body

C. Lower airway foreign body

D. Lobar pneumonia

E. Status asthmaticus

**8-2.** A 3-year-old girl is playing with friends at a birthday party when she suddenly begins coughing and choking. She is rushed to the emergency department, but her distress has resolved by the time of arrival. Wheezing is present over her right lower and middle lung fields, and hyperinflation is present over these areas on expiratory chest films. Which of the following is indicated?

A. Albuterol to relieve her lower airway obstruction

B. Amoxicillin to treat her community-acquired pneumonia

C. Broad-spectrum antibiotics for her epiglottitis

D. Parental reassurance about the benign nature of the episode

E. Rigid bronchoscopy to remove the foreign body

**8-3.** A 26-month-old boy presents to the emergency department after his father witnessed him ingest an object that looked like a nickel. He is playful and in no acute distress. Radiography reveals a circular object in the stomach. The object does not have a double ring. What treatment is indicated?

A. Administer activated charcoal

B. Allow for spontaneous passage of the coin

C. Allow for spontaneous passage of the button battery

D. Perform emergent endoscopic removal of the button battery

E. Induce emesis with syrup of ipecac

**8-4.** A 24-month-old boy presents after ingestion of a foreign body. The child is currently asymptomatic. Which of the following foreign bodies requires immediate removal?

A. Button battery in the esophagus

B. Coin in the lower esophagus

C. Coin in the stomach

D. Marble in the intestine

E. Single magnet in the intestine

**8-5.** An 8-month-old boy is admitted to the hospital with bacterial meningitis. On the night after admission, he has a generalized tonic-clonic seizure. The seizure continues for 5 minutes. He has been persistently febrile and last received acetaminophen 15 minutes ago. He is placed on a non-rebreather. What is the next best step in management?

A. Administer a dose of fosphenytoin

B. Administer a dose of lorazepam

C. Await the resolution of fever after acetaminophen administration

D. Expand antibiotic coverage due to treatment failure

E. Obtain brain imaging to assess for an intracranial abscess

**8-6.** A 3-week-old former full-term neonate presents to the emergency department (ED) with new-onset seizures. She had 2 generalized tonic-clonic seizures at home and has appeared lethargic since that time. She has another seizure in the ED, which abates with intravenous (IV) lorazepam. A small cluster of vesicles is noted over her occiput. Which of the following studies is likely to be positive in this neonate with status epilepticus?

**A.** Gram-positive cocci in Gram stain of cerebrospinal fluid (CSF)

**B.** Maternal herpes simplex virus serologies

**C.** Positive enteroviral polymerase chain reaction (PCR) in the CSF

**D.** Positive urine drug screen

**E.** Subdural hematoma

**8-7.** An 18-month-old girl presents after a first-time seizure. She was in her usual state of health and watching television when she suddenly became sleepy and all of her extremities began shaking. The parents estimate that the episode lasted 12 minutes, but she was becoming more awake by the time of arrival to the hospital. In triage, her temperature is 103.8°F. Bilateral otitis media is present on examination, and the remainder of her examination is normal. What is the most likely cause of this child's prolonged seizure?

**A.** Bacterial meningitis

**B.** Epilepsy

**C.** Fever

**D.** Intracranial abscess

**E.** Traumatic brain injury (TBI)

**8-8.** A 24-month-old boy presents with a first-time seizure in the setting of otitis media. He was febrile upon arrival to the emergency department. His generalized tonic-clonic seizure lasted approximately 10 minutes, and he was sleepy for 5 minutes afterward. Which of the following is true?

**A.** Electroencephalogram and neuroimaging are indicated.

**B.** Lumbar puncture is indicated.

**C.** Scheduled acetaminophen will reduce the risk of another similar episode.

**D.** The child had febrile status epilepticus.

**E.** The child had a simple febrile seizure.

**8-9.** A 4-year-old boy presents with a first-time seizure. He was in his usual state of health when he developed generalized tonic-clonic movements. At the time of arrival of medical transport, the child had been seizing for 10 minutes. Rectal diazepam was administered, and the seizure quickly abated. The child is now somewhat sleepy but answers questions appropriately. His vital signs and neurologic examination are normal. What testing is indicated?

**A.** Emergent electroencephalogram

**B.** Lumbar puncture

**C.** Nonurgent electroencephalogram

**D.** Stat computed tomography (CT) of the brain without contrast

**E.** Serum electrolytes, ammonia, and amino acids

**8-10.** A 24-month-old girl presents with the rapid onset of respiratory distress, wheezing, and facial swelling that developed during dinner at a local seafood restaurant. On examination, her face, lips, tongue, and uvula appear swollen. She is in moderate respiratory distress with diffuse wheezes throughout all lung fields. What is the most likely cause of her signs and symptoms?

**A.** Anaphylaxis

**B.** Familial hereditary angioedema

**C.** Epiglottitis

**D.** Foreign body aspiration

**E.** Status asthmaticus

**8-11.** A 12-year-old girl with a history of asthma develops facial swelling, respiratory distress, and hives during an outdoor dinner this evening. On examination, wheezing is present throughout all lung fields. Which of the following is responsible for her signs and symptoms?

**A.** Excessive bradykinin

**B.** Hyperreactivity of the lower airways due to pollen

**C.** Ingestion of histamine in seafood

**D.** Mast cell degranulation

**E.** Viral infection of the bronchioles

**8-12.** A 14-year-old girl with a history of asthma and food allergies presents to the emergency department after the acute onset of facial swelling, urticaria, and respiratory distress. She is awake but appears distressed. Intramuscular epinephrine is quickly administered upon her arrival. What is the next best step in management?

**A.** Administer dexamethasone

**B.** Administer oral diphenhydramine

**C.** Administer nebulized racemic epinephrine

**D.** Obtain intravenous (IV) access

**E.** Rapid sequence intubation

**8-13.** A 6-year-old boy is admitted with concern for osteomyelitis. During a magnetic resonance imaging (MRI) study with radiocontrast, he acutely develops respiratory distress, wheezing, facial swelling, and a rash. He is awake and alert but appears distressed. What is the next best step in management?

A. Administer diphenhydramine
B. Administer intravenous (IV) epinephrine
C. Begin cardiopulmonary resuscitation
D. Provide a continuous albuterol nebulization
E. Start empirical broad-spectrum antibiotics for sepsis

**8-14.** A 4-year-old boy presents with abdominal pain that began yesterday. The pain is centrally located. He developed nonbloody, nonbilious emesis and a concomitant poor appetite. The pain has markedly increased and has become more localized to the right side of his abdomen. On examination, he demonstrates hypoactive bowel sounds, distension, guarding, and rebound tenderness. Tenderness is most severe in the right lower quadrant. What is the most likely etiology of the child's abdominal pain?

A. Gastroenteritis
B. Intussusception
C. Malrotation with volvulus
D. Perforated appendicitis
E. Pyelonephritis

**8-15.** A 4-year-old girl presents with abdominal pain and vomiting. The pain was initially "all over" but now seems localized to the right lower quadrant. Palpation of the left lower quadrant causes pain in the right lower quadrant. Her emesis is nonbloody and nonbilious. Upon arrival to the emergency department, she is febrile. Which of the following is most likely to resolve the child's abdominal pain?

A. Appendectomy
B. Antibiotics for urinary tract infection
C. Contrast enema
D. Decreased intake of fatty foods
E. Ladd procedure

**8-16.** A 25-day-old former full-term infant presents with persistent emesis and fussiness over the past 12 hours. His emesis appears green, although he has been fed only breast milk. Which of the following is likely to be present?

A. Duodenal obstruction on upper gastrointestinal series
B. Elevated serum lipase
C. Enlarged appendix on abdominal ultrasonography
D. Hyperglycemia and elevated β-hydroxybutyrate
E. Hypertrophy of the pylorus on abdominal ultrasonography

**8-17.** A 16-month-old boy presents with 4 hours of emesis and episodes of crying. During the episodes, he flexes his hips and turns red with crying. The episodes have become more frequent. He initially appeared normal between episodes but now appears lethargic. What is the most likely diagnosis?

A. Appendicitis
B. Brief resolved unexplained event (BRUE)
C. Gastroenteritis
D. Intussusception
E. Malrotation with volvulus

**8-18.** A 15-month-old girl presents with abdominal pain and emesis. The symptoms began this morning with no precipitating factors. The pain occurs in waves that are characterized by crying and "curling up in a ball." Between episodes, she was initially awake and alert, but now she appears more tired. She has also had a stool that appeared darker than normal. Which of the following is indicated for treatment of her condition?

A. Appendectomy
B. Bowel rest
C. Contrast enema
D. Intravenous (IV) antibiotics
E. Ladd procedure

**8-19.** A 28-month-old boy presents with fever and lethargy. He was in his usual state of health until last evening, when he became febrile and complained of headache. He refused dinner and went to bed early. This morning, he was again febrile and hard to awaken, refused breakfast, and vomited. On examination, purpura are present on his distal lower extremities. He is disoriented and only intermittently follows commands. What is the most likely cause of his altered mental status?

A. Abusive head trauma
B. Accidental ingestion of diphenhydramine
C. Enteroviral meningitis
D. Meningococcal meningitis
E. Status epilepticus

**8-20.** A 2-week-old infant presents with fever, lethargy, and seizure. She was in her usual state of health until yesterday when she developed irritability and poor feeding. Today, she has been lethargic and developed a fever. En route to the hospital, she developed a generalized tonic-clonic seizure that lasted for 2 minutes. On arrival to the emergency department, she is unarousable, febrile, tachycardic, and tachypneic. Examination reveals vesicles on the mucous membranes and a cluster of ulcerated lesions on the occipital scalp. Which of the following is true about this child's disease?

- **A.** Adequate intrapartum penicillin could have prevented this condition.
- **B.** Further febrile seizures can be prevented with acetaminophen.
- **C.** Maternal antiviral prophylaxis may have prevented this condition.
- **D.** The infection was likely transmitted from a sibling with hand, foot, and mouth disease.
- **E.** The viral infection is likely to resolve without treatment.

**8-21.** A 7-month-old male infant presents to the emergency department with lethargy. His father reports that he went to check on him overnight and noted that he was having trouble breathing and would not wake up. On examination, he is lethargic. Vital signs are significant for tachycardia with elevated blood pressure, and respiratory rate is 20 breaths/min with occasional pauses. He has multiple blanching purple macules on his legs, which the father believes are from crawling. Similar lesions are noted on the trunk. Which of the following tests is most likely to reveal the cause of the child's condition?

- **A.** Arterial blood gas
- **B.** Blood culture
- **C.** Coagulation studies and platelet count
- **D.** Computed tomography (CT) of the brain
- **E.** Radiography of the chest

**8-22.** An unvaccinated 13-month-old boy presents to the emergency department with fussiness and difficulty breathing. His father reports that he tripped and fell onto a wood floor while walking. He has just begun walking and is often clumsy. On examination, he is initially irritable and then becomes lethargic. He takes shallow respirations, but breath sounds are clear bilaterally. Computed tomography (CT) of the head reveals a subdural hematoma, and he is taken to the operating room for evacuation. He is also found to have multiple callused ribs. Which of the following is true of this child's condition?

- **A.** Coagulation factors are likely to be abnormal.
- **B.** Gram stain of the cerebrospinal fluid (CSF) is likely to reveal gram-positive cocci.
- **C.** It could have been prevented by routine vaccination.
- **D.** The injury was likely caused by rapid acceleration and deceleration.
- **E.** The patient likely has blue sclera.

**8-23.** An obtunded 11-year-old girl is brought to the emergency department. She has had unexplained weight loss over the past few months and now has had 2 days of abdominal pain and emesis. She has become progressively sleepy throughout the day. Chemistries are significant for a bicarbonate level of 12 mEq/L and blood glucose of 577 mmol/L. Computed tomography (CT) of the head reveals cerebral edema. Which additional tests are likely to be abnormal?

- **A.** Abdominal ultrasound
- **B.** β-Hydroxybutyrate
- **C.** Peripheral blood smear
- **D.** Stool culture
- **E.** Urine drug screen

**8-24.** A 14-year-old boy with a history of depression is brought to the emergency department (ED) by his mother with abdominal pain and multiple episodes of vomiting. The patient admits to having ingested approximately thirty 500-mg acetaminophen tablets in an attempt to end his life. His mother estimates the pills were taken in the last 6 to 8 hours, but she is uncertain of the exact time of the ingestion. The patient denies taking any other medications. Lab values show negative aspirin and ethanol levels, but serum acetaminophen level returns elevated at 165 μg/mL. Urine drugs of abuse screen is negative. Vital signs are within normal limits, and the patient is alert, although he is actively vomiting and complaining of abdominal pain. His weight is 45 kg. What is the next best step in treating this patient in the ED?

- **A.** Orogastric lavage
- **B.** Activated charcoal
- **C.** Repeat serum acetaminophen level in 4 hours to determine initiation of any therapy
- **D.** Intravenous (IV) *N*-acetylcysteine
- **E.** An antiemetic

**8-25.** A 2-year-old girl is brought to the emergency department (ED) for a possible accidental drug ingestion. The father found the patient playing with her grandmother's open pill bottle on the floor with pills scattered about the room. No pill fragments were found in the patient's mouth, and up to this point, the patient has been asymptomatic and acting appropriately. The ingestion occurred approximately 45 minutes ago. The father says the pill bottle contained medication for the grandmother's high blood pressure and depression.

The patient initially is asymptomatic with normal vital signs, but within a few hours of observation in the ED, her heart rate is noted to be 60 bpm at rest and her blood pressure is 75/40 mm Hg. Blood sugar checked on arrival was 95 mg/dL, and at recheck 4 hours later, it is 55 mg/dL. The father notes that the patient appears less active than before.

On exam, the patient is normothermic with other vitals noted as previously described. The patient is sleepy and fusses during the exam. Her pupils are normal in size and reactive. Cardiac exam is significant for bradycardia. Respiratory exam is normal with no bradypnea. Perfusion is normal. Neurologic exam demonstrates normal reflexes and tone, but the patient is drowsy. Electrocardiogram (ECG) shows sinus bradycardia with no other abnormalities. What class of medication is most likely responsible for this patient's altered mental status and hypoglycemia?

- **A.** Calcium channel blocker
- **B.** β-Blocker
- **C.** Tricyclic antidepressant
- **D.** Selective serotonin reuptake inhibitor (SSRI)
- **E.** α-Adrenergic blocker

**8-26.** A 17-year-old boy is brought to the emergency department (ED) with respiratory distress and vomiting. The patient lives in a rural area, and earlier in the day, he had been helping his father apply pesticides without any protective measures. On exam, he is bradycardic but normotensive. He is in some distress, coughing continuously. His pupils are constricted, and he has excessive tearing and salivation. Lung exam reveals wheezing bilaterally. He also complains of abdominal pain and has had multiple episodes of diarrhea and emesis since arrival to the ED. What is the mechanism of toxicity for insecticide poisoning as seen in this patient?

- **A.** Inhibition of the acetylcholinesterase enzyme causing increased cholinergic effects
- **B.** Increased release of norepinephrine causing increased sympathomimetic effects
- **C.** Blockade of the cholinergic receptors causing decreased cholinergic effects
- **D.** Increase in the release of acetylcholine causing increased cholinergic effects
- **E.** Decreased release of norepinephrine causing decreased sympathomimetic effects

**8-27.** A 3-year-old boy presents to the emergency department (ED) after swallowing an unknown amount of paint thinner stored in an old soda bottle in the garage. Parents report the patient vomited almost immediately after the ingestion, and he has been coughing and is complaining of throat pain. In the ED, he is noted to be in mild respiratory distress with a hoarse-sounding cough. He has an oxygen saturation of 91% on room air and mildly elevated respiratory rate and heart rate for age. Exam of his oropharynx reveals mild erythema but no ulcerations or swelling. Lung exam is significant for crackles bilaterally with occasional expiratory wheezing. The remainder of his exam is normal. Which of the following statements is correct regarding hydrocarbon ingestion and toxicity?

- **A.** Hydrocarbons are readily absorbed from the intestine, and risk of systemic toxicity is high.
- **B.** After hydrocarbon ingestion, patients can be observed in the ED for 2 hours and, if asymptomatic, may be safely discharged home.
- **C.** Activated charcoal is not indicated because it has minimal absorptive effect on hydrocarbon substances.
- **D.** Pneumatoceles are usually seen on chest radiograph within 48 to 72 hours after hydrocarbon aspiration.
- **E.** Early initiation of systemic corticosteroids has been shown to decrease pulmonary injury in hydrocarbon aspiration.

**8-28.** A 3-year-old boy is brought to the emergency department (ED) by ambulance after his parents found the boy with altered mental status and vomiting. His father had been working on his car in the garage the night before and left multiple bottles of various car maintenance fluids open. He found his son in the garage this morning with several bottles spilled on the floor around him, so he is unsure what the child may have ingested.

The patient is lethargic but does arouse to sternal rub. Pupils are equal and reactive to light. Oropharynx reveals no ulcerations or edema. Cardiac exam is significant for tachycardia to the 140s but no murmurs. His lungs are clear; however, he is tachypneic and has mild to moderate retractions. Extremities are warm with capillary refill of 2 to 3 seconds without cyanosis. The patient does not arouse to his parent's voice but does cry with the blood draw and intravenous (IV) line placement.

Chemistry reveals the following: bicarbonate 15 mEq/L, blood urea nitrogen (BUN) 20 mg/dL, creatinine 0.8 mg/dL, calcium 7.9 mg/dL, and anion gap of 22; the remaining values are normal. A venous blood gas analysis shows a pH of 7.25, $PCO_2$ of 30 mm Hg, normal lactate level, and serum osmolarity of 315 mOsm/L. Urinalysis shows calcium oxalate crystals. Acetaminophen and ethanol levels are undetectable. What is the best initial treatment to prevent further toxicity of this acute ingestion?

**A.** Alkalinization of the urine

**B.** Gastric lavage

**C.** Activated charcoal

**D.** Hemodialysis

**E.** Fomepizole

**8-29.** A 17-year-old girl is brought to the emergency department (ED) after ingesting approximately 50 to 75 full-strength aspirin tablets. She has vomited several times in the ambulance and is complaining of abdominal pain and ringing in her ears. Her serum salicylate level returns at 35 mg/dL. Her exam reveals a heart rate in the 130s and respiratory rate of 28 breaths/min. Perfusion is delayed at 3 to 4 seconds in her extremities. There is mild tenderness to palpation of the epigastric area, but no rebound or guarding. Mental status is normal. She has received two 1-L normal saline boluses, and her heart rate is now in the 100s with normal perfusion. What is the next best step in the management of this patient?

**A.** Give an additional 1-L normal saline bolus

**B.** Administer multidose activated charcoal

**C.** Perform urinary alkalinization with sodium bicarbonate containing intravenous (IV) fluids

**D.** Consult nephrology for initiation of hemodialysis

**E.** Monitor serial salicylate levels

**8-30.** A 12-year-old boy with a history of 4 previous admissions for diabetic ketoacidosis (DKA) is admitted to the pediatric intensive care unit for altered mental status related to another episode of DKA in the setting of a recent flu-like illness. His hemoglobin A1c on admission is 6.8, which is stable from his 4 previous endocrinology clinic visits over the past 12 months. The patient uses Lantus (insulin glargine) once daily at night and Humalog (insulin lispro) with meals, and his parents report he has been compliant with his insulin regimen. For this patient with known type 1 diabetes, which of the following is a risk factor for recurrent episodes of DKA?

**A.** Frequent clinic appointments

**B.** Male gender

**C.** Use of long-acting insulin

**D.** Previous episodes of DKA

**E.** Low hemoglobin A1c

**8-31.** An 8-year-old boy with no past medical history is admitted to the pediatric intensive care unit with altered mental status and fever. His mother reports he has lost 4 to 5 lb in the past few weeks, and he developed a headache, diarrhea, and malaise 3 days ago. Mother denies any fevers and states that everyone in the family has had nonbloody diarrhea in the past week.

On admission, the patient's vital signs are within normal limits except for elevated respiratory rate of 30 breaths/min. Serum glucose is 450 mg/dL with a hemoglobin A1c of 8.5. His blood work reveals the following: pH 7.15, serum bicarbonate of 10 mEq/L, β-hydroxybutyrate of 3.2 mg/dL, and sodium of 130 mEq/L. He received two 20-mL/kg fluid boluses at the outside hospital emergency department prior to transfer and became more disoriented and thus was transferred for a higher level of care. What is the most likely cause of this patient's altered mental status?

**A.** Bacterial meningitis

**B.** Cerebral edema

**C.** Hyponatremia

**D.** Hypovolemic shock

**E.** Sepsis

**8-32.** A 10-year-old girl presents with 3 weeks of weight loss, polyuria, and polydipsia and is found to have elevated glucose and ketone levels on her urinalysis at her pediatrician's office. She is referred to the emergency department (ED) for further evaluation and is found to have a serum glucose of 390 mg/dL and a pH of 7.25. Which of the following is true regarding diabetic ketoacidosis (DKA)?

**A.** Pancreatic α-cell failure results in a net deficit of insulin production, which is the cause of DKA.

**B.** Hyperglycemia results from increased glucose production by the liver and kidneys stimulated by counterregulatory hormones such as cortisol and glucagon.

**C.** Ketosis leads to an osmotic diuresis, which may lead to volume depletion, dehydration, and subsequent tissue hypoperfusion.

**D.** Metabolic acidosis occurs due to elevated plasma concentrations of the ketoacids acetoacetate and lactic acid.

**E.** Ketosis is caused by counterregulatory hormones, which cause the release of free fatty acids into circulation as well as fatty acid oxidation to ketones, which takes place in the kidneys.

**8-33.** A 7-year-old girl presents to the emergency department (ED) with a chief complaint of acute abdominal pain and vomiting that began earlier today. The patient's parents deny any diarrhea, fevers, or known sick contacts. They also mention that she has started wetting the bed when she was previously continent during the night.

The patient is afebrile with tachycardia to the 130s and tachypnea to the 30s with normal blood pressure. Chart review shows that the patient has lost almost 4 lb since her last well-child visit 1 month ago. Her exam is significant for dry mucous membranes and sunken eyes. Perfusion is delayed at 3 to 4 seconds; however, pulses are strong. Lungs are clear, but she is tachypneic and noted to be breathing quite deeply with moderate subcostal retractions. Abdominal exam shows mild tenderness to palpation, but no rebound or guarding and no organomegaly. Patient is drowsy but follows commands, and otherwise, the neurologic exam is normal. Which of the following tests will reveal the cause of this patient's acute abdominal pain and vomiting?

**A.** Chest radiograph

**B.** Stool culture

**C.** Serum glucose

**D.** Ultrasound of the appendix

**E.** Computed tomography (CT) scan of the head

**8-34.** A 10-month-old male infant born full term presents to urgent care for evaluation of fever and poor feeding. His mother reports some nasal congestion and cough for 3 days; he then developed a fever to 102°F last night. The patient has been refusing to eat overnight and has only had 1 wet diaper in the past 12 hours. The patient attends daycare and is up to date on his vaccinations.

The patient's exam is significant for fever to 101°F, heart rate of 175 bpm, respiratory rate of 46 breaths/min, blood pressure of 85/35 mm Hg, and oxygen saturation of 93% on room air. Pulses are bounding, and perfusion is flash. Lungs reveal diminished breath sounds with crackles to the left base. Heart exam is significant for tachycardia without murmurs, rubs, or gallops. During your time in the room, the patient, who was initially irritable and crying, has become more lethargic, crying weakly during the exam. What is the most important first step in treating this patient?

**A.** Administer broad-spectrum intravenous (IV) antibiotics

**B.** Administer IV isotonic fluid bolus

**C.** Obtain chest radiograph

**D.** Obtain venous blood gas

**E.** Perform endotracheal intubation

**8-35.** An 18-month-old girl is brought to the emergency department (ED) by her parents for vomiting and diarrhea for the past 4 days. Her older brother is in daycare and had similar symptoms 2 days prior to the patient becoming ill. Parents are concerned because she vomits every time she drinks and has not had a wet diaper in > 12 hours.

Patient's vital signs are as follows: temperature 100.4°F, heart rate 170s bpm, blood pressure 98/55 mm Hg, respiratory rate 26 breaths/min, and oxygen saturation of 99% on room air. On exam, the patient is alert but fussy. Mucous membranes are sticky, and there are only scant tears as she cries. Heart rate is 170 bpm with regular rhythm and no murmurs, rubs, or gallops. Abdominal exam reveals hyperactive bowel sounds and no tenderness to palpation or organomegaly. Her feet are cool to the touch with weak pulses, and capillary refill is delayed at 3 to 4 seconds. After two 20-mL/kg boluses of fluid, the patient's heart rate is 135 bpm, and perfusion is approximately 2 seconds. How would you categorize this patient's presentation?

**A.** Neurogenic shock

**B.** Cardiogenic cold shock

**C.** Obstructive cold shock

**D.** Sepsis warm shock

**E.** Hypovolemic cold shock

**8-36.** A 15-year-old boy is brought to the emergency department (ED) complaining of chest pain and difficulties breathing while playing a football game. He suffered a direct hit to the torso by another player's helmet during a tackle. His vital signs show a heart rate of 140 bpm, blood pressure of 90/50 mm Hg, respiratory rate of 30 breaths/min, and oxygen saturation of 93% on 3-L nasal cannula that was started in the ambulance due to hypoxia to 85% in the field. He complains of chest pain to his mid and left chest area. Chest exam reveals tachycardia with regular rhythm and strong heart sounds; however, heart sounds are shifted to the right hemithorax with absent breath sounds and decreased chest wall movement over the left hemithorax. Radial and femoral pulses are weak, and extremities are cool with delayed capillary refill. What is the best explanation of this patient's shock and next best step in management?

**A.** Cardiogenic shock due to arrhythmia. Obtain electrocardiogram (ECG).

**B.** Obstructive shock due to tension pneumothorax. Perform needle decompression.

**C.** Hypovolemic shock due to intra-abdominal hemorrhage. Rapidly administer packed red blood cells (PRBCs).

**D.** Hypovolemic shock due to dehydration. Push 1-L isotonic fluid bolus.

**E.** Obstructive shock due to cardiac tamponade. Consult cardiology for emergent echocardiogram.

**8-37.** A 4-year-old child with a history of persistent asthma is brought into urgent care due to acute onset of difficulty breathing at daycare. The mother states that the daycare worker reported that the breathing difficulties started shortly after the patient woke up from a nap and ate a snack.

Vitals are significant for blood pressure of 83/35 mm Hg, heart rate of 165 bpm, respiratory rate of 50 breaths/min, and oxygen saturation of 89% on room air, which improves only slightly to 92% on a non-rebreather. On exam, the patient is in severe distress with mild swelling around his eyes and lips. He is tachycardic with no murmurs. Lung exam shows diffuse wheezing bilaterally with occasional crackles and mild to moderate subcostal retractions. He appears pale and has a faint raised rash to his back and chest. Mother states that the patient has no known allergies and takes a daily combination long-acting β-agonist-steroid inhaler as well as albuterol as needed for his asthma, as prescribed by his pediatrician. Which of the following is true regarding this patient's shock?

**A.** Delay in administration of epinephrine is associated with increased risk of mortality.

**B.** A risk factor for poor outcomes with this type of shock is use of β-agonists.

**C.** The majority of serious cases of this type of shock are due to exposure to latex and insect stings.

**D.** Measurement of serum histamine is helpful in making the diagnosis.

**E.** Allergen skin testing should be performed as soon as possible to determine the cause of this patient's shock.

**8-38.** A 6-year-old girl with no past medical history presents to the emergency department (ED) with abdominal pain, vomiting, and fatigue. The patient has been sick for about 10 days and has seen her pediatrician several times and was diagnosed with influenza A about 7 days ago. Her fevers have resolved; however, the patient's mother is concerned because her daughter has not yet regained her energy level and only wants to lie on the couch all day. She has also been complaining of abdominal pain and has vomited approximately 5 times in the past 24 hours. Vomiting is nonbloody and nonbilious, and mother denies any diarrhea. No one else has been ill at home.

On exam, vital signs are as follows: temperature 98.5°F, heart rate 140 bpm, respiratory rate 40 breaths/min, blood pressure 90/50 mm Hg, and oxygen saturation 97% on room air. Patient appears tired. Mucous membranes are sticky. Heart exam reveals tachycardia with no murmurs, rubs, or gallops. Breathing is unlabored, but the patient is mildly tachypneic and there are faint wheezes to bilateral bases. The abdomen is mildly tender to palpation with normoactive bowel sounds, but there is no rebound or guarding. Liver edge is palpated 2 to 3 cm below the costal margin, and there is no splenomegaly. Extremities are cool with perfusion of 3 to 4 seconds and slightly diminished pulses. Neurologic exam is nonfocal.

The patient receives a total of 40 mL/kg of normal saline fluid boluses as part of her initial resuscitation; however, her heart rate remains elevated to the 140s, and she now has a diastolic murmur at the left sternal border. Oxygen saturations have now dropped to the high 80s, and her breathing is more labored. Which of the following tests would be most helpful in determining the underlying cause of this patient's presentation?

**A.** Serum lactate

**B.** B-type natriuretic peptide

**C.** Serum creatinine

**D.** Liver transaminases

**E.** Venous blood gas

**8-39.** A 12-year-old boy is brought to the emergency department (ED) by his parents with complaints of headache and mild wrist pain after falling off his bicycle yesterday. The patient reports he hit the right side of his head and body on the concrete. He was wearing a helmet and denies loss of consciousness or vomiting. He endorses right wrist pain as well as a persistent mild headache since the fall that is relieved by acetaminophen.

His exam is notable for mild swelling and bruising of the right wrist without deformity, and he has minimal scattered abrasions and bruising to his right cheek, but otherwise, his exam is unremarkable. Plain films of the wrist show mild soft tissue swelling but no fracture. The patient is anxious because school soccer team tryouts are tomorrow, and he is anxious he will have to miss the chance to play due to his injuries. Which of the following is the best anticipatory guidance for this family regarding this child's injuries and symptoms?

A. The patient should be placed on strict bed rest until his headaches have resolved.

B. Continued helmet use should be encouraged because helmets are designed to prevent traumatic brain injuries (TBIs) in children.

C. After a mild TBI, all physical activity should be avoided for a minimum of 2 weeks regardless of symptoms.

D. The patient is still symptomatic and therefore should not be allowed to participate in soccer tryouts tomorrow.

E. The patient should not return to academic classes at school until his headaches have fully resolved.

**8-40.** A 10-year-old girl is brought via emergency medical services (EMS) to the emergency department (ED) after being in a motor vehicle collision as a passenger. The vehicle was traveling at approximately 45 miles per hour, and the patient was wearing her seat belt. She was found unconscious at the scene still inside the vehicle with contusions and multiple abrasions to her head, face, and upper torso. During extraction from the vehicle by emergency responders, she regained consciousness briefly and was conversant with EMS; however, en route to the hospital, she had a rapid decline in mental status. On arrival to the ED, her Glasgow Coma Scale (GCS) score is 8, and pupils are dilated, unequal, and minimally reactive. She is hypertensive to the 160s/100s, with a heart rate of 55 bpm. What finding on computed tomography (CT) scan of the brain would best explain this patient's clinical picture?

A. Subarachnoid hemorrhage

B. Subdural hematoma

C. Epidural hematoma

D. Intraventricular hemorrhage

E. Ischemic brain infarct

**8-41.** An 18-month-old boy is brought to the emergency department (ED) by emergency medical services (EMS) due to seizure activity and apnea. His parents report he was found in the crib seizing and blue to the face. He was intubated in the field and has received 2 doses of lorazepam intravenous (IV) with cessation of seizure activity. The patient's vital signs reveal a heart rate of 60 bpm, blood pressure of 150/85 mm Hg, respiratory rate of 14 breaths/min, and oxygen saturation of 97% (patient being bagged through endotracheal tube).

Initial workup includes a chest radiograph that shows healing rib fractures and a noncontrast head computed tomography (CT) that shows a parietal skull fracture with multiple subdural hematomas. Which of these interventions is appropriate for the management of this patient's intracranial process?

A. Lumbar puncture

B. IV 3% saline bolus

C. Transfusion of packed red blood cells (PRBCs)

D. Positioning of the patient's head at the level of the heart

E. Antihypertensive medication to lower patient's blood pressure

**8-42.** A 15-month-old boy is brought to the emergency department (ED) by emergency medical services (EMS) after an older sibling tipped over his high chair. The parents are very worried because they said he hit his head "hard" on the concrete kitchen floors and had twitching movements to his entire body for a few seconds before immediately crying. They deny loss of consciousness, but he did vomit once in the ambulance ride to the hospital and 2 more times in the ED. He is fussy on exam and has a large hematoma to his forehead, but no step-offs or obvious skull deformities. Neurologic exam is within normal limits for age. The parents are anxious and are requesting head imaging. Which of the following is an indication for head imaging?

A. Parental concern

B. Vomiting

C. Hematoma to the scalp

D. Fussiness

E. Seizure-like movements

**8-43.** A 3-year-old girl is brought to the emergency department (ED) by her mother with the chief complaint of altered mental status and vomiting. Temperature is 100.6°F with normal heart rate, respiratory rate, and blood pressure. Her exam is significant for icteric sclera, moist mucous membranes with yellow tint to gingiva, jaundice to her face and torso, and hepatomegaly. The patient is drowsy but arousable, and neurologic exam shows hyperreflexia. The patient has been ill for the past week and was diagnosed with influenza A at her primary care physician's office earlier today, and the physician recommended that the patient be evaluated in the ED.

Labs are significant for ammonia of 50 μmol/L, international normalized ratio (INR) of 2.3, total bilirubin of 11 mg/dL, alanine aminotransferase (ALT) of 800 IU/L, aspartate aminotransferase (AST) of 780 IU/L, albumin of 2.5 g/dL, glucose of 85 mg/dL, and hemoglobin of 8.9. Administration of which of the following would most likely help to address the underlying cause of this patient's somnolence?

**A.** Intravenous (IV) antibiotics

**B.** IV dextrose bolus

**C.** Lactulose

**D.** Packed red blood cell (PRBC) transfusion

**E.** 5% albumin bolus

**8-44.** You are working in the intensive care unit (ICU) caring for a 2-year-old boy born at 30 weeks with a history of short gut syndrome and total parenteral nutrition (TPN) dependence who was admitted with fever and presumed septic shock with hypotension requiring multiple vasopressors over the past 24 hours. He has been receiving broad-spectrum antibiotics (vancomycin and cefepime) while awaiting blood cultures from his central line. You are called by the nurse due to concerns about decreased urine output. She reports he has voided 0.3 mL/kg/h in the past 12 hours.

You order labs, which show a blood urea nitrogen (BUN) of 18 mg/dL and creatinine of 0.7 mg/dL, an increase from recent outpatient clinic visit levels of BUN 10 mg/dL and creatinine 0.3 mg/dL. International normalized ratio (INR) has increased from 1.2 on admission to 1.9, with alanine aminotransferase (ALT) and aspartate aminotransferase (AST) rising from just slightly above normal on admission to > 300 IU/L in the past 24 hours. Which of the following is the most important risk factor for the acute kidney injury (AKI) seen in this patient hospitalized in the ICU?

**A.** History of prematurity

**B.** TPN dependence

**C.** Continued fevers

**D.** Use of vancomycin

**E.** Multiorgan failure

**8-45.** A 4-year-old girl is brought to the emergency department by her mother for 7 days of diarrhea that had bright red blood several days ago but that has now resolved. Diarrhea was associated with abdominal pain and occasional nonbloody, nonbilious emesis. Her daughter initially had a fever up to 101°F but has been afebrile for approximately 36 hours. The patient attends daycare, and the family recently traveled to Costa Rica on vacation 2 weeks ago. Mother states that no one else in the family has been ill with diarrhea, and the daycare manager states no other parents of children in the daycare have reported any diarrheal illnesses. The mother has become more concerned because the patient's urine volume has decreased in the past 24 hours, and the color, which was yellow yesterday, has now turned darker.

Labs are significant for white blood cell (WBC) count of 18, hemoglobin of 8.8, mean corpuscular volume (MCV) of 83 fL, and platelets of 90. Chemistry shows sodium of 133 mEq/L, potassium of 3.7 mEq/L, bicarbonate of 18 mEq/L, chloride of 98 mEq/L, blood urea nitrogen (BUN) of 30 mg/dL, and creatinine of 1.2 mg/dL. What other laboratory or radiologic finding would you expect to find if checked in this patient?

**A.** Positive Coombs test

**B.** Schistocytes and helmet cells on blood smear

**C.** Renal scarring on renal ultrasound

**D.** Urinalysis positive for blood but without red blood cells (RBCs) on microscopic exam

**E.** *Klebsiella* species growth on urine culture

**8-46.** A 2-year-old girl with a history of cardiomyopathy presents to the emergency department with increased work of breathing and fever. Parents report that her older brother had upper respiratory symptoms 2 days ago and they think that the patient caught his "cold." The patient is afebrile with a heart rate in the 170s, respiratory rate in the 50s, and oxygen saturation of 88% on room air. The patient has clear rhinorrhea, and lung auscultation reveals crackles with wheezing bilaterally and mild subcostal and intercostal retractions. Cardiac exam is significant for tachycardia with an S4 gallop. Liver edge is palpated 3 cm below the costal margin. Perfusion is 3 seconds distally. The patient is admitted to the cardiovascular intensive care unit (ICU) for further monitoring. Which of the following is best used as a surrogate marker for cardiac output and oxygen delivery in this patient with heart failure?

**A.** B-type natriuretic peptide (BNP)

**B.** Left atrium saturation

**C.** Serum lactate

**D.** Pulmonary venous saturation

**E.** Serum creatinine

**8-47.** An 18-month-old girl is brought to the hospital after being found face down in her family's pool. When she was pulled from the water, she had a pulse but no spontaneous respirations. Bystander cardiopulmonary resuscitation (CPR) was performed, and the patient underwent rapid sequence intubation upon arrival to the emergency department (ED). Which of the following best describes the mechanism of lung injury in the patient?

A. Pneumothorax

B. Pulmonary barotrauma

C. Chemical pneumonitis

D. Surfactant washout and dysfunction

E. Acute interstitial pneumonia

**8-48.** A 17-year-old boy is brought to the hospital after being found by friends face down in a pool during an unsupervised house party at his friend's house. Bystander cardiopulmonary resuscitation (CPR) was performed for 15 minutes before the patient was intubated in the field by emergency medical services (EMS). Upon arrival to the emergency department (ED), his temperature is 37.5°C, pulse is 95 bpm, blood pressure is 100/60 mm Hg, and oxygen saturation is 98% with no spontaneous respirations over the bagged ventilation. Glasgow Coma Scale (GCS) score is 5 and does not improve after administration of naloxone. Which of the following is the most likely cause of this patient's neurologic impairment?

A. Profound electrolyte disturbances

B. Hypoxic-ischemic brain injury

C. Drug overdose

D. Postictal state

E. Traumatic brain injury (TBI)

**8-49.** A 6-year-old child is brought to the emergency department (ED) after falling backward into a campfire and sustaining a deep partial-thickness burn involving 20% of body surface area. Which of the following is true regarding fluid resuscitation for this patient?

A. Hypotonic fluids should be used.

B. Adequate fluid hydration is achieved when urine output is at least 0.5 mL/kg/h.

C. Half of the calculated initial 24-hour fluid resuscitation should be given in the first 4 hours of resuscitation.

D. Underhydration can result in metabolic acidosis.

E. Body surface area is not used in the calculation of fluid resuscitation needs in the first 24 hours.

**8-50.** A 10-year-old boy is rescued from a house fire and brought to the emergency department (ED) for evaluation. He did not sustain any burns. His temperature is 37.5°C, pulse is 146 bpm, blood pressure is 97/65 mm Hg, respiratory rate is 28 breaths/min, and oxygen saturation is 91% on room air. On physical exam, the child appears anxious. Soot is noted in the nares and oropharynx, and there are blisters on the palate. The child has mild inspiratory stridor at rest. Heart is tachycardic but otherwise normal, and the child is warm and well perfused. Transmitted inspiratory upper airway sounds are heard in all lung fields without wheezes, rhonchi, or rales and no increased work of breathing. Capillary refill is 2 seconds. Skin is without evidence of partial-thickness burns. Which of the following is the best next step in management of the child?

A. Administer supplemental oxygen via nasal cannula to maintain oxygen saturation > 95%

B. Discharge child home after monitoring on room air for 4 hours

C. Administer bilevel positive airway pressure (BiPAP)

D. Perform immediate endotracheal intubation

E. Administer nebulized albuterol

**8-51.** An otherwise healthy 14-year-old boy presents 1 hour following a dog bite to his right forearm. The laceration is thoroughly cleaned, debrided, and irrigated, and it is decided to allow the wound to heal by secondary intention. The dog is owned by the patient's neighbors who provided paperwork showing the dog is up to date on rabies vaccination. The patient completed his childhood tetanus immunization series, but his last tetanus vaccine was 10 years ago. The patient does not have any known drug allergies. Which of the following best describes additional management that this patient should be offered?

A. Administer tetanus toxoid and prescribe clindamycin

B. Administer tetanus toxoid and prescribe amoxicillin/clavulanate

C. Administer tetanus immune globulin and prescribe clindamycin

D. Administer tetanus immune globulin and prescribe amoxicillin/clavulanate

E. Administer tetanus toxoid and tetanus immune globulin; antibiotics are not indicated unless signs of infection develop

**8-52.** A 17-year-old boy is brought to the emergency department (ED) after being struck by a vehicle while riding his bicycle. Primary survey is pertinent for patent airway, tachypnea with decreased breath sounds on the right with associated trachea shift toward the left, strong pulses with tachycardia and good distal perfusion, and Glasgow Coma Scale (GCS) score of 14. Based on the primary survey, which of the following conditions does this patient most likely have?

**A.** Hemothorax
**B.** Simple pneumothorax
**C.** Tension pneumothorax
**D.** Atelectasis
**E.** Rib fracture

**8-53.** An 8-year-old girl is brought to the emergency department (ED) after falling 12 feet from a staircase landing to a tiled floor in her family's home. Primary and secondary survey reveal stable airway, breathing, and circulation; Glasgow Coma Scale (GCS) score of 13; and a left radioulnar fracture. Which of the following statements is true in assessing this child for cervical spine injury?

**A.** The child is not old enough to provide a reliable response to questions during physical exam of the cervical spine.
**B.** Magnetic resonance imaging (MRI) of the spine is the preferred test to diagnose a cervical spine injury in this patient.
**C.** Pain with neck movement alone is not an indication of a cervical spine injury.
**D.** Physical examination cannot exclude a cervical spine injury in this child due to her left radioulnar fracture.
**E.** Her cervical spine cannot be assessed until she has received adequate analgesia.

**8-54.** A 4-year-old unvaccinated boy presents to the emergency department (ED) with rapid-onset high fever and respiratory distress. Vitals include temperature of 40°C, heart rate of 152 bpm, respiratory rate of 40 breaths/min, blood pressure of 94/60 mm Hg, and oxygen saturation of 96%. The child appears toxic, with significant drooling and respiratory distress, and is immediately intubated for impending respiratory failure. Which pathogen is most likely responsible for this child's condition?

**A.** *Staphylococcus aureus*
**B.** *Streptococcus pneumoniae*
**C.** *Haemophilus influenzae*, type b
**D.** *H influenzae*, nontypeable
**E.** Parainfluenza virus

**8-55.** A 6-month-old former term male infant presents with 3 days of cough and nasal congestion and now 6 hours of fast, labored breathing. His 2-year-old brother has been sick with a cold. Vitals include temperature of 38.4°C, heart rate of 165 bpm, respiratory rate of 44 breaths/min, blood pressure of 82/54 mm Hg, and oxygen saturation of 96%. On exam, the child appears sick with respiratory distress. He is active and fussy. There is copious nasal discharge and intermittent cough. He is tachypneic with nasal flaring and moderate subcostal retractions. He has rhonchi and transmitted upper airway sounds throughout his chest and intermittent wheezing with good aeration. His capillary refill is 2 seconds. Which of the following is the next best management step for this child?

**A.** Obtain chest radiograph
**B.** Obtain viral testing
**C.** Administer a short-acting β-agonist
**D.** Start supplemental oxygen via nasal cannula
**E.** Suction the nasopharynx

**8-56.** An 18-year-old man with cystic fibrosis (CF) is admitted to the hospital for a pulmonary exacerbation. This is his third pulmonary exacerbation this year, and he was also recently admitted for hemoptysis. Spirometry performed on this patient is likely to reveal which of the following patterns?

**A.** Increased forced expiratory volume in 1 second ($FEV_1$)
**B.** Decreased $FEV_1$
**C.** Restrictive lung disease pattern
**D.** Normal pattern for age
**E.** Increased $FEV_1$

**8-57.** A 4-month-old former term, previously healthy, male infant is currently admitted to the acute care floor for respiratory syncytial virus (RSV) bronchiolitis. He presented with 2 days of nasal congestion and cough, which progressed to rapid, labored breathing and required high-flow nasal cannula supplemental oxygen upon admission. He is now on his second day of admission on maximal support that can be administered via high-flow nasal cannula. When you examine the patient during rounds, you note the patient has head bobbing and marked intercostal retractions; moreover, he appears tired and does not respond vigorously to your exam. What is the best next step in the management of this child?

**A.** Obtain a stat chest radiograph
**B.** Administer ceftriaxone for superimposed bacterial pneumonia
**C.** Administer albuterol and steroids
**D.** Initiate bilevel positive airway pressure (BiPAP)
**E.** Give a hypertonic saline nebulization treatment

**8-58.** A 6-year-old boy with a history of wheezing presents to the emergency department (ED) with cough, wheezing, and labored breathing. He has not had any fevers. His temperature is 37.0°C, heart rate is 127 bpm, respiratory rate is 38 breaths/min, blood pressure is 100/65 mm Hg, and oxygen saturation is 96% on room air. His exam is pertinent for moderate respiratory distress with diffuse wheezing and prolonged expiratory phase on auscultation. During his ED course, he is given supplemental oxygen, albuterol nebulization, ipratropium bromide nebulization, dexamethasone, and magnesium. Which of these therapies causes decreased bronchomotor tone, mucosal edema, and secretions through anticholinergic effects?

**A.** Supplemental oxygen

**B.** Albuterol

**C.** Ipratropium bromide

**D.** Dexamethasone

**E.** Magnesium sulfate

**8-59.** An 8-year-old girl with cerebral palsy, static encephalopathy, and seizure disorder is admitted to the hospital following an aspiration event that occurred at home in the context of an intercurrent illness. Which of the following best describes the basic pathophysiology of lung injury that occurs with aspiration?

**A.** Infiltration of neutrophils with epithelial damage

**B.** Barotrauma resulting in alveolar damage

**C.** Chemical damage to the bronchioles resulting in increased lung compliance

**D.** Air trapping within alveoli due to aspirated material

**E.** Surfactant wash-out leading to decreased lung compliance

**8-60.** A previously healthy, developmentally normal 5-year-old boy presents with acute-onset fever, cough, respiratory distress, and hypoxia. He is admitted to the hospital and placed on supplemental oxygen and started on antibiotics for pneumonia. His family recently went camping in a wooded area along the Mississippi River. He fails to improve despite 4 days of empiric antibiotic therapy for community-acquired pneumonia. Which of the following is the most likely pathogen responsible for the patient's illness?

**A.** *Coccidioides* species

**B.** *Blastomyces* species

**C.** *Aspergillus fumigatus*

**D.** *Mucor* species

**E.** *Histoplasma capsulatum*

**8-61.** A 16-year-old girl with hemoglobin SS sickle cell disease (SCD) presents to the emergency department (ED) with fever, cough, chest pain, and rapid breathing. She denies any chest pain or other pain. She has no ill contacts and no known drug allergies. Her vitals demonstrate a temperature of 39.7°C, heart rate of 120 bpm, blood pressure of 124/68 mm Hg, respiratory rate of 32 breaths/min, and oxygen saturation of 90% on room air. Physical exam is pertinent for adolescent girl in respiratory distress with mild conjunctival pallor and moist mucous membranes. Auscultation reveals tachycardia with normal S1 and S2 and no murmurs or gallops. There is depressed air movement and loud rales and crackles with moderate intercostal retractions and nasal flaring. Spleen is not enlarged. There is no edema. Laboratory evaluation from clinic today demonstrated a hemoglobin of 10 g/dL. What is the best next step in management for this patient?

**A.** Obtain chest radiograph to evaluate for acute chest syndrome

**B.** Transfuse the patient with O-negative packed red blood cells (PRBCs)

**C.** Give a 40-mL/kg normal saline bolus

**D.** Start supplemental oxygen via non-rebreather and prepare bilevel positive airway pressure (BiPAP)

**E.** Administer ampicillin and azithromycin

**8-62.** A 3-month-old term female infant presents to the emergency department (ED) for cough. While there, she has 2 episodes of coughing followed by apnea that resolves with stimulation and administration of blow-by oxygen. She is admitted to the hospital and ultimately diagnosed with pertussis. The location of this infection is best described as which of the following?

**A.** Diffuse involvement of the lungs

**B.** Limited to the ciliated respiratory epithelium

**C.** Patchy airspace disease

**D.** Sloughing of tracheal wall pseudomembranous material

**E.** Upper airway disease

**8-63.** A 2-year-old, previously healthy, fully vaccinated boy presents to the emergency department (ED) with inspiratory stridor, respiratory distress, and a sharp, "barky" cough. Parents report he had rhinorrhea and low-grade fevers for 2 days preceding the onset of stridor. There is no history of foreign body aspiration. He is nontoxic appearing. An anteroposterior neck radiograph is most likely to show which of the following?

**A.** Narrowed subglottic air column

**B.** Widened soft tissue space

**C.** A rounded, thickened epiglottis

**D.** Thickening of the aryepiglottic folds

**E.** Severe tracheal deviation

**8-64.** A 17-year-old boy with known hypertension presents to the emergency department (ED) with severe headache, blurred vision, and nausea. Upon questioning, he reveals he recently stopped taking his antihypertensive medications. His vitals reveal a temperature of 37°C, heart rate of 100 bpm, blood pressure of 190/122 mm Hg, respiratory rate of 22 breaths/min, and oxygen saturation of 100% on room air. Repeat blood pressure is 196/117 mm Hg. Four-extremity blood pressures do not reveal a difference in the legs and the right upper extremity blood pressure. There is no abdominal bruit. He is initially alert and oriented and then becomes lethargic. Which of the following is the best next step in management of this patient?

A. Rest in a quiet room

B. Promptly lower the blood pressure by up to 25% with intravenous (IV) antihypertensives

C. Promptly lower the blood pressure by 50% with IV antihypertensives

D. Restart home oral antihypertensives and discharge home

E. Admit patient for observation

**8-65.** An 18-year-old previously healthy woman presents with markedly elevated blood pressures associated with headache, nausea, and blurred vision. On questioning, she admits to illicit drug use. Which of the following is most likely responsible for the patient's acute severe hypertension?

A. Marijuana

B. Cocaine

C. Phencyclidine (PCP)

D. Oxycodone

E. Acetaminophen with codeine

## ANSWERS

**Answer 8-1.** C

The child's presentation is consistent with a foreign body aspiration into the lower airway. The aspiration event took place while she was at unobserved play, raising suspicion for aspiration of a small toy or part of a toy. The coughing and choking episode had a rapid onset and resolved spontaneously, and focal wheezing is now present over the right lower lobe of the lung. It is likely that the foreign body has lodged into a right-sided bronchus. Notably, most foreign bodies are radiolucent on chest radiography, but chest radiography may reveal other typical radiographic findings such as hyperinflation distal to the site of the foreign body. The hyperinflation is due to air trapping distal to the partially obstructive foreign body. The hyperinflation is best visualized during expiration. The foreign body can be removed via bronchoscopy.

Epiglottitis causes the acute onset of fever, toxic appearance, respiratory distress, stridor, and drooling. Its symptoms progress rapidly and do not self-resolve. Tracheal foreign bodies cause stridor and hoarseness, rather than wheezing, which is a sign of a lower airway obstruction. Lobar pneumonia can result in focal wheezing, but it would not explain the child's rapid onset of coughing and choking. Status asthmaticus results in wheezing, but the wheezing is typically diffuse rather than focal.

(Chapter 118: Acute Upper Airway Obstruction)

**Answer 8-2.** E

The child presents with classic findings of aspiration of a foreign body into the lower airway. The aspiration event is marked by an episode of coughing and choking during unobserved play, raising concern for the aspiration of a small toy or food item. She then has spontaneous resolution of the distress. This resolution of distress is typical of foreign bodies moving from the upper airway into the lower airway. The child now has right-sided wheezing and hyperinflation, consistent with aspiration of the foreign body into a right-sided bronchus. Rigid bronchoscopy can be used to remove the foreign body from the airway.

Albuterol will not reverse a lower airway obstruction that is caused by a foreign body. Although community-acquired pneumonia may cause focal wheezing, its onset is not so rapid, and it more commonly causes a focal lung infiltrate than focal hyperinflation. Epiglottitis causes the rapid progression of respiratory distress, stridor, drooling, and fever, and it does not rapidly self-resolve. Parental reassurance is not indicated for a child with suspected foreign body aspiration, as the child may develop complications of the foreign body such as a distal pneumonia.

(Chapter 118: Acute Upper Airway Obstruction)

**Answer 8-3.** B

The child presents after a witnessed ingestion of a nickel, which now is present in his stomach. Most foreign bodies that have already passed from the esophagus to the stomach will continue through the gastrointestinal tract. They will be passed spontaneously, and the parent can monitor for the presence of the coin in the stool. Objects larger than 4 to 6 cm in length or 2.5 cm in diameter are less likely to pass through the pylorus and may require endoscopic removal.

Administration of activated charcoal is used to prevent absorption of ingested toxins, but it does not play a role in the treatment of most foreign body ingestions. Button batteries are of particular concern in children, as they may cause alkaline injury and perforation of the gastrointestinal tract. Button batteries are characterized by a double ring in anteroposterior radiographs, as well as a step-off in the lateral view. Button batteries require emergent endoscopic removal to prevent perforation of the esophagus, stomach, or intestine. Inducing emesis with syrup of ipecac is not indicated after foreign body ingestions.

(Chapter 390: Other Esophageal Disorders)

**Answer 8-4.** A

Certain types of ingested foreign bodies put the child at risk of bowel perforation and therefore require immediate removal. Button batteries require emergent removal regardless of their location or associated symptomatology. Button batteries may result in alkaline injury and perforation of the esophagus. Esophageal button batteries can be differentiated from coins by the presence of a double ring on anteroposterior radiographs and the presence of a step-off on lateral radiographs.

Ingested coins do not require immediate removal unless the patient is symptomatic. Coins may also require removal from the esophagus if they fail to progress to the stomach within 4 to 6 hours. Coins that have progressed to the stomach are likely to spontaneously pass into the intestine unless they are > 2.5 cm in diameter or 4 to 6 cm in length, which may prevent passage through the pylorus. Small objects in the intestine are also likely to pass spontaneously and do not require removal unless they are sharp or magnetized. A single magnet in the intestine is not an emergency, but multiple magnets may attract each other, resulting in necrosis and perforation of the intervening bowel.

(Chapter 390: Other Esophageal Disorders)

**Answer 8-5.** B

The infant has a generalized tonic-clonic seizure in the setting of bacterial meningitis and fever. Both meningitis and fever are well-recognized causes of seizures. Regardless of the cause, abatement of a prolonged seizure is important in preventing brain injury. Status epilepticus injures the brain through multiple mechanisms, including excitotoxicity, increased cerebral metabolic demand, decreased cerebral perfusion, and decreased cerebral oxygenation. The first-line treatment for status epilepticus is benzodiazepines such as lorazepam, diazepam, or midazolam. In addition, the airway and breathing should be carefully monitored, and supplemental oxygen should be administered.

Fosphenytoin can be administered if benzodiazepines do not result in resolution of seizure activity. The infant's fever may be contributing to the seizure, but awaiting fever control is not appropriate, as the child may develop brain injury in the interim. Expanding antibiotic coverage and obtaining brain imaging can be considered in the treatment and further evaluation of this child's meningitis, but abatement of the seizure takes priority.

(Chapter 553: Status Epilepticus)

**Answer 8-6.** B

The neonate presents with new-onset seizures, lethargy, and a cluster of vesicles over her occiput. Her recurrent seizures without a return to her mental status baseline are consistent with status epilepticus. Seizures abate with administration of a benzodiazepine, which is the first-line treatment for status epilepticus. Status epilepticus may be a manifestation of underlying epilepsy or may be secondary to an underlying condition, such as encephalitis, meningitis, accidental or purposeful ingestion, trauma, or a metabolic derangement. This neonate's age and cluster of occipital vesicles are highly concerning for herpes simplex virus encephalitis. The herpes simplex virus was likely acquired from the neonate's mother at birth, and the cluster of vesicles on the occiput likely reflects the location of a scalp electrode that was used for fetal monitoring during delivery. Maternal serologies for herpes simplex virus are likely to be positive. In addition, the neonate is likely to have herpes simplex isolated from both the occipital wound and CSF. Herpes may also be isolated from the blood.

Gram-positive cocci in the Gram stain of the CSF indicate bacterial meningitis. Although bacterial meningitis is an important consideration in a child with new seizures and lethargy, this child's vesicular rash is highly suggestive of herpes simplex virus encephalitis. Enterovirus may also cause rash, encephalitis, and fevers, but the cluster of vesicles on the occiput is more suggestive of herpes virus than enterovirus. A positive urine drug screen would indicate an intoxication as a cause of the status epilepticus, but an intoxication would not explain the neonate's occipital rash. A subdural hematoma is concerning for abusive head trauma, which is another cause of status epilepticus, but the neonate's vesicular rash makes herpes simplex virus a more likely etiology of the seizures.

(Chapter 553: Status Epilepticus, Chapter 304: Herpes Simplex Virus Infections)

**Answer 8-7.** C

The toddler presents with her first seizure, which occurred in the setting of fever and acute otitis media. Her presentation is consistent with a simple febrile seizure. Simple febrile seizures last < 15 minutes and occur only once in a 24-hour period. Seizure semiology is most often generalized tonic-clonic but may also be tonic or atonic. Conversely, febrile seizures are classified as complex if they last > 15 minutes, occur more than once in 24 hours, or demonstrate focality. Benzodiazepines can be used to treat febrile seizures that last > 5 minutes. Rectal diazepam can be administered by parents at home. Seizure precautions should also be discussed with the child's parents.

New-onset seizures merit consideration of infections of the central nervous system, such as bacterial meningitis and intracranial abscesses. However, this child's otherwise reassuring mental status and nonfocal seizures make febrile seizures more likely. This first-time seizure could be the initial presentation of epilepsy, but the child's fever makes a febrile seizure more likely. TBI may also cause prolonged seizures, but this child does not have a known history of trauma to support an injury. Trauma also would not explain her finding of acute otitis media on examination.

(Chapter 551: Febrile Seizures)

**Answer 8-8.** E

This child had a simple febrile seizure, which is defined by a duration < 15 minutes, a return to baseline within 10 minutes, and occurrence only once in a 24-hour period. Most simple febrile seizures last < 5 minutes. Febrile seizures occur in children aged 3 months to 6 years, but the majority of affected children have their first seizure before the age of 3 years.

Scheduled antipyretics such as acetaminophen and ibuprofen do not decrease the risk of recurrence of febrile seizures. Electroencephalogram, neuroimaging, and lumbar puncture are not routinely indicated in otherwise healthy children with simple febrile seizures if they have returned to their mental status baseline and do not demonstrate other concerning signs for meningitis. Febrile status epilepticus refers to a febrile seizure that lasts > 30 minutes continuously or intermittently without a return to baseline between seizure activity.

(Chapter 551: Febrile Seizures)

**Answer 8-9.** C

The child has a first-time generalized tonic-clonic seizure that abates with administration of rectal diazepam. He is slightly sleepy, but his vital signs and neurologic examination are reassuring. All children with first-time seizures should have an electroencephalogram. However, in a child who has returned to baseline, obtaining an electroencephalogram is not urgent and can be completed in the outpatient setting.

Emergent electroencephalograms are not indicated in a child who responded to benzodiazepines and is returning to baseline. Lumbar puncture is indicated in the setting of a seizure that is suspected to be due to meningitis or encephalitis, but this child's normal examination is not consistent with an intracranial infection. Emergent neuroimaging is not indicated in most children with new-onset seizures unless there is suspicion for an intracranial hemorrhage, such as in the case of known trauma or an unusual clinical course such as a lack of response to antiepileptics. Serum electrolyte, ammonia, and amino acid testing is not routinely indicated for a first-time seizure but may be considered if an underlying genetic etiology is suspected.

(Chapter 552: New-Onset Seizures)

**Answer 8-10.** A

The child presents with classical findings of anaphylaxis, including the acute onset of respiratory distress, lower airway obstruction, and angioedema. It is likely that she will also develop urticaria. Anaphylaxis results from a cross-linking of immunoglobulin E on the surface of mast cells and basophils upon exposure to an allergen. The child's presentation raises concern for exposure to an allergen such as shellfish at dinner. Once immunoglobulin E has been cross-linked on the cell surface, activated cells degranulate, resulting in the release of multiple mediators, including histamine and leukotrienes.

Hereditary angioedema may result in both cutaneous swelling and respiratory distress, but it is a rare disorder. Epiglottitis and foreign body aspirations may result in acute respiratory distress but would not explain the child's wheezing or swelling. Status asthmaticus would explain the child's respiratory distress and diffuse wheezing but not her swelling.

(Chapter 190: Anaphylaxis, Urticaria, and Angioedema)

**Answer 8-11.** D

The adolescent presents with signs of anaphylaxis, including facial swelling, respiratory distress, wheezing, and urticaria. Anaphylaxis results from exposure to an allergen. The allergen results in cross-linking of immunoglobulin E on the surface of mast cells. Mast cells subsequently degranulate, releasing their contents, which include histamine and leukotrienes. The first-line treatment for anaphylaxis is intramuscular or intravenous (IV) epinephrine. The adolescent's respiratory status should also be supported with supplemental oxygen, and IV access should be obtained for hemodynamic support should she develop signs of anaphylactic shock.

Excessive bradykinin is present in patients with hereditary angioedema, but this patient does not have a history to support this chronic and recurrent condition. Children with asthma demonstrate a hyperreactivity of the airways to allergens and irritants such as pollen. Although asthma may explain this child's wheezing and respiratory distress, it would not explain her urticaria or facial swelling. Ingestion of histamine in seafood describes scombroid poisoning. The primary symptoms of scombroid include flushing and diarrhea. Viral infection of the bronchioles describes bronchiolitis, which typically occurs in patients < 24 months of age. Lower respiratory tract disease is usually preceded by symptoms of upper respiratory tract infection.

(Chapter 190: Anaphylaxis, Urticaria, and Angioedema)

**Answer 8-12.** D

The adolescent has a history of food allergies and asthma and presents with signs concerning for anaphylaxis, including facial swelling, urticaria, and respiratory distress. She has appropriately received intramuscular epinephrine, the first-line treatment for anaphylaxis. Airway, breathing, and circulation should be the primary focus in patients who present with suspected anaphylaxis. In addition to epinephrine, patients with anaphylaxis require IV access, as they may develop fatal anaphylactic shock and require support of blood pressure. In addition, supplemental oxygen should be provided. Bronchodilators such as albuterol can be used for patients with persistent bronchospasm.

Glucocorticoids such as dexamethasone may be administered to prevent the second phase of the biphasic reaction of anaphylaxis, but IV access is a higher priority in the management of this adolescent. Similarly, antihistamines such as diphenhydramine can be used to treat urticaria and pruritus, but their administration does not supersede the need for IV access. Nebulized racemic epinephrine plays less of a role in the treatment of anaphylaxis than albuterol, which acts a bronchodilator in the lower airways. Rapid sequence intubation is required for some patients with anaphylaxis. However, this patient is currently awake and can receive supplemental oxygen during the evaluation of the respiratory status after administration of epinephrine.

(Chapter 190: Anaphylaxis, Urticaria, and Angioedema)

**Answer 8-13.** B

The child presents with signs and symptoms concerning for an anaphylactoid reaction to radiocontrast media. In contrast to a true anaphylactic reaction, the reaction to contrast media is thought to be due to direct induction of mast cell degranulation by the contrast media rather than a reaction that is mediated by immunoglobulin E. Despite these different pathophysiologic mechanisms, the first-line therapy for both anaphylaxis and an anaphylactoid reaction is epinephrine. Epinephrine can be administered intravenously or intramuscularly. In addition, the child needs support of his respiratory and cardiovascular status with supplemental oxygen and administration of IV fluids to maintain normotension. Albuterol can also be considered for persistent signs of lower airway obstruction.

Although diphenhydramine may help with pruritus and urticaria, it will not treat this child's respiratory distress. Cardiopulmonary resuscitation is not necessary in a child who is awake and alert. Administration of nebulized albuterol can be considered for children with persistent lower airway obstruction after the administration of epinephrine. However, albuterol will not prevent this child from progressing to anaphylactic shock. The very rapid onset of the child's symptoms after receiving contrast makes anaphylaxis more likely than sepsis as the etiology of the child's decompensation.

(Chapter 190: Anaphylaxis, Urticaria, and Angioedema)

**Answer 8-14.** D

The child presents with abdominal pain, emesis, and anorexia. His pain was initially centrally located, but his tenderness is now most prominent in the right lower quadrant. These findings are highly concerning for acute appendicitis. In addition, he has hypoactive bowel sounds, abdominal distension, guarding, and rebound tenderness. These findings are highly concerning for a perforated appendicitis. The child should receive empirical antimicrobials with coverage for enteric flora and consultation by a pediatric surgeon.

Gastroenteritis results in vomiting and diarrhea but would not explain the migration of this child's pain or surgical abdomen. Enteric obstructions such as intussusception or malrotation with volvulus can cause abdominal pain and emesis and can both progress to bowel necrosis and perforation. However, the migration of this child's pain is more consistent with appendicitis than intussusception or volvulus. Pyelonephritis can cause right-sided abdominal pain and emesis but is typically associated with dysuria, urinary frequency, and urinary urgency. Pain is typically elicited at the costovertebral angle rather than the right lower quadrant.

(Chapter 408: Acute Appendicitis, Chronic Appendicitis, and Typhlitis)

**Answer 8-15.** A

The child presents with classic finding of appendicitis, including migration of abdominal pain to the right lower quadrant, fever, and emesis. The child also demonstrates a positive Rovsing sign, which describes elicitation of pain in the right lower quadrant upon palpation of the left lower quadrant. Other signs of appendicitis include the obturator sign, which is pain with internal rotation of the right hip, and psoas sign, which is right lower quadrant pain in response to extension of the right hip. The latter is a sign of retrocecal appendicitis. The treatment of appendicitis is an appendectomy, which is typically performed laparoscopically.

The child's presentation does not include typical symptoms of a urinary tract infection such as dysuria, urinary frequency, and urinary urgency. A contrast enema can be used for a reduction of an intussusception, which is another cause of abdominal pain and emesis. However, the migration of the child's pain to the right lower quadrant is not consistent with intussusception. Decreased intake of fatty foods may decrease abdominal pain and diarrhea in the setting of pancreatitis, which is another cause of abdominal pain and emesis. The pain of pancreatitis is epigastric rather than located in the right lower quadrant. A Ladd procedure is used in the setting of malrotation with volvulus, which may also cause abdominal pain and emesis. However, the pain of volvulus does not migrate to the right lower quadrant.

(Chapter 408: Acute Appendicitis, Chronic Appendicitis, and Typhlitis)

**Answer 8-16.** A

The neonate presents with bilious emesis and fussiness. His presentation is highly concerning for a gastrointestinal obstruction. In particular, given his age and the bilious nature of his emesis, malrotation with volvulus is of foremost concern. The majority of individuals with malrotation present with volvulus during infancy and most often during the first month of life. An abdominal radiograph may demonstrate signs of obstruction, but the imaging modality of choice for volvulus is an upper gastrointestinal series. The upper gastrointestinal series may demonstrate duodenal obstruction, a misplaced duodenojejunal junction, and a paucity of air in the distal intestines. Air fluid levels and dilated loops of bowel may also be present. Notably, although ultrasound may demonstrate a classic whirlpool sign of twisted mesentery, it is not a highly sensitive or specific test for volvulus. Initial management of volvulus includes intravenous (IV) fluids, IV antibiotics, and placement of a nasogastric tube for decompression. Urgent surgical management is indicated due to the risk of intestinal necrosis.

Elevated serum lipase is associated with pancreatitis, which does not cause bilious emesis. An enlarged appendix on abdominal ultrasound raises concern for appendicitis, which causes abdominal pain, anorexia, fever, and emesis. The emesis associated with appendicitis is nonbilious. Hyperglycemia and elevated β-hydroxybutyrate describe diabetic ketoacidosis, which may cause emesis and abdominal pain. However, diabetes is very rare in this age group, and it would not cause bilious emesis. Hypertrophy of the pylorus results in gastric outlet obstruction and nonbilious emesis in young infants.

(Chapter 392: Malrotation and Volvulus)

**Answer 8-17.** D

Intussusception is a form of gastrointestinal obstruction that results from a telescoping of one portion of bowel into another. It is most common among children aged 6 months to 3 years. It is characterized by emesis and paroxysms of abdominal pain that are characterized by crying and flexion of the hips and knees. Between episodes, the infant may initially appear comfortable, but as the obstruction progresses, the child becomes more lethargic between episodes. The child may develop hematochezia or "currant jelly" stools that contain blood and mucus, but this is a late finding that indicates bowel wall ischemia. On examination, a mass may be palpable in the right lower quadrant over the ileocolic junction, which is the most common site of intussusception. Untreated, the intussusception leads to compression of venous and lymphatic drainage and resultant bowel wall edema. The bowel wall may become ischemic and may necrose. Abdominal radiography may demonstrate signs of obstruction and is also used to evaluate for pneumoperitoneum. Abdominal ultrasound may be used to evaluate for the classic "target sign" of intussusception. Most intussusceptions can be reduced with air or contrast enema.

The pain associated with appendicitis is typically constant and migrates to the right lower quadrant. Tenderness is most prominent in the right lower quadrant, and rebound tenderness or guarding may also be present. A BRUE refers to an event that lasts < 1 minute and includes cyanosis or pallor, abnormal breathing, change in tone, and altered responsiveness. This infant's recurrent episodes are likely explained by intussusception. Gastroenteritis causes both vomiting and diarrhea, rather than vomiting alone, and the associated abdominal pain is not typically so paroxysmal. Malrotation with volvulus causes abdominal pain and bilious emesis. Most cases occur within the first year of life.

(Chapter 384: Gastrointestinal Obstructions, Chapter 399: Intussusception)

**Answer 8-18.** C

The child presents with typical findings of intussusception, a form of gastrointestinal obstruction caused by a telescoping of the bowel into itself. The intussusception results in episodes of abdominal cramping and fussiness. The child may initially appear well between episodes but eventually becomes more lethargic as the bowel wall becomes ischemic. The child may also develop bloody stools. Later in the course of disease, the child may develop "currant jelly" stools, which are characterized by both blood and mucus. The most common location of intussusception is at the ileocolic junction, which may lead to a sausage-shaped mass that is palpable in the right lower quadrant. Abdominal radiography is used to evaluate for obstruction and possible pneumoperitoneum, as the bowel is at risk of perforation. Ultrasonography may reveal a classic "target sign" at the area of intussusception. The treatment of choice for reduction of an intussusception is an air contrast enema.

Prolonged bowel rest is not required for children with intussusception. Once the intussusception has been reduced, many children are able to quickly advance their diet back to normal. IV antibiotics are not needed for uncomplicated intussusception but would be indicated in the setting of perforation. Of note, some children with intussusception are initially evaluated for bacterial meningitis due to their fussiness that progresses to lethargy. If bacterial meningitis is suspected, empirical IV antibiotics are indicated. A Ladd procedure is used in the treatment of malrotation with volvulus, which causes bilious emesis and typically occurs during the first year of life.

(Chapter 384: Gastrointestinal Obstructions, Chapter 399: Intussusception)

**Answer 8-19.** D

The child's findings of fever, altered mental status, headache, and emesis are highly suggestive of meningitis. He lacks typical findings of neck stiffness, although neck stiffness is not a reliable sign of meningitis in children < 2 years of age. His purpuric rash leads to concern for meningococcal meningitis. Meningococcus is well recognized to cause a rash on the extremities that is initially macular and later evolves into purpura, petechiae, and ecchymoses. The involved tissue may become ischemic and necrose. The child requires a lumbar puncture to obtain cerebrospinal fluid (CSF), which should be sent for glucose, protein, cell counts, Gram stain, and culture. Blood cultures should also be obtained. The empirical treatment of choice for bacterial meningitis includes vancomycin and third-generation cephalosporin. Once meningococcus is confirmed on culture, monotherapy with ceftriaxone is appropriate.

Abusive head trauma may result in altered mentation and may be associated with other injuries such as ecchymoses. Purpura on the extremities, however, are not characteristic of abuse. Accidental ingestion of diphenhydramine produces the classic anticholinergic toxidrome "hot as a hare, blind as a bat, dry as a bone, red as a beet, mad as a hatter." This child's fever and altered mental status are consistent with the toxidrome, but he lacks other signs. In addition, the toxidrome does not explain his purpura. *Enterovirus* is a common cause of meningitis, but it does not classically cause purpura. Subclinical status epilepticus may cause altered mental status, but it is less likely than an intracranial infection in the setting of fever, headache, emesis, and purpura.

(Chapter 98: Acute Neurological Dysfunction, Chapter 226: Bacterial Infections of the Central Nervous System)

**Answer 8-20.** C

The neonate presents with fever, poor feeding, irritability that has progressed to lethargy, and a generalized tonic-clonic seizure. Her examination is notable for lethargy, tachypnea, tachycardia, ulcerated lesions on the occiput, and vesicles on the mucous membranes. Her presentation is highly concerning for herpes simplex virus (HSV) meningoencephalitis. The lesions on the occiput are particularly concerning for a fetal scalp electrode as a site of inoculation. The majority of cases of neonatal herpes simplex virus are transmitted during delivery. For mothers with known herpes virus infections, prophylaxis is often administered prior to delivery. Cesarean section is performed for mothers with active lesions at the time of delivery. However, some mothers may be unaware of their infection or may receive inadequate prophylaxis. This neonate requires urgent resuscitation in the setting of hemodynamic instability, respiratory distress, and seizure. Cerebrospinal fluid (CSF) should be obtained for routine studies and cultures, as well as HSV polymerase chain reaction (PCR). The cutaneous and mucous membrane lesions should also be swabbed and sent for culture. Surface specimens of the eyes, mouth, and anus should also be sent for viral culture. Acyclovir is the antiviral of choice.

Intrapartum penicillin is used to prevent early-onset group B streptococcal disease, but it does not prevent the transmission of HSV. This neonate's seizures are related to an intracranial infection. Febrile seizures are not a typical diagnosis in neonates and cannot be prevented with antipyretics. Hand, foot, and mouth disease is caused by coxsackievirus and can be transmitted between siblings. However, this neonate's vesicular rash and ulcerated occipital lesions are more likely a sign of HSV than coxsackievirus. HSV progresses and is often fatal without treatment.

(Chapter 304: Herpes Simplex Virus Infections)

**Answer 8-21.** D

By report, the infant was found lethargic and in respiratory distress and, at the hospital, is found to be lethargic, tachycardic, and hypertensive with irregular respirations. He is currently demonstrating the Cushing triad, which raises concern for elevated intracranial pressure. In addition, he has ecchymoses on his lower extremities and torso. Extremity bruising is rare in infants who are not yet ambulatory, and bruising on the neck, torso, and ears is highly concerning for abuse. This child should undergo stat CT of the brain given the concern for abusive head trauma. Abusive head trauma may occur through direct trauma to the head or through shaking, which results in rapid acceleration and deceleration and tearing of the bridging veins. The child may also develop associated retinal hemorrhages. In addition, infants and children with abusive head trauma may develop hypoxic-ischemic injury that is best detected on magnetic resonance imaging. Of note, the majority of infants and children who undergo abusive head trauma have no disclosed history of trauma at the time of presentation.

An arterial blood gas can be used to evaluate for respiratory failure but will not determine the etiology of the respiratory failure. Sepsis is an important consideration in an obtunded patient, and thus, a blood culture is a reasonable consideration. However, given the constellation of symptoms, abusive head trauma is more likely than sepsis. Coagulation studies and platelet studies may be used to evaluate for a bleeding diathesis. Although this child does have multiple ecchymoses, his presentation is more concerning for abuse than a bleeding diathesis. Radiography of the chest may be used as a part of the evaluation for pulmonary and cardiac pathology, but it is unlikely to be useful in this patient who is demonstrating the Cushing triad and cutaneous manifestations of abuse.

(Chapter 36: Child Maltreatment: Neglect to Abuse)

**Answer 8-22.** D

The child presents with multiple signs that are concerning for child abuse, including a subdural hematoma and multiple calluses of the ribs. The description of falling on a hard surface does not explain his multiple injuries. Subdural hematomas result from tearing of the bridging veins during acceleration and deceleration when a baby is being shaken. Hematomas may also result from direct trauma. In addition, the affected infant may develop hypoxic-ischemic injury secondary to the trauma. Other common injuries that raise concern for abuse include retinal hemorrhages, skull fractures, metaphyseal fractures, unexplained liver or splenic lacerations, abdominal hematomas, burns, and bruising in unusual areas such as the neck, trunk, or ears.

Coagulation abnormalities are much less likely to explain the subdural hematoma than child abuse. In addition, coagulation abnormalities would not explain the child's fractures. A positive Gram stain of the CSF fluid is consistent with bacterial meningitis. Although bacterial meningitis is an important consideration in a child with altered mental status, it would not explain his subdural bleeding or fractures. Vaccination would not have prevented this child's abuse, but routine vaccination should continue to be encouraged. Blue sclerae are associated with osteogenesis imperfecta, which predisposes children to both fractures and bleeding. However, this is a rare disease and is unlikely to explain this child's acute presentation.

(Chapter 36: Child Maltreatment: Neglect to Abuse)

**Answer 8-23.** B

The adolescent presents with classical findings of diabetic ketoacidosis, including recent weight loss, vomiting, abdominal pain, hyperglycemia, metabolic acidosis, and cerebral edema. Other common findings include polyuria, polydipsia, and decreased energy. Diabetic ketoacidosis results from decreased production of insulin from the pancreatic islet cells. Diabetic ketoacidosis is characterized by a serum pH < 7.3, an anion gap metabolic acidosis, production of ketones such as β-hydroxybutyrate, and hyperglycemia. Cerebral edema is an ominous sign because it is associated with significantly increased mortality. The treatment of diabetic ketoacidosis requires both dextrose-containing fluid and insulin. Insulin is initially administered intravenously. Patients with cerebral edema are also treated with mannitol, which has been shown to prevent brain damage and death.

Abdominal ultrasound has no utility in the diagnosis of diabetic ketoacidosis but can be considered in children whose altered mental status is concerning for an acute abdominal process such as appendicitis. A peripheral blood smear is not useful for patients with diabetic ketoacidosis. Although the child does have weight loss, malignancy would not explain her other findings. Stool culture is unlikely to be positive in this child with typical findings of diabetic ketoacidosis. Of note, diabetic ketoacidosis is frequently initially misdiagnosed as gastroenteritis. A urine drug screen is unlikely to be positive. Although ingestions may explain altered mental status, they would not explain this child's hyperglycemia.

(Chapter 537: Diabetes Mellitus)

**Answer 8-24.** D

This adolescent patient's acute ingestion of approximately 10 g of acetaminophen is well above the potentially hepatotoxic ingestion of 150 to 200 mg/kg in children or 7.5 g in adults. Acetaminophen is metabolized in the liver prior to urinary and bile excretion. It is first oxidized by the liver's cytochrome P450 system, generating *N*-acetyl-*p*-benzoquinoneimine (NAPQI), a molecule that acts as an oxidant and thus is highly cytotoxic. NAPQI is normally eliminated by conjugation to the reduced form of glutathione (GSH), which is then eliminated as mercapturic acid and cysteine conjugates. After an acetaminophen overdose, the amount of NAPQI generated can exceed the capacity of this detoxification mechanism, leading to toxic levels in the hepatocytes, and thus can cause severe liver injury.

The antidote for acute acetaminophen toxicity is the drug *N*-acetylcysteine (NAC), which counters NAPQI in several ways. NAC functions both as a glutathione precursor to replenish depleted glutathione stores as well as a glutathione substitute that directly binds to NAPQI. In addition, NAC facilitates the sulfation pathway of acetaminophen metabolism.

Initiation of antidote therapy with NAC for acute acetaminophen toxicity is guided by plotting the serum acetaminophen concentration on the Rumack-Matthew nomogram (see Figure 114-4) at ≥ 4 hours after a single acute

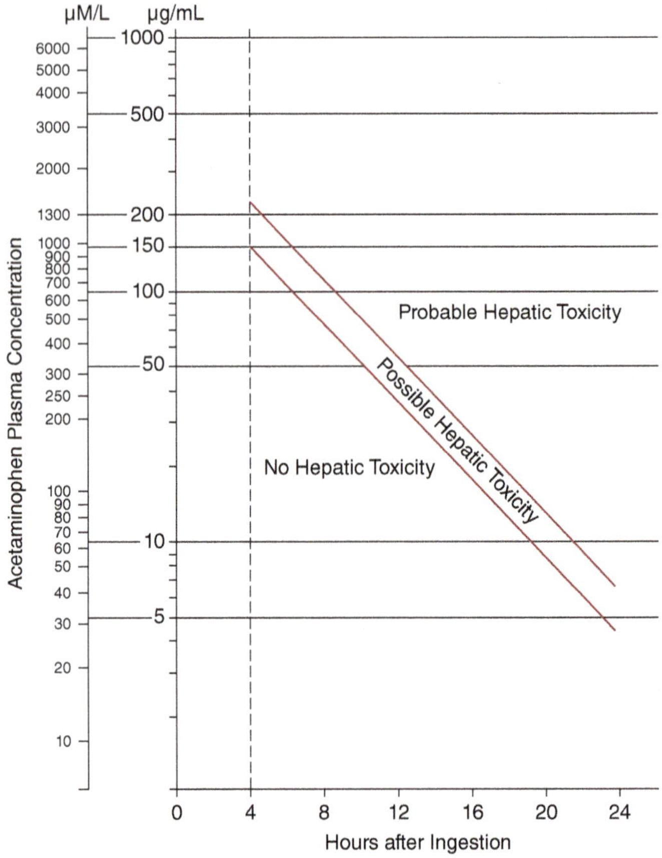


**FIGURE 114-4.** Rumack-Matthews nomogram of hepatotoxicity after acetaminophen ingestion. The Rumack-Matthews nomogram shows the risk of hepatotoxicity based on the relationship between plasma acetaminophen concentration and time after ingestion. The range between the red lines represents a 25% chance of clinically significant disease. (Mark W. Kline, *Rudolph's Pediatrics*, 23rd Edition. Copyright © McGraw-Hill Education. All rights reserved.)

ingestion. The nomogram is not useful in predicting toxicity after subacute overdose or multiple ingestions over a prolonged time period. NAC therapy is initiated if the acetaminophen level is above the lower line (possible hepatotoxicity) on the nomogram. In this case, the patient's serum acetaminophen level of 165 μg/mL is well above the possible hepatotoxicity line at 6 to 8 hours after ingestion. Ideally, NAC therapy should be started within 8 to 10 hours of acetaminophen ingestion because its ability to prevent fulminant hepatic failure decreases after this time frame. In this case, because the exact time of ingestion is unknown, it may be approaching the optimal therapeutic window; therefore, treatment with NAC should not be delayed.

Orogastric lavage is only recommended within 1 to 2 hours after a potentially lethal ingestion, and this patient has presented much later than this window. Additionally, the risk of aspiration during orogastric tube placement in this already vomiting patient outweighs the minimal benefits. Activated charcoal decreases absorption by binding most toxins; however, like orogastric lavage, it is not recommended in patients with active vomiting, as is seen in this case. Delaying initiation of NAC to check another acetaminophen level in this patient who already has a toxic level documented would only delay treatment and increase the chance of hepatic injury in this patient. Administration of an antiemetic for the patient's comfort would be reasonable but is not the next best step to address this possibly life-threatening drug toxicity.

(Chapter 114: Toxic Ingestions and Exposures, section titled "Pharmaceutical Agents")

**Answer 8-25.** B

Although all of the medication classes listed may cause altered mental status, this patient most likely ingested a β-blocker based on her other associated exam and lab findings including bradycardia, hypotension, and hypoglycemia. β-Blockers inhibit the binding of catecholamines to both cardiac and noncardiac β-adrenergic receptors. In the heart, $\beta_1$-adrenergic receptors blockade results in decreased chronotropy and inotropy, and the blockade of noncardiac $\beta_2$-adrenergic receptors antagonizes bronchial and smooth muscle relaxation and also causes hypoglycemia by inhibition of glycogenolysis and gluconeogenesis. The changes in mental status may be attributed to both hypoglycemia and cerebral hypoperfusion caused by the excess β-receptor antagonism and resultant hypotension.

Calcium channel blockers inhibit the influx of calcium through the L-type calcium channels of myocardial cells and, thus, similarly to β-blockers, result in decreased chronotropy and inotropy. However, whereas β-blocker poisoning may cause hypoglycemia, calcium channel blocker overdose typically results in hyperglycemia due to the inhibition of calcium-mediated insulin release from the islet cells of the pancreas. α-Adrenergic blockers such as clonidine mimic the opioid toxidrome including pinpoint pupils, central nervous system (CNS) depression, hypothermia, and respiratory depression, and can lead to eventual apnea and/or coma. Although this patient does have CNS depression, she does not have respiratory depression, and pupils are normal in size. The patient also does not demonstrate the hallmarks of SSRI toxicity, which in addition to altered mental status include hyperthermia, hyperreflexia, muscle rigidity, and diaphoresis. Tricyclic antidepressant toxicity is rapid in onset, usually within an hour, and can result in death in as little as 6 hours. The most common cause of death is cardiovascular toxicity through decreased contractility, widened QRS and QT intervals, and ventricular arrhythmias including torsades de pointes. Cholinergic receptor blockade results in sedation, coma, and myoclonus, as well as tachycardia, hyperthermia, and mydriasis, which does not fit the picture of the patient in this case.

(Chapter 114: Toxic Ingestions and Exposures, section titled "Pharmaceutical Agents")

**Answer 8-26.** A

Organophosphate and carbamate insecticides bind the acetylcholinesterase (AChE) enzyme, preventing the breakdown of acetylcholine in the synaptic cleft and resulting in increased cholinergic effect at the muscarinic, nicotinic, and central nervous system (CNS) receptors. Carbamate toxicity is generally shorter and less serious when compared to organophosphate poisoning because carbamates form reversible bonds to AChE, whereas organophosphates can permanently inhibit AChE, resulting in a more severe and prolonged toxicity. Patients with organophosphate and carbamate toxicity show signs and symptoms of cholinergic excess. Effects include bronchorrhea, bronchospasm (muscarinic receptors), muscle weakness, muscular incoordination, and fasciculations (nicotinic receptors). CNS cholinergic effects can include seizures and coma.

The patient's presentation is consistent with the presence of excess acetylcholine, not increased norepinephrine, which would result in increased sympathetic nervous system stimulation manifested as tachycardia, mydriasis, and bronchodilation.

(Chapter 114: Toxic Ingestions and Exposures, Environmental and Household Toxins)

**Answer 8-27.** C

Activated charcoal has minimal capacity for absorption of hydrocarbon substances and therefore is not recommended. Gastric lavage is also of limited use because most ingestions of hydrocarbons occur in the younger age group and, therefore, the volume of ingestion is small and potential aspiration during lavage outweighs any benefits. Furthermore, most hydrocarbons are poorly absorbed from the intestinal tract after ingestion, and therefore, systemic toxicity from ingestion is rare except in large volumes. The primary concern of hydrocarbon ingestion is pulmonary aspiration resulting in chemical pneumonitis. Patients with suspected hydrocarbon ingestion who are asymptomatic for ≥ 6 hours after ingestion are unlikely to have pulmonary aspiration and may be safely discharged home with detailed follow-up instructions. Symptomatic patients should be admitted to the hospital for further observation and management. Chest radiograph should be obtained for continued cough or tachypnea and will usually show pneumonitis. Pneumatoceles are a late finding of hydrocarbon ingestion, usually appearing on radiographs 1 to 2 weeks after the initial necrotizing pneumonitis, not in the immediate few days after ingestion. Empiric antibiotics are usually not recommended unless fever and leukocytosis develop later in the course, which would suggest superimposed bacterial infection. Corticosteroids have not been shown to prevent pneumonitis.

(Chapter 114: Toxic Ingestions and Exposures, section titled "Environmental and Household Toxins")

**Answer 8-28.** E

This patient's labs and exam are consistent with acute ethylene glycol toxicity, likely due to ingestion of antifreeze found in the garage. Early suspicion for this ingestion is imperative because even a small-volume ingestion of ethylene glycol is potentially lethal. Initial symptoms of toxicity include ataxia, altered level of consciousness, and vomiting as seen in this patient's case. Ethylene glycol initially causes an elevated osmolar gap, followed by the development of an elevated anion gap metabolic acidosis due to the toxic metabolite glycolic acid. Ethylene glycol is metabolized into this and other toxic metabolites by aldehyde dehydrogenases. Fomepizole acts to block alcohol dehydrogenases, thus slowing further toxicity, and is the initial treatment of choice for ethylene glycol poisoning. Because the turnaround time for ethylene glycol blood levels may be long, the decision to start treatment with fomepizole often must be based on clinical presentation along with labs demonstrating an elevated osmolar gap or an elevated anion gap metabolic acidosis.

Other clues to this patient's ingestion are his Kussmaul respirations, similar to what is seen in diabetic ketoacidosis, as his body works to compensate for the acute metabolic acidosis by blowing off carbon dioxide. Low serum calcium may also be seen due to another toxic metabolite, oxalic acid, which causes calcium to precipitate into calcium oxalate crystals in the kidneys.

Alkalinization of the urine is the treatment for salicylate toxicity and does not have a role in the initial management of ethylene glycol toxicity. Gastric lavage and activated charcoal would also not be indicated in this case. Hemodialysis does have a role in ethylene glycol toxicity if fomepizole is not readily available and may be considered for very high serum levels of ethylene glycol, severe metabolic acidosis, worsening renal failure, or severe neurologic disturbances.

(Chapter 114: Toxic Ingestions and Exposures, section titled "Environmental and Household Toxins")

**Answer 8-29. B**

The next best step in this patient's management would be administration of activated charcoal. Activated charcoal binds salicylate, preventing systemic absorption, and thus has an important role in the prevention of further toxicity. Typically, multiple-dose activated charcoal is recommended in salicylate poisoning because of the potential for delayed systemic absorption due to salicylate concretions that can form in the gastrointestinal tract or due to sustained-release salicylate preparations. Volume resuscitation is an important part of the initial management of salicylate toxicity because patients often present with severe volume depletion due to vomiting as well as increased insensible losses secondary to hyperventilation as a result of stimulation of the medullary respiratory center.

The patient in this case initially appears to be hypovolemic with tachycardia and delayed perfusion; however, she has already received 2 IV fluid boluses with improved heart rate and perfusion. Additional fluid boluses are unwarranted and excessive hydration should be avoided because it increases the risk of pulmonary and cerebral edema. Urinary alkalinization is indicated in patients who are symptomatic with serum salicylate levels > 40 mg/dL. Sodium bicarbonate functions to increase the serum pH, which favors movement of salicylate from the central nervous system (CNS) and other organs into the serum. Alkalinization of the urine also favors excretion and enhanced elimination of salicylate. The target for urinary pH is 7.5 to 8, with a serum pH of 7.4 to 7.5. In our patient's case, her serum salicylate level is < 40 mg/dL, and although certainly serial salicylate levels will need to be monitored to assure that levels are not increasing, gastrointestinal decontamination should not be delayed while awaiting these repeat levels. Hemodialysis does have a role in salicylate overdose by helping to directly eliminate salicylate from the blood as well as to correct fluid overload and electrolyte and acid-base disturbances; however, it is usually reserved for the most severe ingestions where serum salicylate levels exceed 100 mg/dL and therefore would not yet be indicated in this patient's case.

(Chapter 114: Toxic Ingestions and Exposures, section titled "Pharmaceutical Agents")

**Answer 8-30. D**

For patients with known type 1 diabetes, the risk of recurrent DKA includes previous episodes of DKA, as our patient's history reveals. Other risk factors for recurrent DKA include female gender (peripubertal or adolescent), poor glycemic control (higher hemoglobin A1c), psychiatric disorders, unstable social situations, limited access to medical services, and possible use of insulin pump, because only fast- or short-acting insulin is used; therefore, any interruption of insulin delivery via the pump results in insulin deficiency, which can then trigger DKA. Risk factors for DKA at diagnosis of type 1 diabetes are age < 5 years, ethnic minority status, lower socioeconomic status, and lack of health insurance.

(Chapter 537: Diabetes Mellitus)

**Answer 8-31. B**

This patient is likely presenting with diabetic ketoacidosis (DKA), as evidenced by his metabolic acidosis and elevated serum glucose and hemoglobin A1c. Cerebral edema accounts for 60% to 100% of mortality related to DKA. The exact mechanism of cerebral edema in DKA is unknown; however, several mechanisms have been suggested, and it is likely that different mechanisms affect different individuals. Vasogenic cerebral edema may occur because cerebral microvascular endothelium is directly affected by elevated ketones in the blood, thus causing alteration in permeability of the blood-brain barrier. It is also thought that serum levels of proinflammatory cytokines may be elevated in patients being treated for DKA. These cytokines may affect cerebral capillary function and contribute to cerebral edema. It has also been proposed that excessive intravenous (IV) fluids cause a decline in serum osmolality, leading to an influx of free water into brain cells; however, studies have not clearly defined the association between IV fluid volume, tonicity, and rate of infusion.

It is unlikely that the cause of the patient's fever is bacterial meningitis because this patient has been symptomatic for multiple days and bacterial meningitis is usually quite fulminant in presentation. Also, the history that multiple family members have had nonbloody diarrhea suggests a possible viral etiology. Serum sodium measurement in the setting of hyperglycemia is not accurate due to hyperglycemia-induced dilutional hyponatremia. Serum sodium may be calculated using the correction of adding 1.6 mEq of sodium for every 100 mg/dL of blood glucose above normal, so in our patient's case, serum sodium is likely around 135 mEq/L (assuming a normal blood glucose is 100 mg/dL). Although this patient is at risk for hypovolemic shock due to both his acute diarrheal illness as well as increased fluid losses due to hyperglycemia-driven polyuria, the patient's heart rate and blood pressure are normal, so he has likely been adequately resuscitated with the 2 fluid boluses he already received. Sepsis can cause cerebral hypoperfusion and should be considered as a cause of altered mental status; however, it is less likely the cause of altered mental status in this afebrile patient.

(Chapter 537: Diabetes Mellitus)

**Answer 8-32.** B

DKA is caused by a relative or absolute deficiency of insulin due to pancreatic β-cell failure. This deficiency of insulin prevents glucose from entering cells, causing a "starvation state," and thus stimulates the release of the counterregulatory hormones glucagon (by the pancreatic α cells), catecholamines, cortisol, and growth hormone. These hormones then stimulate hepatic and renal glucose production. They also act on insulin-dependent peripheral tissues (muscle, liver, adipose) to reduce glucose utilization. All of these counterregulatory hormone effects act to raise serum glucose.

Other effects of the counterregulatory hormones include the release of free fatty acids into the circulation through lipolysis as well as fatty acid oxidation to ketone bodies in the liver, not the kidneys. The metabolic acidosis seen in DKA is caused by elevated plasma concentrations of the ketoacids acetoacetate and β-hydroxybutyrate. Lactic acid may accumulate as a result of tissue hypoperfusion secondary to dehydration from a hyperglycemia-driven osmotic diuresis; ketosis does not contribute directly to relative volume-depleted state. Although lactic acid may contribute to the metabolic acidosis seen in DKA, it is not a ketoacid.

(Chapter 537: Diabetes Mellitus)

**Answer 8-33.** C

Vomiting in the absence of diarrhea should always raise a red flag and warrants further evaluation. The best test to obtain in this case would be a serum glucose to look for hyperglycemia because this patient is likely presenting with diabetic ketoacidosis (DKA). Clues to this diagnosis include the patient's recent unintentional weight loss and new-onset nocturnal enuresis caused by glucose spilling into the urine and subsequent hyperglycemic-osmotic diuresis. Her exam shows Kussmaul respirations (deep and rapid breathing) as her body works to compensate for the metabolic acidosis created by ketoacids in the blood.

Although acute viral or bacterial gastroenteritis can initially present with vomiting prior to onset of diarrhea, this patient's lack of fever, no exposure to sick contacts, and no diarrhea make gastroenteritis less likely, and regardless, stool culture would not be indicated after only 1 day of symptoms. Pneumonia can present with vomiting and referred pain to the abdomen, but again, lack of fever and this patient's clear lung exam should lead you to examine other diagnoses. Acute appendicitis would typically present with fever and with evidence of acute peritonitis on exam; however, this patient has no evidence of rebound or guarding, making this diagnosis also unlikely. Central nervous system (CNS) hemorrhage, mass, or other causes of increased intracranial pressure can be causes of vomiting alone; however, the patient has a normal neurologic exam, and other aspects of her history and exam should lead you to check a serum glucose rather than obtain a head CT as the best test to make the diagnosis.

(Chapter 537: Diabetes Mellitus)

**Answer 8-34.** B

This patient is presenting in septic shock, specifically warm shock as evidenced by his altered mental status, flash capillary refill, widened pulse pressure, and decreased urine output. Based on the unilateral crackles on exam, he likely has a bacterial pneumonia with possible bacteremia as a source of his infection. The American College of Critical Care-Pediatric Advanced Life Support (ACCM-PALS) guidelines recommend implementing 5 key elements during the first hour of managing pediatric septic shock: (1) recognition, (2) establishing IV access, (3) starting IV fluids and resuscitation as needed, (4) administering antibiotics, and (5) starting vasoactive agents as needed. In this case, after recognizing that the patient is in warm shock, IV access should be established and fluid boluses should be rapidly administered. Broad-spectrum antibiotics, chest radiograph, and obtaining a venous blood gas are all reasonable steps in this patient's care; however, these interventions are not the most important first step in this case. Endotracheal intubation may be needed if the patient's mental status continues to deteriorate; however, at this time, he is protecting his airway. Administration of supplemental oxygen via nasal cannula or facemask would be appropriate in the management of septic shock as well.

(Chapter 97: Pathophysiology of Sepsis)

**Answer 8-35.** E

Shock is the reduction in oxygen delivery to tissues. In cold shock, this reduction in oxygen delivery occurs as a result of intravascular hypovolemia and/or myocardial dysfunction. On exam, the patient will appear similar to the patient in the case, presenting with cool extremities due to blood vessel constriction as the body attempts to maintain blood pressure and oxygen delivery to vital organs. This patient's history of decreased intake and increased fluid losses through emesis and diarrhea as well as decreased urine output also alert you to her hypovolemic state as a cause of cold shock. If a patient in cold shock is not adequately resuscitated, the resultant hypoxia to peripheral tissues leads to organ dysfunction and metabolic acidosis. Pediatric cold shock responds well to volume resuscitation with intravenous (IV) fluid boluses, as seen in this case, and patients with myocardial dysfunction respond well to ionotropic support with peripheral epinephrine. Warm shock is less common in children than in adults, with only 20% of septic children presenting in warm shock. Warm shock presents with warm extremities, bounding pulses, and flash capillary refill due to excessive vasodilation. Neurogenic shock results in a warm shock picture with hypotension due to some neurologic injury.

Cardiogenic shock may result from decreased cardiac output resulting in decreased oxygen delivery to peripheral tissues and vital organs. Exam findings such as cardiac gallop, hepatomegaly, and crackles over the lung fields may be present initially but can also develop after aggressive fluid resuscitation as the heart ineffectively handles an increase in circulating volume. Examples of obstructive shock include cardiac tamponade and tension pneumothorax, both of which would be expected to have distinct exam findings not present in our patient.

(Chapter 97: Pathophysiology of Sepsis, Chapter 544: Trauma to the Nervous System)

**Answer 8-36. B**

Shock is the reduction in oxygen delivery to tissues. This patient is presenting with obstructive shock due to tension pneumothorax. Obstructive shock may occur when extracardiac diseases lead to impaired cardiac output and is usually secondary to tension pneumothorax and cardiac tamponade. Clues to tension pneumothorax include patient's history of trauma to the chest with hypotension and hypoxia. Exam findings consistent with tension pneumothorax include shift of the trachea away from the side of absent breath sounds in the setting of hemodynamic instability, and tension pneumothorax warrants emergent treatment by insertion of a needle into the pleural space through the second intercostal space at the midclavicular line. This allows relief of the tension and provides time to place a chest tube for continued evacuation of air.

Blunt trauma to the abdomen may cause intra-abdominal bleeding and present with findings suggestive of hypovolemic shock; however, this patient is complaining of chest pain, and his exam findings suggest pathology in the chest. Cardiac tamponade could present after severe trauma to the chest; however, exam findings would include muffled heart sounds and possible jugular venous distension. Cardiac arrhythmia has been reported after blunt chest trauma; however, this patient's exam is more concerning for tension pneumothorax and treatment should address this emergency first.

(Chapter 116: Trauma, Burns, and Bites)

**Answer 8-37. A**

Anaphylactic shock is a life-threatening process caused by the sudden release of histamine, leukotrienes, and other mast cell– and basophil-mediated substances. It is a type I hypersensitivity reaction driven by immunoglobulin E after exposure to an allergen. Anaphylaxis results in systemic symptoms involving the skin, respiratory, gastrointestinal, and cardiovascular systems. Severe anaphylaxis can lead to hypotension and ultimately shock with compensatory tachycardia, as seen in this patient. The most important initial treatment is intramuscular epinephrine within 30 minutes of onset of symptoms. Delay in administration of epinephrine is associated with increased mortality. The most common causes of anaphylaxis include food, medications, insect bites, latex, and blood products. Of these, foods and medications cause the majority of serious anaphylactic reactions requiring emergency department care. Serum histamine levels are usually not helpful in the diagnosis of anaphylaxis because histamine only stays elevated for 15 to 30 minutes after onset of symptoms. Serum tryptase, a protease specific to mast cells, may stay elevated for up to 6 hours after an anaphylactic reaction and therefore may be helpful in demonstrating mast cell activation; however, a normal serum tryptase does not exclude anaphylaxis as it may be normal, especially in food antigen-triggered anaphylaxis. Risk factors for poor outcomes in anaphylaxis including preexisting diagnosis of asthma, use of β-adrenergic or α-adrenergic antagonists (not β-agonists), and use of angiotensin-converting enzyme (ACE) inhibitors. These medications interfere with the body's compensatory mechanisms and can lead to severe and protracted anaphylaxis. After an episode of anaphylaxis, follow-up with an allergy-immunology specialist and skin testing or serum immunoglobulin E testing are reasonable; however, skin testing should be performed at least 6 weeks after an anaphylactic event to avoid false-negative results.

(Chapter 190: Anaphylaxis, Urticaria, and Angioedema)

**Answer 8-38. B**

This patient is presenting in shock likely due to poor cardiac output, or cardiogenic shock. The patient's preceding viral symptoms may clue the examiner to a diagnosis of viral myocarditis. Cardiogenic shock may be difficult to diagnose due to subtle and nonspecific complaints such as fatigue, abdominal pain, anorexia, vomiting, and respiratory complaints such as cough and wheezing. Cardiogenic shock is often misdiagnosed as hypovolemic shock as a cause for tachycardia, leading to continued fluid administration, which may then result in further decompensation, as is seen in this case. Other misdiagnoses include asthma or pneumonia as an explanation for the common findings of respiratory distress, wheezing, and crackles. Abdominal pain and hepatomegaly are often present due to hepatic congestion.

Evaluation of the patient with suspected cardiogenic shock should include basic labs including a chemistry, which may reveal an anion gap acidosis due to elevated serum lactate;

however, serum lactate may also be normal in cardiogenic shock. Furthermore, serum lactate is often elevated in other forms of shock including hypovolemic or septic shock; therefore, it does not point to a specific diagnosis. Poor kidney perfusion from decreased cardiac output may result in elevated serum creatinine level; however, serum creatinine usually lags behind any acute kidney injury, so again, it may not be helpful in the initial diagnosis of cardiogenic shock. Elevated B-type natriuretic peptide (BNP), indicative of cardiac distension, is a useful biomarker in the presence of cardiogenic shock. Although BNP cannot point the clinician to the specific cause of the underlying cardiac insult that led to cardiogenic shock, it can provide a surrogate for the progression of the clinical course.

(Chapter 107: Cardiogenic Shock)

**Answer 8-39.** D

Mild TBI, or concussion, is most often managed in the outpatient setting. Children with mild TBI should avoid further risk of head injury, including contact sports, until symptoms have resolved and until after evaluation and clearance by a medical professional to reduce the risk of second-impact syndrome (SIS). SIS results in diffuse cerebral edema after a second concussion in a child still symptomatic from a prior concussion. In this case, our patient should not be allowed to participate in soccer tryouts because he is still symptomatic as he is complaining of headaches. Although the patient and parents should be encouraged to continue safety helmet use while bike riding, helmets are designed to prevent skull fractures, not TBIs. Strict bed rest and severe limitation in all physical activities are not warranted, and more recent research actually shows a role for noncontact, subsymptomatic exercise in recovery from mild TBI. Similarly, the patient may return to academic classes as his symptoms allow, and it is not necessary for his headaches to be completely resolved if they are not interfering with his academic tasks.

(Chapter 544: Trauma to the Nervous System)

**Answer 8-40.** C

Primary brain injury occurs from several mechanisms, including direct injury to brain parenchyma from penetrating injuries, skull fractures, or hematomas as well as through the initial acceleration-deceleration and rotational forces that cause axonal shearing injury. Direct injury can occur at 2 sites: the site of direct impact (coup) and the brain opposite the site of injury (countercoup). Epidural hematomas (EDHs) usually result from shearing of the meningeal arteries, and these patients classically present with initial loss of consciousness, followed by a brief lucid period, and finally show acute signs of increased intracranial pressure (ICP) and deterioration in mental status. Signs of increased ICP are evident in this patient's exam and vital signs, including her dilated and minimally reactive pupils and elevated systemic blood pressure, the body's compensatory mechanism to maintain cerebral perfusion pressure (CPP = MAP [mean arterial pressure] – ICP). In children, EDHs may also occur due to disruption of venous sinuses between the skull and dura. These children usually have a more subtle presentation followed by rapid and potentially fatal deterioration. The remaining answer choices all could be seen on CT as a result of a severe traumatic brain injury (TBI); however, they are not as likely to explain the patient's initial loss of consciousness followed by a lucid period and subsequent rapid deterioration.

(Chapter 544: Trauma to the Nervous System)

**Answer 8-41.** B

This patient's vital signs are consistent with the Cushing triad (bradycardia, irregular and slow breathing, and hypertension), which is indicative of cerebral edema likely as a result of nonaccidental trauma. IV hypertonic saline 3% 5 to 10 mL/kg should be administered to help acutely with brain edema. The effects of hypertonic saline are fleeting as sodium equilibrates across the blood-brain barrier within a few hours and loses its effectiveness unless the elevated serum sodium level is continuously maintained. Caution should be used in inducing a hypernatremic state because hypernatremia is associated with renal failure and acute respiratory distress syndrome in children treated for intracranial hypertension. The use of hypertonic saline should be limited to the minimum amount required to maintain intracranial pressure (ICP) < 20 mm Hg rather than used to target a certain serum sodium level. Another option for acute cerebral edema is IV mannitol 0.25 to 1 g/kg; however, mannitol can induce an osmotic diuresis and increase the risk of hypotension and thus should be used cautiously.

Lumbar puncture is contraindicated in patients who show signs of increased ICP because it can lead to brain herniation. Transfusion of PRBCs may be indicated if the patient's hemoglobin is low to assure adequate oxygen-carrying capacity; however, this is not the first intervention for management of acute brain injury with increased ICP. The head of the patient should be maintained at 30 degrees of elevation, not level with the heart. The patient's hypertension is a compensatory mechanism to maintain cerebral perfusion pressure in the setting of increased ICP; therefore, the blood pressure should not be lowered acutely, or it may precipitate further hypoxic injury to the brain.

(Chapter 105: Management of Acute Brain Injury)

**Answer 8-42.** B

Indications for neuroimaging include persistent altered level of consciousness, new focal neurologic deficit, severe headache, vomiting, amnesia, exam findings concerning for skull fracture or penetrating skull injury, and seizures with atypical or concerning features. This patient has vomiting and thus should have imaging to identify any serious pathology.

Head computed tomography (CT) is the initial imaging modality of choice because it can be performed rapidly. CT is adequate for identification of intracranial lesions such as hemorrhage, mass lesions, and obstructive hydrocephalus, and it is also sensitive for the identification of skull and cervical spine fractures. Dose-reduction CT scanning protocols have become standard for children; however, there is still radiation exposure. CT scans obtained in the first 24 hours should be interpreted cautiously because certain pathology such as strokes, demyelination, or global ischemia may not be readily seen.

(Chapter 105: Management of Acute Brain Injury)

**Answer 8-43.** C

The clinical findings of acute liver failure (ALF) are a result of the impairment of the liver's synthetic, excretory, and detoxifying functions and include coagulopathy, jaundice, and hepatic encephalopathy. The Pediatric Acute Liver Failure (PALF) study group defines ALF as follows: (1) biochemical evidence of acute liver injury; (2) no evidence of chronic liver disease; and (3) hepatic-based uncorrectable coagulopathy with an INR ≥ 1.5 (approximate to a prothrombin time [PT] ≥ 15 seconds) with clinical hepatic encephalopathy or an INR ≥ 2.0 (approximate to PT ≥ 20 seconds) without encephalopathy due to a liver cause, not correctable by IV vitamin K. Although there is no specific blood test that correlates with the degree of hepatic encephalopathy, elevated serum ammonia levels should alert the physician to consider it in the differential of altered mental status such as in this patient's case.

This patient's encephalopathic picture is most likely due to her elevated ammonia level, perhaps precipitated by an acute viral illness with a fulminant viral hepatitis. Lactulose works to lower ammonia level by inducing bowel movements and by increasing the excretion of ammonium in the stools. Repeated doses of lactulose will be needed to reduce the serum ammonia; however, it is an effective therapy. Other treatments for hyperammonemia include branched-chain amino acids, IV L-ornithine, L-aspartate, probiotics, and rifaximin, although most treatments have limited proven efficacy.

Hypoglycemia should be always be considered in a patient with ALF and altered mental status because the liver is responsible for maintaining appropriate blood glucose levels during fasting through glycogenolysis. However, this patient's glucose is within normal range, so IV dextrose is unlikely to improve her mental status. Her hemoglobin, although low, would not be expected to cause this degree of mental status changes. Anemia in the setting of liver failure should prompt the physician to consider sources of bleeding such as esophageal varices secondary to increased portal hypertension usually seen in more long-standing liver disease. An isotonic fluid or 5% albumin bolus would be appropriate if the patient has evidence of volume depletion; however, she has normal heart rate and no evidence of dehydration on exam.

(Chapter 419: Acute Liver Failure, Chapter 420: End-Stage Liver Disease)

**Answer 8-44.** E

AKI is a spectrum of diminished kidney function ranging from subclinical renal injury to complete renal failure with total loss of kidney function. AKI may be defined in several ways, including an abrupt (usually within 48 hours) reduction in kidney function defined by absolute increase in serum creatinine of > 0.3 mg/dL or a relative increase of > 50% from baseline or oliguria of < 0.5 mL/kg for > 6 hours. The patient in this case meets several of these criteria for AKI. In adult literature, it has been noted that even small increases in serum creatinine (as little as 0.3 mg/dL) have been associated with increased mortality rates. Similar findings have been seen in the pediatric heart failure literature where patients with a ≥ 0.3 mg/dL rise in serum creatinine have a 7-fold increased risk of mortality.

Severity of illness and other organ involvement are the most important risk factors associated with development of AKI in critically ill children. In this patient's case, he has multiorgan involvement in the form of acute liver failure (ALF) as evidenced by an abnormal INR and rising liver transaminases. He likely had poor organ perfusion due to hypotension as a result of his sepsis. This patient previously had normal kidney function based on outpatient lab values, so his prematurity and TPN dependence do not appear to have affected his baseline kidney function. Use of nephrotoxic medications has been shown to be a risk factor for development of AKI in patients hospitalized in the ICU; however, in this case, the patient's initial kidney injury is unlikely to be due to vancomycin because he has only been receiving the medication for 24 hours. Nevertheless, vancomycin levels should be monitored closely, and this and other medications cleared by the kidneys should be renally dosed, and further nephrotoxic medications such as nonsteroidal anti-inflammatory drugs should be avoided if possible.

(Chapter 467: Acute Kidney Injury)

**Answer 8-45.** B

This patient has hemolytic-uremic syndrome (HUS), historically the most common glomerular disease to cause severe acute kidney injury (AKI) in a previously healthy young child. Most children with HUS (90%) have a preceding diarrheal illness caused by Shiga-like toxin producing *Escherichia coli* (usually *E coli* 0157:H7), otherwise known as Shiga toxin-producing *E coli*-associated (STEC+) HUS. The onset of HUS usually occurs 5 to 10 days after the onset of the diarrhea, as the gastrointestinal symptoms are beginning to resolve. The severity of the AKI is variable, but up to 60% of patients may develop oliguria or anuria and require dialysis. Hypertension is also variable but may be severe. The mean duration of AKI resulting from HUS is 2 weeks.

The pathophysiology of HUS is rooted in damage to the endothelium with formation of microthrombi, leading to the characteristic diagnostic triad of microangiopathic hemolytic anemia, thrombocytopenia, and AKI. Shiga-like toxin can bind to a receptor that is expressed on human glomerular endothelial and mesangial cells and on tubular epithelial cells. Once the toxin damages glomerular endothelial cells, a thrombotic microangiopathic reaction occurs, which is characterized by depositions of fibrin and damage to RBCs and platelets. Peripheral blood smear will show schistocytes and helmet cells. Coombs testing is negative in STEC+ HUS but can be positive in atypical forms of HUS. Renal ultrasound during the acute stages of AKI is not likely to show scarring, which would be present after a more subacute chronic injury to the kidneys. Urinalysis in HUS would show hematuria and proteinuria with RBCs seen on microscopic exam due to the renal glomerular damage. Urinalysis positive for blood but negative for red blood cells on microscopic exam is characteristic of myoglobinuria and may be seen in acute rhabdomyolysis. Other strains of Shiga toxin-producing *E coli* (0103:H2) have been associated with HUS after causing a urinary tract infection, but HUS is not typically seen in urinary tract infections caused by *Klebsiella* species.

(Chapter 468: Glomerular Diseases)

**Answer 8-46. C**

Mixed venous oxygen saturation can be indicative of cardiac output and systemic oxygen extraction and is useful in the management of patients with heart failure or low cardiac output syndrome. In patients without any intracardiac left-to-right shunt, the pulmonary artery oxygen saturation is the true "mixed" venous oxygen saturation and can be measured by a thermodilution catheter; however, the pulmonary artery is not practical to access in infants and children and cannot be used in children with structural anomalies that involve left-to-right shunting. The superior vena cava (SVC) saturation approximates the pulmonary artery saturation well enough that many routinely use the SVC saturation as a surrogate for the mixed venous saturation in pediatric patients. Saturations obtained from a catheter in the SVC or right atrium provide an indirect assessment of cardiac output and oxygen delivery and are useful to trend in patients with heart failure. Even more easily assessed and still useful as a surrogate marker of adequate oxygen delivery is serum lactate. Serum lactate rises as the body shifts to anaerobic metabolism, indicating inadequate oxygen delivery or impaired oxygen utilization. Multiple studies have shown the usefulness of serum lactate in predicting outcome in children as well as adults after cardiac surgery or trauma.

Serum BNP is secreted in response to ventricular strain. BNP and its N-terminal pro-hormone NT-proBNP are useful markers to trend in adults and children with heart failure as a way to measure response to therapy; however, serum BNP is not a true surrogate for oxygen delivery to tissues. Serum creatinine certainly will rise over time with inadequate kidney perfusion as a result of heart failure; however, early in the course of acute kidney injury (AKI), for whatever underlying reason, changes in creatinine do not provide an accurate reflection of perfusion and therefore would not be the best marker of true oxygen delivery.

(Chapter 491: Heart Failure, Chapter 467: Acute Kidney Injury)

**Answer 8-47. D**

When a child aspirates water during drowning, water enters the alveoli. Aspiration of either salt or fresh water leads to surfactant dysfunction and washout, disrupting the alveolar-capillary membrane, with ensuing noncardiogenic pulmonary edema and acute respiratory distress syndrome. The acute lung injury can progress over the initial 24-hour period. Other common respiratory complications of nonfatal drowning include aspiration pneumonia, due to aspiration of regurgitated stomach contents, pathogens present in water, or polluted water. Secondary nosocomial pneumonias can also occur.

(Chapter 115: Submersion Injuries)

**Answer 8-48. B**

The patient described underwent a prolonged hypoxia, resulting in hypoperfusion of organs, including the brain. Following respiratory failure, neurologic failure is the next most common cause of organ failure among drowning victims. Profound hypoxia causes a hypoxic-ischemic brain injury or sometimes even brain death. Posthypoxic encephalopathy is the most common cause of death in patients who are hospitalized due to drowning. Brain injury is the most common long-term sequela of drowning. Other predisposing causes of neurologic disease include drug overdose, a seizure that caused loss of consciousness prior to drowning, and trauma to the head or spinal cord injury from striking head or neck on pool or rock but are less likely in this patient. It is reasonable to administer a dose of naloxone if opioid intoxication is suspected; however, there was no improvement in this patient. Among children and adolescents, the 1- to 4-year-old age group has the highest risk of drowning, followed by the adolescent age group, which is usually related to high risk-taking behaviors.

(Chapter 115: Submersion Injuries)

**Answer 8-49. D**

Fluid resuscitation during the first 24 hours after a burn is paramount, and metabolic acidosis can occur as a result of inadequate perfusion and can usually be treated by increasing fluid volume. The volume of fluid to be given during the initial 24 hours is calculated based on body weight and percent body surface area burned. Crystalloid, crystalloid and colloid, or hypertonic saline fluids are preferred. In general, half of the calculated initial 24-hour fluid requirements should be given over the first 8 hours, and the second half should be given between hours 9 and 24. Urine output of at least 1 mL/kg/h in young children and at least 30 to 50 mL/h in older adolescents is an indicator of adequate fluid resuscitation; a Foley catheter should be placed to monitor urinary output. Note that patients with partial-thickness burns over > 10% body surface area should be treated at a burn center.

(Chapter 116: Trauma, Burns, and Bites)

**Answer 8-50.** D

The child in the vignette has suffered a smoke inhalation injury and is at risk for airway compromise and poor gas exchange. Physical exam clues of airway injury include carbonaceous material (soot) in the nasopharynx and oropharynx, blistering in the pharynx, stridor at rest, and decreased oxygen saturation levels. Because airway edema can be progressive in the first 36 hours after smoke inhalation injury, early intubation is recommended in children who have signs of impending airway compromise. Children in house fires are at risk for smoke inhalation injury even if they do not sustain any burns.

(Chapter 116: Trauma, Burns, and Bites)

**Answer 8-51.** B

Eighty to 90% of pediatric bites are inflicted by dogs. The upper extremities are the most common site injured by dog bites in older children, whereas the head and neck are more common sites in children < 4 years of age. Dog bites should be cleaned, debrided, and irrigated and can be managed with primary, delayed, or secondary closure, depending on the time elapsed since bite, degree of wound contamination, amount of tissue loss, and cosmetic considerations. Prophylactic antibiotics are recommended in most cases, with amoxicillin/clavulanate being the drug of choice to cover the most common pathogens. In penicillin-allergic children, clindamycin plus trimethoprim/sulfamethoxazole is an alternative prophylactic antibiotic regimen. Postexposure prophylaxis for rabies and tetanus should be considered. In this case, rabies immunization is not necessary because there is documentation of up-to-date rabies immunization in the offending dog. For patients whose most recent tetanus immunization was > 5 years ago or who have an unknown immunization history, active immunization with tetanus toxoid is indicated. If a patient never received the primary 3-dose immunization, passive immunization with tetanus immune globulin should also be given.

(Chapter 116: Trauma, Burns, and Bites)

**Answer 8-52.** C

The child described in the vignette most likely has a tension pneumothorax, as evidenced by decreased breath sounds with contralateral trachea shift in the setting of hemodynamic instability. It is important to recognize and emergently treat tension pneumothoraces because these patients may not be stable enough for a chest radiograph. Emergent treatment of a tension pneumothorax involves inserting a needle at the second intercostal space at the midclavicular line into the pleural space, allowing evacuation of accumulated gas; this emergent air evacuation is followed by chest tube placement. Hemothorax and simple pneumothorax would not be expected to cause a trachea shift. Children with contiguous rib fractures may have paradoxical inward movement of the involved portion of the chest while they inspire ("flail chest").

(Chapter 116: Trauma, Burns, and Bites)

**Answer 8-53.** D

Every trauma patient should be presumed to have a cervical spine injury until proven otherwise, and immobilization of the cervical spine should be continued until a cervical spine injury has been excluded. In many cases, a physical exam can exclude injury if there is no pain with full-range neck mobilization. Pain with movement of the neck, cervical vertebral body tenderness to palpation, obvious deformity, and neurologic abnormalities arising from the neck are signs of possible cervical spine injury. A cervical spine injury cannot be excluded by physical exam when a patient is uncooperative or unresponsive, is too young to give reliable responses to questions, or has a distracting injury. The patient described in the vignette has a distracting painful injury, so the physical exam cannot reliably rule out a spinal cord injury.

(Chapter 116: Trauma, Burns, and Bites)

**Answer 8-54.** C

The child in the vignette presents with a constellation of findings consistent with acute upper airway obstruction secondary to swelling of the epiglottis and supraglottic tissue, known as epiglottitis. *H influenzae*, type b (Hib) is the most common cause of epiglottitis, which is now a rare disease due to widespread immunization against Hib. In the prevaccine era, invasive Hib disease (including epiglottitis and meningitis) was common and affected about 1 in 200 children aged 0 to 5 years. Although the other pathogens listed can cause epiglottitis, they are far less common than Hib, especially in an unvaccinated child such as the one in the vignette. Nontypeable *H influenzae* more typically causes noninvasive disease such as acute otitis media and conjunctivitis. Parainfluenza virus is a common cause of croup, which typically presents with fever, barky cough, and stridor following a viral prodrome.

(Chapter 258: Haemophilus influenzae)

**Answer 8-55.** E

The vignette describes an infant with classic presentation of viral bronchiolitis, which involves peribronchial inflammation and airway plugging with mucus. Bronchiolitis is the most common lower respiratory tract infection in children < 2 years old. Respiratory syncytial virus (RSV) is the most common pathogen responsible for lower respiratory tract infections in this age group. The child described in the vignette demonstrates evidence of lower respiratory tract infection, and the diagnosis of bronchiolitis can be made clinically without any viral testing or imaging. The infant described is exhibiting respiratory distress, as evidenced by tachypnea, nasal flaring, and retractions, but would not warrant immediate intubation at present. The primary treatment for viral bronchiolitis is supportive, including suctioning. Supplemental oxygen is not indicated in this patient who is not hypoxic and may respond to suctioning alone. Although the infant does have wheezing on exam, short-acting β-agonists have not been shown to be helpful in the treatment of viral bronchiolitis.

(Chapter 96: Acute Respiratory Dysfunction, Chapter 236: Viral Respiratory Infections Including Influenza)

**Answer 8-56.** B

Typically, patients with CF demonstrate an obstructive airway pattern. Their spirometry will demonstrate a decreased $FEV_1$. The $FEV_1$ measure is a marker of lung function and also predicts survival. The adolescent patient described in the vignette with a history of multiple exacerbations and hemoptysis likely has a decreased $FEV_1$.

(Chapter 507: Cystic Fibrosis)

**Answer 8-57.** D

The infant described in the vignette has impending respiratory failure in context of RSV bronchiolitis and is currently on day 3 to 4 of his admission, which corresponds with the expected peak of illness for RSV bronchiolitis. The patient has maxed out support on high-flow nasal cannula, and the next step should be initiation of noninvasive positive-pressure ventilation with BiPAP. BiPAP provides continuous positive airway pressure throughout the respiratory cycle and also gives pressure or volume support during inspiration.

(Chapter 104: Respiratory Support)

**Answer 8-58.** C

Ipratropium bromide is an inhaled anticholinergic that is often used in conjunction with a short-acting β-agonist for treatment of an acute asthma exacerbation. Ipratropium bromide blocks cholinergic receptors, causing decreased bronchomotor tone, mucosal edema, and secretions. When used together with a short-acting β-agonist, it can improve lung function and decrease hospitalization rates. Albuterol is a short-acting $\beta_2$-agonist that works by relaxing smooth muscles in the airway, causing bronchodilation. Dexamethasone is a systemic corticosteroid that has broad anti-inflammatory properties, including decreasing inflammation in the airways. Magnesium sulfate is an adjunct therapy that is used in patients with severe asthma exacerbations that causes smooth muscle relaxation.

(Chapter 505: Childhood Asthma)

**Answer 8-59.** A

Pulmonary aspiration occurs when foreign bodies or fluid (including gastric contents and saliva) enters the lungs during inspiration. Certain clinical states and conditions are risk factors for aspiration, including cerebral palsy and developmental delay. Although a single small-volume aspiration event can be cleared without sequelae, large-volume aspiration and/or recurrent small-volume aspiration trigger an inflammatory response dominated by neutrophilic infiltration. Regardless of the acidity of the aspirate material, neutrophilic infiltration ensues. Migration, activation, and sequestration of neutrophils cause epithelial damage, increased permeability, decreased compliance, and eventual scarring.

(Chapter 504: Aspiration Syndromes)

**Answer 8-60.** B

The boy's failure to improve with appropriate antibiotic coverage for community-acquired pneumonia should prompt further evaluation, including possibility of a fungal respiratory infection. Endemic mycoses, including *H capsulatum*, *Blastomyces* species, *Coccidioides* species, and *Paracoccidioides* species, can cause respiratory infection in immunocompetent hosts after inhalation of infectious conidia from fungi in the soil. Of the endemic mycoses listed, pulmonary blastomycosis commonly has an acute presentation following exposure to the fungi in wooded areas near bodies of water in the Ohio and Mississippi River Valley areas. In contrast, pulmonary histoplasmosis and pulmonary coccidioidomycosis usually present subacutely over the course of weeks. *Aspergillus* and *Mucor* species are unlikely causes because they predominantly cause disease in immunocompromised individuals.

(Chapter 237: Fungal Respiratory Infections)

**Answer 8-61.** D

Acute chest syndrome (ACS) is a serious complication of SCD and a top cause of mortality among children and young adults with SCD. It is defined by a combination of clinical signs and symptoms (fever, cough, chest pain, tachypnea, hypoxia) plus a pulmonary infiltrate on chest radiograph. The patient's presentation described in the vignette is consistent with ACS; however, a chest radiograph should not be obtained until the patient has stable airway, breathing, and circulation. The best next step in the management of this child is to start supplemental oxygen as a higher level of support such as BiPAP is set up, because the patient demonstrates severe respiratory distress characterized by tachypnea, hypoxia, accessory muscle use, and decreased aeration with adventitious sounds. In patients with ACS, maintaining adequate hydration status is important, but one should avoid overhydration. Anti-infectious agents that cover pneumococcus, *Mycoplasma*, and *Chlamydia* should be started promptly (often a third-generation cephalosporin plus a macrolide), as well as coverage for influenza if suspected.

(Chapter 430: Hemoglobinopathies)

**Answer 8-62.** C

*Bordetella pertussis* is gram-negative coccobacillus that causes pertussis, or whooping cough. It involves a toxin-mediated infection of the ciliated epithelium of the respiratory tract.

The bacterial toxin allows bacteria to attach to the respiratory epithelium, causing inflammation and toxin-mediated paralysis of cilia, which hinders pulmonary clearance. The bacteria are spread through aerosolized droplets, with an incubation period typically in the 7- to 10-day range. The natural history of the disease follows 3 stages: the catarrhal stage characterized by mild, nonspecific symptoms such as rhinorrhea, cough, and low-grade fevers; the paroxysmal stage characterized by coughing fits followed by an inspiratory "whoop"; and the convalescent stage where the paroxysmal cough diminishes. Paroxysmal symptoms can last weeks to months, earning whooping cough the nickname of the "100-day cough." In infants and young children who are often not yet fully vaccinated against pertussis, the characteristic "whoop" may be absent because they do not have the strength to create one. Rather, they may present with coughing bouts followed by choking, gasping, apnea, and/or cyanosis or pallor and often followed by posttussive emesis and exhaustion.

(Chapter 497: The Global Burden of Lower Respiratory Tract Infections and Mucosal Immunology of the Lower Respiratory Tract in Children)

**Answer 8-63.** A

The patient described has a classic presentation of viral laryngotracheobronchitis, commonly known as croup. Croup, the most common infectious cause of acute stridor in children, is commonly characterized by stridor, fever, and barky cough following onset of viral upper respiratory infection symptoms. Common viral etiologies of croup include parainfluenza types I to III, respiratory syncytial virus (RSV), and adenovirus. The infection causes edema of the airway, particularly in the supraglottic region. Although neck films are not indicated to diagnose croup, an anteroposterior neck film would be likely to demonstrate narrowing of the supraglottic air column, classically known as the "steeple sign." Corticosteroids such as dexamethasone decrease the severity of symptoms.

(Chapter 118: Acute Upper Airway Obstruction, Chapter 96: Acute Respiratory Dysfunction)

**Answer 8-64.** B

The patient described has severe acute hypertension with evidence of end-organ damage (lethargy), sometimes also described as a hypertensive emergency. By contrast, severe acute hypertension without evidence of end-organ damage is also known as hypertensive urgency. The patient's hypertensive crisis was likely triggered by stopping his home antihypertensives. Abrupt stops of clonidine or β-blockers are known to trigger hypertensive crises. Given evidence of end-organ damage, efforts should be made to decrease the patient's blood pressure promptly; however, the decrease should not be too great or there is risk for permanent end-organ damage due to hypertension-induced dysregulation. The goal should be to lower the blood pressure promptly by no more than 25% within the first 8 hours of treatment.

(Chapter 475: Systemic Hypertension)

**Answer 8-65.** B

Cocaine and amphetamines are illicit drugs known to cause severe acute hypertension. In addition to hypertension, these drugs cause other signs of sympathetic system overactivity, including hyperthermia and tachycardia. The other drugs listed are not stimulants and therefore would not cause acute hypertension.

(Chapter 475: Systemic Hypertension)

# CHAPTER 9 Infectious Diseases

Omar Jaber, Charu J. Sehgal, Padma Swamy, Galit Holzmann-Pazgal, Elisha Acosta, Lynda Chima Aririguzo, Anna Rueda, Jennifer Benjamin, Judy Kim, Margaret Wood, Andria Tatem, Wallis Molchen, and Shailendra Das

**9-1.** A 2-year-old boy presents to the emergency department (ED) with cough for 2 days. His mother describes the cough as barky, almost seal-like. Mom reports that the cough was preceded by a couple of days of runny nose. He is not ill appearing and currently does not have a fever. What is the most common cause of the patient's symptoms?

**A.** *Staphylococcus aureus*

**B.** Respiratory syncytial virus (RSV)

**C.** *Haemophilus influenzae* type b

**D.** Parainfluenza virus (PIV)

**E.** Adenovirus

**9-2.** A 3-year-old girl, who was previously healthy, presents to your clinic with a 3-day history of fever (maximum temperature of 103°F) and wet-sounding cough. On exam, she is tachypneic, with a respiratory rate of 32 breaths/min; no retractions are seen, and you note crackles on the right anterior chest. Pulse oximetry reveals oxygen saturation of 94% on room air. A chest radiograph (CXR) confirms a right middle lobe infiltrate. What is the best first-line treatment option for this patient?

**A.** Oral azithromycin

**B.** Intravenous (IV) ceftriaxone

**C.** Oral amoxicillin

**D.** Oral ciprofloxacin

**E.** Supportive care (no antibiotics)

**9-3.** A 16-year-old previously healthy male from Tennessee presents with fever, malaise, progressive dyspnea, and dry cough for 6 weeks. He reports no recent travel, 2 months prior, he did go camping and cave exploring with some friends. Chest radiograph (CXR) reveals 2 small pulmonary nodules in the right lower lobe and hilar lymphadenopathy. What is the most likely etiology?

**A.** *Histoplasma capsulatum*

**B.** *Blastomyces* species

**C.** *Coccidioides* species

**D.** *Cryptococcus* species

**E.** *Paracoccidioides* species

**9-4.** You are rounding on a 7-year-old girl with acute lymphoblastic leukemia who received an allogenic hematopoietic stem cell transplantation 6 months ago. The patient is admitted for nonproductive cough and tachypnea. Pulse oximetry reveals an oxygen saturation of 88% on room air. Upon further questioning, the mom states she forgot to refill 2 of the child's medications last week. The patient is not allergic to any medications. Polymerase chain reaction (PCR) testing on sputum confirms your suspicion of an infectious etiology. What is the best treatment for the suspected etiology?

**A.** Dapsone

**B.** Clindamycin

**C.** Amoxicillin-clavulanic acid

**D.** Trimethoprim-sulfamethoxazole

**E.** Ciprofloxacin

**9-5.** A 14-year-old boy with cystic fibrosis (CF) is admitted for a pulmonary exacerbation. His cultures on this admission grow *Pseudomonas aeruginosa*. Reviewing the previous hospital records, it is noted that the patient previously grew *Pseudomonas* as well. What is the most accurate statement regarding *Pseudomonas* eradication in patients with CF?

**A.** It is easy to eradicate *P aeruginosa* from the lower airways because the organism is so rare.

**B.** It is difficult to eradicate *Pseudomonas* because it has a high incidence of person-to-person transmission within the general population.

**C.** It is difficult to eradicate *Pseudomonas* because the organisms can develop biofilms, making them hard to penetrate by antibiotics and immune phagocytosis.

**D.** It is easy to eradicate *Pseudomonas* due to high susceptibility of most antibiotic classes.

**E.** It is difficult to eradicate *Pseudomonas;* however, by about age 18, only a small percentage (< 5%) of CF patients have acquired *Pseudomonas*.

**9-6.** Based on the American Academy of Pediatrics (AAP) guidelines, which of the following patients would qualify for palivizumab?

**A.** A 35-week premature infant who is on room air and whose parents both smoke

**B.** A term baby born with Tetralogy of Fallot who recently underwent Blalock-Taussig shunt and is being discharged on furosemide

**C.** A 6-week-old infant born at 30 weeks of gestation, who was on continuous positive airway pressure for the first 3 weeks of life and was discharged on room air and no medications

**D.** A term baby with Down syndrome with no cardiac disease

**E.** A 16-month-old baby, born at 24 weeks of gestation, currently on room air, who received 5 doses of palivizumab last season

**9-7.** You are seeing a 6-year-old boy with chronic sinus issues (congestion and headaches). The parents report that his nose is "always congested," and he has green nasal discharge. In addition, he has chronic productive cough and recurrent ear infections. The parents believe their son's symptoms are related to bad allergies. The patient is noted to have normal growth. On exam, you auscultate heart sounds on the right side of the chest. What is the most likely cause of this patient's symptoms?

**A.** Hypersensitivity to aeroallergens

**B.** Defect in a protein regulating chloride transport

**C.** Ultrastructural defect in motile cilia

**D.** Chronic colonization of fungus

**E.** Typical infections for a healthy 6-year-old boy

**9-8.** A 16-year-old boy with moderate persistent asthma presents to your clinic with functional decline. He reports coughing up brown sputum and a feeling of malaise. Computed tomography (CT) of the chest reveals central bronchiectasis. Lab findings demonstrate a serum IgE of 1250 IU/mL and positive immediate cutaneous hypersensitivity to *Aspergillus* antigen. What is the primary treatment of choice in this patient?

**A.** Itraconazole

**B.** Amphotericin B

**C.** Inhaled fluticasone

**D.** Azithromycin

**E.** Oral prednisone

**9-9.** An 8-year-old girl presents to the urgent care center due to dry cough for 1 week associated with low-grade temperature (maximum temperature of 100.2°F) and malaise. The patient's mother reports the cough is worse at night, and the patient complains her chest is hurting due to the cough. The mother states that her daughter's school teacher told her that several other children in the class have recently missed school due to similar symptoms. Chest radiograph (CXR) demonstrates diffuse interstitial infiltrates. What is the treatment of choice for this patient?

**A.** Amoxicillin-clavulanic acid

**B.** Azithromycin

**C.** Oseltamivir

**D.** Cefdinir

**E.** Trimethoprim-sulfamethoxazole

**9-10.** An 8-month-old infant presents with chief complaint of vomiting and diarrhea. He has been having 6 to 8 watery, nonbloody, large-volume stools daily for 2 days with several episodes of emesis. His father notes that he has also felt warm but he did not check a temperature. He does not attend daycare, but his older sibling who is in daycare recently developed diarrhea that resolved after 48 hours. His immunizations are up to date. On exam, his temperature is 38.3°C, heart rate is 160 bpm, and respiratory rate is 40 breaths/min. He is alert but slightly fussy, and abdomen is soft, nontender, and nondistended. Capillary refill is 3 seconds. Fecal leukocyte test is negative. What test is most likely to yield the etiology of his illness?

**A.** *Clostridium difficile* toxin polymerase chain reaction (PCR)

**B.** Stool ova and parasite

**C.** Stool culture

**D.** Norovirus PCR

**E.** Rotavirus enzyme immunoassay (EIA)

**9-11.** A 9-year-old boy living in Texas presents in July with a 10-day history of fever. His mother states that he began having fevers up to 40°C 10 days ago, associated with headache, nausea, and body aches. He has vomited several times. About 3 days prior to presentation, he developed a diffuse rash, involving his trunk and extremities without oral involvement. He has multiple animal exposures including playing with a stray cat about 3 weeks ago, a recently adopted shelter dog, and a visit to a petting zoo 6 weeks ago. On exam, he is tired but alert and cooperative, smiles occasionally, and is non–toxic appearing. His temperature is 39.8°C, there are bilateral shotty anterior cervical lymph nodes, and he has a normal-appearing oropharynx, normal abdominal exam, and a faint diffuse erythematous maculopapular rash on his back and extremities. His complete blood count (CBC) demonstrates a white blood cell (WBC) count of 6000/μL with 20% neutrophils, 10% bands, 60% lymphocytes, and 10% monocytes. Platelet count is 120,000/μL. Complete metabolic panel is normal except for sodium of 132 mEq/L, aspartate aminotransferase (AST) of 111 IU/L, and alanine aminotransferase (ALT) of 67 IU/L. Coagulation panel is normal. What is the most likely diagnosis in this patient?

**A.** Meningococcemia

**B.** Typhus

**C.** *Bartonella*

**D.** Enterovirus

**E.** Epstein-Barr virus (EBV)

**9-12.** A 17-year-old African American boy presents to the emergency department (ED) with complaints of fever, bilateral knee and ankle pain, and a rash. He reports that he has some nausea and vomiting but no diarrhea. His head hurts, and he feels some fatigue. Otherwise his review of systems is negative. He denies any animal exposures or travel, and his immunizations are all up to date. He is sexually active with female partners. On exam, overall, he is nontoxic, alert, and relatively well appearing. His rash involves his legs, back, and shoulders and is erythematous and papulopustular with some areas appearing petechial/nonblanching. His knees and ankles bilaterally are very tender to palpation but not swollen. Otherwise, his physical exam is normal. CBC demonstrates white blood cell (WBC) count of 22,000/μL with 20% bands and 66% segmented neutrophils. Platelet count is 150,000/μL. Hemoglobin is normal. Aspartate aminotransferase (AST) and alanine aminotransferase (ALT) are 23 IU/L and 13 IU/L, respectively. Sodium is 140 mEq/L. Blood cultures are drawn, and the patient is discharged home. You are called 24 hours later and told that his blood cultures are positive for a gram-negative organism. What is the most likely pathogen in this case?

**A.** *Salmonella*

**B.** *Neisseria meningitidis*

**C.** *Shigella*

**D.** *Haemophilus ducreyi*

**E.** *Neisseria gonorrhoeae*

**9-13.** You are called to the emergency department (ED) to see an 8-month-old patient with 3 days of fever and 1 day of rash. His rash began on his face and spread distally. Additional symptoms include fussiness, conjunctivitis, barky cough, and rhinorrhea. On exam, his temperature is 39°C, and he has a diffuse erythematous maculopapular rash from head to extremities. It is blanching. His immunizations are up to date for age. The child recently traveled internationally and was well until 6 days after returning home. What isolation precautions should immediately be taken in the ED?

**A.** Droplet precautions

**B.** Contact precautions

**C.** Airborne precautions

**D.** Contact and airborne precautions

**E.** Standard precautions

**9-14.** Which of the following is the most common route of transmission of infectious agents in the healthcare setting?

**A.** Droplet transmission

**B.** Contact transmission

**C.** Airborne transmission

**D.** Contaminated food or water

**E.** Contaminated intravenous (IV) infusate

**9-15.** A 3-year-old girl is presenting to the clinic for her well-child check. She is currently 16 kg and has normal growth and development. Your exam is unremarkable. Her parents report that they are leaving in 3 weeks for a trip to Mumbai, India, lasting for 5 weeks. The parents are wondering if the child needs any prophylaxis for malaria. What is your next step in management?

**A.** Doxycycline 2.2 mg/kg daily (35.2 mg daily): Start 1 day prior to trip and continue for 4 weeks after last exposure

**B.** Atovaquone/proguanil (62.5 mg/25 mg) pediatric tablet (1 pediatric tablet daily): Start 1–2 days prior to trip and continue for 7 days after last exposure

**C.** Chloroquine phosphate (one-half pediatric tablet by mouth weekly): Start 2 weeks prior to trip and continue for 4 weeks after last exposure

**D.** Mefloquine (one-fourth tablet by mouth weekly): Start 2 weeks prior to trip and continue for 4 weeks after last exposure

**E.** Artemether/lumefantrine (2 tablets by mouth): Take 2 tablets once arrived every 8 hours for 2 doses and then every 12 hours for 2 doses

**9-16.** An 18-month-old girl presents to the clinic with 6 episodes of bloody stools for 2 days. The child attends daycare. On examination, her weight is 12 kg, temperature is 38.9°C, the mucous membranes are moist, and the child is making tears. The abdominal exam consists of a soft abdomen, without any guarding or rebound and with increased bowel sounds. Stool culture shows *Salmonella typhi*. What is the next step in management?

**A.** Oral hydration with oral rehydration solution

**B.** Loperamide 1 mg by mouth 3 times a day until diarrhea ceases

**C.** Ciprofloxacin 120 mg by mouth 2 times a day for 7 days

**D.** Metronidazole 120 mg by mouth 3 times a day for 7 days

**E.** BRAT (bananas, rice, applesauce, and toast) diet

**9-17.** A 6-month-old male infant, traveling to Nigeria in 1 month, comes for his general well-child exam. He has received all of his immunizations on time thus far. His exam is unremarkable. After you complete the visit, you prescribe antimalarial medication for him given that malaria is endemic to Nigeria. What vaccines should you order for him?

**A.** Diphtheria, tetanus, and pertussis (DTaP), *H influenzae* type b (HiB), inactivated polio vaccine (IPV), hepatitis (Hep) B, rotavirus, 13-valent pneumococcal vaccine (PCV13)

**B.** DTaP, HiB, IPV, Hep B, Hep A, rotavirus, PCV13

**C.** DTaP, HiB, IPV, Hep B, rotavirus, PCV13, measles-mumps-rubella (MMR)

**D.** DTaP, HiB, IPV, Hep B, rotavirus

**E.** DTaP, HiB, IPV, Hep A, rotavirus, PCV13

**9-18.** A 12-month-old male infant adopted from the Democratic Republic of Congo presents with his adoptive parents for his well-child checkup. The adoptive parents deny any known significant past medical history or biologic family history. The family shares the vaccination card with you, and you note that he had the bacillus Calmette-Guérin (BCG) vaccine at birth, and the DTP/Hep B/HiB and polio vaccines at 4, 10, and 14 weeks. Examination is unremarkable. What tuberculosis (TB) screening would you conduct?

**A.** Interferon-γ release assay (IGRA)

**B.** Tuberculin skin test (TST)

**C.** This child does not need screening because he is well appearing.

**D.** Induced sputum

**E.** Early morning nasogastric aspirates

**9-19.** A 5-year-old boy adopted from Vietnam presents to your clinic with his adoptive parents. His growth, development, and past medical history are unremarkable. His physical exam is unremarkable. The parents present you with his vaccine record (see following table). In addition to routine screening lab work, what vaccine does he need?

| Vaccine Given | Age of Patient at Different Vaccination Doses |
|---|---|
| Bacillus Calmette-Guérin | Birth |
| Hepatitis B | Birth, 2 months, 6 months |
| DTP | 2 months, 4 months, 6 months, 4 years |
| Hepatitis A | 12 months, 18 months |
| Measles, mumps, rubella | 12 months, 3 years |
| Varicella | 12 months, 3 years |
| Oral polio vaccine | 2 months, 4 months, 6 months, 12 months |

**A.** Diphtheria, tetanus, and pertussis (DTaP)

**B.** *Human influenzae* type b (HiB)

**C.** 13-valent pneumococcal vaccine (PCV13)

**D.** Measles-mumps-rubella (MMR)

**E.** Inactivated polio vaccine (IPV)

**9-20.** A 7-year-old boy recently arrived from Venezuela is seen in your clinic. Parents report that he has had the following symptoms for about 1 week: fever, body aches, and facial swelling. On physical exam, you note that he has left-sided periorbital edema, with conjunctivitis and preauricular lymphadenitis. What treatment can be offered to this child?

**A.** Supportive therapy for presenting symptoms

**B.** Benznidazole (5–7.5 mg/kg/d) twice daily for 60 days

**C.** Nifurtimox (15–20 mg/kg/d) 3 times a day for 90 days

**D.** Itraconazole (10 mg/kg/d) twice daily for 6 months

**E.** Albendazole 400 mg as a 1-time dose

**9-21.** A 4-year-old child from Tanzania presents for her first visit to the clinic with her adoptive parents about 2 weeks after arrival to the United States. Per the paperwork, the child does not have any significant medical or familial history. The adoptive parents report that she is doing well and is developing normally. Physical exam is unremarkable. The parents present you with the following vaccine record (see following table). What vaccines should you order today?

| Vaccine Given | Age of Patient at Different Vaccination Doses |
|---|---|
| Bacillus Calmette-Guérin | Birth |
| Hepatitis B | Birth, 2 months, 6 months |
| DTP | 2 months, 4 months, 6 months |
| Measles, mumps, rubella | 12 months |
| Varicella | 12 months |
| Oral polio vaccine | 2 months, 4 months, 6 months, 12 months |
| Yellow fever | Day prior to arrival in United States |

**A.** Hepatitis A, diphtheria, tetanus, and pertussis (DTaP), inactivated polio vaccine (IPV)

**B.** Hepatitis A, measles-mumps-rubella (MMR), varicella, DTaP, IPV

**C.** MMR, varicella, DTaP, IPV

**D.** Hepatitis A, MMR, varicella, DTaP

**E.** Hepatitis A, MMR, varicella, IPV

**9-22.** A 2-year-old girl presents to the clinic with wheezing per her mother's report. The mother is concerned that the child is also eating dirt as well. She states that the child has been spending a lot of time with a puppy that they got about 6 months ago. You notice that the lab work from the well-child check shows marked eosinophilia. You draw an erythrocyte sedimentation rate (ESR), which is elevated. Physical exam reveals rales and hepatomegaly on exam. What is your next step in eliciting the diagnosis?

**A.** Stool ova and parasites

**B.** Pulmonary function testing

**C.** Immunoglobulin testing

**D.** Interferon-γ release assay (IGRA)

**E.** Radioallergosorbent test (RAST)

**9-23.** A 10-year-old boy with no prior medical history presents to the emergency department (ED) in September with the complaint of fever, headache, muscle pain, fatigue, nausea/vomiting, and abdominal pain. On physical exam, you notice that this child, although in no distress, has neck stiffness and photophobia. You perform a lumbar puncture, which is clear with 5 WBCs/μL (mild lymphocytic pleocytosis), normal glucose, and slightly elevated protein in the cerebrospinal fluid (CSF). CSF culture is pending. What would be your next step in the care of this patient?

**A.** Amoxicillin (80 mg/kg/d) by mouth twice daily

**B.** Ceftriaxone (100 mg/kg/d) IV once daily for 14 days

**C.** Acyclovir (30 mg/kg/d) IV 3 times a day

**D.** Acetaminophen 10 mg/kg per dose by mouth every 4 hours as needed for fever and Ceftriaxone (100 mg/kg/d) IV once daily, to be discontinued if the CSF culture is negative

**E.** Hydrocortisone (1 mg/kg/d) IV every 12 hours and Ceftriaxone (100 mg/kg/d) IV once daily, to be discontinued if the CSF culture is negative

**9-24.** A 15-year-old girl presents to the clinic with weakness and trouble walking. She states these symptoms started about 1 day prior to the visit. On exam, you note that she has hyporeflexia of the patellar and Achilles tendons. She later reports that she traveled to Brazil and that, 3 weeks ago, she had a fever with rash on the palms and soles of her hands and feet, joint pain, and red eyes. What test would you use to determine the etiology of her presentation?

**A.** *Campylobacter jejuni* stool culture

**B.** Rapid influenza A testing using immunofluorescence

**C.** Monospot testing for Epstein-Barr virus (EBV)

**D.** *M pneumoniae* polymerase chain reaction (PCR)

**E.** Zika IgM using Dengue plaque reduction neutralization test

**9-25.** A previously healthy, normally developing, 15-month-old girl presents to the outpatient clinic with 2 days of fussiness, pulling at her right ear, and fever to 101°F. She has no allergies and is not taking any medications. On exam, she is alert and well hydrated. Both of her tympanic membranes are erythematous and bulging and have effusions. This is her fourth episode of acute otitis media (AOM) in the past 6 months. She finished her most recent course of amoxicillin 8 weeks ago. What is the best treatment plan for this patient?

**A.** Plan to observe for 48 hours and start amoxicillin if her symptoms worsen or fail to improve.

**B.** Start a 10-day course of amoxicillin and refer to otorhinolaryngology (ENT) for evaluation of pressure equalization tube (PET) placement due to recurrent AOM.

**C.** Start a 10-day course of amoxicillin–clavulanic acid and refer to ENT for evaluation of PET placement due to recurrent AOM.

**D.** Start a 10-day course of amoxicillin and plan to switch to amoxicillin–clavulanic acid if her symptoms worsen or fail to improve after 72 hours of initial antibiotic therapy.

**E.** Start a 10-day course of amoxicillin–clavulanic acid for recurrent AOM and refer her to audiology for a formal hearing screen.

**9-26.** The father of a 5-year-old boy brings his son to the emergency department (ED) due to concern that he is refusing to walk since he awoke this morning. The father has noted that he will not bear weight on his right foot. He has had no recent trauma or illness, he has no significant past medical history, and his immunizations are up to date. His vitals in clinic show an axillary temperature of 101.5°F, heart rate of 90 bpm, respiratory rate of 24 breaths/min, and blood pressure of 1005/65 mm Hg. On physical exam, he is alert and in mild distress, and he guards with attempted manipulation of his right leg. He is holding his right hip in a flexed, abducted, externally rotated position. On palpation, the hip is found to be warm to touch and erythematous. On skin exam, he has a 2-cm scab overlying his right knee. The remainder of his exam is normal. A joint aspirate of his right hip is performed by orthopedic surgery, and results show > 50,000 WBCs/μL, with predominance of neutrophils. What is the most common etiologic agent in this patient's case?

**A.** *Pseudomonas aeruginosa*

**B.** *Neisseria gonorrhoeae*

**C.** *Kingella kingae*

**D.** *Human influenzae* type b (HiB)

**E.** *Staphylococcus aureus*

**9-27.** A 17-year-old girl presents for an appointment today after being asked to return to clinic. Her recent urine specimen indicates a positive chlamydia test diagnosed by a nucleic acid amplification test (NAAT) collected 2 days ago. At the prior visit, she reported sexual activity with one 16-year-old male partner. Her last sexual encounter was 1 week ago. She currently has an intrauterine device (IUD) for contraception but does not routinely use condoms. The remainder of tests for human immunodeficiency virus (HIV), gonorrhea, and syphilis performed 2 days ago are negative. In clinic, the patient was prescribed and observed taking azithromycin 1 g orally. Of the following choices, what is the appropriate counseling to provide this patient?

**A.** Return for a routine test of cure in 2 weeks.

**B.** Abstain from further sexual activity for at least 48 hours.

**C.** Return in 3 months for repeat testing.

**D.** The IUD should be removed due to the high risk of pelvic inflammatory disease.

**E.** All of her sexual partners in the past 90 days should also be treated.

**9-28.** A patient with which of the following medical conditions would qualify for at least 1 dose of 23-valent pneumococcal polysaccharide vaccine (PPSV23)?

**A.** Neurofibromatosis

**B.** Mild intermittent asthma

**C.** Severe peanut allergy

**D.** Diabetes mellitus

**E.** Recurrent urinary tract infections

**9-29.** Which of the following is the correct pairing of an infectious disease with the necessary isolation precautions for use in the hospital setting?

**A.** Airborne precautions for varicella-zoster virus

**B.** Contact precautions for influenza

**C.** Droplet precautions for *Mycobacterium tuberculosis*

**D.** Airborne precautions for norovirus

**E.** Droplet precautions for vancomycin-resistant *Enterococcus*

**9-30.** A 4-year-old boy with a history of an orthotopic heart transplant was recently discharged from the hospital after a 14-day admission for the treatment of respiratory failure due to pneumonia. A few days after discharge, he presents to the clinic with concern for new-onset fever, watery diarrhea, nausea, and loss of appetite. His stool studies return positive for *Clostridium difficile*. Of the following, which is true of this patient's diagnosis?

**A.** Due to the sporicidal properties, an alcohol-based hand hygiene product is recommended to prevent person-to-person spread of *C difficile*.

**B.** Asymptomatic colonization is common in young children, and current guidelines recommend not testing children < 5 years old.

**C.** Oral metronidazole given for 10 days of therapy is the appropriate choice for initial treatment.

**D.** It is uncommon for a patient to have a repeat *C difficile* infection if the initial antibiotic course was completed.

**E.** Only a single course of therapy is usually needed for *C difficile*, as only 1% of patients experience a relapse.

**9-31.** A 21-month-old girl presents with a 1-day history of fever, fussiness, poor oral intake, and crusting around her eyes and mouth. She has no known history of allergies. She has taken no medications or supplements other than acetaminophen for fever. On exam, she is febrile and ill appearing. She has tachycardia and normal heart rhythm with no murmur, rub, or gallop. She has clear breath sounds with symmetric air entry. She has notable perioral and periocular crusted yellow discharge (Figure 362-8). Her skin is erythematous, tender, and desquamating under her neck, in her axilla, and in the flexural aspect of her arms and legs. What is her diagnosis?

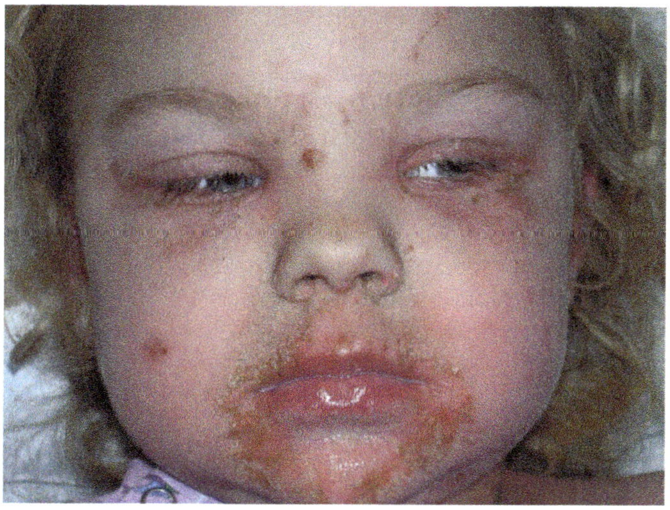

**FIGURE 362-8.** (Mark W. Kline, *Rudolph's Pediatrics*, 23rd Edition. Copyright © McGraw-Hill Education. All rights reserved.)

**A.** Erythema multiforme

**B.** Staphylococcal scalded skin syndrome

**C.** Toxic epidermal necrolysis

**D.** Kawasaki disease

**E.** Stevens-Johnson syndrome

**9-32.** A 16-year-old previously healthy boy presents to the emergency department (ED) with acute onset of fever to 104°F and severe headache starting 2 days ago. He reports that today he noted the appearance of small red bumps on his wrists and ankles that are now spreading to his arms and legs. He denies sore throat, cough, nasal congestion, vomiting, and diarrhea. He has no allergies and is taking no medication. He has no other past medical history except for an appendectomy 3 years ago. He lives with his parents, a brother, and a dog in Houston, Texas. He and his family recently hiked part of the Appalachian Trail in North Carolina and returned home from their trip 1 week ago. On exam, he is mildly dehydrated, tired appearing, and febrile. He has small 1- to 4-mm erythematous macules that blanch on his upper and lower extremities that involve the palms and soles. What is the next best step in the evaluation and treatment for this patient?

**A.** Confirm the diagnosis with specific serologic antibody testing

**B.** Obtain further history to determine whether the patient had a tick exposure

**C.** Order laboratory testing including a complete blood count (CBC) and complete metabolic panel

**D.** Start antibiotic treatment with doxycycline immediately

**E.** Place the patient on airborne precautions in isolation

**9-33.** A 9-year-old girl presents to urgent care with a 4-day history of a red, painful, swollen inguinal lymph node, low-grade fever, malaise, and decreased appetite. On exam, she is overall well appearing and afebrile, and her vital signs are normal. She has a 2-cm mobile, tender lymph node with overlying erythema in her left inguinal region. She has no rash and no other lymphadenopathy elsewhere. On further questioning, mom reports that they recently adopted a kitten and her daughter has spent a lot of time playing with the kitten at home. What is the best test to confirm this patient's diagnosis?

**A.** Biopsy of the affected lymph node

**B.** Ultrasound of the affected lymph node

**C.** Polymerase chain reaction (PCR) of lymph node or pus aspirate

**D.** IgG-based immunofluorescent antibody test (IFAT)

**E.** Enzyme immunoassay (EIA) test

**9-34.** A 10-day-old female infant presents to clinic for a well-child exam. Her mother reports that she has noted thick yellow eye discharge from both eyes that started 2 days ago and has been worsening since initial symptoms began. The mother states that her baby has been fussier but denies fever, cough, trouble breathing, poor feeding, decreased wet diapers, or lethargy. On exam, the baby is afebrile, alert, well hydrated, and active. She has purulent discharge noted on bilateral upper and lower eyelids, mild erythema and edema of bilateral upper eyelids, and conjunctival injection. Cardiac and lung exams are normal. There are no rashes or other abnormal skin findings. When asked for further history, the mother reports that she has a history of a chlamydia infection that was treated shortly after the birth of this child. Of the following, which is true of this patient's diagnosis?

- **A.** This infection has an incubation period of 2 to 5 days.
- **B.** Point-of-care testing in clinic can confirm the diagnosis of this bacterial pathogen.
- **C.** Topical erythromycin shortly after birth has been highly effective to prevent conjunctivitis in exposed infants.
- **D.** The treatment of choice is oral erythromycin.
- **E.** Warm compresses and massage of the nasal bridge should be recommended.

**9-35.** In clinic today, a teenage boy presents with a fever of 102°F and sore throat for 2 days. No vomiting, diarrhea, or rashes have been noted. There is no cough or congestion, but the patient experienced some rhinorrhea a few days ago. He feels tired and is not sleeping well due to headaches and throat discomfort. His friends have been ill as well, and one was diagnosed with strep throat via a rapid strep test. Exam is significant for a slightly ill-appearing boy with erythematous oropharynx and fairly enlarged tonsils without exudates but who has some postnasal drip. His lymph nodes are shotty and diffuse, but you feel a slightly larger one that is submandibular on the anterior left side. You do a rapid test for strep in the office; it is negative, so you send a throat culture. The patient has no allergies, and the pharmacy is out of penicillin VK. Which is the first medication you would pick for treatment pending the culture?

- **A.** Amoxicillin
- **B.** Azithromycin
- **C.** Vancomycin
- **D.** Cefdinir
- **E.** Clindamycin

**9-36.** A teenage boy presents in clinic with a fever of 102°F and sore throat. No vomiting, diarrhea, or rashes have been noted. There is no cough or congestion. He feels tired and is not sleeping well due to headaches and throat discomfort. Exam is significant for a slightly ill-appearing boy with erythematous oropharynx and fairly enlarged tonsils without exudates but who has some postnasal drip. His lymph nodes are shotty and diffuse, but you feel a slightly larger one that is submandibular on the anterior left side. A rapid test and a throat culture come back negative for strep. The patient has no allergies, but the pharmacy is out of penicillin, so you give him amoxicillin and send him home. The same patient comes to see you 1 week later. His chief complaint is now extreme fatigue, a rash, and persistent sore throat. He has been taking his prescribed antibiotic and is almost finished with the course. His temperature is now 99°F to 100°F. The rash has become more significant in the past 2 days. Upon exam today, you note that the patient's tonsils are still erythematous and covered with a whitish film. His lymph nodes, especially posterior, have increased in size. However, his rash is most dramatic—erythematous, maculopapular, and blanching; it is generalized in distribution from the trunk/back to extremities. His liver also seems to be enlarged, and you can feel the splenic tip well below the costal margin. What is your most likely diagnosis now based on these findings?

- **A.** Roseola
- **B.** Rubella
- **C.** Infectious mononucleosis
- **D.** Group A β-hemolytic streptococcal infection
- **E.** Amoxicillin/penicillin reaction

**9-37.** A healthy 5-year-old boy presents to the clinic with a 2-week history of an enlarged lymph node on the right side of his neck. His mother states that, at first, it did not seem to be too significant, but it has grown in the past 2 weeks significantly and also appears to be draining. The boy states that the lesion is not painful. He has had no fever, weight loss, or night sweats. He likes to play outside, especially with dogs and cats. The family has recently started feeding a small stray kitten outside their house. When the boy was asked if he touched the cat, he replied that he did not; his mother did not look so sure. Exam shows a solitary lesion on the right mid neck, about 1.5 inches in diameter and slightly hard to palpation. There seems to be a head on it, but no pus is seen or expressed and it is not painful to touch. Otherwise, his exam is normal, except for faint tiny lacerations on his fingers. What is the most likely pathogen causing this presentation?

- **A.** Infectious mononucleosis
- **B.** *Streptococcus pyogenes*
- **C.** *Francisella tularensis*
- **D.** *Bartonella henselae*
- **E.** *M tuberculosis*

**9-38.** A mother comes in with her 6-year-old daughter for a complaint of a bump on the child's neck. The mother noticed the bump about 3 days ago. The patient has had a bit of congestion, mostly in the mornings, but no fever and is attending school. No vomiting or diarrhea and no rash are present. The bump seems just a bit tender, per mom, and is located in the left neck, is submandibular, and looks to be about 1.5 cm across. It feels smooth and mobile. The mother of the patient is not sure if it has grown. What would be the next step in management of this patient?

**A.** Lymph node biopsy

**B.** Antibiotic treatment

**C.** Chest radiograph (CXR)

**D.** Blood work to include complete blood count (CBC), sedimentation rate, blood cultures, and serologic testing

**E.** Observation and follow-up in 1 to 2 weeks

**9-39.** A newborn infant presents for his 2-week well-child check. Mom had inconsistent prenatal care, as she emigrated here from El Salvador during her pregnancy with this child. The infant is solely nursing, has regained his birth weight, and is having normal newborn stools. Mom notes a rash on his scalp, which she thinks is cradle cap. Upon exam, you note 2 to 3 small round vesicular lesions on the patient's scalp. The vesicles do not appear to be pustular or painful, but there is a small amount of erythema surrounding them and clear fluid inside. What should be the next step in treatment?

**A.** Intravenous (IV) acyclovir for 14 days, followed by oral acyclovir for 6 months

**B.** IV acyclovir for 21 days, followed by oral acyclovir for 6 months

**C.** Observation only; it turned out to be seborrhea after all

**D.** Topical mupirocin

**E.** Clindamycin for possible methicillin-resistant *Staphylococcus aureus* (MRSA)

**9-40.** A 17-year-old male college student presents to your student health clinic. He discloses that he is human immunodeficiency virus (HIV) positive, is sexually active, and is concerned about a painful genital ulcer that has developed over the past few days. His genitourinary exam is significant for a 2-cm, tender, erythematous ulcer near the corona of the penis, as well as enlarged inguinal lymph nodes that are tender and fluctuant upon palpation. If the ulcer exudates test negative for herpes simplex virus (HSV), which of the following would be the most appropriate treatment?

**A.** Metronidazole 2 g orally once

**B.** Clindamycin 300 mg orally twice a day for 7 days

**C.** Azithromycin 1 g orally once

**D.** Podofilox 0.5% topical gel

**E.** Erythromycin base 500 mg orally once

**9-41.** You are the attending on service for the general pediatric hospitalist team. Before rounding, your intern privately discloses that she was seen at an urgent care clinic last night for new-onset vesicles on her lower back and was diagnosed with shingles. Your intern is worried if this will affect her care of patients both today and in 2 days when she will switch to the hematology-oncology service. She asks you what she should do. Regarding hospital infection control and prevention, which of the following would be the best recommendation?

**A.** She should practice standard hand hygiene. She should keep lesions covered until lesions crust over. She should be allowed to care for all patients.

**B.** She should practice standard hand hygiene. She should keep lesions covered until lesions crust over. She may care for immunocompetent patients but not for immunocompromised patients.

**C.** She should practice standard hand hygiene. She should keep lesions covered until treated for 24 hours. She may care for all patients after 24 hours of treatment.

**D.** She should practice standard hand hygiene at home. However, she should not be allowed to care for any patients until lesions crust over, no matter the location of the lesions.

**E.** She should practice standard hand hygiene. She should keep lesions covered until lesions crust over. She should only care for patients in an outpatient setting and should avoid inpatient care.

**9-42.** A 7-month-old female infant presents to your clinic as a referral from a local ophthalmologist to establish care. She was born in Liberia and came to the United States with her mother about 1 month ago to visit relatives. Given concerns for the child's vision, her family took her to the ophthalmologist, where she was diagnosed with chorioretinitis. You note the child to have hypotonia, hepatomegaly, delayed motor and speech milestones, and a head circumference greater than the 99th percentile. The mother discloses that she had minimal prenatal care and that the child had a diffuse, purplish, maculopapular rash at birth. You then order a magnetic resonance imaging (MRI) scan of the brain, which shows intraparenchymal calcifications and obstructive hydrocephalus. What is the most likely cause of this patient's findings?

**A.** Congenital cytomegalovirus (CMV) infection

**B.** Congenital rubella infection

**C.** Congenital Zika virus infection

**D.** Congenital toxoplasmosis infection

**E.** Congenital syphilis

**9-43.** A 17-year-old, previously healthy boy born and raised in the United States presents to your clinic. He is a senior in high school and plans to participate in his school's healthcare program, which would allow him to shadow and assist medical personnel in the nearby hospital. Before starting, the program requires tuberculosis (TB) screening. A tuberculin skin test (TST) was placed in clinic 2 days ago. Today, his area of erythema spans 16 mm, and his area of induration spans 3 mm. He reports no travel outside of the United States and has had no known contact with persons suspected to have TB. What is the most appropriate next step?

**A.** Obtain a chest radiograph (CXR) to examine for latent or active TB

**B.** Repeat TST in 1 month to verify results

**C.** Send interferon-γ release assay (IGRA) to verify results

**D.** Start isoniazid therapy for suspected latent TB

**E.** Medically clear him for the healthcare program

**9-44.** A 16-year-old girl presents with her mother to your clinic due to 1 week of illness. The illness started with fatigue, headache, and abdominal pain. Over the past 3 days, the girl has developed sore throat, fever, generalized abdominal pain, and fever of 102.2°F orally. While in her grandmother's care yesterday, she was given acetaminophen and amoxicillin. She experienced no major improvement, but this morning, she developed a diffuse red rash. On exam today, the teenager appears tired but nontoxic and in no acute distress. She has enlarged tonsils with white exudates, fine petechiae on the soft palate, and enlarged lymph nodes located in the bilateral cervical changes. Her rash is diffuse, blanching, erythematous, and maculopapular, and her spleen is palpable 3 cm below the left costal margin. The most common cause of this patient's clinical syndrome is also associated with which of the following conditions?

**A.** Postinfectious glomerulonephritis (group A β-hemolytic *Streptococcus*)

**B.** Congenital microcephaly (caused by congenital cytomegalovirus [CMV])

**C.** Keratoconjunctivitis (adenovirus)

**D.** Burkitt lymphoma

**E.** Superficial pyoderma

**9-45.** A 4-month-old infant is being seen in the emergency department (ED) for parental concerns of poor feeding and weakness. The parents report that the baby has been afebrile but has had several days of constipation and is now no longer finishing bottles. They also report that the baby is not as energetic as before. On your exam, you note an infant who is alert but whose physical exam is notable for ptosis, mild dehydration, symmetric hypotonia, and diminished deep tendon reflexes. To confirm the diagnosis, what is the appropriate test?

**A.** Stool specimen for toxin assay

**B.** Rectal biopsy

**C.** Magnetic resonance imaging (MRI) of brain and spine

**D.** Blood culture

**E.** Thyroid-stimulating hormone (TSH) and free thyroxine ($T_4$)

**9-46.** A 5-year-old child presents to your clinic with history of 3 days of cough, fever, temperatures to 40°C, congestion, myalgia, and conjunctivitis. The child was previously healthy but unvaccinated due to parental hesitancy. The family recently traveled to visit relatives in Switzerland. On exam, you note a cough without wheeze, mild conjunctivitis, generalized lymphadenopathy, and small (~1-mm) bluish-white spots with surrounding erythema on the buccal mucosa opposite his lower molars. What is the most appropriate treatment for this patient's diagnosis?

**A.** Intravenous (IV) immunoglobulin

**B.** Supportive care alone

**C.** Vitamin A supplementation

**D.** Doxycycline

**E.** Penicillin

**9-47.** You are seeing a 5-week-old infant in the emergency department (ED) in December for concern for apnea at home. The patient's mother describes 2 episodes of pauses in breathing that occurred today. The infant has had some congestion and cough but has not had a fever and has been eating normally. The infant is previously healthy and has a 4-year-old sibling who attends daycare and has had a cough with rhinorrhea and some wheezes for the past 5 days. On your exam, the infant is mildly tachypneic (respiratory rate, 40 breaths/min) and has scattered wheezes and rales but is otherwise awake and alert. What is the most likely diagnosis?

**A.** Seasonal influenza infection

**B.** Respiratory syncytial virus (RSV) infection

**C.** Nonaccidental trauma

**D.** Gastroesophageal reflux

**E.** Asthma

**9-48.** You are seeing a 2-day-old infant in the newborn nursery. The baby girl was born full term to a G2P2 mother who has a healthy 3-year-old son who attends daycare. The pregnancy was uncomplicated, mother received all recommended prenatal care, and neither parent has traveled outside the United States. The baby has been breastfeeding well since birth and has normal weight, length, and head circumference. The mother and newborn were preparing for discharge; however, there is now a concern for a failed hearing screen. What is the most likely infectious cause for hearing loss in this baby?

**A.** Congenital Zika virus infection

**B.** Congenital toxoplasmosis infection

**C.** Congenital rubella infection

**D.** Group B *Streptococcus* meningitis

**E.** Congenital cytomegalovirus (CMV) infection

**9-49.** A 3-year-old boy presents to the clinic for perianal pruritus. He was previously healthy and attends daycare. The father reports that he is complaining of his bottom itching at bedtime. He is otherwise asymptomatic. On physical exam, there is trace perianal erythema, no abdominal tenderness, and no other physical exam findings. You would like to confirm the diagnosis prior to treatment. What would be the best test to confirm the diagnosis?

**A.** Stool examination for ova and parasites

**B.** Early morning cellophane tape microscopy

**C.** Culture of the anal canal

**D.** Serum IgE food allergy panel

**E.** Serum eosinophil count

**9-50.** You are seeing a 12-year-old boy with a history of mild intermittent asthma and morbid obesity (body mass index > 99% for age) in clinic in January. His mother reports that he was in his usual state of health until yesterday when he began to complain of a sore throat, nonproductive cough, and fatigue. She gave him albuterol via inhaler with spacer per his asthma action plan with some improvement in his cough. He also complained of chills, and when she checked his temperature, it was 39°C. Your exam today is notable for fever to 39.2°C, cough, biphasic wheezing on exam without increased work of breathing, and mild erythema of the posterior oropharynx in a child who appears tired. Mother reports that she has heard of multiple children home sick at his school. What is the best treatment for this child?

**A.** Supportive care alone (encouraging fluids, rest, antipyretics)

**B.** Scheduled albuterol every 4 hours via metered-dose inhaler and spacer

**C.** Oral oseltamivir treatment course and albuterol prn via metered-dose inhaler and spacer

**D.** Oral amantadine treatment course and albuterol prn via metered-dose inhaler and spacer

**E.** Oral amoxicillin treatment course and albuterol prn via metered-dose inhaler and spacer

**9-51.** You are evaluating a term baby girl born approximately 48 hours ago to a 24-year-old mother who is a refugee recently arrived in the United States. On your exam, the baby is small for gestational age, has scattered red-purple macules throughout her skin, and has a loud, machine-like murmur. You are concerned that the disease process you identify in this infant has the potential to lead to poor developmental outcomes. Which of the following strategies is effective in preventing deafness and disability from this infant's disease?

**A.** Prenatal screening and intrapartum penicillin for at-risk mothers

**B.** Prenatal screening and regular immunoglobulin infusions for at-risk mothers

**C.** Postnatal course of valganciclovir for the infant

**D.** Universal immunization coverage for children and women of childbearing age prior to conception

**E.** Phototherapy combined with double volume exchange transfusion for the infant

**9-52.** You are evaluating a term infant in the newborn nursery who was born yesterday to a 32-year-old mother with a past medical history of human immunodeficiency virus (HIV) infection. The baby is doing well, but you are worried about the infant's risk of perinatal HIV infection. Which of the following interventions would be associated with the largest reduction in risk of mother-to-child transmission of HIV infection?

**A.** Delivery via scheduled cesarean section at 38 weeks' gestation

**B.** Exclusive formula feeding from birth

**C.** Infant prophylaxis with 6 weeks of zidovudine

**D.** Intrapartum intravenous (IV) zidovudine treatment for the mother

**E.** Combined antiretroviral therapy of the mother with suppression of viral load

**9-53.** You are seeing a previously healthy, 8-year-old boy in clinic who presents with complaints of 2 weeks of copious, watery diarrhea, intermittent/crampy abdominal pain, and subjective weight loss. He has not had any fevers and has not noticed any blood or mucus in his stools. He typically eats an appropriate, well-rounded diet, but has not been as hungry as usual in the past few weeks. His parents report that the entire family went on an extended backpacking and camping trip about 1 month ago. Which test is the most appropriate to confirm this child's likely diagnosis?

**A.** Stool microscopy for ova and parasites

**B.** Specific stool antigen test

**C.** Intestinal biopsy of small bowel

**D.** Stool culture

**E.** Serum erythrocyte sedimentation rate (ESR) and C-reactive protein (CRP) level

**9-54.** You are seeing a 17-year-old girl in the emergency department (ED). She is presenting for a fall from her horse while barrel racing. She fell against a wooden fence and sustained deep abrasions to her hip, thigh, and arm. She was previously healthy, and in the electronic medical record, you can confirm that she is up to date on all her immunizations, including primary 3-dose series of DTaP immunization and Tdap booster at age 11 years. In addition to proper cleansing of the wounds and care for her injuries, what would be the most appropriate plan for prevention of tetanus?

**A.** Booster dose of Tdap or Td alone.

**B.** Tetanus immune globulin (TIG) alone.

**C.** Booster dose of Tdap or Td and TIG.

**D.** Booster dose of Tdap or Td, TIG, and metronidazole.

**E.** No additional tetanus prevention is necessary because she is up to date on vaccines.

**9-55.** A mother delivers a baby with severe malformations including microcephaly and arthrogryposis. Further testing reveals infection with Zika virus. Which of the following diseases follows the same common mode of transmission by which the mother likely acquired Zika?

**A.** Kawasaki disease

**B.** Rheumatic fever

**C.** Poststreptococcal glomerulonephritis

**D.** Malaria

**E.** Hand-foot-mouth disease

**9-56.** A 7-year-old girl is complaining that her butt itches. Her mother is mortified that the child won't stop scratching her bottom. The girl is having trouble sleeping at night. On exam, she has perianal excoriations but is otherwise normal. A test tape specimen indicates small, pearly white, threadlike objects. The cause of this child's symptoms is most likely due to which of the following?

**A.** *Ascaris lumbricoides*

**B.** *Enterobius vermicularis*

**C.** *Entamoeba histolytica*

**D.** *Diphyllobothrium latum*

**E.** *Strongyloides stercoralis*

**9-57.** A 6-year-old boy comes to the clinic with the rapid onset of fever, muscle pain, and rash. The rash is maculopapular, beginning on the flexor surfaces of the wrist and evolving to a hemorrhagic-type appearance. You learn that he went on a camping trip with his Boy Scout troop 9 days prior to presentation. Which of the following findings can best be used to differentiate Rocky Mountain spotted fever (RMSF) from Kawasaki disease?

**A.** Thrombocytopenia is specific to Kawasaki disease and not RMSF.

**B.** The rash for RMSF spares the trunk.

**C.** The rash in RMSF does not involve the palms and soles.

**D.** Fever in RMSF is lower than in Kawasaki disease.

**E.** Patients with Kawasaki disease are more likely to have conjunctivitis, mucous membrane involvement, and extremity changes.

**9-58.** A 17-year-old adolescent presents to clinic for evaluation. He confidently admits to having 6 sexual partners in the past 2 weeks, stating that he had an "eventful" vacation over spring break. Which of the following findings is consistent with the diagnosis of gonorrhea?

**A.** Painless ulcer, with painful swelling of the groin and painful suppurative inguinal lymphadenopathy

**B.** Painful papulopustule on prepuce, with painful supportive inguinal lymphadenopathy

**C.** Inflamed, hyperkeratotic, whitish plaques on penis accompanied by purulent discharge

**D.** Painless, mucosal, and warty erosions that are flat, velvety, moist, and broad based

**E.** Flat, smooth, or pedunculated papules

**9-59.** Ten days ago, a 4-year-old boy developed nonbloody diarrhea that has continued despite dietary management. His stools have been pale, watery, and frothy. He remains afebrile. Microscopic examination of his stools is likely to show which of the following?

**A.** *Toxoplasma gondii*

**B.** *Sporothrix schenckii*

**C.** *Enterobius vermicularis*

**D.** *Shigella sonnei*

**E.** *Cryptosporidium*

**9-60.** A 17-year-old girl comes to the office with complaints of vaginal discharge for 3 days. She has no significant past medical history. She uses a copper IUD for contraception and does not take any medications. She has had 2 consensual sexual partners in the past 3 months and had consensual sex 1 week ago with a boy from her school. On physical exam, she has a temperature of 37.1°C, heart rate of 76 bpm, respiratory rate of 14 breaths/min, and blood pressure of 112/70 mm Hg. She has no abdominal tenderness. On pelvic examination, she has a friable cervix with purulent cervical discharge and no cervical motion tenderness. Gram stain and culture of the discharge shows multiple white blood cells (WBCs) and gram-negative intracellular diplococci. What organism is most likely the cause of her symptoms?

**A.** *Treponema pallidum*
**B.** *Gardnerella vaginalis*
**C.** Human papillomavirus (HPV)
**D.** *Neisseria gonorrhoeae*
**E.** Herpes simplex virus (HSV)

**9-61.** A 6-year-old boy who recently emigrated from India is brought to hospital with a complaint of fever, back pain, abdominal pain, and lethargy. On physical examination, his temperature is 39.6°C, heart rate is 140 bpm, respiratory rate is 30 breaths/min, and blood pressure is 95/65 mm Hg. He is ill appearing and thin. He has pale conjunctiva and mucous membranes. Capillary refill is 2 seconds. There is a II/VI vibratory systolic ejection murmur. His lungs are clear to auscultation. His abdomen is diffusely tender to palpation, and the liver and spleen are palpated 5 cm and 6 cm below the costal margins, respectively. Examination of the spine and paraspinal muscles is normal.

A complete blood count (CBC) shows the following: white blood cell (WBC) 5000/μL, 30% neutrophils, 50% lymphocytes, and 20% monocytes; hemoglobin 8.5 g/dL, hematocrit 26.2%, and platelet count 120 × $10^3$/μL. Additionally, you send a peripheral smear to pathology, which shows a crescent-shaped gametocyte above a ring-form trophozoite (Figure 347-4). This child's illness was most likely caused by which of the following?

**A.** A bite from an *Anopheles* mosquito
**B.** A bite from an *Ixodes* tick
**C.** A bite from a reduviid bug
**D.** A bite from an *Aedes* mosquito
**E.** A bite from a *Dermacentor* tick

**9-62.** A mother brings in a 4-year-old boy after 5 days of greasy, foul-smelling diarrhea. His mom also reports nausea, weight loss, and abdominal cramps. There is no blood in the stool. He is afebrile and normotensive, with heart rate of 80 bpm and respiratory rate of 16 breaths/min. Physical exam shows a well-appearing boy with mild abdominal discomfort but no tenderness or organomegaly. He went camping about 2 weeks ago and had been drinking water from a stream near the cabin. Which test will most help determine the most likely cause of his symptoms?

**A.** Stool guaiac
**B.** Stool white blood cell (WBC) count
**C.** Stool test for secretory IgA antibodies against gliadin and human tissue transglutaminase
**D.** Stool-reducing substances
**E.** Test for stool oocyte and parasite

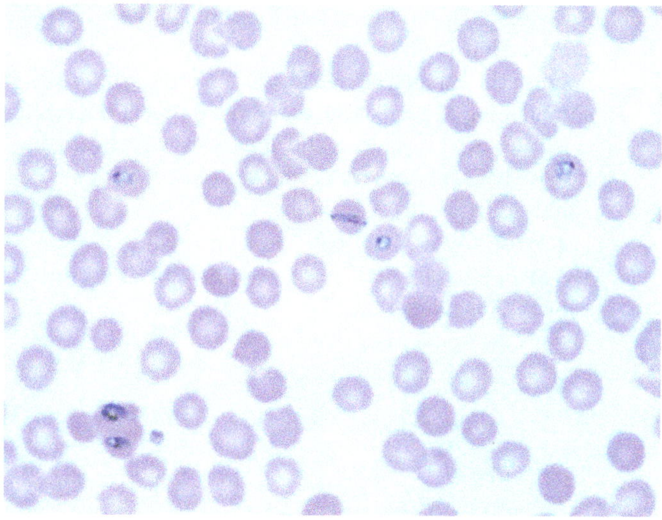

**FIGURE 347-4.** Crescent-shaped gametocyte above a ring-form trophozoite (center of slide). (Reproduced with permission from the Centers for Disease Control and Prevention [CDC]. Photo contributor Dr. Earl Long.)

**9-63.** A 10-year-old girl is brought by her mother for evaluation of a new rash in August. Her mother noted a red circular lesion approximately 2 cm in diameter 3 days ago. It has increased in size slowly and now has central clearing. The girl has been outside a lot this summer but does not recall any tick bites. She is afebrile and has no other symptoms. You suspect Lyme disease. What is the next most appropriate step in management?

**A.** Order Lyme disease IgM
**B.** Treat with doxycycline
**C.** Order rapid strep test
**D.** Order complete blood count (CBC)
**E.** Refer to rheumatology for further evaluation

**9-64.** A 5-year-old girl is brought to the clinic in the summertime in Arkansas. Her mother is concerned because she has had a fever for 2 days and started complaining of a headache today. On physical exam, she is febrile and tachycardic, and you observe a petechial rash on her arms and legs with involvement of the palms and soles that her mother had not noticed before. Last week, she took a trip to a nearby lake to go fishing. Her symptoms are most likely due to an infection with which of the following?

**A.** *Borrelia burgdorferi*

**B.** *Rickettsia rickettsii*

**C.** *Trypanosoma cruzi*

**D.** *Streptococcus pyogenes*

**E.** Cytomegalovirus (CMV)

**9-65.** You are treating a previously healthy 4-year-old boy who was brought in by his mother with high fever with unclear focus for 3 days. He is not immunized. He was recently toilet trained in preparation for preschool attendance. He has been febrile despite acetaminophen and ibuprofen given regularly. His mother states that he has not been himself since the start of the illness with reduced oral intake. She noticed that since his admission to the hospital, he had 1 episode of incontinence and has had difficulty walking. On examination, you see an alert, oriented, well-hydrated child with normal ear, nose, and throat (ENT) exam and normal chest, abdominal, and joint exam. He is noted to have reduced vision on confrontation, complains of pain behind his neck, and keeps his legs folded when lying down. What is the next best step in managing this patient?

**A.** Obtain a complete blood count (CBC), C-reactive protein (CRP) level, and blood and urine cultures

**B.** Assess for papilledema and perform a lumbar puncture

**C.** Send blood cultures when he spikes his next temperature

**D.** Start on empiric broad-spectrum antibiotics

**E.** Treat with aspirin

**9-66.** A previously healthy 4-year-old boy was brought in with high fever with unclear focus for 3 days. He has been febrile despite acetaminophen and ibuprofen given regularly. His mother states that he has not been himself since the start of the illness with reduced oral intake. Since his admission to the hospital, he had 1 episode of incontinence and has had difficulty walking. On examination, you see an alert, oriented, well-hydrated child with normal ENT exam and normal chest, abdominal, and joint exam. You find no evidence of papilledema. He is noted to have reduced vision on confrontation, complains of pain behind his neck, and keeps his legs folded when lying down. You perform a lumbar puncture, which shows gram-negative coccobacillus, suggestive of *Haemophilus influenzae*. Which of the following is correct regarding this particular type of meningitis?

**A.** It is rare for children to have seizures during the course of the illness.

**B.** Administration of corticosteroids with antibiotics is effective in reducing the incidence of hearing loss.

**C.** Polycythemia and stroke are common due to decreased red blood cell destruction and increased blood viscosity.

**D.** Bacteremia with this organism is not associated with a petechial rash.

**E.** Approximately 75% to 95% of survivors can have sensorineural hearing loss.

**9-67.** You are seeing a recently adopted 1-year-old child for a well-child check with her new caregivers. Her parents do not report any complications with the birth; she was born at term and has been medically cleared to travel to the United States with vaccinations and screening complete blood count (CBC) and lead, which are both normal. Which of the following is true for testing for tuberculosis (TB)?

**A.** A tuberculin skin test (TST) is indicated if the incidence of TB in her country of origin is $< 20$ cases per 100,000.

**B.** A TST reaction of 6 mm is negative in a child with immunosuppression.

**C.** In children $< 2$ years old, chest radiograph (CXR) is more useful to detect disease than TST.

**D.** American Academy of Pediatrics recommends routine testing of interferon-$\gamma$ for children $< 2$ years old.

**E.** TST is required for children with known human immunodeficiency virus (HIV) infection or those with history of previous TB disease.

**9-68.** You are seeing a 4-month-old infant who was born at 35 weeks for a well-child visit. She is moving all her extremities and attempting to roll over. She is fixing and following objects past midline and is smiling. Her mother reports that she is not making any cooing sounds. She is playing with her hands and has recently started reaching for her toes. Her birth history was significant for jaundice and a rash, which improved in the first week after birth. What is the next best step in management of this child?

**A.** Follow in 2 months to ensure normal development and for vaccinations

**B.** Immediately refer for auditory brainstem response (ABR) testing

**C.** Refer to early childhood intervention (ECI)

**D.** Refer to ECI and perform an audiogram

**E.** Refer to speech therapy

**9-69.** A 16-year-old female patient undergoes liver transplantation for autoimmune hepatitis. Her initial postoperative course is uncomplicated. However, she returns to the hospital 9 months after transplant with fever and chills. Family reports a maximum temperature of 103°F. The patient reports nonspecific malaise and mild abdominal pain. Patient and family report adherence to all medications. Exam in the emergency department (ED) reveals a moderately ill-appearing adolescent woman febrile to 102.6°F with clear oropharynx, tachycardia with regular rhythm, tachypnea with clear lung exam, soft abdominal exam with mild generalized tenderness, and no peripheral edema. Chest x-ray (CXR), complete blood count (CBC), complete metabolic panel, urine culture, and blood cultures are ordered. Which additional test is most warranted in the initial workup of this patient?

**A.** Echocardiogram

**B.** Galactomannan assay

**C.** Magnetic resonance imaging (MRI) of the brain

**D.** Liver biopsy

**E.** Interleukin-6 levels

**9-70.** A 16-year-old boy from the northwest region of New Mexico presents to a local emergency department (ED) with right upper quadrant abdominal pain. Evaluation reveals cystic echinococcosis with a single large cyst in the liver. Cyst rupture can most commonly lead to which of the following?

**A.** Anaphylaxis

**B.** Hepatocellular carcinoma

**C.** Hepatitis A infection

**D.** Hemorrhage

**E.** Pancreatitis

**9-71.** A 34-year-old primigravida woman who works in a daycare gives birth to a small-for-gestational-age infant with jaundice and a petechial rash throughout his body. Which intrauterine infection is the most likely culprit?

**A.** Herpes simplex virus (HSV)

**B.** *Enterovirus*

**C.** Cytomegalovirus (CMV)

**D.** Group B *Streptococcus*

**E.** *Escherichia coli*

**9-72.** A 4-year-old boy from southern California is brought to the emergency department (ED) by his grandmother for 3 days of fever and cough. Grandmother reports the boy developed fever 3 days prior to presentation with a maximum temperature of 104°F on the morning of the presentation. He has also been complaining of generalized discomfort and headache. He has a worsening cough and eye redness. This morning, he was noted to have a rash behind his ears and neck. On exam, the boy is ill appearing. He is awake but irritable. He has mild tachypnea with intermittent cough. Oral exam reveals white dots with surrounding erythema on his buccal mucosa and injected conjunctiva with swelling of his eyelids. The boy's parents work as missionaries in sub-Saharan Africa and are currently not reachable, and his immunization status is unknown. This clinical presentation is most consistent with which viral illness?

**A.** Varicella

**B.** Coxsackie

**C.** Rubella

**D.** Mumps

**E.** Measles

**9-73.** An unvaccinated 8-year-old boy presents to the emergency department (ED) with fever and increasingly painful muscle spasms. On exam, a healing abrasion is noted on his right shoulder, which the family reports was obtained when the patient was scraped by a rake about 10 days ago while helping his family clean up leaves in the yard. The family considered seeking medical care at the time of injury to see whether stitches were needed as the wound was fairly deep, but bleeding stopped with pressure, so they chose to monitor at home. Tetanus is suspected. Which of the following treatments should be initiated?

**A.** Vancomycin plus a fourth-generation cephalosporin

**B.** Cyclobenzaprine

**C.** Tetanus immune globulin (TIG)

**D.** Dantrolene

**E.** DTaP

**9-74.** A 14-year-old Hispanic boy presents to your office with a 3-day history of fever, headache, and myalgias. He returned from a camping trip in the Smoky Mountains 10 days ago and denies any injury or exposures to wildlife. He has had fevers up to 104°F, diffuse myalgias, and severe headaches not responsive to analgesics. On exam, he appears generally fatigued and has a faint petechial rash on his ankles. Labs are notable for thrombocytopenia and hyponatremia. What is true about this patient's diagnosis?

**A.** Diagnosis is made based on history and clinical findings.

**B.** Specific serologic testing should be used to confirm diagnosis prior to initiating treatment.

**C.** Polymerase chain reaction (PCR) testing should be ordered to confirm diagnosis.

**D.** Immunofluorescent staining of skin biopsy specimens at the site of the rash has poor specificity and sensitivity for diagnosis.

**E.** Stool ova and parasite tests can confirm the diagnosis.

**9-75.** Which of the following is true regarding recommended screening for sexually transmitted infections (STIs)?

**A.** Routine annual screening for chlamydia, gonorrhea, and human immunodeficiency virus (HIV) should be offered to all sexually active females < 25 years of age.

**B.** Routine annual screening for infections such as syphilis, herpes simplex virus (HSV), and *Trichomonas* is recommended for females with high-risk sexual activity, even if asymptomatic.

**C.** At least 1-time screening for chlamydia and gonorrhea is recommended for all sexually active males < 25 years of age.

**D.** Routine annual screening for pharyngeal gonorrhea is recommended for men who have sex with men who have had receptive oral intercourse in the preceding year.

**E.** Routine annual screening for HIV is recommended for all sexually active males < 25 years of age.

**9-76.** A 5-year-old girl with history of renal transplant 2 years ago for end-stage renal disease from congenital nephrotic syndrome presents to the emergency department (ED) with a 2-day history of fever, chills, and complaints of pain with urination. Vital signs are temperature of 101.6°F, heart rate of 110 bpm, blood pressure of 99/62 mm Hg, respiratory rate of 16 breaths/min, and oxygen saturation of 98% on room air. Her medications include prednisone, tacrolimus, and mycophenolate. Initial lab work is notable for an absolute neutrophil count of 495; urinalysis shows > 50 WBCs and 2+ blood. She has history of prior febrile urinary tract infection. Last urine culture grew > 100,000 colony-forming units/mL of *Klebsiella*. While additional labs and urine culture are pending, which of the following would be the most appropriate empiric antibiotic regimen for this patient?

**A.** Vancomycin plus piperacillin-tazobactam

**B.** Meropenem

**C.** Cefepime

**D.** Ceftazidime

**E.** Vancomycin

**9-77.** A 3-year-old boy is brought to your office by his mother for concern of exposure to pulmonary tuberculosis (TB). The mother reports that the boy's grandfather, who had been visiting from Bangladesh until 2 weeks ago, was recently diagnosed with pulmonary TB. Your patient overall feels well and has no respiratory signs or symptoms. He was born in the United States and has never received the bacille Calmette-Guerin (BCG) vaccine. He has no known medical issues. Which of the following should be recommended for this patient?

**A.** Perform tuberculin skin test (TST) and initiate treatment with isoniazid if reactive area is at least 5 mm

**B.** Order an interferon-γ release assay (IGRA) (eg, QuantiFERON-TB) and initiate treatment with isoniazid if positive

**C.** Obtain chest radiograph (CXR) and initiate treatment if radiographic findings are suggestive of TB

**D.** Start isoniazid therapy for a minimum of 3 months

**E.** Start isoniazid therapy for a minimum of 9 months

**9-78.** Which of the following medications is generally recommended by experts as most effective for prevention of disseminated *Mycobacterium avium* complex (MAC) disease in human immunodeficiency virus (HIV) patients with CD4+ counts of < 100 cells/μL?

**A.** Azithromycin or clarithromycin

**B.** Rifabutin

**C.** Rifabutin plus clarithromycin

**D.** Ethambutol plus azithromycin

**E.** Isoniazid

**9-79.** A 14-year-old boy is brought in by his mother with a 4-day history of cough. He states that he occasionally feels warm. He last took acetaminophen 2 hours ago. Chest radiograph (CXR) shows hilar adenopathy but no focal consolidation. He recently returned from a camping trip to Tennessee and states he enjoyed exploring caves with his father. Which of the following fungal infections is he most likely to have?

**A.** Histoplasmosis

**B.** Mycobacteria

**C.** Coccidiomycosis

**D.** Blastomycosis

**E.** *Coccidioides*

**9-80.** A 12-year-old boy is seen in clinic to follow up on a bump on his right hand that has not improved since his last visit. He initially noticed the bump 2 weeks ago after gardening with his grandmother. On today's examination, his temperature is 37°C. Since his last visit, he has developed an additional bump and a red streak extending proximally from the bump. The bump is firm, mobile, and nontender. What treatment do you recommend?

**A.** Clindamycin

**B.** Itraconazole

**C.** Bacitracin

**D.** Close observation

**E.** Vancomycin

**9-81.** A 2-year-old girl presents with a neck mass that has been present for many weeks. Her mother is very worried because the mass has not improved. She recently completed a course of amoxicillin. On examination, she is a very active toddler. Her oropharynx is clear. There is no rhinorrhea or cough. A single, firm, nonmobile anterior cervical lymph node is palpated without pain. The overlying skin has a purplish hue. What is the treatment of choice?

**A.** Incisional biopsy

**B.** Clindamycin

**C.** Initiate RIPE therapy (rifampin, isoniazid, pyrazinamide, and ethambutol)

**D.** Continue amoxicillin

**E.** Excisional biopsy

**9-82.** You are in the nursery and caring for a 2-day-old female infant who was born at 37 weeks' gestation. She fails her hearing test. The medical student asks you if the baby could have congenital cytomegalovirus (CMV). Which of the following statements about CMV is correct?

**A.** Less than 5% of the population is seropositive.

**B.** CMV can only be acquired during the first trimester of pregnancy.

**C.** Children with CMV cannot transmit the infection to their parents.

**D.** Transmission occurs by direct or indirect contact with infected secretions.

**E.** Animals are its only reservoir.

**9-83.** A 10-day-old neonate presents to the pediatrician's office due to poor feeding. The mother states that the baby is sleeping more and she is having difficulty waking her up to feed. She was born full term via an uncomplicated spontaneous vaginal delivery. Her hospital course was notable for hyperbilirubinemia requiring 36 hours of phototherapy. On examination, her temperature is 36.4°C, she appears lethargic, her anterior fontanel is bulging, and her weight is down 14% from her birth weight. Additionally, you note a small blister on her scalp. You refer the baby to the emergency department (ED) for further evaluation. Which of the following is the most appropriate empiric treatment of choice?

**A.** Ampicillin and gentamicin

**B.** Ampicillin and ceftriaxone

**C.** Acyclovir alone

**D.** Acyclovir and cefotaxime

**E.** Ampicillin, gentamicin, and acyclovir

**9-84.** A baby is being examined in the newborn nursery following delivery. The neonate appears very small for gestational age. The baby is noted to have a "blueberry muffin" rash, jaundice, and hepatomegaly on examination. Which of the following is the best preventative measure against rubella?

**A.** Good handwashing

**B.** Vaccination

**C.** Administering hyperimmune globulin to pregnant women

**D.** Cesarean delivery

**E.** Intrapartum chemoprophylaxis of pregnant women

**9-85.** A 6-year-old boy presents with his mother to the clinic for evaluation of his abdominal pain. You send the eager medical student in to take a history and see the patient. She exits the room and comes to find you. She is concerned because while she was talking to the mother, the boy was crying and curled up in the fetal position. By the time you enter the room, the boy is sitting in the exam room comfortably. The mother states that he has been vomiting and not wanting to eat. The family recently emigrated from East Asia. Which of the following tests is most likely to confirm the etiology of the boy's symptoms?

**A.** Complete blood count (CBC)

**B.** Sputum sample

**C.** Stool sample

**D.** Abdominal ultrasound

**E.** Liver function tests

**9-86.** You are seeing a 3-year-old girl on the inpatient floor who was admitted due to dehydration. At handoff, you are told that she presented to the emergency department (ED) with fever, abdominal pain, and watery diarrhea. Mother reports that other children at daycare have been sick with similar symptoms. Initial laboratory tests reveal a sodium of 162 mEq/L, potassium of 3.1 mEq/L, and blood glucose of 54. She is on intravenous (IV) fluids. Stool culture results are positive for *Shigella dysenteriae*. Which of the following complications is she at risk of developing?

**A.** Hemorrhagic shock

**B.** Liver abscess

**C.** Sensorineural hearing loss

**D.** Irritable bowel syndrome

**E.** Hemolytic-uremic syndrome

**9-87.** Which of the following statements concerning gastrointestinal infections is correct?

**A.** The incidence of norovirus has greatly diminished secondary to routine vaccination.

**B.** *Clostridium difficile* diarrhea is commonly associated with daycare centers.

**C.** Viral agents are the most frequent cause of infectious diarrhea in children in developed countries.

**D.** Waterborne outbreaks are frequently caused by *Campylobacter* species.

**E.** *Listeria monocytogenes* is associated with ingestion of undercooked pork.

**9-88.** A 4-year-old previously healthy boy is admitted to the pediatric intensive care unit with respiratory failure.

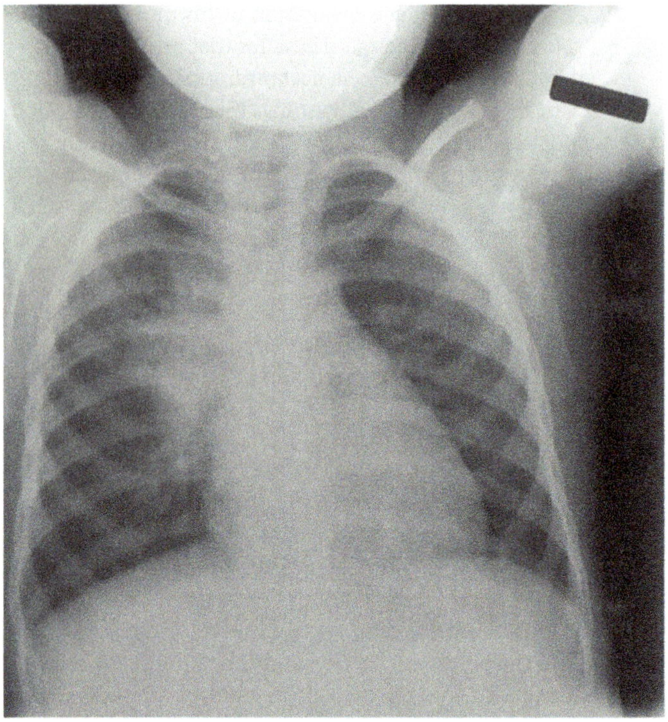

**FIGURE 264-2.** A chest radiograph from a child with early pulmonary tuberculosis demonstrating hilar adenopathy and perihilar infiltrate. (Mark W. Kline, *Rudolph's Pediatrics*, 23rd Edition. Copyright © McGraw-Hill Education. All rights reserved.)

His initial chest radiograph (CXR) is shown in Figure 264-2. The acid-fast stain of his gastric fluid is positive. The mother asks you how her son got sick. Which of the following is the most likely source?

**A.** Family member recently released from prison

**B.** Prior lung infection

**C.** The nurse caring for him in the hospital

**D.** Daycare

**E.** Travel to Puerto Rico

**9-89.** A 12-year-old girl presents with a rash on her upper body for the past 2 weeks. The rash is described as hypopigmented macules that coalesce on her chest, back, and upper arms. A skin scraping is obtained and examined under a microscope with potassium hydroxide (KOH). Microscopic examination reveals a "spaghetti and meatballs" appearance. What would you recommend as treatment to this patient?

**A.** Topical 2.5% corticosteroids

**B.** Topical 2.5% selenium sulfide shampoo

**C.** Oral cephalexin

**D.** Oral terbinafine

**E.** Topical emollients

**9-90.** A 2-month-old male infant presents to the emergency department (ED) because of poor feeding for the past week. He was born at term with an uncomplicated pregnancy and delivery course. His grandmother bought him a honey pacifier that he loves. He has not been sucking his pacifier or bottle as usual. His cry seems weak. He has not been moving as much. There is no report of a bowel movement in the past week. He has not had a fever. On examination, he has a weak cry and is hypotonic. He has a poor suck reflex. Deep tendon reflexes are normal. The examination is otherwise normal. What is most likely causing this infant's condition?

**A.** Hypothyroidism
**B.** Poliomyelitis
**C.** *Clostridium botulinum*
**D.** Guillain-Barré syndrome
**E.** Hirschsprung disease

**9-91.** You are called to examine an infant in the newborn nursery. On examination, the infant was found to have low birth weight, hepatosplenomegaly and cataracts. Multiple red-purple macular "blueberry muffin" lesions were all over the infant's body. The patient was diagnosed with congenital rubella. Which clinical scenario would be most consistent with an infant born with congenital rubella?

**A.** The mother was diagnosed with human immunodeficiency virus (HIV) at the time of delivery and found to have syphilis.
**B.** The mother was diagnosed with mononucleosis during pregnancy.
**C.** The mother received no prenatal care.
**D.** The mother has multiple cats in the home and was treated for lymphadenitis during the third trimester.
**E.** The mother was noted to have vesicular lesions on her genitals at the time of vaginal delivery.

**9-92.** A 3-year-old boy presents with a rash on his stomach for the past week. The rash started as 1 lesion on his stomach, and he now has multiple lesions on his stomach and chest. On physical examination, the lesions are flesh-colored, dome-shaped papules with an umbilicated center. What advice would you give for treatment?

**A.** Referral to dermatology
**B.** Topical hydrocortisone ointment
**C.** Topical ketoconazole cream
**D.** Reassurance that the condition is self-limited
**E.** Zinc pyrithione shampoo

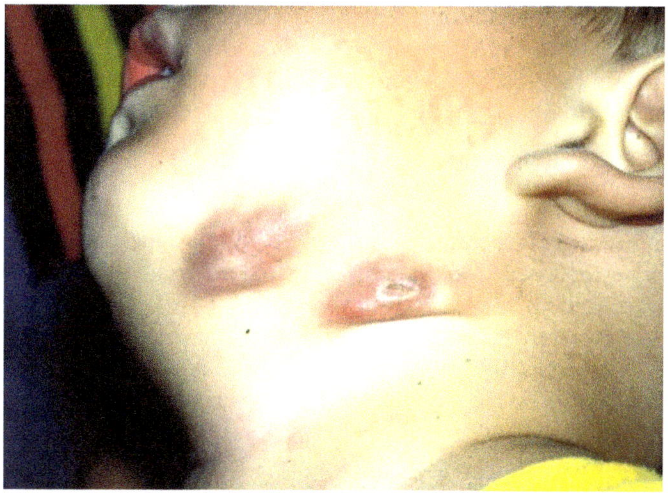

**FIGURE 265-1.** Cervical lymph nodes in a young child. (Mark W. Kline, *Rudolph's Pediatrics*, 23rd Edition. Copyright © McGraw-Hill Education. All rights reserved.)

**9-93.** A 2-year-old girl presents with new-onset fever and 1 month of neck swelling. She has no significant past medical history and no prolonged illnesses or hospitalizations. She has not been around any animals. On examination, she has a temperature of 102.3°F. There are 2 enlarged lymph nodes on the left submandibular area. They are nontender to touch, firm, and immobile. The skin overlying the nodes is a reddish-purple color (Figure 265-1). You have a high level of suspicion for your diagnosis. Which of the following tests should you order to confirm your diagnosis?

**A.** Group A streptococcal (GAS) rapid antigen detection test
**B.** *Bartonella henselae* polymerase chain reaction (PCR) test
**C.** Fluorescent antibody staining for *Yersinia pestis*
**D.** Serology testing for *Francisella tularensis*
**E.** Interferon-γ release assay (IGRA)

## ANSWERS

**Answer 9-1. D**

The patient has infectious croup (laryngotracheobronchitis); PIV is the most common cause of infectious croup in young children. There are 4 serotypes, with PIV-3 being the most prevalent. Other viruses may be involved less commonly, including RSV and adenovirus. With croup, PIV causes inflammation, edema, and necrosis of epithelium of the subglottic tissues. This results in the classic "barky" cough;

the cough is usually preceded by a few days of rhinorrhea and nasal congestion. In more severe cases, stridor, nasal flaring, and suprasternal or subcostal retractions may be observed. Corticosteroids are the mainstay of therapy, reducing severity and duration of symptoms.

*S aureus* is associated with bacterial tracheitis. With bacterial tracheitis, patients present with high fever and are ill appearing. Tracheoscopy usually demonstrates large amounts of mucopurulent secretions and subglottic edema, along with tracheal sloughing.

Now rarely seen due to widespread routine immunization, *H influenzae* type b was a common cause of epiglottitis, a life-threatening emergency due to inflammation and swelling of the epiglottis. In contrast to croup, patients appear severely ill, with fever, stridor, drooling, and often a "tripod" appearance (leaning forward and extending the neck to open the airway and increase air entry).

(Section 17: Infectious Diseases, Chapter 236: Viral Respiratory Infections Including Influenza)

**Answer 9-2.** C

The patient presents with community-acquired pneumonia. Although she presents with fever and cough, she is breathing comfortably (without retractions) and is not hypoxemic. Thus, an oral antibiotic prescribed in the outpatient setting is appropriate.

Differentiating between bacterial and viral pneumonia is often difficult. The patient in the vignette has a lobar consolidation, which correlates more with a bacterial pneumonia; mild interstitial and perihilar changes are more likely seen in viral pneumonia.

The Pediatric Infectious Diseases Society, in conjunction with the Infectious Diseases Society of America, has published guidelines addressing the approach to community-acquired pneumonia, including criteria for admission, diagnostic testing, and treatment options. Amoxicillin is the first-line oral antibiotic choice for uncomplicated community-acquired pneumonia in patients < 5 years old. This is targeted at *Streptococcus pneumoniae*, the most common bacterial etiology. In patients > 5 years of age, one must also take into consideration atypical pathogens, such as *Mycoplasma pneumoniae* or *Chlamydia pneumoniae*. In this case, azithromycin may be an appropriate option.

Although supportive care is appropriate in cases of viral pneumonia (which is more common than bacterial pneumonia), the focal findings on exam and lobar infiltrate on CXR suggest a bacterial etiology.

(Section 17: Infectious Diseases, Chapter 235: Community-Acquired Pneumonia in Children)

**Answer 9-3.** A

*H capsulatum* is an endemic dimorphic fungi that, in the United States, lives in the soil mainly in the areas around the Ohio and Mississippi River valleys. Respiratory infection related to histoplasmosis usually presents over the course of weeks with fever, malaise, cough, dyspnea, and lymphadenopathy. Lung cavitation may occasionally be seen. Diagnostic methods include culture of tissue or bronchoalveolar lavage fluid, histopathology of a lymph node, or antigen detection in urine or serum. Itraconazole is first-line treatment for pulmonary histoplasmosis.

Pulmonary blastomycosis tends to cause more acute symptoms, similar to bacterial pneumonia. *Coccidioides* is found mainly in the southwestern United States, including Arizona, New Mexico, and California. *Cryptococcus* causes opportunistic infections in immunocompromised patients. *Paracoccidioides* is endemic to Central and South America.

(Section 17: Infectious Diseases, Chapter 295: Histoplasmosis)

**Answer 9-4.** D

The patient in the vignette has *Pneumocystis jirovecii* pneumonia (PJP), evidenced by nonproductive cough, tachypnea, and hypoxemia. PJP occurs in immunocompromised hosts (patients with AIDS, malignancy, or primary immunodeficiency or on immunosuppressive agents). Patients who are immunocompromised should be on PJP prophylaxis, with the first-line agent being trimethoprim-sulfamethoxazole. Diagnosis is made by obtaining sputum or bronchoalveolar lavage fluid and involves cytologic staining (Grocott's methenamine silver staining), direct fluorescent antibody testing, or molecular testing (polymerase chain reaction [PCR]). First-line treatment for PJP is intravenous (IV) trimethoprim-sulfamethoxazole. Alternative (but possibly less effective) agents include pentamidine, dapsone, atovaquone, or clindamycin-primaquine.

(Section 17: Infectious Diseases, Chapter 237: Fungal Respiratory Infections)

**Answer 9-5.** C

*P aeruginosa* is a non–lactose-fermenting, oxidase-positive, gram-negative rod that is frequently multidrug resistant. It plays an important role in patients with CF, causing more rapid decline in lung function once acquired. By about age 18, 50% of CF patients have acquired *Pseudomonas*; by adulthood, it is the highest prevalent organism. Other populations at risk for acquiring *Pseudomonas* infection include immunosuppressed or immunocompromised patients, patients with tracheostomy tubes, and diabetics. In CF, a "mucoid" form can predominate. Development of biofilms can make the organism difficult to eradicate, evading immune responses such as phagocytosis and resisting antimicrobial killing. Person-to-person transmission can occur, and contact isolation precautions are recommended for caregivers of patients with CF. Due to the relative multidrug resistance of the organism, it is sometimes recommended to choose 2 antibiotics simultaneously for treatment for CF exacerbation. There are 4 general classes of antibiotics used to treat exacerbations: β-lactams, aminoglycosides, fluoroquinolones, and colistin.

(Section 17: Infectious Diseases, Chapter 244: Anaerobic Infections)

**Answer 9-6.** B

Respiratory syncytial virus (RSV) is the leading cause of viral lower respiratory tract disease in infants, and RSV bronchiolitis is the most common cause of hospitalization in infants. Passive immunoprophylaxis is available for those at highest risk of severe morbidity, in the form of a monoclonal antibody. Palivizumab is a humanized mouse monoclonal immunoglobulin. The AAP routinely updates its guidelines regarding who should receive palivizumab. Current recommendations include the following:

- In the first year of life, palivizumab is recommended for infants born at < 29 weeks 0 days of gestation.
- In the first year of life, palivizumab prophylaxis is recommended for preterm infants born at < 32 weeks, 0 days of gestation with a requirement for > 21% oxygen for at least 28 days after birth.
- In the first year of life, palivizumab prophylaxis is recommended for infants with hemodynamically significant congenital heart disease.
- In the second year of life, palivizumab prophylaxis is not recommended, except for children who required at least 28 days of supplemental oxygen after birth and who continue to require medical intervention (supplemental oxygen, chronic corticosteroid, or diuretic therapy).
- Monthly prophylaxis should be discontinued in any child who experiences a breakthrough RSV hospitalization.
- RSV prophylaxis may be considered in other pulmonary diseases; however, there are insufficient data to recommend routine prophylaxis in Down syndrome or cystic fibrosis (CF).

(Section 26: Disorders of the Cardiovascular System, Chapter 481: Cardiovascular Issues in the Child and Adolescent)

**Answer 9-7.** C

The patient in the vignette has primary cilia dyskinesia (PCD), evidenced by chronic sinusitis, recurrent otitis media, chronic productive cough, and situs inversus (with heart sounds on the right). The primary defect in most patients with PCD is a structural defect in the motile cilia. Motile cilia have a classic "9+2" configuration. Cilia line the nasal tract, tracheobronchial tree, and reproductive tract. Recurrent sinopulmonary infections are a result of immotile or malfunctioning cilia.

Allergic rhinitis results from hypersensitivity to aeroallergens. Allergic rhinitis usually has a temporal association and does not result in daily symptoms. Cystic fibrosis (CF) is caused by a genetic defect that results in abnormalities in the structure and function of the cystic fibrosis transmembrane conductance regulator (CFTR) protein, which regulates chloride and sodium transport. This leads to a net increase in water absorption, with reduction in the airway surface liquid and the mucus in the airways becoming stickier. Due to the effects of dysfunctional CFTR in the pancreas, the majority of patients with CF will have problems with malabsorption of nutrients and poor weight gain.

(Section 27: Disorders of the Respiratory System, Chapter 503: Disorders Causing Airway Obstruction)

**Answer 9-8.** E

The patient meets criteria for allergic bronchopulmonary aspergillosis (ABPA). ABPA is a hypersensitivity reaction to *Aspergillus fumigatus* antigens colonizing the respiratory tract. It is seen in roughly 10% of patients with cystic fibrosis (CF) or steroid-dependent asthma. Clinically, patients present with productive cough, wheezing, and dyspnea as a result of mucus plugging. Bronchiectasis, along with central nodules, may be seen on CT scan. Criteria for ABPA include elevated serum IgE and at least 2 of the following: specific antibodies to *A fumigatus*, radiographic findings consistent with ABPA, and peripheral eosinophilia. The key to therapy is treating the immune response; thus, corticosteroids are the mainstay treatment. Antifungals (ie, itraconazole), used adjunctively, have been shown to improve outcomes and possibly lessen the duration of steroid therapy.

(Section 17: Infectious Diseases, Chapter 237: Fungal Respiratory Infections)

**Answer 9-9.** B

The child has *M pneumoniae*, which causes "walking pneumonia." The most common route of transmission of *M pneumoniae* from person to person is by inhalation of respiratory droplets expelled through coughing. It is commonly seen in closed settings, such as school, daycare, or college dormitories. *M pneumoniae* is a common cause of community-acquired pneumonia. The treatment of choice is oral azithromycin.

(Section 17: Infectious Diseases, Chapter 268: *Mycoplasma* Infections)

**Answer 9-10.** D

Based on the history and physical exam, the child is most likely to have norovirus infection. Since introduction of the rotavirus vaccine, norovirus has emerged as the leading cause of infectious enteritis in children < 5 years of age in the United States. Norovirus is highly contagious and easily spreads among daycare and household contacts. It typically causes vomiting and watery diarrhea and resolves with supportive care. Young children are more susceptible to dehydration due to fluid losses.

There are 2 oral live attenuated rotavirus vaccines licensed in the United States. The vaccine schedule depends on product used. RV5 vaccine is administered as a 3-dose series for infants at age 2 months, 4 months, and 6 months. RV1 vaccine is administered as a 2-dose series with doses given at ages 2 months and 4 months. The 8-month-old infant in the vignette should be fully immunized against rotavirus because he is up to date on his vaccinations.

*Shigella* can be associated with daycare attendance but typically results in frequent small-volume stools with mucus and blood associated with abdominal cramping and tenderness. Fecal leukocytes are 90% specific in differentiating bacterial from nonbacterial causes of enteritis and would be expected to be positive with gastroenteritis due to *Shigella*. Infected infants are more likely to be severely dehydrated and hypothermic.

*C difficile* is a spore-forming, obligate anaerobic, gram-positive bacillus. Manifestations of disease are mediated by toxins A and B. *C difficile* is typically associated with antimicrobial use. Infants and children are more likely to carry *C difficile* in the gastrointestinal tract asymptomatically. Up to 33% of infants and children < 2 years of age are asymptomatic carriers. Fecal leukocytes would also be expected to be positive.

Ova and parasite infections typically do not present with acute symptom onset or fever. For patients with watery diarrhea who are ≤ 5 years old (or their contacts) or who are involved in daycare outbreaks, *Cryptosporidium* and *Giardia* antigen testing can be considered. Traditional ova and parasite examination should be considered for patients who are residents of or visitors from developing countries or areas of North America where infections caused by worms are reported with some frequency.

(Section 17: Infectious Diseases, Chapter 221: Diagnostic Approaches to Infectious Diseases, Chapter 231: Gastrointestinal Infections, Chapter 278: Salmonella, Shigella, and Escherichia coli, Chapter 245: Clostridial Infections)

**Answer 9-11. B**

Endemic typhus (also known as murine typhus or flea-borne typhus) is caused by *Rickettsia typhi* or *Rickettsia felis* transmitted to humans via infected feces from the rat or cat flea. Infection can occur via a flea bite or by inoculation of flea feces into the skin by scratching or through broken skin. The incubation period is 1 to 2 weeks and symptoms include abrupt onset of fever, headaches, chills, nausea, myalgias, and emesis. A rash occurs in 20% to 80% of patients and can appear 6 to 7 days after fever onset. The rash is typically macular or maculopapular. Associated laboratory findings can include hyponatremia, thrombocytopenia and elevation of liver transaminases. The patient's exposure to a stray cat is consistent with likely exposure to the cat flea, as is the timing of the exposure. Thrombocytopenia and elevation of liver transaminases are also consistent laboratory findings. Recommended treatment for all ages includes doxycycline.

*Neisseria meningitidis* are gram-negative aerobic diplococci that can be found in the human respiratory tract. Infection can lead to respiratory tract infection or pneumonia, with invasive disease leading to bacteremia and/or meningitis. Peak colonization occurs in adolescents and young adults. Risk factors for invasive disease include smoking, crowded living conditions, underlying immune defects, and concurrent viral respiratory tract infection. Meningitis without sepsis can occur in 50% of cases, with symptoms including fever, headache, and neck stiffness. Sepsis occurs in 5% to 10% of patients and presents with petechial or purpuric rash with fulminant presentation of circulatory collapse, coagulopathy, and disseminated intravascular coagulation.

Cat scratch disease, caused predominately by *Bartonella henselae*, is typically associated with a prolonged regional lymphadenitis, often associated with an inoculation site papule, after a cat scratch or bite. *Bartonella* are fastidious, slow-growing, pleomorphic, gram-negative Proteobacteria. Cats, especially kittens < 1 year of age, are the major reservoir and tend to have prolonged, asymptomatic intraerythrocytic bacteremia. They infect humans by scratch, bite, or mucous membrane (conjunctival, respiratory) inoculation.

EBV (a member of the family Herpesviridae) is the major cause of infectious mononucleosis. Most EBV infections are thought to be spread through saliva. EBV is excreted in oropharyngeal secretions and is transmitted by contact with saliva via kissing or other mucosal contact with contaminated objects. The incubation period of EBV infectious mononucleosis is 30 to 50 days. The clinical syndrome of EBV infectious mononucleosis is usually preceded by a 3- to 5-day prodrome of malaise, fatigue, headache, nausea, abdominal pain, or some combination of these symptoms. Over the next 7 to 20 days, sore throat and fever gradually increase. The triad of fever, sore throat, and posterior cervical adenopathy occurs in > 80% of symptomatic patients. Sore throat is often accompanied by evidence of moderate-to-severe pharyngitis, with marked tonsillar enlargement. A blanching, erythematous, maculopapular exanthema occurs in about 5% to 15% of patients, but as many as 80% develop this rash if treated with ampicillin or other β-lactam antibiotics.

Enteroviruses constitute a genus within the Picornaviridae family of viruses. Infection occurs via fecal–oral or respiratory route. The onset of the illness is typically abrupt with fever (≥ 38°C) in combination with 1 or multiple signs and symptoms: poor feeding, lethargy, irritability, emesis, diarrhea, abdominal pain, and upper respiratory tract symptoms. Approximately 25% of patients develop an exanthem. Undifferentiated febrile illness typically lasts < 5 days. In *Enterovirus* infections, fever may be biphasic in nature with an intervening period of euthermia. On physical examination, findings are absent or minimal and may consist of mild pharyngeal and conjunctival injection, lymphadenopathy, and exanthems. Illness may involve respiratory, gastrointestinal, neurologic (ie, meningitis), or cardiac manifestations. Other than a rash, this patient's clinical course and exam findings lack typical characteristics of *Enterovirus* infection.

(Section 17: Infectious Diseases, Chapter 289: Rickettsial Infections, Chapter 270: Neisseria Meningitides, Chapter 252: Cat Scratch Disease (Bartonella henselae), Chapter 306: Epstein-Barr Virus Mononucleosis, Chapter 301: Enterovirus and Parechovirus Infections)

**Answer 9-12.** E

*N gonorrhoeae* is the second most commonly reported bacterial sexually transmitted infection (STI) in the United States. *N gonorrhoeae* is a gram-negative bacterium that typically appears as diplococci on Gram stain. The majority of gonorrhea infections in men and women are asymptomatic and found on routine screening. Endocervicitis is the most common clinical manifestation of gonorrhea in women. Urethritis is another clinical presentation in women but is often associated with endocervicitis. In men, urethritis is the most common clinical manifestation of gonorrhea. Of particular note is the serious condition of disseminated gonococcal infection (DGI), a bloodborne infection that has been classically described as a triad of petechial or pustular skin lesions, polyarthralgia, and tenosynovitis but may also manifest as septic arthritis alone (culture-positive joint fluid in approximately 50% of cases only), which occurs in 2% to 5% of gonorrhea-infected individuals, or involvement of joint and skin alone, known as the arthritis-dermatitis syndrome. Complications of DGI include meningitis and endocarditis, which are very rare. DGI is more common in African Americans than in other race/ethnicity groups. Direct diagnosis of gonorrhea by nucleic acid amplification tests (NAATs) is the preferred method because NAAT sensitivity is superior to culture but varies by the type of NAAT. US Food and Drug Administration (FDA)–approved NAATs are available for vaginal, endocervical, and urine testing for women, and urine and urethral testing for men. Culture retains an important role in gonorrhea management due to antimicrobial resistance issues. Treatment of DGI, including arthritis and tenosynovitis, includes ceftriaxone 1 g intravenous (IV) or intramuscularly (IM) every 24 hours along with azithromycin (empirically for chlamydia). Treatment should continue for a minimum of 7 days.

*N meningitidis* would not be distinguishable on Gram stain from *N gonorrhoeae* and should be considered initially in this patient. Meningococci are transmitted by aerosol or contact with secretions and colonize the respiratory mucosa. Focal spread can lead to respiratory tract infection, including pneumonia. Invasion through epithelial surfaces leads to bloodstream dissemination, allowing the bacteria to seed the meninges, pericardium, or large joints. Meningitis without shock occurs in about 50% of cases (higher in developing countries) and is indistinguishable from other forms of purulent meningitis. Bacteria are isolated from the blood in up to 75% of cases. Meningococcal sepsis occurs in 5% to 10% of patients and is characterized by fever and petechial or purpuric rash. This can progress to fulminant meningococcal septicemia (purpura fulminans) and is associated with rapid growth of meningococci in the bloodstream. Patients present with severe, persistent shock with little or no signs of meningitis. Focal infections occur less frequently and include septic arthritis, purulent pericarditis, conjunctivitis, urethritis, osteomyelitis, primary peritonitis, and endophthalmitis.

Although also sexually transmitted, *H ducreyi*, a small, fastidious, gram-negative rod, causes chancroid and typically presents with painful genital ulcer(s) and tender suppurative inguinal lymphadenopathy. It does not cause diffuse rash or arthritis/arthralgias.

Among the Enterobacteriaceae, *Salmonella* and *Shigella* are important causes of gastroenteritis. In addition, they can cause extraintestinal disease. Most illness begins with fever, malaise, anorexia, and occasionally vomiting or headache. Diarrhea usually begins as watery diarrhea and may progress within hours or days to dysentery. Physical findings include fever, systemic toxicity, increased bowel sounds, and lower abdominal tenderness. The white blood cell (WBC) count is usually elevated. Leukemoid reactions with as many as 50,000 cells/μL occasionally occur. A variety of complications of shigellosis occur. Dehydration, hypoglycemia, hyponatremia, hypernatremia, and hypokalemia can occur; hypoglycemia and hyponatremia are associated with an increased mortality rate. Seizures are a common extraintestinal manifestation and occur exclusively in children. Bacteremia is uncommon in healthy children but is more common with human immunodeficiency virus (HIV) infection and severe malnutrition. In about half of bacteremic children, there may be polymicrobial bacteremia caused by other organisms that have traversed the injured gut. Extraintestinal suppurative complications such as osteomyelitis, meningitis, septic arthritis, and splenic abscess are rare. The lack of diarrhea and patient's age make *Shigella* unlikely.

Bacteremia and mesenteric adenitis are the rule with *Salmonella typhi* but much less common with other nontyphoid *Salmonella*. Nontyphoidal *Salmonella* is one of the most commonly reported bacterial causes of foodborne outbreaks in the United States. *S typhi* is very rare in developed countries. In the United States, the highest incidence of nontyphoid *Salmonella* infection is in the first year of life. Thereafter, rates of infection decline rapidly by age 5 years and remain constant throughout adulthood. The range of clinical manifestations of *Salmonella* infection includes asymptomatic infection, gastroenteritis, bacteremia, focal infection, urinary tract infection, and enteric fever. Diarrhea is the most common manifestation of salmonellosis. This patient's lack of diarrhea and age make *Salmonella* bacteremia and invasive disease less likely. Lack of travel outside the United States would also make *S typhi* infection extremely unlikely.

(Section 17: Infectious Diseases, Chapter 228: Sexually Transmitted Infections, Chapter 278: Salmonella, Shigella, and Escherichia coli; Chapter 270: Neisseria meningitidis)

**Answer 9-13.** D

This patient is at high risk for measles infection. Risk factors include presumed lack of immunity (< 12 months so would not have received measles-mumps-rubella [MMR] vaccine) and recent international travel. Symptoms and time of onset are also consistent with potential measles infection.

The incubation period for measles, the time from infection to clinical disease, is approximately 10 days to the onset of fever and 14 days to the onset of rash, but can range from 8 to 21 days from exposure to rash onset.

The rash initially presents as discrete, irregular, erythematous macules behind the ears, on the neck, and along the hairline. The rash then spreads caudal over the ensuing 24 hours to involve the face, trunk, and arms. Persons with measles are infectious for several days before and after the onset of rash, when levels of measles virus in blood and body fluids are highest and when the symptoms of cough, coryza, and sneezing are most severe. These symptoms facilitate virus spread. Measles can also lead to complications including otitis media, bronchopneumonia, laryngotracheobronchitis (croup), and diarrhea, as well as acute encephalitis. Measles virus can be isolated from urine as late as 1 week after rash onset, and viral shedding may be prolonged in children with impaired cell-mediated immunity.

Measles virus is transmitted primarily by respiratory droplets over short distances and, less commonly, by small-particle aerosols that remain suspended in the air for long periods of time. Airborne transmission appears to be important in certain settings, including schools, pediatricians' offices, hospitals, and enclosed public places, and infectious droplets may persist for several hours after an infected child has left a pediatrician's office.

In addition to standard precautions, airborne transmission precautions are indicated for 4 days after the onset of rash in otherwise healthy children and for the duration of illness in immunocompromised patients.

Additional infectious etiologies to consider in this patient include respiratory virus infections such as parainfluenza and adenovirus.

Parainfluenza virus (PIV) symptoms can range from upper respiratory infection to croup, bronchiolitis, and pneumonia, depending on the serotype. Overall, croup is the most common associated diagnosis. Croup begins with an upper respiratory infection of several days in duration, followed by hoarseness and a "barking seal" croupy cough. Inspiratory stridor and marked retractions are evident in more severe infections. Fever is usually mild. Most children recover after 48 to 72 hours, but some children progress to severe airway obstruction. Person-to-person transmission of PIV occurs via direct contact with large-droplet aerosols or fomites, and illness follows an incubation period of 2 to 6 days. Interestingly, about 25% of children with measles have co-infection with PIV.

In addition to standard precautions, contact precautions are recommended for hospitalized infants and young children diagnosed with parainfluenza for the duration of illness.

Adenoviruses are some of the most common viruses that cause febrile respiratory illnesses in children. The incubation period for respiratory tract infection varies from 2 to 14 days. The usual duration of illness is then 5 to 7 days, although symptomatology can last up to 2 weeks. Infants and children most commonly manifest upper respiratory infection symptoms with conjunctivitis, otitis media, coryza, or pharyngitis, and less commonly manifest croup or a pertussis-like syndrome. Adenovirus disease can also present with exanthem.

In addition to standard precautions for young children with respiratory tract infections, contact and droplet precautions are indicated for the duration of hospitalization in children with respiratory adenoviral infection.

(Section 17: Infectious Diseases, Chapter 220: Infection Control and Prevention, Chapter 311: Measles, Chapter 236: Viral Respiratory Infections Including Influenza)

**Answer 9-14.** **B**

The most common route of transmission of pathogens in the healthcare setting is via contact with contaminated hands, body sites, or objects. Organisms are carried from the hands of one person to another and are frequently implicated in the transmission of bacteria, fungi, parasites, and viruses. Proper hand hygiene removes most organisms transiently carried on the hands and is therefore the key component of all infection prevention programs.

A variety of fomites can be involved in the transmission of infectious agents, including stethoscopes, patient care equipment, and toys. All have been cultured and shown to harbor pathogens. These pathogens can then be spread from the fomites to the hands of healthcare providers or body surfaces of patients. These fomites serve as potential reservoirs of pathogens if not disinfected appropriately between patients.

Direct contact between children and caregivers transmits skin organisms such as bacteria, fungi, and mites.

Some pathogens are aerosolized in small or large droplets. Small droplets can be carried by air currents, remain suspended, and infect persons at longer distances than large droplets, which require relatively close contact (within a few feet) in order for the droplet to move from one person to the next.

Transmission of pathogens by food or water is rare in the healthcare setting; however, outbreaks related to contaminated foods, products, or medications have been reported. Intrinsic or extrinsic contamination of IV fluids, oral or tube feedings, and medications is an occasional cause of healthcare-associated infection.

(Section 17: Infectious Diseases, Chapter 220: Infection Control and Prevention)

**Answer 9-15.** **D**

A child traveling to a malaria-endemic area with chloroquine resistance should not be placed on chloroquine. Because this child is < 8 years of age, doxycycline is not a recommended source of prophylaxis. Artemether/lumefantrine is prescribed for treatment of malaria, not used for prophylaxis. Although atovaquone/proguanil can be prescribed, given the daily dose and the longer length of travel, mefloquine is preferred. Mefloquine is the prophylaxis of choice for adults and children traveling to a *Plasmodium falciparum* chloroquine-resistant area for > 4 weeks.

(Section 17: Infectious Diseases, Chapter 347: Malaria)

**Answer 9-16.** A

Loperamide, which is an antimotility drug, should not be used in children for the treatment of acute diarrhea. This child can be treated with oral hydration to prevent dehydration because she is well appearing. Given that this child is well-hydrated, supportive therapy with oral hydration is recommended. Antibiotics are not indicated in uncomplicated gastroenteritis with *Salmonella* because treatment with antibiotics may result in prolonged shedding or a carrier state. After rehydration, children should be given an unrestricted age-appropriate diet; hence, the BRAT diet is not recommended.

(Section 17: Infectious Diseases, Chapter 231: Gastrointestinal Infections)

**Answer 9-17.** C

Routine vaccination with DTaP, HiB, IPV, Hep B, rotavirus, and PCV13 is recommended. Hep A is contraindicated for children under the age of 12 months. MMR is recommended for this patient given that there is travel outside of the United States. Because this dose is administered before 12 months of age, it will not count as part of the 2-dose series.

(Section 17: Infectious Diseases, Chapter 239: Immunizations)

**Answer 9-18.** B

Because this child is under the age of 5 years and is from a TB-endemic region, he would need screening for *Mycobacterium tuberculosis* infection. Furthermore, because he is under the age of 5, the preferred testing methodology consists of TST (Figure 264-7). The IGRA is not recommended to be used for screening in children under the age of 2 years. Induced sputum and early morning nasogastric aspirates are techniques used to obtain sputum for culture. Culture is used for diagnosis of TB disease and not infection.

(Section 17: Infectious Diseases, Chapter 264: Tuberculosis (Mycobacterium tuberculosis))

**Answer 9-19.** E

Because this child is 5 years of age and is relatively healthy, he does not need HiB or PCV13 vaccination. Because he received 4 doses of DTaP with the fourth dose after his fourth birthday he does not need an additional DTaP. DTP is different from DTaP in that it contains whole-cell pertussis versus the acellular version that is used in the United States. He does not need MMR because he has received 2 doses of MMR both above the age of 12 months, with the doses being at least 1 month apart. He does need a polio dose because he did not receive a dose after his fourth birthday.

(Section 17: Infectious Diseases, Chapter 239: Immunizations)

**Answer 9-20.** B

This child is presenting with the Romaña sign (unilateral periorbital edema, conjunctivitis, and preauricular lymphadenitis), which is a clinical manifestation of acute Chagas disease. Chagas disease is caused by the protozoa *Trypanosoma cruzi* (Figure 350-5).

*T cruzi* has the highest prevalence of infection in Bolivia, Argentina, Venezuela, and Brazil. Chagas disease can occur in 3 phases: acute, latent, and chronic. In many patients (~95%), the acute infection symptoms can be mild or even absent. The presenting symptoms of acute infection can include a chagoma (nodular skin reaction) or the Romaña sign. With severe acute infection, children can present with myocarditis or meningoencephalitis. The acute phase lasts about 2 to 3 months, and then the patient can enter the latent phase, which can last anywhere from 10 to 40 years with good health. Chronic cardiomyopathy is the most common symptom of chronic Chagas disease followed by digestive tract disorders.

First-line treatment for *T cruzi* consists of benznidazole given that it is better tolerated. Nifurtimox can also be used for the treatment of Chagas disease, although it is less well tolerated. Both drugs need to be obtained through the Centers for Disease Control and Prevention (CDC) because neither drug has been approved through the US Food and Drug Administration (FDA). Treatment is indicated for those under the age of 18 years. Treatment can reduce parasitemia and reduce the severity and length of illness, which is why supportive therapy alone is not indicated.

Albendazole is indicated for nematode, cestode, or trematode infection and not for protozoan infection (Chapter 318). Itraconazole is used for fungal infections and not for the treatment of protozoan infections (Chapter 242).

(Section 17: Infectious Diseases, Chapter 350: Trypanosomiases, Chapter 318: Antiparasitic Therapy, Chapter 242: Antifungal Therapy)

**Answer 9-21.** A

Because this child is 4 years of age and has not had her hepatitis A, she should receive her first dose of hepatitis A during this visit. Because she is also 4 years of age, she needs her 4-year-old DTaP and IPV booster doses at this visit. Yellow fever vaccine is a live vaccine virus, and this child received a dose 2 weeks prior, so this child should not receive the MMR or varicella vaccination at this visit. Two live vaccines can be given on the same day, but if not given on the same day, then the 2 live vaccines need to be 4 weeks apart. This is because if there is active circulating antibody, then it can interfere with the replication of the live vaccine, leading to a subpar immune response.

(Section 17: Infectious Diseases, Chapter 239: Immunizations, Chapter 302: Viral Hemorrhagic Fevers)

**Answer 9-22.** C

This child likely has visceral larva migrans due to *Toxocara* given the hepatomegaly, eosinophilia, dog exposure, and wheezing. Toxocariasis can occur covertly without visceral or ocular involvement. Given the pica, this is less likely to be

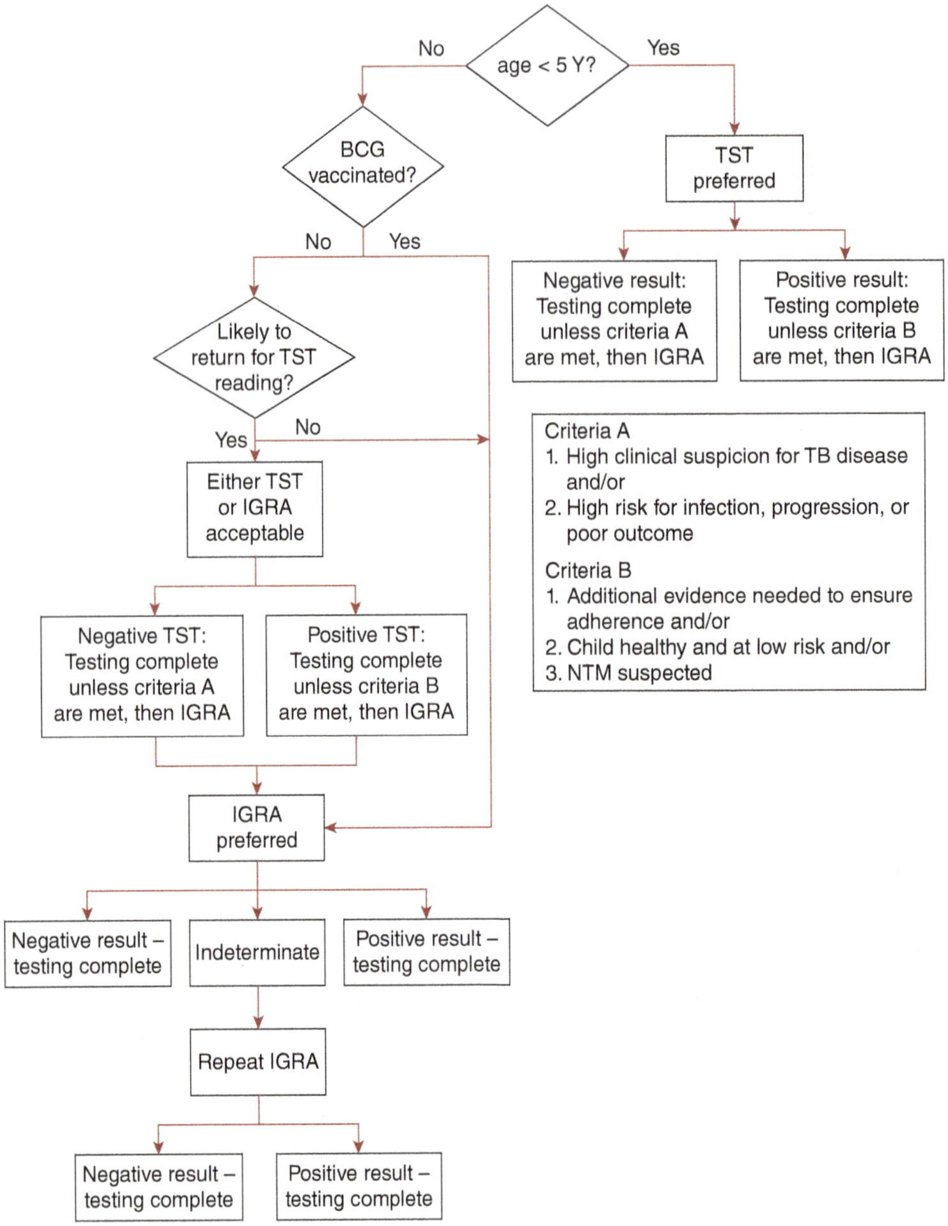


**FIGURE 264-7.** An algorithm provided for the use of tuberculin skin tests (TSTs) and interferon-γ release assays (IGRAs) in children with at least 1 risk factor for tuberculosis (TB) infection. BCG, bacille Calmette-Guérin; NTM, nontuberculous *Mycobacterium*. *New data may allow lowering the age for use of IGRAs to children as young as 2 years. Readers should consult a current edition of the American Academy of Pediatrics Red Book for best advice. (Reproduced with permission from Starke JR; Committee On Infectious Diseases. *Pediatrics*: Interferon-γ release assays for diagnosis of tuberculosis infection and disease in children, 2014 Dec;134(6):e1763-e1773.)

allergic, and RAST is not indicated. Stool ova and parasites is not indicated because *Toxocara* larvae cannot complete their life cycle in humans and will not secrete eggs. Pulmonary function testing will give the function, but not the etiology of the wheezing. IGRA is used for tuberculosis (TB) testing, which is less likely given the presentation. Persistent eosinophilia, hypergammaglobulinemia, and elevated ESR support the diagnosis of *Toxocara*.

(Section 17: Infectious Diseases, Chapter 326: Toxocariasis (Visceral and Ocular Larva Migrans))

**Answer 9-23. D**

This child likely has aseptic meningitis secondary to West Nile virus (WNV). The bulk of the transmission occurs during August to September, with the season starting in July and ending in December. Given the aseptic meningitis picture, a full 14-day course of antibiotics is probably not necessary. It is reasonable to treat with antibiotics until the CSF culture results are confirmed as negative. Given the clinical presentation, the patient is less likely to have herpes simplex virus (HSV) and more likely to have WNV. Most likely, this child will have

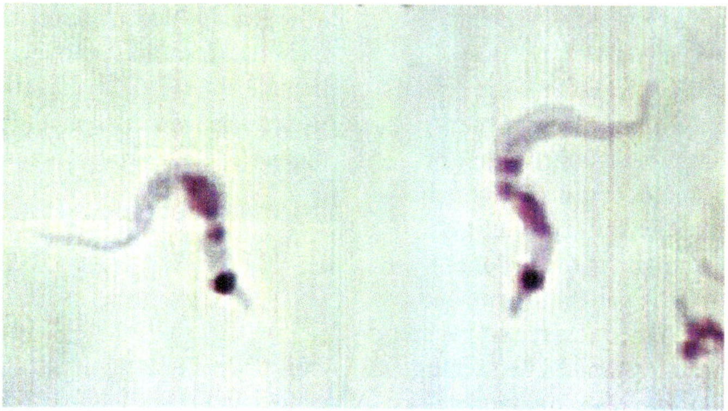

**FIGURE 350-5.** *Trypanosoma cruzi* in peripheral blood smear. (Mark W. Kline, *Rudolph's Pediatrics*, 23rd Edition. Copyright © McGraw-Hill Education. All rights reserved.)

a self-limited disease and will improve. However, children or adults who present with WNV encephalitis (eg, altered sensorium, seizures, parkinsonian and other movement disorder features) are more likely to have residual symptoms.

(Section 17: Infectious Diseases, Chapter 300: Arboviruses)

**Answer 9-24.** E

This 15-year-old girl likely presents with Guillain-Barré syndrome after Zika infection. Although Zika virus has been associated with congenital defects, there also has been an association with Guillain-Barré. Her recent travel to Brazil and her symptoms are concerning for Zika virus infection. Although *C jejuni*, EBV, *M pneumoniae*, and influenza A are all associated with Guillain-Barré, the presenting symptoms are more consistent with Zika. The rash associated with Zika typically is noted on the trunk and can spread to the arms, face, legs, soles, and palms.

(Section 17: Infectious Diseases; Chapters 300, 561, and 268 and https://www.cdc.gov/pregnancy/zika/testing-follow-up/testing-and-diagnosis.html)

**Answer 9-25.** B

Based on the history and physical, this patient has bilateral otitis media without severe symptoms. Severe symptoms are defined as a toxic-appearing child, fever ≥ 39°C in the past 48 hours, persistent otalgia for > 48 hours, and unreliable follow-up. Therefore, because the patient is < 2 years old and she has bilateral AOM, the most appropriate antibiotic treatment is amoxicillin. Any patient who is 6 months to < 2 years old with bilateral AOM with or without severe symptoms qualifies for antibiotic treatment. Initial observation would not be appropriate. She has not taken any antibiotics in the past 30 days, which makes the first-line choice of antibiotics amoxicillin in this case. If the patient had taken amoxicillin in the past 30 days or was presenting with otitis-conjunctivitis syndrome, then amoxicillin–clavulanic acid would have been the first-line choice for antibiotic treatment. Additionally, this patient meets criteria for recurrent AOM and should be referred to ENT for evaluation for PETs. The definition of recurrent AOM is ≥ 3 separate well-documented episodes of AOM in the past 6 months or ≥ 4 episodes in a 12-month period with at least 1 episode in the preceding 6 months. This child would benefit from a hearing screen, but it would be more appropriate to refer after recovering from her current illness and the ENT evaluation.

(Section 17: Infectious Diseases, Chapter 238: Infection of the Middle Ear)

**Answer 9-26.** E

The patient in this vignette has the diagnosis of right hip septic arthritis. It is considered an orthopedic emergency due to the risk of long-term orthopedic complications. Joint aspiration is the most important part of the diagnostic evaluation. Synovial fluid should be sent for Gram stain, aerobic cultures, and cell count with a leukocyte differential. The most common organism causing septic arthritis in all age groups is *S aureus*, both methicillin-sensitive *S aureus* and methicillin-resistant *S aureus* (MRSA). In children < 4 years old, *S aureus*, *Streptococcus pyogenes*, *K kingae*, and *S pneumoniae* are the most common causes. In children > 4 years, *S aureus* and *S pyogenes* are the most common pathogens. *N gonorrhoeae* is more commonly found in neonates or sexually active adolescents. *Pseudomonas* can cause septic arthritis in the case of a penetrating injury with a nail. In the past, HiB was the most prominent causative agent, but now it is rare due to routine vaccination with the HiB vaccine.

(Section 17: Infectious Diseases, Chapter 229: Bone, Joint, and Soft Tissue Infections)

**Answer 9-27.** C

The correct counseling for a patient with a chlamydia infection is to return 3 months after treatment for repeat testing. This testing will allow detection of reinfection of this patient if there has been repeated exposure to an infected partner. Test of cure within a few weeks after treatment is not routinely performed except in cases of questionable adherence to treatment, persistent symptoms, or repeat exposure to chlamydia. In fact, a NAAT can remain positive for up to 3 weeks after successful treatment due to nonviable chlamydia organisms, and this can cause false-positive results. Any patient who has been treated for chlamydia should be advised to abstain from sexual activity for at least 7 days after a single-dose azithromycin treatment or until he or she has completed a 7-day course of one of the alternative antibiotic treatment options. Treatment for chlamydia and screening for other sexually transmitted infections (STIs) are recommended for any of the patient's sexual partners in the past 60 days. If the patient has not had sexual activity in the past 60 days, then the most recent partner beyond that time should receive treatment and STI screening. IUDs are not considered a risk factor for pelvic inflammatory disease.

(Section 17: Infectious Diseases, Chapter 228: Sexually Transmitted Infections)

**Answer 9-28.** **D**

The 23-valent pneumococcal polysaccharide vaccine (PPSV23) is used for children at least 2 years of age who are at high risk of invasive pneumococcal disease. Children aged 2 to 18 years old with chronic heart disease, chronic lung disease, diabetes mellitus, cerebrospinal fluid (CSF) leak, and cochlear implants should receive the recommended series of 13-valent pneumococcal vaccine (PCV13) first and then a total of 1 dose of PPSV23 at least 8 weeks after the most recent PCV13. Children aged 2 to 18 years old with sickle cell and other hemoglobinopathies, anatomic or functional asplenia, congenital or acquired immunodeficiency, human immunodeficiency virus (HIV) infection, chronic renal failure, nephrotic syndrome, malignant neoplasms, leukemia, lymphoma, Hodgkin disease, other diseases treated with immunosuppressive drugs or radiation therapy, solid organ transplantation, or multiple myeloma all require the recommended series of PVC13 and then 2 doses of PPSV23. The first dose of PPSV23 should be given at least 8 weeks after the most recently administered PCV13, and the second dose should be given at least 5 years after the first dose of PPSV23.

(Section 17: Infectious Diseases, Chapter: 239 Immunizations)

**Answer 9-29.** **A**

Airborne precautions require a fit-tested N95 or higher-level respirator for healthcare personnel and a single room with negative airflow for isolation of the patient. The air comes from the hallway into the room and exits to the outdoors to a high-efficiency particulate air filtration system. Airborne precautions are used to prevent the transmission of pathogens such as *M tuberculosis*, measles virus, and varicella-zoster virus. For droplet precautions, patients are placed in a single room or placed together in one room if they have the same infection. Masks should be worn when entering the room to provide patient care. Droplet precautions are required for illnesses transmitted by droplets such as influenza, pertussis, or adenovirus. Contact precautions include wearing gloves and gowns to prevent transmission of pathogens spread by contact as well as for patients colonized with multidrug-resistant bacteria. Common pathogens requiring contact precautions include enteric pathogens (eg, norovirus, rotavirus, *Shigella*, *Clostridium difficile*), methicillin-resistant *Staphylococcus aureus* (MRSA), and vancomycin-resistant *Enterococcus*.

(Section 17: Infectious Diseases, Chapter 220: Infection Control and Prevention)

**Answer 9-30.** **C**

This patient is at high risk of developing a *C difficile*–associated disease (CDAD) due to his immunocompromised state, recent treatment with antibiotics, and prolonged hospitalization. The diagnosis is made by detecting the *C difficile* toxin in the stool. Asymptomatic colonization occurs frequently in neonates and young infants, and current guidelines recommend not testing children < 1 year of age. A 10-day course of metronidazole is the best choice for initial treatment in most patients. Up to 40% of patients experience a relapse after discontinuing initial therapy with metronidazole; however, a second course of the same antibiotic treatment will cure up to 90%. Patients with hypoalbuminemia or severe manifestations (ie, toxic megacolon, intestinal perforation, or bacteremia) should receive vancomycin as the first-line treatment for CDAD. Those who have failed treatment with metronidazole twice also should receive vancomycin. Fecal transplantation has been used successfully in refractory cases. In the hospital, contact precautions should be used for patients with *C difficile*. Alcohol-based hand hygiene products are not sporicidal and should not be used to prevent spread of this illness. Hand washing with soap and water and glove use are the most effective means to prevent transmission.

(Section 17: Infectious Diseases, Chapter 245: Clostridial Infections)

**Answer 9-31.** **B**

This patient has staphylococcal scalded skin syndrome. It is caused by exfoliative toxins, enterotoxins A and B, produced by *Staphylococcus aureus*. Patients present with fever, irritability, and tender erythema of the skin, most marked in the flexural areas and around the mouth and nose. Additionally, perioral and periocular crusting with radial fissures is a characteristic feature. Within 12 to 24 hours of the onset, flaccid blisters and superficial erosions form, which may be followed by widespread superficial peeling of the skin, most often seen in infants. Erythema multiforme is a hypersensitivity reaction confined to the skin and/or mouth, with the most common cause being herpes simplex virus (HSV). Typical lesions begin as erythematous macules that rapidly change into erythematous edematous plaques. In Stevens-Johnson syndrome (SJS) mucosal lesions are most prominent. Painful erosions occur on the lips and mucous membranes including ocular, genital, and anal mucosae. Extensive eruption of erythematous macules and papules with superimposed blisters and erosions on the face, trunk, extremities, and genitalia is associated with SJS and typically involves 10% of the body surface area. Toxic epidermal necrolysis is similar to SJS with full-thickness epidermal necrosis but involves > 30% of body surface area. Kawasaki disease is a vasculitis with systemic inflammation defined by fever of at least 5 days in duration and 4 of the following features: changes in extremities, polymorphous exanthem, bilateral conjunctival injection, changes in lips and oral cavity, and cervical lymphadenopathy.

(Section 17: Infectious Diseases, Chapter 279: Staphylococcal Infections; Section 18: Disorders of the Skin, Chapter 362: Skin Infections and Exanthems)

**Answer 9-32. D**

This patient has Rocky Mountain spotted fever (RMSF) based on his presentation with the classic triad of fever, headache, and centrifugal petechial rash. The fever is usually abrupt in onset and high grade. The skin rash begins to appear on average 2 to 3 days after the onset of illness. However, only 50% of people have a rash during the first 3 days of illness, and 5% of children never develop a rash. The history of exposure to ticks is present in only 3% to 18% of patients at their initial evaluation. In this patient, determining whether there was tick exposure is not necessary to start the appropriate treatment. A clinician who suspects this diagnosis based on history and exam should not delay treatment. Doxycycline and tetracycline are the agents of choice for RMSF and other rickettsial infections and can be given to treat patients of all ages. It is not advisable to wait to start treatment until the rash appears or to exclude this possible diagnosis based on lack of tick exposure or exposure to the geographically endemic areas. The diagnosis of RMSF must be based on only the history and physical exam findings because specific laboratory tests may not become positive until the second week of infection. Specific serologic testing should be performed to confirm a diagnosis of RMSF but would not be positive at the time of this patient's presentation. Some laboratory abnormalities that can be seen, but are not diagnostic for this illness, are thrombocytopenia, hyponatremia, leukopenia, and elevated liver enzymes. This illness is not transmitted from person to person via airborne transmission and does not require airborne precautions or isolation. Instead, it is transmitted by ticks. The tick must be attached to the human host for at least 6 hours to transmit the disease.

(Section 17: Infectious Diseases, Chapter 289: Rickettsial Infections)

**Answer 9-33. C**

This patient has cat scratch disease caused by *Bartonella henselae*. Cutaneous inoculation of *B henselae* is cat (especially kitten) related in 90% of cases, 50% to 75% of which occur via a scratch or bite. The typical cat scratch disease presentation involves a tender solitary lymph node or group of nodes at a single site with overlying skin erythema. These nodes appear from 1 week to 1 to 2 months after inoculation. Between 30% and 50% of patients will have an elevated temperature, which can be accompanied by malaise, anorexia, night sweats, and headache. The nodes involved usually are the ones that drain the upper extremities, head, neck, and groin. PCR of the lymph node or pus aspirate, primary skin lesion, or other tissue is a highly sensitive and specific diagnostic tool. It is particularly useful when serology is negative and a diagnosis is urgent. Biopsy of the lymph node shows a characteristic but nondiagnostic histologic picture with epithelioid granuloma and Langerhans giant cells. Imaging such as ultrasound is also nonspecific. Serologies are likely to be negative in this patient because she is early in her disease course. Both IFAT and EIA antibodies develop slowly; thus, seroconversion may occur only after ≥ 3 weeks of illness.

(Section 17: Infectious Diseases, Chapter 252: Cat Scratch Disease [Bartonella henselae])

**Answer 9-34. D**

This infant has acute purulent chlamydial neonatal conjunctivitis. The treatment of choice is oral erythromycin 50 mg/kg/d in 4 divided doses daily for 14 days. Topical treatment of chlamydia-associated neonatal conjunctivitis is not recommended because local eye treatment does not prevent or clear nasopharyngeal carriage and thus results in further risk of developing pneumonia or repeat episodes of conjunctivitis. For this reason, prophylaxis with topical erythromycin or tetracycline regimens applied to the eyes shortly after delivery has not been highly effective because it does not eliminate nasopharyngeal colonization and increases the risk for pneumonia.

The typical incubation period is 5 to 12 days, in comparison to *Neisseria gonorrhoeae* conjunctivitis, which typically occurs in the first 2 to 5 days after birth. This chlamydial infection may be diagnosed by culture, immunofluorescence, or enzyme-linked immunosorbent assay. Nucleic acid amplification tests (NAATs) are not an approved diagnostic tool, and point-of-care testing does not currently exist for this illness. Warm compresses and massage are indicated in the treatment of eye discharge related to nasolacrimal duct stenosis.

(Section 17: Infectious Diseases, Chapter 254: Chlamydia)

**Answer 9-35. A**

Not being able to use penicillin as the first-line drug complicates matters, but there are several options available. Amoxicillin is readily available and close in function to penicillin, although it has more drug resistance. Because our patient does not have documented penicillin allergy, it would be appropriate to start the amoxicillin while throat culture is pending. Azithromycin is often used in the treatment of group A β-hemolytic *Streptococcus*, but mostly for those allergic to penicillin or who would like the course over with in a timely fashion; it is very important to finish the course. Vancomycin is available oral and IV but is used for more serious bacterial infections such as pneumonia or meningitis; oral vancomycin is given in *Clostridium difficile* infection. A third-generation cephalosporin, such as cefdinir, would also cover for strep throat and provide broader coverage of other upper respiratory infections. Clindamycin may be an option for recurrent strep infection or if concerned about abscess formation.

(Section 17: Infectious Diseases, Chapter 280: Streptococcus Group A Infections)

**Answer 9-36.** C

Roseola and rubella are viral exanthems. Roseola infantum is a common acute febrile illness of infants and young children characterized by 3 to 5 days of fever followed by rapid defervescence and the appearance of an erythematous macular or maculopapular rash. The patient in the clinical scenario is a teenager and still had an elevated temperature upon re-presentation. Rubella is quite uncommon in the United States now due to the available vaccine but presents with low-grade fevers, sore throat, malaise, and coryza. Patients may also have joint involvement and paresthesia, neither of which our patient has described. A rash is also present but is slighter than the one that may present in infectious mononucleosis.

The incubation period of Epstein-Barr virus (EBV) infectious mononucleosis is 30 to 50 days. The clinical syndrome of EBV infectious mononucleosis is usually preceded by a 3- to 5-day prodrome of malaise, fatigue, headache, nausea, abdominal pain, or some combination of these symptoms. Over the next 7 to 20 days, sore throat and fever gradually increase. The triad of fever, sore throat, and posterior cervical adenopathy occurs in > 80% of symptomatic patients. Sore throat is often accompanied by evidence of moderate-to-severe pharyngitis, with marked tonsillar enlargement that may be covered with shaggy gray or white exudate. Throat cultures are positive for group A β-hemolytic streptococci in about 30% of patients, which may represent accompanying disease or pharyngeal colonization in patients with EBV infectious mononucleosis. Fever is present in 85% to 95% of patients, from 39°C (102°F) up to 40.5°C (105°F), and on average lasts 10 days but may persist for weeks. Fatigue and lymphadenopathy may persist longer. Adenopathy most often involves only the bilateral posterior cervical nodes but may involve any node, including anterior cervical, epitrochlear, or even generalized lymph nodes. Enlarged lymph nodes may be affected singly or in groups (not necessarily symmetrical) and may be very large or small (the size of grapes); they are most often firm, discrete, and moderately tender to palpation. Splenomegaly, defined as the largest dimension greater than the 95th percentile per age, often results in a spleen that is palpable 2 to 3 cm below the costal margin, and this occurs in about 50% of patients with EBV infectious mononucleosis. Massive splenomegaly may occur, usually defined operatively as a spleen extending well into the left lower quadrant or pelvis or that has crossed the midline of the abdomen and that weighs at least 500 to 1000 g. Rupture is rare but can be a potentially fatal complication. Hepatomegaly occurs in 10% to 30% of patients, but < 5% of patients develop jaundice. Serum aspartate aminotransferase (AST) and serum lactate dehydrogenase (LDH) are mildly elevated in the majority of patients and may persist for weeks to months. A blanching, erythematous, maculopapular exanthema occurs in about 5% to 15% of patients, but as many as 80% develop this rash if treated with ampicillin or other β-lactam antibiotics.

There is an approximate 30% chance that the patient presenting with mononucleosis also has strep throat, either concurrently or via colonization with group A β-hemolytic *Streptococcus* bacteria. However, this patient has been treated appropriately for at least a week with antibiotics without much change in status; in fact, it seems he is clinically progressing now with rash, splenomegaly, fatigue, and exudative pharyngitis. In a patient with infectious mononucleosis, β-lactam antibiotics can increase the chance of the morbilliform rash described in the vignette to 85%.

Penicillin/amoxicillin reactions, if significant, will usually present immediately, around day 4 of therapy, or around day 8. This could theoretically be one of those situations if it were not for the other symptoms described, and the patient would likely be clinically improved while on the therapy for diagnosis.

(Section 17: Infectious Diseases, Chapter 306: Epstein-Barr Virus Mononucleosis)

**Answer 9-37.** D

Besides lymphadenopathy, infectious mononucleosis usually presents with fever, malaise, and sore throat. The child in the vignette did not have any of these symptoms. In addition, the lymph nodes are usually not draining in infectious mononucleosis.

*S pyogenes* would present with acute pharyngitis symptoms rather than an enlarged cervical lymph node alone. There usually would be fever, sore throat, and physical findings of erythematous and enlarged tonsils along with cervical lymphadenopathy. It usually would not present as a single node either, but rather a collection of lymph nodes. The child in the vignette did not have findings other than that of the single enlarged lymph node.

Glandular tularemia is reported more commonly in children, who often present with tender lymphadenopathy and no history of ulceration or other skin lesion. In some cases, the ulcer is not recognized before it heals spontaneously and patients present with lymphadenopathy alone. The regional lymphadenopathy in both ulceroglandular and glandular tularemia is very tender, with erythema of the overlying skin and eventual suppuration in some cases. Young children commonly have involvement of the lymph nodes in the neck. This child's lymph nodes were not tender, and he had no history of contact with ticks.

Typical cat scratch disease, caused by *B henselae*, is probably the most common cause of prolonged subacute regional lymphadenitis in children. Cutaneous inoculation of *B henselae* is cat (especially kitten) related in 90% of cases, 50% to 75% of which occur via scratch or bite. A few days to a few weeks later, often unrecognized by the patient, a 2- to 5-mm erythematous, nonpainful papule appears at the inoculation site in up to two-thirds of patients and persists for a few weeks;

*B henselae* can be found in these lesions. When inoculation is presumably respiratory and involves mucous membranes (especially about the head and neck), inoculation lesions are absent. The hallmark of typical cat scratch disease is chronic regional lymphadenitis in a node or nodes draining the site of inoculation. Most frequently, cat scratch disease involves a solitary lymph node or a group of nodes at a single site, while only rarely will cat scratch disease manifest as generalized adenopathy. Usually tender initially and often remaining tender, these nodes appear from 1 week to 1 to 2 months after inoculation. Size may vary from 1 to 2 cm to 5 to 10 cm, and erythema of the overlying skin may occur. Suppuration occurs in 10% to 20% of cases, and drainage of pus due to breakdown of overlying skin may persist for weeks. Cat scratch disease usually involves the nodes draining the upper extremity, head, neck, and groin, but any lymph node location is possible. Epitrochlear lymphadenopathy with or without axillary adenopathy is typical, although not pathognomonic, of cat scratch disease.

Tuberculosis (TB) of the superficial lymph nodes is the most common form of extrapulmonary TB in children. Most cases occur within 6 to 9 months of the initial infection, although some cases appear years later. The tonsillar, anterior cervical, and submandibular nodes become involved secondary to extension of a primary lesion of the upper lung fields or abdomen. Disease is most often unilateral, but bilateral involvement may occur. As infection progresses, multiple nodes are affected, resulting in a mass of matted nodes. Systemic signs and symptoms other than low-grade fever are usually absent. The chest radiograph is usually normal, although adenopathy in the chest may be apparent.

(Section 17: Infectious Diseases, Chapter 252: Cat Scratch Disease [Bartonella Henselae])

**Answer 9-38.** E

Lymph node biopsies are called for if the patient has had the lesion for about 4 weeks or it enlarges rapidly, even with intervention such as antibiotics. Biopsies are recommended if blood work and CXR do not provide an etiology. If the patient in the question had prolonged fevers, weight loss, night sweats, fatigue, bone pain, or abnormal labs, this would also indicate the need for a biopsy. This patient could be given antibiotics for treatment, but it is often not needed and the lesion has only been noted for 3 days. CXR and blood work could be done if the lesion is growing, painful, or troublesome in any way or for the parent's peace of mind. However, at 3 days, it is perfectly reasonable to wait and see if it resolves on its own. Therefore, observation would be the most correct next step.

(Section 23: Disorders of the Blood, Chapter 436: The Spleen and Lymph Nodes)

**Answer 9-39.** A

The difference between length of therapy depends on whether the patient has herpes simplex virus (HSV) infection limited to the skin/eye/mouth (SEM) or central nervous system (CNS)/neurologic manifestations of disease. Clinical manifestations of CNS disease include seizures (focal or generalized), lethargy, irritability, tremors, poor feeding, temperature instability, and bulging fontanel. Between 60% and 70% of babies classified as having CNS disease have associated skin vesicles at some point in the disease course. Patients with SEM disease receive 2 weeks of IV acyclovir, and those with CNS disease receive 21 days of IV acyclovir; they both need to continue afterward with oral acyclovir treatment for 6 months. Our infant in the clinical scenario does not present with neurologic difficulties. The diagnosis of neonatal HSV infection requires that conjunctivae, oral, and anal swabs (surface specimens) be sent for HSV culture, along with an additional swab of any cutaneous lesion. Cerebrospinal fluid (CSF) and whole blood should be obtained and sent for HSV polymerase chain reaction (PCR) as well. In addition, surface swabs may be sent for HSV PCR. The diagnosis of SEM disease is determined by the recovery of HSV from the surface swabs with or without positive blood PCR, normal CSF indices, negative CSF HSV PCR, and no evidence of disseminated disease (eg, no thrombocytopenia, elevated alanine aminotransferase [ALT], coagulopathy, or pneumonitis).

Observation in this case can delay care and have lasting negative effects on this patient. The description of the lesions does not depict a bacterial infection, and the infant has no signs of fever, spreading erythema, or induration, so clindamycin and mupirocin for this reason would not be warranted.

(Section 17: Infectious Diseases, Chapter 304: Herpes Simplex Virus Infections)

**Answer 9-40.** C

Based on history and physical exam, this patient most likely has chancroid, a sexually transmitted infection (STI) caused by *Haemophilus ducreyi*. Although HSV is a more common cause of genital ulcers among sexually active youth in the United States, chancroid can occur, particularly in association with sporadic outbreaks. Clinical manifestations of chancroid include painful genital ulcer and tender suppurative lymphadenopathy. Patients with chancroid also have a higher prevalence of HIV and syphilis. Presumptive diagnosis of chancroid can be made when all of the following criteria are met:

- One or more painful genital ulcers
- Negative dark-field examination of the ulcer exudate or negative syphilis serology within 7 days
- Regional inguinal adenopathy
- Negative HSV test from ulcer exudates

Current treatment options for chancroid are any of the following:

- Azithromycin 1 g orally once
- Ceftriaxone 250 mg intramuscular (IM) once
- Ciprofloxacin 500 mg orally twice a day for 3 days
- Erythromycin base 500 mg orally 3 times a day for 7 days

A single dose of azithromycin would be the appropriate choice for this patient. Erythromycin could also be prescribed, but single dosing of erythromycin would not be appropriate, as stated earlier. Clindamycin can be an option for other infections, including bacterial vaginosis, but is not appropriate for chancroid. Podofilox gel can be used for topical treatment of condyloma acuminatum, the skin lesions caused by human papillomavirus (HPV).

Although this patient is already aware of his HIV status, he should also be tested for syphilis. A syphilis chancre is typically a painless, indurated ulcer (instead of the painful chancroid seen in this patient). Penicillin is the treatment of choice for syphilis.

(Section 17: Infectious Diseases, Chapter 228: Sexually Transmitted Infections, Chapter 283: Syphilis)

**Answer 9-41.** B

Work restrictions for illness in healthcare personnel vary according to the condition. The intern has been diagnosed with shingles, or herpes zoster, with lesions located on her lower back. Zoster is a reactivation of the varicella-zoster virus. Unlike primary varicella-zoster virus infection (chickenpox), which is typically transmitted via aerosolized nasopharyngeal secretions or direct contact with skin lesions, zoster is largely transmitted via direct contact with skin lesions. Therefore, if the zoster lesions in a healthcare worker can be covered, the worker may continue to care for immunocompetent patients while practicing standard hand hygiene. He or she should continue to cover the lesions until they crust over. Despite covering the lesions, the healthcare worker should be restricted from care of immunocompromised patients. If the lesions cannot be covered, the worker should be restricted from all patient care. Immunocompromised patients can present in the hospital or the outpatient setting. In this scenario, the intern has lesions localized to her back, which she can keep covered. Therefore, the correct answer is B.

(Section 17: Infectious Diseases, Chapter 220: Infection Control and Prevention, Table 220-2)

**Answer 9-42.** D

This child was born in Liberia, West Africa, after minimal prenatal care. She presents with chorioretinitis, obstructive hydrocephalus, intraparenchymal calcifications, hepatomegaly, hypotonia, and history of a "blueberry muffin–like" rash. The most likely diagnosis for this patient is congenital toxoplasmosis infection, caused by the coccidian parasite *Toxoplasma gondii*. The classic triad of congenital toxoplasmosis is chorioretinitis, intracranial calcifications (often intraparenchymal), and obstructive hydrocephalus. This triad is most commonly found in children who were not treated prenatally and/or in other countries that have more virulent strains of *T gondii*. The seroprevalence rates of *T gondii* range from < 10% in some European countries to 60% to 80% in South America and Africa, where this child was born. Other clinical manifestations of congenital toxoplasmosis include rashes (maculopapular rash, petechiae, purpura, and "blueberry muffin" rash), hepatosplenomegaly, myocarditis, pneumonitis, thrombocytopenia, anemia, hepatitis, and cholestasis. Neurologic manifestations vary and can include hypotonia, seizures, sensorineural hearing loss, lethargy, and other motor abnormalities.

Microcephaly, which can be seen in congenital Zika virus infection, congenital rubella syndrome, and congenital CMV infection, is not typically seen in congenital toxoplasmosis infection.

Although congenital CMV can manifest with sensorineural hearing loss, "blueberry muffin" rash, and hepatosplenomegaly, the intracranial calcifications are typically periventricular. In the patient described, the calcifications are intraparenchymal.

Congenital rubella syndrome can also present with delayed milestones and "blueberry muffin" rash. However, it is often associated with cataracts and congenital heart defects, which are not seen in this patient.

(Section 17: Infectious Diseases, Chapter 349: Toxoplasmosis, Chapter 305: Cytomegalovirus, Chapter 315: Rubella)

**Answer 9-43.** E

It is important to understand how to screen for TB and interpret results. Screening in asymptomatic individuals can be done with either a TST or an IGRA. A TST involves intradermal injection of 0.1 mL of purified protein derivative; the results are interpreted 48 to 72 hours after injection. To interpret the results, the transverse diameter of induration is measured. The diameter of erythema is not used to interpret results. Once the diameter of induration is measured, the patient's risk factors are considered when interpreting a result as positive or negative. See Table 264-1.

In this scenario, the patient is 17 years old, previously healthy, asymptomatic, and born in the United States; has no known infectious contacts; and has not started working in the healthcare setting yet. He has no risk factors, and his area of induration is < 5 mm. Therefore, his TST is negative. He does not need follow-up tests at this time. There are no concerns for TB infection. Therefore, he may participate in the school's healthcare program.

(Section 17: Infectious Diseases, Chapter 264: Tuberculosis [Mycobacterium tuberculosis], Table 264-1)

**Answer 9-44.** D

This adolescent's clinical presentation is consistent with infectious mononucleosis, which is most commonly caused by Epstein-Barr virus (EBV). Infectious mononucleosis typically presents clinically with a 3- to 5-day period of fatigue, headache, abdominal pain, and/or nausea. Sore throat and fever gradually occur and increase over the next 7 to 20 days. Infectious mononucleosis has a classic triad of sore throat, fever, and bilateral posterior cervical lymphadenopathy and is seen in > 80% of symptomatic patients. Pharyngitis

**TABLE 264-1.** Amount of Induration that Defines a Positive Mantoux Tuberculosis Skin Test

| Reaction Size | Risk Factors |
|---|---|
| 5 mm | Contacts of infectious cases |
| | Abnormal chest radiograph |
| | Human immunodeficiency virus infection or other immunocompromised state |
| ≥ 10 mm | Birth or previous residence in a high-prevalence country |
| | Certain medical risk factors: diabetes mellitus, silicosis, renal disease |
| | Occupation in healthcare field; exposure to tuberculosis patients |
| | Member of a locally defined high-risk group |
| | Close contact of a high-risk adult (except healthcare workers) |
| | Age < 4 years |
| ≥ 15 mm | No risk factors |

Mark W. Kline, *Rudolph's Pediatrics*, 23rd Edition. Copyright © McGrawHill Education. All rights reserved.

often is characterized by tonsillar enlargement, tonsillar exudates, and occasionally fine petechiae along the soft palate and uvula. Splenomegaly can occur, although splenic rupture is rare. Approximately 80% of individuals with infectious mononucleosis who are treated with a β-lactam (eg, amoxicillin) develop a blanching, morbilliform rash, as seen in this scenario. EBV is the major cause of infectious mononucleosis. EBV can also cause Burkitt lymphoma, a fast-growing lymphoma of B cells that can involve the abdomen, lymph nodes, head and neck, bone marrow, and/or central nervous system (CNS).

CMV can also cause infectious mononucleosis and can be clinically indistinguishable from EBV IM. However, EBV is the most common cause of infectious mononucleosis in this age group. Congenital CMV infection can cause congenital microcephaly.

Group A β-hemolytic *Streptococcus* can also cause pharyngitis with tonsillar exudates and palatal petechiae, fever, malaise, and abdominal pain. However, it is not typically associated with splenomegaly. Group A β-hemolytic *Streptococcus* can also cause superficial pyoderma (impetigo), as well as precipitate a postinfectious glomerulonephritis.

Upper respiratory viruses, such as adenovirus, can also cause fever, pharyngitis, and enlarged cervical lymph nodes. However, this adolescent's presentation is more consistent with infectious mononucleosis. Adenovirus can cause keratoconjunctivitis.

(Section 17: Infectious Diseases, Chapter 306: Epstein-Barr Virus Mononucleosis, Chapter 236: Viral Respiratory Infections Including Influenza, Chapter 280: Streptococcus Group A Infections, Chapter 305: Cytomegalovirus)

**Answer 9-45. A**

This presentation is consistent with infant botulism, which is caused by the release of neurotoxin from ingested spores of *Clostridium botulinum* that germinate in the colon. This toxin binds and produces a presynaptic blockade at the peripheral cholinergic junctions, preventing release of acetylcholine. This causes flaccid paralysis that is symmetric. The toxin does not, however, cross the blood–brain barrier, so infants will have a paradoxical alertness. The ingested spores are usually from an unidentified source; however, spores have been identified in corn syrup and honey. Honey is not recommended for infants under the age of 12 months. The median age at presentation is 16 weeks, and diagnosis is made by identifying the toxin in the stool. Early treatment of infant botulism maximizes efficacy. As a result, the decision to treat should be based on clinical presentation, not laboratory test results. A stool or enema specimen can eventually be submitted to a state laboratory or the Centers for Disease Control and Prevention (CDC). Treatment is BabyBIG®, a human botulism antitoxin/IgG. The Infant Botulism Treatment and Prevention Program (IBTPP) can be contacted at 510-231-7600 to consult with an IBTPP clinical specialist, who is available 24 hours/day.

Blood cultures are not routinely recommended for diagnosis of infant botulism. Blood cultures would be appropriate to diagnose sepsis or another bacterial infection; however, the characteristic paralysis and lack of fever point away from sepsis as a cause of weakness and poor feeding.

MRI of brain and spine would be normal in an infant with botulism, as the toxin does not cross the blood–brain barrier, but could identify another neurologic cause of weakness.

Rectal biopsy would be the diagnostic test if the cause of this infant's constipation was suspected to be Hirschsprung disease; however, the poor feeding and weakness are not consistent with that diagnosis.

Congenital hypothyroidism could cause weakness but would usually have been diagnosed by a newborn screen.

(Section 17: Infectious Diseases, Chapter 245: Clostridial Infections)

**Answer 9-46. C**

This case is a classic presentation of measles virus infection. The patient presents with fever, cough, coryza, and conjunctivitis, along with pathognomonic Koplik spots on the buccal mucosa. Measles is a highly infectious virus, and lack of vaccination along with international travel are important risk factors. The virus also presents with a characteristic maculopapular rash that progresses caudal to cephalic and usually follows behind the presentation of fever, cough, coryza, and Koplik spots.

There is no specific antiviral therapy for measles; however, vitamin A deficiency is associated with increased morbidity and mortality, and the World Health Organization endorses vitamin A supplementation for all children with acute infection, regardless of country. Supportive care alone would be the appropriate treatment for many other viruses that cause febrile illness with similar presentation to this case.

IV immunoglobulin would be appropriate therapy for Kawasaki disease. The diagnosis of Kawasaki disease requires fever along with 4 out of the 5 following criteria: (1) nonpurulent conjunctivitis, (2) mucosal changes, (3) cervical lymphadenopathy, (4) polymorphous rash on the trunk, and (5) extremity changes. The child in the case could have been confused to have Kawasaki disease due to the conjunctivitis and mucosal changes; however, the characteristic Koplik spots along with cough and coryza make the diagnosis of measles.

Penicillin would be appropriate therapy for scarlet fever, and doxycycline would be the appropriate therapy for Rocky Mountain spotted fever (RMSF), or another rickettsial illness; however, this child has no known tick exposures and a more consistent presentation for measles infection.

(Section 17: Infectious Diseases, Chapter 311: Measles)

**Answer 9-47. B**

RSV infection is the most common cause of lower respiratory tract infection in infants and young children. Most children with RSV infection will present with a clinical picture indistinguishable from other viral upper respiratory tract infection; however, about 20% to 30% of infants will develop lower respiratory tract infection due to the smaller size of bronchioles and immature immune system. This can manifest as wheezing, tachypnea, rales, and increased work of breathing with subcostal retractions, abdominal breathing, nasal flaring, and grunting. In young infants, < 8 weeks old, especially those with history of prematurity, apnea can be a common presentation. This apnea may be present even without other symptoms of disease.

Seasonal influenza infection is another common cause of severe lower respiratory tract infection, but it typically presents with fever and systemic symptoms and later in the winter season than RSV.

Nonaccidental trauma, especially abusive head trauma, can cause apnea, and pediatricians should have a high index of suspicion in young infants; however, this infant's presentation of cough and apnea is much more suggestive of an infectious etiology.

Gastroesophageal reflux is common in infants and is often found in association with apnea or other apparent life-threatening event, but it is not typically associated with cough and wheeze. In addition, the history of a close contact (older sibling) with viral upper respiratory tract symptoms is more consistent with an infectious etiology.

Asthma rarely presents with wheezing in such a young infant and does not typically cause apnea.

(Section 17: Infectious Diseases, Chapter 236: Viral Respiratory Infections Including Influenza)

**Answer 9-48. E**

CMV infects 30,000 to 40,000 infants annually in the United States and is the most common infectious cause of hearing loss. Only about 10% of infected infants are symptomatic at birth, with the most severe form of disease being cytomegalic inclusion disease. In the case of infants born with asymptomatic infection, about 15% will be at risk of subsequent sensorineural hearing loss. Many asymptomatic infections occur in pregnancies where the mother had recurrent CMV infection. Many infants who have asymptomatic infection will have normal initial hearing screen but be at risk of subsequent hearing loss due to the infection, leading to some consideration of the utility of universal screening for congenital CMV. Mothers frequently acquire CMV infection during pregnancy from an older sibling who is in preschool or daycare.

Congenital Zika virus infection can cause a similar spectrum of neurologic manifestations; however, there is not currently ongoing transmission within the United States. Infection from a partner who traveled to a Zika-endemic area within the past 6 months could be a source for infection.

Toxoplasmosis is a less common cause of congenital infection with neurologic manifestations, often presenting with chorioretinitis. Congenital rubella would be more common in the infant of a mother who was a recent immigrant or had been unvaccinated because routine vaccination prevents the disease.

Meningitis is a common infectious cause of hearing loss; however, infants with postnatal meningitis are typically seriously ill and would not be asymptomatic.

(Section 17: Infectious Diseases, Chapter 305: Cytomegalovirus, Section 12: Clinical Genetics and Dysmorphology, Chapter 174: Hearing Loss)

**Answer 9-49. B**

This child is presenting with profound perianal pruritus, which can be caused by nonspecific dermatitis, infection, medication, or other irritant. *Enterobius vermicularis*, or pinworm, is a common parasitic infection in preschool-age children. The eggs can survive several days in the environment, and reinfection through autoinoculation is common. The pruritus is caused by the migration of the female worms out of the anal canal to deposit their eggs on the perianal skin. This occurs at nighttime, and the eggs can cause profound pruritus. Reinfection can occur through ingestion of the eggs.

Early morning cellophane tape application to the perianal skin can demonstrate eggs on microscopic examination. The eggs of *E vermicularis* have a characteristic appearance, being flat on one side and convex on the other, and are 35 to 55 μm in size.

The eggs are not shed in the intestinal lumen, and so are not generally visualized on study of ova and parasites in the stool.

Perianal strep infection can present with profound perianal erythema and occasionally pruritus and can present with concomitant strep pharyngitis. It would best be diagnosed with anal canal culture. Food allergy would be an uncommon cause of perianal pruritus, although certain foods can cause histamine release and pruritus.

Although eosinophilia can be present with a variety of parasitic infections, the degree of eosinophilia does not correlate well with the diagnosis of *E vermicularis* infestation.

(Section 17: Infectious Diseases, Chapter 322: Enterobiasis [Pinworm], Section 21: Disorders of the Gastrointestinal System, Chapter 411: Other Anorectal Disorders)

### Answer 9-50. C

This child is demonstrating signs and symptoms of seasonal influenza virus infection, which is characterized by sudden onset of fever, malaise, sore throat, and respiratory symptoms, during the characteristic time period. The mother also reports sick contacts at school, which is potentially indicative of a local outbreak. Treatment for influenza includes supportive care with antipyretics and antiviral pharmacotherapy in children at high risk of complication. It is unknown whether this child received the annual influenza vaccine; however, in the case of a likely diagnosis, antiviral treatment is recommended regardless of vaccine status.

Supportive care alone could be the correct treatment in a child of this age absent any risk factors; however, given his 2 risk factors for serious complication—morbid obesity and asthma—he should receive antiviral treatment. In the United States, oral oseltamivir is the treatment of choice because it has activity against both influenza A and B strains and a generally well-tolerated side effect profile. Amantadine is only active against influenza A, and recent seasonal strains isolated in the United States have demonstrated resistance.

Scheduled albuterol alone could be appropriate treatment for an acute asthma exacerbation; however, the fever is suggestive of an infectious process.

Oral amoxicillin could be an appropriate treatment for community-acquired pneumonia; however, the lack of localized findings on exam and seasonal presentation make influenza a more likely diagnosis than bacterial pneumonia.

(Section 17: Infectious Diseases, Chapter 236: Viral Respiratory Infections Including Influenza)

### Answer 9-51. D

This infant is demonstrating signs and symptoms of congenital rubella syndrome. The red-purple macules are the so-called "blueberry muffin" rash of neonatal thrombocytopenic purpura. The baby also has a patent ductus arteriosus and is small for gestational age, which are among the possible consequences of congenital rubella syndrome. There are no pharmacologic treatments for congenital rubella syndrome, and the disease can cause a spectrum of morbidity and mortality including deafness and intellectual disability.

Prevention of congenital rubella syndrome is accomplished through vaccinations to prevent infection in pregnant women. Because it is a live vaccine, it must be given at least 1 month prior to pregnancy. In the United States, rubella is a universally recommended child vaccine; however, unimmunized individuals exist, as a consequence of vaccine refusal or recent immigration from a country where coverage is not adequate. This mother is at risk of not being immunized due to her refugee status. Although mothers can be tested for rubella immune status during pregnancy, there is not adequate evidence that treatment with immunoglobulin during pregnancy prevents infection.

Intrapartum penicillin would be an appropriate treatment for prevention of early-onset group B streptococcal infection in mothers identified as group B *Streptococcus* carriers; however, this infant does not demonstrate signs of sepsis.

Valganciclovir is an appropriate treatment for congenital cytomegalovirus (CMV) infection and can prevent progression of sensorineural hearing loss in those infants.

Kernicterus from neonatal hyperbilirubinemia, which causes visible jaundice, can cause deafness and neurologic injury. Kernicterus and its developmental sequelae can be prevented by treating elevated bilirubin with phototherapy and exchange transfusion; however, this infant does not have jaundice.

(Section 17: Infectious Diseases, Chapter 315: Rubella)

### Answer 9-52. E

Prevention of mother-to-child transmission of HIV infection is important both for individual patients and as part of the public health strategy to address the global HIV/AIDS pandemic. In the United States, reduction in perinatal transmission is being achieved through screening and identification of pregnant women with HIV infection and appropriate treatment strategies. The administration of zidovudine alone from weeks 14 to 32 of gestation reduces perinatal transmission from 25% to < 8%. Treatment with combined antiretroviral therapy (cART) and viral load monitoring further reduce risk of transmission to < 1%.

There is evidence that cesarean section mode of delivery reduces risk of transmission; however, the amount of risk reduction is minimal for women who have viral loads < 1000 copies/mL, and therefore, it is not routinely recommended. Similarly, intrapartum zidovudine is recommended for women with detectable viral loads > 1000 copies/mL or who have not been receiving cART during pregnancy.

Because there is an association between breastfeeding and transmission of HIV, it is recommended to avoid breastfeeding in areas where there are readily available safe alternatives; however, in resource-limited settings, the World Health Organization recommends exclusive breastfeeding for at least 12 to 24 months with maternal cART. In those settings, the risk of HIV transmission is lower with exclusive breastfeeding than with combination of some formula and some breastfeeding.

Infants with perinatal HIV exposure are routinely treated with 6 weeks of oral zidovudine therapy to further reduce the risk of transmission. If the mothers had received cART and had suppressed viral loads, there is some consideration for a shorter course (4 weeks) of zidovudine therapy for infants.

If infants are born to mothers who had not received cART or did not have suppressed viral loads at the time of delivery, they should receive at least 2 drug treatments with zidovudine and nevirapine for prophylaxis.

It is important for pediatricians caring for infants at risk of perinatal HIV to understand the risks of mother-to-child transmission and the prevention strategies. The latest guidelines for treatment and prevention of HIV infection are available at http://www.aidsinfo.nih.gov/.

(Section 17: Infectious Diseases, Chapter 310: Human Immunodeficiency Virus Type 1 Infection)

**Answer 9-53. B**

This child is presenting with signs and symptoms of giardiasis caused by the parasite *Giardia intestinalis* (formerly *Giardia lamblia* or *Giardia duodenalis*). This is a flagellated protozoa that is the most frequent cause of waterborne diarrhea and can cause disease in both developed and developing countries. It is frequently associated with camping or daycare, and infections can be symptomatic (with copious, watery diarrhea, crampy abdominal pain, anorexia, vomiting, or weight loss) or asymptomatic. The cysts can be visualized in stool and the trophozoites in watery stool samples; however, microscopy is of lower sensitivity than stool antigen testing. The antigen test is available in commercial kits, sometimes with simultaneous *Cryptosporidium* testing.

Microscopy for ova and parasites could detect the *Giardia* cysts; however, it is less sensitive and would be an appropriate test for concerns for ascariasis or other nematode infection.

Intestinal biopsy is appropriate to confirm a diagnosis of celiac disease, a malabsorption diarrhea caused by an autoimmune reaction to dietary gluten. However, celiac disease presents typically in children with failure to thrive, abdominal pain and bloating with gluten ingestion, and extraintestinal manifestations (including rash).

Stool culture is an appropriate test for dysentery caused by bacterial pathogens. *Giardia* can be differentiated from bacterial dysentery as there is typically no fever or blood or mucus in the stool.

Serum inflammatory markers would be a nonspecific finding but can be useful in the evaluation of chronic diarrhea where inflammatory bowel disease is suspected.

(Section 17: Infectious Diseases, Chapter 344: Giardiasis, Section 21: Disorders of the Gastrointestinal System, Chapter 380: Diarrhea)

**Answer 9-54. A**

Tetanus is an acute and life-threatening disease caused by production of an exotoxin from the *Clostridium tetani* bacteria (an obligate anaerobe). These bacteria are ubiquitous throughout the world in soil and feces, but prevention through immunization has resulted in few cases annually in the United States. The disease occurs when *C tetani* spores contaminate a wound and the production of tetanospasmin toxin occurs, without any overt signs of infection at the wound. The toxin spreads through local diffusion and the bloodstream. It binds at the neuromuscular junction and prevents acetylcholine release. This results in a presentation of muscle spasm and stiffness, with potential progression to seizures, difficulty swallowing, and respiratory failure.

Prevention of disease is accomplished by active or passive immunization. Active immunization with tetanus toxoid via DTaP, Tdap, or Td with a primary series of 3 doses produces levels of circulating antitoxin. Passive immunization is accomplished through intramuscular (IM) administration of human TIG.

It is possible for *C tetani* to infect any wound; however, wounds that are contaminated by soil or feces or complicated by crush, deep puncture, or restricted blood flow are at an increased risk. Guidelines for prevention of tetanus recommend that no further immunization is required for any type of wound if a primary 3-dose series of Td, DTaP, or Tdap has been completed and a booster has been received within the past 5 years. If a wound is clean and uncomplicated, a booster is required only if it has been > 10 years since the primary series or most recent booster. If a wound is dirty or complicated and the patient has never completed a 3-dose tetanus toxoid series, passive immunization with TIG is also recommended.

In this case, the patient has a dirty wound and has completed the primary series, although it has been > 5 years since her last tetanus toxoid booster, so she requires active immunization with either Tdap or Td. The addition of metronidazole or penicillin would be appropriate for treatment of fulminant tetanus but is not necessary for prevention.

(Section 17: Infectious Diseases, Chapter 284: Tetanus)

**Answer 9-55. D**

Zika is a flavivirus transmitted through humans via a mosquito bite, similar to malarial transmission. Imported cases in North America have been widely reported, as well as sexual transmission from imported cases to their nontraveling partners. Spread in the Americas has been attributed to expansion of *Aedes albopictus* and *Aedes aegypti* mosquito populations, which are competent vectors for transmission. Two major complications of Zika infection are postinfectious Guillain-Barré syndrome and congenital infection, most notably microcephaly. Other symptoms include intracranial calcifications, ventriculomegaly, reduced brain volume, polymicrogyria, or other brain malformation; sensorineural hearing loss; chorioretinitis, optic nerve hypoplasia, macular atrophy, or other eye abnormalities; clubfoot; and arthrogryposis.

Kawasaki disease has an unknown etiology, although the current belief is that it occurs through an immunologic process and is not transmitted by an insect vector. Rheumatic fever is an immune process following infection with group A *Streptococcus*. Poststreptococcal glomerulonephritis is an immune process following infection with group A

*Streptococcus.* Hand-foot-mouth disease is a vesicular rash directly caused by *Enterovirus*, commonly coxsackie.

(Section 17: Infectious Diseases, Chapter 300: Arboviruses)

**Answer 9-56.** B

*E vermicularis* is a pinworm parasite that infects the gastrointestinal tract. Pinworms rarely produce serious pathology, and many infections are asymptomatic. The most common presentation is perianal and perineal pruritus that is typically worse at night. Pruritus may provoke such severe scratching that local bleeding, secondary pyogenic infection, and lichenification can occur.

Nocturnal perianal pruritus strongly suggests pinworm infection, especially in children. Thin, creamy-white worms are often found if the perianal region is examined when the child is awakened by itching. Because no egg shedding occurs inside the intestinal lumen, ova are not often seen in stools, so examination of stool specimens for ova and parasites is not recommended. The cellophane tape swab technique is the diagnostic method of choice.

Albendazole is the treatment of choice. Mebendazole is as effective but is available in the United States only through compounding pharmacies. Pyrantel pamoate is the most frequently used medication in the United States because it is inexpensive and available without a prescription. However, it has greater toxicity, with side effects including anorexia, nausea, vomiting, abdominal cramps, diarrhea, neurotoxic effects, and transient increases in hepatic enzymes. Therefore, a second dose is given 2 weeks after the initial dose to reduce the risk of autoinoculation from previous unhatched *E vermicularis* eggs. Repeated infections are common and should be treated in the same fashion as initial infections.

*A lumbricoides* is a roundworm infection. Symptoms are usually weight loss and digestive issues. *E histolytica* is a cause of liver cysts. *D latum* is a tapeworm infection from raw or undercooked fish. Symptoms are generally mild and can include diarrhea, abdominal pain, vomiting, and weight loss. Severe vitamin $B_{12}$ deficiency can occur due to the parasite absorbing 80% or more of the host's $B_{12}$ intake, leading to megaloblastic anemia. *S stercoralis* is a roundworm that most commonly causes dermatitis. Infection can occur in the gastrointestinal tract, leading to burning pain, tissue damage, sepsis, and ulcers.

(Section 17: Infectious Diseases, Chapter 322: Enterobiasis [Pinworm])

**Answer 9-57.** E

Most of the initial symptoms of RMSF are nonspecific, but the classic triad of fever, headache, and rash, seen in this patient, is found in the minority of patients when they first present for medical care. After an incubation of 2 to 14 days, patients often present with high fever exceeding 38.9°C, which is usually the earliest sign. Fever may be accompanied by severe myalgias and malaise. Headache is commonly frontal in location and is likely secondary to inflammation and increased intracranial pressure related to vasculitis. The maculopapular rash usually starts on the second to fourth day of illness on the flexor surfaces of the wrists and ankles before moving in a central direction. Typically, the palms and soles are also involved. Patients with Kawasaki disease are more likely to have conjunctivitis, mucous membrane involvement, and extremity changes.

Kawasaki disease will usually cause a thrombophilia, not thrombocytopenia. The rash for RMSF can involve the trunk, genitalia, palms, and soles. Both Kawasaki disease and RMSF are associated with high fevers.

(Section 17: Infectious Diseases, Chapter 289: Rickettsial Infections)

**Answer 9-58.** C

*Neisseria gonorrhoeae* is the second most commonly reported bacterial sexually transmitted infection (STI) in the United States. In men, urethritis is the most common clinical manifestation of gonorrhea. Symptomatic men report dysuria and/or discharge that appears as soon as 2 to 4 days after urethral exposure. The discharge may be scant, or mucus may be present as a profuse purulent discharge. The hyperkeratotic whitish plaques are consistent with balanitis seen with gonorrhea.

Answer choice A is a description of lymphogranuloma venereum caused by *Chlamydia trachomatis*. Ulcers are generally not seen with gonococcal infections. Answer choice B is a description of a chancroid caused by *Haemophilus ducreyi*. Again, ulcers are generally not seen with gonococcal infections. Answer choice D is the description of the condyloma lata of syphilis caused by *Treponema pallidum*. Answer choice E is the description of the condyloma acuminata seen in human papillomavirus (HPV) infections.

(Section 17: Infectious Diseases, Chapter 269: Neisseria gonorrhoeae)

**Answer 9-59.** E

*Cryptosporidium* species are obligate intracellular parasites that primarily infect the gastrointestinal tract of humans. Symptoms generally persist for 1 to 2 weeks. Occasionally, patients recover and then experience a recurrence of symptoms before the illness ends.

Severe cryptosporidiosis occurs in immunosuppressed patients, including those with advanced AIDS, cancer, hypogammaglobulinemia, severe combined immunodeficiency, and bone marrow and solid organ transplants. Such patients may have severe, life-threatening illness with intractable diarrhea and severe volume loss. Symptoms often last for months to years; wasting, hypovolemia, and weight loss are common. In general, the severity of the diarrheal illness correlates with the severity of immunosuppression. None of the other organisms cause the symptoms seen in this child.

*Toxoplasma* infection is usually associated with fever, myalgia, and encephalitis. *S schenckii* is a fungus that causes a cutaneous infection. It does not cause diarrhea. *E vermicularis* is a pinworm associated with perianal itching and rarely causes diarrhea. Microscopy will not be helpful in diagnosis of shigellosis. Furthermore, the child would present with bloody diarrhea.

(Section 17: Infectious Diseases, Chapter 340: Cryptosporidiosis)

**Answer 9-60.** D

The patient in this vignette has symptoms of cervicitis that include mucopurulent cervical discharge, intermenstrual bleeding, cervical friability, and lower abdominal pain. *N gonorrhoeae* are gram-negative diplococci that present with leukocytes and cervical discharge, consistent with the patient's symptoms.

*T pallidum* is the organism responsible for syphilis, which is characterized by a painless, indurated chancre in its primary stage. This patient does not exhibit the typical symptoms of syphilis (Chapter 283).

*G vaginalis* is the cause of bacterial vaginosis and can be diagnosed using the Amsel clinical criteria, which require the presence of 3 of the following 4 factors: (1) homogenous, thin white discharge that coats the vaginal walls; (2) > 20% of squamous cells with a clue cell appearance (vaginal epithelial cells studded with adherent coccobacilli, giving it a stippled appearance); (3) pH of vaginal fluid > 4.5; and (4) fishy odor before or after addition of 10% potassium hydroxide (KOH) (whiff test). They are nonmotile, non–spore-forming coccobacilli (Chapter 228).

HPV is a member of the papillomavirus family capable of infecting humans. It is a closed, circular, double-stranded DNA virus. HPV infection typically manifests with genital warts. Genital HPV types also often appear as flat, smooth, or pedunculated papules, specifically on mucosal surfaces. These lesions can also occur on conjunctival, nasal, oral, respiratory, gastrointestinal, and bladder mucosa (Chapter 228).

Genital lesions from HSV evolve from vesicles and pustules to ulcers over the first week and a half and then crust and heal during the subsequent 10 days. Lesions are distributed over the labia majora, labia minora, mons pubis, vaginal mucosa, and cervix in women.

(Section 17: Infectious Diseases, Chapter 269: Neisseria gonorrhoeae)

**Answer 9-61.** A

The patient in the vignette has *Plasmodium falciparum* (malaria) infection visualized in the image showing a crescent-shaped *P falciparum* gametocyte above a ring-form trophozoite. This infection is transmitted by the *Anopheles* mosquito throughout the tropical areas of the world, including sub-Saharan Africa and the Indian subcontinent, as identified in the vignette.

Patients with malaria typically present with fever, chills, rigors, and headache, which may be paroxysmal. Nausea, vomiting, diarrhea, abdominal pain, arthralgias, myalgias, and respiratory symptoms can occur. Hepatosplenomegaly is common. Typical laboratory findings include anemia and thrombocytopenia.

The *Ixodes* tick is the common vector for *Borrelia burgdorferi*, which is the cause of Lyme disease (Chapter 262), an illness characterized by a target rash (erythema migrans) accompanied by fever, arthralgias, myalgias, headache, and fatigue. The diagnosis of Lyme disease can be made clinically or serologically. Blood smears can show the spirochete but will not have the crescent-shaped gametocyte seen with *Plasmodium*. It is most commonly found in the wooded areas of the northeastern United States.

The reduviid bug (also known as triatomine or "kissing bug") is the vector for the parasite *Trypanosoma cruzi*, which causes Chagas disease. Most patients with Chagas disease are asymptomatic, although young children are more likely to display symptoms. A red, indurated nodule may form at the inoculation site on the face or arms. If the site of entry is the conjunctiva, unilateral eyelid edema (Romaña sign) may occur. Fever, malaise, hepatomegaly, and generalized lymphadenopathy may develop acutely, but resolve without treatment within 3 months. Chagas cardiomyopathy is a late complication that occurs years to decades after the initial infection. *T cruzi* are flagellated parasites that may be observed in blood smears during the acute phase of infection (Chapter 350).

The *Aedes* mosquito is the known vector for the yellow fever virus. The period of infection is characterized by sudden onset of fever, headache, malaise, musculoskeletal pain, low back pain, and nausea. Physical signs include injected conjunctiva, flushing of the skin, and relative bradycardia despite fever, known as Faget sign. Patients are typically dehydrated with hypotension, reduced urinary output, and, frequently, proteinuria. Myocarditis, azotemia, encephalopathy, progressive liver damage, bleeding, and shock can occur; mortality rates in patients who progress to the period of intoxication range from 20% to 50% (Chapter 302).

The *Dermacentor* tick is the vector for *Rickettsia rickettsii*, the cause of Rocky Mountain spotted fever (RMSF). Most of the initial symptoms are nonspecific, and the classic triad of fever, headache, and rash is found in the minority of patients when they first present for medical care. Patients will often present with high fever exceeding 38.9°C, usually accompanied by severe myalgias and malaise. The patient can also have abdominal pain, which may be severe enough to suggest an acute surgical abdomen and can be associated with vomiting or diarrhea (Chapter 289).

(Section 17: Infectious Diseases, Chapter 347: Malaria)

**Answer 9-62.** E

*Giardia intestinalis* (former names: *Giardia lamblia* or *Giardia duodenalis*) is a protozoan flagellate that is one of the most common disease-causing parasites in both developed and developing countries. It is one of the most frequently identified agents of waterborne diarrhea and common among campers.

The exact pathophysiology of the diarrhea is not known. The most severe cases are characterized by malabsorption and lactose intolerance, with varying degrees of inflammation and villous blunting. Although giardiasis affects persons of all age groups, children 0 to 5 years of age are at highest risk. In the United States and other developed countries, *Giardia* is prevalent in childcare centers and custodial institutions, among backpackers and others spending time in wooded areas, and among travelers to disease-endemic areas.

Symptoms include watery, foul-smelling diarrhea that can be sudden in onset and accompanied by abdominal distension, epigastric cramping, flatus, nausea, vomiting, anorexia, and fatigue. Systemic symptoms such as fever and chills are uncommon. Blood and mucus in the stools do not occur in giardiasis.

Giardiasis is confirmed by detecting the parasite or its antigens in the stool or intestinal lining. Cysts are the most commonly detected form present in the feces, and trophozoites are almost entirely limited to liquid stools.

Although blood can be present in many infectious causes of diarrhea, such as *Shigella*, *Salmonella*, and *E coli*, *Giardia* does not cause a bloody diarrhea.

Stool WBC count is a nonspecific test to detect inflammatory diarrhea. This type of diarrhea may be a symptom of an infection caused by bacteria such as *Shigella*, *Clostridium difficile*, *Campylobacter*, or *Salmonella*, but may also be related to inflammatory bowel disease. It is unlikely to help diagnose a parasitic infection.

Secretory IgA antibodies against gliadin and human tissue transglutaminase are tests for gluten-sensitivity celiac disease. The patient in the vignette does not have symptoms of gluten sensitivity (Chapter 403).

Measurement of stool-reducing substances tests for carbohydrate malabsorption. Given the child's age and sudden onset, this is an unlikely cause of the diarrhea (Chapter 403).

(Section 17: Infectious Diseases, Chapter 344: Giardiasis)

**Answer 9-63.** B

Erythema migrans (EM) is the trademark feature of Lyme disease. It starts as a small red bump and then grows to form a large annular erythematous lesion with a central clearing to form the characteristic "bull's eye." For patients who present with an EM rash (80%–90% of patients), the diagnosis of Lyme disease should be based on the clinical presentation alone and treatment with antibiotics, usually a tetracycline, may begin. For patients who do not have EM, support by laboratory tests is likely necessary to confirm the diagnosis. Laboratory confirmation depends on serologic testing for antibodies to *Borrelia burgdorferi*. Because the rash usually develops before antibodies to the bacteria are detectable, antibody test results in most patients with EM will be negative early on, and testing should be delayed. Although sensitivity and specificity of tests for antibodies may vary, by far the most important factor that determines the predictive value of a test result is the prior probability that the patient has Lyme disease.

However, a major problem in diagnosing Lyme disease is the widespread practice of ordering serologic tests in patients with only nonspecific symptoms (eg, fatigue, arthralgia), virtually all of whom will have a low pretest probability of having Lyme disease, which can lead to an increased incidence of false positives. Patients with Lyme disease almost always have specific signs (eg, EM, facial nerve palsy, arthritis). Although nonspecific symptoms, such as fever and malaise, commonly accompany these specific signs, such symptoms are extremely common in the general population and almost never will be the only clinical manifestation of Lyme disease. Ordering IgM is unnecessary given the patient's clinical presentation with EM. Additionally, there is risk for IgM to return as negative due to early presentation of the patient because the body has not yet produced antibodies at this time. The erythema marginatum rash seen in rheumatic fever can be confused with EM. The characteristic rash of erythema marginatum consists of an evanescent, pink, erythematous macule, with a clear center and serpiginous outline (Chapter 230). Additionally, this patient has not had symptoms of strep throat warranting the need for a strep test and does not exhibit any other symptoms of rheumatic disease.

(Section 17: Infectious Diseases, Chapter 262: Lyme Disease)

**Answer 9-64.** B

Most of the initial symptoms of Rocky Mountain spotted fever (RMSF) are nonspecific, but the classic triad of fever, headache, and rash, seen in this patient, is found in patients when they first present for medical care. Patients often present with high fever exceeding 38.9°C, accompanied by severe myalgias and malaise. Headache is commonly frontal in location and is likely secondary to inflammation and increased intracranial pressure related to vasculitis. Abdominal pain may be present and severe enough to suggest an acute surgical abdomen and can be associated with vomiting or diarrhea. *B burgdorferi* is the cause of Lyme disease. Although the patient in the vignette may have nonspecific symptoms similar to Lyme disease, like fever and malaise, the rash found in Lyme disease is typically the characteristic "target" rash. Additionally, Lyme disease is predominantly found in the Northeast and Midwestern United States, not in Arkansas (Chapter 262).

*T cruzi* is the cause of Chagas disease, which usually presents with nonspecific symptoms or no symptoms at all. The rash seen in this patient is not typically seen with Chagas disease (Chapter 350). *S pyogenes* is the most common cause of streptococcal pharyngitis. Although headache, fever, and rash can be seen in rheumatic fever, a complication of streptococcal pharyngitis, the patient in the vignette did not express any sore throat symptoms. In addition, the rash does not involve the palms and soles. CMV infections usually present with nonspecific malaise and flu-like illness. Congenital infection can present with a "blueberry muffin" rash and ocular symptoms. Given the age of the patient, the geographic location, and the triad of fever, headache, and petechial rash, RMSF is the most likely cause.

(Section 17: Infectious Diseases, Chapter 289: Rickettsial Infections)

**Answer 9-65.** B

The patient in this scenario is demonstrating signs of reduced functioning with unstable gait, reduced vision, and meningeal irritation (by keeping his legs flexed so as to avoid irritation). As a result, assessment for papilledema and a lumbar puncture are indicated to assess for bacterial causes of meningitis (Table 226-1).

(Section 17: Infectious Diseases, Chapter 258: *Haemophilus influenzae*)

**TABLE 226-1.** Bacterial Causes of Meningitis

| Relative Frequency | 0–1 Month | > 1 Month |
|---|---|---|
| Common | *Streptococcus agalactiae* | *Streptococcus pneumoniae* |
| | *Escherichia coli* | *Neisseria meningitidis* |
| | *Listeria monocytogenes* | |
| | *Klebsiella species* | |
| | *Enterobacter species* | |
| Uncommon | *Staphylococcus aureus*[a] | *Streptococcus pyogenes* |
| | Coagulase-negative staphylococci[a] | Gram-negative bacilli |
| | Enterococcal species | *Haemophilus influenzae* type b[b] |
| | *Pseudomonas aeruginosa* | |
| Rare | *S pneumoniae* | *L monocytogenes* |
| | *Streptococcus pyogenes* | *S aureus*[a] |
| | *Citrobacter diversus* | Coagulase-negative staphylococci[a] |
| | *H influenzae* non–type b | |
| | *Salmonella* species | |

[a]Usually associated with neurosurgical procedures.

[b]Common where *Haemophilus influenzae* type b vaccine is unavailable.

Mark W. Kline, *Rudolph's Pediatrics*, 23rd Edition. Copyright © McGrawHill Education. All rights reserved.

**Answer 9-66.** B

The sequelae from Hib meningitis differ from those of other bacterial meningitides (Table 226-1).

- Approximately 30% of children will have seizures at some point in the course of Hib meningitis.
- Hib bacteremia can have a petechial rash similar to meningococcemia.
- Patients can also have a secondary site of infection, such as a septic arthritis or facial cellulitis. Shock is present in approximately 20% of cases.
- Anemia is common, the result of a combination of accelerated red blood cell destruction and diminished erythropoiesis.
- Complications include subdural effusion or empyema, ischemic or hemorrhagic cortical infarction, cerebritis, ventriculitis, intracerebral abscess, and hydrocephalus.
- Mortality is approximately 5%.
- Long term, 15% to 30% of patients can have sensorineural hearing loss, language disorders, and developmental disorders.
- A meta-analysis of randomized controlled trials in children has shown that the incidence of severe hearing loss due to *H influenza* decreased by the administration of corticosteroids with antibiotics.

(Section 17: Infectious Diseases, Chapter 258: *Haemophilus influenzae*)

**Answer 9-67.** E

International adoptees should be screened for illnesses of public health importance. The condition of most relevance to international adoptees is TB. *Mycobacterium tuberculosis* is transmitted via inhalation of droplets nuclei. A TST is routinely performed in children aged 2 to 14 years of age who are examined in countries where the incidence is > 20 per 100,000 population. Patients who have signs or symptoms suggestive of TB or have HIV should have a TST or an interferon-γ assay. A reaction of ≥ 5 mm is considered to be a positive test for patients with HIV (Table 264-1). Interferon-γ is increasingly used in children with previous bacille Calmette-Guerin (BCG) immunizations but is not recommended for routine testing because there is a lack of data on reliability of a negative interferon-γ release assay (IGRA) result. CXR is often used in addition to IGRA and TST testing in those with positive test results to identify TB disease.

(Section 17: Infectious Diseases, Chapter 264: Tuberculosis (*Mycobacterium tuberculosis*)

**Answer 9-68.** D

Congenital cytomegalovirus (CMV) is the most common cause of congenital infection and leading cause of sensorineural hearing loss. CMV can be transmitted through most body fluids, including saliva, urine, human milk, genital secretions, and blood. Pregnant women with primary CMV have a 30% to 40% risk of transmission to the fetus. Perinatal transmission can happen when exposed to genital secretions, and postnatal transmission occurs commonly through breast milk. Human milk–associated CMV is usually asymptomatic, although preterm and very-low-birth-weight infants are at risk for developing disease. Congenital CMV presents with petechial rash, purpura, jaundice, elevated direct bilirubin, hemolysis, and thrombocytopenia, which is probably the case in this child with the history of jaundice. However, most infants with CMV-associated sensorineural hearing loss may be asymptomatic at birth. An elevated aspartate aminotransferase (AST), elevated conjugated bilirubin, hemolysis, and thrombocytopenia are the most common laboratory abnormalities. Confirmation of congenital CMV is by isolation of the virus in saliva or urine, by culture, or by polymerase chain reaction (PCR). In infants with symptomatic CMV (with multisystem involvement of central nervous system (CNS), visual system, and auditory system), there is a clear benefit with regard to hearing and neurodevelopmental outcomes in treating patients with 6 months of valganciclovir.

(Section 17: Infectious Diseases, Chapter 305: Cytomegalovirus)

**Answer 9-69.** B

This patient returns to the hospital during the late solid organ transplant period. During this phase, immunosuppressive medications have usually been decreased from the intense early (< 1 month) and intermediate (1–6 months) posttransplant periods. However, host susceptibility remains high for several uncommon pathogens including *Listeria*, *Nocardia*, invasive fungal infections, and late viral infections with cytomegalovirus (CMV), herpes simplex virus (HSV), and John Cunningham (JC) polyomavirus. Therefore, early investigation for fungal infection with serum galactomannan assay should be considered. Echocardiogram, MRI of brain, and liver biopsy may be necessary but would not be warranted as part of the early workup. Interleukin-6 levels are considered a nonspecific test of inflammation and have not been widely adopted in the evaluation of fever in a solid organ transplant recipient due to problems with sensitivity and specificity.

(Section 17: Infectious Diseases, Chapter 224: Fever and Infection in the Immunocompromised Patient)

**Answer 9-70.** A

The release of antigenic cyst fluid can cause severe allergic reactions including anaphylaxis. Cyst rupture also predisposes patients to spread of disease with secondary infection of the peritoneal cavity and development of multiple secondary cysts. There is no association described between cystic echinococcosis and hepatocellular carcinoma or hepatitis A infection. Similarly, life-threatening blood loss or hemorrhage from cyst rupture is not considered a common risk factor. A small proportion of cysts (5%–15%) rupture into the biliary tree, leading to jaundice; however, pancreatitis is not expected.

(Section 17: Infectious Diseases, Chapter 333: Echinococcosis)

**Answer 9-71.** C

Neonates can become infected by pathogens through transplacental or ascending transmission prenatally, at delivery by passage through an infected birth canal, or through exposure/infection in the first few weeks of life. CMV affects 0.5% of all live births, making it the most common congenital infection in humans. Only about 10% of infected fetuses will be symptomatic at birth. CMV is ubiquitous, and the majority of adults eventually become infected. Transmission occurs by contact of infected secretions including tears, oropharyngeal secretions, cervical and vaginal secretions, breast milk, semen, urine, blood, and transplanted organs. Children in group childcare have been noted to have increased rates of viral excretion, presumably due to child-to-child transmission from saliva on hands and toys. Classic symptoms of congenital CMV infection include being small for gestational age, microcephaly, hepatosplenomegaly, jaundice, and petechiae over the body. Additionally, laboratory studies will show thrombocytopenia and elevated liver function tests. Many of these babies will have complications throughout their lifetimes, including vision loss, sensorineural hearing loss, and intellectual disability. HSV and *Enterovirus* are more classically associated with perinatal or postnatal infection leading to symptoms shortly after birth. HSV infection is associated with a vesicular rash instead of a petechial rash. *Enterovirus* typically presents with fever, emesis, diarrhea, seizures, apnea, and/or a bulging anterior fontanelle. Group B *Streptococcus* and *E coli* are bacterial infections that can present in the early postnatal period with signs of sepsis.

(Section 17: Infectious Diseases, Chapter 225: Therapy for Perinatal and Neonatal Infections)

**Answer 9-72.** E

Limited outbreaks of vaccine-preventable diseases continue to occur in the United States due to communities opposed to vaccination for a variety of reasons including religious and philosophical objections or unfounded concerns for serious adverse effects. Measles virus is among the most contagious human pathogens, leading to outbreaks even in communities where the majority of people have immunity. Classically, symptoms start 10 days after infection, beginning with progressive fever, conjunctiva, and coryza. Cough quickly develops as well, along with Koplik spots on the buccal mucosa. An erythematous rash of discrete macules develops approximately 14 days after infection, starting at the hairline/neck and progressing caudally. Varicella is characterized by a vesicular rash. Coxsackie is an *Enterovirus* associated with buccal ulcerations and vesicular or painful macular lesions on the hands and feet. Congenital and postnatal rubella infections are particularly rare in the United States consisting of adenopathy and a macular rash that starts on the face and spreads caudally. Mumps is characterized by fever and parotid swelling.

(Section 17: Infectious Diseases, Chapter 311: Measles)

**Answer 9-73.** C

Although rare in the United States, with an average of 29 cases per year, global morbidity and mortality from tetanus remain quite high, with approximately 49,000 infants dying from tetanus in 2013. Mean incubation of tetanus is 5 to 12 days, and onset is often slow with progressive stiffness of muscles particularly in the neck, jaw, and large muscles of the back and legs. Due to trismus (marked stiffness and spasms of the jaw and neck), swallowing may become difficult. Soon after initial onset of symptoms, any stimulation or attempt at voluntary movement can lead to full-body contractions that last 5 to 10 seconds, with the entire body becoming rigid, with head retracted, back arched, extremities extended, and fists clenched. The majority of treatment for tetanus involves supportive care; however, TIG should be administered as soon as possible based on severity of disease in doses of 3000 to 6000 units IM. A portion of the TIG should be infiltrated around the wound. This prevents unbound toxin from reaching the central nervous system (CNS). Tetanus infection does not confer immunity to tetanus. However, DTaP is for children < 7 years of age. Instead of broad-spectrum antibiotics, metronidazole at 30 mg/kg/d is recommended to decrease the number of toxin-producing organisms. Benzodiazepines or neurologic blocking agents are used in many centers to assist with anxiety and spasms. Cyclobenzaprine, a muscle relaxant, and dantrolene, which is approved for the treatment of spasticity and malignant hyperthermia, are not a part of the standard treatment of tetanus.

(Section 17: Infectious Diseases, Chapter 284: Tetanus)

**Answer 9-74.** A

This patient most likely has the *Rickettsia rickettsii* infection Rocky Mountain spotted fever (RMSF) based on his clinical presentation and probable exposure to ticks in an endemic region. The incubation period is typically 7 days but can range from 1 to 14 days. Symptoms of RMSF are usually prodromal headache, malaise, and myalgias. This is typically then followed by a skin rash 2 to 3 days later, most classically a centrifugal petechial rash starting in the wrists and ankles. The absence of a rash, however, should not delay diagnosis or treatment because up to 20% of adults and 5% of children may never develop a rash. Major complications of RMSF are usually a result of vasculitic injury. Severe illness may result in encephalitis, meningitis, pulmonary edema, respiratory distress syndrome, cardiac arrhythmias, gastrointestinal bleeding, hepatitis, skin necrosis, and coagulopathy.

Diagnosis is based on history and physical exam findings because specific lab testing may not be positive until the second week of infection. Serologic testing is available for RMSF, but most patients will have negative antibody testing at time of clinical presentation. PCR testing can detect *R rickettsii* in the blood and biopsy specimen in the acute phase of illness, but this testing is not yet widely available. Immunofluorescent staining of skin biopsy specimens at the site of the rash has 70% sensitivity and 100% specificity for detecting *R rickettsii*. Nonspecific lab abnormalities that may be seen in RMSF include thrombocytopenia, hyponatremia, leukopenia, and elevated liver enzymes. Empiric treatment should be initiated if RMSF is suspected.

(Section 17: Infectious Diseases, Chapter 289: Rickettsial Infections)

**Answer 9-75.** D

Recommendations for sexually active females age < 25 years are as follows:

- Routine annual screening for chlamydia and gonorrhea is recommended.
- HIV screening should be offered. Frequency of screening should be based on risk factors.
- Routine screening for other infections (syphilis, HSV, *Trichomonas*, bacterial vaginosis) is not recommended in asymptomatic females.
- Pap smears are recommended starting at age 21.

Recommendations for sexually active males age < 25 are as follows:

- There is insufficient evidence to recommend routine screening of all males for chlamydia and gonorrhea. Screening for chlamydia and gonorrhea should be considered in high-prevalence areas or in men with risk factors for infection.
- HIV screening should be offered. Frequency of screening should be based on risk factors.

Recommendations for men who have sex with men (MSM) are as follows:

- Routine annual screening for HIV and syphilis is recommended.
- Routine annual screening for urethral chlamydia and gonorrhea is recommended for MSM who have had insertive anal intercourse in the preceding year.
- Routine annual screening for rectal chlamydia and gonorrhea is recommended for MSM who have had receptive anal intercourse in the preceding year.
- Routine annual screening for pharyngeal gonorrhea is recommended for MSM who have had receptive oral intercourse in the preceding year.

(Section 17: Infectious Diseases, Chapter 228: Sexually Transmitted Infections)

**Answer 9-76.** B

This patient presents to the ED with neutropenic fever, and history and urinalysis are suggestive of underlying urinary tract infection. In general, empiric antibiotic treatment for febrile neutropenia should ensure broad coverage for gram-negative organisms, including *Pseudomonas*, and some coverage for *Staphylococcus aureus* Empiric single-agent regimens for neutropenic fever include ceftazidime, cefepime, and carbapenems (eg, meropenem or imipenem). If *Klebsiella* infection is suspected, as in this patient, or if local rates of extended-spectrum β-lactamase–positive strains are high, then carbapenems are preferred. In absence of clinical instability or hypotension, monotherapy is recommended, as combination antimicrobial therapy has not been shown to have marked difference in outcomes compared to monotherapy. Given the potential risks of vancomycin, including selection for vancomycin-resistant *Enterococcus*, vancomycin should be added to empiric therapy only if patients have hypotension, signs of sepsis, obvious catheter-related infection, severe mucositis, or known colonization with methicillin-resistant *Staphylococcus aureus* (MRSA).

(Section 17: Infectious Diseases, Chapter 224: Fever and Infection in the Immunocompromised Patient)

**Answer 9-77.** D

In the United States, children who are < 5 years old or who have risk factors for rapid development of TB disease should be started on isoniazid after exposure to potentially infectious adults with pulmonary TB. The incubation time of pulmonary TB may be shorter than development of positive testing, and therefore, children may potentially develop severe TB even before testing becomes positive. About 10% of immunocompetent children with TB disease do not react initially to a TST, but most become reactive after several months of treatment. Therefore, the child should be treated for a minimum of 3 months after contact with the infectious case has broken. The test of infection should then be repeated. If repeat testing is positive, then infection of TB is documented and isoniazid should be continued for a total of 9 months. If repeat testing is negative, treatment can be stopped.

(Section 17: Infectious Diseases, Chapter 264: Tuberculosis [Mycobacterium tuberculosis])

**Answer 9-78.** A

In general, most experts recommend that patients with HIV who have CD4+ counts of < 100 cells/μL be started on prophylactic medication for prevention of disseminated MAC. Azithromycin and clarithromycin are more effective than rifabutin. Rifabutin can be used, but *Mycobacterium tuberculosis* infection must first be excluded. Prophylaxis combination therapy is not recommended due to lack of cost effectiveness and increased adverse events.

(Section 17: Infectious Diseases, Chapter 265: Nontuberculous Mycobacterial Infections)

**Answer 9-79.** A

The spore-bearing mold form of *Histoplasma capsulatum* grows in the environment at temperatures < 35°C, occurs worldwide, and is most commonly found in the United States in the Mississippi River and Ohio River basins. Infections occur as sporadic cases in communitywide outbreaks when dry, windy conditions facilitate aerosolization of spores and as localized clusters caused by disturbance of heavily contaminated microenvironments. Such hyperendemic foci include soil in sites of bird roosts, including stream banks; bat-infested caves; rotting logs; and the attics, wall insulation, and fireplaces of old structures. Infection is symptomatic in about half of otherwise normal patients who are more heavily exposed. In these patients, fever, cough, and chest pain are common symptoms; chest radiographs often show focal pneumonitis and/or hilar adenopathy. Symptoms are almost always self-limited in otherwise healthy patients and resolve within 2 weeks without treatment. Pulmonary nodules (histoplasmomas) from such infections may persist indefinitely and develop radiographically visible calcifications over months to years. Infrequently, the fever, weight loss, and fatigue persist unabated for > 4 weeks, and antifungal therapy then may be required. Intense exposure of immunocompetent hosts can cause severe, life-threatening illness characterized by persistent fever, respiratory distress, diffuse reticulonodular chest infiltrates, and sometimes progressive fungal dissemination.

(Section 17: Infectious Diseases, Chapter 295: Histoplasmosis)

**Answer 9-80.** B

Lymphocutaneous sporotrichosis accounts for 75% of infections. Following inoculation, the average incubation period is 3 weeks but ranges from 5 days to 6 months. Lesions usually involve the upper extremities but may occur on the face and trunk. The primary lesion is a firm, mobile, nontender subcutaneous nodule that enlarges and becomes discolored. After 2 weeks, it undergoes necrosis, leaving a painless ulcer. During the next several weeks, additional lesions develop along the proximal lymphatics; intervening lymphatic channels become thickened, with overlying cutaneous erythema. Lesions can persist for months to years. Few heal spontaneously, with scarring of the ulcers. Systemic symptoms are absent or mild.

Painless papulovesicular, ulcerative, or nodular lesions that fail to respond to antibiotics should prompt consideration of sporotrichosis. The differential diagnosis includes infection with *Nocardia* species, *Francisella tularensis*, nontuberculous mycobacteria, *Treponema pallidum*, and *Leishmania*. Nodular lymphangitis can also be seen with infections caused by some pyogenic bacteria such as *Pseudomonas* species, *Bacillus anthracis*, and other mycoses, including blastomycosis, chromoblastomycosis, coccidioidomycosis, cryptococcosis, and histoplasmosis. Nodular lymphangitis can be seen with mycetoma, which may be caused by bacteria or fungi. A careful travel and exposure history may help differentiate these entities.

(Section 17: Infectious Diseases, Chapter 298: Sporotrichosis)

**Answer 9-81.** E

The natural history of nontuberculous mycobacterial (NTM) cervical adenitis is resolution over many months, although the patient is commonly left with significant scarring and, occasionally, chronic sinus tract formation. In general, excisional biopsy remains the treatment of choice for cervical lymphadenitis caused by NTM. Incisional biopsy should not be performed because it frequently leads to development of a draining sinus tract or recurrent disease. Total excision of the inflammatory mass usually precludes persistence or recurrence. However, removal of all involved lymph nodes may be impossible due to the close proximity of vital structures. Excision is best performed early, in order to improve the cosmetic outcome before extension of disease into the subcutaneous structures occurs. Chemotherapy is not generally necessary for children with NTM lymphadenitis if surgical excision can be achieved safely. If tuberculosis (TB) cannot be reasonably excluded, an initial course of anti-TB therapy should be considered. Many cases of cervical adenitis caused by the *Mycobacterium avium* complex (MAC) resolve during treatment with standard anti-TB medications, although no controlled trials have been reported. In a small percentage of cases in which complete surgical excision is not possible, recurrence of adenitis is a problem. Chemotherapy may be helpful; the purpose is to prevent extension of recurrence so that a second surgical procedure is not necessary. The most commonly used regimen is a combination of at least 2 drugs, including clarithromycin, rifampin, or rifabutin and ethambutol.

(Section 17: Infectious Diseases, Chapter 265: Nontuberculous Mycobacterial Infections)

**Answer 9-82.** D

CMV is a ubiquitous virus, and humans are its only reservoir. In populations with higher socioeconomic conditions, approximately 40% of adolescents are seropositive, with another 1% seroconverting annually thereafter. Approximately 70% of adults from higher socioeconomic strata and 90% from lower socioeconomic strata eventually become infected with CMV.

Transmission of CMV occurs by contact with infected secretions via direct (including sexual) contact or indirect contact. Sources of virus include tears, oropharyngeal secretions, cervical and vaginal secretions, breast milk, semen, urine, blood, and transplanted organs. Intrauterine transmission of CMV is especially important. Spread among children in group childcare facilities is the result of horizontal transmission from child to child through saliva on hands and toys. This mode of viral transmission is so efficient that it is not unusual to find excretion rates as high as 20% to 40% in young toddlers attending group childcare. Young children acquiring primary CMV infection at childcare facilities are at risk of transmitting CMV to their seronegative parents, which in turn can lead to intrauterine transmission should a mother be pregnant at the time. Seronegative caretakers working in daycare centers are also at increased risk for acquisition of CMV infection.

(Section 17: Infectious Diseases, Chapter 225: Therapy for Perinatal and Neonatal Infections)

**Answer 9-83.** E

Neonatal herpes simplex virus (HSV) disease is treated with parenteral acyclovir administered at 60 mg/kg/d in 3 divided doses. Duration of therapy is 21 days for babies with disseminated and central nervous system (CNS) disease and 14 days for babies with skin, eyes, and mouth (SEM) disease. All babies with CNS involvement should have a repeat lumbar puncture near the end of intravenous (IV) therapy to document polymerase chain reaction (PCR) negativity prior to stopping parenteral therapy; in the unlikely event that the PCR remains positive near the end of the 21-day treatment course, IV acyclovir should be administered for another week, with repeat cerebrospinal fluid (CSF) PCR assay performed near the end of the extended treatment period and another week of parenteral therapy if it remains positive. Consultation with an infectious diseases specialist is warranted in these cases. Oral acyclovir suppressive therapy (300 mg/m$^2$/dose administered 3 times per day) should be administered to all babies following completion of parenteral therapy and continued for 6 months; patients with CNS disease benefit from suppressive therapy in terms of neurodevelopmental outcomes, while all disease classifications of neonatal HSV benefit in terms of preventing cutaneous recurrences.

Infants are more susceptible to serious infections and infections by organisms that are much less common in older children or adults. Group B *Streptococcus*, *Escherichia coli*, *Listeria monocytogenes*, *Enterococcus*, *Staphylococcus aureus*, and HSV can cause sepsis in the first 2 months of life. In the first month of life, most experts believe that a full septic workup should be performed, including blood and urine cultures as well as a lumbar puncture. Given her age, she will also need to be treated empirically with ampicillin and gentamicin while awaiting culture results.

(Section 17: Infectious Diseases, Chapter 225: Therapy for Perinatal and Neonatal Infections, Chapter 222: Acute Fever Without a Focus)

**Answer 9-84.** B

Rubella and congenital rubella syndrome prevention is one of the hallmark successes of the vaccination programs of the United States. By 2005, endemic transmission of rubella was eliminated in the United States, and cases of rubella and congenital rubella syndrome in the United States in 2007 were 99.9% and 99.3% lower, respectively, compared to the prevaccine era. Less than 10 rubella cases have been reported each year in the United States since its elimination was declared, and only 7 cases of congenital rubella syndrome were reported from 2005 through 2013. Rubella vaccination coverage is at least 95% among school-aged children. An estimated 91% of the US population is immune to rubella. The remarkable success in decreasing the incidence of rubella in this country and others has led scientists and international organizations to consider the goal of rubella eradication.

(Section 17: Infectious Diseases, Chapter 225: Therapy for Perinatal and Neonatal Infections)

**Answer 9-85.** C

*Ascaris* should be considered in children from endemic regions presenting with acute abdominal pain, signs of bowel obstruction, nonspecific abdominal symptoms, poor growth, asthma, or eosinophilia. In children, the most frequently noted symptoms are vague epigastric pains, nausea, vomiting, and anorexia. Severe, intermittent, colicky abdominal pain may result from partial intestinal obstruction, which is more common in children than in adults, because children have smaller intestinal lumens. The more serious problems encountered with *Ascaris* infection result from migration of adult worms into the bile and pancreatic ducts, where they may cause biliary stone formation, pancreatitis, cholangitis, small bowel perforation, and complete intestinal obstruction, volvulus, or intussusception. Worms occasionally may migrate upward and emerge through the mouth or nose or migrate downward and pass through the rectum. Heavy infections may also lead to malabsorption, malnutrition, poor growth, and cognitive impairment.

The diagnosis of ascariasis is made using a combination of clinical, epidemiologic, and microbiologic information. In a region where *Ascaris lumbricoides* is endemic, the differential diagnosis of a child presenting with fever, respiratory symptoms, and pulmonary infiltrates should include bacterial or viral pneumonia, tuberculosis (TB), and *Ascaris*, especially if associated with eosinophilia. *Ascaris* should also be considered in children from endemic regions presenting with acute abdominal pain, signs of bowel obstruction, nonspecific abdominal symptoms, poor growth, asthma, or eosinophilia.

The diagnosis of *Ascaris* is generally confirmed by identifying typical eggs in the feces through light microscopy. Ascaris eggs are usually abundant, and stool concentration is rarely needed to see them. Examining stools from consecutive days increases sensitivity of microscopy. Adult worms can also be passed from the rectum or nose. If a patient brings a spontaneously passed worm to the clinic, a stool should be examined to ascertain whether any other worms remain. Abdominal computed tomography (CT) scans or ultrasonography may be useful to visualize adult worms in the abdomen or biliary tract.

(Section 17: Infectious Diseases, Chapter 319: Ascariasis)

**Answer 9-86.** E

*Shigella* should be suspected in children with fever and diarrhea, particularly if there are seizures, or in children with small-volume diarrhea with abdominal cramping, blood, white blood cells (WBCs), or mucus in the stool. Many patients with *Shigella sonnei*, however, do not have bloody diarrhea. The diagnosis hinges on the recovery of *Shigella* from a fresh stool specimen or a rectal swab.

A variety of complications of shigellosis occur. Dehydration, hypoglycemia, hyponatremia, hypernatremia, and hypokalemia can occur; hypoglycemia and hyponatremia are associated with an increased mortality rate. Seizures are a common extraintestinal manifestation and occur exclusively in children. Isolated seizures are usually not associated with any long-term neurologic sequelae. Ekiri syndrome, a severe toxic encephalopathy with seizures, rapid progression, and high mortality, is a rare complication of shigellosis. Bacteremia is uncommon in healthy children but is more common with human immunodeficiency virus (HIV) infection and severe malnutrition. In about half of bacteremic children, there may be polymicrobial bacteremia caused by other organisms that have traversed the injured gut. Extraintestinal suppurative complications such as osteomyelitis, meningitis, septic arthritis, and splenic abscess are rare. Hemolytic-uremic syndrome is an important complication of *S dysenteriae* type 1 infection, reported in 1% to 4% of children; it is seen occasionally with *Shigella flexneri*. Reactive arthritis and Reiter syndrome (arthritis, urethritis, and iritis in conjunction with HLA-B27) are unusual postinfectious complications of *Shigella*, usually occurring in adolescents or adults.

(Section 17: Infectious Diseases, Chapter 278: Salmonella, Shigella, and Escherichia coli)

**Answer 9-87.** C

In cases of suspected infectious enteritis, epidemiologic risk factors may allow consideration of a specific pathogen. Exposures to animals (eg, reptiles), contaminated water, travel to endemic areas, recent receipt of antibiotics, and attendance at a childcare center are important risk factors. For example, *Giardia* and *Cryptosporidium* are the most common gastrointestinal infections reported with waterborne outbreaks. Outbreaks of enteric infections in children attending childcare centers have included bacteria (*Shigella*, *E coli* including O157:H7), viruses (adenovirus, astrovirus, norovirus, and rotavirus), and parasites (*Cryptosporidium parvum* and *G intestinalis*). National outbreaks of infectious bacterial enteritis have followed ingestion of undercooked ground beef, chicken, or pork (*Escherichia coli* O157:H7 and other Shiga-toxin–producing *E coli* [STEC], *Salmonella* species), raw fish (*Salmonella* species), milk products (*L monocytogenes*), nuts (*E coli* O157:H7, *Salmonella* species), and raw fruits or vegetables (*E coli* O157:H7, *L monocytogenes*, *Salmonella* species).

In developed countries, viral agents are the most frequent cause of infectious diarrhea in children. In the United States, rotavirus was the most common cause of gastroenteritis before the introduction of routine rotavirus vaccination in 2006. Currently, human caliciviruses such as norovirus are the most frequent cause of infectious enteritis in children < 5 years of age. The most commonly isolated bacteria causing acute infectious enteritis are *Campylobacter* and *Salmonella* species, followed by *Shigella* and *E coli* O157:H7 and other STEC. An increasing incidence of antimicrobial-associated

*C difficile*–associated disease (CDAD) in hospitalized children has been reported.

(Section 17: Infectious Diseases, Chapter 231: Gastrointestinal Infections)

**Answer 9-88.** A

Children acquire *Mycobacterium tuberculosis* from adults in their environment. Environmental risk factors include those characteristics that make it more likely that the child shares the air with an adult with infectious tuberculosis (TB). Factors that increase the risk of a child being infected with *M tuberculosis* include (1) birth or travel/residence in a country in which TB is endemic; (2) early childhood environments with exposures to multiple high-risk caregivers, for example, some orphanages; or (3) contact with high-risk adults who have had previous residence in a jail, prison, or high-risk nursing home, and homelessness in some communities. Also included are use of illegal drugs, experience as a healthcare worker who cares for high-risk patients, having unscreened foreign visitors stay in the home, and locally defined risk factors. Factors that increase the risk of developing disease once infected include age < 2 years, co-infection with human immunodeficiency virus (HIV), other immunocompromising diseases or treatments (corticosteroids, tumor necrosis factor-α inhibitors), and malnutrition.

Most children in the United States are infected with *M tuberculosis* in the home, but outbreaks of childhood TB centered in elementary and high schools, nursery schools, family daycare homes, churches, school buses, and stores have occurred. Childhood TB case rates in the United States and in other developed countries are strikingly higher among ethnic and racial minority groups and among the poor. In the United States, approximately 85% of TB cases in children occur among African American, Hispanic, Asian, and Native American children.

(Section 17: Infectious Diseases, Chapter 264: Tuberculosis (Mycobacterium tuberculosis))

**Answer 9-89.** B

Based on the history and microscopic examination of skin scrapings, this patient most likely has tinea versicolor caused by *Malassezia*. Tinea versicolor is caused by *Malassezia* species, which is a fungus that most commonly causes skin diseases. These lesions are most commonly seen on the chest, back, and upper arms. The incidence is highest in adolescents and young adults. Skin scrapings with KOH show a "spaghetti and meatballs" appearance. Treatment of tinea versicolor is typically managed with topical 2.5% selenium sulfide, zinc pyrithione, or azole creams.

Topical corticosteroids would be used to treat seborrheic dermatitis caused by *Malassezia*. Oral cephalexin would be more appropriate to treat bacterial cellulitis. Topical terbinafine can be used to treat tinea versicolor, but oral terbinafine is not effective for the treatment of *Malassezia*. Topical emollients would be appropriate for treatment of cradle cap or atopic dermatitis.

(Section 17: Infectious Diseases, Chapter 296: Malassezia)

**Answer 9-90.** C

Infant botulism is caused by ingesting spores of *C botulinum* that germinate in the colon and produce a neurotoxin. The neurotoxin travels in the blood to the peripheral cholinergic synapses and irreversibly binds. This leads to a flaccid paralysis preventing the release of acetylcholine. Infant botulism is the most common form of botulism reported in the United States. The median age of presentation is 16 weeks. There are no clear epidemiologic risk factors for the development of infant botulism. Possible spore sources include foods, dust, and soil. A history of honey ingestion is present in a minority of cases, and honey is not recommended for children < 12 months of age.

The other answer choices could be included in the differential for a child presenting with hypotonia. Congenital hypothyroidism can have a subtle presentation but can include lethargy, hoarse cry, feeding problems, constipation, macroglossia, umbilical hernia, large fontanels, hypotonia, dry skin, hypothermia, and prolonged jaundice. Poliomyelitis is usually asymptomatic. Less than 1% of children with poliomyelitis have flaccid paralysis. Classic presentation of Guillain-Barré syndrome is a previously well child who develops acute progressive ascending weakness and is areflexic or hyporeflexic. The age range is typically older children. Hirschsprung disease is a motor disorder of the bowel that causes a functional obstruction in the neonatal period with abdominal distention and failure to pass meconium.

(Section 17: Infectious Diseases, Chapter 245: Clostridial Infections)

**Answer 9-91.** C

The patient has a congenital infection that was caused by a maternal disease process during pregnancy. The most common congenital infections include toxoplasmosis, syphilis, rubella, cytomegalovirus (CMV), and herpes simplex virus (HSV). Rubella is also called German measles and is no longer endemic in the United States. However, there are still some cases worldwide among those who are unimmunized. Infants with congenital rubella syndrome are typically born to mothers who are recent immigrants to the United States or have not been immunized against rubella.

Congenital syphilis is usually asymptomatic at birth. When there are findings, they are hepatomegaly, profuse rhinitis ("syphilitic snuffles"), and a maculopapular rash that leads to desquamation on the soles of the feet. The mother diagnosed with mononucleosis during pregnancy most likely had CMV. In newborns, CMV often presents with intrauterine growth retardations, hepatosplenomegaly, and a "blueberry muffin" rash. The mother with cats who was treated for lymphadenitis most likely had toxoplasmosis. Congenital toxoplasmosis has a classic triad of chorioretinitis, intracranial calcifications, and obstructive hydrocephalus. The mother with genital vesicular lesions most likely had HSV. In neonates, disseminated HSV can often present similar to bacterial sepsis. Infants present with fever, lethargy, irritability, and seizures.

(Section 17: Infectious Diseases, Chapter 315: Rubella)

**Answer 9-92.** D

The patient presents with molluscum contagiosum. This is a common cutaneous viral infection caused by the poxvirus *Molluscipoxvirus.* This virus replicates in the human epidermis and is spread by direct contact. It can present at any age, with a peak incidence between 0 and 4 years. Lesions are most commonly seen on the trunk, extremities, and face. Molluscum contagiosum is typically asymptomatic. Diagnosis is usually based on clinical examination. Molluscum is a self-limited condition, and the lesions generally regress spontaneously. Reassurance of the parents is generally the first-line treatment for uncomplicated cases.

Referral to dermatology would be appropriate if the lesions have persisted despite conservative management. Topical hydrocortisone ointment would be an appropriate treatment for atopic dermatitis. Topical ketoconazole cream would be an appropriate treatment if the patient presented with seborrheic dermatitis or fungal infections such as tinea. Zinc pyrithione shampoo is used to treat seborrheic dermatitis or tinea versicolor.

(Section 17: Infectious Diseases, Chapter 312: Molluscum Contagiosum)

**Answer 9-93.** E

These lesions are most likely caused by nontuberculous mycobacteria (NTM), leading to NTM adenitis. Although most patients with NTM disease have immunosuppressing conditions, most children with NTM adenitis are immunologically normal. The key to diagnosis of an NTM infection is a high level of suspicion based on epidemiologic factors and clinical presentation. Before a diagnosis of NTM adenitis can be made, tuberculosis (TB) needs to be ruled out. This should be done by obtaining an epidemiologic history and testing for TB infection. Testing can either be done by tuberculin skin test (TST) and/or an IGRA.

The GAS rapid antigen detection test would be used if the patient was suspected to have GAS pharyngitis. The other tests are used to detect other organisms that cause lymphadenitis in children. *B henselae* is known to cause cat scratch disease; *Y pestis* is known to cause plague; *F tularensis* is known to cause tularemia. These organisms are zoonotic infections that are spread via contact with infected animals. This patient had no contact with animals.

(Section 17: Infectious Diseases, Chapter 265: Nontuberculous Mycobacterial Infections)

# CHAPTER 10 Oncology

Frank Y. Lin and Priya Mahajan

**10-1.** The parents of a 3-year-old girl who recently completed treatment for unilateral retinoblastoma are expecting a second child. They are concerned that this new child will also develop retinoblastoma. There is no other family history of cancer, and both parents are healthy. You counsel the parents that the risk this second child will develop retinoblastoma is which of the following?

**A.** < 5%

**B.** 25%

**C.** 50%

**D.** 75%

**E.** 90%

**10-2.** A 4-month-old boy is found to have bilateral leukocoria and strabismus at his well-child exam. He is diagnosed with bilateral retinoblastoma after an evaluation by a pediatric ophthalmologist and a brain magnetic resonance imaging (MRI) scan. Which of the following tumors is he also at risk for?

**A.** Neuroblastoma

**B.** Hepatoblastoma

**C.** Hodgkin lymphoma

**D.** Osteosarcoma

**E.** Wilms tumor

**10-3.** Exam of a term newborn male reveals absence of irises and mild hypospadias. The patient's siblings and parents are healthy with no known medical conditions. Which tumor is the patient at most risk of developing?

**A.** Medulloblastoma

**B.** Wilms tumor

**C.** Adrenocortical carcinoma

**D.** Retinoblastoma

**E.** Renal angiomyolipoma

**10-4.** A 12-year-old boy has recently been diagnosed with osteosarcoma of the left distal femur. On family history, you learn that his mother died from breast cancer at age 35 and his maternal grandfather had leukemia and now has colon cancer. What is the most likely germline genetic alteration you expect to find in this patient?

**A.** Inactivating mutation in *TP53*

**B.** *APC* mutation

**C.** Mutation of *NF1*

**D.** Mutation of *VHL*

**E.** *DICER1* mutation

**10-5.** A 17-year-old girl with a history of acute myeloid leukemia presents to your clinic with new onset of swollen ankles, nighttime cough, and preference for sleeping propped up with pillows. Chest radiograph demonstrates enlarged cardiac borders, and echocardiogram reveals a left ventricular ejection fraction of 30% (normal, 50%–65%). On review of her cancer treatment, she completed chemotherapy 2 years ago and achieved sustained remission. Which of the following chemotherapy agents is most likely to contribute to her new symptoms?

**A.** Vincristine

**B.** Etoposide

**C.** Daunorubicin

**D.** Cytarabine

**E.** Methotrexate

**10-6.** A 15-year-old boy completed chemotherapy and radiation therapy for Ewing sarcoma of the left pelvis 2 years ago. At a routine clinic visit, he feels fatigued. A complete blood count reveals a white blood cell count of 35,000/μL, hemoglobin of 8.3 g/dL, and platelet count of 33,000/μL. Peripheral blasts are present. Which of the following chemotherapy agents is most likely to be responsible for these new findings?

**A.** Vincristine

**B.** Etoposide

**C.** Doxorubicin

**D.** Ifosfamide

**E.** Cyclophosphamide

**10-7.** Which of the following statements about phase 3 clinical trials is correct?

**A.** They are designed to identify the appropriate dose and dosing schedule of a therapeutic agent.

**B.** They are designed to identify toxicities of a therapeutic agent at various doses.

**C.** They typically use the recommended adult phase 2 dose in children.

**D.** They are designed to compare the current best available therapy to a novel treatment approach, typically in a randomized fashion.

**E.** They are designed to determine whether or not a novel agent can produce an objective response against a particular tumor.

**10-8.** What is the most common solid tumor of childhood?

**A.** Central nervous system (CNS) tumors

**B.** Wilms tumor

**C.** Neuroblastoma

**D.** Osteosarcoma

**E.** Hodgkin lymphoma

**10-9.** A 17-year-old girl presents to the emergency department with a 4-week history of fatigue, fever, cough, night sweats, and swollen lymph nodes in her neck. A mononuclear spot test is negative. You notice that the patient has increased work of breathing when supine. The complete blood count reveals a white blood cell count of 4000/μL, hemoglobin of 9 g/dL, and platelet count of 55,000/μL. Your differential diagnosis includes leukemia and lymphoma. Which of the following is the next best test to order?

**A.** Lumbar puncture

**B.** Bone marrow aspirate

**C.** Lymph node biopsy

**D.** Chest radiograph (CXR)

**E.** Blood culture

**10-10.** A 7-year-old girl presents to the emergency department with a 3-week history of fever, pallor, bruising, and fatigue. A complete blood count reveals a white blood cell count of 87,000/μL, hemoglobin of 6 g/dL, and platelet count of 17,000/μL, and peripheral smear demonstrates 70% blasts. Chemistries reveal potassium of 5.2 mmol/L (normal 3.5–5.5 mmol/L), creatinine of 0.7 mg/dL (0.3–0.6 mg/dL), ionized calcium of 1.1 mmol/L (normal 1.1–1.3 mmol/L), phosphorus of 5.5 mg/dL (normal 2.5–5 mg/dL), and uric acid of 10 mg/dL (normal 2–6.2 mg/dL). You have started intravenous (IV) hydration and placed the patient on monitors. Which of the following is the next best step in management?

**A.** Administration of IV hydrocortisone

**B.** Administration of rasburicase (urate oxidase)

**C.** Administration of calcium gluconate

**D.** Bone marrow biopsy

**E.** Replete potassium

**10-11.** A 6-month-old female infant presents to your clinic with a firm, purpuric, and violaceous mass of the upper extremity that the parents report is rapidly growing. You suspect that this patient has a kaposiform hemangioendothelioma. What is the next best step in caring for this patient?

**A.** Obtain a complete blood count with differential

**B.** Order magnetic resonance imaging (MRI) of the brain

**C.** Start steroids

**D.** Give intravenous (IV) vincristine

**E.** Plan for immediate surgical resection

**10-12.** A 10-year-old girl presents to the emergency department with a 4-week history of intermittent fevers and worsening leg pain. Her temperature is 38.4°C. Her heart rate is 110 bpm, and respiratory rate and blood pressure are normal. On physical exam, she is awake and alert. She has mild petechiae and diffuse lymphadenopathy. She has splenomegaly. Her complete blood count reveals a white blood cell count of 72,000/μL, hemoglobin of 8.0 g/dL, and platelet count of 35,000/μL. What is the next best step in her evaluation?

**A.** Perform a bone marrow aspirate and biopsy

**B.** Administer a normal saline bolus

**C.** Start steroids immediately

**D.** Transfuse blood products

**E.** Obtain a chest radiograph (CXR), blood cultures, and chemistries

**10-13.** Which of the following chemotherapeutic agents is classified as an alkylating agent?

**A.** Etoposide

**B.** Cyclophosphamide

**C.** Methotrexate

**D.** Vincristine

**E.** Cytarabine

**10-14.** A 17-year-old male athlete presents to the emergency department with a 2-week history of left thigh pain and swelling. Pain is progressively worse despite rest, ice, and elevation. He has no history of fevers. On exam, you palpate a mass in his distal thigh. A plain radiograph of the leg demonstrates a mixed pattern of bone lysis and sclerosis, with disruption of the bone cortex in the distal femur. There is periosteal new bone formation in a "sunburst" pattern. A complete blood count with differential is normal. What is the most likely diagnosis associated with this classic radiographic appearance?

**A.** Rhabdomyosarcoma

**B.** Acute lymphoblastic leukemia

**C.** Langerhans cell histiocytosis

**D.** Osteosarcoma

**E.** Osteomyelitis

**10-15.** A 16-year-old girl was recently diagnosed with osteosarcoma of the right proximal tibia. You are completing her staging evaluation. What is the best next test to evaluate for pulmonary metastases?

**A.** Computed tomography (CT) of the chest

**B.** Magnetic resonance imaging (MRI) of the chest

**C.** Chest radiograph (CXR)

**D.** Chest ultrasound

**E.** Bone scan

**10-16.** An 18-month-old girl presents to your clinic with 3 weeks of twitching of her arms and legs. Parents report that her gait has become unsteady in the past few weeks. On physical exam, you notice involuntary rapid horizontal eye movements, and you palpate an abdominal mass. What tumor is this patient most likely to have?

**A.** Hepatoblastoma

**B.** Leukemia

**C.** Brain tumor

**D.** Neuroblastoma

**E.** Wilms tumor

**10-17.** A 14-year-old girl presents with 2 weeks of progressively worsening abdominal pain. Vital signs are stable, and on physical exam, her abdomen is mildly distended and tender to palpation. Abdominal ultrasound demonstrates a large, complex, solid, cystic pelvic mass likely arising from the right ovary. Serum α-fetoprotein (AFP), β-human chorionic gonadotropin (β-hCG), inhibin, and CA-125 were normal. Computed tomography (CT) of the abdomen and pelvis confirmed a large, predominantly cystic mass with fat and solid components likely arising from the right ovary. No lymphadenopathy was seen. The patient underwent an exploratory laparotomy and right salpingo-oophorectomy. Pathology is consistent with a mature teratoma. What treatment do you recommend?

**A.** Observation only

**B.** Chemotherapy alone

**C.** Chemotherapy plus radiation

**D.** Radiation alone

**E.** Immunotherapy

**10-18.** Among the following categories, more children die from which group of childhood cancers?

**A.** Pediatric leukemias

**B.** Pediatric lymphomas

**C.** Pediatric central nervous system (CNS) tumors

**D.** Nephroblastomas

**E.** Pediatric thyroid cancers

**10-19.** You are consulted to see an 11-month-old girl admitted with prolonged fever of unknown origin. On physical exam, you note an ill-appearing child with generalized adenopathy, and you palpate her spleen 3 cm below her left costal margin. Laboratory results reveal hemoglobin of 8.2 g/dL, absolute neutrophil count of 800/μL, and fibrinogen of 52 mg/dL. You suspect a diagnosis of hemophagocytic lymphohistiocytosis (HLH). Which of the following studies would meet the HLH diagnostic criteria for this child?

**A.** Low serum sodium level

**B.** Elevated ferritin level

**C.** White matter changes on brain magnetic resonance imaging (MRI)

**D.** Elevated transaminases

**E.** Elevated erythrocyte sedimentation rate

**10-20.** A 15-month-old girl presents to the emergency department (ED) with several days of irritability and morning vomiting. Further history reveals that during the past couple months, she has no longer been taking independent steps and appears to have poor balance when cruising. She has not experienced recent head trauma or injury. Exam in the ED reveals papilledema and dysconjugate gaze. Complete blood count, serum chemistries, and liver function tests are within normal limits. What is the next best test to perform?

**A.** Lumbar puncture

**B.** Serum tumor markers (AFP and β-hCG)

**C.** Electroencephalogram (EEG)

**D.** Magnetic resonance imaging (MRI) of the brain

**E.** Blood cultures

**10-21.** A 6-week-old full-term female infant presents to your clinic with a small 2-cm vascular lesion of the neck. The lesion is bright red, raised, and rubbery. Her parents report that this lesion was first noted 3 weeks ago and was not present at birth. Clinically, the patient is doing well. You suspect that this is the most common benign vascular tumor of infancy. You counsel the parents that this lesion will continue to proliferate in the next 6 months and then involute over time. Complications include ulceration of the lesion. What does this patient have?

**A.** Infantile hemangioma

**B.** Congenital hemangioma

**C.** Venous malformation

**D.** Lymphatic malformation

**E.** Angiosarcoma

**10-22.** A 3-year-old boy presents to your office for follow-up. He has a 4-week history of a scaly, waxy, red-to-brown papular rash. The rash did not respond to common topical treatments, and immunostains on recent skin biopsy were positive for CD1a and CD207. He now presents with a 1-week history of low-grade fevers and decreased energy and is having excessive thirst and urination. You order a complete blood count (CBC) and differential, liver function tests, and a skeletal survey. What additional assessment should be performed?

**A.** Computed tomography (CT) of the brain

**B.** Bilateral bone marrow and aspirate

**C.** Urine specific gravity and urine and serum osmolality

**D.** CT of the chest

**E.** No other workup is needed

**10-23.** A 3-year-old boy is admitted with a left-sided abdominal mass and blood pressure of 100/65 mm Hg. Ultrasound and computed tomography (CT) scan demonstrate a left renal mass suspected to be Wilms tumor. The pediatric surgery service is preparing a left radical nephrectomy to remove the neoplasm. Which of the following studies should be considered prior to surgical resection?

**A.** Urine catecholamines

**B.** Coagulation studies

**C.** Urinalysis

**D.** Electrocardiogram

**E.** No other workup needed

**10-24.** A 2-week-old full-term male infant presents to your clinic for a well-child examination. Parents report he is breastfeeding well and is making good wet diapers. They have noticed recent abdominal distension. Pulse and blood pressure are normal. On physical examination, he is well appearing. You palpate a firm abdominal mass. You order an abdominal ultrasound, which shows a large echogenic left renal mass. What is the most likely diagnosis?

**A.** Rhabdoid tumor

**B.** Renal cell carcinoma

**C.** Congenital mesoblastic nephroma

**D.** Clear cell carcinoma of the kidney

**E.** Wilms tumor

**10-25.** A 4-year-old girl presents to the emergency department with new-onset hematuria. Parents report 1-week history of constipation and abdominal pain. Her blood pressure is 128/76 mm Hg. On exam, you palpate an abdominal mass, and abdominal ultrasound reveals a mass arising from the right kidney. Computed tomography (CT) of the abdomen reveals a right renal mass and a characteristic "claw sign." You suspect that the patient has the most common pediatric renal tumor. What is the most likely diagnosis?

**A.** Renal cell carcinoma

**B.** Clear cell sarcoma of the kidney

**C.** Mesoblastic nephroma

**D.** Wilms tumor

**E.** Rhabdoid tumor

**10-26.** A 20-month-old boy presents with abdominal distension. He is otherwise asymptomatic. On physical examination, he is noted to have an abdominal mass. Abdominal ultrasound reveals an echogenic liver mass. You suspect that he has the most common malignant tumor of the liver. What tumor marker is important to obtain in children with liver tumors?

**A.** α-Fetoprotein (AFP)

**B.** Carcinoembryonic antigen (CEA)

**C.** β-Human chorionic gonadotropin (β-hCG)

**D.** Lactate dehydrogenase (LDH)

**E.** Cancer antigen 125 (CA-125)

**10-27.** You are consulted on a newborn male infant with a white blood cell count of 30,000/µL with peripheral blasts. On physical examination, you note that he has upward-slanting, almond-shaped eyes, a flattened facial profile, small ears, and a single palmar crease of the hand. He is clinically well appearing and stable on room air. No hepatosplenomegaly is noted on examination. Which of the following is the most appropriate management for this patient?

**A.** Plan for immediate bone marrow transplant

**B.** Start steroids immediately

**C.** Evaluate liver and renal function and observe closely

**D.** Perform leukapheresis

**E.** Start increased hydration and anticipate chemotherapy

**10-28.** A 22-month-old girl presents with a 1-week history of worsening abdominal pain and distension. A palpable abdominal mass is appreciated on physical examination. A computed tomography (CT) of the abdomen reveals a large right-sided adrenal mass. You suspect she has the most common extracranial solid tumor of childhood. What is the most appropriate tumor marker or ancillary diagnostic test to assess in this patient?

**A.** Urine homovanillic acid (HVA) and vanillylmandelic acid (VMA)

**B.** β-Human chorionic gonadotropin (β-hCG)

**C.** α-Fetoprotein (AFP)

**D.** Cancer antigen 125 (CA-125)

**E.** Inhibin

## ANSWERS

**Answer 10-1.** A

Genetic counseling for patients with retinoblastoma is based on the proband's presentation, family history, and genetics. The 3-year-old girl described in the question stem likely had sporadic, non-hereditary retinoblastoma due to her unilateral disease and older age of presentation. With no family history of cancer, the risk for the sibling is 1% if the affected proband has unilateral retinoblastoma. The risk is 2% if the proband has bilateral disease. These risks remain for future siblings due to the possibility of gonadal mosaicism.

(p. 2070, Section 24: Neoplastic Disorders; Part 3: Solid Tumors; Chapter 457)

**Answer 10-2.** D

This young infant with bilateral retinoblastoma most likely has a germline alteration in one copy of the tumor suppressor gene *RB1*. Approximately 95% of children with bilateral retinoblastoma carry a germline mutation in the *RB1* gene. Individuals with *RB1* gene abnormalities are at increased risk for developing secondary cancers, particularly sarcomas, such as osteosarcoma, and melanomas. Neuroblastoma, hepatoblastoma, Hodgkin lymphoma, and Wilms tumor have not been specifically identified as *RB1*-dependent tumors.

(p. 1992: Section 24: Neoplastic Disorders; Part 1: Principles of Oncology; Chapter 439; p. 2070: Section 24: Neoplastic Disorders; Part 3: Solid Tumors; Chapter 457)

**Answer 10-3.** B

This patient most likely has WAGR syndrome: Wilms tumor, aniridia, genitourinary anomalies, and mental retardation. WAGR syndrome is characterized by a microdeletion of 11p13. Patients with deletion of *WT1* as part of the deletion are at a significantly increased risk of developing Wilms tumor and require close surveillance with serial abdominal ultrasounds. Molecular diagnosis is performed by array comparative genomic hybridization. Medulloblastoma can be associated with Gorlin syndrome and Lynch syndrome. Adrenocortical carcinoma is described in Li-Fraumeni syndrome. Retinoblastoma can be associated with *RB1* alterations. Renal angiomyolipoma is described in tuberous sclerosis.

(p. 1944: Section 24: Neoplastic Disorders; Part 1: Principles of Oncology; Chapter 439)

**Answer 10-4.** A

This 12-year-old boy's diagnosis and family history meet several clinical diagnostic criteria for Li-Fraumeni syndrome, which is found in individuals with inactivating germline mutations in the *TP53* tumor suppressor gene. Classic tumor types seen in Li-Fraumeni syndrome include early-onset breast cancer, sarcomas, brain tumors, leukemia, and adrenocortical carcinoma. Intensive cancer surveillance (the Toronto Protocol) has been demonstrated to reduce cancer mortality in these patients. *APC* mutations are found in patients with familial adenomatous polyposis who are at increased risk for tumors of the colon, thyroid, stomach, and small intestine. Mutations of *NF1* are described in neurofibromatosis type 1 (von Recklinghausen disease), and affected individuals are at increased risk for neurofibromas, low-grade gliomas, and malignant peripheral nerve sheath tumors. Mutations of *VHL* cause the Von Hippel–Lindau syndrome, in which patients are at increased risk for developing retinal and central nervous system (CNS) hemangioblastomas, pheochromocytomas, and renal cell carcinomas. *DICER1* mutations are associated with pleuropulmonary blastoma, ovarian sex cord stromal tumors, pinealoblastoma, and Wilms tumor.

(p. 1995: Section 24: Neoplastic Disorders; Part 1: Principles of Oncology; Chapter 439)

**Answer 10-5. C**

Specific late effects of chemotherapy can be associated with certain classes of drugs. Cardiac toxicities are strongly associated with anthracyclines, such as doxorubicin and daunorubicin, and typically in a dose-dependent manner. Anthracycline-induced cardiotoxicities include arrhythmias and heart failure due to cardiomyopathy. Risk for anthracycline-induced cardiomyopathy significantly increases after a cumulative dose of 450 mg/m$^2$ but can occur at lower doses, particularly when combined with other risk factors such as radiation therapy. Cytarabine, etoposide, vincristine, and methotrexate are not associated with significant cardiotoxicity.

(p. 2006: Section 24: Neoplastic Disorders; Part 1: Principles of Oncology; Chapter 441; p. 2017: Section 24: Neoplastic Disorders; Part 1: Principles of Oncology; Chapter 444)

**Answer 10-6. B**

Chemotherapeutic agents, including alkylating agents and topoisomerase II inhibitors, particularly epipodophyllotoxins such as etoposide, have been clearly linked with an increased risk for secondary (or therapy-related) acute myeloid leukemia (AML). Secondary AML associated with epipodophyllotoxins typically occurs 2 to 4 years after initial treatment, whereas secondary leukemia associated with alkylating agents, such as cyclophosphamide, typically occurs 4 to 10 years after initial exposure. Secondary AML portends a poor prognosis.

(p. 2017: Section 24: Neoplastic Disorders; Part 1: Principles of Oncology; Chapter 444; p. 2026: Section 24: Neoplastic Disorders; Part 2: Hematologic Malignancies; Chapter 446)

**Answer 10-7. D**

Phase 3 clinical trials compare the current best available therapy to a new treatment approach for which there is a body of evidence supporting potential superiority. These trials enroll large numbers of patients and typically compare the efficacy of 2 or more therapeutic regimens. Phase 1 clinical trials are designed to identify the appropriate dose and dosing schedule of a novel chemotherapeutic agent as well as to define the toxicities of a novel chemotherapeutic agent at various doses. Phase 1 clinical trials are typically conducted in children with resistant or refractory disease and begin at a dose near the recommended adult phase 2 dose in the children. Phase 2 clinical trials attempt to determine whether or not a novel chemotherapeutic agent can produce an objective response against the tumor.

(p. 2014: Section 24: Neoplastic Disorders; Part 1: Principles of Oncology; Chapter 443)

**Answer 10-8. A**

CNS tumors are the most common solid tumors of childhood and overall the second most common childhood malignancy (second to leukemia). Brain tumors occur at an incidence of 3.1 per 100,000 children per year. Pediatric CNS tumors are now the leading cause of cancer-associated mortality.

(p. 2062: Section 24: Neoplastic Disorders; Part 3: Solid Tumors; Chapter 456)

**Answer 10-9. D**

This patient presents with fever, lymphadenopathy, night sweats, and pancytopenia, which are concerning for lymphoma or T-cell lymphoblastic leukemia. These patients may present with a large mediastinal mass, subsequently putting them at risk for respiratory compromise. It is critical to obtain a CXR to evaluate for a mediastinal mass prior to allowing them to undergo anesthesia and testing for further disease evaluation. A large mediastinal mass is considered a medical emergency and involves multidisciplinary care and high-level medical monitoring.

(p. 2059: Section 24: Neoplastic Disorders; Part 2: Hematologic Malignancies; Chapter 445)

**Answer 10-10. B**

The child in this vignette is presenting with a new diagnosis of acute leukemia and is at very high risk for tumor lysis syndrome (TLS). TLS is caused by the release of intracellular by-products of leukemic cells, including potassium, phosphorus, and uric acid. Management of TLS includes IV hydration and careful management of electrolyte disturbances. For patients with high tumor burden and elevated uric acid, such as the child in this vignette, rapid degradation of uric acid with rasburicase (urate oxidase) is indicated. Allopurinol, an inhibitor of xanthine oxidase, may be an alternative option for management of hyperuricemia; however, its effect is not immediate. In TLS, patients are at risk for hyperkalemia; therefore, repletion of potassium is typically not necessary. Due to increased binding of extracellular calcium with phosphorus, serum calcium may decrease and lead to precipitation of calcium phosphate in renal tubules. Other malignancies with significant tumor burden and increased risk for TLS include Burkitt lymphoma and lymphoblastic lymphoma.

(p. 2022: Section 24: Neoplastic Disorders; Part 2: Hematologic Malignancies; Chapter 445)

**Answer 10-11. A**

Kaposiform hemangioendothelioma (KHE) is a rare vascular tumor typically present during infancy or early childhood. Lesions are often firm, indurated, and purpuric. KHE is frequently associated with Kasabach-Merritt phenomenon (KMP), occurring in 70% of KHE cases. KMP is characterized by a consumptive coagulopathy associated with profound thrombocytopenia, hypofibrinogenemia, and elevated fibrin split products. The mortality associated with KHE is largely due to the extensive coagulopathy. Surgical excision with or without embolization is the most effective treatment for KHE. However, with large lesions or in the presence of KMP, multimodality treatment is often necessary. Therapeutic modalities include steroids, α-interferon, antifibrinolytic agents, and chemotherapy, including vincristine and sirolimus. Many clinicians often use sirolimus as first-line therapy. An MRI of the lesion may be helpful in characterizing the extent of involvement.

(p. 2072: Section 24: Neoplastic Disorders; Part 3: Solid Tumors; Chapter 458)

**Answer 10-12.** E

The girl in this vignette likely has newly diagnosed leukemia or lymphoma. These patients can present with mediastinal involvement, and it is important to assess respiratory status and obtain a baseline CXR. Evaluating for a mediastinal mass is critical prior to sedating the patient for any procedure, such as a bone marrow aspirate and biopsy. If the girl in this case has a significant mediastinal mass, the diagnosis of leukemia can be obtained by flow cytometry of peripheral blood. Patients with newly diagnosed leukemia and lymphoma can present with infections and metabolic abnormalities, such as tumor lysis syndrome (TLS), and therefore, blood cultures and chemistries are important in the initial evaluation in this patient. Although this patient will likely need blood products, she does not currently have active bleeding and remains hemodynamically stable. The patient is currently hemodynamically stable, and normal saline boluses are not currently warranted. Steroids ideally should be started after making a definitive bone marrow diagnosis unless necessary for urgent airway or central nervous system (CNS) compromise.

(p. 2022: Section 24: Neoplastic Disorders; Part 2: Hematologic Malignancies; Chapter 445)

**Answer 10-13.** B

Cyclophosphamide is an example of an alkylating agent. Alkylating agents are chemically reactive compounds that nonspecifically damage DNA by forming covalent bonds to cross-linking nucleobases, resulting in cytotoxicity. Other alkylating agents include ifosfamide and melphalan. Etoposide is a topoisomerase inhibitor, which causes DNA strands to break. Methotrexate and cytarabine are antimetabolites. Methotrexate inhibits dihydrofolate reductase, thereby interfering with cell repair and replication. Vincristine is a vinca alkaloid that inhibits tubulin by blocking microtubule polymerization.

(p. 2003: Section 24: Neoplastic Disorders; Part 1: Principles of Oncology; Chapter 441)

**Answer 10-14.** D

The appearance of lytic and blastic lesions described as a "sunburst" is classic for osteosarcoma. A plain radiograph is an appropriate initial test if a malignant bone neoplasm is suspected. On plain radiographs, osteosarcoma typically has a mixed pattern of bone lysis and sclerosis. Osteoid formation within the tumor results in calcification in the bony and soft tissue areas of the tumor. In osteosarcoma, periosteal new bone formation can appear in a "sunburst" pattern. It is less likely that this patient has rhabdomyosarcoma (a soft tissue sarcoma), acute lymphoblastic leukemia (normal complete blood count and may have marrow involvement seen on magnetic resonance imaging [MRI]), Langerhans cell histiocytosis (osteolytic bone lesions), or osteomyelitis (no history of fever).

(p. 2039: Section 24: Neoplastic Disorders; Part 3: Solid Tumors; Chapter 449)

**Answer 10-15.** A

The lungs are the most frequent site of metastases for patients with osteosarcoma. Staging typically requires a bone scan to evaluate for bony metastases and a CT scan of the chest to assess for pulmonary metastatic disease. Although an MRI of the chest, CXR, or ultrasound may show metastases to the lungs, a chest CT is more sensitive and remains the radiographic choice for evaluation of pulmonary metastases.

(p. 2039: Section 24: Neoplastic Disorders; Part 3: Solid Tumors; Chapter 449)

**Answer 10-16.** D

Neuroblastoma is a tumor of the sympathetic nervous system and most commonly arises in the adrenal gland or along the sympathetic chain. Paraneoplastic syndromes, such as opsoclonus-myoclonus-ataxia syndrome (OMAS), occur in approximately 5% of patients with neuroblastoma. Signs and symptoms of OMAS include cerebellar ataxia, myoclonic jerks, sudden muscle spasms, and involuntary, rapid eye movements. Children with neuroblastoma and OMAS usually have favorable outcomes.

(p. 2052: Section 24: Neoplastic Disorders; Part 3: Solid Tumors; Chapter 453)

**Answer 10-17.** A

Mature teratomas are the most common histologic subtype of childhood germ cell tumor. Ovarian germ cell tumors often present with onset of abdominal distention and discomfort. Histology includes teratoma, dysgerminoma, yolk sac tumor, or mixed germ cell tumor. Surgical resection alone is the management for mature teratomas. Current treatment for malignant germ cell tumors is based on risk classification.

(p. 2062: Section 24: Neoplastic Disorders; Part 3: Solid Tumors; Chapter 455)

**Answer 10-18.** C

Advances in multimodal therapies, including surgery, chemotherapy, radiotherapy, and stem cell transplantation, have significantly improved the overall survival rate of childhood cancers combined. The 5-year survival rate for all pediatric cancers combined was only 58% between 1975 and 1977, compared with 85% between 2006 and 2012. However, this improved survival varies across childhood cancer types. At this time, more children will die from pediatric CNS tumors than any other type, despite being the second most common cancer in children.

(p. 2000: Section 24: Neoplastic Disorders; Part 1: Principles of Oncology; Chapter 440, p. 2062: Section 24: Neoplastic Disorders; Part 3: Solid Tumors; Chapter 456)

**Answer 10-19.** B

HLH is a syndrome of uncontrolled immune activation leading to pathologic levels of extreme inflammation. HLH represents a wide spectrum of conditions that result in a common end point of multisystem organ failure mediated by pathologic inflammation. Currently, the diagnosis of HLH is made by the presence of 5 of the following 8 diagnostic criteria: (1) fever, (2) splenomegaly, (3) cytopenias of at least 2 lineages in the peripheral blood, (4) elevated triglycerides or low fibrinogen, (5) evidence of hemophagocytosis in tissue (ie, bone marrow, spleen, lymph nodes), (6) low or absent natural killer cell activity, (7) high ferritin level, and (8) elevated soluble interleukin-2 receptor levels. Central nervous system (CNS) involvement may occur at the time of diagnosis, manifested by meningeal signs, altered mental status, and/or seizures. Cerebrospinal fluid studies may reveal an elevated protein concentration, moderate pleocytosis, and occasionally hemophagocytosis on cytologic evaluation. MRI of the brain may reveal subdural effusions or hemorrhages, parameningeal infiltration, or areas of hypodensity or necrosis, but these are not diagnostic criteria for HLH.

(p. 2079: Section 24: Neoplastic Disorders; Part 4: Mononuclear Phagocytic System Disorders, Chapter 459)

**Answer 10-20.** D

Presenting signs and symptoms of children with brain tumors vary according to numerous factors, including tumor size, rate of growth, and location; presence or absence of increased intracranial pressure (ICP); effect on normal brain structures; and the age of the child. The child in the vignette most likely has a posterior fossa tumor causing her presenting symptoms due to obstructive hydrocephalus and mass effect against brain stem structures. Classic symptoms of increased ICP due to obstructive hydrocephalus include morning headaches that improve during the day and vomiting. The finding of dysconjugate gaze may manifest from cranial nerve 6 palsy due to increased ICP or tumor mass effect. In very young children, a bulging fontanelle or separation of cranial sutures may be observed.

The next best step in the evaluation of this child includes head imaging with an MRI of the brain with and without gadolinium contrast, if clinically safe to do so. Computed tomography (CT) scan can be performed rapidly if the child is medically unstable and can assess for evidence of obstructive hydrocephalus, herniation of cranial contents, or intracranial hemorrhage. Lumbar puncture is part of the metastatic workup of certain pediatric brain tumors such as medulloblastoma or ependymoma but is not indicated at this time, particular with concern for increased ICP. An EEG can be performed as part of a seizure evaluation. The tumor markers AFP and β-hCG can be sent from markers serum and cerebrospinal fluid (CSF) as part of a diagnostic evaluation of intracranial germ cell tumors.

(p. 2063: Section 24: Neoplastic Disorders; Part 3: Solid Tumors, Chapter 456)

**Answer 10-21.** A

Infantile hemangiomas are the most common benign vascular tumor of infancy, presenting in 3% to 10% of infants. They are typically not present at birth and most often appear in the first few weeks of life. Infantile hemangiomas usually grow in the first 3 to 4 months of life and generally begin to involute around 6 to 18 months of age. Treatment of infantile hemangiomas includes observation and/or a β-blocker, such as propranolol. Congenital hemangiomas, in contrast, are rare and are completely developed at birth. They are benign vascular tumors that proliferate in utero. Venous and lymphatic malformations are both vascular malformations and not tumors. They result from the abnormal development of venous and lymphatic vessels, respectively. Angiosarcomas are rare, aggressive neoplasms that can occur in any region of the body but are more frequent in skin and soft tissue. Treatment includes chemotherapy.

(p. 2071: Section 24: Neoplastic Disorders; Part 3: Solid Tumors; Chapter 458)

**Answer 10-22.** C

This patient has multiorgan Langerhans cell histiocytosis (LCH). LCH has a wide spectrum of clinical presentations and can often be challenging to diagnose. Cutaneous lesions occur in up to 50% of patients, and skin biopsy is consistent with LCH. Given low-grade fevers, fatigue, polyuria, and polydipsia, further workup is warranted. Patients should be evaluated with a CBC and differential, skeletal survey, and liver function tests to evaluate for cytopenias, bony lesions, and liver dysfunction, respectively. Diabetes insipidus can be a complication of LCH. Clinical assessment for polyuria and polydipsia is important in all patients affected by LCH because it can develop at any time and has been found in up to 20% of all patients with LCH and 50% of patients with central nervous system (CNS) lesions. If clinical history suggests the possibility of diabetes insipidus, screening labs with urine specific gravity, urine osmolality, and serum osmolality should be obtained, as well as brain magnetic resonance imaging (MRI). A bilateral bone marrow is performed in the presence of cytopenias. A chest CT is recommended in patients with respiratory symptoms.

(pp. 2075–2076: Section 24: Neoplastic Disorders; Part 4: Mononuclear Phagocytic System Disorders; Chapter 459)

**Answer 10-23.** B

Approximately 80% of renal neoplasms in children are Wilms tumor (or nephroblastoma), and renal neoplasms occur predominantly in children < 5 years of age. Coagulation studies should be performed prior to surgical intervention because Wilms tumor has been associated with acquired von Willebrand disease, a bleeding disorder that affects primary hemostasis. The timing of surgical resection of Wilms tumor varies. In North America, where Children's Oncology Group guidelines are generally followed, upfront nephrectomy is recommended if clinically possible, and knowledge of the patient's coagulation profile is important. By contrast, guidelines in Europe from the Société Internationale d'Oncologie Pédiatrique (SIOP) include 4 to 6 weeks of preoperative chemotherapy followed by nephrectomy. Acquired von Willebrand disease typically resolves during upfront chemotherapy. Urinalysis may reveal hematuria but does not alter the initial management plan. Urine catecholamine levels are negative in Wilms tumor but are often positive in neuroblastoma, which is included in the differential of a pediatric abdominal mass.

(pp. 2048–2049: Section 24: Neoplastic Disorders; Part 3: Solid Tumors; Chapter 452)

**Answer 10-24.** C

Congenital mesoblastic nephroma, although rare, is the most common renal neoplasm diagnosed in the first 3 months of life. Congenital mesoblastic nephroma originates from the mesenchymal tissue in the embryonic kidney and is frequently associated with the translocation t(12;15), which results in the fusion protein ETV6-NTRK3. This tumor is generally nonaggressive, and surgical removal is the treatment of choice. Wilms tumor is the most common pediatric renal tumor, and the median age at diagnosis is 3.5 years. Although Wilms tumor is more common in younger children, renal cell carcinoma occurs more frequently in individuals aged 15 to 19 years. Other kidney tumors include clear cell sarcoma (3% of pediatric renal tumors) and rhabdoid tumor of the kidney (2% of pediatric renal tumors). Patients with renal cell carcinoma, clear cell carcinoma, and rhabdoid tumor of the kidney have considerably worse outcomes compared to patients with Wilms tumor.

(p. 2048: Section 24: Neoplastic Disorders; Part 3: Solid Tumors; Chapter 452)

**Answer 10-25.** D

Renal tumors account for approximately 7% of all pediatric cancers. A majority of these tumors are Wilms tumors (80%). Other childhood kidney tumors are rarer and include renal cell carcinoma (~4%), clear cell sarcoma of the kidney (~3%), congenital mesoblastic nephroma (~2%), and rhabdoid tumor of the kidney (~2%). The median age at diagnosis of Wilms tumor is approximately 3.5 years, and a majority of Wilms tumor cases occur before the age of 5. The classic presentation of a child with Wilms tumor is the presence of an abdominal mass. Other associated symptoms can include constipation, abdominal distension/pain, hematuria, and hypertension.

(p. 2046: Section 24: Neoplastic Disorders; Part 3: Solid Tumors; Chapter 452)

**Answer 10-26.** A

AFP levels should be obtained in patients with liver tumors. High AFP can be seen in malignant liver tumors. Hepatoblastoma is the most common malignant tumor of the liver and typically occurs in young children, with a mean age of onset between 18 and 20 months. Approximately 95% of cases of hepatoblastoma occur before age 5. Liver tumors in children most commonly present as an asymptomatic mass. Levels of AFP are elevated in most patients with hepatoblastoma. Patients with hepatoblastoma who have a > 90% decline of elevated AFP over the course of therapy have an improved outcome. Levels of AFP are elevated in half of hepatocellular carcinoma patients at diagnosis and can be elevated in some germ cell tumors. CEA is a marker followed in colorectal cancers. β-hCG is a marker used in choriocarcinomas and germ cell tumors. LDH is a nonspecific marker used in germ cell tumors, lymphoma, and leukemia. CA-125 is a nonspecific marker and may be elevated in some ovarian cancers.

(p. 2057: Section 24: Neoplastic Disorders; Part 3: Solid Tumors; Chapter 454)

**Answer 10-27.** C

This newborn has transient myeloproliferative disorder (TMD). He also has characteristic clinical features of Down syndrome (DS). Children with DS are at greater risk for developing TMD, and children with DS also have a 10- to 20-fold higher incidence of leukemia. TMD is transient in nature, and often affected individuals experience a spontaneous resolution. Close observation is recommended for patients who are clinically stable. TMD may be progressive such that patients have side effects of leukostasis and hepatosplenomegaly with multiorgan compromise. These patients may benefit from chemotherapy. Bone marrow transplant is reserved for particular malignant and nonmalignant disorders; however, it is not indicated in a stable patient with TMD. Leukapheresis may be beneficial in patients with marked leukocytosis and/or in patients with symptoms secondary to leukostasis.

(p. 2027: Section 24: Neoplastic Disorders; Part 2: Hematologic Malignancies; Chapter 446)

**Answer 10-28.** A

This patient has neuroblastoma. Approximately 90% of neuroblastomas produce catecholamines, resulting in increased urinary metabolites. Neuroblastoma is a tumor of the sympathetic nervous system and represents approximately 5% of childhood cancers overall. Approximately 90% of affected children are diagnosed before the age of 5. A majority of neuroblastomas arise in the adrenal gland or along the sympathetic chain. Extra-abdominal disease also can occur. Dihydroxyphenylalanine (DOPA) and dopamine convert primarily to HVA, and norepinephrine and epinephrine convert primarily to VMA. Urine HVA and VMA are useful ancillary diagnostic tests when neuroblastoma is suspected. Urine HVA and VMA can also be followed to assess disease response and activity. β-hCG and AFP are tumor markers commonly assessed in germ cell tumors. AFP can also be helpful in certain liver tumors, such as hepatoblastoma. CA-125 and inhibin are markers of ovarian tumors.

(pp. 2052–2053: Section 24: Neoplastic Disorders; Part 3: Solid Tumors; Chapter 453)

# CHAPTER 11 Disorders of the Blood

Mona D. Shah

**11-1.** The mother of a 4-year-old patient calls to report that she noticed he has developed red spots and purplish bruises on both of his legs, some of which are firm and palpable, even though he denies any history of trauma. Moreover, he told his mother that his most recent stool appeared bloody. You ask that they go to the emergency department (ED), where a complete blood count (CBC) reveals that his platelet count is $397 \times 10^9$/L. You suspect Henoch-Schönlein purpura (HSP). Which of the following findings would be consistent with your diagnosis?

**A.** Decreased factor VIII level

**B.** Wet purpura (purpura in the oral mucosa)

**C.** Elevated blood pressure

**D.** Hypofibrinogenemia

**E.** Prolonged prothrombin time

**11-2.** You are asked to evaluate a 5-year-old boy with persistently elevated hemoglobin. The $p_{50}$ (the partial pressure of oxygen at which the patient's hemoglobin is 50% saturated with oxygen) is 20 mm Hg (normal is 26 mm Hg), and his hemoglobin saturation curve is left shifted. This suggests that his polycythemia is due to which of the following?

**A.** Chuvash polycythemia

**B.** Presence of a *JAK2* mutation

**C.** Living at high altitude

**D.** Cyanotic cardiac disease

**E.** Higher-affinity hemoglobin

**11-3.** A neonate's blood differs from that of older children and adults in many respects. Which of the following correctly describes a characteristic that is particular to the neonate?

**A.** The red blood cell (RBC) of the neonate has a low mean corpuscular volume (MCV) that increases as the patient ages.

**B.** Newborns have a high hemoglobin concentration that declines over the first 2 days of life.

**C.** Neonatal RBCs contain primarily embryonic hemoglobin.

**D.** Newborn blood has higher oxygen affinity than that of a 1-year-old.

**E.** The neonate has higher levels of protein C than a 1-year-old.

**11-4.** You are counseling a family about iron supplementation after their son was found to have iron-deficiency anemia on routine screening at his 1-year well-child visit. Which of the following is true about supplementation for iron deficiency?

**A.** All iron supplementation, regardless of formulation, should be taken with milk.

**B.** Proton pump inhibitors can improve the absorption of iron supplementation.

**C.** To avoid gastrointestinal pain, iron should always be taken with food.

**D.** The hemoglobin begins to rise within 1 week of starting iron supplementation.

**E.** Taking iron supplementation with orange juice can improve absorption.

**11-5.** Which of the following correctly orders the sequence with which the laboratory findings of iron deficiency become evident?

**A.** Decreased iron stores and decreased ferritin → decreased transferrin saturation, increased ratio of zinc protoporphyrin to heme → anemia, microcytosis

**B.** Decreased transferrin saturation, increased ratio of zinc protoporphyrin to heme → decreased iron stores and decreased ferritin → anemia, microcytosis

**C.** Decreased iron stores and decreased ferritin → anemia, microcytosis → decreased transferrin saturation, increased ratio of zinc protoporphyrin to heme

**D.** Increased iron stores and increased ferritin → decreased transferrin saturation, increased ratio of zinc protoporphyrin to heme → anemia, microcytosis

**E.** Decreased iron stores and decreased ferritin → decreased transferrin saturation, decreased ratio of zinc protoporphyrin to heme → anemia, microcytosis

**11-6.** A patient with juvenile rheumatoid arthritis is found to be mildly anemic, with a hemoglobin of 10.5 g/dL. His iron studies show normal transferrin saturation and an elevated ferritin level. You suspect that he has anemia of chronic disease. Which of the following is likely to have contributed to his anemia?

**A.** Decreased hepcidin levels

**B.** Increased ferroportin expression

**C.** Decreased intestinal iron absorption

**D.** Enhanced release of iron from macrophages

**E.** Increased renal iron excretion

**11-7.** A 2-year-old boy presents to your office with pallor and fatigue. His mother tells you that he is a picky eater who drinks at least 32 oz of milk each day. His laboratory studies reveal a hemoglobin of 4.8 g/dL and a mean corpuscular volume (MCV) of 51 fL. You suspect iron-deficiency anemia. In counseling the mother, what do you tell her?

**A.** The patient should drink milk when taking the iron you are prescribing.

**B.** The patient should continue to drink milk because it is a good source of iron.

**C.** Milk should be avoided because it contains phytates that chelate iron.

**D.** Milk proteins can irritate the gastrointestinal tract and lead to microscopic blood loss.

**E.** The patient will require iron therapy for 1 month.

**11-8.** A 4-year-old girl presented to your office with fever and dysuria 1 week ago. Her urinalysis is positive for leukocyte esterase and nitrites. Her urine culture eventually grew out > 100,000 colonies of *Escherichia coli*. You started her on a course of trimethoprim-sulfamethoxazole (TMP-SMX). Her fever and dysuria resolved completely, but the mother returns to the clinic today for the development of a rash. On examination, the child is well appearing, but there are multiple punctate nonblanching macular purplish spots on her arms, legs, and trunks. You obtain a complete blood count (CBC) that shows a white blood cell (WBC) count of $1.7 \times 10^9$/L, hemoglobin of 7 g/dL, and platelets of $25 \times 10^9$/L. What is the most likely cause of her laboratory findings?

**A.** Acute lymphoblastic leukemia

**B.** Drug effect

**C.** Viral suppression

**D.** Congenital bone marrow failure syndrome

**E.** Aplastic anemia

**11-9.** A 9-month-old previously healthy male infant is brought to your office by his mother for decreasing activity levels. He has not had any fevers or complaints of pain. He has marked pallor, but the rest of his examination, including an abdominal examination, is normal. The mother tells you that he drinks 10 oz of milk a day and is not a picky eater. You obtain a complete blood count (CBC) that shows a white blood cell (WBC) count of $12 \times 10^9$/L, hemoglobin of 5 g/dL, and platelets of $273 \times 10^9$/L. His differential is normal, with no blasts. His mean corpuscular volume (MCV) is 86 fL, and his reticulocyte count is < 1%. A test for parvovirus is negative. Of the following, which test will likely be helpful in rendering a diagnosis?

**A.** Serum iron level

**B.** Hemoglobin electrophoresis

**C.** Erythrocyte adenosine deaminase

**D.** Glucose-6-phosphate dehydrogenase (G6PD) enzyme levels

**E.** Lead level

**11-10.** You are seeing a 3-year-old patient new to your practice who has had long-standing mild pancytopenia and macrocytosis. You entertain the diagnosis of an inherited bone marrow failure syndrome that is associated with pancytopenia. Your leading considerations are congenital amegakaryocytic thrombocytopenia, Diamond-Blackfan anemia, dyskeratosis congenita, Fanconi anemia, and Shwachman-Diamond syndrome. These syndromes also have in common what other feature?

**A.** Increased risk of malignancy

**B.** Absent thumb

**C.** Pancreatic insufficiency

**D.** Mutation in *cMPL*, the thrombopoietin (TPO) receptor

**E.** Elevated erythrocyte adenosine deaminase activity

**11-11.** You are seeing a 2-year-old boy whose family has recently moved to your area for his initial visit. His past medical history is notable for bilateral pollicization surgeries (surgery to create thumbs from fingers) for his congenitally absent thumbs. The parents also report that at the time of surgery, he was found to have a slightly low platelet count, but he did not need a transfusion before the surgery. In addition to repeating the complete blood count (CBC), you decide to order an abdominal ultrasound. Which of the following tests will confirm the diagnosis that you suspect?

**A.** Bone marrow aspirate and biopsy

**B.** Radiographs of forearms

**C.** Telomere length assays for leukocyte subsets

**D.** Chromosome fragility test with diepoxybutane (DEB)

**E.** Erythrocyte adenosine deaminase levels

**11-12.** A newborn female infant develops jaundice at 12 hours of life. Her indirect bilirubin is 21.2 mg/dL. Her mother's blood type is AB+; her blood type is A+. Her direct Coombs test is negative. Her complete blood count (CBC) results are as follows: white blood cell (WBC) $15.2 \times 10^9$/L, hemoglobin 10 g/dL, hematocrit 30%, mean corpuscular volume (MCV) 98 fL, mean corpuscular hemoglobin concentration (MCHC) 37 g/dL, and platelets $275 \times 10^9$/L. What is the next best step?

**A.** Glucose-6-phosphate dehydrogenase (G6PD) enzyme activity in erythrocytes

**B.** Hemoglobin electrophoresis

**C.** *UGT1A1* activity

**D.** Osmotic fragility

**E.** Abdominal ultrasound

**11-13.** A 2-year-old girl is being evaluated for persistent anemia. She was a term newborn who was found to be jaundiced on the first day of life. Blood type of both the mother and the patient is O+. The father has had mild anemia all of his life, and he reports that his father (the paternal grandfather) had a splenectomy for an unspecified blood disorder. The patient's current labs show a hemoglobin of 10.9 g/dL, mean corpuscular hemoglobin concentration (MCHC) of 38 g/dL (normal, 31 36 g/dL), reticulocyte count of $300 \times 10^9$/L, and total bilirubin of 1.8 mg/dL, and the peripheral blood smear is shown in Figure 429-2A. What do you tell the parents?

**A.** The patient has normal blood because she is not anemic.

**B.** The patient's condition will improve after treatment with steroids.

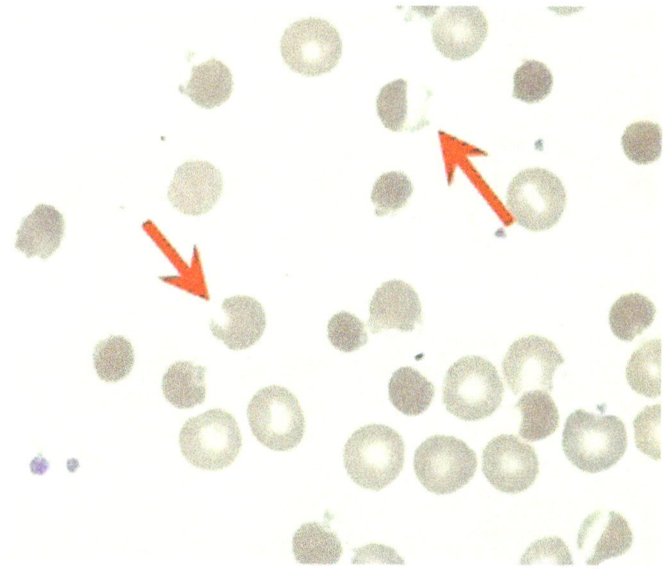

**FIGURE 429-2A.** Acute intravascular hemolysis triggered by infection in child with glucose-6-phosphate dehydrogenase (G6PD) deficiency, with blister and bite cells present (*arrows*). (Mark W. Kline, Rudolph's Pediatrics, 23rd Edition. Copyright © McGraw-Hill Education. All rights reserved.)

**C.** The patient needs iron supplementation.

**D.** The patient likely has a defect in the red blood cell (RBC) membrane–cytoskeletal complex.

**E.** The patient likely has an autosomal recessively inherited hemolytic anemia.

**11-14.** A 15-month-old boy is brought to your office with a fever. He is well appearing without any localizing signs. You order a urinalysis that is positive for leukocyte esterase and nitrites. You start him on trimethoprim-sulfamethoxazole (TMP-SMX). The urine culture eventually grows out 100,000 colonies of *E coli*. Two days later, his mother returns to your office. She reports that he has been irritable and his eyes have turned a yellow color. She also reports that his urine has turned a dark brown color. His urinalysis is positive for blood, although there are only a few red blood cells (RBCs) on microscopic analysis. You check his hemoglobin and find that it is 8.5 g/dL. What is the best test to diagnose the etiology of this patient's illness?

**A.** Parvovirus antibody

**B.** Glucose-6-phosphate dehydrogenase (G6PD) enzyme testing

**C.** Allergy testing

**D.** Creatine kinase levels

**E.** Serum creatinine

**11-15.** A 5-year-old boy with a history of hereditary spherocytosis presents with pallor and fatigue. One week ago, he was seen by his primary care doctor for a fever and runny nose. He was diagnosed with an upper respiratory tract infection at that time. His mother reports that his fevers and runny nose resolved, but over the past several days, he has developed progressive fatigue and pallor. His vital signs are as follows: temperature 36.7°C, heart rate 160 bpm, respiratory rate 26 breaths/min, and blood pressure 110/54 mm Hg. On examination, you note an extremely pale child. A complete blood count (CBC) reveals the following: white blood cell (WBC) count 13 × $10^9$/L, hemoglobin 5.4 g/dL, hematocrit 16.2%, platelets 164 × $10^9$/L, and reticulocyte count < 1%. What test will likely reveal an underlying etiology?

**A.** Parvovirus B19 polymerase chain reaction (PCR)
**B.** Direct antibody testing
**C.** Stool blood testing
**D.** Activated partial thromboplastin time (aPTT)
**E.** Bone marrow biopsy

**11-16.** A 5-year-old boy presents with pallor and fatigue. Two weeks ago, he was seen by his primary care doctor for a fever and runny nose. He was diagnosed with an upper respiratory tract infection at that time. His mother reports that his fevers and runny nose resolved, but over the past several days, he has developed progressive fatigue and pallor. On examination, you note an extremely pale child. Temperature is 36.7°C, heart rate is 160 bpm, respiratory rate is 26 breaths/min, and blood pressure is 110/54 mm Hg. A complete blood count (CBC) reveals the following: white blood cell (WBC) count 13 × $10^9$/L, hemoglobin 5.4 g/dL, hematocrit 16.2%, platelets 134 × $10^9$/L, and reticulocyte count 210 × $10^9$/L. Direct antiglobulin test is positive for immunoglobulin G (IgG). What is the best treatment for this patient?

**A.** Plasmapheresis
**B.** Corticosteroids
**C.** Intravenous immunoglobulin (IVIG)
**D.** Splenectomy
**E.** Antithymocyte antiglobulin

**11-17.** A 14-year-old boy presents with sudden onset of left upper quadrant abdominal pain. Doppler ultrasound reveals a hepatic vein thrombosis. His past medical history is significant for aplastic anemia, which was diagnosed at age 10. He was treated with antithymocyte antiglobulin and cyclosporine, with good recovery of his counts. His current blood counts are all within normal ranges. What laboratory test will likely reveal an etiology for his thrombosis?

**A.** Protein C
**B.** Factor V Leiden
**C.** Bone marrow biopsy
**D.** Homocysteine levels
**E.** Flow cytometry

**11-18.** A 16-year-old girl with a history of systemic lupus erythematosus presents with a temperature of 38.8°C. Her heart rate is 125 bpm, blood pressure is 145/85 mm Hg, respiratory rate is 16 breaths/min, and oxygen saturations is 100% on room air. When you examine her, she is uncooperative and combative. Her cardiovascular examination is notable for a systolic murmur heard best at the left lower sternal border. Her lungs are clear to auscultation bilaterally. Her abdomen is soft and nontender; she has no hepatosplenomegaly. Her laboratory results are as follows: white blood cell (WBC) count 16.5 × $10^9$/L, hemoglobin 7 g/dL, hematocrit 21%, platelets 72 × $10^9$/L, smear notable for schistocytes, sodium 135 mmol/L, potassium 4.1 mmol/L, chlorine 108 mmol/L, bicarbonate 25 mmol/L, blood urea nitrogen 35 mg/dL, and creatinine 2.25 mg/dL. What is the best diagnostic test for this patient?

**A.** ADAMTS13 levels
**B.** Stool culture for *E coli* O157:H7
**C.** Bone marrow biopsy
**D.** Direct Coombs test
**E.** Blood culture

**11-19.** A 4-year-old boy presents with petechiae after a diarrheal illness and is found to have thrombocytopenia and hypertension. His stool studies are positive for *E coli* 0157:H7. Which of the following lab results would be expected?

**A.** Normal red blood cells (RBCs)
**B.** Positive direct Coombs test
**C.** High haptoglobin
**D.** Low lactate dehydrogenase (LDH)
**E.** Elevated creatinine

**11-20.** A newborn whose mother is known to have sickle cell trait and whose father has β-thalassemia trait has a newborn screen from day of life 1 that reveals the presence (in alphabetical order) of hemoglobin A, hemoglobin F, and hemoglobin S. You make which of the following conclusions?

**A.** The patient has sickle cell anemia.
**B.** The patient has hereditary persistence of fetal hemoglobin.
**C.** The patient has 1 normal β-globin gene.
**D.** The patient has sickle cell trait.
**E.** The patient has β-thalassemia trait.

**11-21.** Although sickle hemoglobin is present only in red blood cells (RBCs), patients with sickle cell anemia are at risk of having multiple organs damaged as a consequence of either hemolysis or vaso-occlusion arising from sickled RBCs. Which of the following studies is routinely performed to assess the likelihood of damage to a target organ?

**A.** Audiology examination to assess the risk of hearing loss

**B.** Renal ultrasound to assess the risk of hyposthenuria

**C.** Bone density scan to assess bone damage from vaso-occlusive crises

**D.** Chest radiograph to assess the risk of pulmonary hypertension

**E.** Transcranial Doppler ultrasound to assess the risk of stroke

**11-22.** A 5-year-old girl with a history of sickle cell anemia comes to the emergency department (ED) with fever and a cough. She looks otherwise well, but her chest x-ray (CXR) shows a right lower lobe pneumonia. Which of the following would be the best antibiotic regimen for this patient?

**A.** Amoxicillin and clavulanic acid

**B.** Amoxicillin and clindamycin

**C.** Ceftriaxone and azithromycin

**D.** Ceftriaxone and vancomycin

**E.** Ciprofloxacin monotherapy

**11-23.** A 5-year-old African American boy with human immunodeficiency virus (HIV) is taking dapsone for *Pneumocystis* pneumonia prophylaxis due to a sulfa allergy. He presents with tachypnea and fatigue and appears cyanotic, but his oxygen saturation does not improve with supplemental oxygen. You suspect pseudocyanosis from methemoglobinemia as a complication of dapsone therapy. Before you treat him with methylene blue, you ask about the family history or personal history of which of the following disorders?

**A.** Cyanotic heart disease

**B.** Glucose-6-phosphate dehydrogenase (G6PD) deficiency

**C.** Pyruvate kinase deficiency

**D.** Scott syndrome

**E.** Hereditary spherocytosis

**11-24.** Which of the following is frequently observed in patients with sickle cell *trait*?

**A.** Microcytic anemia

**B.** Priapism

**C.** Hematuria

**D.** Stroke

**E.** Normal hemoglobin electrophoresis

**11-25.** You are seeing a 15-month-old patient who has microcytosis (mean corpuscular volume [MCV] 55 fL), mild anemia (hemoglobin 10 g/dL), and normal serum iron. You recall that his newborn screen showed a small amount of abnormal hemoglobin (hemoglobin Barts), so you order a repeat hemoglobin electrophoresis. The results are normal. You suspect he has which of the following?

**A.** Silent carrier for α-thalassemia

**B.** α-Thalassemia trait

**C.** β-Thalassemia trait

**D.** Hemoglobin H disease

**E.** α-Thalassemia major

**11-26.** A baby is born to parents who are both known to have β-thalassemia minor due to heterozygosity for $\beta^0$ mutations. The baby is found to have a normal hematocrit at birth. You make which of the following conclusions?

**A.** The patient does not have thalassemia major.

**B.** A diagnosis for thalassemia cannot be made until 6 months of age.

**C.** Hemoglobin electrophoresis should be done now.

**D.** The patient has a 25% chance of having thalassemia trait.

**E.** The patient has a 50% chance of having thalassemia major.

**11-27.** You are seeing a 3-year-old Vietnamese girl for the first time. The mother reports that she has a history of iron-deficiency anemia, which was originally diagnosed around 1 year of age when routine screening revealed a hemoglobin of 10.5 g/dL. The mother admits that it is often difficult to get her daughter to take the iron regularly and that it often gives her constipation. You send for more blood work, which shows the following: white blood cell (WBC) count $6.8 \times 10^9$/L, hemoglobin 10.6 g/dL, platelets $302 \times 10^9$/L, mean corpuscular volume (MCV) 59 fL, red blood cell (RBC) count $5.41 \times 10^{12}$/L, ferritin 45 ng/mL (normal, 12–160 ng/mL), transferrin saturation 35% (normal, 20%–50%), and serum iron 35 μg/dL (normal, 26–170 μg/dL). A hemoglobin electrophoresis shows hemoglobin A 98%, hemoglobin A2 2%, and no hemoglobin S or F. The smear shows many hypochromic microcytic cells noted. Multiple target cells are noted. Given these lab findings, what is the most likely diagnosis?

**A.** Iron deficiency

**B.** β-Thalassemia major

**C.** α-Thalassemia trait

**D.** Intestinal malabsorption

**E.** β-Thalassemia intermedia

**11-28.** You are counseling a father about the treatment options for his child with β-thalassemia major. In addition to the increased risk of infection, splenectomized patients are at an increased risk of which of the following?

**A.** Aplastic anemia
**B.** Increased bleeding
**C.** Cancer
**D.** Renal failure
**E.** Thrombosis

**11-29.** Based on a screening transcranial Doppler, it is determined that your patient with sickle cell disease (SCD) is at high risk for stroke. You are counseling the family on starting chronic transfusion therapy. After hearing of the risk of iron overload, the parents ask you to anticipate when he will need to start chelation therapy. You tell them chelation will start when?

**A.** Only if he has the mutations for hereditary hemochromatosis
**B.** As soon as he starts the transfusions
**C.** Only if he shows symptoms of iron overload
**D.** After he has received approximately 200 mL/kg of packed red blood cells (PRBCs)
**E.** As soon as his ferritin is above the normal range

**11-30.** A healthy newborn is circumcised in the nursery prior to discharge. After the circumcision, his wound continues to ooze blood despite pressure and bandaging. His laboratory studies reveal the following: prothrombin time (PT) is 15.9 seconds (normal, 12.2–15.8 seconds), activated partial thromboplastin time (aPTT) is 80 seconds (normal, 25–60 seconds), and platelet count is $200 \times 10^9$/L (normal, $145–450 \times 10^9$/L). Factor VII is 35% (normal, 40%–150%), factor VIII is 12% (normal, 43%–168%), factor IX is 30% (normal, 60%–160%), and von Willebrand factor (vWF) antigen is 150% (normal, 42%–190%). You conclude that the patient likely has which of the following?

**A.** Factor VII deficiency
**B.** Hemophilia A
**C.** Hemophilia B
**D.** von Willebrand disease type 3
**E.** A platelet defect

**11-31.** You are evaluating a patient with hereditary hemorrhagic telangiectasia (HHT), and you note multiple punctate telangiectasias on his lips and tongue. Which of the following is true regarding this patient's disorder?

**A.** Although this syndrome is characterized by telangiectasias, these are benign entities that do not need to be investigated further.
**B.** The most common presenting symptom is frequent epistaxis.
**C.** Telangiectasias only form on the viscera.
**D.** Bleeding into the joints is common, leading to arthritis and limited mobility.
**E.** Patients frequently have soft tissue hypertrophy of 1 extremity.

**11-32.** A 2-year-old boy is being evaluated for easy bruising and epistaxis. His family history is notable for his mother who had heavy menstrual periods as a teenager but has not had any formal evaluation. On examination, his skin is doughy and elastic, and he has increased joint mobility. There are no telangiectasias in his nares or on his skin. His laboratory studies reveal a normal prothrombin time (PT)/activated partial thromboplastin time (aPTT) and complete blood count (CBC), his ristocetin cofactor level is 98%, his von Willebrand antigen level is 110%, and his factor VIII level is 90%. You suspect that he has which of the following?

**A.** A mutation in the endoglin gene (*HHT1*)
**B.** von Willebrand disease (vWD) type 1
**C.** vWD type 2
**D.** vWD type 3
**E.** Ehlers-Danlos syndrome

**11-33.** You are counseling a 17-year-old boy with mild hemophilia A and his parents about the use of desmopressin (DDAVP) prior to his upcoming wisdom teeth extraction. In discussing the possible complications associated with DDAVP, you tell them that DDAVP may lead to which of the following?

**A.** Hypernatremia
**B.** Flushing
**C.** Thrombocytopenia
**D.** Inhibitor development
**E.** Diuresis

**11-34.** You are evaluating a boy who has frequent nosebleeds and a prolonged activated partial thromboplastin time (aPTT). His family history is notable for a maternal uncle and a first cousin (the son of mom's sister) who have been diagnosed with "hemophilia." You find that he has a factor VIII level of 120%. You suspect he most likely has which condition?

**A.** Type 2N von Willebrand disease (vWD)
**B.** Type 3 vWD
**C.** Type 1 vWD
**D.** Hemophilia A
**E.** Hemophilia B

**11-35.** You are evaluating a 15-year-old girl from the Aland Islands, an autonomously governed Swedish-speaking part of Finland, for her menorrhagia. She has had heavy periods since the onset of her menses and reports that she also bruises easily, has frequent nosebleeds, and had prolonged bleeding after a tooth extraction. There is a history of menorrhagia for many of the women on her maternal side, beginning with her great grandmother who was diagnosed with "pseudohemophilia" by Dr. Erick von Willebrand. Her mother tells you that the family's diagnosis has since been reclassified as von Willebrand disease (vWD). Her laboratory studies show a platelet count of 180 × $10^9$/L, von Willebrand factor (vWF) activity (ristocetin cofactor, vWF:RCof) of 40%, von Willebrand antigen (vWF:Ag) of 35%, normal distribution of vWF multimers, and factor VIII activity of 70%. You conclude that she has type 1 vWD. What is the most important criterion used in establishing this diagnosis?

**A.** Clinical history and family history

**B.** Ristocetin cofactor level

**C.** von Willebrand antigen level

**D.** Factor VIII level

**E.** vWF multimer

**11-36.** You are evaluating an 8-year-old, premenarchal girl with a history of easy bruising. Her mother is concerned about the possibility of her daughter having von Willebrand disease (vWD) because the mother has been diagnosed with vWD type 2B. The patient has no prior surgeries and no history of frequent nosebleeds. Which of the following set of labs would be most consistent with the patient having the same diagnosis as her mother?

**A.** Platelet count, 180 × $10^9$/L; von Willebrand factor (vWF) activity (ristocetin cofactor, vWF:RCof), 28%; von Willebrand antigen (vWF:Ag), 30%; factor VIII activity, 50%; slightly decreased but normal distribution of vWF multimers; no platelet aggregation in response to low-dose ristocetin

**B.** Platelet count, 200 × $10^9$/L; vWF activity (vWF:RCof), 10%; von Willebrand antigen (vWF:Ag), 32%; factor VIII activity, 50%; absent high- and intermediate-sized vWF multimers; no platelet aggregation in response to low-dose ristocetin

**C.** Platelet count, 0 × $10^9$/L; vWF activity (vWF:RCof), 40%; von Willebrand antigen (vWF:Ag), 45%; factor VIII activity, 80%; absent high-molecular-weight multimers; platelets do aggregate in response to low-dose ristocetin

**D.** Platelet count, 200 × $10^9$/L; vWF activity (vWF:RCof), 10%; von Willebrand antigen (vWF:Ag), 32%; factor VIII activity, 50%; slightly decreased but normal distribution of vWF multimers; no platelet aggregation in response to low-dose ristocetin

**E.** Platelet count, 180 × $10^9$/L; vWF activity (vWF:RCof), 40%; von Willebrand antigen (vWF:Ag), 45%; factor VIII activity, 8%; slightly decreased but normal distribution of vWF multimers; no platelet aggregation in response to low-dose ristocetin

**11-37.** A 14-year-old girl is being seen for menorrhagia. She has always bruised easily and has a past history of frequent nosebleeds that have since resolved. Her mother reports that she also has heavy periods, and her mother, the patient's grandmother, is reported to have had a hysterectomy because of heavy periods. The patient's laboratory studies are as follows: hemoglobin 10.5 g/dL, platelets 300 × $10^9$/L, normal prothrombin time (PT) and activated partial thromboplastin time (aPTT), von Willebrand activity (ristocetin cofactor, vWF:RCof) 28% (normal, > 50%), von Willebrand antigen (vWF:Ag) 30% (normal, > 50%), factor VIII activity 55% (normal, > 50%), and normal distribution but slightly diminished amounts of von Willebrand factor (vWF) multimers. You conclude that the patient has which condition?

**A.** von Willebrand disease (vWD) type 1

**B.** vWD type 2A

**C.** vWD type 2M

**D.** vWD type 2N

**E.** vWD type 3

**11-38.** A 2-year-old boy with severe hemophilia A, who has not had any hemarthroses since starting prophylaxis 1 year ago, begins to have knee bleeds that are refractory to his usual treatment dose of recombinant factor VIII. Laboratory studies reveal an inhibitor of 11 Bethesda units (BUs). What do you tell his parents?

**A.** Inhibitors occur in 90% of severe hemophilia A patients.

**B.** It is not possible to eradicate the inhibitor.

**C.** His titer of 11 BU is considered a low-titer inhibitor.

**D.** Immune tolerance induction may eradicate the inhibitor.

**E.** The inhibitor is likely to spontaneously resolve.

**11-39.** An 18-year-old patient with type 1 von Willebrand disease (vWD) is planning to undergo wisdom teeth extraction. Because he has previously been shown to respond well to intranasal desmopressin (DDAVP), he will be using DDAVP and aminocaproic acid (an antifibrinolytic) as coverage for his procedure. You remind him of which of the following?

**A.** DDAVP may result in retention of free water.

**B.** He should use DDAVP daily for 7 days.

**C.** He should increase his daily intake of fluids.

**D.** DDAVP will decrease factor VIII levels.

**E.** DDAVP should be used 4 times a day.

**11-40.** A newborn baby is noted to have profuse bleeding after circumcision, requiring urologic intervention. On further questioning, the mother reports that she has a history of heavy periods and that she recalls an aunt who needed a transfusion after childbirth. You send off some preliminary lab work that shows a white blood cell (WBC) count of $12 \times 10^9$/L, hemoglobin of 9 g/dL, platelets of $372 \times 10^9$/L, activated partial thromboplastin time (aPTT) of 37 seconds, prothrombin time (PT) of 13.1 seconds, and fibrinogen of 202 mg/dL. Factor VIII activity is 9%, and factor IX activity is 35%. Of the following choices, what is the most likely diagnosis?

**A.** von Willebrand disease (vWD)

**B.** Disseminated intravascular coagulation

**C.** Hemophilia B

**D.** Afibrinogenemia

**E.** Vitamin K deficiency

**11-41.** A 12-year-old girl presents with menorrhagia and a history of significant bleeding 4 days after a tonsillectomy. Her family history is notable for her having a brother who had an intracranial hemorrhage in the newborn period as a full-term newborn and for her mother having had 3 miscarriages. Her prothrombin time (PT), activated partial thromboplastin time (aPTT), platelet count, and peripheral smear are all normal, as is her von Willebrand panel. You suspect which of the following?

**A.** Decreased clot solubility

**B.** Increased clot solubility

**C.** Elevated factor XIII level

**D.** Decreased factor V level

**E.** Increased protein C level

**11-42.** A 2-year-old boy is brought to the emergency department (ED) after being found playing with a rodenticide. His international normalized ratio is 3.5, and you suspect that he has ingested a vitamin K antagonist commonly used in rodenticides. Which of the following factors is expected to be normal?

**A.** Factor II

**B.** Factor V

**C.** Factor VII

**D.** Factor IX

**E.** Factor X

**11-43.** A 1-week-old presents to your office with bruising and coffee-ground emesis. She was a term baby who was born at home and is now exclusively breastfed. Her prothrombin time (PT) is > 100 seconds, and her activated partial thromboplastin time (aPTT) is 160 seconds. This patient has which of the following?

**A.** Low factor VIII level

**B.** Low factor V level

**C.** Factor V Leiden

**D.** Low factor VII level

**E.** Cystic fibrosis

**11-44.** Which of the following is associated with an increased risk of thrombosis?

**A.** Thrombocytopenia

**B.** Prothrombin gene mutation

**C.** Factor V deficiency

**D.** Nephritic syndrome

**E.** Homocysteine deficiency

**11-45.** A 16-year-old girl was started on oral contraceptive pills for acne 2 months ago. She presents with a swollen and painful left leg. Doppler ultrasound reveals a thrombus in her left iliac and femoral veins. She is placed on anticoagulation with subsequent resolution of her clot. You obtain studies after stopping anticoagulation 6 months after her presentation. Which of the following suggests that she has a higher risk of thrombosis than the normal population?

**A.** Protein C activity of 165% (normal, 76%–146%)

**B.** Antithrombin activity of 102% (normal, 79%–120%)

**C.** Factor VIII activity level of 97% (normal, 43%–168%)

**D.** Factor V that is resistant to cleavage by activated protein C (APC)

**E.** Plasma homocysteine level of 7 μmol/L (normal, 4–14 μmol/L)

**11-46.** A 6-year-old boy is brought into your clinic because his mother has noticed increased bruising. She reports that he has been otherwise doing well with no fevers and normal appetite and activity levels. He is well appearing, but you note multiple bruises on his trunk and legs. The rest of his examination is unremarkable. You obtain labs that show the following: white blood cell (WBC) 8.4 × $10^9$/L, hemoglobin 13 g/dL, and platelets 15 × $10^9$/L. You suspect immune thrombocytopenic purpura. Which of the following is true about this disease?

**A.** The diagnosis must be confirmed by a bone marrow biopsy.

**B.** He should be given platelet transfusions to minimize his bleeding risk.

**C.** Laboratory testing for platelet autoantibodies should be performed by the blood bank.

**D.** Most patients will have resolution of their symptoms within 3 months.

**E.** Once this episode resolves, the patient will be at an increased risk to develop leukemia.

**11-47.** You are asked to evaluate a term newborn, born to a healthy G1P1 mother after an uncomplicated pregnancy and delivery, who is noted to have petechiae and prolonged oozing after a heel stick for the newborn screen. Aside from petechiae over his face and chest, he is a well-appearing newborn. Of note, he has normal thumbs and forearms and no hepatosplenomegaly. A complete blood count (CBC) is obtained from his cord blood that is normal except for a platelet count of 12 × $10^9$/L. His mother has a normal platelet count. In addition to a head ultrasound to evaluate for the possibility of intracranial hemorrhage, which of the following is the most appropriate next step?

**A.** Transfusion of maternal platelets because the patient may have neonatal alloimmune thrombocytopenia (NAIT)

**B.** Abdominal ultrasound to evaluate for renal anomalies because Fanconi anemia is in the differential

**C.** Intravenous immunoglobulin (IVIG) because the patient may have maternally derived neonatal autoimmune thrombocytopenia

**D.** Toxoplasma, syphilis, rubella, cytomegalovirus, and herpes simplex (TORCH) titers to evaluate for the possibility that his symptoms are due to cytomegalovirus (CMV) infection during the pregnancy

**E.** Platelet aggregation studies to rule out the possibility of Glanzmann thrombasthenia

**11-48.** A full-term infant is admitted to the nursery after an uncomplicated delivery to a G1P1 mother. He is noted to have multiple bruises. A complete blood count (CBC) shows a white blood cell (WBC) count of 17 × $10^9$/L, hemoglobin of 15 g/dL, and platelets of 24 × $10^9$/L. The mother's platelet count is normal, and the infant's human platelet antigen (HPA)-1a testing is positive. You diagnose neonatal alloimmune thrombocytopenia (NAIT). What is the next best course of action?

**A.** Transfusion of maternal platelets

**B.** Transfusion of random donor platelets

**C.** Observation

**D.** Intravenous immunoglobulin (IVIG)

**E.** Steroids

**11-49.** You are asked to evaluate an otherwise well term newborn baby boy who presented with petechiae at birth and was found to have a platelet count of 70 × $10^9$/L. His physical examination is normal, and no infectious source is identified. His family history is notable for his mother and a maternal aunt and uncle with hearing loss and easy bruising. Additionally, his uncle is on dialysis for renal failure. Which test would you order next?

**A.** X-rays of his forearms

**B.** Diepoxybutane (DEB) chromosome breakage test

**C.** Examination of his peripheral blood smear

**D.** Bone marrow aspirate and biopsy

**E.** Platelet aggregation studies

**11-50.** A 17-year-old girl on the varsity cross-country team presents with menorrhagia for her last 2 periods. Prior to this, she has had normal periods since menarche at age 12. There is no family history of bleeding symptoms or a bleeding disorder. She does report frequent use of ibuprofen following long training runs. Laboratory studies show hemoglobin of 11.5 g/dL, platelet count of 170 × $10^9$/L, a peripheral smear that is normal in appearance, normal prothrombin time (PT) and activated partial thromboplastin time (aPTT), and a normal von Willebrand panel with von Willebrand activity (ristocetin cofactor, vWF:RCof) of 55%, von Willebrand antigen (vWF:Ag) of 60%, factor VIII activity of 76%, and normal von Willebrand factor (vWF) multimers. You suspect that the patient has which of the following conditions?

**A.** von Willebrand disease (vWD) type 1

**B.** Acquired cyclooxygenase deficiency

**C.** May Hegglin anomaly (a myosin heavy chain 9 [MYH9]-related disorder)

**D.** Factor VII deficiency

**E.** Immune thrombocytopenia

**11-51.** You are seeing a 1-year-old boy for a well-child visit. In reviewing his history, you note that he has had 4 episodes of otitis media and 1 hospitalization for pneumonia and has had eczema since 4 months of age. You obtain a screening complete blood count (CBC) and note that he has a hemoglobin of 11 g/dL, white blood cell (WBC) of $6 \times 10^9$/L, and a platelet count of $47 \times 10^9$/L. The pathologist notes that the platelets appear small. You suspect that this patient has which condition?

**A.** Thrombocytopenia absent radius

**B.** Wiskott-Aldrich syndrome

**C.** Fanconi anemia

**D.** Congenital amegakaryocytic thrombocytopenia

**E.** Hyper-immunoglobulin E (IgE) syndrome

**11-52.** A 1-year-old girl is brought to the emergency department (ED) by her mother with fever and irritability for 1 day. On examination, you find a toxic-appearing infant, with a temperature of 39.5°C, heart rate of 168 bpm, blood pressure of 108/68 mm Hg, and a respiratory rate of 34 breaths/min. She has no abnormal lymphadenopathy. You hear clear breath sounds in both lung fields, and she is tachycardic with a systolic flow murmur. Her abdomen is nontender with no hepatosplenomegaly. You do not note any rashes. You obtain labs, including a complete blood count (CBC), and blood and urine cultures. The CBC shows a white blood cell (WBC) count of $17 \times 10^9$/L, hemoglobin of 13 g/dL, and platelets of $1105 \times 10^9$/L. Her blood culture eventually grows out *Streptococcus pneumoniae*. She is admitted and treated with antibiotics. What is the most likely cause of her high platelet count?

**A.** Familial thrombocytosis

**B.** Essential thrombocytosis

**C.** Iron-deficiency anemia

**D.** Reactive thrombocytosis

**E.** Kawasaki disease

**11-53.** A 4-year-old boy presents with epistaxis and a history of easy bruising. There is no family history of bleeding problems. The patient's laboratory studies are as follows: normal prothrombin time (PT) and activated partial thromboplastin time (aPTT); normal von Willebrand panel with von Willebrand activity (ristocetin cofactor, vWF:RCof) of 85%, von Willebrand antigen (vWF:Ag) of 90%, factor VIII activity of 105%, and normal von Willebrand factor (vWF) multimers. A complete blood count (CBC) shows a hemoglobin of 12 g/dL, white blood cell (WBC) count of $6.5 \times 10^9$/L, and platelet count of $140 \times 10^9$/L, and large platelets were noted on the smear. Platelet aggregation studies showed a lack of response to ristocetin. What is the most likely diagnosis?

**A.** Bernard-Soulier syndrome

**B.** Glanzmann thrombasthenia

**C.** Shwachman-Diamond syndrome

**D.** Kostmann disease

**E.** Pearson syndrome

**11-54.** A 3-year-old boy presents with prolonged epistaxis and a history of easy bruising. There is no family history of bleeding problems. The patient's laboratory studies show a normal complete blood count (CBC) and smear, normal von Willebrand panel, and normal prothrombin time (PT) and activated partial thromboplastin time (aPTT), but platelet aggregation shows no response to adenosine diphosphate (ADP), thrombin, and epinephrine, and platelets are found to lack glycoprotein (GP) IIb/IIIa. What is the most likely diagnosis?

**A.** Bernard-Soulier syndrome

**B.** Glanzmann thrombasthenia

**C.** Shwachman-Diamond syndrome

**D.** Kostmann disease

**E.** Pearson syndrome

**11-55.** A 13-year-old African American girl comes to your clinic. A routine blood count done to screen for iron deficiency reveals an absolute neutrophil count of $900 \times 10^6$/L. The rest of her blood count is normal. She has been healthy all her life, with no hospitalizations or serious infections. She denies any mouth ulcers or gingivitis. She is not on any medications. As far as the family knows, there is no history of inherited bone disorders or children who died at young ages. Which of the following is the most likely diagnosis?

**A.** Myelokathexis

**B.** Reticular dysgenesis

**C.** Kostmann syndrome

**D.** Ethnic pseudoneutropenia

**E.** Glycogen storage disease type Ib

**11-56.** You obtain a complete blood count (CBC) that shows a white blood cell (WBC) count of 5.4 × $10^9$/L, a hemoglobin of 13 g/dL, and platelets of 350 × $10^9$/L. His absolute neutrophil count is 3500 cells/μL. What further evaluation would be needed to establish a diagnosis?

**A.** Complete blood counts (CBCs) 2 times a week
**B.** Quantitative immunoglobulin levels
**C.** Bone marrow biopsy
**D.** Human immunodeficiency virus (HIV) testing
**E.** No further testing needed

**11-57.** You are asked to see an 8-month-old infant who is hospitalized for pneumonia and failure to thrive. The child has a history of steatorrhea and pancreatic insufficiency. His laboratory studies show a white blood cell (WBC) of 4.1 × $10^9$/L with an absolute neutrophil count of 900 × $10^6$/L, hemoglobin of 10.5 g/dL, mean corpuscular volume (MCV) of 92 fL, and platelets of 102 × $10^9$/L. His sweat test is normal. You suspect that he has a mutation in which of the following genes?

**A.** *TERT* associated with dyskeratosis congenita
**B.** *CFTR* associated with cystic fibrosis
**C.** *RMRP* associated with cartilage-hair hypoplasia
**D.** *SBDS* associated with Shwachman-Diamond syndrome
**E.** *TP53* associated with Li-Fraumeni syndrome

**11-58.** Shwachman-Diamond syndrome, Chediak-Higashi syndrome, severe congenital neutropenia, cyclic neutropenia, and cartilage-hair hypoplasia all have which of the following in common?

**A.** Increased risk of malignancy
**B.** *ELA2* mutations
**C.** Ribosome dysfunction
**D.** Neutropenia
**E.** Platelet dysfunction

**11-59.** A 6-year-old girl is admitted for fever and pneumonia. The mother reports that she has been admitted several times for various bacterial infections. On physical examination, her vital signs are temperature of 40.2°F, heart rate of 190 bpm, respiratory rate of 50 breaths/min, and blood pressure of 70/38 mm Hg; oxygen saturation level is 92% on room air. She is ill-appearing. Her heart rate is tachycardic, and a systolic murmur is appreciated. Her abdomen is soft and nontender. See the figure for further clinical findings. Of the following options, which is mostly likely to be true regarding this patient?

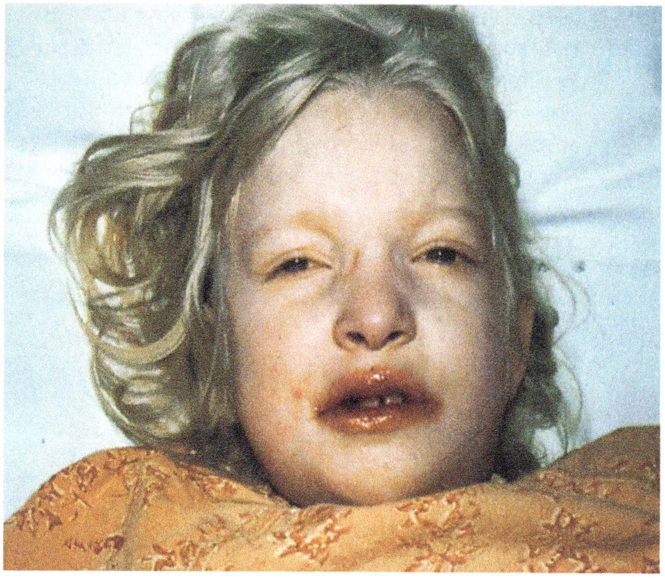

(Reproduced, with permission, from Prose NS, Kristal L. *Weinberg's Color Atlas of Pediatric Dermatology.* 5th ed. New York: McGraw-Hill, 2017.)

**A.** She has pancreatic insufficiency.
**B.** She has nail dystrophy.
**C.** She has triphalangeal thumbs.
**D.** She has peripheral neuropathy.
**E.** She has elevated immunoglobulin E (IgE) levels.

**11-60.** A 3-month-old male infant is admitted for pneumonia after presenting with a 1-day history of fever and increased work of breathing. In taking his history, his mother notes that his umbilical cord did not fall off until about a month of age. On physical examination, his vital signs are temperature of 40.2°C, heart rate of 180 bpm, respiratory rate of 50 breaths/min, blood pressure of 70/38 mm Hg, and oxygen saturation of 92% on 1 L of oxygen. He is sleepy and ill appearing. His head is normocephalic, his pupils are reactive, and his tympanic membranes are well visualized with a good light reflex. His heart rate is tachycardic, and a systolic murmur is appreciated. He is tachypneic with crackles and decreased breath sounds on the right side. His abdomen is soft and nontender with no hepatosplenomegaly. He has normal tone and bulk. You obtain labs and start him on antibiotics. His complete blood count (CBC) shows a white blood cell (WBC) count of 32,000 × $10^6$/L, a hemoglobin of 12.5 g/dL, and platelets of 550 × $10^9$/L. His absolute neutrophil count is 29,000 × $10^6$/L. What is the most likely diagnosis?

**A.** Leukemoid reaction
**B.** Acute leukemia
**C.** Leukocyte adhesion deficiency-1 (LAD-1)
**D.** Drug reaction
**E.** Myeloproliferative disease

**11-61.** A 10-year-old boy is admitted for osteomyelitis of his right fourth metatarsal after presenting with pain and swelling of his foot. He has had a history of multiple skin abscesses that were drained. Cultures from these abscesses grew out *Staphylococcus aureus.* When he was 5 years old, he also had an episode of lymphadenitis requiring antibiotics. Given this patient's history, what test is most likely to reveal a diagnosis?

**A.** Bone marrow biopsy
**B.** Dihydrorhodamine test
**C.** Immunoglobulin E (IgE) levels
**D.** Skin biopsy
**E.** Lymphocyte subsets

**11-62.** You are evaluating a 3-year-old boy who has an eczematous rash. His past medical history is notable for a hospitalization at 8 months of age for pneumonia and 15 episodes of otitis media in the first year of life. His physical examination is unremarkable except for a pruritic, papular rash on his face and extremities. His complete blood count (CBC) reveals a white blood cell (WBC) count of $7 \times 10^9$/L, hemoglobin of 11 g/dL, and platelet count of $150 \times 10^9$/L. His serum immunoglobulin G (IgG) level is 600 IU/mL, and his immunoglobulin E (IgE) level is 3000 IU/mL. You conclude that he has which condition?

**A.** Wiskott-Aldrich syndrome
**B.** Hyper-IgE syndrome
**C.** Thrombocytopenia absent radii
**D.** Leukocyte adhesion defect
**E.** Milk protein allergy

**11-63.** A 16-year-old girl with menorrhagia presents to the emergency department (ED) with fatigue and is found to have a hemoglobin level of 6.2 g/dL. She is transfused 2 units of packed red blood cells (PRBCs). This episode is her first transfusion. Within minutes of starting the transfusion, she develops shortness of breath, her oxygen saturation drops to 80%, and her blood pressure is 70/30 mm Hg. Her temperature is 37°C. The transfusion is immediately stopped, and she is given diphenhydramine, hydrocortisone, and epinephrine. What test should be included in the evaluation of her transfusion reaction?

**A.** Chest x-ray (CXR)
**B.** Immunoglobulin E (IgE) levels
**C.** Immunoglobulin A (IgA) levels
**D.** Skin allergy testing
**E.** Early morning cortisol level

**11-64.** A 12-year-old boy who is undergoing chemotherapy for acute lymphoblastic leukemia has chemotherapy-induced pancytopenia, for which he receives a blood transfusion. After the transfusion starts, he develops vomiting, fever, and chills. He does not have any rash or shortness of breath. His blood transfusion is stopped, with rapid resolution of his symptoms. Shortly afterward, his urine turns a dark color and is cloudy. What other findings are consistent with the patient's clinical picture?

**A.** New infiltrate on chest radiograph (CXR)
**B.** Metabolic alkalosis
**C.** Hypocalcemia
**D.** Low haptoglobin
**E.** Polycythemia

**11-65.** One of your patients is going to the operating room tomorrow for cardiac surgery. The surgeon asks you to get consent from the family for possible blood transfusion. Which of the following is not routinely screened at the blood bank?

**A.** Hepatitis A
**B.** Hepatitis B
**C.** Hepatitis C
**D.** Human immunodeficiency virus (HIV)
**E.** Human T-lymphotropic virus-1 (HTLV-1)

## ANSWERS

**Answer 11-1.** C

Patients with HSP may have renal involvement, which may lead to hypertension. Therefore, evaluation of patients suspected of having HSP should include careful attention to vital signs for evidence of renal involvement, including close attention to evidence of hypertension. The petechiae and purpura associated with HSP are characteristically in the lower extremities rather than mucosal. Although patients have petechiae and purpura, the lesions arise from vasculitis and are not due to coagulopathy, so fibrinogen and clotting factor levels and prothrombin time are normal.

(p. 1905, Section 23: Disorders of the Blood, Part 1: Principles of Blood Disorders, Chapter 424: Approach to Suspected Hematologic Disorders; pp. 938–939, Section 15: Rheumatology, Chapter 200: Vasculitides)

**Answer 11-2.** E

A leftward-shifted oxygen dissociation curve and a lower-than-normal $p_{50}$ are consistent with an increased hemoglobin

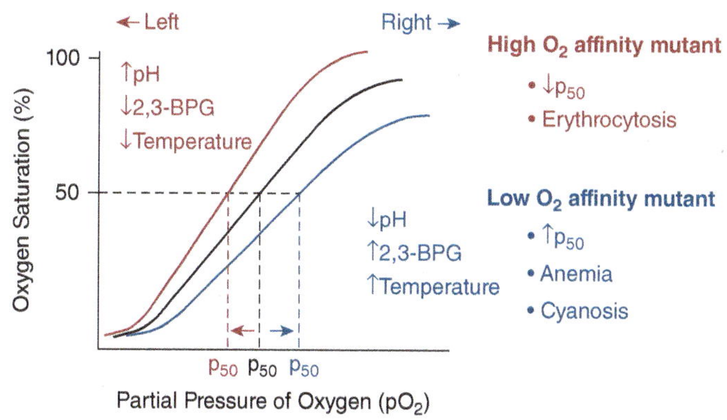


**FIGURE 430-2.** The oxyhemoglobin dissociation curve and its physiologic modulation. Hemoglobin tetramers with increased oxygen affinity cause decreased oxygen delivery to tissues, with a resultant erythrocytosis, while tetramers with low affinity cause cyanosis that is usually clinically insignificant. 2,3-BPG, 2,3-bisphosphoglycerate; $p_{50}$, partial pressure of oxygen at which hemoglobin is 50% saturated with oxygen. (Mark W. Kline, *Rudolph's Pediatrics*, 23rd Edition. Copyright © McGraw-Hill Education. All rights reserved).

oxygen affinity. This results in less oxygen release to the tissues and thus a compensatory increase in hemoglobin. Figure 430-2 shows a graphic display of effects of pH, 2,3-bisphosphoglycerate (2,3-BPG), and temperature on oxygen affinity. Chuvash polycythemia is due to mutations in the von Hippel-Lindau gene, which is part of the oxygen-sensing apparatus. *JAK2* mutations are associated with polycythemia vera. Patients living at high altitude and with cyanotic cardiac disease have increased red blood cell mass due to chronic hypoxia but have normal hemoglobin oxygen affinity.

(pp. 1907–1910, Section 23: Disorders of the Blood, Part 1: Principles of Blood of Disorders, Chapter 425: Hematopoiesis; pp. 1932–1934, Section 23: Disorders of the Blood, Part 2: Disorders of Red Blood Cells and Anemia, Chapter 430: Hemoglobinopathies)

## Answer 11-3. D

Fetal hemoglobin has higher oxygen affinity than hemoglobin A. Newborn RBCs have high levels of fetal hemoglobin (α2γ2)—approaching 70%. After birth, the percentage of fetal hemoglobin decreases after synthesis of γ-globin is replaced by β-globin synthesis. At 4 months of age, fetal hemoglobin accounts for 40% of the total hemoglobin, and by 1 year of age, hemoglobin A (α2β2) is predominant (98%). The higher oxygen affinity of fetal hemoglobin is due to its relative decrease in affinity for 2,3-BPG compared with hemoglobin A. The RBC of the neonate has a high MCV (on average 107 fL) that decreases in the first year of life and then rises with age. Newborns have a high hemoglobin level that then rises in the first 2 days of life as plasma volume initially decreases postnatally. Protein C levels are low at birth and rise with age, reaching adult levels by adolescence.

(pp. 1907–1910, Section 23: Disorders of the Blood, Part 1: Principles of Blood Disorders, Chapter 425: Hematopoiesis)

## Answer 11-4. E

Iron deficiency is the most common global nutritional deficiency, and iron-deficiency anemia is the most common hematologic disease of infancy and childhood. Non-heme dietary iron comes primarily in the ferric state ($Fe^{3+}$) and is reduced to the ferrous state ($Fe^{2+}$) in an acidic environment. Ascorbic acid can therefore improve the absorption of iron. Iron supplementation should never be taken with milk, food, or proton pump inhibitors as these all inhibit the absorption of iron. Hemoglobin is one of the last indices to improve, although reticulocytosis can be seen within 1 week of starting iron supplementation.

(pp. 1914–1917, Section 23: Disorders of the Blood, Part 2: Disorders of Red Blood Cells and Anemia, Chapter 427: Iron Deficiency)

## Answer 11-5. A

Anemia and microcytosis are late findings in iron deficiency. First, in the prelatent phase, iron stores are depleted and ferritin levels are typically low. Importantly, ferritin levels can remain normal or elevated if there is concurrent inflammation. This is followed by latent iron deficiency, which is evident in a decrease in transferrin saturation. The final step of heme formation is the incorporation of an iron molecule into the porphyrin ring. As the amount of iron being transported in the plasma decreases, there is less iron available to be incorporated into the porphyrin ring and a resulting rise in the ratio of zinc protoporphyrin to heme. Finally, with overt iron-deficiency anemia, there is a diminution in red blood cell (RBC) volume and quantity. See Table 427-1 for laboratory values associated with different stages of iron deficiency.

**TABLE 427-1.** Stages of Iron Deficiency

| | Normal | Prelatent | Latent | Iron Deficiency Anemia |
|---|---|---|---|---|
| Iron stores | Present | Decreased | Absent | Absent |
| Serum ferritin (ng/mL) | > 40 | < 20 | < 10 | < 10 |
| Transferrin saturation (%) | 35 | 35 | < 16 | < 16 |
| Free erythrocyte protoporphyrin (ng/dL) | 10 | 10 | > 35 | > 35 |
| Hemoglobin (g/dL) | 12 | 12 | 12 | < 11 |
| Mean corpuscular volume (fL) | 80 | 80 | 80 | < 70 |

Mark W. Kline, *Rudolph's Pediatrics*, 23rd Edition. Copyright © McGraw-Hill Education. All rights reserved.

(pp. 1914–1917, Section 23: Disorders of the Blood, Part 2: Disorders of Red Blood Cells and Anemia, Chapter 427: Iron Deficiency)

**Answer 11-6.** C

Anemia of chronic disease is multifactorial and likely due to impaired iron mobilization and decreased intestinal absorption of iron. As in this vignette, the anemia is usually mild to moderate, normocytic, and normochromic. Serum iron levels are low, but transferrin saturation is normal and serum ferritin is typically elevated due to the inflammatory state. Additionally, in anemia of chronic inflammation, production of hepcidin, a peptide hormone synthesized by the liver, is increased. Hepcidin acts as a negative regulator of iron release by acting to decrease ferroportin expression. Because ferroportin is required for both intestinal transport of iron and macrophage release of iron, the decrease in ferroportin leads to decreased iron absorption and decreased release of iron from macrophage stores. Humans do not have a mechanism of active iron excretion.

(pp. 1914–1917, Section 23: Disorders of the Blood, Part 2: Disorders of Red Blood Cells and Anemia, Chapter 427: Iron Deficiency)

**Answer 11-7.** D

Milk can contribute to the development of iron deficiency in multiple ways. It is a poor source of iron, so toddlers who rely primarily on milk for nutrition have insufficient iron intake. Milk contains proteins that can irritate the gastrointestinal tract of some patients and lead to microscopic blood loss, and milk inhibits the absorption of iron. Phytates are compounds found in plants; they can chelate iron and inhibit its absorption. Typical therapy for iron-deficiency anemia continues for several months after the anemia is corrected in order to replenish iron stores.

(pp. 1914–1917, Section 23: Disorders of the Blood, Part 2: Disorders of Red Blood Cells and Anemia, Chapter 427: Iron Deficiency)

**Answer 11-8.** B

The patient developed pancytopenia after a course of TMP-SMX, which is known to cause bone marrow suppression. Other than the petechiae, she is well appearing with no fevers, hepatosplenomegaly, or pain that would point toward an underlying leukemia. The patient had a bacterial urinary tract infection, with no other signs of a concurrent viral infection. Although this could be the first presentation of an acquired aplastic anemia or congenital bone marrow failure syndrome, these are relatively rare diseases, and drug effect is more likely.

(pp. 1917–1921, Section 23: Disorders of the Blood, Part 2: Disorders of Red Blood Cells and Anemia, Chapter 428: Anemia Due to Diminished Red Blood Cell Production)

**Answer 11-9.** C

The patient has anemia with a low reticulocyte count, indicating that the anemia resulted from a production failure. Erythrocyte adenosine deaminase levels help distinguish between Diamond-Blackfan anemia and transient erythrocytopenia of childhood (TEC), both of which can present with pure red blood cell (RBC) aplasia. Diamond-Blackfan anemia is a bone marrow failure syndrome that results from a defect in ribosome biosynthesis, causing RBCs to be sensitive to death by apoptosis. Patients have elevated levels of erythrocyte adenosine deaminase. Most patients can be treated with steroids, but some will need chronic transfusions. TEC is a diagnosis of exclusion that describes the temporary and spontaneous cessation of erythropoiesis. Patients are managed with supportive care and eventually recover. Anemia in hemoglobinopathies and RBC enzyme mutations results from increased RBC turnover of the abnormal cells. Patients typically have high reticulocyte counts. Although the anemia seen in lead toxicity or iron deficiency is also from ineffective erythropoiesis and patients can also have a low reticulocyte count, it is typically a microcytic anemia.

(pp. 1917–1921, Section 23: Disorders of the Blood, Part 2: Disorders of Red Blood Cells and Anemia, Chapter 428: Anemia Due to Diminished Red Blood Cell Production)

**Answer 11-10.** A

Many inherited bone marrow failure syndromes are classically associated with a defect in one cell line; however, many progress to pancytopenia and aplastic anemia. Congenital amegakaryocytic thrombocytopenia, Diamond-Blackfan anemia, dyskeratosis congenita, Fanconi anemia, and Shwachman-Diamond syndrome all are associated with an increased risk of malignancy. Additionally, patients with thrombocytopenia absent radii, which is not a bone marrow failure syndrome, have an increased risk of leukemia, although aplastic anemia has not been reported. Thrombocytopenia absent radii patients may have hypoplastic or misplaced thumbs, but not the absent thumbs that are associated only with Fanconi anemia patients. Pancreatic insufficiency is a feature of Shwachman-Diamond syndrome as well as Pearson syndrome, which is another bone marrow failure syndrome and arises from mitochondrial DNA deletion. Mutations in *cMPL* are specific to congenital amegakaryocytic thrombocytopenia, and elevated erythrocyte adenosine deaminase is a diagnostic test for Diamond-Blackfan anemia.

(pp. 1917–1921, Section 23: Disorders of the Blood, Part 2: Disorders of Red Blood Cells and Anemia, Chapter 428: Anemia Due to Diminished Red Blood Cell Production)

**Answer 11-11.** D

The patient's thumb abnormalities and thrombocytopenia are symptoms frequently seen in patients with Fanconi anemia. Although patients with thrombocytopenia absent radii may have misplaced or hypoplastic thumbs, they are distinguished from Fanconi anemia patients who may have absent thumbs. Although the bone marrow of Fanconi anemia patients is often abnormal, the diagnostic test is confirmation of increased chromosomal fragility in the presence of DNA cross-linking agents such as DEB or mitomycin C. Telomere length assays are useful in the diagnosis of dyskeratosis congenita, which is classically characterized by a triad of lacy pigmentation, oral leukoplakia, and dysplastic nails. Erythrocyte adenosine deaminase levels are elevated in Diamond-Blackfan anemia patients. Although patients with Diamond-Blackfan anemia may have hypoplastic thumbs, the hallmark of the disease is red blood cell (RBC) aplasia, not thrombocytopenia.

(pp. 1917–1921, Section 23: Disorders of the Blood, Part 2: Disorders of Red Blood Cells and Anemia, Chapter 428: Anemia Due to Diminished Red Blood Cell Production)

**Answer 11-12.** D

The patient has hereditary spherocytosis, which can be confirmed by osmotic fragility testing. This patient's jaundice is not consistent with physiologic jaundice given the elevated bilirubin level within the first 24 hours of life. In this setting, with an MCHC of > 36 g/dL, the most likely diagnosis is hereditary spherocytosis in the newborn period. Outside the newborn period, this typically presents as intermittent jaundice and palpable splenomegaly. Neonates with G6PD deficiency can also present with nonphysiologic jaundice; however, G6PD deficiency is X-linked, and this patient is a female. In addition, the MCHC is normal in patients with G6PD. Hemoglobin electrophoresis would delineate the type of hemoglobin present (ie, hemoglobin A, S, or C). *UGT1A1* activity is useful in the diagnosis of Gilbert syndrome, and an abdominal ultrasound would not be clinically useful at this time.

(pp. 1922–1926, Section 23: Disorders of the Blood, Part 2: Disorders of Red Blood Cells and Anemia, Chapter 429: Hemolytic Anemia)

**Answer 11-13.** D

The patient's elevated reticulocyte count indicates that her RBC turnover is increased, even though her anemia is mild. Further, her increased MCHC, the presence of spherocytes on her smear, and elevated total bilirubin level all indicate a hemolytic anemia. While patients with autoimmune hemolytic anemia can also have spherocytes, the family history is suggestive of an autosomal dominantly inherited hemolytic anemia such as hereditary spherocytosis. Hereditary spherocytosis is a defect in the erythrocyte membrane that decreases the ability of the cell to deform and it becomes trapped in the sinusoids of the spleen, resulting in extravascular hemolysis. In iron-deficiency anemia, the RBCs are microcytic and hypochromic with a low MCHC. Autoimmune-mediated hemolytic anemia can be treated with corticosteroids. The treatment for hereditary spherocytosis is primarily supportive.

(pp. 1922–1926, Section 23: Disorders of the Blood, Part 2: Disorders of Red Blood Cells and Anemia, Chapter 429: Hemolytic Anemia)

**Answer 11-14.** B

This patient has signs of intravascular hemolysis with a low hemoglobin and hemoglobinuria. In the setting of a recent exposure to a sulfa-based antibiotic, the patient likely has G6PD deficiency. G6PD is an X-linked disorder. Although many patients are asymptomatic, they can present with intravascular hemolysis after exposure to certain triggers including infections, sulfa drugs, fava beans, or mothballs. Although parvovirus can lead to anemia, this is due to acute aplasia from destruction of early RBC precursors in the bone marrow. It does not lead to jaundice and hemoglobinuria. The reaction to sulfa drugs in patients with G6PD deficiency is not an immunoglobulin E (IgE)-mediated allergy. Creatine kinase and creatinine levels would not be helpful in diagnosing the underlying etiology of this patient's hemolysis.

(pp. 1922–1926, Section 23: Disorders of the Blood, Part 2: Disorders of Red Blood Cells and Anemia, Chapter 429: Hemolytic Anemia)

**Answer 11-15.** A

In patients with high rates of red blood cell (RBC) turnover, such as patients with hemoglobinopathies, enzymopathies, hemolytic anemias, or erythrocyte membrane defects, infections with parvovirus B19 cause a low hemoglobin with a low reticulocyte count. The infection destroys early RBC precursors and causes RBC aplasia for about a week. Because RBCs last approximately 120 days, most children are able to maintain adequate hemoglobin levels and are asymptomatic. However, patients who have higher rates of RBC turnover may not be able to maintain their levels and can develop severe anemia. Direct antibody testing and stool blood testing would be negative because this patient's anemia is due to decreased production of RBCs. His aPTT should be normal. A bone marrow biopsy would reveal decreased erythrocyte precursors; however, this would not reveal the underlying etiology.

(pp. 1903–1907, Section 23: Disorders of the Blood, Part 1: Principles of Blood of Disorders, Chapter 424: Approach to Suspected Hematologic Disorders; pp. 1917–1921, Section 23: Disorders of the Blood, Part 2: Disorders of Red Blood Cells and Anemia, Chapter 428: Anemia Due to Diminished Red Blood Cell Production)

**Answer 11-16.** B

Given the presence of IgG on the red blood cells (RBCs), this patient has warm-reactive autoimmune hemolytic anemia (AIHA). The IgG autoantibodies bind to RBC antigens; these opsonized cells are then cleared by the spleen, leading to the anemia and clinical symptoms described in this vignette. Warm-reactive AIHA is responsive to corticosteroids. Splenectomy is used to treat refractory AIHA; it is only used after other treatment options have been exhausted because postsplenectomy patients are at an increased risk for infection. Plasmapheresis is only effective in cold-reactive AIHA, where circulating immunoglobulin M (IgM) antibodies can be cleared. IVIG and antithymocyte antiglobulin have not been shown to be effective.

(pp. 1922–1926, Section 23: Disorders of the Blood, Part 2: Disorders of Red Blood Cells and Anemia, Chapter 429: Hemolytic Anemia)

**Answer 11-17.** E

Idiopathic thrombosis in males is extremely rare. The differential diagnosis includes underlying genetic thrombophilias and drug effects, but should also include paroxysmal nocturnal hemoglobinuria (PNH), a clonal disease characterized by chronic intravascular hemolysis and recurrent thrombosis. This patient most likely has PNH. Only about 25% of patients present with classic nocturnal hemoglobinuria. Patients with aplastic anemia and thromboses involving unusual sites should all be screened for PNH. In particular, PNH has been shown to develop more commonly in patients successfully treated with an antithymocyte antiglobulin and cyclosporine. Diagnosis has traditionally been made with a Ham acid test, which detects complement-mediated hemolysis. However, flow cytometry has become the standard for diagnosis. Protein C, factor V Leiden, and homocysteine levels are associated with prothrombotic states; however, given this patient's history of aplastic anemia, PNH is the more likely diagnosis.

(pp. 1917–1921, Section 23: Disorders of the Blood, Part 2: Disorders of Red Blood Cells and Anemia, Chapter 428: Anemia Due to Diminished Red Blood Cell Production; pp. 1922–1926, Section 23: Disorders of the Blood, Part 2: Disorders of Red Blood Cells and Anemia, Chapter 429: Hemolytic Anemia; pp. 1956–1961, Section 23: Disorders of the Blood, Part 3: Disorders of Coagulation and Platelets, Chapter 434: Diagnosis and Management of Thrombosis)

**Answer 11-18.** A

The patient has anemia, thrombocytopenia, and schistocytes, which indicate a microangiopathic hemolytic anemia. The pentad of fever, microangiopathic hemolytic anemia, thrombocytopenia, renal disease, and neurologic disease is diagnostic of thrombotic thrombocytopenic purpura (TTP). Endothelial cells typically release large von Willebrand factor (vWF) multimers; these multimers are cleaved by a metalloproteinase, ADAMTS13. However, in patients with TTP, this metalloproteinase is absent, often because an antibody binds to ADAMTS13, rendering it inactive. The increased number of circulating vWF multimers promotes the formation of microthrombi, consuming platelets. Patients with autoimmune disorders, such as systemic lupus erythematosus, can develop a specific autoantibody inhibitor to ADAMTS13. More rarely, this can be caused by a germline genetic mutation in the *ADAMTS13* gene.

The differential diagnosis for microangiopathic hemolytic anemia includes hemolytic-uremic syndrome, as seen with infection from *E coli* O157:H7, but these patients often present with bloody diarrhea and do not typically have neurologic changes. A bone marrow biopsy would not be useful in the diagnosis of TTP. A direct Coombs test would be helpful in patients with autoimmune hemolytic anemia (AIHA); however, this does not present with schistocytes, and patients do not develop neurologic changes or renal dysfunction. ADAMTS13 levels would be more specific than blood cultures in making the diagnosis of TTP.

(pp. 1922–1926, Section 23: Disorders of the Blood, Part 2: Disorders of Red Blood Cells and Anemia, Chapter 429: Hemolytic Anemia; p. 1966; Section 23: Disorders of the Blood, Part 3: Disorders of Coagulation and Platelets, Chapter 435: Disorders of Platelets)

**Answer 11-19.** E

This child has hemolytic-uremic syndrome (HUS) secondary to enterotoxic *E coli*. Children will present with abdominal pain and fever. HUS is characterized by the triad of microangiopathic hemolytic anemia, thrombocytopenia, and acute renal failure. Given this patient's hypertension, it is likely he has laboratory evidence of acute renal injury as seen with an elevated creatinine. HUS leads to intravascular hemolysis; therefore, the RBC count is expected to be low, and RBC fragments (schistocytes) are often seen on a blood smear. The hemolysis often leads to low haptoglobin because it is bound with hemoglobin from hemolyzed cells and an elevated LDH due to the cell lysis. The direct Coombs test, however, would be negative because patients with HUS do not have an antibody-mediated hemolysis.

(pp. 1922–1926, Section 23: Disorders of the Blood, Part 2: Disorders of Red Blood Cells and Anemia, Chapter 429: Hemolytic Anemia)

**Answer 11-20.** D

The presence of hemoglobin A and hemoglobin S allows us to infer that the patient synthesizes both normal β-globin and $\beta^S$-globin chains. This indicates that one of her β-globin alleles makes wild-type β-globin and the other β-globin allele makes sickle β-globin. Hence, the patient has sickle cell trait and not sickle cell anemia, where both β-globin alleles are $\beta^S$. Without information on the relative abundance of the hemoglobin A versus hemoglobin S, there is insufficient information to know whether the allele making β-globin is a wild-type allele or an allele that has diminished β-globin synthesis (a $\beta^+$), so no conclusion can be drawn as to whether the patient has a normal β-globin gene or has β-thalassemia. The major form of hemoglobin present in all newborns (except those with γ-chain mutations) is fetal hemoglobin, so no conclusion can be drawn

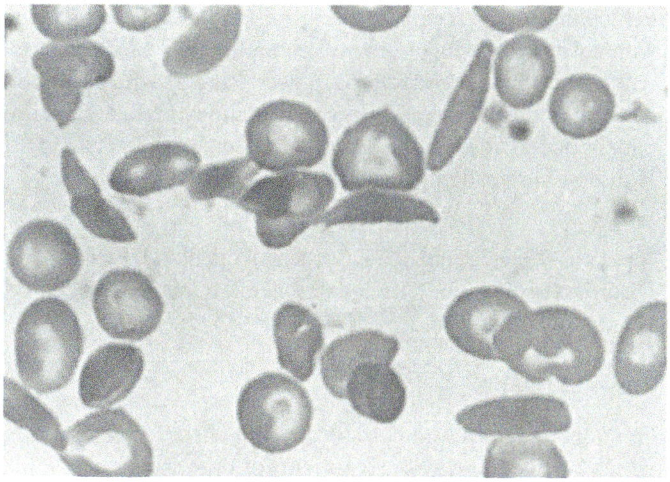

**FIGURE 430-1.** Peripheral blood film in sickle cell anemia (Hb SS). There are numerous irreversibly sickled cells visible, as well as variability in size and shape of erythrocytes (anisocytosis) and significant reticulocytosis. (Mark W. Kline, *Rudolph's Pediatrics*, 23rd Edition. Copyright © McGraw-Hill Education. All rights reserved.)

as to whether the patient has persistence of fetal hemoglobin from a newborn screen done on the first day of life.

(pp. 1926–1939, Section 23: Disorders of the Blood, Part 2: Disorders of Red Blood Cells and Anemia, Chapter 430: Hemoglobinopathies)

**Answer 11-21.** E

Hemolysis and vaso-occlusion are the 2 main causes of complications from sickle cell disease (SCD) (Figure 430-1). Transcranial Doppler ultrasounds are used to screen for SCD patients who are at increased risk of stroke. Clinical strokes occur in 11% of patients with SCD by the age of 18 years if they do not receive primary stroke prophylaxis, and of those patients who have a clinically overt stroke, 50% to 90% have an additional stroke. Transcranial Dopplers are used to detect stenosis in the major cerebral arteries. Children with stenosis begin chronic transfusions to maintain their hemoglobin S concentration at < 30% to decrease their stroke risk.

While SCD patients are at risk for renal dysfunction and pulmonary hypertension and can have vaso-occlusive crises that cause bone damage, renal ultrasound, chest radiograph, and bone density scanning are not used to screen for these disorders, respectively. Screening for hearing loss is typically only used in SCD patients who are being chelated due to iron overload, as hearing loss is not linked directly to SCD.

(pp. 1926–1939, Section 23: Disorders of the Blood, Part 2: Disorders of Red Blood Cells and Anemia, Chapter 430: Hemoglobinopathies)

**Answer 11-22.** C

This patient meets the criteria for acute chest syndrome, defined as fever and changes on CXR. Acute chest syndrome is the leading cause of mortality for patients with sickle cell disease (SCD). There are many causes of acute chest syndrome, including infarction, atelectasis, pulmonary edema, bronchospasm, and infection. Although an infectious agent is often not identified, empiric antibiotic therapy with ceftriaxone and azithromycin is necessary to cover the usual respiratory pathogens, such as pneumococcus, as well as atypical bacteria such as *Mycoplasma* and *Chlamydia pneumoniae*. Supplemental oxygen and hydration are also mainstays of treatment.

(pp. 1926–1939, Section 23: Disorders of the Blood, Part 2: Disorders of Red Blood Cells and Anemia, Chapter 430: Hemoglobinopathies)

**Answer 11-23.** B

Methemoglobin is created when the iron component of hemoglobin is in the ferric state ($Fe^{3+}$), which cannot bind oxygen. This occurs throughout the red blood cell (RBC) life cycle, but is typically reduced through an intracellular cytochrome $b_5$ reductase enzyme. There are congenital and acquired causes of methemoglobinemia, which occurs when the intracellular reductase pathways are overwhelmed or dysfunctional. In acquired methemoglobinemia, methylene blue is the treatment of choice. Methylene blue reduces methemoglobin via an alternative NADPH–flavin pathway. Importantly, the NADPH–flavin pathway requires G6PD to generate glutathione. In patients with G6PD deficiency, methylene blue is ineffective and may cause hemolysis.

Patients with cyanotic heart disease are not pseudocyanotic. Both pyruvate kinase deficiency and hereditary spherocytosis are hemolytic anemias that do not affect the use of methylene blue. Scott syndrome is a qualitative platelet defect.

(pp. 1933–1934, Section 23: Disorders of the Blood, Part 2: Disorders of Red Blood Cells and Anemia, Chapter 430: Hemoglobinopathies)

**Answer 11-24.** C

Hematuria is often seen in patients with sickle cell trait. Sickle cell trait is the heterozygous state for the $\beta^S$ gene. It is relatively common, affecting 1 in 12 African Americans. Although the red blood cells (RBCs) do not typically sickle, sickling can be observed in the renal medulla, which is a relatively acidic and hypertonic environment. This can lead to renal papillary necrosis and intermittent episodes of gross hematuria. Patients with sickle cell trait typically have about 30% to 40% hemoglobin S, which can be seen in hemoglobin electrophoresis. These patients otherwise have normal RBC indices and do not typically suffer the vaso-occlusive complications of sickle cell disease (SCD).

(pp. 1926–1939, Section 23: Disorders of the Blood, Part 2: Disorders of Red Blood Cells and Anemia, Chapter 430: Hemoglobinopathies)

**Answer 11-25.** B

Hemoglobin Barts is a tetramer of 4 γ-globin chains. The presence of hemoglobin Barts in the neonatal period indicates that there is an excess of γ-globin chains relative to α-globin chains. (Remember, fetal hemoglobin is made up of $\alpha_2 \gamma_2$.) Once γ-chain synthesis is turned off and replaced by β-globin chains, a similar excess of β-globin would result in the formation of hemoglobin H (a tetramer of 4 β-globin chains). Since the repeat hemoglobin electrophoresis does not show the presence of hemoglobin H, the decrease in the amount of α-globin is not as severe as that seen in hemoglobin H disease (3 α-globin gene mutations), but since the patient is slightly anemic and microcytic, the patient is not a silent carrier (single α-globin gene mutation). Hence, the patient likely has α-thalassemia trait (2 α-globin gene mutations). Patients with β-thalassemia trait have a relative excess of α-globin chains compared with β-globin chains.

(pp. 1926–1939, Section 23: Disorders of the Blood, Part 2: Disorders of Red Blood Cells and Anemia, Chapter 430: Hemoglobinopathies)

**Answer 11-26.** C

β-Thalassemia is caused by mutations in the β-globin gene. Heterozygosity for the β-thalassemia gene results in a mild reduction of β-globin synthesis and a mild reduction in hemoglobin A production. Children born to parents who are both heterozygous for β-globin thalassemic mutations have a 50% chance of inheriting 1 mutant thalassemic allele and a 25% chance of inheriting both mutated alleles. Depending on the degree of compromise in synthesis of β-globin chains associated with the mutated alleles, these children may exhibit either the thalassemia intermedia or thalassemia major phenotype. However, because fetal hemoglobin ($\alpha_2 \gamma_2$) is the major hemoglobin at birth, patients who have no functioning β-globin alleles can have normal hematocrits at birth and do not become anemic until γ-globin chain synthesis is turned off. A hemoglobin electrophoresis should be done at birth. The hemoglobin electrophoresis will identify β-thalassemia major patients who synthesize no β-globin chains because it would show only the presence of hemoglobin F, without any hemoglobin A.

(pp. 1926–1939, Section 23: Disorders of the Blood, Part 2: Disorders of Red Blood Cells and Anemia, Chapter 430: Hemoglobinopathies)

**Answer 11-27.** C

Microcytic anemia that is "refractory" to iron supplementation is most often caused by poor compliance. However, other causes must be considered, and in this patient, microcytic anemia with normal iron indices is most likely caused by an underlying thalassemia. This patient has a Mentzer index (mean corpuscular volume [MCV]/red blood cell [RBC]) of < 13, which is indicative of an underlying thalassemia. A patient with β-thalassemia major or intermedia would have increased hemoglobin A2 percentage. There are 4 α-globin genes. Patients with deletion of a single gene are asymptomatic "silent carriers" with no abnormal hematologic indices. Patients with a 2-gene deletion often have an asymptomatic microcytic anemia, as this patient does. Patients with 3 genes deleted have hemoglobin H disease, and patients with a 4-gene deletion have hydrops fetalis.

(pp. 1926–1939, Section 23: Disorders of the Blood, Part 2: Disorders of Red Blood Cells and Anemia, Chapter 430: Hemoglobinopathies)

**Answer 11-28.** E

Splenomegaly can be a complication of chronic transfusions, which is the mainstay of treatment for thalassemia major. Chronic transfusions can decrease extramedullary hematopoiesis and prolong and improve quality of life. However, patients who develop splenomegaly have an increased transfusion requirement due to the associated hypersplenism and increased red blood cell (RBC) clearance. As a result, splenectomy can be recommended. It is well known that asplenic patients are at higher risk of infection from encapsulated organisms and should be immunized prior to splenectomy. However, these patients are also at higher risk for thrombosis and pulmonary hypertension. There is no known association between splenectomy and renal failure, malignancy, aplastic anemia, or increased bleeding.

(pp. 1926–1939, Section 23: Disorders of the Blood, Part 2: Disorders of Red Blood Cells and Anemia, Chapter 430: Hemoglobinopathies)

**Answer 11-29.** D

Because there is no physiologic mechanism for iron excretion, patients on chronic transfusion regimens inevitably develop iron overload, whether or not they have a genetic predisposition. However, chelation starts only after sufficient chelatable iron has accumulated, which usually occurs after approximately 200 mL/kg of PRBCs. The goal of chelation is to prevent the organ damage that gives rise to the symptoms of iron overload. These include endocrinopathies, cardiac dysfunction, and liver dysfunction. While ferritin is used to monitor the iron stores, it is not a precise measure because it fluctuates with inflammation as well. Hence, while it is useful to monitor trends, it should only be used in conjunction with more precise quantitation by liver biopsy or radiologic imaging methods.

(pp. 1926–1939, Section 23: Disorders of the Blood, Part 2: Disorders of Red Blood Cells and Anemia, Chapter 430: Hemoglobinopathies)

**Answer 11-30.** B

The levels of a number of procoagulant and antithrombotic factors are different in the neonate when compared with adult values. Notably, the vitamin K–dependent coagulation factors (II, VII, IX, and X) are approximately half the adult values in the healthy newborn and rise to 80% by 6 months of age. Therefore, the factor VII and IX levels in this clinical scenario are normal for age. Factor VIII levels, however, are comparable to adult values in the healthy newborn. Thus, this patient's factor VIII level is abnormally low, even for a newborn. While low factor VIII levels can be seen in von Willebrand disease (vWD), von Willebrand antigen is absent in type 3 vWD patients. A qualitative platelet disorder is not ruled out by a normal platelet count; however, the presence of a low factor VIII in this patient makes hemophilia A (mild) the most likely diagnosis.

(pp. 1944–1950, Section 23: Disorders of the Blood, Part 3: Disorders of Coagulation and Platelets, Chapter 432: Inherited Bleeding Disorders)

**Answer 11-31.** B

HHT, also known as Osler-Weber-Rendu syndrome, is most frequently present with epistaxis, and any patient presenting with frequent nosebleeds should be examined for mucosal telangiectasias leading to their symptoms. HHT is characterized by the cutaneous and visceral vasculopathies, including telangiectasias and arteriovenous malformations, which can lead to potentially life-threatening bleeding. This genetic disorder has been associated with mutation of the endoglin gene (*HHT1*) or of the activin receptor-like kinase 1 (alk1) gene (*HHT2*). Although synovial hemangiomas have been described in this syndrome, they are quite rare, and HHT patients generally do not have problems with joint bleeding and motility. Port wine stains, varicose veins, and soft tissue hypertrophy of 1 extremity are characteristic of Klippel-Trenaunay-Weber syndrome.

(p. 1941, Section 23: Disorders of the Blood, Part 3: Disorders of Coagulation and Platelets, Chapter 431: Normal and Abnormal Hemostasis)

**Answer 11-32.** E

Because collagen is an integral component of blood vessels, collagen disorders can also present with bleeding symptoms. This patient's elastic skin and hypermobility is suggestive of Ehlers-Danlos syndrome. The endoglin gene is mutated in hereditary hemorrhagic telangiectasia (HHT) (Osler-Weber-Rendu syndrome), which is characterized by the presence of skin and mucosal telangiectasias. His von Willebrand activity and antigen levels are well matched and within the normal range, making type 2 and 3 vWD unlikely. Although these levels may be seen in vWD type 1 patients under certain circumstances, the lack of a clear family history and the presence of other clinical signs consistent with a collagen defect favor Ehlers-Danlos syndrome.

(pp. 1941–1942, Section 23: Disorders of the Blood, Part 3: Disorders of Coagulation and Platelets, Chapter 431: Normal and Abnormal Hemostasis)

**Answer 11-33.** B

Flushing is a common side effect from DDAVP. DDAVP is a synthetic form of vasopressin (antidiuretic hormone). It can cause retention of free water, leading to hyponatremia and oliguria. In type 2B von Willebrand disease (vWD) patients, DDAVP can cause thrombocytopenia because the defective von Willebrand factor (vWF) has an increased affinity for the platelet glycoprotein (GP) Ib/IX/V binding site. This leads to an apparent thrombocytopenia as the platelets are now bound to vWF. Inhibitor formation is most likely in severe hemophilia A patients who are exposed to exogenous factor. As DDAVP causes release of endogenous factor VIII and vWF from storage pools, there is no exposure to exogenous factor.

(p. 1949, Section 23: Disorders of the Blood, Part 3: Disorders of Coagulation and Platelets, Chapter 432: Inherited Bleeding Disorders)

**Answer 11-34.** E

Hemophilia B, also known as Christmas disease, is an X-linked recessive trait that results in the congenital deficiency of factor IX. This patient's prolonged aPTT and his family history, which is consistent with an X-linked disorder, point to hemophilia B as the most likely diagnosis. Type 2N and type 3 vWD patients and hemophilia A patients would all have low factor VIII levels, and hence, these answers are incorrect. Although type 1 vWD patients can have normal factor VIII levels, the aPTT would also be normal.

(pp. 1944–1950, Section 23: Disorders of the Blood, Part 3: Disorders of Coagulation and Platelets, Chapter 432: Inherited Bleeding Disorders)

**Answer 11-35.** A

The diagnosis for vWD rests on a combination of personal and family bleeding history and supportive laboratory studies. The patient's von Willebrand activity and antigen levels are in a range that does not clearly distinguish between type 1 patients and healthy controls, because many factors can modulate vWF levels. Most individuals have antigen, ristocetin cofactor, and factor VIII activity > 50%. However, levels between 30% and 50% can be normal because blood type, thyroid state, and other factors can modulate these lab values. Therefore, personal bleeding history and family history are critical to diagnosing vWD.

(pp. 1944–1950, Section 23: Disorders of the Blood, Part 3: Disorders of Coagulation and Platelets, Chapter 432: Inherited Bleeding Disorders)

**Answer 11-36.** C

Patients with type 2B vWD have increased affinity of the abnormal vWF for platelet glycoprotein Ib (GPIb). Hence, they have a positive response in low-dose ristocetin-induced platelet aggregation and have diminished high-molecular-weight vWF multimers and thrombocytopenia because of clearance of the vWF-bound platelets. Answer choice A contains the expected findings in a patient with type 1 vWD. Answer choice B contains the findings in type 2A vWD, as the activity-to-antigen ratio is decreased and high and intermediate multimers are absent. Answer choice D represents type 2M because the activity-to-antigen ratio is decreased, but the multimer distribution is normal. Answer E suggests either type 2N vWD or mild hemophilia A (in a female patient, this may occur due to extreme lyonization, Turner syndrome, or, rarely, coinheritance of 2 mutated factor VIII alleles).

(pp. 1944–1950, Section 23: Disorders of the Blood, Part 3: Disorders of Coagulation and Platelets, Chapter 432: Inherited Bleeding Disorders)

**Answer 11-37. A**

The patient's proportionally low vWF activity and antigen levels, the appearance of her multimers, and her family history and personal bleeding history are all consistent with type 1 vWD. More than 75% of patients with vWD have type 1. Type 2A is ruled out by the normal activity-to-antigen ratio and the presence of normal distribution of multimers. Type 2M is ruled out by the activity-to-antigen ratio. Type 2N is characterized by low factor VIII levels due to a mutation that selectively inactivates the factor VIII binding site on the vWF; therefore, type 2N is ruled out by the normal factor VIII level. The patient's vWF activity and antigen levels are too high to be type 3, which is characterized by complete absence of vWF.

(pp. 1944–1950, Section 23: Disorders of the Blood, Part 3: Disorders of Coagulation and Platelets, Chapter 432: Inherited Bleeding Disorders)

**Answer 11-38. D**

Inhibitors occur in approximately 30% of patients with severe hemophilia A, usually within the first 20 exposures; however, they can occur at any age. Inhibitors can be eradicated with repeated exposure to factor VIII concentrate (immune tolerance induction); however, this may take months to years. If a patient with a known inhibitor is actively bleeding, treatment with recombinant factor VIIa or a prothrombin complex concentrate may be needed. Inhibitor titers $\leq 5$ BU are considered low titers and more likely to be transient. Given that the patient in this vignette has a titer $> 5$, it is not likely to spontaneously resolve.

(p. 1947, Section 23: Disorders of the Blood, Part 3: Disorders of Coagulation and Platelets, Chapter 432: Inherited Bleeding Disorders)

**Answer 11-39. A**

DDAVP (a synthetic form of vasopressin, or antidiuretic hormone) use can lead to fluid retention and hyponatremia. Patients should therefore limit fluid intake, and serum sodium needs to be monitored. As tachyphylaxis occurs, the dosing is typically daily to every 2 days, and treatment is generally limited to 3 consecutive days. Factor VIII levels rise with the release of von Willebrand factor (vWF) that results from DDAVP use.

(p. 1949, Section 23: Disorders of the Blood, Part 3: Disorders of Coagulation and Platelets, Chapter 432: Inherited Bleeding Disorders)

**Answer 11-40. A**

This patient's bleeding history, family history, and laboratory evaluation are most consistent with vWD type 2N. In type 2N, factor VIII is low due to an autosomal recessive mutation that selectively inactivates the factor VIII binding site on von Willebrand factor (vWF). A low factor VIII level could also be indicative of hemophilia A; however, a deficiency of factor VIII is caused by mutations on the X chromosome, and in general, females are unaffected carriers. Therefore, this patient's family history is not consistent with hemophilia A. Moreover, it is not an answer choice. Patients with vWD type 2N are often misdiagnosed as having hemophilia A. Hemophilia B is a bleeding disorder caused by low factor IX levels, and this patient's levels are within normal range for age. The patient has a normal fibrinogen level and normal platelets, which is not consistent with disseminated intravascular coagulation or afibrinogenemia. Vitamin K deficiency would lead to abnormal coagulation studies.

(pp. 1944–1950, Section 23: Disorders of the Blood, Part 3: Disorders of Coagulation and Platelets, Chapter 432: Inherited Bleeding Disorders)

**Answer 11-41. B**

Factor XIII deficiency is an autosomal recessive disorder associated with excessive bruising, muscle and joint bleeding, menorrhagia, delayed postsurgical bleeding, umbilical stump bleeding, and intracranial hemorrhage. In its activated form, factor XIII is responsible for cross-linking the fibrin clot. Therefore, in a factor XIII–deficient patient, clot solubility is increased. Increased factor XIII would result in decreased clot solubility. The normal PT makes factor V deficiency unlikely, and increased protein C level does not cause increased bleeding symptoms.

(p. 1943, Section 23: Disorders of the Blood, Part 3: Disorders of Coagulation and Platelets, Chapter 431: Normal and Abnormal Hemostasis)

**Answer 11-42. B**

Synthesis of factors II, VII, IX, and X requires vitamin K as a cofactor. Factor V is a liver-synthesized factor that is not vitamin K dependent. Therefore, it is useful in distinguishing liver failure from vitamin K deficiency.

(pp. 1939–1944, Section 23: Disorders of the Blood, Part 3: Disorders of Coagulation and Platelets, Chapter 431: Normal and Abnormal Hemostasis)

**Answer 11-43.** D

Classical vitamin K deficiency bleeding in newborns presents in the first week of life. Typical symptoms include easy bruising, mucus membrane bleeding, and hematemesis. Risk factors include babies who have not been given vitamin K treatment, are breastfed, or are poor feeders. Such patients will have low levels of vitamin K–dependent factors: II, VII, IX, and X. Factor V and VIII levels are unaffected. Factor V Leiden is a prothrombotic mutated factor V that is resistant to degradation by activated protein C. While neonates with pancreatic disease such as cystic fibrosis are at risk for vitamin K deficiency bleeding due to poor absorption of fat-soluble vitamins, this is an unlikely presentation of cystic fibrosis during the first week of life. Of note, early-onset vitamin K deficiency bleeding occurs in the first 24 hours of life due to placental transfer of antibodies that interfere with vitamin K. Late-onset vitamin K deficiency bleeding presents at 2 weeks to 6 months.

(pp. 1939–1944, Section 23: Disorders of the Blood, Part 3: Disorders of Coagulation and Platelets, Chapter 431: Normal and Abnormal Hemostasis)

**Answer 11-44.** B

Prothrombin G20210A mutation occurs in approximately 3% of the general population and increases the risk for thrombosis mainly by causing excess prothrombin production. Factor V deficiency is associated with increased bleeding, not with increased thrombosis. (Factor V Leiden is the most common inherited thrombophilia, and the mutation causes a resistance of factor V to inactivation by activated proteins C and S.) Patients with nephrotic syndrome, not nephritic syndrome, are at an increased risk of thrombosis due to loss of clotting factors in the urine. Hyperhomocysteinemia is a risk factor of stroke in children. See Table 434-2 for the differential diagnosis for thrombophilia.

(pp. 1956–1961, Section 23: Disorders of the Blood, Part 3: Disorders of Coagulation and Platelets, Chapter 434: Diagnosis and Management of Thrombosis)

**Answer 11-45.** D

Factor V resistance to cleavage by APC is known as factor V Leiden. Cleavage of factor V inactivates this clotting factor; therefore, in factor V Leiden, factor V is unable to be inactivated by APC. Heterozygotes for this mutation have a 5- to 8-fold increase in thromboembolic disease, and homozygotes have an 80-fold increase in lifetime risk. Protein C is an anticoagulant; therefore, a slightly elevated level would not increase her risk of thrombosis. The antithrombin, factor VIII, and plasma homocysteine levels are normal.

(pp. 1956–1961, Section 23: Disorders of the Blood, Part 3: Disorders of Coagulation and Platelets, Chapter 434: Diagnosis and Management of Thrombosis)

**TABLE 434-2.** Inherited and Acquired Thrombophilia

| **Inherited** | **Acquired** |
|---|---|
| High Risk of Thrombosis | Lupus anticoagulant |
| *Severe deficiencies* | Antiphospholipid antibodies |
| Protein C | Deficiencies of protein C |
| Protein S | Deficiency of protein S |
| Antithrombin | Deficiency of antithrombin |
| *Combined genetic mutations* | Elevated factor VIII activity |
| Heterozygous for both factor V Leiden and prothrombin G20210A | |
| Homozygous for factor V Leiden | |
| Homozygous for prothrombin G20210A | |
| Moderate Risk of Thrombosis | |
| Heterozygous for factor V Leiden | |
| Heterozygous for prothrombin G20210A | |
| Elevated factor VIII | |
| Hyperhomocysteinemia | |
| Elevated lipoprotein | |
| Dysfibrinogenemia | |
| Dysplasminogenemia/ hypoplasminogenemia | |

Mark W. Kline, *Rudolph's Pediatrics*, 23rd Edition. Copyright © McGraw-Hill Education. All rights reserved.

**Answer 11-46.** D

Isolated thrombocytopenia in a well-appearing child points toward immune thrombocytopenic purpura, an autoimmune-mediated process leading to increased destruction of platelets. Although patients have circulating autoantibodies, there is no standardized laboratory test to identify these antibodies, and in otherwise healthy-appearing children with no other concerning findings (eg, fevers, hepatosplenomegaly, red blood cell [RBC] or WBC abnormalities on the smear), a bone marrow biopsy is not needed. Over 75% of patients will have resolution of their symptoms within 3 months with no further sequelae. Many patients can be observed without treatment, but those with active bleeding and platelet counts < 10,000 can be treated with steroids, intravenous immunoglobulin (IVIG), or anti-D immunoglobulin (in Rh-positive patients). Platelet transfusions are not indicated except in cases of severe or life-threatening bleeding, because the circulating antibodies will also destroy transfused platelets.

(pp. 1961–1970, Section 23: Disorders of the Blood, Part 3: Disorders of Coagulation and Platelets, Chapter 435: Disorders of Platelets)

**Answer 11-47.** A

NAIT arises from a mismatch between maternal and paternal platelet antigens, most often human platelet antigen (HPA)-1. Maternal immunoglobulin G (IgG) antibodies against HPA1 cause peripheral platelet destruction in the newborn. Unlike Rh incompatibility, NAIT can present in the firstborn child and presents typically with petechiae, purpura, or mucosal bleeding immediately after birth. Treatment is to transfuse maternal platelets. However, it is acceptable to transfuse random platelets as well. Intracranial hemorrhage can occur in 10% to 20% of infants. The normal maternal platelet count rules out maternally derived neonatal autoimmune thrombocytopenia. Although IVIG may also provide some benefit in NAIT, it is not the first choice for treatment. The uncomplicated pregnancy with a well-appearing newborn makes a TORCH infection unlikely. Glanzmann thrombasthenia is a functional platelet disorder and is not associated with thrombocytopenia. Other causes of thrombocytopenia to be considered in a neonate, including Fanconi anemia, thrombocytopenia absent radii, and congenital amegakaryocytic thrombocytopenia, are also in the differential, but given the patient's low counts, transfusion should be prioritized over additional diagnostic testing.

(pp. 1961–1970, Section 23: Disorders of the Blood, Part 3: Disorders of Coagulation and Platelets, Chapter 435: Disorders of Platelets)

**Answer 11-48.** A

Although NAIT is self-limited with resolution within 2 to 6 weeks, 10% to 20% of patients have intracranial hemorrhage while the platelet count is low. Treatment is a temporizing measure aimed at raising the platelet count to reduce the risk of intracranial hemorrhage. The *best* choice for transfusion is maternal platelets that lack HPA-1a, and therefore, will not be cleared by the circulating alloantibodies. Often, these platelets are not available, and a random donor unit will be used instead. IVIG can also be used but takes 24 to 72 hours to take effect and should be given in conjunction with platelet support. Steroids have not been shown to be beneficial, and observation is unacceptable given the high rate of intracranial hemorrhage (10%–20%).

(pp. 1961–1970, Section 23: Disorders of the Blood, Part 3: Disorders of Coagulation and Platelets, Chapter 435: Disorders of Platelets)

**Answer 11-49.** C

The vignette describes a classic autosomal dominant pattern of inheritance. The thrombocytopenia and family history of easy bruising associated with hearing loss and renal disease suggest an MYH9-related disorder. MYH9-related disorders are caused by mutation in the nonmuscle myosin heavy chain II, leading to pathognomonic Dohle-like bodies in neutrophils that can be seen on light microscopy. Examination of the peripheral blood smear would show macrothrombocytopenia. X-ray of the forearms is useful in diagnosing thrombocytopenia absent radii. The diagnosis of Fanconi anemia is made using the DEB chromosome breakage test. A bone marrow biopsy would show congenital amegakaryotic thrombocytopenia. Bernard-Soulier syndrome is associated with macrothrombocytopenia; however, it is an inherited disorder of platelet function and not associated with hearing loss and renal failure.

(pp. 1961–1970, Section 23: Disorders of the Blood, Part 3: Disorders of Coagulation and Platelets, Chapter 435: Disorders of Platelets)

**Answer 11-50.** B

Nonsteroidal anti-inflammatory drugs such as ibuprofen inhibit cyclooxygenase activity, leading to platelet dysfunction that can manifest as increased mucosal bleeding or menorrhagia. Although patients with type 1 vWD can present with relatively normal von Willebrand activity and antigen levels, the lack of a family history and the recent onset of her symptoms suggest that vWD is unlikely. Because she has a normal smear, an MYH9-related disorder is also unlikely, because this is an autosomal dominant macrothrombocytopenia. Given this patient's normal PT, factor VII deficiency is also unlikely. Her normal platelet count also eliminates immune thrombocytopenia from consideration.

(pp. 1961–1970, Section 23: Disorders of the Blood, Part 3: Disorders of Coagulation and Platelets, Chapter 435: Disorders of Platelets; pp. 1971–1974, Section 23: Disorders of the Blood, Part 4: Disorders of the Spleen and Lymph Nodes, Chapter 436: The Spleen and Lymph Nodes)

**Answer 11-51.** B

Wiskott-Aldrich syndrome, and the related entity X-linked thrombocytopenia (XLT), should be suspected in any male patient with thrombocytopenia and small platelets. Wiskott-Aldrich syndrome differs from XLT in that patients with Wiskott-Aldrich syndrome have impaired immunity and are at risk for infections and lymphoreticular malignancies. Patients typically present to medical attention due to bleeding during infancy. Although thrombocytopenia absent radius, Fanconi anemia, and congenital amegakaryocytic thrombocytopenia are all associated with thrombocytopenia, the presence of small platelets and frequent infections in this patient is more suggestive of Wiskott-Aldrich syndrome. Patients with hyper-IgE syndrome are also likely to have infections and eczema but do not have small and decreased numbers of platelets.

(pp. 1961–1970, Section 23: Disorders of the Blood, Part 3: Disorders of Coagulation and Platelets, Chapter 435: Disorders of Platelets)

**Answer 11-52.** D

Thrombocytosis in children is almost always reactive to an underlying condition; in this patient's case, the elevated platelet count is a response to the patient's bacteremia. Importantly, thrombocytosis under these circumstances is not associated with an increased risk of thrombosis. Essential thrombocythemia, a clonal disorder, and familial thrombocytosis are extremely rare and would not be the most likely diagnoses. Reactive thrombocytosis is more common, with a series reporting it in 15% of hospitalized patients. The patient does not meet any of the other criteria for Kawasaki disease.

(pp. 1967–1968, Section 23: Disorders of the Blood, Part 3: Disorders of Coagulation and Platelets, Chapter 435: Disorders of Platelets)

**Answer 11-53.** A

Glycoprotein (GP) Ib/IX/V is defective or deficient in patients with Bernard-Soulier syndrome. Because it is the platelet receptor for vWF, the patient's platelets are unable to aggregate in response to ristocetin. The von Willebrand activity, antigen, and multimer are normal. See Figure 435-3 for a schematic representation of other inherited platelet function disorders. Patients with Glanzmann thrombasthenia lack GP IIb/IIIa, which is required for bridging platelets. Unlike those of patients with Bernard-Soulier syndrome, platelets from patients with Glanzmann thrombasthenia do respond to ristocetin. Shwachman-Diamond syndrome is a congenital neutropenia syndrome arising from mutations in the *SBDS* gene. Pearson syndrome is a similar disorder arising from deletions of mitochondrial DNA. Kostmann disease is an autosomal recessive form of severe congenital neutropenia.

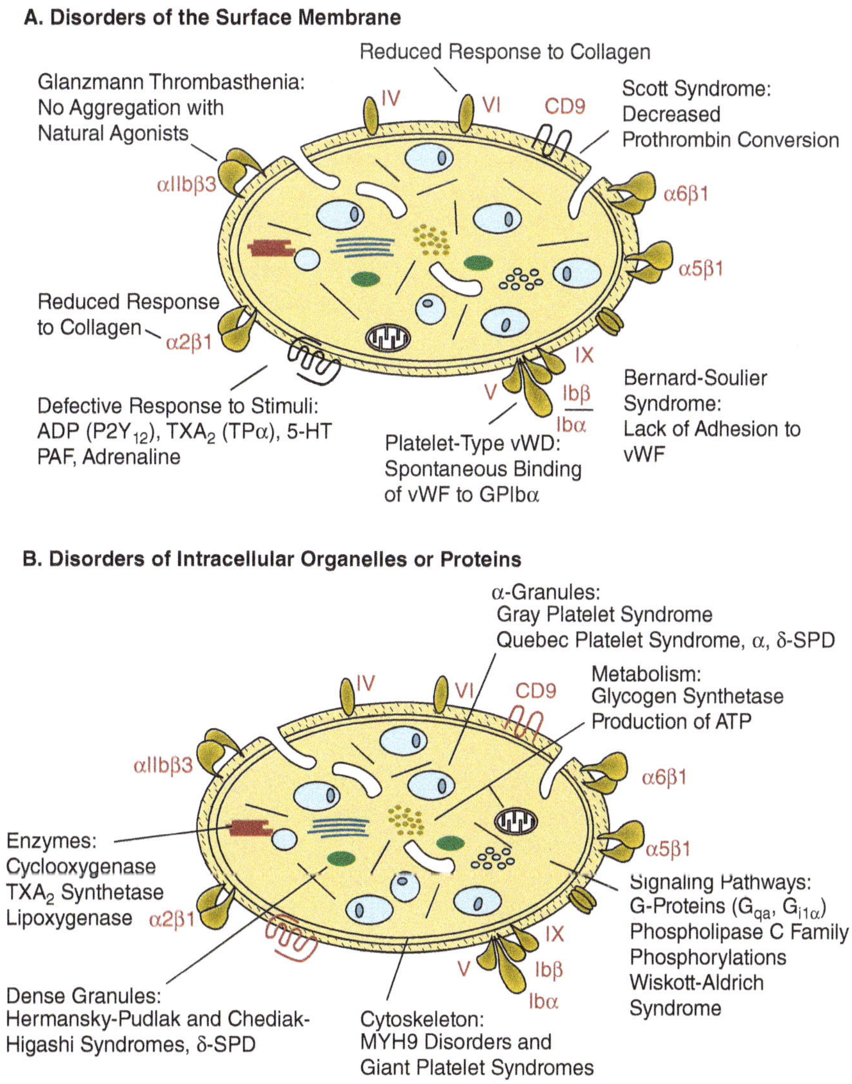


**FIGURE 435-3.** Schematic showing recognized inherited qualitative platelet disorders and their sites of dysfunction. **A:** Disorders of the surface membrane. **B:** Disorders of intracellular constituents of platelets. 5-HT, 5-hydroxytryptamine; ADP, adenosine diphosphate; δ-SPD, delta storage pool deficiency; PAF, platelet activating factor; $TXA_2$, thromboxane $A_2$; vWF, von Willebrand factor. (Reproduced with permission from Nurden AT. Qualitative disorders of platelets and megakaryocytes, *J Thromb Haemost.* 2005;3(8):1773-1782.)

(pp. 1968–1970, Section 23: Disorders of the Blood, Part 3: Disorders of Coagulation and Platelets, Chapter 435: Disorders of Platelets)

**Answer 11-54.** B

Patients with Glanzmann thrombasthenia lack GP IIb/IIIa, which is required for bridging platelets. Platelets are activated by ADP, serotonin, and thromboxane $A_2$. GP IIb/IIIa activation follows platelet activation from these agonists. Platelets lacking GP IIb/IIIa do not aggregate in response to these agonists. Platelets of patients with Bernard-Soulier syndrome are only defective in response to ristocetin because they lack GP Ib/IX/V, the von Willebrand factor (vWF) receptor. Shwachman-Diamond syndrome is a congenital neutropenia syndrome arising from mutations in the *SBDS* gene. Pearson syndrome is a similar disorder arising from deletions of mitochondrial DNA. Kostmann disease is an autosomal recessive form of severe congenital neutropenia.

(pp. 1968–1970, Section 23: Disorders of the Blood, Part 3: Disorders of Coagulation and Platelets, Chapter 435: Disorders of Platelets; pp. 1971–1974, Section 23: Disorders of the Blood, Part 4: Disorders of the Spleen and Lymph Nodes, Chapter 436: The Spleen and Lymph Nodes; pp. 1974–1982, Section 23: Disorders of the Blood, Part 5: Disorders of White Blood Cells, Chapter 437: Disorders of Granulocytes)

**Answer 11-55.** D

Persons of African ancestry may have a lower normal range for neutrophil counts. The mechanism of this phenomenon is still unclear. Patients with myelokathexis, reticular dysgenesis, and Kostmann syndrome would all have had a history of infections. Patients with glycogen storage disease type Ib have other associated problems, including hypoglycemia, growth delay, and hyperlipidemia. In this otherwise healthy patient, ethnic pseudoneutropenia is the best answer.

An 18-month-old male presents to your clinic to establish care. His mother reports that he has been hospitalized multiple times. He was hospitalized at 2 months of age for *E coli* urosepsis. He was hospitalized again at 9 months of age for pneumonia. She reports that since then, he seems to have fevers on a monthly basis but has not needed to be hospitalized. She reports that he occasionally has "cold sores" around the time of his febrile episodes but otherwise has been doing well.

On physical examination, his vital signs are temperature of 37.6°C, heart rate of 110 bpm, respiratory rate of 16 breaths/min, and blood pressure of 90/58 mm Hg; weight is 10 kg. He is well appearing and active in your office. His head is normocephalic, pupils are reactive, and tympanic membranes are well visualized with a good light reflex. Cardiac examination reveals no heart murmurs. Lungs are clear to auscultation bilaterally. Abdomen is soft and nontender with no hepatosplenomegaly. He has normal tone and bulk.

(pp. 1974–1982, Section 23: Disorders of the Blood, Part 5: Disorders of White Blood Cells, Chapter 437: Disorders of Granulocytes)

**Answer 11-56.** A

The history of serious recurrent infections and cyclic fevers is concerning for cyclic neutropenia. Cyclic neutropenia is caused by a mutation in *ELA2*, the gene encoding for neutrophil elastase, and is inherited in an autosomal dominant pattern. Patients with cyclic neutropenia have nadir neutrophil counts that can be < 200 cells/μL approximately every 3 weeks. During these nadirs, patients may have aphthous ulcers, gastroenteritis, and cervical lymphadenopathy. Patients will also be susceptible to life-threatening infections from *Clostridium perfringens* and gram-negative organisms. In between episodes, patients will have normal neutrophil counts and normal examinations. Therefore, a single normal neutrophil count is not sufficient to rule out cyclic neutropenia. The diagnosis is made by monitoring neutrophil counts twice a week over 6 to 8 weeks. Quantitative immunoglobulin levels and bone marrow biopsy would not be useful in the diagnosis of cyclic neutropenia. This recurrent, cyclic pattern of illness is not consistent with HIV infection.

(pp. 1974–1982, Section 23: Disorders of the Blood, Part 5: Disorders of White Blood Cells, Chapter 437: Disorders of Granulocytes)

**Answer 11-57.** D

The differential for neutropenia with concurrent pancreatic insufficiency is Shwachman-Diamond syndrome and Pearson syndrome. Shwachman-Diamond syndrome is an autosomal recessive disorder; the vast majority of patients have mutations in the *SBDS* gene on chromosome 7. Shwachman-Diamond syndrome patients may also have anemia and thrombocytopenia and usually present like the child in the vignette with failure to thrive and steatorrhea. Patients with Pearson syndrome have mitochondrial DNA mutations (not a choice given here). They also present with lactic acidosis and sideroblastic anemia. *CFTR* mutations are seen in cystic fibrosis patients. Interestingly, one of the first cohorts of identified patients with Shwachman-Diamond syndrome was found in cystic fibrosis clinics because they also had pancreatic insufficiency and pulmonary infections (due to their neutropenia). *TERT* mutations are seen in some patients with dyskeratosis congenita, and *RMRP* mutations are found in cartilage-hair hypoplasia patients. Although both of these disorders are associated with neutropenia, neither is associated with pancreatic insufficiency. *TP53* mutation is a gene that codes for a protein that regulates the cell cycle and hence functions as a tumor suppressor. Inherited *TP53* mutations are seen in Li-Fraumeni syndrome, which can have increased risks of breast cancer, bone cancer, leukemia, and soft tissue cancers (eg, sarcomas). Li-Fraumeni syndrome is not associated with pancreatic insufficiency.

(pp. 1974–1982, Section 23: Disorders of the Blood, Part 5: Disorders of White Blood Cells, Chapter 437: Disorders of Granulocytes)

**Answer 11-58.** D

All of these disorders share the finding of neutropenia. Most, but not all, also have an increased risk of malignancy. Cartilage-hair hypoplasia, a rare autosomal recessive disorder characterized by dwarfism, fine hair, and immunodeficiency, has an increased risk of cancer, particularly non-Hodgkin lymphoma and basal cell carcinoma. Patients with Chediak-Higashi syndrome are at an increased risk of developing lymphomas, whereas patients with severe congenital neutropenia and Shwachman-Diamond syndrome have an increased risk of developing myelodysplastic syndrome and acute myeloid leukemia. However, patients with cyclic neutropenia do not have an increased risk of cancer despite having mutations on the same gene (*ELA2*) as patients with severe congenital neutropenia. Among this group, only Shwachman-Diamond syndrome has been associated with ribosomal defects and Chediak-Higashi syndrome with platelet defects.

(pp. 1974–1982, Section 23: Disorders of the Blood, Part 5: Disorders of White Blood Cells, Chapter 437: Disorders of Granulocytes)

**Answer 11-59.** D

This patient has Chediak-Higashi syndrome. Patients with Chediak-Higashi syndrome have partial oculocutaneous albinism and silvery hair. They are also at risk for recurrent bacterial infections due to neutrophil dysfunction. They also have peripheral neuropathy and prolonged bleeding times. Chediak-Higashi syndrome is caused by a defect in granule formation, leading to the formation of giant granules with impaired chemotactic activity and intracellular killing. This picture depicts an ill-appearing child with the light skin and silvery hair associated with the disease. Pancreatic insufficiency is seen in Shwachman-Diamond syndrome, which is not associated with oculocutaneous albinism. Nail dystrophy is a characteristic of patients with dyskeratosis congenita, along with lacy reticulated pigmentation, dysplastic nails, and oral leukoplakia. Triphalangeal thumbs are seen in a number of genetic disorders including Diamond-Blackfan syndrome, Fanconi syndrome, and Holt-Oram syndrome, but are not typically found in patients with Chediak-Higashi syndrome. Elevated IgE levels are found in hyper-IgE syndrome, which is associated with coarse facial features and hyperextensible joints.

(pp. 1974–1982, Section 23: Disorders of the Blood, Part 5: Disorders of White Blood Cells, Chapter 437: Disorders of Granulocytes)

**Answer 11-60.** C

Although both acute leukemia and leukemoid reactions can present with high WBC counts, the patient's overall picture is more consistent with leukocyte adhesion deficiency. LAD-1 is a rare autosomal recessive congenital immunodeficiency caused by a deficiency of the $\beta_2$ subunit of the leukocyte adhesion molecule. As a result, neutrophils are produced but cannot migrate to sites of infection. LAD-1 is characterized by recurrent infections, marked leukocytosis, and delayed umbilical cord separation. Older patients have recurrent episodes of periodontitis. In leukemoid reactions, high leukocyte counts are seen in response to severe bacterial infections and are usually marked by increased numbers of myelocytes, metamyelocytes, and bands (not seen in this patient). More immature precursors are seen in acute leukemias. There are drugs that can cause leukocytosis—for example, steroids are known to cause a transient increase in the WBC count due to de-margination of the neutrophils—but this response would not be the best answer in a patient with severe infection and a history of delayed cord separation. Myeloproliferative disease can also present with leukocytosis but, again, does not present with a history of delayed cord separation.

(pp. 1974–1982, Section 23: Disorders of the Blood, Part 5: Disorders of White Blood Cells, Chapter 437: Disorders of Granulocytes)

**Answer 11-61.** B

This patient's history is consistent with chronic granulomatous disease (CGD), a defect in phagocytes that renders them unable to kill microbes with the reactive oxygen species. Patients with CGD do not produce hydrogen peroxide, and as a result, patients often get recurrent infections with catalase-positive organisms (eg, *S aureus*, *Klebsiella*, *Salmonella*) and fungi. Specifically, patients with a history of recurrent bacterial infections with catalase-positive organisms or who have osteomyelitis at multiple sites or in the small bones of the hands or feet (as in this patient) should be evaluated for CGD. The classic test for CGD is the nitro blue tetrazolium dye test. Patients with CGD are unable to activate the NADPH oxidase system; therefore, the neutrophils cannot reduce the yellow water-soluble tetrazolium dye to an insoluble blue formazan pigment. Newer diagnostic methods include the dihydrorhodamine test, which is a flow cytometric approach that measures the conversion of dihydrorhodamine to rhodamine on neutrophil activation. Patients with hyper-IgE also have recurrent *Staphylococcus* infections but have other clinical features including chronic eczema, retention of primary dentition, and a coarse facial appearance. Bone marrow biopsy, skin biopsy, and lymphocyte subsets would not be helpful in the diagnosis of CGD.

(pp. 1974–1982, Section 23: Disorders of the Blood, Part 5: Disorders of White Blood Cells, Chapter 437: Disorders of Granulocytes)

**Answer 11 62.** B

This patient's history of infection, eczematoid rash, and increased IgE levels is most consistent with hyper-IgE syndrome. By school age, patients have a history of recurrent skin abscesses, pneumonias, and chronic otitis media. Although patients with Wiskott-Aldrich syndrome or milk protein allergy also may have eczema, neither of these is associated with the degree of elevation in IgE in this vignette. Patients with hyper-IgE syndrome typically have IgE levels exceeding 2500 IU/mL. Patients with thrombocytopenia absent radii have a high frequency of cow's milk allergy but do not have elevated IgE levels. Patients with leukocyte adhesion defect may have similar infections as in this patient but have an elevated WBC count.

(pp. 1974–1982, Section 23: Disorders of the Blood, Part 5: Disorders of White Blood Cells, Chapter 437: Disorders of Granulocytes; pp. 1961–1970, Section 23: Disorders of the Blood, Part 3: Disorders of Coagulation and Platelets, Chapter 435: Disorders of Platelets)

**Answer 11-63.** C

Anaphylaxis is a dramatic but extremely rare adverse reaction to blood products. However, patients with IgA deficiency are at risk of an anaphylactic reaction during the first blood transfusion due to the presence of circulating anti-IgA antibodies. IgA deficiency is one of the most common immunodeficiencies, affecting approximately 1 in 600 individuals. Many of these patients are asymptomatic but are often diagnosed during routine blood donation. Future transfusions should be with units donated by other IgA-deficient individuals. Routine testing for transfusion reactions involves a clerical review of the unit and computer records and posttransfusion direct antibody testing, as well as bilirubin, haptoglobin, and urinalysis if hemolysis is suspected. A CXR is not required in a patient whose respiratory symptoms have resolved. Although anaphylaxis is generally caused by IgE-mediated mast cell degranulation, anaphylaxis in blood transfusion is usually due to IgG anti-IgA antibodies circulating in an IgA-deficient patient. Early morning cortisol levels are used to check for adrenal insufficiency after long-term steroids and are not necessary for doses given during an anaphylactic episode.

(pp. 1982–1990, Section 23: Disorders of the Blood, Part 6: Principles of Transfusion, Chapter 438: Transfusion Medicine)

**Answer 11-64.** D

The patient is having an acute hemolytic reaction. This is a noninfectious reaction that results from the transfusion of ABO-incompatible red blood cells (RBCs). These patients

**TABLE 438-6.** Clinical Service and Blood Bank Approach to Acute Transfusion Reactions

| Clinical Service | Blood Bank | Clinical Service and Blood Bank |
|---|---|---|
| Terminate transfusion and maintain IV access with normal saline (0.9% sodium chloride) | Clerical check of unit, requisition, and computer records | Review blood bank results before subsequent transfusions |
| Examine patient for severe reaction and closely monitor symptoms, vital signs, and urine output | DAT (purple top, EDTA tube) on post-transfusion specimen | Investigate possible risks to other patients who may have been affected by patient-identification error |
| Provide other supportive measures for patient if appropriate and send blood culture from patient if deemed necessary | Visual check of post-transfusion specimen plasma for hemolysis (pink color) | • If allergic reaction assessed, then no testing is indicated<br>• If anaphylaxis is diagnosed, accompanied by hypotension or angioedema, patient or donor should be tested for IgA deficiency and anti-IgA antibodies |
| Repeat bedside check of the patient's identification wristband against blood component label | Additional testing on the pre- and post-transfusion specimens if acute hemolysis expected:<br>• Repeat ABO and Rh testing<br>• Repeat crossmatch with implicated units<br>• Repeat antibody screen<br>• Repeat DAT and antibody screen on additional specimens obtained at intervals after the transfusion reactions | If pulmonary complications are suspected:<br>• Fluid overload should be considered<br>• Testing the patient and donor for anti-WBC antibodies and anti-HLA antibodies should be performed |
| Return unit(s) to blood bank along with patient's post-transfusion blood samples and completed transfusion record | | |

DAT, direct antiglobulin test; EDTA, ethylenediaminetetraacetic acid; HLA, human leukocyte antigen; Ig, immunoglobulin; IV, intravenous; WBC, white blood cell.

Mark W. Kline, *Rudolph's Pediatrics*, 23rd Edition. Copyright © McGraw-Hill Education. All rights reserved.

have signs of intravascular hemolysis with evidence of hemoglobin in their urine. A low serum haptoglobin is also indicative of intravascular hemolysis as the release of free hemoglobin binds to haptoglobin, causing a drop in serum haptoglobin levels. Additionally, due to active hemolysis, patients will have a lower-than-expected rise in posttransfusion hemoglobin levels. Occasionally, these patients may develop renal failure, shock, and disseminated intravascular coagulation if a large volume is transfused. Transfusion-related acute lung injury is another noninfectious complication of transfusion and is confirmed by CXR findings, but it is not consistent with this patient's clinical picture. Hypocalcemia and metabolic alkalosis are often signs of citrate toxicity, which is a complication of massive transfusion (defined as greater than the patient's blood volume in 24 hours). See Table 438-6 for the blood bank approach to acute complications of transfusions.

(pp. 1982–1990, Section 23: Disorders of the Blood, Part 6: Principles of Transfusion, Chapter 438: Transfusion Medicine)

**Answer 11-65. A**

Hepatitis A is not tested routinely in blood banks in the United States and is rarely transmitted through blood products. It is most often transmitted through the fecal–oral route. All blood products undergo testing for hepatitis B surface antigen (HBsAg), hepatitis B core antibody (HBcAb), hepatitis C antibody (HepCAb), and HIV antibody. Improved testing for HIV has reduced the risk of transmission to 1 in 3 million. HTLV-1 is a retrovirus that is implicated in causing T-cell leukemia and has been screened by blood banks since the late 1980s.

(p. 1989, Section 23: Disorders of the Blood, Part 6: Principles of Transfusion, Chapter 438: Transfusion Medicine, Table 438-5)

# CHAPTER 12 Allergy and Immunology

Alan Baptist, Madeleine B. Chollet, Elise Coulson, and Sherry Zhou

**12-1.** A 14-year-old boy presents to your clinic with year-round symptoms of sneezing, congestion, nasal discharge, and watery eyes. His symptoms seem to be worse after spending extended periods of time in his bedroom. He is healthy otherwise. On physical exam, he has pale nasal turbinates and moderate clear rhinorrhea. Skin prick shows a positive reaction to dust mite. What would you recommend to him initially?

**A.** Oral antihistamine

**B.** Oral leukotriene receptor antagonist

**C.** Intranasal steroids

**D.** Avoidance measures, frequent vacuuming, dust mite pillow and mattress encasement, washing beddings weekly, and an oral antihistamine

**E.** Immunotherapy to dust mite

**12-2.** A 4-year-old boy with allergic rhinitis (AR) and sensitivities on skin-prick testing to tree, grass, ragweed, and dust mite presents to clinic for follow-up. His parents report that avoidance measures, antihistamines, and intranasal steroids have not been sufficient to control his symptoms. He has missed multiple days of school due to his symptoms. The family is interested in immunotherapy. What advice might you provide to the family?

**A.** He is not a good candidate for immunotherapy because patients need to demonstrate at least 5 environmental allergens to receive benefit.

**B.** He qualifies for sublingual immunotherapy because he is allergic to grass and ragweed.

**C.** Immunotherapy will not be very helpful in long term because it is only effective while the patient is receiving the shots.

**D.** He is too young for immunotherapy because it is only effective in children older than the age of 6.

**E.** His risk of developing asthma is increased once he starts immunotherapy.

**12-3.** Which of the following medications should be avoided in a 12-year-old child with severe constipation?

**A.** Loratadine

**B.** Levocetirizine

**C.** Chlorpheniramine

**D.** Fexofenadine

**E.** Cetirizine

**12-4.** An 18-year-old woman is referred to your clinic due to chronic severe nasal congestion, rhinitis, and itchy eyes. Most of her symptoms are worst in the spring, although she has year-round nasal congestion that she finds very bothersome. Exam reveals pale nasal turbinates, congestion, and rhinorrhea. She is currently taking fexofenadine daily, phenylephrine daily, and intermittent nasal saline rinse. What do you recommend?

**A.** Stop phenylephrine and add an intranasal steroid

**B.** Stop fexofenadine and switch to cetirizine

**C.** Keep current medications and add an intranasal steroid

**D.** Keep current medications and add an oral decongestant

**E.** Keep current medications and add a leukotriene receptor antagonist

**12-5.** A 5-year-old boy is referred to your clinic for evaluation of rhinitis. Mom states that for the past 2 weeks, his symptoms seem to have worsened. He constantly has a runny nose, mostly with clear drainage but sometimes with a yellow tint. He also seems to have itchy eyes, and the right eye seems to be redder than the left. He is otherwise active and growing well. Examination of his nasal cavity reveals erythematous mucosa with crusty secretion and some clear rhinorrhea. What is the most likely diagnosis?

**A.** Allergic rhinoconjunctivitis

**B.** Nonallergic rhinoconjunctivitis

**C.** Viral rhinoconjunctivitis

**D.** Chronic sinusitis

**E.** Adenoidal hypertrophy

**12-6.** Which of the following statements is correct about the different families within the order Hymenoptera?

**A.** Africanized honeybees (*Apis mellifera scutellata*) have more potent venom than other honeybees (*Apis mellifera*).

**B.** Paper wasps are the most aggressive family within the order Hymenoptera.

**C.** Yellow jackets are less aggressive than paper wasps but tend to build their nests near buildings, making them more likely to encounter people and cause stings.

**D.** Hornets only sting in self-defense, such as when they are accidentally grabbed or stepped on.

**E.** As many as 50% of people living in areas infested with fire ants (*Solenopsis invicta*) get stung each year.

**12-7.** An 8-year-old girl is stung by a bee, and she develops tongue swelling, shortness of breath, and generalized hives. Which of the following statements about allergy testing is true?

**A.** Either intradermal venom testing or measurement of serum immunoglobulin E (IgE) to venoms can be used to identify venom-specific IgE antibodies.

**B.** Her honeybee IgE level will be very high because she had a severe reaction to the honeybee sting.

**C.** If her allergy testing is positive, she has a 5% chance of having a systemic reaction to a future sting.

**D.** She does not need allergy testing because there are no therapies to prevent a future reaction to a bee sting.

**E.** She should never have allergy testing because she had anaphylaxis.

**12-8.** A 15-year-old girl is stung on her left hand while mowing the grass. Her hand becomes red and swollen at the site of the sting. Over the next 24 hours, her left wrist and forearm become swollen and red. She does not have any other symptoms including dyspnea, diarrhea, vomiting, palpitations, chest pain, or lightheadedness. Which of the following is appropriate advice to give to the patient?

**A.** She has developed cellulitis from her Hymenoptera sting, and she should be prescribed antibiotics.

**B.** She is at high risk of developing anaphylaxis in the next 24 hours, and she should be prescribed an epinephrine autoinjector.

**C.** She is currently having anaphylaxis and should call 911.

**D.** She has developed a large local reaction that will resolve over the course of 5 to 10 days.

**E.** She is experiencing swelling that will typically resolve completely after 1 to 2 doses of diphenhydramine.

**12-9.** A 16-year-old boy with a history of migraine headaches comes to the allergy clinic to discuss venom immunotherapy. He was stung by a yellow jacket a month ago and developed redness and pain at the site of the sting that lasted a couple hours. His sister has an allergy to wasps, and he is worried that he has an allergy to them as well. He is currently taking propranolol for migraine prophylaxis. Which of the following is true about venom immunotherapy?

**A.** Using a standard schedule, he can achieve protection from systemic reactions to stings in 1 to 2 weeks.

**B.** Venom immunotherapy is not indicated because he did not have an allergic systemic reaction to the sting.

**C.** β-Blockers are an absolute contraindication to venom immunotherapy.

**D.** He is not eligible for the rush schedule because of his family history of a vespid allergy.

**E.** There is a high frequency of adverse effects associated with venom immunotherapy.

**12-10.** A 10-year-old boy is stung by multiple fire ants while running barefoot outside. He develops wheezing, an itchy throat, and hives. His mother calls 911. Which of the following medications should be administered first to the patient?

**A.** Diphenhydramine

**B.** Cetirizine

**C.** Prednisone

**D.** Epinephrine

**E.** Venom immunotherapy

**12-11.** An 8-year-old girl has mouth pruritus and describes a "prickly" sensation when eating kiwi and banana. She has noticed these symptoms before when eating bananas, but the symptoms seem to be worsening. Her father reports that when she was younger she never liked bananas, but he never noticed any reactions when she ate them. She has spina bifida with neurogenic bladder and asthma. She is allergic to latex but has no other known drug allergies. Physical exam is notable only for lower extremity neurologic deficits. What is the most likely cause of her current oral symptoms?

**A.** A primary immunoglobulin E (IgE)-mediated allergy to kiwi that cross-reacts with banana

**B.** Oral candidiasis

**C.** Eosinophilic esophagitis

**D.** Contact irritant dermatitis

**E.** Latex-fruit syndrome

**12-12.** A 10-year-old boy with spina bifida undergoes a bladder augmentation cystoplasty. Ten minutes into the procedure, the anesthesiologists note profound hypotension. On further inspection, the patient's skin appears blotchy and erythematous. The procedure is aborted, and with supportive therapy, the boy recovers within several hours. In addition to consideration of anesthetic allergy, which of the following would be the most appropriate evaluation to investigate for a possible cause?

**A.** Evaluation for type I hypersensitivity reaction to latex

**B.** Evaluation for mastocytosis

**C.** Evaluation for side effects of the sedatives used

**D.** Evaluation of kidney and liver function

**E.** Evaluation for type IV hypersensitivity to chlorhexidine antiseptic scrub

**12-13.** An 18-year-old nursing assistant comes to see you about reactions at work. These reactions occurred while he was taking vital signs on patients at a skilled nursing facility. A coworker at the facility recommended he be evaluated for a latex allergy, and now he would like your opinion. What is the next best diagnostic or therapeutic step?

**A.** Prescribe epinephrine autoinjectors and then instruct him to conduct a latex challenge at work

**B.** Take a thorough clinical history followed by serum fluorescence enzyme-linked immunosorbent assay (ELISA) testing if appropriate

**C.** Reassure him that if he has been able to conduct his job thus far the reactions are unlikely to be dangerous, but you will send serum fluorescence ELISA testing just to be sure

**D.** Recommend allergy skin testing followed by a latex challenge if negative

**E.** Prescribe epinephrine autoinjectors and give him an anaphylaxis action plan

**12-14.** A 12-year-old girl is diagnosed with latex allergy following an anaphylactic episode that occurred while playing with a balloon at a friend's birthday party. Which of the following actions should she and her parents be instructed to take in the future?

**A.** Avoid all fruits and vegetables that could cause latex-fruit syndrome, even if she has previously tolerated them

**B.** Avoid annual influenza vaccine, if possible, because the needles and vials may contain latex

**C.** Avoid measles-mumps-rubella (MMR) vaccination, if possible, because the vaccine contains proteins that may contain latex

**D.** Carry self-injectable epinephrine at all times

**E.** Frequently eat the fruits and vegetables that could cause latex-fruit syndrome to decrease the likelihood of developing an immunoglobulin E (IgE)-mediated allergy to these foods

**12-15.** A 16-year-old girl has a job at a veterinary office and has been experiencing a patchy pruritic erythematous rash on her hands and wrists. It first appeared 5 weeks ago after her office changed the brand of gloves in the exam rooms, and the onset was somewhat insidious. The appearance has waxed and waned over the past 5 weeks. Which of the following is the most likely explanation of her symptoms and the correct next diagnostic or therapeutic intervention?

**A.** This is likely a type I immunoglobulin E (IgE)-mediated hypersensitivity reaction to the new gloves; conduct skin-prick testing and ask her to carry an epinephrine autoinjector in case the reaction becomes more severe.

**B.** This is likely a type II hypersensitivity reaction mediated by antibodies caused by cross-reactivity between the latex in the glove and self-antigens; ask her to strictly avoid contact with the gloves and prescribe her a topical steroid ointment.

**C.** This is likely a type III serum sickness reaction caused by the nonhuman proteins she is exposed to in her daily work; treat her with a prednisone taper and encourage her to wash her hands frequently.

**D.** This is likely a type IV hypersensitivity reaction to the gloves mediated by T cells; perform patch testing to determine which component of the gloves is the culprit, and treat the current dermatitis with a topical steroid ointment.

**E.** This is likely a type V hypersensitivity reaction to the gloves mediated by autoantibodies binding to cell surface receptors; treat her with a prednisone taper and encourage her to complete further workup for autoimmune diseases such as lupus.

**12-16.** A 2-month-old female infant presents for her routine follow-up appointment. She was born at full term via a normal spontaneous vaginal delivery and has been healthy since birth. You are working with a medical student, and she asks why so many early vaccines are important in a healthy baby. Which of the following explanations is true regarding the importance of vaccinations?

**A.** Infants are not born with a fully functional immune system, and their adaptive immune system is characterized by a low number of memory B cells. They are at particular risk for dangerous infection by encapsulated bacteria. Multiple and early vaccines are necessary to sustain and maintain immunologic memory against these bacteria.

**B.** Infants are not born with a fully functional immune system, and toll-like receptor expression is decreased; therefore, they are at particular risk for infection from nonencapsulated bacteria. Multiple and early vaccines are necessary to facilitate recognition of a variety of pathogen-associated molecular patterns (PAMPs).

**C.** The adaptive immune system is characterized by low numbers of regulatory T cells in early infancy, which leads to lower responses to infection, making infants at particular risk for dangerous infection by encapsulated bacteria. Multiple and early vaccines are necessary to sustain and maintain immunologic memory against these bacteria.

**D.** The innate immune system is characterized by decreased numbers of neutrophils in early infancy, which leads to decreased effectiveness in response to infection, making infants at particular risk for infection by encapsulated bacteria. Multiple and early vaccines are necessary to shift the response toward the Th1 phenotype, which favors responses to these pathogens.

**E.** Lymphoid organs are less mature in early infancy. The maturation of paracortex is poor, and therefore, multiple and early vaccines are necessary to sustain and maintain immunologic memory against encapsulated bacteria, which cause particularly dangerous infections in early infancy.

**12-17.** Which of the following statements regarding the innate immune system is correct?

**A.** Antiviral responses typically induce activation of a class of transcription factors called nuclear factor-κB (NF-κB).

**B.** Tissue macrophages recognize pathogen-associated molecular patterns (PAMPs), which facilitates recruitment of other cells to clear the bacteria.

**C.** Most responses to bacteria lead to activation of a class of transcription factors called interferon response factors (IRFs)

**D.** The most critical cells for the clearance of cells infected by viruses are neutrophils.

**E.** Activated neutrophils kill certain pathogens, such as *Mycobacteria* and fungi, that are resistant to macrophage killing.

**12-18.** Which of the following statements about T-cell maturation and function is correct?

**A.** Functional recombination of the T-cell receptor genes is controlled by the autoimmune regulator (*AIRE*) gene family.

**B.** Maturation of T cells occurs mainly in the germinal center of lymph nodes.

**C.** In the medulla of the thymus, T cells become positive for CD4 and CD8.

**D.** During positive selection, T cells with strong affinity for self are signaled to undergo apoptosis.

**E.** Double-positive T cells exit the thymus to circulate in the periphery.

**12-19.** Which of the following statements about antigen-presenting cells (APCs) is correct?

**A.** APCs are essential for B-cell function.

**B.** After dendritic cells are activated, they migrate to the bone marrow where they present antigen to T cells.

**C.** APCs stimulate naïve CD4-positive cells in the context of major histocompatibility complex (MHC) class I molecules.

**D.** Dendritic cells work independently from the ensuing T-cell response and interact only when they are presenting their antigens.

**E.** Macrophages are less potent APCs but exhibit similar characteristics as dendritic cells.

**12-20.** Which of the following statements about human immunoglobulin is correct?

**A.** Initially, all mature B cells express immunoglobulin M (IgM) and immunoglobulin A (IgA) on their cell surface.

**B.** On exposure to a new antigen, isotype switching can occur and antigen specificity is altered.

**C.** IgM is the first immunoglobulin to be generated and is secreted as a pentamer.

**D.** Immunoglobulin E (IgE) is the most abundant immunoglobulin in human serum and mediates allergic reactions.

**E.** Immunoglobulin G (IgG) is the major immunoglobulin at mucosal surfaces and can be found in breast milk.

**12-21.** A 2-year-old boy with a past medical history of frequent otitis media infections, oral candidiasis, and failure to thrive is admitted to the hospital for a fever and cough. He quickly progresses to respiratory failure. He is intubated, and *P jiroveci* is found in his bronchoalveolar lavage. What test would you order next?

- **A.** Quantitative serum immunoglobulin levels
- **B.** Human immunodeficiency virus (HIV) serology
- **C.** Neutrophil oxidative burst
- **D.** Gene sequencing analysis
- **E.** Sweat chloride test

**12-22.** Which of the following scenarios would most likely precipitate a workup for frequent infections?

- **A.** A 3-year-old girl with a peanut allergy who has a history of *Escherichia coli* meningitis at 3 weeks of age and had 2 viral upper respiratory infections (URIs) over the past year
- **B.** A 7-year-old boy with asthma who has a history of neonatal sepsis and an episode of otitis media at age 4
- **C.** A 5-year-old girl with molluscum contagiosum who has a history of 9 viral URIs over the past year
- **D.** A 5-month-old boy with eczema who has a history of food protein–induced enterocolitis and 2 episodes of bilateral otitis media
- **E.** A 2-year-old girl with spina bifida who has a history of an *E coli* urinary tract infection and perioral impetigo

**12-23.** A 4-year-old boy presents for routine follow-up. His mother reports she is concerned because he is constantly sick. He has been hospitalized twice for pneumonia and has had multiple ear infections every year. On exam, you notice that, although he has no surgical history, his tonsils are absent. What recommendations do you give his mother in terms of preventive care and further diagnosis of his condition?

- **A.** He should hold off on getting his measles, mumps, and rubella (MMR) booster because live vaccine may not be safe for him. He should get his immunoglobulin levels checked.
- **B.** He should get his MMR vaccine now, but he may need an additional booster later because he may not respond sufficiently to the usual number of doses. He should get his immunoglobulin levels checked.
- **C.** He should follow a normal vaccine schedule now to protect him from any further infection. He should get specific antibody titers to tetanus toxoid and to pneumococcal serotypes.
- **D.** He will need specific antibody titers to tetanus toxoid and to pneumococcal serotypes to see if he responded to prior vaccines. He will need interferon-γ treatment.
- **E.** He should get his MMR vaccine now, but he may need an additional booster later because he may not respond sufficiently to the usual number of doses. He should wear a mask when he is in public and should be kept out of preschool if possible.

**12-24.** A 4-year-old boy presents for follow-up after hospital discharge from *Klebsiella* pneumonia. He has a past medical history of 2 *Candida* skin infections. What laboratory test would you send to evaluate for chronic granulomatous disease (CGD)?

- **A.** Quantitative immunoglobulin levels
- **B.** *TLR3* gene sequencing
- **C.** Dihydrhodamine (DHR) assay
- **D.** Nitroblue tetrazolium test
- **E.** Flow cytometry analysis of T-lymphocyte markers

**12-25.** An 8-month-old boy with past medical history of frequent respiratory illnesses presents with a fever and respiratory distress. He was found to have *P jiroveci* pneumonia and a primary immunodeficiency. Which of the following gene defects would most likely be associated with *P jiroveci* infection?

- **A.** *MYD88*
- **B.** *C5-9*
- **C.** *CXCR4*
- **D.** *CD40*
- **E.** *XIAP*

**12-26.** Severe combined immunodeficiency disease (SCID) is defined by which of the following specific criteria?

- **A.** Presence of a *DCLRE1C* gene defect
- **B.** Positive dihydrhodamine (DHR) assay
- **C.** Absence or very low number of T cells and no or very low T-cell function
- **D.** Absence or very low number of B cells and no or very low B-cell function
- **E.** Positive nitroblue tetrazolium test

**12-27.** A 6-month-old girl is admitted to the hospital for fever, cough, and shortness of breath. She has a history of chronic diarrhea and failure to thrive. Physical exam is notable for a lack of tonsils and thrush. There is no thymic shadow on the chest x-ray. She is diagnosed with *Pneumocystis jiroveci*. Human immunodeficiency virus (HIV) testing is negative. This child most likely has which of the following conditions?

**A.** Hemophagocytic lymphohistiocytosis

**B.** Selective immunoglobulin A (IgA) deficiency

**C.** Wiskott-Aldrich syndrome

**D.** Severe combined immunodeficiency disease (SCID)

**E.** Autoimmune lymphoproliferative syndrome

**12-28.** A 12-month-old boy with a history of recurrent otitis media is seen in the emergency department (ED) for his third skin abscess since birth. His mother reports that he has had intermittent rashes and skin infections for most of his life. His physical exam is notable for a broad nasal bridge and hyperextensible joints. His immunoglobulin E (IgE) is elevated to 3000 IU/mL. A mutation in which of the following genes is responsible for his condition?

**A.** *STAT3*

**B.** *BTK*

**C.** *FOXP3*

**D.** *AIRE*

**E.** *IKBKG*

**12-29.** A 3-year-old boy is admitted to the pediatric intensive care unit for a lung abscess. He has a history of recurrent infections including skin abscesses, pneumonia, and a perirectal abscess. Genetic analysis reveals a mutation in *CYBB*, and he is diagnosed with chronic granulomatous disease (CGD). Which of the following is a true statement about CGD?

**A.** Individuals with CGD are at a decreased risk of developing inflammatory bowel disease.

**B.** Individuals with CGD do not generate the respiratory burst needed for killing catalase-negative microbes.

**C.** Female carriers of a *CYBB* mutation are at increased risk of developing autoimmune arthritis and discoid lupus erythematosus.

**D.** Some individuals with CGD have the McLeod blood phenotype, which means that they can only receive transfusions with immunoglobulin A (IgA)-deficient blood.

**E.** The nitroblue tetrazolium test is the gold standard for diagnosis.

**12-30.** A 5-year-old girl is seen in clinic. She is asymptomatic, and her past medical history is unremarkable. Laboratory tests reveal a decreased serum immunoglobulin A (IgA) level of 1 mg/dL. Her serum immunoglobulin G (IgG), immunoglobulin M (IgM), and immunoglobulin E (IgE) levels are within the normal range. Which of the following statements about her condition is true?

**A.** Selective IgA deficiency is a contraindication for blood transfusion with IgA-containing blood products.

**B.** Nearly all children with selective IgA deficiency will go on to develop common variable immunodeficiency (CVID).

**C.** She requires IgG replacement therapy for treatment of her condition.

**D.** Selective IgA deficiency is protective against developing an autoimmune condition.

**E.** Approximately one-fifth of children with selective IgA deficiency will have normal IgA levels as an adolescent.

**12-31.** Which of the following is the first immunologic disorder in which clinical trials of gene therapy were attempted?

**A.** X-linked severe combined immunodeficiency

**B.** Adenosine deaminase deficiency

**C.** Wiskott-Aldrich syndrome

**D.** X-linked chronic granulomatous disease (CGD)

**E.** Artemis deficiency

**12-32.** Potential barriers to hematopoietic cell transplantations (HCTs) for primary immune deficiencies include all the following except:

**A.** Drug toxicity

**B.** Graft rejection

**C.** Graft-versus-host disease

**D.** Immune dysregulation

**E.** Adequate number of human leukocyte antigen (HLA)-matched donors

**12-33.** Why is there a potential risk of insertional mutagenesis with gene therapy?

**A.** Because the expression of therapeutic transgene is controlled by homologous promoters

**B.** Because homologous recombination cannot always replace the DNA fragment containing the mutation

**C.** Because by integrating an additional normal copy of the gene of interest into the patient's cell using viral vectors, the gene is integrated randomly into the DNA

**D.** Because homologous recombination occurs at a very low frequency

**E.** Because insulator sequences in the vector are not effective in shielding cellular genes from viral transcriptional elements

**12-34.** Which of the following cytokines is correctly matched with the T-helper cell that produces it?

**A.** IL-2 – TH2

**B.** IL-4 – TH1

**C.** IL-5 – TH2

**D.** IL-13 – TH1

**E.** Interferon-γ –TH2

**12-35.** Antigen-presenting cells (APCs) present peptide fragments from allergens to T cells as part of the allergic response. Which of the following types of APCs is the most efficient at presenting allergenic peptides?

**A.** Dendritic cells

**B.** Macrophages

**C.** B cells

**D.** Mast cells

**E.** Neutrophils

**12-36.** A 15-year-old boy with a history of asthma and allergies to cats and peanuts is seen in your clinic. He is told to avoid cats and peanuts. He is started on an inhaled corticosteroid and is told to take antihistamines before any known exposures to cats. He is given epinephrine for his history of a peanut allergy. Which of the following statements about allergy therapies is correct?

**A.** Scrupulous allergen avoidance can result in symptomatic relief but has no long-term effects.

**B.** Antihistamines counteract anaphylaxis by dilating smooth muscle and causing cutaneous vasoconstriction.

**C.** Anti–IL-5 therapy is being used in the treatment of severe eosinophilic asthma.

**D.** Antihistamines are more useful than steroids for managing chronic allergic inflammation.

**E.** Anti-immunoglobulin E (IgE) monoclonal antibodies work by cross-linking IgE to T cells.

**12-37.** An 8-month-old girl is seen in clinic for patches of dry erythematous skin on her cheeks, neck, elbows, and knees. The girl's father says that his daughter cannot sleep from the itching and has been scratching at night. Her father bathes her every day in a bubble bath. A mutation in which of the following would be most consistent with her diagnosis?

**A.** Filaggrin

**B.** *TSLP*

**C.** *ADAM33*

**D.** *FAS*

**E.** *SH2D1A*

**12-38.** Which of the following is true regarding immunoglobulin E (IgE) production and signaling?

**A.** The first signal required for class-switch recombination is provided by the TH1 cytokines IL-4 or IL-13.

**B.** The second signal for class-switch recombination is from the interaction of CD40 and CD23.

**C.** FCεRI is a high-affinity IgE receptor that is found only on mast cells.

**D.** IgE remains permanently bound to FCεRI until it is internalized.

**E.** Binding of IgE to FCεRI initiates a signal transduction cascade that causes mast cells to release stored granules.

**12-39.** Immunoglobulin E (IgE)-induced immediate hypersensitivity reaction often is followed by a late-phase or delayed reaction. Which of the following statements is true about a late-phase reaction?

**A.** Late-phase or delayed reaction can occur within 2 hours of the acute reaction.

**B.** Late-phase or delayed reaction can occur 4 to 24 hours after the acute reaction has subsided.

**C.** Late-phase or delayed reaction can occur several days to weeks after the acute reaction has subsided.

**D.** The late-phase reaction manifests only as gastrointestinal symptoms.

**E.** The late-phase reaction arises from the recruitment to the allergen challenge site of an inflammatory cellular infiltrate that includes lymphocytes.

**12-40.** Which of the following cytokine or transcription factors is closely associated with TH1 cells?

**A.** Interferon-γ

**B.** GATA-3

**C.** IL-4

**D.** IL-13

**E.** IL-5

**12-41.** What of the following is true regarding late-phase reactions?

**A.** They usually occur > 24 hours after the initial exposure to an allergen.

**B.** They are mostly mediated by mast cell products.

**C.** Only T lymphocytes are involved in the inflammatory process.

**D.** Anaphylaxis does not occur with late-phase reactions.

**E.** Symptoms of late-phase reactions are generally less severe.

**12-42.** A 2-year-old boy presents with his parents for evaluation of possible allergy to egg. He was never exposed to egg because his older brother has an egg allergy. The parents would like to perform every test possible to assess for food allergy. Which of the following statements is appropriate to tell his parents?

**A.** It is reasonable to do an extended panel of food testing given his family history of food allergies.

**B.** Blood immunoglobulin E (IgE) test is superior than skin-prick test to confirm food allergies.

**C.** Blood IgE and skin-prick tests have high negative predictive value.

**D.** Blood IgE and skin-prick tests are not practical to obtain in the outpatient clinical setting.

**E.** Positive skin-prick test means the child is allergic to eggs and should strictly avoid them.

**12-43.** A 12-year-old girl presents for evaluation of seasonal allergies. She shows multiple aeroallergen sensitivities on skin test. What is the most effective monotherapy for her?

**A.** Intranasal corticosteroids

**B.** Leukotriene receptor antagonist

**C.** Oral antihistamines

**D.** Oral steroids

**E.** A combination of a leukotriene receptor antagonist and oral antihistamines

**12-44.** A 16-year-old boy presents for follow-up. He is allergic to multiple seasonal and perennial allergens. He has tried oral antihistamines and intranasal steroids, but his symptoms are still not controlled. He is interested in starting allergy shots. Which of the following statements is true regarding allergen-specific immunotherapy?

**A.** Immunotherapy can be used to treat allergic airway diseases but not insect venom allergy.

**B.** The benefit of immunotherapy lasts years after discontinuation of treatment.

**C.** A minimum of 5 years of treatment is required.

**D.** Immunotherapy only treats current allergens but does not decrease the risk of developing new allergen sensitization.

**E.** Immunotherapy has no effect on asthma risk in children with allergic rhinitis (AR).

**12-45.** A 10-year-old girl presents to the emergency department (ED) with rapid onset of diffuse hives, wheezing, and vomiting after eating cookies at her friend's birthday party. Treatment should *not* be delayed for laboratory confirmation; however, theoretically, which of the following tests would confirm the most likely diagnosis?

**A.** Histamine level 2 hours after the episode

**B.** Tryptase level 2 hours after the episode

**C.** Complete blood count (CBC) with differential 2 hours after the episode

**D.** Erythrocyte sedimentation rate (ESR) 2 hours after the episode

**E.** C-reactive protein (CRP) 2 hours after the episode

**12-46.** A 6-year-old boy presents to the emergency department (ED) with generalized hives and lethargy. The symptoms occurred 20 minutes after taking amoxicillin for an ear infection. He was noted to be pale, diaphoretic, and hypotensive. What is the most important initial treatment for him?

**A.** Intravenous (IV) normal saline bolus (20 mL/kg)

**B.** IV diphenhydramine

**C.** IV methylprednisolone

**D.** Inhaled bronchodilator

**E.** Intramuscular (IM) epinephrine

**12-47.** In patients with urticaria, how long must they exhibit near-daily symptoms of the condition to be considered as having chronic disease?

**A.** 4 weeks

**B.** 6 weeks

**C.** 2 months

**D.** 3 months

**E.** 6 months

**12-48.** Which of the following conditions is primarily mediated by the kinin pathway?

**A.** A patient with hereditary angioedema

**B.** A patient with itchy eyes and rhinitis in the spring

**C.** A patient who develops generalized hives and wheezing after eating peanuts

**D.** A patient who passes out after being stung by a yellow jacket

**E.** A patient who develops trouble breathing and generalized urticaria after receiving intravenous (IV) ceftriaxone

**12-49.** You are seeing a 3-year-old boy who is not vaccinated due to his parents' fear of vaccine reactions. Which of the following statements regarding vaccine allergy is true?

- **A.** True immunoglobulin E (IgE)-mediated anaphylaxis to immunization is quite common.
- **B.** Vaccine reaction usually involves activation of IgE in response to the immunizing antigen, rather than a vaccine component.
- **C.** Gelatin has been implicated in anaphylactic reactions to the measles, mumps, and rubella (MMR), varicella, and influenza vaccines.
- **D.** An egg allergy is an absolute contraindication to receiving the influenza vaccine.
- **E.** Diphtheria and tetanus vaccine have the highest rates of IgE-mediated reaction compared to other vaccines.

**12-50.** Which of the following statements correctly describes angioedema?

- **A.** Angioedema, commonly called *hives*, involves extravasation of fluid in the superficial dermis.
- **B.** Angioedema always appears with urticaria.
- **C.** Edematous swelling associated with angioedema usually resolves within 2 hours.
- **D.** Angioedema is characterized by well-circumscribed, pruritic, raised, erythematous skin wheals.
- **E.** Angioedema typically involves the periorbital tissues, lips, tongue, posterior oropharynx, larynx, hands, feet, or genitals.

**12-51.** A 2-year-old girl developed hives and vomiting after eating scrambled egg. She also had wheezing and hives after eating peanut butter. Which of the following is true regarding her food allergies?

- **A.** She is more likely to outgrow her peanut allergy than her egg allergy.
- **B.** She may be able to tolerate baked egg but is unlikely to tolerate baked peanut.
- **C.** The severity of her food allergic reaction is expected to increase with each exposure.
- **D.** Her little brother has the same risk as the general population of developing a peanut allergy.
- **E.** Waiting to introduce peanuts until after 1 year of age reduces the risk of developing a peanut allergy.

**12-52.** A 14-year-old boy develops an itchy mouth and throat when he eats raw apples; however, he does not have any symptoms when he eats apple pie. Which of the following is the correct diagnosis for his condition?

- **A.** Atopic dermatitis
- **B.** Food protein–induced enterocolitis
- **C.** Eosinophilic esophagitis
- **D.** Oral allergy syndrome
- **E.** Alpha-gal allergy

**12-53.** A 2-month-old girl who is exclusively breastfed is seen in the clinic for the passage of frequent mucousy and sometimes bloody stools. She is otherwise well and has been gaining weight appropriately. Which of the following statements is true about her condition?

- **A.** The most commonly implicated foods for this condition are wheat and fish.
- **B.** She likely became sensitized via maternally ingested proteins excreted in breast milk.
- **C.** Her mother must stop breastfeeding and switch to infant formula.
- **D.** She has food protein–induced enterocolitis.
- **E.** Colonoscopy would show diffuse inflammation of the gastrointestinal tract and crypt abscesses.

**12-54.** An 18-month-old boy developed a rash around his mouth after eating lobster. Which of the following is the gold standard for diagnosing food allergy?

- **A.** Clinical history
- **B.** Skin-prick testing
- **C.** Measurement of serum food-specific immunoglobulin E (IgE) antibodies
- **D.** Double-blind placebo-controlled oral food challenge
- **E.** Patch test

**12-55.** A 2-year-old boy develops hives, wheezing, and nausea within 10 minutes of eating cashews for the first time. Which of the following is true about preventing and treating food allergies?

- **A.** His symptoms can be managed with an oral $H_1$ or $H_2$ antihistamine alone.
- **B.** Glucocorticoids are first-line agents for management of anaphylaxis.
- **C.** His parents should carry a single dose of epinephrine at all times.
- **D.** Avoidance of food allergens can be challenging because of cross-contamination in food-processing facilities.
- **E.** Children should be observed by a physician for 2 hours after a severe food allergic reaction.

**12-56.** A 1-year-old girl with a past medical history of anaphylaxis to egg presents for routine follow-up and immunizations. It is currently peak influenza season. She is well appearing on physical exam. Which of the following is the next step in regard to her immunization schedule?

**A.** Immunize her against influenza now and measles, mumps, and rubella (MMR) in 1 year.

**B.** Immunize her against influenza only.

**C.** Immunize her against MMR only.

**D.** Do not immunize her against either MMR or influenza.

**E.** Immunize her against both MMR and influenza now.

**12-57.** Which of the following represents an immunologically mediated drug reaction?

**A.** An 18-year-old boy with a soft tissue infection who develops acute kidney injury (AKI) while receiving vancomycin

**B.** A 17-year-old girl with trichomoniasis who develops a metallic taste and abdominal pain after receiving metronidazole

**C.** A 6-year-old boy with otitis media who develops abdominal pain after receiving penicillin

**D.** A 3-year-old girl with vesicoureteral reflux who develops fever, rash, and liver failure while receiving daily sulfamethoxazole-trimethoprim

**E.** A 1-week-old boy with sepsis who develops deafness after receiving gentamicin

**12-58.** A 4-year-old boy presents for routine follow-up. He has a past medical history of wheezing with viral infections as an infant. He is well appearing on initial exam and weighs 14.2 kg. During the visit, he receives the measles, mumps, and rubella (MMR) vaccine, and within 10 minutes, he develops a diffuse urticarial rash and wheezing. You administer one autoinjector containing 0.15 mg of epinephrine. After 5 minutes, his breathing still remains labored and his blood pressure is 62/45 mm Hg. While you are waiting for emergency medical services (EMS) transport to the hospital, what is the immediate next best step?

**A.** Administer an albuterol nebulizer treatment

**B.** Administer a second dose of 0.15 mg intramuscular (IM) epinephrine

**C.** Administer diphenhydramine 15 mg intravenous (IV)

**D.** Administer methylprednisolone 30 mg IV

**E.** Administer oxygen by face mask

**12-59.** A 16-year-old girl has the following adverse drug reactions listed on her chart:

- Vancomycin caused flushing and warmth 20 minutes into the second infusion.
- Ciprofloxacin caused nausea and diarrhea on the first day of the course.
- Metronidazole caused metallic taste and abdominal pain after the first dose.
- Cephalexin caused a lacy macular rash 2 days into the course.
- Penicillin caused a pruritic urticarial rash 20 minutes after the second dose.

She would like clarification on her allergies. What testing would you advise she needs?

**A.** Patch testing to vancomycin

**B.** Serum immunoglobulin E (IgE) antibody assay to ciprofloxacin

**C.** Drug challenge to metronidazole

**D.** Desensitization to cephalexin

**E.** Skin-prick testing to penicillin

**12-60.** Which of the children in the following scenarios is most likely to have an allergic reaction to amoxicillin?

**A.** A 5-year-old girl with past medical history of asthma and anaphylaxis to the influenza vaccine

**B.** A 17-year-old boy with past medical history of atopic dermatitis and severe allergic rhinitis (AR)

**C.** An 8-year-old girl with a tic disorder and a family history of mother and aunt who have penicillin allergy

**D.** A 14-year-old boy with past medical history of attention-deficit/hyperactivity disorder and anaphylaxis to cefadroxil

**E.** A 12-year-old girl with past medical history of anaphylaxis to peanuts and sulfamethoxazole

## ANSWERS

**Answer 12-1. D**

The patient has perennial allergic rhinitis (AR) from dust mite allergy based on the history and skin test result. Optimal management of AR requires preventative measures to minimize exposure to allergens together with judicious use of pharmacologic agents to alleviate symptoms. Avoidance measures, such as dust mite mattress and pillow encasements, controlling humidity at home, frequent vacuuming, and washing bedding weekly, as well as use of a high-efficiency particulate arrestance (HEPA) filter, can be part of this first step.

Histamine is produced by mast cells and mediates many allergic symptoms, including AR. Antihistamines are generally safe and can be used in children. It is recommended to use preventative measures together with pharmacologic agents, such as antihistamines, as the optimal management to treat AR in children.

Leukotrienes are involved in allergic inflammation. They are comparable in terms of effectiveness as oral antihistamines. They are also generally safe to use in children.

Intranasal steroids are very effective anti-inflammatory drugs used to treat AR. They are more effective than antihistamines and leukotriene receptor antagonist. However, their side effects make them less attractive for use in children.

Immunotherapy is a very effective therapy for AR. However, this is a time-consuming therapy that requires a lot of commitment. It is recommended for patients who have failed avoidance measures and medications to treat AR.

(p. 900, Section 14: Allergic Disorders, Chapter 189: Allergic Rhinitis and Conjunctivitis)

**Answer 12-2.** B

This patient qualifies for sublingual immunotherapy given he has demonstrated sensitivity to grass and ragweed. Sublingual immunotherapy is safe and effective in children as young as 3 years of age. There is no requirement regarding the number of aeroallergen sensitivities one needs to demonstrate to receive immunotherapy. Most patients will receive benefits years after discontinuation of treatment. Allergen immunotherapy has been shown to reduce the risk of development of asthma in children with AR.

Most patients will receive benefit and remain on immunotherapy for 3 to 5 years. Subcutaneous immunotherapy is relatively safe, and severe systemic reactions occur in < 1% of patients.

(p. 901, Section 14: Allergic Disorders, Chapter 189: Allergic Rhinitis and Conjunctivitis)

**Answer 12-3.** C

Second-generation oral antihistamines, such as loratadine, desloratadine, fexofenadine, cetirizine, and levocetirizine, are preferred over first-generation medications, such as diphenhydramine, chlorpheniramine, and hydroxyzine, because of their reduced tendency to cause sedation and/or anticholinergic effects. This patient already has severe constipation at baseline, so it is important to avoid first-generation antihistamines that might worsen his symptoms.

(p. 901, Section 14: Allergic Disorders, Chapter 189: Allergic Rhinitis and Conjunctivitis)

**Answer 12-4.** A

Topical nasal decongestants, such as phenylephrine, oxymetazoline, xylometazoline, and naphazoline nasal sprays, work by constricting blood vessels lining the nose. They may provide temporary relief, but their longer-term use should be strongly discouraged due to the risk of rebound nasal congestion that can set in within 5 to 7 days of repeated use.

Intranasal corticosteroids are the most effective monotherapy to treat allergic rhinitis (AR). They can provide substantial relief even when used on an as-needed schedule. Their side effects include burning and stinging. When used appropriately, they are generally not associated with alterations in the hypothalamic-pituitary-adrenal axis, ocular pressure or cataract formation, or changes in bone density.

Fexofenadine and cetirizine are both second-generation oral antihistamines. They are effective in the management of the ocular and nasal symptoms associated with seasonal allergies. Switching from one to the other is an option, although in this case, topical decongestants need to be stopped first.

Oral decongestants are not recommended due to their cardiovascular and central nervous system side effects.

The effectiveness of leukotriene receptor antagonists in the treatment of AR is comparable to that of oral antihistamines. They should be considered in patients with concomitant asthma. The combination of a leukotriene receptor antagonist and an antihistamine does not provide added benefit.

(p. 901, Section 14: Allergic Disorders, Chapter 189: Allergic Rhinitis and Conjunctivitis)

**Answer 12-5.** C

Viral rhinoconjunctivitis is characterized by erythematous mucosa with either purulent or crusty secretion. This is suggestive of an acute infection. This diagnosis is also supported by the unilateral eye erythema. Allergic rhinoconjunctivitis is associated with frequent sneezing, nasal congestion, and discharge. Exam usually reveals pale, enlarged nasal turbinates with clear rhinorrhea. Nonallergic rhinoconjunctivitis has many causes, such as irritants, toxins, temperature change, and ingestion of certain foods. The history does not support this diagnosis. Chronic sinusitis commonly has copious thick nasal drainage and sinus pain that lasts 12 weeks or more. Patients often have other systemic symptoms, such as headache, fever, cough, facial pain, and low energy. This child does not have symptoms to suggest adenoidal hypertrophy such as mouth breathing, sleep disturbance, or ear effusions.

(p. 900, Section 14: Allergic Disorders, Chapter 189: Allergic Rhinitis and Conjunctivitis)

**Answer 12-6.** E

Imported fire ants are native to Central and South America. They are present throughout the Gulf Coast and southeastern United States. Fire ant stings are common, especially for children who play outdoors in these areas. Epidemiologically, up to 50% of people living in infested areas get stung each year.

Venom potency does not differ between Africanized honeybees and other honeybees. Paper wasps are less aggressive than the vespids (yellow jackets and hornets), but they build their nests near buildings, making them more likely to encounter people. Yellow jackets and hornets are more aggressive and will sting with less provocation.

(p. 908, Section 14: Allergic Disorders, Chapter 192: Insect Sting Allergy)

**Answer 12-7.** A

Specific IgE antibodies can be demonstrated by intradermal venom skin test or by measurement of serum IgE to venoms. These 2 tests correlate closely but not perfectly, and the 2 test methods can be complementary. The specific IgE level does not correlate with the severity of the reaction. She had a systemic reaction to the honeybee sting, and if her testing is positive, she will have a 20% to 70% chance of having a systemic reaction in the future. Patients with anaphylaxis are eligible for allergy testing. Furthermore, allergy testing is indicated for patients with systemic reactions because they may be eligible for venom immunotherapy. Protection from systemic reactions to stings can be achieved with 8 weeks of venom immunotherapy in 80% to 90% of patients using a standard schedule.

(p. 908, Section 14: Allergic Disorders, Chapter 192: Insect Sting Allergy)

**Answer 12-8.** D

The patient has developed a large local reaction to her Hymenoptera sting. She is not experiencing anaphylaxis. Large local reactions cause prolonged swelling contiguous with the sting site approximately 6 to 12 hours after the initial sting. Large local reactions do not progress to anaphylaxis and resolve over the course of 5 to 10 days without intervention. Large local reactions do not resolve completely with antihistamines, although antihistamines can help to reduce some symptoms. Cellulitis is often confused with an infection, but infections rarely occur from insect stings, and antibiotics are not recommended.

(p. 908, Section 14: Allergic Disorders, Chapter 192: Insect Sting Allergy)

**Answer 12-9.** B

Venom immunotherapy is only offered to patients with a history of an immunoglobulin E (IgE)-mediated reaction to venom. This patient's reaction is not consistent with a venom allergy. It is normal to have some pain and redness at a site of a sting. He did not have a large local reaction because large local reactions are defined as a reaction that causes prolonged swelling contiguous with the sting site with delayed onset 6 to 12 hours after the sting.

Venom immunotherapy is primarily offered to patients who have had a systemic reaction, although some patients with only cutaneous manifestations or large local reaction would be offered this therapy based on other factors. The standard schedule takes approximately 8 weeks to achieve protection from a systemic reaction. Venom immunotherapy has a relatively low risk of adverse effects. β-Blockers are not an absolute contraindication, but these patients have a slightly increased risk of adverse effects. A family history of a vespid (eg, any wasp from the family Vespidae) allergy does not play a role in the decision of whether to pursue standard or rush therapy for patients needing venom immunotherapy.

(p. 908, Section 14: Allergic Disorders, Chapter 192: Insect Sting Allergy)

**Answer 12-10.** D

This boy has developed anaphylaxis from being stung by fire ants. He should be administered epinephrine as soon as possible. Antihistamines and steroids can be administered after epinephrine, but epinephrine is the only effective treatment for anaphylaxis and should be given first. There is no role for venom immunotherapy in the treatment of anaphylaxis.

(p. 908, Section 14: Allergic Disorders, Chapter 192: Insect Sting Allergy)

**Answer 12-11.** E

The vignette in this question is an example of latex-fruit syndrome. It occurs frequently in individuals who have a latex allergy. It is caused by a sensitization to the major latex allergen proteins (*Hevea brasiliensis* allergen Hev b 5, Hev b 6, and Hev b 7), which are similar to proteins found in various fruits and vegetables including avocado, kiwi, banana, potato, tomato, chestnut, and papaya.

A primary IgE-mediated food allergy to kiwi is an example of a type I hypersensitivity reaction and would result in more systemic symptoms including urticaria/rash, rhinitis, conjunctivitis, bronchospasm, and/or anaphylaxis usually within minutes to hours after the exposure. There is no cross-reaction typically between kiwi and banana.

Oral candidiasis can sometimes happen with inhaled corticosteroid use for asthma; however, this child complains of oral irritation only in the setting of eating certain foods, which would be unlikely to be caused by thrush.

Eosinophilic esophagitis is a chronic disease of the esophagus characterized histologically by eosinophilic inflammation. It is increasing in prevalence and can happen in both young children and adults. In children, symptoms most often start out as vomiting and abdominal pain, which then progress to dysphagia and can eventually cause food impaction. Eosinophilic esophagitis is thought to have a component of delayed-type hypersensitivity to foods.

Perioral irritant dermatitis happens frequently in babies from saliva or moist foods irritating the skin. It is not necessarily secondary to an allergy to these foods. It is treated with application of an emollient barrier prior to eating. The description of the girl's symptoms is not consistent with irritant dermatitis, which manifests as a rash rather than mouth pruritus.

(p. 909, Section 14: Allergic Disorders, Chapter 193: Latex Allergy)

**Answer 12-12.** A

Type I hypersensitivity reactions are mediated primarily by mast cells and typically occur within minutes to 2 hours after exposure to the offending agent. This type of life-threatening allergic reaction can be the presenting symptom in as many as 30% of latex-allergic children, and children with spina bifida have the highest prevalence of latex allergy (18%–73%). Latex can be found in many medical supplies and is an important culprit of perioperative anaphylaxis. For children with spina bifida, it is recommended that evaluation for latex allergy be conducted prior to surgery.

Mastocytosis is a disorder of clonal mast cell deposition in organs, which predisposes patients to severe anaphylaxis, including in a perioperative setting. Children with mastocytosis often have characteristic skin findings called *urticaria pigmentosa*, which are depositions of mast cells in the skin. Urticaria pigmentosa appears as fixed dark patches that can develop over hives if the skin is disturbed. Given this boy's known spina bifida, latex allergy is more likely in this scenario.

Hypotension is a known side effect of sedative medications. Anesthesiologists are adept at identifying and treating this hypotension, and there is no specific test to rule out this type of reaction. Additionally, the skin findings in the clinical scenario in this question make an anaphylactic reaction more likely.

Medications are cleared by the liver and/or the kidney. With organ dysfunction, certain medication levels can build up and cause increased adverse reactions. However, this scenario is not consistent with this explanation.

Contact allergy to chlorhexidine antiseptic scrub does occur frequently; however, this scenario would not be expected to cause the severe and immediate systemic reaction described in the question. Type IV reactions are delayed-type hypersensitivity reactions typically appearing 48 to 72 hours after exposure to the offending agent; these reactions are mediated by T cells.

(p. 909, Section 14: Allergic Disorders, Chapter 193: Latex Allergy)

**Answer 12-13.** B

The first step in diagnosing any allergy is taking a good clinical history. Clinical features that would be consistent with an immediate immunoglobulin E (IgE)-mediated hypersensitivity to latex could include urticarial rash, angioedema, acute rhinitis or conjunctivitis, bronchospasm, and hypotension that occur within 2 hours of exposure to the offending agent. If the history is consistent with an IgE-mediated allergy to latex, then the next step is confirmatory testing. In the United States, there is no commercially available standardized latex reagent for skin testing; therefore, serum testing with fluorescence ELISA is recommended.

In this clinical scenario, it is unclear what this patient's "reactions" consist of; however, it is common for healthcare workers to be exposed to latex through medical supplies such as catheters, gloves, and blood pressure cuffs, and it is always appropriate to begin by taking a thorough clinical history. It is not appropriate to reassure this patient or have him test his tolerance of latex on his own. Once the allergy is clarified and confirmed, it would be appropriate to prescribe epinephrine autoinjectors and give him an anaphylaxis action plan.

(pp. 909–910, Section 14: Allergic Disorders, Chapter 193: Latex Allergy)

**Answer 12-14.** D

Patients with any form of immediate hypersensitivity reaction that could cause anaphylaxis should always carry 2 epinephrine autoinjectors at all times.

Long-term management of patients with latex allergy consists of strict avoidance of latex-containing products. Patients should inform all healthcare providers and caretakers of their allergy and should wear a medic alert bracelet. Additionally, even though most healthcare settings now use only latex-free products, it is recommended that patients have a personal supply of nonlatex gloves for use when required.

There have been some anecdotal reports of latex-allergic patients developing reactions from injection of medications through latex ports in intravenous tubing; however, flu and MMR vaccines are not known to contain latex, and latex-allergic patients should be encouraged to receive them as any other patient would.

Patients diagnosed with a latex allergy should discuss eating the foods associated with latex-fruit syndrome with their doctor. In general, if a patient already tolerates these foods without symptoms, then there is no reason for them to be avoided; however, latex-allergic individuals should be cautious when eating these foods for the first time.

(p. 910, Section 14: Allergic Disorders, Chapter 193: Latex Allergy)

**Answer 12-15.** D

This reaction description is most consistent with either allergic or irritant contact dermatitis. Allergic contact dermatitis is a type IV immunologic reaction. Type IV hypersensitivity reactions are mediated by helper T cells and are often termed *cell-mediated reactions*. Examples of cell-mediated reactions include contact dermatitis and chronic transplant rejection. Contact dermatitis may be caused by any number of chemical accelerators or other additives in the rubber mixture. Because this type of reaction is distinct from type I hypersensitivity, which may cause a life-threatening reaction, it is important to distinguish true latex allergy from sensitization to other chemicals in rubber products. Patch testing can be conducted to evaluate which products are causing the type IV reaction. Topical steroids may be prescribed for bothersome contact dermatitis rashes.

Type I hypersensitivity reactions are mediated by antigen-specific IgE, which triggers mast cell degranulation upon exposure to the offending agent. For a latex allergy, the sensitization will happen when the patient is exposed to latex in some way, usually mucosally, cutaneously, or in an intraoperative setting where the latex antigens can be leached from the rubber products by moisture. It has also been reported that latex antigen may be adsorbed into cornstarch powder in gloves, thereby causing respiratory exposure via inhalation. After this initial exposure, the sensitized individual will generate latex-specific IgE. Subsequently, the antigen will cause crosslinking of the specific IgE bound to mast cells, thereby activating the mast cells and causing release of their mediators. These mediators cause typical immediate hypersensitivity symptoms including urticaria/rash, rhinitis, conjunctivitis, bronchospasm, and/or anaphylaxis, usually within minutes to hours after the exposure.

A type II hypersensitivity reaction is sometimes called *antibody dependent* or *cytotoxic* and is an autoimmune reaction. This type occurs when immunoglobulin M (IgM) or immunoglobulin G (IgG) binds to the host antigen, leading to cellular destruction. This is tested via the Coombs test. An example of type II hypersensitivity is autoimmune hemolytic anemia.

Type III hypersensitivity reactions are also called *immune complex disease*. This type of reaction occurs when IgG binds to an antigen and forms immune complexes that are deposited elsewhere, causing diseases such as serum sickness and membranous nephropathy.

Type V hypersensitivity reactions are not typically differentiated in the United States and are similar to type II reactions, except that the antibodies bind to the cell surface receptor, thereby preventing its intended ligand from binding. Graves disease would be an example of this phenomenon.

(p. 110, Section 14: Allergic Disorders, Chapter 193: Latex Allergy)

**Answer 12-16.** A

Infants are born with the capacity to defend against many infections, but their immune system is not fully functional. They are at risk of a range of infections but particularly to encapsulated organisms such as *Streptococcus pneumoniae* and *Haemophilus influenzae*. This susceptibility is driven by a number of factors, including their low number of memory B cells, which are needed to execute a speedy immune response. In infants, regulatory T cells dominate to prevent reactions against maternal antigens. Additionally, T-cell response is qualitatively skewed toward a Th2 response, which does not favor a response to pathogens. Although toll-like receptor expression and response to pathogens by neutrophils are intact, cytokine secretion and complement production are diminished in infants compared to adults. Finally, germinal centers in lymphoid organs are not mature until 4 months of age in humans. Altogether, these factors make it necessary for young infants to receive multiple vaccine boosters to sustain immune responses and maintain immunologic memory.

(p. 869, Section 13: Immunological Disorders, Chapter 182: Overview of the Immune System)

**Answer 12-17.** B

The innate immune system is composed of both mechanical barriers and certain cellular defenses. Tissue macrophages recognize PAMPs, which are highly conserved structures expressed in many microorganisms but not humans. Many of these PAMPs are recognized by toll-like receptors, which leads to secretion of cytokines and ultimately recruitment of additional cells to participate in clearance of the pathogen.

Most responses to bacteria lead to activation of transcription factors called NF-κB, whereas response to infection by viruses leads to activation of a class of transcription factors called IRFs. Natural killer cells selectively identify and kill virally infected cells and tumor cells using cytotoxic mechanisms. The most critical cell responsible for clearance of conventional bacterial infections is the neutrophil. Certain pathogens, such as *Mycobacteria* and fungi, are resistant to killing by neutrophils and are instead killed by activated macrophages.

(pp. 870–871, Section 13: Immunological Disorders, Chapter 182: Overview of the Immune System)

**Answer 12-18.** C

Thymocytes undergo a rearrangement of genes that will eventually form their T-cell receptors; these events are partially dependent on functional recombinase-associated genes. Maturation of T cells starts in the thymic cortex. Here, positive selection occurs; this is a process where T cells that cannot bind major histocompatibility complex (MHC) are eliminated. The T cells then migrate to the thymic medulla, where they become positive for CD4 and CD8. Negative selection occurs in the medulla and is when T cells with high-affinity self-reactivity are eradicated. Self-antigen expression in the thymus is controlled at least partly by the *AIRE* gene. Finally, single positive cells exit to the periphery.

(p. 872, Section 13: Immunological Disorders, Chapter 182: Overview of the Immune System)

**Answer 12-19.** E

APCs are essential for T-cell function. Dendritic cells, macrophages, and B cells can all act as APCs, but dendritic cells are the most potent. Dendritic cells first capture antigen by sampling their surroundings by various mechanisms. After an antigen is internalized and the dendritic cells are activated, they migrate to the draining lymph nodes, where they present their antigen to T cells. Dendritic cells can produce cytokines, which can greatly influence the ensuing T-cell response. APCs stimulate naïve CD4+ cells in the context of MHC class II molecules and naïve CD8+ cells in the context of MCH class I molecules.

(pp. 873–874, Section 13: Immunological Disorders, Chapter 182: Overview of the Immune System)

**Answer 12-20.** C

Initially, all mature B cells express IgM and immunoglobulin D (IgD) on their cell surface. Class switching can occur after exposure to an antigen or under the influence of certain cytokines, but antigen specificity is preserved (the type of immunoglobulin is different, but the antigen it responds to is the same). IgM is the first to be generated in an immune response; it is secreted as a pentamer. IgG is the most abundant and is 80% of the total immunoglobulin. IgG is the only class of antibody that can significantly cross the placenta. IgA is the major immunoglobulin at mucosal surfaces and is found in secretions such as tears, sweat, saliva, and colostrum. IgE plays a role in eradication of helminths and mediation of allergic reactions.

(p. 874, Section 13: Immunological Disorders, Chapter 182: Overview of the Immune System)

**Answer 12-21.** B

In general, cellular immunodeficiency is associated with recurrent and disseminated viral, atypical mycobacterial, and fungal infections. Pneumonia caused by *P jiroveci* and other opportunistic infections and oral candidiasis are highly suggestive of T-cell immunodeficiency. In children, it is important not to forget to evaluate for secondary immunodeficiencies such as HIV, which can be acquired vertically prenatally or through breastfeeding. Pediatric patients with HIV can present in early childhood with common bacterial infections that are more frequent or more severe than those in their peers.

Quantitative immunoglobulin levels are used to evaluate for hypogammaglobulinemia, which can be found in a number of immunodeficiency disorders including X-linked agammaglobulinemia or common variable immunodeficiency (CVID). Neutrophil oxidative burst tests such as dihydrhodamine (DHR) assay are used to evaluate for chronic granulomatous disease (CGD). Patients with CGD have a phagocytic cell defect and, as such, typically present with recurrent pyogenic and fungal infections. Patients with cystic fibrosis (CF) are particularly susceptible to respiratory infections with *Pseudomonas aeruginosa, Burkholderia* species, and *Staphylococcus aureus*. CF can be confirmed with a sweat chloride test. Gene sequencing analysis is not typically used until after other, more basic evaluation of the immune system has been performed.

(p. 875, Section 13: Immunological Disorders, Chapter 183: Increased Susceptibility to Infections)

**Answer 12-22.** C

A thorough and detailed history is important in deciding whether and when to work up a child with frequent infections. The threshold to define a high frequency of infections may vary somewhat depending on clinical context; however, the following guidelines are suggested: 2 or more systemic bacterial infections at any time (eg, sepsis, deep-seated abscesses, or meningitis), 3 or more bacterial infections, or 6 to 8 or more URIs in 1 year. Other factors that may play a role in clinical decisions regarding workup of frequent infections are the severity of infections and the organism present. Finally, history should include questions about associated conditions such as autoimmunity, failure to thrive, and pertinent family history.

(p. 875, Section 13: Immunological Disorders, Chapter 183: Increased Susceptibility to Infections)

**Answer 12-23.** A

This patient's presentation is consistent with X-linked agammaglobulinemia (Bruton agammaglobulinemia). Because it is X-linked, it is much more common in males. These children often have a lack of tonsil development and an almost complete lack of immunoglobulins. They are at risk for frequent respiratory infections and/or chronic diarrhea with pathogens such as *Giardia lamblia.*

Children with serious immunodeficiency should not receive live vaccines because these vaccines could potentially cause disease. As soon as immunodeficiency is suspected, a targeted workup should be initiated. In this case, the patient has history and exam findings concerning for a humoral immune deficiency, and he should undergo testing for quantitative immunoglobulin levels as well as flow cytometry of lymphocyte subsets. Once these tests are performed, genetic testing can be pursued, and if this is not fruitful, eventually whole-genome sequencing should be done. Genetic tests are rarely used initially. Specific antibody titers to tetanus toxoid and to pneumococcal serotypes can be used to evaluate the functional antibody response; these are helpful in patients with known mild hypogammaglobulinemia. This patient needs immunoglobulin levels first. Interferon-γ treatment is used in patients with chronic granulomatous disease (CGD) to reduce infections. Patients with hypogammaglobulinemia or agammaglobulinemia are treated with immunoglobulin replacement therapy in the form of intravenous immunoglobulin or subcutaneous immunoglobulin infusions.

(pp. 875–876, Section 13: Immunological Disorders, Chapter 183: Increased Susceptibility to Infections)

**Answer 12-24.** C

CGD is caused by a defect in phagocytic cells, resulting in their inability to produce the superoxide anions required to kill fungi and bacteria. It is usually diagnosed before the age of 5 years. Children with CGD have frequent fungal and bacterial infections with species such as *Aspergillus, Candida, Klebsiella, Nocardia, Serratia,* and *Staphylococcus.* The DHR assay is the newer and preferred test to diagnose CGD because it produces fewer false-negative tests when compared to nitroblue tetrazolium. Quantitative immunoglobulin levels can be used to rule out hypogammaglobulinemia; these levels vary by age. Defects in the *TLR3* gene are seen in patients who are susceptible to herpes simplex encephalitis. Flow cytometry analysis for T-lymphocyte markers can be used to diagnose defects in cellular immunity.

(p. 875, Section 13: Immunological Disorders, Chapter 183: Increased Susceptibility to Infections)

**Answer 12-25.** D

The baby in this scenario has a hyper-immunoglobulin M (IgM) syndrome, which is a group of primary immunodeficiencies associated with defects in the *CD40* and *CD40L* genes. This syndrome can be X-linked or autosomal recessive.

**TABLE 183-2.** Genetic Defects Associated with Susceptibility to Specific Pathogens

| Gene Defect | Pathogen |
|---|---|
| *CD40LG, CD40* | *Pneumocystis jiroveci*, *Cryptosporidium*, *Toxoplasma*, parvovirus |
| *IL12B, IL12RB1, IFNGR1/2, STAT1, IKBKG* | Mycobacteria |
| *MYD88, IRAK4* | Pyogenic and encapsulated organisms |
| *SH2D1A (SAP), XIAP* | Epstein-Barr virus |
| *TLR3, UNC93B1* | Herpes simplex virus encephalitis |
| *C5-9* | *Neisseria* species |
| *EVER1/2, CXCR4* | Human papillomavirus |

Mark W. Kline, *Rudolph's Pediatrics*, 23rd Edition. Copyright © McGraw-Hill Education. All rights reserved.

It often manifests in the first year of life when the child becomes sick with opportunistic infections such as *P jiroveci*. See Table 183-2 for genetic defects associated with specific pathogens.

*MYD88* is a gene that is integral for making an adaptor protein that is involved in signaling within immune cells. Defects in *MYD88* cause increased susceptibility to pyogenic and encapsulated bacterial infections.

Defects in the terminal complement pathway such as deficiencies of C5, C6, C7, C8, or C9 result in susceptibility to meningococcal infection with *Neisseria* species. CH50 and serum levels of individual complements should be measured when this is suspected.

*CXCR4* is an α-chemokine receptor; defects in this gene are associated with infection with human papillomavirus.

*XIAP* (X-linked inhibitor of apoptosis) is a rare primary immunodeficiency associated with hemophagocytic lymphohistiocytosis triggered by Epstein-Barr virus.

(p. 875, Section 13: Immunological Disorders, Chapter 183: Increased Susceptibility to Infections)

**Answer 12-26.** C

Children with SCID are born with marked susceptibility to pathogens that typically results in death by 1 to 2 years of age in the absence of treatment. The diagnosis represents a true pediatric emergency.

SCID is defined by specific criteria: absence or very low number of T cells (< 300 CD3+ T cells/μL) and no or very low T-cell function (< 10% of lower limit of normal) as measured by response to phytohemagglutinin or presence of T cells of maternal origin. At least 16 molecular defects are recognized as causes of SCID (Table 184-1) and can often be distinguished by absence or presence of B cells or natural killer (NK) cells.

The DHR assay is the newer and preferred test to diagnose chronic granulomatous disease (CGD) because it produces fewer false-negative tests when compared to nitroblue tetrazolium. A *DCLRE1C* gene defect is one of the 16 different molecular defects recognized as a cause of SCID.

(Section 13: Immunological Disorders, Chapter 184: Primary Immunodeficiency Diseases)

**Answer 12-27.** D

The patient's clinical picture is consistent with SCID. Children with SCID classically present with a history of recurrent infections including opportunistic infections such as thrush and *P jiroveci* pneumonia, lymphopenia, hypogammaglobulinemia, absence of tonsils on physical exam, and lack of a thymic shadow on chest radiograph.

Children with hemophagocytic lymphohistiocytosis present with fever, splenomegaly, cytopenias, hypertriglyceridemia, low or absent natural killer (NK) cell activity, and hemophagocytosis in the bone marrow, spleen, or lymph nodes. Individuals with IgA deficiency are often asymptomatic, but some develop recurrent respiratory or gastrointestinal infections. Children with Wiskott-Aldrich syndrome present with recurrent infections, eczema, and thrombocytopenia. Classic signs of autoimmune lymphoproliferative syndrome include splenomegaly, autoimmune cytopenias, increased levels of vitamin $B_{12}$ and interleukin-10 (IL-10), and a high percentage of αβ T cells that do not express either CD4 or CD8.

(p. 877, Section 13: Immunological Disorders, Chapter 184: Primary Immunodeficiency Diseases)

**Answer 12-28.** A

This boy has hyper-IgE syndrome as evidenced by his high IgE level, history of recurrent skin infections, and classic physical exam findings including a broad nasal bridge and hyperextensible joints. The most common cause of hyper-IgE syndrome is an autosomal dominant deleterious mutation in *STAT3*.

A mutation in *BTK* causes X-linked agammaglobulinemia, which presents as recurrent otitis media, sinusitis, pneumonia, and diarrhea. Individuals with X-linked agammaglobulinemia are at increased risk for development of enteroviral meningoencephalitis, not skin abscesses. A mutation in *FOXP3* causes immune dysregulation-polyendocrinopathy-enteropathy X-linked syndrome (IPEX), which manifests clinically as enteropathy, type 1 diabetes, eczema, recurrent infections, thyroid disease, and cytopenias. Autoimmune polyendocrinopathy-candidiasis-ectodermal dystrophy (APECED) is caused by a deficiency in *AIRE*. APECED presents with chronic mucocutaneous candidiasis, hyperparathyroidism, and Addison disease. Children with a deficiency in *IKBKG* present with recurrent pyogenic and

**TABLE 184-1.** Examples of Combined Cellular and Humoral Immunodeficiencies

| Features | | Associated Gene Defect(s) | Mode of Inheritance |
|---|---|---|---|
| Severe Combined Immunodeficiency Disease (SCID) | | | |
| $T^-B^+NK^-$ | | *IL2RG* | XR |
| | | *JAK3* | AR |
| $T^-B^-NK^+$ | | *RAG1* | AR |
| | | *RAG2* | AR |
| | Radiosensitivity | *DCLRE1C* | AR |
| | Radiosensitivity | *PRKDC* | AR |
| | Radiosensitivity, microcephaly | *LIG4* | AR |
| | Radiosensitivity, microcephaly | *NHEJ1* | AR |
| $T^-B^+NK^+$ | | *IL7R* | AR |
| | | *CD3D* | AR |
| | | *CD3E* | AR |
| | | *CD247* | AR |
| | | *PTPRC* | AR |
| | Thymic shadow present | *CORO1A* | AR |
| $T^-B^-NK^-$ | | *ADA* | AR |
| | Neutropenia, deafness | *AK2* | AR |
| Combined Immunodeficiencies | | | |
| Distinctive clinical features absent | | | |
| | MHC[a] class I deficiency | *TAP1, TAP2, TAPBP, B2M* | AR |
| | Other CD8+ T-cell deficiency | *ZAP70* | AR |
| | MHC class II deficiency | *CIITA, RFX5, RFXANK, RFXAP* | AR |
| | Other CD4+ T-cell deficiency | *MAGT1, LCK, UNC119* | XR (*MAGT1*), AR (*LCK*), AD (*UNC119*) |
| | Others | *CD3G, DOCK2, CARD11, MAP3K14, IKBKB, MALT1, BCL10* | AR |

[a]Major histocompatibility complex.

AD, autosomal dominant; AR, autosomal recessive; XR, X-linked recessive.

Mark W. Kline, *Rudolph's Pediatrics*, 23rd Edition. Copyright © McGraw-Hill Education. All rights reserved.

mycobacterial infections, elevated serum immunoglobulin M (IgM) levels, and ectodermal dysplasia.

(p. 878, Section 13: Immunological Disorders, Chapter 184: Primary Immunodeficiency Diseases)

**Answer 12-29.** C

CGD is caused by defects in the NADPH oxidase complex. Individuals with CGD are particularly susceptible to infections by catalase-positive microbes because defects in the NADPH oxidase complex result in an inability to generate the respiratory burst necessary for killing phagocytized microbes. Female carriers of the *CYBB* mutation are at increased risk for autoimmune and inflammatory conditions including photosensitivity, arthritis, discoid lupus, Raynaud phenomenon, inflammatory colitis, and chorioretinitis.

Individuals with X-linked CGD are at increased risk of developing an inflammatory bowel disease that is similar to Crohn disease. X-linked CGD is associated with the McLeod blood phenotype, which makes cross-matching difficult but does not require the patient to only receive IgA-deficient blood. The nitroblue tetrazolium test is no longer used routinely; instead, CGD is diagnosed using a flow cytometry–based dihydrhodamine (DHR) assay.

(p. 880, Section 13: Immunological Disorders, Chapter 184: Primary Immunodeficiency Diseases)

**Answer 12-30.** E

Approximately 20% of children aged 4 to 10 years who meet the criteria for selective IgA deficiency will have a normal IgA level by adolescence. As such, physicians should be cautious about diagnosing children with selective IgA deficiency.

Only some children with IgA deficiency will go on to develop CVID. Mutations in *TNFRSF13B* and inducible costimulator (*ICOS*) increase an individual's risk of developing CVID. Individuals with IgA deficiency do not need to receive IgG replacement. Although individuals with IgA deficiency carry a slightly increased risk for anaphylaxis during blood transfusions, blood transfusions are not contraindicated in this population. Individuals with IgA deficiency are at an increased risk for developing autoimmune diseases.

(p. 879, Section 13: Immunological Disorders, Chapter 184: Primary Immunodeficiency Diseases)

**Answer 12-31.** B

Because of the strong selective advantage for genetically intact progenitor cells to differentiate into T lymphocytes, severe combined immunodeficiency represents an ideal group of disorders to be treated by gene therapy. Adenosine deaminase deficiency was the first disorder in which clinical trials of gene therapy were attempted.

(p. 889, Section 13: Immunological Disorders, Chapter 186: Gene Therapy for Primary Immune Deficiencies)

**Answer 12-32.** E

HCTs have significant treatment-related morbidity and mortality, particularly those caused by drug toxicity, graft rejection and failure, graft-versus-host disease, incomplete immune reconstitution, and immune dysregulation. HCT from HLA-matched related donors is available to only about 15% of patients with primary immune deficiencies, which is far from adequate.

(p. 889, Section 13: Immunological Disorders, Chapter 186: Gene Therapy for Primary Immune Deficiencies)

**Answer 12-33.** C

In gene therapy, where stable integration of an additional normal copy of the gene of interest is inserted into a patient's cells using viral vectors, the gene is integrated randomly into the DNA, which has a potential risk of insertional mutagenesis. Expression of the therapeutic transgene is controlled by heterologous promoters, which can lead to dysregulated expression of the gene, and the physiologic control of gene expression may not be maintained.

New viral vectors with insulator sequences in the vector should shield cellular genes from viral transcription elements and reduce the risk of insertional mutagenesis.

In gene editing, homologous recombination allows the donor template to incorporate into the DNA, replacing the DNA fragment containing the mutation. This is an approach to avoid insertional mutagenesis. However, one of the challenges is low frequency of homologous recombination.

(pp. 889, 891, Section 13: Immunological Disorders, Chapter 186: Gene Therapy for Primary Immune Deficiencies)

**Answer 12-34.** C

TH2 cells produce IL-5, which promotes eosinophil production in the bone marrow. TH2 cells also produce IL-4 and IL-13, which promote immunoglobulin E (IgE) production. TH1 cells produce IL-2 and interferon-γ (Figure 182-6).

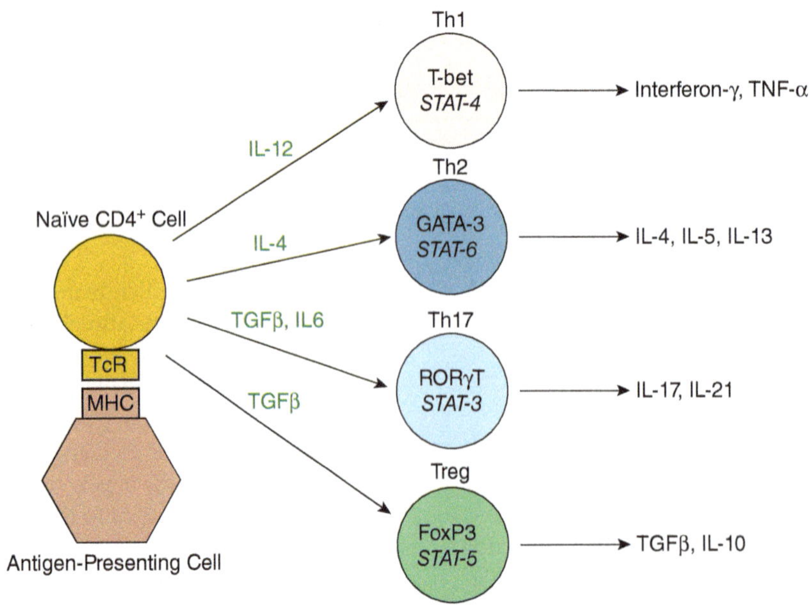


**FIGURE 182-6.** T-cell lineage commitment. Naïve CD4+ T cells are stimulated by peptide presented on an antigen-presenting cell in the context of a class II HLA (major histocompatibility complex [MHC]) molecule. Cytokines direct intracellular expression of lineage-specific transcription factors, resulting in acquisition of different T-helper cell phenotypes. (Mark W. Kline, *Rudolph's Pediatrics*, 23rd Edition. Copyright © McGraw-Hill Education. All rights reserved.)

(p. 893, Section 14: Allergic Disorders, Chapter 187: Allergic Disease and Atopy)

**Answer 12-35.** A

Dendritic cells are the most efficient of the APCs. In atopic individuals, the number and phenotype of dendritic cells are altered in such a way as to favor a TH2 response.

(p. 893, Section 14: Allergic Disorders, Chapter 187: Allergic Disease and Atopy)

**Answer 12-36.** C

Treatment of allergic conditions requires a multimodal approach. Anti–IL-5 therapy is used in the treatment of hypereosinophilic syndrome and eosinophilic asthma.

Avoidance of allergens not only provides symptomatic relief but also can result in hyposensitization in the long term. Some allergic conditions, including asthma, are treated with anti-IgE monoclonal antibodies. Anti-IgE monoclonal antibodies bind free IgE in the blood, thereby blocking the binding of IgE to FcεRI. Epinephrine—not antihistamines—counteracts anaphylaxis by dilating smooth muscle and causing cutaneous vasoconstriction. Antihistamines are useful for immediate hypersensitivity reactions but ineffective for chronic inflammation. Steroids are much better at managing chronic inflammation.

(p. 893, Section 14: Allergic Disorders, Chapter 187: Allergic Disease and Atopy)

**Answer 12-37.** A

This child has atopic dermatitis. Mutations in filaggrin are found in as many as 40% of patients with atopic dermatitis of European descent. Filaggrin is important for maintaining the skin-barrier function.

Homozygosity in *TSLP* is found in some patients with eosinophilic esophagitis. *ADAM33* polymorphisms have been implicated in asthma. Defects in *FAS* result in autoimmune lymphoproliferative syndrome. X-linked lymphoproliferative syndrome is caused by mutations in *SH2D1A*.

(p. 894, Section 14: Allergic Disorders, Chapter 187: Allergic Disease and Atopy)

**Answer 12-38.** D

Class-switch recombination is the name for the process in which B cells shift immunoglobulin production from immunoglobulin M (IgM) to IgE. Two signals are required for this process. The first signal is provided by the TH2 cytokines IL-4 and IL-13. The second signal is provided by the interaction of CD40, which is a B-cell protein, and CD40L, which is expressed on the surface of activated T-helper cells. CD23 is another name for FCεRII, which is an IgE receptor expressed on B cells. IgE also interacts with the high-affinity IgE receptor FCεRI, which is found on a variety of cells including mast cells, basophils, dendritic cells, eosinophils, platelets, and monocytes. The binding affinity of FCεRI is 2 to 4 logs stronger than the binding affinity of other immunoglobulin receptors, which means that when IgE attaches to FCεRI, it remains attached permanently until it is internalized. This interaction between IgE and FCεRI is not sufficient to cause release of the mast cell granules; IgE bound to FCεRI must cross-link with an allergic protein to initiate this signaling cascade.

(p. 894, Section 14: Allergic Disorders, Chapter 187: Allergic Disease and Atopy)

**Answer 12-39.** B

An IgE-induced immediate hypersensitivity reaction often is followed by a late-phase or delayed reaction, a second wave of hypersensitivity responses occurring several hours after the acute reaction has subsided. The late-phase reaction may manifest as decreased airflow in asthmatics, gastrointestinal symptoms, skin inflammation, anaphylaxis, or recurrence of sneezing and rhinorrhea in patients with allergic rhinitis (AR) from 4 to 24 hours after the initial allergen contact. The late-phase reaction arises from the recruitment to the allergen challenge site of an inflammatory cellular infiltrate that includes neutrophils, T lymphocytes, basophils, monocytes, and eosinophils.

(Section 14: Allergic Disorders, Chapter 187: Allergic Disease and Atopy)

**Answer 12-40.** A

TH1 cells express the transcription factor T-bet and produce interferon-γ, which serves a critical role in immunity against intracellular microbes. TH1 cells also produce tumor necrosis factor to promote inflammation. TH2 cells play an essential role in host defenses against helminthic infections and are defined by the transcription factor GATA-3. They produce IL-4 and IL-13, which are essential cellular elements of the innate immune response. TH2 cells also produce IL-5, which is a key factor for eosinophil development and survival.

(Section 14: Allergic Disorders, Chapter 188: Clinical Aspects of Allergic Diseases)

**Answer 12-41.** B

In some patients, the early-phase reaction is followed by a late-phase reaction, which is mediated by mast cell products in conjunction with T-cell–derived cytokines and chemokines. Late-phase reactions occur within 6 to 24 hours of exposure to an allergen. Chemokines promote the infiltration of the mucosa with eosinophils, neutrophils, basophils, T lymphocytes, and macrophages. Late-phase reactions can be as severe or more severe than early-phase reactions.

(Section 14: Allergic Disorders, Chapter 188: Clinical Aspects of Allergic Diseases)

**Answer 12-42.** C

Laboratory tests are useful only when there is a history and presenting symptoms suggestive of an IgE-mediated allergic condition. It is not appropriate to screen multiple foods without appropriate clinical history. Allergen-specific blood IgE tests are comparable to skin-prick tests to confirm allergies. A positive test (ie, sensitization) does not always correlate with clinical allergy and should be regarded as confirmatory only in the context of highly probable or documented reaction. The positive predictive value is about 40%, whereas the negative predictive value is about 90%, which makes it far more useful for ruling out a particular allergen.

(Section 14: Allergic Disorders, Chapter 188: Clinical Aspects of Allergic Diseases)

**Answer 12-43.** A

The development of highly effective topical steroids with minimal systemic effects has been instrumental in the treatment of common allergic disorders such as allergic rhinitis (AR). As monotherapy, intranasal corticosteroids are more efficacious than either leukotriene receptor antagonists or antihistamines or their combination. Oral steroids are not indicated to treat allergic rhinoconjunctivitis.

(Section 14: Allergic Disorders, Chapter 188: Clinical Aspects of Allergic Diseases)

**Answer 12-44.** B

Allergen-specific immunotherapy has proven to be clearly effective therapy for allergic airway diseases and insect venom allergy. Clinical benefits of immunotherapy may be sustained for years after discontinuation of treatment. Allergen immunotherapy for AR has reduced the risk of developing new allergen sensitizations and has reduced the risk of asthma in children with AR. Immunotherapy is time and resource consuming because it requires a minimum 3-year commitment on the part of the patient.

(Section 14: Allergic Disorders, Chapter 188: Clinical Aspects of Allergic Diseases)

**Answer 12-45.** B

This patient has symptoms consistent with acute anaphylaxis, most likely from components in the cookie. Anaphylaxis is a clinical diagnosis, with symptoms occurring within minutes of allergen exposure. Treatment should not be delayed for laboratory confirmation, but confirmatory testing would show systemic mast cell activation.

Tryptase is a protease specific to mast cells, and it reaches serum peak 30 to 120 minutes after the event and remains elevated for 6 hours. It is helpful to confirm systemic mast cell activation. Although histamine can be useful to confirm systemic mast cell activation, it is detectable in plasma for only 15 to 30 minutes after the anaphylactic event. CBC with differential is helpful to assess other conditions, such as bacterial infections, but would not confirm the diagnosis of mast cell activation. ESR and CRP are acute-phase reactants and markers for inflammation and would not be useful to confirm acute mast cell activation.

(Section 14: Allergic Disorders, Chapter 190: Anaphylaxis, Urticaria, and Angioedema)

**Answer 12-46.** E

This patient is having anaphylaxis from amoxicillin use. The approach to treating anaphylaxis should focus on maintaining the airway, breathing, and circulation. The most important initial clinical treatment is epinephrine, which is most effective when administered IM within 30 minutes of onset of symptoms.

After IM epinephrine is administered, volume resuscitation with IV fluids is indicated for persistent hypotension. In the presence of bronchospasm, inhaled bronchodilators, such as albuterol, should be administered. Antihistamines without epinephrine are insufficient to adequately treat anaphylaxis. Corticosteroids are frequently given to attenuate the potential late-phase inflammatory response and prevent recurrence of symptoms 8 to 12 hours after the initial onset. However, they are not effective for the initial acute phase.

(p. 903, Section 14: Allergic Disorders, Chapter 190: Anaphylaxis, Urticaria, and Angioedema)

**Answer 12-47.** B

Urticaria or angioedema with near-daily symptoms lasting > 6 weeks is considered chronic, and a more thorough diagnostic evaluation may be indicated. Thirty to 50% of patients with chronic urticaria demonstrate mast cell–stimulating autoantibodies, suggesting an autoimmune mechanism. Over two-thirds of urticaria or angioedema cases are self-limited, with symptoms resolving in < 6 weeks.

(Section 14: Allergic Disorders, Chapter 190: Anaphylaxis, Urticaria, and Angioedema)

**Answer 12-48.** A

Acute angioedema, urticaria, and anaphylaxis are most often the result of activation of mast cells, which releases histamine, leukotrienes, and other mediators into the superficial dermis (urticaria) and deep dermis (angioedema). Activation of mast cells may be the result of specific immunoglobulin E (IgE) cross-linking from exposure to allergens, such as food, drugs, aeroallergens, or insect venom. Hereditary angioedema is mediated by kinin, with bradykinin as the most important mediator in this condition. Treatment of kinin-related angioedema is distinct because these conditions do not respond to antihistamines and corticosteroids.

(Section 14: Allergic Disorders, Chapter 190: Anaphylaxis, Urticaria, and Angioedema)

**Answer 12-49.** C

In the pediatric population, anaphylactic reactions to vaccines are a concern. True IgE-mediated anaphylactic reaction to immunizations is rare and more commonly involves activation of IgE in response to vaccine components rather than the immunizing antigen itself. Gelatin is a stabilizing agent added to vaccines. It has been implicated in anaphylactic reactions to MMR, varicella, influenza, and Japanese encephalitis vaccines.

Children with a history of egg allergy should be seen by an allergist prior to receiving influenza vaccine, but egg allergy is not an absolute contraindication to influenza vaccine. IgE-mediated reaction to vaccine antigen is very rare for diphtheria and tetanus.

(Section 14: Allergic Disorders, Chapter 190: Anaphylaxis, Urticaria, and Angioedema)

**Answer 12-50.** E

Urticaria and angioedema are characterized by localized swelling of the skin and/or mucous membranes. Urticaria, commonly called *hives*, involves extravasation of fluid in the superficial dermis. It is characterized by well-circumscribed, pruritic, raised, erythematous skin wheals, often with central pallor and blanching with applied pressure. Individual urticarial lesions typically disappear within 24 hours without any residual skin changes, unless from excoriation.

Angioedema results from similar vasopermeability in the deeper layers of the dermis and subcutaneous tissue. Angioedema may appear associated with urticaria, but it occasionally presents as an isolated symptom. Angioedema typically involves the periorbital tissues, lips, tongue, posterior oropharynx, larynx, hands, feet, or genitals. Less commonly, angioedema may involve the gastrointestinal tract, resulting in abdominal pain, nausea, vomiting, and diarrhea. Edematous swelling of angioedema may take 24 to 72 hours or, in some instances, longer to fully resolve.

(Section 14: Allergic Disorders, Chapter 190: Anaphylaxis, Urticaria, and Angioedema)

**Answer 12-51.** B

This girl has an allergy to egg and peanut. The severity of a food allergic reaction varies for similar exposures both between individuals and for the same individual. Children often outgrow allergies to milk, egg, wheat, and soy, but allergies to tree nuts, peanuts, shellfish, and fish tend to be lifelong. Some allergens, including egg and milk, are heat labile, whereas others, such as peanut, are heat resistant. As such, she may be able to tolerate baked egg even if she has a reaction to unbaked (scrambled) eggs. Peanut allergenicity is not affected by baking, so she is unlikely to tolerate baked peanut. Food allergies have a strong genetic component, and siblings of peanut-allergic children are 7 times more likely to develop a peanut allergy than children in the general population. Introducing allergenic foods by 6 months of age, rather than waiting until a child is older, reduces the likelihood of a child developing food allergies.

(Section 14: Allergic Disorders, Chapter 191: Food Allergy)

**Answer 12-52.** D

This boy has oral allergy syndrome. Oral allergy syndrome occurs in older children or teenagers who have prior pollen sensitization. He is reacting to the pollen antigen on the apple, not the apple itself. The pollen antigen is heat labile, meaning that it is destroyed when baked, which is why he can eat baked apples in apple pie without symptoms.

Food protein–induced enterocolitis is present in infants and presents with vomiting and diarrhea several hours after ingestion of the allergenic food. Eosinophilic esophagitis presents with food impaction, dysphagia, recurrent vomiting, and abdominal pain. Atopic dermatitis is a skin condition that presents with dry, red, itchy patches of skin. Alpha-gal allergy is a delayed reaction to mammalian meat.

(p. 906, Section 14: Allergic Disorders, Chapter 191: Food Allergy)

**Answer 12-53.** B

This baby has allergic proctocolitis, not food protein–induced enterocolitis. Whereas babies with allergic proctocolitis present with frequent mucousy and sometimes bloody stools, babies with food protein–induced enterocolitis present with profuse vomiting and diarrhea within a few hours of ingestion of an allergenic food. Cow's milk and soy are commonly implicated in both of these conditions. In exclusively breastfed babies, babies become sensitized to maternally ingested proteins that are excreted in the breast milk. Mothers of babies with allergic proctocolitis do not necessarily need to stop breastfeeding. Elimination of allergenic foods from the mom's diet usually resolves the baby's symptoms. Food protein–induced enterocolitis, not allergic proctocolitis, causes diffuse inflammation of the gastrointestinal tract and crypt abscesses.

(p. 906, Section 14: Allergic Disorders, Chapter 191: Food Allergy)

**Answer 12-54.** D

The gold standard for diagnosing food allergy is a double-blind placebo-controlled oral food challenge. Oral food challenges are typically performed in an allergist's office. A complete history and physical exam are vital components to the diagnosis of food allergy and can help distinguish some cases of food allergy from other disorders. The timing of symptoms, quantity of food, and exposure history to a particular food are all important pieces of the clinical history. Skin-prick testing and measurement of serum food-specific IgE antibodies are used routinely in the diagnosis of food allergy. The sensitivity of these 2 tests is approximately 85%, but because the specificity is only 40%, neither skin-prick testing nor serum food-specific IgE is the gold standard for diagnosis. Patch tests are not routinely used in the diagnosis of food allergies.

(p. 907, Section 14: Allergic Disorders, Chapter 191: Food Allergy)

**Answer 12-55.** D

This boy is experiencing anaphylaxis from eating cashews. Epinephrine is the appropriate treatment for anaphylaxis. A child's parents should carry 2 doses of self-injectable epinephrine at all times because one dose may not halt the progression of symptoms and because biphasic reactions can occur in up to 6% of cases. A child should be observed by a physician for a period of 4 to 6 hours after a severe food allergic reaction in order to monitor for a biphasic reaction. Oral $H_1$ and $H_2$ antihistamines can be used alone in milder cases where only the skin or gastrointestinal system is involved but should not be used alone in cases of anaphylaxis. Similarly, glucocorticoids and albuterol are second-line agents and should not be used alone to treat an allergic reaction to a food. Avoidance of an offending food is critical to preventing symptoms of food allergy but can be challenging because there can be cross-contamination in food-processing facilities. Children and parents should be instructed on how to read labels and may benefit from education by a registered dietitian.

(p. 907, Section 14: Allergic Disorders, Chapter 191: Food Allergy)

**Answer 12-56.** E

Influenza vaccines are often incubated in egg cells and contain residual egg protein. Historically, people with serious egg allergies were advised to see an allergist before receiving the influenza vaccine. However, recent data have shown that it is safe for even severely egg allergic people to receive the influenza vaccine. The MMR vaccine does not contain egg protein. This 1-year-old girl should receive both the MMR and influenza vaccine now at her routine visit.

(p. 912, Section 14: Allergic Disorders, Chapter 194: Drug and Vaccine Allergy)

**Answer 12-57.** D

Adverse reactions to drugs can be classified as immunologic or nonimmunologic. Most adverse drug reactions are predictable nonimmunologic events caused by overdose, toxicity, pharmacologic side effects, and drug–drug interactions.

Drug rash with eosinophilia and systemic symptoms (DRESS) syndrome is an immunologically mediated reaction to medications that is characterized by a latency period of 2 to 6 weeks. It typically presents with eosinophilia and a variety of clinical manifestations including rash, lymphadenopathy, and kidney or liver injury. Although any drug can cause DRESS syndrome, certain drugs such as antiepileptic drugs, allopurinol, and sulfonamides (eg, sulfamethoxazole-trimethoprim) are the most frequent culprits.

Nephrotoxicity and ototoxicity are known dose-dependent effects of vancomycin and gentamicin, respectively, and are not classified as immunologic reactions.

(p. 911, Section 14: Allergic Disorders, Chapter 194: Drug and Vaccine Allergy)

**Answer 12-58.** B

The boy in this scenario is having an anaphylactic reaction to the MMR vaccine. Anaphylaxis occurs promptly after exposure to the culprit medication (several minutes to 2 hours). Symptoms are multisystem and often include a combination of stuffy or runny nose, sneezing, itchy or watery eyes, swelling of tongue or throat, cough, wheeze, shortness of breath, chest tightness, nausea, vomiting, cramps, palpitations, lightheadedness, and loss of consciousness. The most life-threatening and serious symptoms of anaphylaxis are bronchospasm and hypotension, which are reversed by the timely administration of epinephrine. Epinephrine also stabilizes mast cells to prevent further release of histamine. Once an appropriate dose of epinephrine is given, additional doses can be administered at 5- to 10-minute intervals if life-threatening symptoms persist, such as in this scenario.

Additionally, early treatment includes establishment of IV access and resuscitation of fluids, albuterol and oxygen administration, and recumbent positioning. Antihistamines such as diphenhydramine can be given in addition to epinephrine, but they should never be given in place of epinephrine when life-threatening symptoms are present. Administration of IV steroids is not necessary for early treatment; they are given with the intention of decreasing the likelihood of a biphasic reaction and decreasing the airway inflammation in patients with asthma who have an anaphylactic episode.

(p. 911, Section 14: Allergic Disorders, Chapter 194: Drug and Vaccine Allergy)

**Answer 12-59.** E

One of the keys to making a diagnosis of a serious drug allergy is taking an excellent clinical history. It is important to get an accurate timeline of the reaction. Type I immediate hypersensitivity reactions occur within several hours of the first or second dose of a course of medication and would be much less likely to occur several days into the course or many hours after taking the medication. These reactions are multisystem and can be life threatening, so accurate diagnosis is important. Most immune-mediated drug reactions do manifest clinically, at least in part, as a rash. Urticarial rashes are classically associated with anaphylactic reactions. However, urticaria alone is often coincidental and can cause mislabeling of allergies, especially if not taken within the rest of the clinical context. If the clinical history is consistent with a type I hypersensitivity reaction, skin-prick testing can be conducted; however, penicillin is the only medication with validated skin testing protocols. There are published nonirritating concentrations, and many allergists will conduct skin-prick testing to other medications, but these may be harder to interpret. Drug challenges are often used to confirm a negative skin and intradermal test.

Type IV hypersensitivity reactions are delayed cell-mediated reactions, such as allergic contact dermatitis. These can be investigated with patch testing. In this procedure, small quantities of the test substances are placed in plastic wells and taped to the patient's skin for 3 days to 1 week.

Desensitization is used when a person needs to take a medication to which he or she is known to have had a type I hypersensitivity reaction. This is a procedure in which the person is given escalating doses of the medication starting at extremely low amounts. Through unknown mechanisms, this allows tolerance, but only when the medication is taken in an uninterrupted fashion.

In the above scenario, penicillin is the only reaction that is consistent with a type I hypersensitivity reaction necessitating investigation with skin-prick testing.

The reaction to vancomycin is most likely "red man" syndrome. The lacy rash described as a reaction to cephalexin could be a delayed drug rash; however, there is no testing for this type of reaction. The reactions to metronidazole and ciprofloxacin are known side effects of the medications and are not likely to be immune mediated; therefore, testing would not be helpful in these cases.

(p. 911, Section 14: Allergic Disorders, Chapter 194: Drug and Vaccine Allergy)

**Answer 12-60.** **D**

Most penicillin-allergic patients have sensitivity to the central β-lactam portion of the molecule and therefore are likely to be allergic to a number of different penicillins. However, some penicillin-allergic patients have antibodies directed against a side chain. There is overlap between various cephalosporin and penicillin side chains, thereby creating cross-reactivity between these 2 classes of medication. Amoxicillin shares an identical side chain with cefadroxil, and therefore, out of the scenarios in the question, this would be most concerning.

Although type I hypersensitivity reactions involve immunoglobulin E (IgE) antibodies, people with other atopic diseases are not at increased risk of having a drug allergy. Drug allergies do not run in families; therefore, there is not increased risk of a drug allergy in a patient with a family history of drug allergies.

(p. 912, Section 14: Allergic Disorders, Chapter 194: Drug and Vaccine Allergy)

# CHAPTER 13 | Endocrinology

Anisha Gohil and Todd D. Nebesio

**13-1.** A 16-year-old boy presents to his primary care physician after noticing an asymmetric enlargement in his neck. On exam, several masses are noted on his tongue. He also has a Marfanoid body habitus. The tongue masses are later identified as neuromas. Thyroidectomy reveals medullary thyroid cancer. What is the most likely genetic cause of this child's disorder?

**A.** Multiple endocrine neoplasia 2B (MEN2B) due to a gain-of-function mutation in the *RET* proto-oncogene

**B.** Multiple endocrine neoplasia 1 (MEN1) due to an inactivating mutation in the *RET* proto-oncogene

**C.** MEN1 due to a germline mutation in the *MEN1* gene

**D.** MEN2B due to a mutation in the *PRKARIA* gene

**E.** McCune-Albright syndrome due to activating mutations of the G-protein subunit of adenyl cyclase system

**13-2.** A 12-year-old boy is seen in clinic for a well-child visit. On exam, he has adult body odor, scant axillary hair, Tanner stage 3 pubic hair, and 8-mL testes bilaterally. Which of the following statements about normal male puberty is correct?

**A.** The onset of puberty in males is defined as an increase in testicular volume to 8 mL.

**B.** The serum concentration of prolactin increases in normal male puberty.

**C.** The circulation of luteinizing hormone (LH) stimulates testosterone secretion by Leydig cells.

**D.** The circulation of follicle-stimulating hormone (FSH) stimulates spermatogenesis in Leydig cells.

**E.** The circulation of inhibin stimulates FSH secretion.

**13-3.** Which of the following scenarios depicts abnormal pubertal development?

**A.** A 14-year-old girl who grows 2 inches after menarche

**B.** A 14-year-old girl with Tanner stage 1 breast development

**C.** A 12-year-old boy with 3-mL testicles bilaterally

**D.** A 13-year-old girl with Tanner stage 2 breast development on the right and Tanner stage 3 breast development on the left

**E.** A 10-year-old girl who has achieved menarche

**13-4.** A 5-year-old girl presents to clinic for concerns about breast development that began 1 year ago. On exam, she has Tanner stage 3 breasts, estrogenization of her vaginal mucosa, and Tanner stage 2 pubic hair. Since her last well-child visit, she has developed a seizure disorder. A bone age reveals that her skeletal age is closest to 8 years. A brain magnetic resonance imaging (MRI) scan reveals a pedunculated mass in the region of the posterior hypothalamus that projects into the suprasellar cistern. What is the most likely diagnosis for this patient?

**A.** Optic glioma

**B.** Craniopharyngioma

**C.** Ependymoma

**D.** Astrocytoma

**E.** Hamartoma of the tuber cinereum

**13-5.** Which of the following is true in familial male limited precocious puberty?

**A.** Affected girls achieve menarche before age 7.

**B.** Fertility is negatively affected in adulthood.

**C.** Testicular enlargement is more pronounced than penile enlargement.

**D.** The condition results from an activating mutation of the luteinizing hormone (LH) receptor.

**E.** Elevated testosterone with elevated gonadotropin concentrations is common.

**13-6.** A 5-year-old girl has had recent concerns of weight loss, restlessness, and difficulty going to sleep at night. Laboratory testing reveals that she has a suppressed thyroid-stimulating hormone (TSH) level. On exam, she has multiple jagged hyperpigmented macules on her trunk that do not cross the midline. She also has Tanner stage 2 breast development. What is her most likely diagnosis?

**A.** Peutz-Jeghers syndrome

**B.** McCune-Albright syndrome

**C.** Classic congenital adrenal hyperplasia (CAH)

**D.** Familial gonadotropin-independent puberty

**E.** Granulosa cell tumor

**13-7.** Which of the following statements is true regarding premature thelarche?

**A.** Small for gestational age is a risk factor.

**B.** Gonadotropin levels are in pubertal ranges.

**C.** Most cases are self-limited and benign.

**D.** Patients are at an increased risk for polycystic ovarian syndrome in adulthood.

**E.** Most cases occur after the age of 4 years.

**13-8.** A 16-month-old African American male is seen in clinic for a well-child visit. On history, his mother states that he has not started to walk and was exclusively breastfed until 14 months. On physical exam, his anterior fontanelle is open and his wrists appear thickened, and he is below the third percentile for both length and weight. Which of the following sets of laboratory results is most consistent with his diagnosis?

**A.** Decreased calcium, increased phosphate, normal alkaline phosphatase, normal parathyroid hormone

**B.** Decreased calcium, decreased phosphate, increased alkaline phosphatase, increased parathyroid hormone

**C.** Increased calcium, decreased phosphate, decreased alkaline phosphatase, increased parathyroid hormone

**D.** Decreased calcium, decreased phosphate, decreased alkaline phosphatase, decreased parathyroid hormone

**E.** Increased calcium, increased phosphate, increased alkaline phosphatase, increased parathyroid hormone

**13-9.** A 4-day-old infant presents for his first clinic visit after birth. The child was born full term to a healthy mother with no significant past medical history. The child was diagnosed with congenital hypothyroidism by the newborn screen. On exam, heart rate and blood pressure are normal, and no goiter or neck masses are appreciated. What is the most common reason for congenital hypothyroidism in this child?

**A.** Thyroid dysfunction due to prematurity

**B.** Maternal antithyroid antibodies

**C.** Ingestion of goitrogenic substances by the mother

**D.** Inborn defects in thyroid hormone synthesis or action

**E.** Defect in thyroid embryogenesis

**13-10.** Which statement is true regarding congenital hypothyroidism?

**A.** Three to 5% of infants with the disorder are not detected on the newborn screen.

**B.** The incidence of congenital hypothyroidism is 1 in 200 to 1 in 400 births.

**C.** Preferred thyroid hormone preparation for therapy is triiodothyronine ($T_3$).

**D.** Physical growth and development are not normalized by early and adequate therapy.

**E.** The diagnosis is confirmed by serum measurements of thyroid-stimulating hormone (TSH) and $T_3$.

**13-11.** An 8-year-old boy presents to clinic for concerns about early pubertal development. On history, his father notes testicular and penile enlargement without pubic hair development in the past year along with intermittent fatigue. On exam, he has a slightly enlarged thyroid and delayed relaxation phase of his patellar reflexes, and his growth channel has fallen from the 50th to the 10th percentile on the height chart. A bone age assessment is interpreted as being at 4 years. Which laboratory value is most likely seen in this patient?

**A.** Normal thyroid-stimulating hormone (TSH) of 1.0 mU/L

**B.** Elevated free thyroxine ($T_4$) of 7.0 ng/dL

**C.** Elevated TSH of 600 mU/L

**D.** Normal free $T_4$ of 1.8 ng/dL

**E.** Mildly elevated TSH 6.0 mU/L

**13-12.** A 9-year-old healthy girl presents for her yearly well-child visit. On physical exam, her thyroid is full, smooth, symmetric, and easily palpable. Blood tests reveal that her thyroid-stimulating hormone (TSH) is mildly elevated at 9.8 μU/mL and total thyroxine ($T_4$) is normal at 6.5 μg/dL. Which of the following is the best additional test to perform to confirm the diagnosis?

**A.** Magnetic resonance imaging (MRI) of the brain

**B.** Thyroid ultrasound

**C.** TSH receptor antibody

**D.** Thyroid peroxidase antibody

**E.** Total triiodothyronine ($T_3$) level

**13-13.** A 14-year-old girl presents to clinic for the second time in 3 months for concerns about depression and declining school performance. She has been on an antidepressant for the past 2 months without improvement of her symptoms. On physical exam, her pulse rate is 144 bpm and blood pressure is 154/68 mm Hg. Proximal muscle weakness is detected on exam. Of the following hormones, which is most likely to be elevated?

**A.** Thyroid-stimulating hormone (TSH)

**B.** Estradiol

**C.** Luteinizing hormone (LH)

**D.** Tetraiodothyronine ($T_4$)

**E.** Follicle-stimulating hormone (FSH)

**13-14.** A 17-year-old boy was diagnosed with Graves' disease 2 years ago and has been on antithyroid medication (methimazole) since diagnosis. What clinical prognostic sign is most likely to suggest remission of his Graves' disease when antithyroid medication is discontinued?

**A.** Resolution of orbitopathy

**B.** Resolution of goiter

**C.** Resolution of widened pulse pressure

**D.** Resolution of muscle weakness

**E.** Maintenance of a normal body mass index

**13-15.** Which statement is true regarding the metabolism and action of thyroid hormones?

**A.** Triiodothyronine ($T_3$) and reverse $T_3$ ($rT_3$) are produced at different rates.

**B.** The thyroid gland is the sole source of $T_3$.

**C.** Deiodination is the main pathway of thyroid hormone metabolism.

**D.** The concentration of tetraiodothyronine ($T_4$) is 50 to 100 times less than that of $T_3$.

**E.** $T_4$ is more potent than $T_3$.

**13-16.** Of the following conditions, which are associated with an increased prevalence of autoimmune thyroid disease and require periodic screening for hypothyroidism?

**A.** Type 1 diabetes, Turner syndrome, and Down syndrome

**B.** Turner syndrome, Prader-Willi syndrome, and McCune-Albright syndrome

**C.** Down syndrome, type 1 diabetes, and congenital adrenal hyperplasia (CAH)

**D.** Prader-Willi syndrome, Down syndrome, and CAH

**E.** McCune-Albright syndrome, type 1 diabetes, and CAH

**13-17.** A 39-week-gestation infant was born after an uneventful pregnancy. Following delivery, the infant has respiratory distress and is found to have truncus arteriosus. Further examination reveals a low calcium (6.0 mg/dL) and low parathyroid hormone. What is this child's most likely diagnosis?

**A.** Williams syndrome

**B.** DiGeorge syndrome

**C.** Neonatal Graves' disease

**D.** Beckwith-Wiedemann syndrome

**E.** Congenital hypothyroidism

**13-18.** An 11-year-old boy presents to clinic for concerns about short stature. He has been consistently growing at the third percentile for the past 10 years. On exam, his weight is at the 75th percentile. He has a round face with a flattened nasal bridge. Brachydactyly and small cutaneous nodules are felt beneath the skin of his fingertips. Which of the following laboratory results are the most representative of this child's diagnosis?

**A.** Low parathyroid hormone, low calcium, low phosphorous

**B.** Elevated parathyroid hormone, elevated calcium, elevated phosphorous

**C.** Elevated parathyroid hormone, low calcium, elevated phosphorous

**D.** Low parathyroid hormone, elevated calcium, elevated phosphorous

**E.** Elevated parathyroid hormone, elevated calcium, low phosphorous

**13-19.** A 10-year-old boy presents to an emergency department (ED) with fever and dehydration. During the evaluation, a basic metabolic panel is drawn and reveals a total calcium level of 11.3 mg/dL. After recovering from his illness, he has further testing for hypercalcemia, which reveals a total calcium of 11.4 mg/dL and hypocalciuria with a low calcium/creatinine clearance ratio of < 0.01. Which of the following statements is most likely true about his diagnosis?

**A.** Treatment with aggressive hydration is indicated.

**B.** Most patients with this disorder have symptoms of hypercalcemia.

**C.** Vitamin D levels should be obtained before a definitive diagnosis is made.

**D.** This disorder is inherited in an X-linked recessive pattern.

**E.** This is a benign disorder and no treatment is indicated.

**13-20.** Which of the following statements is true regarding hormone effects on the skeleton?

**A.** Glucocorticoids accelerate osteoblast formation and enhance bone formation.

**B.** Thyroid hormone increases bone resorption by increasing the number of osteoclasts.

**C.** Estrogens and androgens suppress maturation of chondrocytes.

**D.** Growth hormone decreases the synthesis of type I collagen and bone-specific alkaline phosphatase.

**E.** Insulin-like growth factor-1 (IGF-1) decreases bone mineral content and density.

**13-21.** An 11-year-old boy presents to clinic for a well-child exam. During the encounter, his family asks if his final adult height can be estimated. His biological mother is 166 cm tall and his father is 183-cm tall. What is his mean parental height?

**A.** 174 cm

**B.** 181 cm

**C.** 168 cm

**D.** 183 cm

**E.** 178 cm

**13-22.** A 15-year-old boy presents to clinic for concerns of lack of pubertal development. On exam, he has 3-mL testes bilaterally, which are not firm. Review of systems is significant for the inability to smell coffee brewing. Follicle-stimulating hormone (FSH), luteinizing hormone (LH), and testosterone levels are low. What is the child's most likely diagnosis?

**A.** Klinefelter syndrome

**B.** Noonan syndrome

**C.** Prader-Willi syndrome

**D.** Turner syndrome

**E.** Kallmann syndrome

**13-23.** Growth hormone has been approved by the US Food and Drug Administration (FDA) for the treatment of which disorders?

**A.** Noonan syndrome, cystic fibrosis (CF), Turner syndrome

**B.** CF, Down syndrome, Prader-Willi syndrome

**C.** Turner syndrome, Prader-Willi syndrome, Down syndrome

**D.** Idiopathic short stature, CF, Turner syndrome

**E.** Prader-Willi syndrome, Noonan syndrome, idiopathic short stature

**13-24.** Which of the following statements about childhood growth is true?

**A.** Supine measurement of length should be used for children younger than 36 months.

**B.** Height velocity should be calculated using measurements taken at least 6 weeks apart.

**C.** Height growth occurs primarily as a continuous linear process.

**D.** Growth velocity during the first 2 years of life averages 15 cm per year.

**E.** A device with a flexible mounted arm should be used to obtain standing height measurements.

**13-25.** A 6-year-old girl presents to clinic for concerns about short stature and a decline in her linear growth and growth velocity. Two years ago, her height plotted at the 25th percentile, and at today's clinic visit, her height is at less than the third percentile for her age or at 3 standard deviations below the mean. Her weight is proportional to her height. Previous workup has included a normal female karyotype (46,XX). A bone age radiograph indicates that her skeletal maturity is 2 years delayed. Growth hormone deficiency is suspected. What biochemical evaluation should be sent to screen for growth hormone deficiency?

**A.** Growth hormone level

**B.** IGF-1 and insulin-like growth factor binding protein-3 (IGFBP-3)

**C.** Free thyroxine ($T_4$) and thyroid-stimulating hormone (TSH)

**D.** Immunoglobulin A (IgA) level and tissue transglutaminase IgA antibody

**E.** Complete blood cell count and erythrocyte sedimentation rate (ESR)

**13-26.** A 16-year-old girl presents as a new patient for concerns of primary amenorrhea. On physical exam, she is tall for her family background. She has normal adult breast development, and her vaginal mucosa appears pink, dull, and thick. Her physical exam is otherwise normal with the exception of minimal pubic hair and axillary hair. She is on no medications and her past medical history is unremarkable. Family history reveals that her younger sister presented in early infancy with an inguinal hernia. What test would be most helpful in establishing a diagnosis?

**A.** Testosterone

**B.** Luteinizing hormone (LH)

**C.** Follicle-stimulating hormone (FSH)

**D.** Estradiol

**E.** Karyotype

**13-27.** A 14-year-old girl has recently moved and presents for a well-child visit before she starts at her new school. She has always been one of the shortest children in her class. She has a B average in school, but she struggles in mathematics. Past medical history reveals that she has had frequent ear infections and has had bilateral myringotomy tubes placed as a young child. Her height is 134 cm, which is less than the third percentile or at −4 standard deviations. Findings on physical exam include a high-arched palate, low-set ears, ptosis, and multiple nevi. Breast development is Tanner stage 2 on the right and Tanner stage 1 on the left. Besides a karyotype, what additional test will likely be elevated and suggestive of the diagnosis?

**A.** Thyroid-stimulating hormone (TSH)

**B.** Insulin-like growth factor 1 (IGF-1)

**C.** Follicle-stimulating hormone (FSH)

**D.** Estradiol

**E.** Tissue transglutaminase immunoglobulin A (IgA) antibody

**13-28.** Which of the following statements about Klinefelter syndrome is correct?

**A.** Klinefelter syndrome is a rare cause of primary gonadal failure.

**B.** The most common karyotype found in individuals with Klinefelter syndrome is 47,XYY.

**C.** Individuals with Klinefelter syndrome often have problems with deviant and criminal behavior.

**D.** Gynecomastia commonly occurs in adolescent males with Klinefelter syndrome.

**E.** Testosterone replacement in Klinefelter syndrome corrects the symptoms of androgen deficiency and reverses infertility.

**13-29.** Which of the following is the most common cause of ambiguous genitalia in a newborn?

**A.** Turner syndrome

**B.** Congenital adrenal hyperplasia (CAH)

**C.** Noonan syndrome

**D.** 5α-Reductase deficiency

**E.** Klinefelter syndrome

**13-30.** A 5-year-old boy presents with Tanner 3 pubic hair, oily skin, and acne. A bone age radiograph of his left hand and wrist is advanced at 9 years. There is concern that the child may have nonclassic congenital adrenal hyperplasia (CAH). Which of the following would be the best laboratory test to evaluate for CAH?

**A.** Cortisol

**B.** Testosterone

**C.** Adrenocorticotropic hormone (ACTH)

**D.** 17-Hydroxyprogesterone

**E.** Dehydroepiandrosterone sulfate (DHEA-S)

**13-31.** A 14-year-old girl presents to her primary care physician with increased fatigue, weakness, abdominal pain, and nausea. She has no significant past medical history. Growth and development have been normal, and she is fully pubertal. Physical exam is remarkable for orthostatic hypotension and darkening of the creases on her hands. Which of the following is the most likely diagnosis?

**A.** Addison disease

**B.** Adrenoleukodystrophy

**C.** Salt-wasting congenital adrenal hyperplasia (CAH)

**D.** Nonclassic CAH

**E.** Brain tumor with subsequent adrenocorticotropic hormone (ACTH) deficiency

**13-32.** Which of the following is the best initial test to screen for adrenal insufficiency?

**A.** Dexamethasone suppression test

**B.** 12-Hour urine cortisol collection

**C.** Cortisol level drawn at 4:00 PM

**D.** Adrenocorticotropic hormone (ACTH) level drawn at any time

**E.** Cortisol level drawn at 8:00 AM

**13-33.** Which of the following are the earliest and most commonly seen signs and symptoms in children with Cushing syndrome?

**A.** Hypertension and weight gain

**B.** Buffalo hump and striae

**C.** Weight gain and growth failure

**D.** Depression and acne

**E.** Headache and weight gain

**13-34.** Which of the following children has the highest likelihood of developing glucocorticoid withdrawal?

**A.** A 5-year-old girl with a brain tumor who was treated with 2 mg of dexamethasone every 6 hours for 6 weeks, after which the medication was stopped

**B.** An 8-year-old boy with asthma who was treated with 2 mg/kg of prednisolone for 5 days, after which the medication was stopped

**C.** A 14-year-old boy with Crohn disease who was treated with 60 mg of prednisone per day for a week, after which the dose was gradually weaned over 2 months and then stopped

**D.** A 6-year-old girl with asthma who was treated with 2 mg/kg of prednisolone for 5 days, after which the dose was weaned over another 5 days and then stopped

**E.** A 12-year-old girl with a severe allergic skin reaction who received a 6-day methylprednisolone dose pack where she took 4 pills the first day and then the dose was decreased daily

**13-35.** A 12-year-old boy presents with a 3-week history of fatigue as well as increased thirst, increased urination, and a 15-pound weight loss. On physical exam, his blood pressure is 115/82 mm Hg and pulse is 108 bpm. A complete blood count (CBC) reveals a normal hemoglobin and hematocrit, but his white blood cell (WBC) count is elevated at 25,000/μL. A comprehensive metabolic profile reveals a sodium of 127 mEq/L, potassium of 5.9 mEq/L, chloride of 92 mEq/L, bicarbonate of 16 mEq/L, and glucose of 892 mg/dL. His venous pH is 7.32. Urinalysis shows > 1000 mg/dL of glucose and large ketones. Which of the following is the most likely explanation for this patient's hyponatremia?

**A.** Hyperkalemia

**B.** Hyperglycemia

**C.** Leukocytosis

**D.** Syndrome of inappropriate antidiuretic hormone (SIADH)

**E.** Acidosis

**13-36.** A previously healthy 10-year-old boy presents with a 2-day history of abdominal pain and vomiting. His mother thought that he had the flu since his older brother was recently diagnosed with a viral illness. On exam, he is afebrile but appears ill because he is tachypneic and tachycardic. Laboratory testing reveals a plasma glucose of 745 mg/dL. His bicarbonate level is 6 mEq/L and venous pH is 7.10. A urinalysis is positive for glucose and large ketones. The most appropriate first step in this patient's management is which of the following?

**A.** Start an insulin drip at 0.1 units/kg/h

**B.** Start maintenance intravenous (IV) fluids

**C.** Bolus with insulin at 0.1 units/kg

**D.** Bolus with normal saline at 20 mL/kg

**E.** Administer bicarbonate

**13-37.** A 4-year-old girl is admitted to the hospital in diabetic ketoacidosis (DKA). Her weight is 20 kg. She received 2 L of intravenous (IV) fluids initially when she arrived in the emergency department (ED) 6 hours ago. She had been feeling better and was conversational, but now she is more somnolent and difficult to arouse. Her blood sugar is 214 mg/dL, and she is on an insulin drip and IV fluids at 2 times maintenance. Which of the following is the most appropriate step in the management of this patient?

**A.** Order a stat head computed tomography (CT) scan

**B.** Administer bicarbonate

**C.** Intubate and hyperventilate

**D.** Administer mannitol

**E.** Increase the IV fluid rate

**13-38.** A 5-year-old girl with known type 1 diabetes presents with a 2-day history of fever and diarrhea. She has not vomited, and her mother has been monitoring blood sugars and checking for ketones in her urine. On exam, she appears to be well hydrated, and the remainder of her exam is unremarkable. A urinalysis reveals positive glucose and moderate ketones. Additional laboratory studies show that her complete blood count (CBC) is normal. Her electrolytes are unremarkable, including a bicarbonate of 23 mEq/L. The only abnormality is a serum blood glucose of 315 mg/dL. In addition to giving her extra insulin, what else would be recommended?

**A.** Encourage sugar-free fluid intake

**B.** Admit to the hospital for observation

**C.** Monitor her blood sugar twice a day

**D.** Place an intravenous (IV) line and give a 20 mL/kg bolus of normal saline

**E.** Check her urine ketones twice a day

**13-39.** Which of the following scenarios has the highest likelihood for the development of ketones?

**A.** A 12-year-old boy with type 1 diabetes goes to a birthday party and eats 2 pieces of cake and a bowl of ice cream. He does not give himself insulin to cover his food intake.

**B.** A 16-year-old girl with type 1 diabetes spends the weekend at her grandmother's house. She received her long-acting insulin each day but only intermittently took her short-acting insulin.

**C.** A 10-year-old girl with type 1 diabetes is on an insulin pump. She takes her pump off during a tennis match and then reattaches it an hour later.

**D.** A 14-year-old girl with type 1 diabetes is playing in a soccer tournament and has 2 games today. She decides to decrease the amount of short-acting insulin she receives at breakfast and lunch.

**E.** A 15-year-old boy with type 1 diabetes is on an insulin pump. He changes his pump site at bedtime. When he wakes up 8 hours later, he discovers that his pump site has fallen off.

**13-40.** A 12-year-old boy has type 1 diabetes diagnosed 4 years ago. He is on multiple daily injections, and his recent hemoglobin A1c was 8.4%. His mother reports frustration in trying to gain better blood sugar control. She reviews his blood sugar records weekly and makes insulin dose adjustments based on the trends in his numbers. He checks his blood sugar 4 to 6 times a day, and he receives his insulin injections in his abdomen, upper arms, and thighs. On exam, there is evidence of blood sugar testing on several of his fingers. His exam is otherwise unremarkable with the exception of 2 small lumps on either side of his umbilicus consistent with lipohypertrophy. Which of the following recommendations would likely lead to improved blood sugar control and a lower hemoglobin A1c?

**A.** Switch to a different type of insulin

**B.** Rotate his insulin injection sites

**C.** Change to an insulin pump

**D.** Check his blood sugar more often

**E.** Refer him to a dermatologist

**13-41.** Which of the following is a true statement about type 2 diabetes?

**A.** Elevated insulin levels are commonly seen in obese adolescents and should initially be treated with metformin.

**B.** Diabetic ketoacidosis (DKA) cannot occur in type 2 diabetics because β cells are still able to produce insulin.

**C.** The average age at diagnosis of type 2 diabetes in children is 10 years old, which corresponds to the onset of puberty.

**D.** Genetics plays a larger role in the development of type 2 diabetes than in type 1 diabetes in children.

**E.** Type 2 diabetes is more commonly seen in non-Hispanic whites than other ethnic groups in the United States.

**13-42.** A 15-year-old obese African American girl has struggled with weight gain for many years. She presents with concerns of fatigue and lack of energy. Other review of systems is positive for increased thirst and urination over the past few weeks. Her weight is 120 kg, and she has lost 5 kg in the past 2 months. On exam, she has darkening of the skin on the back and sides of her neck. She also has a vaginal yeast infection. A urinalysis reveals > 1000 mg/dL of glucose and moderate ketones. Additional tests show that her plasma glucose is 256 mg/dL, bicarbonate is 26 mEq/mL, and hemoglobin A1c is 9.8%. Which of the following would be the most appropriate treatment?

**A.** Refer her to a diabetes specialist to start insulin injections

**B.** Refer her to a dietitian to start a calorie-restricted diet

**C.** Refer her to a diabetes specialist to start metformin

**D.** Refer her to a diabetes specialist to start a sulfonylurea

**E.** Admit her to the hospital for intravenous (IV) fluids and an insulin drip

**13-43.** Which of the following tests is the most helpful in differentiating between new-onset type 1 and type 2 diabetes?

**A.** Blood glucose

**B.** C-peptide

**C.** Hemoglobin A1c

**D.** Urine ketones

**E.** Glutamic acid decarboxylase antibody

**13-44.** A 2-year-old girl presents to the emergency department (ED) with decreased feeding, tachycardia, and lethargy. Her blood glucose is found to be low at 25 mg/dL. Her weight is 12 kg. She is admitted to the hospital for intravenous (IV) fluids and observation. A sepsis workup is negative. She has no low blood sugars for the first 48 hours while she is on IV fluids of 0.9% NaCl with 5% dextrose at 20 mL/h. As she has been stable, it is decided to wean off her IV fluids. However, as the IV fluid rate is decreased, her blood glucose drops. A critical sample is drawn during an episode of hypoglycemia, which shows a plasma glucose of 21 mg/dL, elevated growth hormone of 20 μg/L, elevated cortisol of 38 μg/dL, undetectable C-peptide, and elevated insulin level of 42 μU/mL. Urine ketones are negative. What is the most likely reason for the child's hypoglycemia?

**A.** Insulinoma

**B.** Growth hormone deficiency

**C.** Sulfonylurea ingestion

**D.** Cortisol deficiency

**E.** Exogenous insulin

**13-45.** A term 36-hour-old male infant is hypoglycemic in the nursery with a plasma glucose of 18 mg/dL. His birth weight was 7 pounds 2 ounces. On exam, he has a midline cleft lip and palate and a micropenis with a stretched penile length of 1.8 cm and bilaterally descended testes. Which of the following is the most likely cause of his hypoglycemia?

**A.** Congenital hyperinsulinism

**B.** Growth hormone deficiency

**C.** Small for gestational age

**D.** Gonadotropin deficiency

**E.** Beckwith-Wiedemann syndrome

**13-46.** An 8-day-old infant was born full term, and the pregnancy was complicated by the mother having eclampsia and hypertension. He has had problems with hypoglycemia and is on intravenous (IV) fluids with a glucose infusion rate of 15 mg/kg/min. During one episode of hypoglycemia, the blood glucose was 28 mg/dL. Glucagon was administered, and the blood glucose rose to 65 mg/dL. Which of the following medications would be the initial drug of choice for this infant?

**A.** Growth hormone

**B.** Nifedipine

**C.** Diazoxide

**D.** Hydrocortisone

**E.** Octreotide

**13-47.** A 4-year-old girl presents for her well-child visit in August. Her linear growth and development appear to be normal. The mother's primary concern is that her daughter has had increased thirst and urination over the summer. She was toilet trained at 3 years old, but over the past 2 months, she has needed to use pull-up diapers at night to prevent accidents. She wakes up every 2 hours during the night to drink and urinate. She carries a water bottle with her during the day, and her mother refills it at least 8 times throughout the day. Her mother has tried to restrict water intake. However, when fluids have been restricted, she gets upset but calms after she is allowed to drink. Which of the following details from the history is most concerning for a pathologic condition?

**A.** She was previously toilet trained during the night.

**B.** She carries a water bottle with her during the day.

**C.** She wakes up at night to drink and urinate.

**D.** She is drinking 8 or more bottles of water per day.

**E.** She gets upset when fluids are restricted.

**13-48.** A 15-year-old girl presents to her physician's office with increased thirst and increased urination for the past 3 months. She drinks up to 8 L of water per day as she constantly feels thirsty, and she urinates 10 times or more a day. Her height, weight, and vital signs are all normal. Her physical exam is unremarkable. Electrolyte panel shows a serum sodium of 135 mEq/L, potassium of 4.2 mEq/L, calcium of 9.3 mg/dL, and glucose of 89 mg/dL. Her thyroid-stimulating hormone (TSH) is normal at 1.35 mU/mL. Urinalysis reveals a specific gravity of 1.002 and no glucosuria. She is admitted to the hospital for a water deprivation test. After 12 hours, her sodium is 137 mEq/L, serum osmolality is 286 mOsm/kg, and her urine specific gravity is 1.025. Which of the following is the most likely diagnosis?

**A.** Syndrome of inappropriate antidiuretic hormone (SIADH)

**B.** Compulsive water drinking

**C.** Nephrogenic diabetes insipidus

**D.** Central diabetes insipidus

**E.** Cerebral salt wasting

**13-49.** A 13-year-old boy was a restrained backseat passenger in a motor vehicle accident 2 days ago. He sustained an injury to his brain and is on a ventilator. For the first 24 hours after the accident, his urine output was 3 mL/kg/h. His urine output has subsequently decreased. Laboratory studies now reveal that his serum sodium is 129 mEq/L, serum osmolality is 281 mOsm/kg, and urine sodium is 40 mEq/L. Which of the following would be the most appropriate management at this time?

**A.** Decrease the intravenous (IV) fluid rate

**B.** Start oral salt supplementation

**C.** Bolus with furosemide

**D.** Start a vasopressin drip

**E.** Bolus with hypertonic (3%) saline

**13-50.** A 16-year-old boy is an unrestrained front seat passenger in a motor vehicle accident. He has suffered extensive trauma to his body. Head imaging reveals that he has significant disruption of the pituitary stalk. Of the following hormones, which would most likely be expected to be elevated?

**A.** Growth hormone

**B.** Prolactin

**C.** Insulin-like growth factor 1 (IGF-1)

**D.** Free thyroxine ($T_4$)

**E.** Testosterone

**13-51.** A 13-year-old boy is seen in clinic and noted to have short stature. Review of his growth records show that he has consistently grown along the third percentile for height since the age of 2 years. His mid-parental height prediction is at the 25th percentile. Review of systems is negative. Physical exam reveals no evidence of puberty. His father remembers growing in height after high school. A bone age radiograph reveals a skeletal age of 10 years. Which of the following is the most likely diagnosis?

**A.** Growth hormone deficiency

**B.** Constitutional delay

**C.** Familial short stature

**D.** Hypothyroidism

**E.** Idiopathic short stature

**13-52.** A 10-year-old girl with persistent headaches presents to the emergency department (ED). The headaches have been present for the past 6 months and are worsening in severity and frequency, now waking her up at night from sleep. For the past 3 days, she has been vomiting. On review of systems, her mother notes increased thirst and urination for the past month and poor linear growth for the past year. Due to these worrisome features, a head computed tomography (CT) is ordered, which reveals a sellar mass with calcification, multiple cystic lesions, and some solid components. Which of the following is the most likely diagnosis?

**A.** Germinoma

**B.** Glioma

**C.** Craniopharyngioma

**D.** Meningioma

**E.** Rathke's cleft cyst

**13-53.** A 12-year-old girl is seen for a yearly well-child visit. Her mother states that her daughter is one of the tallest girls in her class and is concerned that there is something wrong. You review her growth records and see that she has grown consistently around the 97th percentile for height. Her mother is 175 cm tall and father is 188 cm tall. Her body mass index (BMI) is at the 70th percentile. She is Tanner stage 3 for breast development. Her review of systems is negative with no abnormalities seen on physical exam. You obtain a bone age, which is read as 12 years. What is the most likely cause of her tall stature?

**A.** Hyperthyroidism

**B.** Obesity

**C.** Precocious puberty

**D.** Constitutional tall stature

**E.** Marfan syndrome

**13-54.** A 4-year-old girl with a 6-month history of polyuria and polydipsia underwent a water deprivation test in the hospital and was found to have central diabetes insipidus. Treatment with oral desmopressin has been started. Which of the following is the next best step?

**A.** Institute a daily fluid restriction

**B.** Obtain a renal ultrasound

**C.** Order an antidiuretic hormone level

**D.** Obtain a brain magnetic resonance imaging (MRI)

**E.** Discharge home with no further workup

**13-55.** A 5-month-old male infant presents to his doctor's office with concerns of poor linear growth. His weight has been following the 25th percentile, but his length has fallen from the 25th to the 3rd percentile. His mother states that he has not started cooing or reaching for objects. His bowel movements are infrequent, dry, and hard. On exam, you notice nystagmus. Birth history is remarkable for prolonged jaundice. There is no history of hypoglycemia. His newborn screen was normal. What is the most likely diagnosis?

**A.** Growth hormone deficiency

**B.** Inadequate caloric intake

**C.** Celiac disease

**D.** Hyperthyroidism

**E.** Hypothyroidism

**13-56.** A 17-year-old girl presents to her pediatrician's office with fatigue. She has done some reading online and would like to be checked for low thyroid hormone. She has no family history of thyroid disease. Her medications include an oral contraceptive pill and loratadine. Other than fatigue, she has no other symptoms. Lab testing reveals a normal thyroid-stimulating hormone (TSH) and an elevated thyroxine ($T_4$). What is the most likely cause of her abnormal thyroid labs?

**A.** Increased thyroxine-binding globulin (TBG)

**B.** Decreased TBG

**C.** Subclinical hyperthyroidism

**D.** Hypothyroidism secondary to Hashimoto thyroiditis

**E.** Hyperthyroidism secondary to Graves' disease

**13-57.** A 2-month-old male infant is admitted with abdominal distention, tachypnea, and persistent vomiting. Abdominal imaging reveals multiple large hepatic hemangiomas. What endocrine abnormality should he be screened for?

**A.** Adrenal insufficiency

**B.** Growth hormone deficiency

**C.** Hypothyroidism

**D.** Diabetes mellitus

**E.** Hypoglycemia

**13-58.** An 11-year-old girl presents to clinic because she noticed a lump on the front of her neck. She has trouble falling asleep, but otherwise feels fine. She denies heart palpitations, and bowel movement frequency is once per day. Her vital signs are normal. On exam, she has a smooth, symmetrically enlarged, and nontender thyroid gland. There are no nodules and no cervical lymphadenopathy. The rest of her physical exam is normal, including eye exam, reflexes, heart exam, strength testing, and no tremor. Laboratory studies show a low thyroid-stimulating hormone (TSH) and normal thyroxine ($T_4$). You obtain further lab testing that shows a positive thyroid peroxidase and antithyroglobulin antibodies and a negative TSH receptor antibody. What is the most likely diagnosis?

**A.** Subacute thyroiditis

**B.** Hashitoxicosis

**C.** Acute suppurative thyroiditis

**D.** Thyroglossal duct cyst

**E.** Graves' disease

**13-59.** You are rounding on a 3-day-old healthy male neonate whose mother has Graves' disease and had a positive thyroid-stimulating hormone (TSH) receptor antibody during the third trimester. The neonate's cord blood was also positive for this antibody. You obtain a TSH, free thyroxine ($T_4$), and total triiodothyronine ($T_3$) from the neonate, and the results are all normal. The baby is feeding well, is asymptomatic, and is discharged home. When should thyroid function tests be rechecked in this infant?

**A.** 2 weeks of life

**B.** 2 months of life

**C.** 6 months of life

**D.** 12 months of life

**E.** No further testing required

**13-60.** A 14-year-old girl presents with an enlarging mass on the right side of her neck. The mass is painless and she has no sweating, weight loss, anxiety, palpitations, or fatigue. There is no known family history of thyroid disease. Her heart rate is 90 bpm, and blood pressure is 105/72 mm Hg. A thyroid-stimulating hormone (TSH) and total thyroxine ($T_4$) level are normal. A thyroid ultrasound shows a solid nodule in the right thyroid gland that is hypoechoic with microcalcifications. What is the next best step in the management of this patient?

**A.** Neck magnetic resonance imaging (MRI)

**B.** Thyroidectomy

**C.** Fine-needle aspiration (FNA)

**D.** Start levothyroxine

**E.** Thyroid uptake scan

**13-61.** You suspect that a 10-year-old female patient may have Cushing syndrome. Her linear growth has stalled, but she has continued to gain weight and is now obese. She has purple striae on her arms, legs, and abdomen that are > 1 cm wide. She also has extreme fatigue. Her blood pressure is 130/90 mm Hg, and she has a plethoric appearance. Which of the following tests is the next best step in her evaluation?

**A.** Adrenocorticotropic hormone (ACTH) level

**B.** Low-dose ACTH stimulation test

**C.** High-dose ACTH stimulation test

**D.** Low-dose dexamethasone suppression test

**E.** High-dose dexamethasone suppression test

**13-62.** A male neonate's newborn screen is positive for congenital adrenal hyperplasia (CAH). The diagnosis is confirmed with an elevated serum 17-hydroxyprogesterone level. Of the following, what is the most likely physical exam feature in this patient?

**A.** Ambiguous genitalia

**B.** Body odor

**C.** Normal exam

**D.** Pubic hair

**E.** Testicular enlargement

**13-63.** A 16-year-old boy presents with persistent hypertension, palpitations, flushing, and headaches. You want to evaluate him for a pheochromocytoma. Of the following, which is the best test to order?

**A.** Chromogranin A

**B.** Urine homovanillic acid

**C.** Urine vanillymandelic acid

**D.** 24-hour urinary creatinine

**E.** Plasma free metanephrines

**13-64.** You are screening a patient with Crohn disease for nutritional deficiencies. Which of the following is the best test to screen for vitamin D deficiency?

**A.** Calcium

**B.** Phosphorus

**C.** 1,25-Dihydroxyvitamin D

**D.** 25-Hydroxyvitamin D

**E.** Parathyroid hormone

**13-65.** After sleeping in, a previously healthy 3-year-old boy appears pale, sweaty, shaky, and irritable. His worried parents bring him to the emergency department (ED) for evaluation. A point-of-care blood sugar is 35 mg/dL. Serum laboratory studies as part of a critical sample are obtained, and the child is given 2 mL/kg of 10% dextrose. The child's symptoms gradually resolve, and he is back to baseline after 30 minutes. A repeat point-of-care blood glucose level is 82 mg/dL. He has been growing and developing normally. He has no history of previous hypoglycemic episodes. He recently had an upper respiratory infection associated with a decreased appetite, and he did not eat much at supper last evening. Which of the following tests can help you confirm your suspected diagnosis while waiting for results of the critical sample to return?

**A.** Urine ketones

**B.** Hemoglobin A1c

**C.** Antibodies for type 1 diabetes mellitus

**D.** Free thyroxine ($T_4$)

**E.** Insulin-like growth factor 1 (IGF-1)

## ANSWERS

**Answer 13-1.** A

With the patient's history of medullary thyroid cancer combined with neuromas on his tongue and Marfanoid body habitus, the patient most likely has MEN2B (Table 530-2). MEN2 syndromes, which are inherited in an autosomal dominant pattern, are caused by a gain-of-function mutation in the *RET* proto-oncogene, not an inactivating mutation of the gene.

*MEN1*, which encodes the tumor suppressor gene *MENIN*, is mutated in MEN1. The parathyroid glands, pituitary gland, and pancreatic islet cells are most often affected in MEN1. The most common endocrine abnormality in MEN1 involves hypercalcemia due to hyperparathyroidism. Pancreatic tumors, including gastrinomas and insulinomas, are the second most common endocrine problem in MEN1. Pituitary tumors occur in > 40% of MEN1 patients; prolactinomas are the most common, followed by tumors secreting growth hormone and adrenocorticotropic hormone (ACTH). The *PRKARIA* gene is responsible for Carney complex, which involves pituitary-independent Cushing syndrome along with an association of heart myxomas and lentigines. Activating mutations of the G-protein alpha subunit are associated with McCune-Albright syndrome, which presents with autonomous endocrine function, fibrous dysplasia, and/or café-au-lait macules.

(Section 28 – Chapter 530: Endocrine Neoplasia Syndromes – Heading: Multiple Endocrine Neoplasia 2 (MEN2), Subheading: Pathogenesis and Epidemiology; Section 28 – Chapter 534: Abnormal Pubertal Development, Heading: Causes of GnRH-Independent Sexual Precocity Among Boys and Girls)

**Answer 13-2.** C

Normal male pubertal development (Figure 533-1B) occurs between the ages of 9 and 14 years, with the average age being approximately 11.5 years. In males, the testicular Leydig cells produce testosterone as a result of stimulation of receptors by circulating LH. The onset of central male puberty is defined as an increase in testicular volume ≥ 4 mL or 2.5 cm in testicular length. This is followed by penile enlargement, pubic hair development, and lastly, a linear growth spurt.

The serum concentration of prolactin increases in normal female puberty, but it does not change in normal male puberty. The circulation of FSH stimulates spermatogenesis by attaching to the FSH receptors of seminiferous tubules. Inhibin, which is produced by the testicular Sertoli cells, suppresses FSH secretion in normal male puberty.

(Section 28 – Chapter 533: Normal Pubertal Development, Heading: Hypothalamic-Pituitary-Gonadal Hormones)

**Answer 13-3.** B

Breast development is the first sign of central puberty in girls, and testicular enlargement (≥ 4 mL in volume) is the first sign of central puberty in boys. Puberty is delayed if a girl has not entered puberty by age 13 years and delayed in a boy if he has not entered puberty by age 14 years.

Following menarche, girls grow approximately 2 to 7 cm (or 0.8 inches to 2.8 inches). Breast development may begin unilaterally, and asymmetric breast growth is not uncommon. The average age of menarche is approximately 12.5 years in girls. Menarche occurs

**TABLE 530-2.** Disease Associations in the Multiple Endocrine Neoplasia Syndromes

| | |
|---|---|
| **Multiple Endocrine Neoplasia Type 1** | *Von Hippel-Lindau syndrome* |
| Parathyroid hyperplasia or adenoma | Pheochromocytoma |
| Islet cell hyperplasia, adenoma, or carcinoma | Islet cell tumor |
| Pituitary hyperplasia or adenoma | Renal cell carcinoma |
| Less common: carcinoid, pheochromocytoma, subcutaneous or visceral lipomas, cutaneous lichen amyloidosis | Hemangioblastoma of central nervous system |
| | Retinal angiomas |
| **Multiple Endocrine Neoplasia Type 2** | *Neurofibromatosis* |
| *MEN2A* | Skin findings: Café-au-lait spots, axillary or inguinal freckling, cutaneous neurofibromas |
| Medullary thyroid carcinoma | Plexiform neurofibroma |
| Pheochromocytoma | Bony lesions (pseudoarthrosis, sphenoid wing hypoplasia) |
| Parathyroid hyperplasia or adenoma | Optic glioma |
| *MEN2B* | Iris Lisch nodules |
| Medullary thyroid carcinoma | Pheochromocytoma |
| Pheochromocytoma | Neuroendocrine tumors of the duodenum |
| Mucosal and gastrointestinal neuromas | *Carney triad* |
| Intestinal neuronal dysplasia (presents like Hirschsprung disease) | Gastrointestinal stromal tumor |
| Marfanoid features | Pulmonary chondroma |
| Mixed Syndromes | Paraganglioma |
| *Carney complex* | *Carney-Stratakis syndrome* |
| Myxomas of heart, skin, and breast | Gastrointestinal stromal tumor |
| Spotty cutaneous pigmentation | Paraganglioma |
| Testicular, adrenal, and growth hormone–producing pituitary tumors | *3PAS* |
| | Pituitary adenoma |
| Peripheral nerve schwannomas | Paraganglioma/pheochromocytoma |

Mark W. Kline, *Rudolph's Pediatrics*, 23rd Edition. Copyright © McGraw-Hill Education. All rights reserved.

about 2 years after the onset of breast development. Although there is controversy surrounding when puberty is precocious, most agree that puberty that begins before the age of 8 years in girls and before the age of 9 years in boys is early.

(Section 28 – Chapter 533: Normal Pubertal Development, Heading: Age of Normal Puberty)

**Answer 13-4.** E

The patient has evidence of central precocious puberty with breast and pubic hair development, estrogenization of her vaginal mucosa, and advanced skeletal maturation. The patient in the scenario mostly likely has a hamartoma of the tuber cinereum, which is associated with gelastic seizures, precocious puberty, and a characteristic appearance of the hamartoma on brain imaging. On MRI, the hamartoma appears as a pedunculated or sessile mass attached to the posterior hypothalamus. The hamartoma is not malignant and may have gonadotropin-releasing hormone (GnRH)-synthesizing neurons.

Optic gliomas, craniopharyngiomas, ependymomas, and astrocytomas can cause central precocious puberty, but they are not classically associated with seizures and the described characteristic appearance on MRI.

(Section 28 – Chapter 534: Abnormal Pubertal Development, Heading: Central (Complete or True) Precocious Puberty, Subheading: Central Nervous System Disorders)

**Answer 13-5.** D

Familial male limited precocious puberty (also known as testotoxicosis) is caused by an activating mutation of the LH receptor. Due to this mutation, which is inherited in an autosomal dominant pattern, testosterone is constantly produced. This disorder manifests clinically only in males. Fertility is normal in adulthood. Boys with this condition have minimal enlargement of the testes because the Leydig cells are predominantly stimulated and not the seminiferous tubules. Therefore, penile enlargement, pubic hair, growth

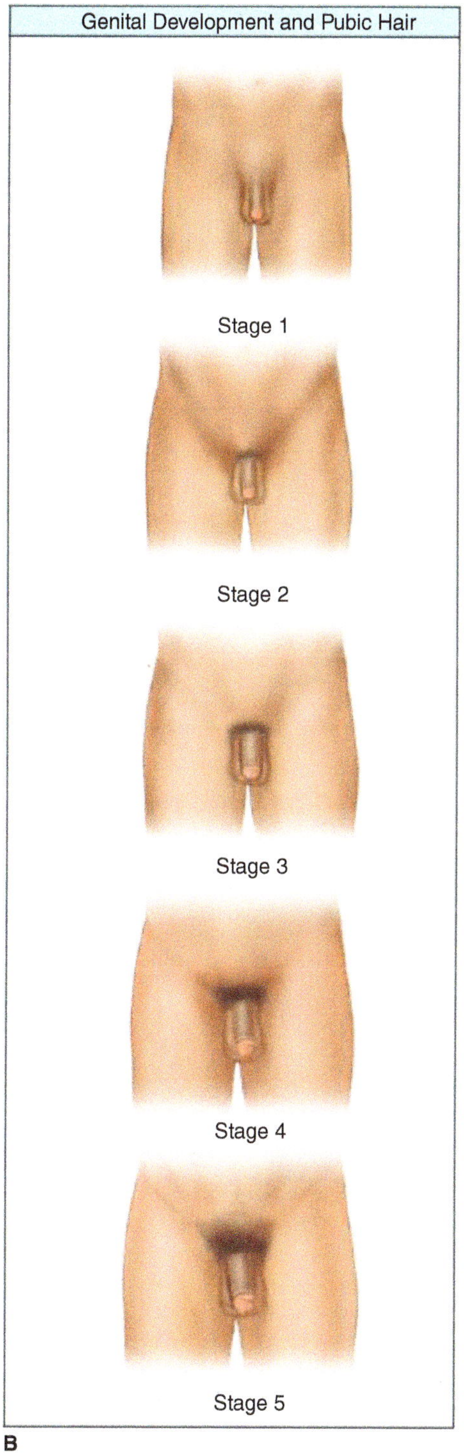


**FIGURE 533-1B.** Genital development and pubic hair growth in boys. Stage G1, prepubertal. Stage G2, enlargement of testis to > 2.5 cm, appearance of scrotal reddening, and increase in rugations. Stage G3, increase in length and to a lesser extent breadth of penis, with further growth of testes and darkening of scrotal skin. Stage G5, adult genitalia. Stage P1, no pubic hair. Stage P2, sparse growth of slightly pigmented, slightly curved pubic hair, mainly at the base of the penis. Stage P3, thicker curlier hair spread laterally. Stage P4, adult-type hair that does not yet spread to the medial thighs. Stage P5, adult type hair spread to medial thighs. (Reproduced with permission from Styne DM: *Pediatric Endocrinology. A Clinical Handbook*. New York: Springer International Publishing; 2016.)

acceleration, and acne are seen, but testicular volume is disproportionately small. Biochemical testing reveals elevated testosterone levels with low gonadotropin concentrations.

(Section 28 – Chapter 534: Abnormal Pubertal Development, Heading: Peripheral Precocious Puberty, Subheading: Boys)

**Answer 13-6.** B

This child has precocious puberty, hyperthyroidism, and café-au-lait spots. This clinical presentation is most consistent with McCune-Albright syndrome. The classic triad of McCune-Albright syndrome is polyostotic fibrous dysplasia, irregular or jagged bordered café-au-lait macules, and autonomous endocrine function. The most common endocrinopathy is GnRH-independent precocious puberty followed by hyperthyroidism. However, all 3 entities of the classic triad do not need to be apparent to make the diagnosis of McCune-Albright syndrome. Activating mutations of the stimulatory G-protein of the adenyl cyclase system are responsible for the autonomous activity in endocrine glands. Cushing syndrome, acromegaly, and hyperparathyroidism can also occur.

Peutz-Jeghers syndrome presents with nasal polyps, hyperpigmentation of the lips, and macules on the buccal mucosa. This autosomal dominant condition can also present with gynecomastia and precocious puberty with Sertoli cell tumors in boys and ovarian cysts in girls. Classic CAH is an autosomal recessive disorder most commonly due to 21-hydroxylase deficiency and presents at birth with ambiguous genitalia in females. Familial male limited precocious puberty is a disorder seen only in males and is caused by an activating mutation of the luteinizing hormone (LH) receptor. Affected males present with signs of virilization and penile enlargement with only a small and disproportionate increase in testicular volume. Granulosa cell tumors are a rare functional neoplasm that can manifest as gonadotropin-independent premature puberty. Peutz-Jeghers syndrome, CAH, familial gonadotropin-independent puberty, and granulosa cell tumors are not associated with café-au-lait macules or hyperthyroidism.

(Section 28 – Chapter 534: Abnormal Pubertal Development, Heading: Causes of GnRH-Independent Sexual Precocity Among Boys and Girls)

**Answer 13-7.** C

Premature thelarche is usually best managed with reassurance because it is a benign, self-limited condition that is considered a normal variant in development.

Girls most often present with premature thelarche before 2 years of age and almost always before 4 years of age. The majority of cases regress within 6 months of onset, but breast tissue may persist. In girls with premature thelarche, no other signs of pubertal development are present. There is no nipple or areolar complex development. Girls with premature thelarche have normal linear growth and normal skeletal maturation. The differential diagnosis of breast development in young girls includes exogenous estrogen exposure, estrogen-secreting

**TABLE 536-2.** Laboratory Data for Rickets of Different Causes

| Type | Calcium | Phosphate | Alkaline Phosphatase | Calcidiol | Calcitriol | Parathyroid Hormone |
|---|---|---|---|---|---|---|
| Calcium deficiency | ↓↑ | ↓ | ↑↑ | N | ↑ | ↑ |
| Phosphate deficiency | N, ↑ | ↓↓ | ↑↑ | N | ↑ | N, ↓ |
| Vitamin D deficiency | | | | | | |
| Mild | N, ↓ | N, ↓ | ↑ | ↓ | N | N |
| Moderate | N, ↓ | ↓ | ↑↑ | ↓ | ↓, N, ↑ | ↑ |
| Severe | ↓ | ↓ | ↑↑ | ↓↓ | ↓ | ↑↑ |
| Loss-of-function *CYP2R1* (25-hydroxylase) | ↓ | ↓ | ↑ | ↓ | ↓ | ↑ |
| Loss-of-function *CYP27B1* (25OHD-1α-hydroxylase) | ↓↓ | ↓↓ | ↑↑↑ | N | ↓↓↓ | ↑↑↑ |
| Loss-of-function *VDR* (resistance to calcitriol) | ↓↓ | ↓↓ | ↑↑↑ | N | ↑↑↑ | ↑↑↑ |
| Loss-of-function *PHEX* (X-linked hypophosphatemic rickets) | N | ↓↓ | ↑ | N | N, ↓ | N |
| Hypophosphatasia | N, ↑ | N, ↑ | ↓ | N | N | N, ↓ |

N, normal; ↓, low; ↑, high.

Reproduced with permission from Sperling MA, ed. *Pediatric Endocrinology*, 4th ed. Philadelphia: Saunders/Elsevier; 2014.

tumor, McCune-Albright syndrome, or central precocious puberty.

In premature thelarche, gonadotropin levels are in the prepubertal range. Small for gestational age is a risk factor for premature adrenarche (but not thelarche). Some girls with premature adrenarche are at an increased risk for polycystic ovary syndrome and insulin resistance as adults.

(Section 28 – Chapter 534: Abnormal Pubertal Development, Heading: Premature Thelarche)

**Answer 13-8.** B

This child has rickets, which is most likely due to decreased vitamin D intake. Breast milk is deficient in vitamin D, and recommendations state that breastfeeding mothers should take 1000 IU of vitamin D daily while their infant should receive 400 IU of vitamin D per day. Individuals with darkly pigmented skin are at an increased risk for vitamin D deficiency. Because the child in this case is black and was exclusively breastfed, he is at high risk for vitamin D deficiency. In children with rickets, delayed closure of fontanelles can be seen along with short stature, poor weight gain, and delayed walking. Common findings on radiographs include cupping and fraying of the metaphyses of the long bones and demineralization. In mild vitamin D–deficient rickets, laboratory abnormalities are more subtle, and calcium, phosphate, and parathyroid levels may be normal with an increased alkaline phosphatase (Table 536-2). In more severe cases, calcium and phosphate are low, with a notable increase in alkaline phosphatase and parathyroid hormone.

(Section 28 – Chapter 536: Disorders of Bone Formation, Heading: Rickets and Osteomalacia)

**Answer 13-9.** E

The most common reason for congenital hypothyroidism is a defect in thyroid embryogenesis with > 95% of cases being idiopathic or sporadic. The prevalence of congenital hypothyroidism is approximately 1 in 2000 to 1 in 4000 newborns.

The remaining answers are also reasons for congenital hypothyroidism (Table 520-1); however, they are less likely in this case. The child is not premature, and therefore, dysfunction due to prematurity would be unlikely. Premature infants may have an immature hypothalamic-pituitary-thyroid axis and are predisposed to thyroid dysfunction. The child's mother is healthy and has no history of thyroid disease, which makes the transplacental acquisition of maternal thyroid-stimulating hormone (TSH) receptor blocking antibodies unlikely. Ingestion of a goitrogenic substance, such as iodines or sulfonamides, by the mother was not given in the history but could cause hypothyroidism and a neonatal goiter. Thyroid dyshormonogenesis can occur from a variety of enzymatic defects, including organification and thyroid iodide transport defects. However, cases of thyroid dyshormonogenesis are less common than defects in thyroid embryogenesis. Infants with thyroid dyshormonogenesis have a normal-appearing thyroid gland in the normal location on ultrasound, and they may have a goiter on exam.

(Section 28 – Chapter 520: Hypothyroidism in the Infant, Heading: Thyroid Dysgenesis)

**TABLE 520-1.** Causes of Hypothyroidism in Infants

| |
|---|
| Thyroid dysgenesis |
| Thyroid aplasia |
| Thyroid hypoplasia |
| Thyroid ectopy |
| Thyroid dyshormonogenesis |
| Resistance to thyroid-stimulating hormone |
| Defect in thyroid hormone transport |
| Resistance to thyroid hormone action |
| Central hypothyroidism |
| Transient hypothyroidism |
| Thyroxine-binding globulin deficiency |
| Hypothyroxinemia of prematurity |
| Nonthyroidal illness |

Mark W. Kline, *Rudolph's Pediatrics*, 23rd Edition. Copyright © McGraw-Hill Education. All rights reserved.

**Answer 13-10.** A

Methods of thyroid testing in newborn screening programs vary from state to state, but screening is commonly conducted with either TSH only or a combination of TSH and thyroxine ($T_4$). The majority of infants with congenital hypothyroidism have primary thyroid disease and an elevated TSH. Approximately 15% of infants with congenital hypothyroidism can have a normal $T_4$ level. Although newborn screening detects the great majority of affected infants, 3% to 5% of infants with congenital hypothyroidism may not be detected by newborn screening.

The incidence of congenital hypothyroidism is approximately 1 in 2000 to 1 in 4000 newborns. Preferred thyroid hormone replacement therapy is $T_4$, and the goal is to start thyroid hormone replacement no later than 2 weeks of life because thyroid hormone is critically important for normal brain growth and development. Physical growth and development are usually normalized with timely and adequate therapy along with close monitoring of thyroid function tests. Confirmation of the diagnosis of congenital hypothyroidism is made by measuring serum TSH and $T_4$.

(Section 28 – Chapter 520: Hypothyroidism in the Infant, Heading: Newborn Screening Programs)

**Answer 13-11.** C

This child has severe hypothyroidism evidenced by an extremely high TSH value, sexual precocity (pubertal signs before age 9), delayed bone age, goiter, and delayed relaxation of deep tendon reflexes. Pseudoprecocious puberty due to severe hypothyroidism can occur in both boys and girls. Boys exhibit penile and testicular enlargement with lack of androgen-mediated body hair, whereas girls can present with menstruation and breast development. These findings occur due to high levels of TSH cross-reacting with follicle-stimulating hormone (FSH) receptors, as both have identical alpha subunits. Galactorrhea can also occur due to increased thyrotropin-releasing hormone production from the hypothalamus, which stimulates both TSH and prolactin from the pituitary gland. The bone age delay reflects the duration of the hypothyroidism. Once a child receives treatment, the signs and symptoms of pseudoprecocious puberty regress.

Normal thyroid function levels are not linked to precocious puberty. A markedly elevated free $T_4$ value (with an accompanying low TSH value) would suggest hyperthyroidism. Unlike this patient, the bone age would not be markedly delayed, and the patient would be hyperreflexive if he was hyperthyroid. A mildly elevated TSH of 6.0 mU/L would not explain this clinical scenario.

(Section 28 – Chapter 521: Acquired Hypothyroidism, Heading: Diagnosis and Management of Acquired Hypothyroidism, Subheading: Clinical Features; Section 28, Chapter 534: Abnormal Pubertal Development, Heading: Causes of GnRH-Independent Sexual Precocity Among Boys and Girls)

**Answer 13-12.** D

Hashimoto thyroiditis is the most common cause of goiter and hypothyroidism in a 9-year-old child. It is an autoimmune condition and is more common in females than males. The onset of Hashimoto thyroiditis is usually insidious, and some children may have no signs or symptoms of hypothyroidism. Most children with Hashimoto thyroiditis and autoimmune hypothyroidism have detectable levels of circulating antithyroid antibodies, which are markers of inflammation in the thyroid gland. A thyroid peroxidase antibody is more often detected compared to an antithyroglobulin antibody.

A goiter and elevated TSH level establishes that the disease originates in the thyroid gland. An MRI of the brain with specific emphasis on the hypothalamus and pituitary gland would only be necessary in cases of central (not primary) hypothyroidism. An enlarged thyroid on physical exam would not be present in cases of central hypothyroidism. A thyroid ultrasound would be helpful if there was thyroid asymmetry or a nodule present. However, in this case, the patient has a thyroid gland that is enlarged but smooth and symmetric. A TSH receptor antibody and total $T_3$ would be helpful in the evaluation of hyperthyroidism and Graves' disease (Figure 521-1).

(Section 28 – Chapter 521: Acquired Hypothyroidism, Heading: Autoimmune (Hashimoto) Thyroiditis, Subheading: Clinical Features and Diagnosis)

**Answer 13-13.** D

This child has hyperthyroidism, which is most commonly due to Graves' disease. Other causes of hyperthyroidism in children include Hashimoto thyrotoxicosis (or hashitoxicosis),

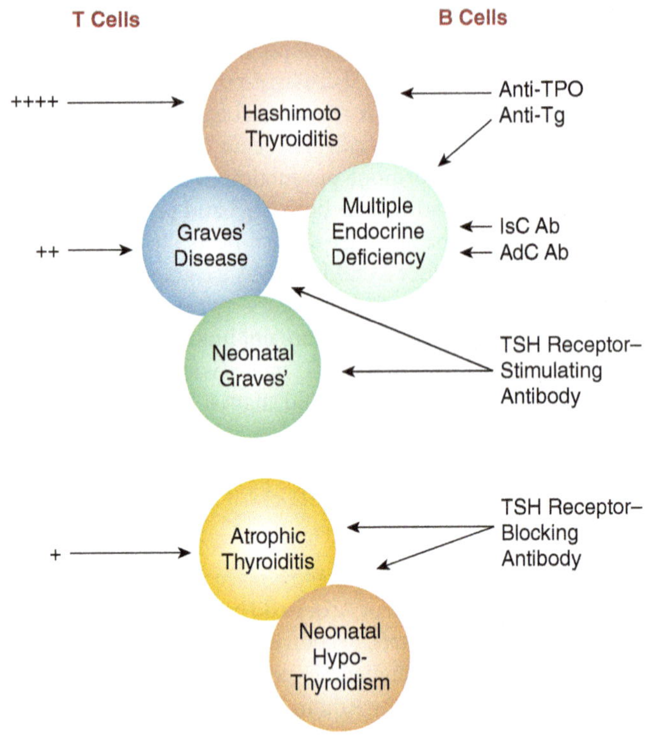


**FIGURE 521-1.** Relationship of T-cell infiltrate of thyroid tissue and B-cell antibody production to clinical autoimmune thyroid disease phenotypes. The extent of lymphoid infiltration is shown as ++++ to +. Antibody types are antithyroid peroxidase (TPO), antiperoxidase antibody, and antithyroglobulin antibody (Tg); IsC Ab and AdC Ab are islet cell and adrenal antibodies. The correlations are only approximate. TSH, thyroid-stimulating hormone. (Mark W. Kline, *Rudolph's Pediatrics*, 23rd Edition. Copyright © McGraw-Hill Education. All rights reserved.)

hyperfunctioning thyroid nodule, or ingestion of thyroid hormone. Classically, the diagnosis of hyperthyroidism is confirmed with a low or suppressed TSH level, elevated $T_4$ and/or free $T_4$, and an elevated $T_3$. TSH receptor antibody, which is also called a thyroid-stimulating immunoglobulin, is positive in Graves' disease. Clinical features of hyperthyroidism include muscle weakness, behavioral problems, frequent or loose stools, declining school performance, and emotional lability. Cardiovascular signs of hyperthyroidism include a widened pulse pressure, tachycardia, and exercise intolerance. Weight loss in conjunction with an increased appetite is also common.

Estradiol, LH, and FSH are hormones that are important in pubertal development but are not associated with hyperthyroidism.

(Section 28 – Chapter 522: Hyperthyroidism, Heading: Graves' Disease, Subheading: Diagnostic Evaluation)

## Answer 13-14. B

The incidence of Graves' disease sharply increases as children approach adolescence. Graves' disease is 6 to 8 times more common in girls than boys. Treatment options include thyroidectomy, radioactive iodine ablation, and antithyroid drugs. In this scenario, the patient is taking methimazole, which inhibits the oxidation of iodine and blocks the production of thyroid hormones. Side effects of methimazole include rash, arthralgia, and agranulocytopenia. Due to the risk of agranulocytopenia, it is recommended that patients have a complete blood count (CBC) during times of illness to document their white blood cell (WBC) count. If it is suppressed, the patient should stop methimazole and be evaluated. Drug therapy is typically continued for 1 to 2 years before a trial off is recommended. The best clinical prognostic sign for determining if the patient has gone into remission is the size of the thyroid gland. Most patients with a persistent goiter will relapse when the medication is discontinued.

Orbitopathy, widened pulse pressure, muscle weakness, and weight loss are all clinical features of Graves' disease. Other clinical signs include emotional lability, tremor, fatigability, and rapid tendon reflex relaxation. However, the resolution of these signs does not suggest that the patient has gone into remission.

(Section 28 – Chapter 522: Hyperthyroidism, Heading: Graves' Disease, Subheading: Medical Management)

## Answer 13-15. C

Thyroid hormone metabolism is mediated by iodothyronine monodeiodinase (MDI) enzymes (Figure 519-3). $T_4$ is progressively deiodinated by MDI-1, MDI-2, and MDI-3. In the first step of thyroid hormone metabolism, $T_4$ is deiodinated

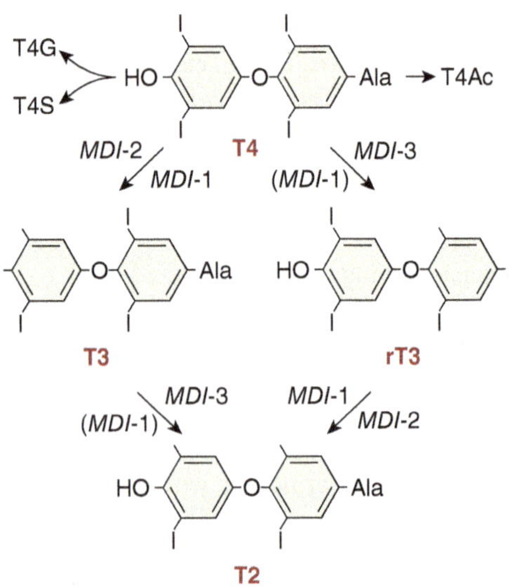


**FIGURE 519-3.** Structure of $T_4$ and $T_3$. $T_4$, tetraiodothyronine, serves largely as a prohormone. Thyroid hormone actions are largely mediated by $T_3$, triiodothyronine, which is derived by monodeiodination from $T_4$ via 2 monodeiodinase enzymes, iodothyronine monodeiodinase (MDI)-1 and MDI-2. Both $T_4$ and T3 are inactivated by MDI-3, which deiodinates $T_4$ to inactive reverse $T_3$ ($rT_3$) and $T_3$ to inactive $T_2$. The iodothyronines are also metabolized to inactive glucuronides and sulfates, shown here as $T_4G$ and $T_4S$. The alanine (Ala) side chain is subject to transamination forming acetic acid analogs, here shown as tetrac or $T_4Ac$, which have some activity but are rapidly degraded. $T_3Ac$ (not shown) has been used to treat thyroid hormone resistance. (Mark W. Kline, *Rudolph's Pediatrics*, 23rd Edition. Copyright © McGraw-Hill Education. All rights reserved.)

to either active $T_3$ or to inactive $rT_3$. Normally, $T_3$ and $rT_3$ are produced at the same rate, although $rT_3$ is produced in greater quantity in sick euthyroid syndrome. $T_4$ is produced only by the thyroid gland, whereas $T_3$ is produced by the thyroid gland and in other tissues, including the liver, brain, and placenta. $T_4$ is deiodinated in these peripheral tissues to $T_3$. The concentration of $T_4$ is 50 to 100 times greater than that of $T_3$, but $T_3$ is more potent than $T_4$. As $T_3$ is the active and biologically relevant hormone, it binds with greater affinity to nuclear receptors in comparison to $T_4$.

(Section 28 – Chapter 519: The Thyroid – Heading: Metabolism of Thyroid Hormones)

**Answer 13-16. A**

Disorders associated with autoimmune hypothyroidism include type 1 diabetes, Turner syndrome, and Down syndrome. In children with type 1 diabetes, it is estimated that about 30% have detectable thyroid autoantibodies (thyroid peroxidase or antithyroglobulin) and about 10% have an elevated thyroid-stimulating hormone (TSH). In Turner syndrome, up to 30% of adults may become hypothyroid, and as many as 50% have detectable thyroid autoantibodies. Periodic screening for thyroid disease is recommended in children with type 1 diabetes as well as in girls with Turner syndrome. In Down syndrome, autoimmune thyroid disease is more common than in the general population. Besides the newborn screen, thyroid studies should be checked at 6 months of life and then yearly thereafter.

CAH is not associated with an increased prevalence of autoimmune thyroid disease. Greater than 95% of CAH cases are caused by an autosomal recessive deficiency of 21 alpha-hydroxylase (mutations of *CYP21A2* gene). Prader-Willi syndrome is also not associated with autoimmune hypothyroidism, but it can be associated with central hypothyroidism. Other pituitary hormone deficiencies seen in Prader-Willi syndrome include growth hormone deficiency and central adrenal insufficiency. Other endocrine issues associated with Prader-Willi syndrome include hypogonadism and type 2 diabetes. Prader-Willi syndrome is the most common cause of syndromic obesity. In McCune-Albright syndrome, defined as the classic triad of gonadotropin-independent precocious puberty, fibrous dysplasia, and café-au-lait macules, there is no association with hypothyroidism. However, the mutation associated with this disorder can cause continued stimulation of endocrine function, leading to hyperthyroidism, Cushing syndrome, and/or growth hormone excess.

(Section 28 – Chapter 521: Acquired Hypothyroidism, Heading: Other Disorders Associated with Hypothyroidism)

**Answer 13-17. B**

This child has DiGeorge syndrome as evidenced by the conotruncal defect of the heart and hypocalcemia due to hypoparathyroidism. The classic presentation for this syndrome includes conotruncal heart defect (eg, tetralogy of Fallot, truncus arteriosus, aberrant right subclavian artery, and interrupted or right aortic arch), hypoplastic thymus, and hypocalcemia secondary to hypoparathyroidism. The hypoparathyroidism is not due to an autoimmune process but is secondary to defects in the development of the third and fourth pharyngeal pouches, which causes parathyroid gland dysgenesis. Incidence ranges from 1 in 4000 to 1 in 10,000 births, with approximately 70% having isolated hypoparathyroidism. Partial or complete absence of the thymus can result in an increased frequency of viral and fungal infections due to impaired cell-mediated immunity and defects in T lymphocyte function. Other features include cleft palate (may be submucosal) and velopharyngeal incompetence (Figure 166-6). The most common genetic cause of sporadic DiGeorge syndrome is a microdeletion in chromosome 22q11.2.

Williams syndrome is associated with idiopathic hypercalcemia, which is self-limited and not related to increased parathyroid hormone secretion. Neonatal Graves' disease, congenital hypothyroidism, and Beckwith-Wiedemann syndrome are not associated with hypocalcemia or hypoparathyroidism.

(Section 28 – Chapter 535: Calcium, Phosphorous, and Magnesium Metabolism: Normal Mineral Homeostasis, Heading: Parathyroid Dysgenesis)

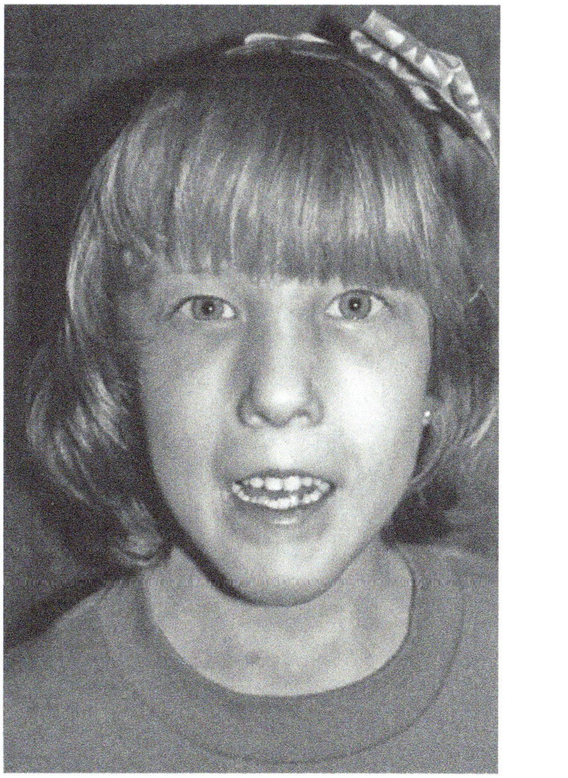

**FIGURE 166-6.** Child with DiGeorge syndrome. Note the tall nasal root and bridge with a bulbous nasal tip and small mouth. (Reproduced with permission from Jorde LB, Carey JC, Bamshad MJ, White RL. *Medical Genetics*. St. Louis: Mosby; 2000.)

**Answer 13-18.** C

This child has Albright hereditary osteodystrophy and pseudohypoparathyroidism type IA. Clinically, these children are short and often obese (see figure). Short stature may not be apparent in childhood but is nearly universal in adults. Typically, patients have developmental delay, round face, subcutaneous calcifications/ossifications, brachydactyly, and flattened nasal bridge. Lab abnormalities include hypocalcemia, hyperphosphatemia, and elevated parathyroid hormone. This disorder is classified by its lack of response to parathyroid hormone and is inherited in an autosomal dominant pattern. Inactivating mutations in *GNAS* cause resistance to parathyroid hormone and other hormones, such as thyroid-stimulating hormone (TSH). When exogenous parathyroid hormone is administered to these patients, it does not improve the hypocalcemia or hyperphosphatemia.

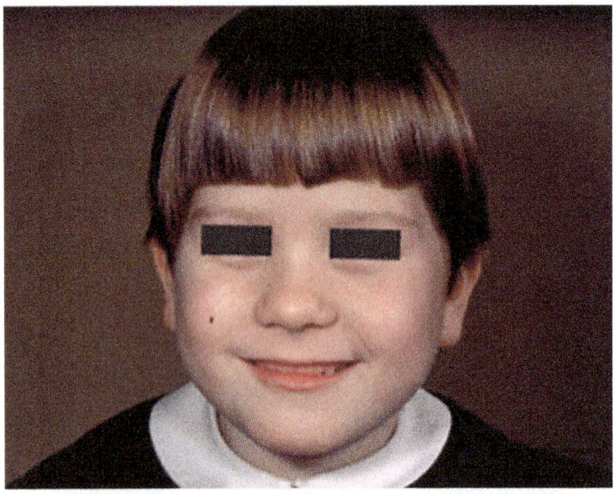

A

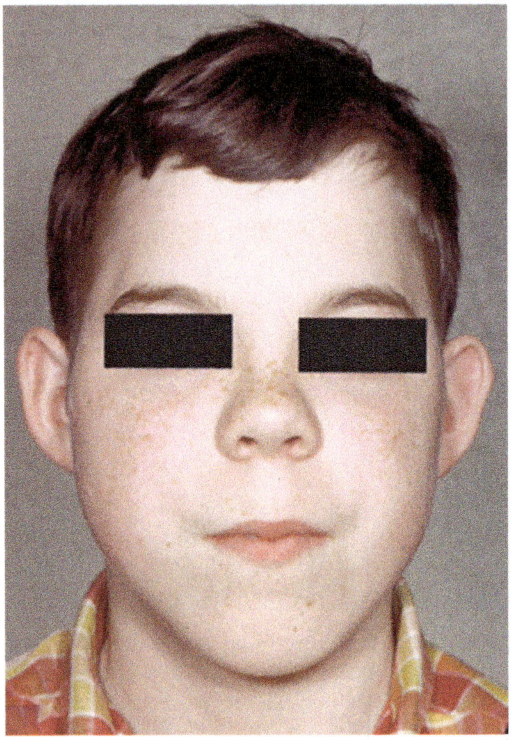

B

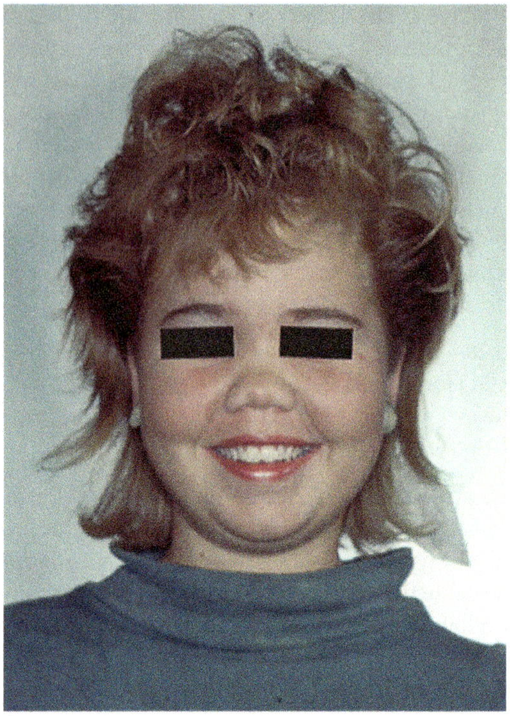

C

Spectrum of characteristics found in pseudohypoparathyroidism. Patients with pseudohypoparathyroidism have the characteristic Albright hereditary osteodystrophy (AHO) phenotype. **A–C.** *Craniofacial:* Round facies with full cheeks, short neck, depressed nasal bridge. (Reproduced with permission from Sarafoglou K, Hoffmann G, Roth K. *Pediatric Endocrinology and Inborn Errors of Metabolism*. New York: McGraw Hill; 2017.)

(Section 28 – Chapter 535: Calcium, Phosphorous, and Magnesium Metabolism: Normal Mineral Homeostasis, Heading: Disorders Associated with Neonatal Hypocalcemia, Subheading: Other Genetic Causes)

**Answer 13-19.** E

This child has hereditary hypocalciuric hypercalcemia type 1, which is also known as familial hypocalciuric hypercalcemia. This benign disorder is characterized by asymptomatic hypercalcemia (11–12 mg/dL) with hypocalciuria (calcium/creatinine clearance ratio < 0.01). This condition is autosomal dominant and is usually discovered incidentally. Due to a heterozygous loss-of-function defect in the calcium-sensing receptor (CaSR), documentation of mild hypercalcemia with hypocalciuria in one parent solidifies the diagnosis.

No treatment is indicated in this disorder, and patients are asymptomatic. They do not have typical symptoms of hypercalcemia, such as polyuria, fatigue, anorexia, irritability, hypertension, behavioral changes, or constipation. Vitamin D levels are not necessary because definitive diagnosis is made through parental testing since it is inherited in an autosomal dominant fashion.

(Section 28 – Chapter 535: Calcium, Phosphorous, and Magnesium Metabolism: Normal Mineral Homeostasis, Heading: Hereditary Hypocalciuric Hypercalcemia Type 1)

**Answer 13-20.** B

Various hormones and growth factors have profound effects on the growing skeleton, especially during childhood. Sixty percent of total body bone mineral content is accrued during puberty. Thyroid hormone increases bone resorption and bone remodeling. Hyperthyroidism results in a generalized net loss of bone. Glucocorticoids suppress osteoblast formation and accelerate osteoblast death, which leads to impaired bone formation. Glucocorticoid excess can also disrupt growth hormone/IGF-1 action as well as alter vitamin D and calcium metabolism. Estrogen and testosterone increase during puberty and promote the proliferation and maturation of chondrocytes. These pubertal hormones promote long bone growth and are necessary for bone mineral accrual. Growth hormone increases osteoblast proliferation, which leads to increased synthesis of bone-specific alkaline phosphatase, IGF-1, and type I collagen. IGF-1 increases both bone mineral content and bone mineral density.

(Section 28 – Chapter 536: Disorders of Bone Formation, Heading: Effects of Hormones and Growth Factors on the Skeleton)

**Answer 13-21.** B

Most children establish a pattern of growth by about 2 to 3 years old, and they do not deviate from this growth channel until puberty. Genetic potential is a significant factor in a child's growth, and the mean parental height (also termed mid-parental or target height) should be considered when evaluating a child's growth pattern. Mean parental height is calculated for boys by averaging parental height and adding 6.5 cm. For girls, mean parental height is calculated by averaging parental heights and subtracting 6.5 cm. Two standard deviations for the calculated mean parental height is approximately 10 cm. Final adult height typically falls within 2 inches above or below the mean parental height.

(Section 28 – Chapter 515: Growth and Growth Impairment, Heading: The Genetic Potential)

**Answer 13-22.** E

This patient has Kallmann syndrome based on his clinical findings of hyposmia (or anosmia) and hypogonadotropic hypogonadism based on his pubertal exam and laboratory studies. Although he is 15 years old, this patient has no evidence of central puberty, as evidenced by his small testicular volume. In Kallmann syndrome, gonadotropin-releasing hormone (GnRH) neurons do not migrate correctly from the olfactory placode to the hypothalamus and the olfactory bulbs do not develop, which results in hypogonadotropic hypogonadism and hyposmia/anosmia. Because there is a deficiency of GnRH (from the hypothalamus), this leads to a deficiency of luteinizing hormone (LH) and follicle-stimulating hormone (FSH) (from the pituitary gland), and central puberty does not proceed normally. Kallmann syndrome occurs more commonly in males.

Klinefelter syndrome affects males, and the most common karyotype is 47,XXY. Gonadotropin levels are elevated at the time of normal pubertal development, and it is not associated with hyposmia. Noonan syndrome, which is an autosomal dominant disorder, is often associated with short stature and cardiac defects. Delayed puberty and cryptorchidism can be seen in Noonan syndrome, and it is not associated with hyposmia. Hypogonadism frequently occurs in Prader-Willi syndrome and is characterized by hypothalamic dysfunction (low LH) along with primary gonadal dysfunction (high FSH). Many boys also have cryptorchidism. Hyposmia is not associated with Prader-Willi syndrome. Turner syndrome is seen only in females, and many have primary gonadal failure, illustrated by an increased FSH level. Turner syndrome is not associated with hyposmia.

(Section 28 – Chapter 534: Abnormal Pubertal Development, Heading: Kallmann Syndrome)

**Answer 13-23.** E

The FDA has approved the use of growth hormone in the treatment of various disorders in children, including growth hormone deficiency, Turner syndrome, chronic renal insufficiency, children born with intrauterine growth restriction (or small for gestational age) who do not have catch-up growth by the age of 2 years, Prader-Willi syndrome with growth failure, Noonan syndrome, and idiopathic short stature. Children with idiopathic short stature are defined as those with a height that is > 2.25 standard deviations below the mean for sex and age and whose epiphyses are not closed. Growth hormone is approved in children with idiopathic short stature who have a growth rate that is unlikely to attain a final adult height within the normal range, which is at least 63 inches (160 cm) for boys and 59 inches (150 cm) for girls.

Although children with Down syndrome are typically short, growth hormone is not approved for this syndrome. Research suggests that growth hormone therapy may improve lung function and have other positive benefits in CF, but it is considered experimental and has not been approved in the treatment of children with CF.

(Section 28 – Chapter 516: Endocrine Abnormalities Causing Growth Impairment, Heading: Other Indications for GH Therapy)

**Answer 13-24.** D

A child's growth pattern is an important indicator of the child's overall general health. Therefore, height measurements need to be accurately obtained and plotted on appropriate growth charts at each clinic visit. During the first 2 years of life, growth velocity averages 15 cm per year and decreases to an average of 6 cm per year later in childhood. During the pubertal growth spurt, peak growth velocity is between 7 and 11 cm per year. Because boys usually begin and complete puberty later than girls and thus stop growing later, this leads to a 13-cm final height difference between males and females. Supine length measurements should be used for children younger than

2 years, and standing height measurements are recommended thereafter. To calculate an accurate height velocity, 2 measurements of height should be made at least 4 months apart, although measurements taken 9 to 12 months apart minimize error. Typically, growth occurs as periodic bursts followed by times of growth arrest; in some children, growth may occur as a continuous process. Devices with a flexible arm mount are often inaccurate because the measurement arm does not always remain in a perpendicular plane. Wall-mounted devices are more accurate, and when taking an upright height measurement, the child should be standing with heels together with the thoracic spine, buttocks, and heels touching the measuring device.

(Section 28 – Chapter 515: Growth and Growth Impairment, Heading: Normal Growth)

**Answer 13-25.** B

A diagnostic evaluation for growth failure should be pursued in a child whose height percentile differs largely from that of his or her mid-parental height, in a child who is falling from his or her growth channel, or in a child whose height is > 3 standard deviations below the mean height for age. Pathologic causes of poor growth and short stature include various endocrinopathies, including growth hormone deficiency, thyroid hormone deficiency, and glucocorticoid excess. IGF-1 and IGFBP-3 are the screening laboratory tests of choice in the evaluation of growth hormone deficiency. IGF-1 and IGFBP-3 are proteins made by the liver and are growth hormone dependent. Growth hormone levels can be measured during provocative stimulation testing to evaluate for growth hormone deficiency. However, random growth hormone levels should not be drawn as a screen for growth hormone deficiency since growth hormone is secreted in a pulsatile manner.

The rest of the choices are various screening tests that may be done during the evaluation of a child with growth failure and short stature (Table 515-2). Thyroid function testing (free $T_4$ and thyroid-stimulating hormone [TSH]) should be drawn to screen for hypothyroidism. Children with celiac disease can sometimes present with no gastrointestinal symptoms (eg, diarrhea, constipation, or abdominal pain) but only with poor growth and short stature. A tissue transglutaminase IgA antibody should be obtained to screen for celiac disease. A sedimentation rate and complete blood cell count are useful to screen for anemia and inflammatory bowel disease. The patient has already had a normal female karyotype, which rules out the diagnosis of Turner syndrome.

(Section 28 – Chapter 515: Growth and Growth Impairment, Heading: The Diagnostic Evaluation of a Child with Short Stature)

**TABLE 515-2.** Screening Tests for Children with Growth Failure

| Test | Purpose |
|---|---|
| Complete blood cell count with erythrocyte sedimentation rate (ESR) | Screening test for inflammatory bowel disease with anemia and elevated ESR |
| Renal function tests (urine, pH, and specific gravity; urea nitrogen; serum creatinine; carbon dioxide; and electrolytes) | Exclude chronic renal failure with acidosis; exclude renal tubular disease |
| Serum calcium, phosphorus, and alkaline phosphatase | Screening tests for rickets |
| Serum free thyroxine and thyroid-stimulating hormone | Exclude hypothyroidism not apparent at physical examination |
| Insulin-like growth factor-1 and insulin-like growth factor-binding protein-3 | Growth hormone deficiency unlikely if normal |
| Tissue transglutaminase IgA antibody; IgA level | Exclude celiac disease |
| Karyotype (done in all short girls) | Excludes Turner syndrome not apparent at physical examination |
| Radiographs of hand and wrist | Determine bone age, which is delayed in hypopituitarism and most other causes of growth failure; not delayed in bone dysplasia |

Mark W. Kline, *Rudolph's Pediatrics*, 23rd Edition. Copyright © McGraw-Hill Education. All rights reserved.

**Answer 13-26.** E

Based on the family history and physical exam, the patient most likely has complete androgen insensitivity syndrome (Table 532-1). Females with this condition have a mutation in the androgen receptor. Therefore, testosterone levels are elevated, but affected individuals lack physical signs of androgen exposure, such as acne, oily skin, pubic hair, and axillary hair. Testosterone is aromatized to estrogen, which results in normal breast development. This patient has signs of estrogen exposure but not androgen exposure. The karyotype in individuals with complete androgen insensitivity is 46,XY. Patients with complete androgen insensitivity syndrome are phenotypically female and identify themselves as female. Amenorrhea occurs due to lack of a uterus, which does not develop due to production of anti-Müllerian hormone from the intra-abdominal testicles. Infants with complete androgen insensitivity syndrome may present with an inguinal hernia. Because it is X-linked, her younger sister may also have this condition. Individuals with partial androgen insensitivity have a wide clinical phenotype with variable degrees of masculinization.

Testosterone would be elevated for a female but normal for a male, and estradiol would be at a normal pubertal level for a female. LH and FSH are helpful in evaluating for primary

**TABLE 532-1.** Classification of Disorders of Sexual Development (DSD)

| |
|---|
| **46,XX DSD–Disorders of Ovarian Development** |
| XX ovotesticular DSD |
| 46,XX testicular DSD (*SRY* gene translocation, duplicate *SOX9*) |
| 46,XX gonadal dysgenesis |
| **46,XX DSD–Androgen Excess** |
| Congenital adrenal hyperplasia (21-hydroxylase deficiency, 11-hydroxylase deficiency, 3β-hydroxysteroid dehydrogenase deficiency) |
| Aromatase deficiency |
| P450 oxidoreductase deficiency |
| Maternal source (ingestion of progestins or androgens, virilizing adrenocortical tumors, ovarian tumors, luteomas) |
| **46,XY DSD–Disorders of Testicular Development** |
| Complete gonadal dysgenesis (Swyer syndrome) |
| Partial gonadal dysgenesis (including camptomelic dysplasia, Denys-Drash, Frasier syndrome) |
| Gonadal regression or vanishing testes syndrome |
| XY ovotesticular DSD |
| **46,XY DSD–Disorders of Androgen Synthesis or Action** |
| Complete or partial androgen insensitivity syndrome |
| Testosterone biosynthesis enzyme defects: 7-dehydrocholesterol reductase deficiency–Smith-Lemli-Opitz syndrome, StAR deficiency, P450scc deficiency, 3β-hydroxysteroid dehydrogenase type II deficiency, 17α-hydroxylase deficiency, 17,20-lyase deficiency, type III 17β-hydroxysteroid dehydrogenase deficiency |
| Persistent Müllerian duct syndrome |
| Leydig cell aplasia or hypoplasia |
| 5α-Reductase deficiency |
| Environmental factors |
| Syndromic associations |
| **Sex Chromosome DSD** |
| Turner syndrome (45,X) |
| Klinefelter syndrome (47,XXY) |
| Mosaic karyotypes including 45,X/46,XY, 46,XX/46,XY |

Mark W. Kline, *Rudolph's Pediatrics*, 23rd Edition. Copyright © McGraw-Hill Education. All rights reserved.

versus secondary gonadal problems (elevated in primary gonadal dysfunction and low in secondary causes). However, a karyotype would be the most helpful test in this clinical scenario.

(Section 28 – Chapter 532: Disorders of Sexual Development, Heading: Androgen Receptor Defects)

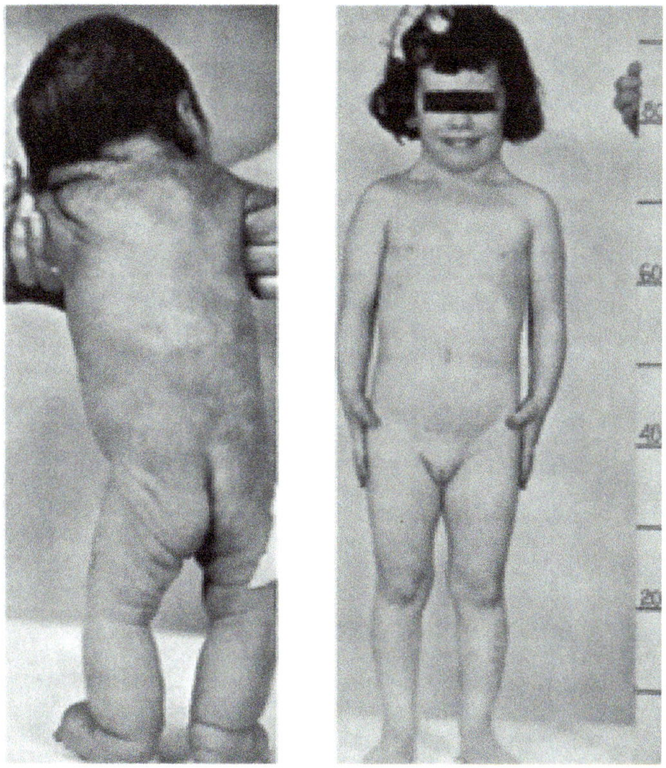

A B

**FIGURE 532-4.** Patient with 45,X Turner syndrome. **A:** Appearance at 7 days of age shows massive lymphedema of lower extremities, webbed neck, puffiness of hands, and loose folds of skin over nape of neck. Dressing covers site of skin biopsy. **B:** At 4 years of age, patient has webbed neck, broad chest, and microthelia. (Reproduced with permission from Grumbach MM, Barr ML. Cytologic tests of chromosomal sex in relation to sexual anomalies in man. *Recent Prog Horm Res.* 1958;14:255-324.)

## Answer 13-27. C

Based on the history and physical exam, the patient has Turner syndrome, which occurs in about 1 in 2000 females. Short stature is universal in this condition, and > 90% of girls require hormone replacement to initiate and progress through puberty due to gonadal dysgenesis. The description of the patient includes many classic features of Turner syndrome. Additional features of Turner syndrome are noted in Figure 532-4 and Figure 532-5. Girls with Turner syndrome are prone to recurrent otitis media and conductive and sensorineural hearing loss. The mean intelligence quotient (IQ) of girls with Turner syndrome is normal, but they often have difficulties in mathematics, multitasking, and social interactions. Because the patient is 14 years old and has Tanner stage 2 breast development on one side, it is likely that she has primary ovarian failure.

Girls with Turner syndrome are at an increased risk for the development of autoimmune conditions, such as hypothyroidism and celiac disease. However, a TSH and tissue transglutaminase IgA antibody may be elevated but would likely not be the reason for delayed pubertal development. An IGF-1 level is an important test to screen for growth hormone deficiency. However, children with Turner syndrome are not growth hormone deficient but are

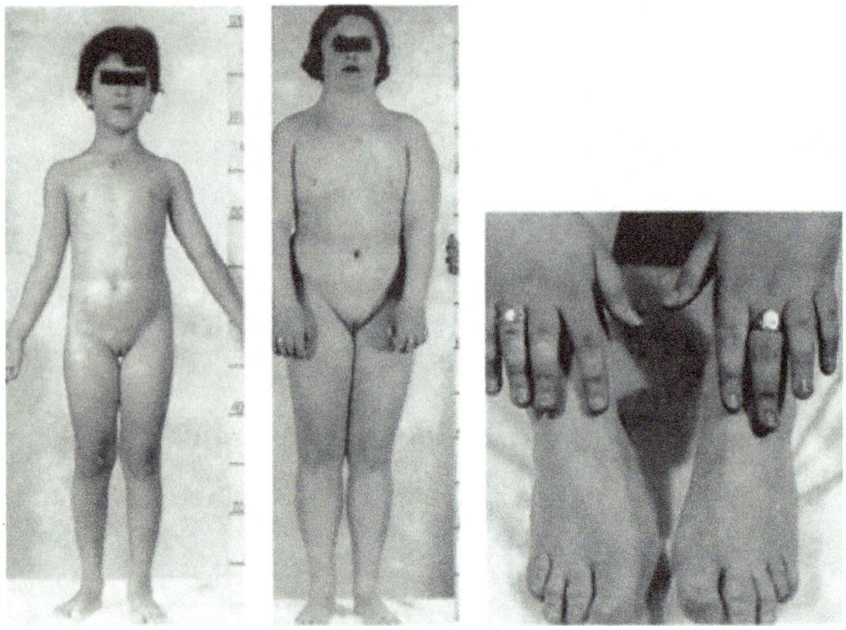

A B C

**FIGURE 532-5.** Two patients with Turner syndrome, chromatin-negative somatic nuclei, and 45,X karyotype. **A:** Age 9 years. Short stature was the presenting problem. **B:** Age 15 years. Classic features of Turner syndrome. **C:** Hands and feet of patient in B show useful clinical signs of conspicuous shortening of fourth digits caused by underdevelopment of metacarpals and metatarsals, puffiness over dorsum of digits between interphalangeal joints, convexity of nails, and prominence of pulp of finger beyond tip of fingernail. (Mark W. Kline, *Rudolph's Pediatrics*, 23rd Edition. Copyright © McGraw-Hill Education. All rights reserved.)

short due to loss of the short stature homeobox (*SHOX*) gene on the distal short arm of the X chromosome. Estradiol produced by the ovaries may be normal or low in cases of ovarian dysfunction. However, an FSH level is a more sensitive indicator of ovarian function. An elevated FSH level due to gonadal dysgenesis is frequently seen in girls with Turner syndrome before the age of 4 years and after the age of 10 years.

(Section 28 – Chapter 532: Disorders of Sexual Development, Heading: Turner Syndrome)

**Answer 13-28.** D

Klinefelter syndrome is the most common cause of primary gonadal failure in males, occurring in about 1 in 500 to 1 in 1000 males. The most common karyotype is 47,XXY. Affected individuals usually enter puberty at a normal age but are not able to progress through and complete puberty. On physical exam, pubic hair development will be normal, but the testes are firm and usually no larger than 6 mL. During puberty, gynecomastia commonly occurs in patients with Klinefelter syndrome (see figure). They may have learning and behavioral problems, but there is a wide clinical spectrum. They are similar to other men with hypogonadism in regard to job status, social adjustment, and criminal behavior. Due to dysgenesis and fibrosis of the seminiferous tubules, infertility occurs. Testosterone replacement results in increased strength, masculinity, and secondary sexual characteristics, but it does not reverse the infertility. By isolating sperm from the testis and using intracytoplasmic sperm injection, fertility can be successful.

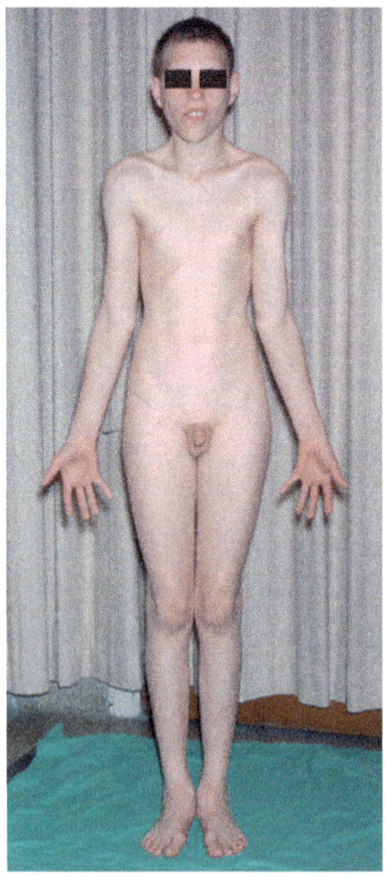

Klinefelter syndrome. (Reproduced with permission from Sarafoglou K, Hoffmann G, Roth K. *Pediatric Endocrinology and Inborn Errors of Metabolism*. New York: McGraw Hill; 2017.)

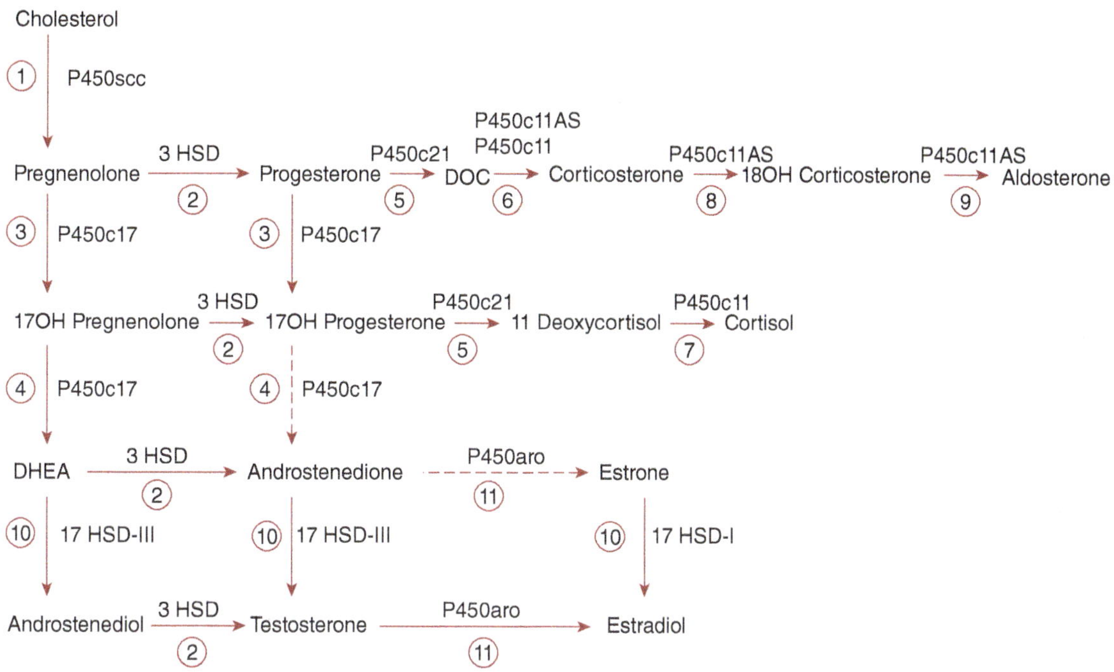


**FIGURE 524-1.** Principal pathways of human adrenal steroidogenesis. Other quantitatively and physiologically minor steroids are also produced. The names of the enzymes are shown by each reaction, and the traditional names of the enzymatic activities correspond to the *circled numbers*. (Mark W. Kline, *Rudolph's Pediatrics*, 23rd Edition. Copyright © McGraw-Hill Education. All rights reserved.)

(Section 28 – Chapter 532: Disorders of Sexual Development, Heading: Klinefelter Syndrome)

**Answer 13-29.** B

CAH due to 21-hydroxylase deficiency accounts for at least half of all cases of ambiguous genitalia in newborns. Male infants appear normal, but females have varying degrees of virilization due to in utero androgen exposure. The appearance of the external genitalia in a girl with 21-hydroxylase deficiency may be indistinguishable from a normal male with the exception of nonpalpable gonads.

Newborns with Turner, Noonan, and Klinefelter syndromes do not have ambiguous genitalia. Individuals with 5α-reductase deficiency may have ambiguous genitalia, but this condition is much less common than CAH.

(Section 28 – Chapter 532: Disorders of Sexual Development, Heading: Congenital Adrenal Hyperplasia)

**Answer 13-30.** D

The best screening test to evaluate for CAH is 17-hydroxyprogesterone. The most common cause of CAH is 21-hydroxylase (p450c21) deficiency. Due to deficiencies in this enzyme, 17-hydroxyprogesterone is not able to be converted to 11-deoxycortisol (Figure 524-1). Testosterone is a less sensitive screening marker of CAH because it may be elevated in other conditions, and it is also produced by the testes. Cortisol may be low and ACTH may be elevated in CAH, but neither are sensitive or specific screening tests to evaluate for CAH. DHEA-S is a good screening test for adrenal activation, but like the other tests, it is not a sensitive or specific test to screen for CAH. DHEA-S levels may be slightly elevated in children with premature adrenarche, and the DHEA-S level corresponds to the Tanner stage of pubertal development. Markedly elevated levels of DHEA-S would be concerning for an adrenal tumor or cancer.

(Section 28 – Chapter 526: Genetic Lesions in Steroidogenesis, Heading: 21-Hydroxylase Deficiency, Subheading: Diagnosis)

**Answer 13-31.** A

The patient is exhibiting many signs and symptoms of primary adrenal insufficiency (Table 527-1). The most common cause of adrenal insufficiency (Table 527-2) at her age is autoimmune adrenalitis or Addison disease. In primary adrenal insufficiency, low levels of cortisol stimulate the pituitary gland to secrete ACTH, which subsequently leads to increased melanocyte-stimulating hormone, causing hyperpigmentation in the creases of the hands, buccal mucosa, knuckles, knees, and old scars.

The most common form of adrenoleukodystrophy is X-linked, and therefore, the disease occurs in males. Adrenal insufficiency occurs due to buildup and deposition of very-long-chain fatty acids in the adrenal glands, which also occurs in the brain, leading to progressive central nervous system (CNS) impairment. Salt-wasting congenital adrenal insufficiency is the most common form of adrenal insufficiency in newborns, but it would not manifest at this age. Girls with nonclassic congenital adrenal insufficiency present with hirsutism, acne, or menstrual irregularities and not symptoms of cortisol deficiency. Children with secondary adrenal insufficiency lack ACTH production. Therefore, signs

**TABLE 527-1.** Signs and Symptoms of Adrenal Insufficiency

| **Features Shared by Acute and Chronic Insufficiency** |
| --- |
| Anorexia |
| Apathy and confusion |
| Dehydration |
| Fatigue |
| Hyperkalemia |
| Hypoglycemia |
| Hyponatremia |
| Hypovolemia and tachycardia |
| Nausea and vomiting |
| Postural hypotension |
| Prolonged neonatal jaundice |
| Salt craving |
| Weakness |
| **Features of Acute Insufficiency (Adrenal Crisis)** |
| Abdominal pain |
| Fever |
| **Features of Chronic Insufficiency (Addison Disease)** |
| Decreased pubic and axillary hair |
| Diarrhea |
| Hyperpigmentation |
| Low-voltage electrocardiogram |
| Small heart on x-ray |
| Weight loss |

Mark W. Kline, *Rudolph's Pediatrics*, 23rd Edition. Copyright © McGraw-Hill Education. All rights reserved.

and symptoms of cortisol deficiency would be present, but hyperpigmentation would not be seen.

(Section 28 – Chapter 527: Adrenal Insufficiency, Heading: Chronic Primary Adrenal Insufficiency)

**Answer 13-32.** E

Plasma concentrations of cortisol and ACTH are highest in the morning and lowest in the evening. ACTH levels peak around 4:00 to 6:00 AM leading to a subsequent cortisol peak at about 8:00 AM. Therefore, a cortisol level drawn at 8:00 AM (not 4:00 PM) is the best choice as an initial screen for adrenal insufficiency. An ACTH level by itself is not helpful. If an ACTH level is elevated and cortisol is low, then this is highly suggestive of primary adrenal insufficiency. Due to the diurnal and episodic nature of ACTH and cortisol secretion, a 12-hour urine collection for cortisol would be inaccurate. A 24-hour urinary free cortisol collection and dexamethasone suppression tests are used to evaluate for cortisol excess or Cushing syndrome.

(Section 28 – Chapter 524: The Adrenal Cortex, Heading: Regulation of Cortisol Secretion; Chapter 525: Evaluation of Adrenal Function, Heading: Plasma Steroids; Chapter 527: Adrenal Insufficiency, Heading: Chronic Primary Adrenal Insufficiency)

**TABLE 527-2.** Causes of Adrenal Insufficiency

| **Primary Adrenal Insufficiency** |
| --- |
| Congenital adrenal hyperplasia (CAH) |
| Autoimmune disorders |
| Autoimmune adrenalitis |
| Autoimmune polyglandular syndromes |
| Adrenal hypoplasia congenita |
| X-linked adrenal hypoplasia |
| Other (*SF1*, IMAGe syndrome) |
| ACTH resistance syndromes |
| Familial glucocorticoid deficiencies, types 1 and 2 |
| Triple A (Allgrove) syndrome |
| Metabolic disorders |
| Adrenoleukodystrophy |
| Peroxisome biogenesis disorders (eg, Zellweger) |
| Cholesterol metabolism (Smith-Lemli-Opitz, Wolman) |
| Mitochondrial (Kearns-Sayre, mitochondrial deletions) |
| Infectious disorders |
| Sepsis |
| Tuberculosis |
| Fungal infections |
| Viral |
| Infiltrative/destructive causes |
| Hemorrhage |
| Amyloidosis, sarcoidosis, metastases |
| Drugs inhibiting steroid biosynthesis |
| **Secondary Adrenal Insufficiency** |
| Hypothalamic tumors, radiation, or surgery |
| Hypopituitarism |
| Isolated ACTH insufficiency |
| Defects in POMC synthesis and processing |
| Withdrawal from glucocorticoid therapy |

ACTH, adrenocorticotropic hormone; POMC, proopiomelanocortin.

Mark W. Kline, *Rudolph's Pediatrics*, 23rd Edition. Copyright © McGraw-Hill Education. All rights reserved.

**Answer 13-33.** C

The 2 most common early signs and symptoms of Cushing syndrome in children are weight gain and growth failure (Table 528-2). The classic cushingoid appearance of cortisol excess described in adults of striae, moon facies, plethora, buffalo hump/fat pad, hypertension, and muscle weakness often take several years to manifest in children. Most children who are overweight are tall, as weight is a very strong driver of linear growth in childhood. Hormone causes of linear growth failure include cortisol excess, growth hormone deficiency, and profound hypothyroidism.

(Section 28 – Chapter 528: Adrenal Excess, Heading: Cushing Syndrome and Disease, Subheading: Clinical Findings and Diagnosis)

**Answer 13-34.** A

It is difficult to predict who may have problems with suppression of the hypothalamic-pituitary-adrenal axis after glucocorticoid therapy. Some individuals are able to recover their hypothalamic-pituitary-adrenal axis quickly after receiving high doses of glucocorticoids over short or long periods of time, whereas others may take several weeks or months to recover. Steroid withdrawal symptoms include lethargy, fatigue, nausea, and anorexia. When glucocorticoids have been used for < 10 days, therapy can typically be discontinued without concern for withdrawal symptoms. However, for the 5-year-old girl with a brain tumor who was treated with dexamethasone for 6 weeks, she will likely have withdrawal symptoms if the glucocorticoid is abruptly stopped without a gradual wean. Furthermore, dexamethasone is a very potent, long-acting glucocorticoid compared to other steroids.

(Section 28 – Chapter 529: Glucocorticoid Therapy and Withdrawal, Heading: Withdrawal of Glucocorticoid Therapy)

**TABLE 528-2.** Signs and Symptoms in Children with Cushing Disease

| Sign/Symptom | % of Patients (n = 39) |
|---|---|
| Weight gain | 92 |
| Growth failure | 84 |
| Osteopenia | 74 |
| Fatigue | 67 |
| Hypertension | 63 |
| Delayed or arrested puberty | 60 |
| Plethora | 46 |
| Acne | 46 |
| Hirsutism | 46 |
| Compulsive behavior | 44 |
| Striae | 36 |
| Bruising | 28 |
| Buffalo hump | 28 |
| Headache | 26 |
| Delayed bone age | 13 |
| Nocturia | 8 |

Mark W. Kline, *Rudolph's Pediatrics*, 23rd Edition. Copyright © McGraw-Hill Education. All rights reserved.

**Answer 13-35.** B

The patient has classic signs and symptoms of new-onset diabetes mellitus, including decreased energy, polydipsia, polyuria, and weight loss. The patient is not in diabetic ketoacidosis, which is defined by hyperglycemia with a venous pH < 7.3 or a serum bicarbonate concentration < 15 mEq/L. Hyperglycemia causes a factitious hyponatremia. The corrected sodium can be estimated by adding 1.6 mEq to the measured value for each 100 mg/dL of blood glucose above normal. With the patient's blood sugar of 892 mg/dL, this is 8 times higher than a normal blood sugar of 100 mg/dL. Therefore, $8 \times 1.6 = 12.8$. If this value is added to the measured sodium of 127 mEq/L, the corrected sodium is normal at 140 mEq/L.

Hyperkalemia is commonly seen in new-onset diabetes and results from hydrogen ions moving intracellularly and displacing potassium to the extracellular space. The hyperkalemia will improve with hydration, insulin, and correction of the acidosis. An elevated WBC count is commonly seen as a stress reaction and positively correlates with the degree of illness. Patients with SIADH will have decreased urine output and not increased urination.

(Section 28 – Chapter 537: Diabetes Mellitus, Heading: Fluid Therapy)

**Answer 13-36.** D

The patient has new-onset diabetes and is presenting in diabetic ketoacidosis (DKA). The goals of treatment of DKA are to restore perfusion, arrest ketone production, replace electrolyte losses, and avoid complications. The first line of treatment is to restore perfusion by giving NaCl (0.9%) at 20 mL/kg in the first 1 to 2 hours. After the initial fluid bolus, IV fluids should be given based on a rehydration plan accounting for the degree of dehydration and maintenance fluid requirement. Insulin should be started as an insulin drip at 0.1 units/kg/h as a continuous infusion only after the initial fluid expansion is completed. A bolus of insulin is unnecessary and should be avoided because this could precipitously drop the serum blood sugar as well as increase the risk of cerebral edema. Bicarbonate is not indicated in this clinical scenario and would increase the potential risk for complications.

(Section 28 – Chapter 537: Diabetes Mellitus, Heading: Fluid Therapy)

**Answer 13-37.** D

A serious and potentially life-threatening complication of DKA is cerebral edema. Because this patient is younger than 5 years old and received a large volume of fluids upon presentation (100 mL/kg), she is at high risk for cerebral edema. Cerebral edema typically occurs 4 to 12 hours after starting treatment, but it can occur later or even before treatment has started. Many, if not all, patients with DKA have some degree of cerebral edema, but most are asymptomatic. Case reports have shown some benefit with mannitol. Close monitoring and rapid recognition of cerebral edema may result in positive outcomes.

Treatment and clinical decision-making should not be delayed for the results of a head CT scan. Bicarbonate is not indicated and would increase the likelihood of cerebral edema. Intubation is not necessary unless respiratory compromise is present. Hyperventilation has been associated with poor outcomes in patients with cerebral edema. Besides mannitol, other early intervention measures include reduction in the IV fluid rate and elevation of the head of the bed.

(Section 28 – Chapter 537: Diabetes Mellitus, Heading: Cerebral Edema in Diabetic Ketoacidosis)

**Answer 13-38.** A

Although her blood sugar is elevated at 315 mg/dL, she is not in diabetic ketoacidosis (DKA) because her bicarbonate level is normal. Because she is not vomiting, she can drink oral sugar-free fluids to hydrate and eliminate the ketones. Supplemental insulin will help her to stop making ketones.

If she was not able to drink or was actively vomiting, then IV fluids or admission to the hospital might be necessary. Children with diabetes should check their blood sugar at least 4 times per day, specifically before breakfast, lunch, supper, and bedtime. Blood sugar testing should be performed more frequently during an illness. When a child with diabetes is ill, ketones should be checked with each void.

(Section 28 – Chapter 537: Diabetes Mellitus, Heading: Sick Day Management)

**Answer 13-39.** E

Diabetic ketoacidosis (DKA) occurs when there is a critical net effective deficit of insulin in the body. Without insulin, counterregulatory hormones rise, adipocytes release free fatty acids, and hepatic fatty acid oxidation increases, resulting in ketone body production. Insulin pumps only deliver short-acting insulin, and there is no long-acting or background insulin present to suppress ketone production. If a patient with diabetes is without insulin for several hours, ketones will be present in the blood and urine. If this is not recognized quickly, ketone bodies will rise and DKA may occur.

Children with diabetes cannot eat themselves into DKA. For the patients in answer choices A and B, their blood sugar will be elevated, but they will not develop ketones as long as they have received their long-acting insulin. For the patient in answer choice C, ketones should not develop if she is off her insulin pump for only 1 hour. Blood sugar is affected by insulin, food, and activity. For the patient in answer choice D, it is appropriate for her to take less insulin to compensate for the increased physical activity. This decrease in insulin will lower her risk of hypoglycemia and should not result in ketone production. Increased physical activity can be countered by either decreasing the insulin dose or increasing carbohydrate consumption.

(Section 28 – Chapter 537: Diabetes Mellitus, Heading: Diabetic Ketoacidosis, Subheading: Pathophysiology )

**Answer 13-40.** B

Lipohypertrophy is due to repeated insulin injections in the same area of the skin. If insulin is injected into areas of lipohypertrophy, absorption of insulin becomes erratic and unpredictable, which leads to inconsistent and difficult-to-regulate blood sugars. Although the patient noted that he is using his abdomen, arms, and legs for insulin injections, he is likely predominantly using just both sides of his abdomen. Lipohypertrophy can be avoided by rotating insulin injection sites and using all available areas, such as the upper arms, thighs, abdomen, hips, and buttocks. The best recommendation for this patient is to rotate his insulin injection sites and avoid the hypertrophied areas until it resolves. Rotation of injection sites will allow for more reliable and predictable insulin absorption.

Switching to a different type of insulin or changing to a pump would not be helpful because all insulin can cause lipohypertrophy due to repeated injections in the same area. The patient is already checking his blood sugar at least 4 to 6 times a day, which is appropriate. Referral to a dermatologist is not necessary. Rare skin findings in a diabetic patient that might be seen by a dermatologist include necrobiosis lipoidica diabeticorum.

(Section 28 – Chapter 537: Diabetes Mellitus, Heading: Skin Problems)

**Answer 13-41.** D

Genetics plays an important role in the risk and development of type 2 diabetes. Siblings of affected individuals with type 2 diabetes have a 3.5 times higher risk of developing diabetes than the general population. In studies of monozygotic twins, there is a concordance of 80% to 100% for type 2 diabetes, which is greater than twice the concordance rate for type 1 diabetes. Obese individuals commonly have elevated insulin levels, but metformin is not always necessary, especially if the patient does not have diabetes. Lifestyle modifications, specifically decreased caloric intake and regular exercise, are the first steps to improve hyperinsulinism, insulin resistance, and obesity. DKA is more commonly seen in type 1 diabetes, but it can also occur in type 2 diabetes due to severe insulin deficiency and β-cell dysfunction from prolonged elevated blood sugar levels. The average age of diagnosis of type 2 diabetes corresponds to the peak of adolescent growth and development, which occurs later than 10 years. Type 2 diabetes is most commonly seen in Native Americans, Asians, African Americans, and Hispanics.

(Section 28 – Chapter 537: Diabetes Mellitus, Heading: Genetic Considerations)

**Answer 13-42.** A

The patient has new-onset diabetes based on her symptoms and elevated random plasma glucose. The diagnostic criteria for diabetes includes symptoms of diabetes and a casual plasma glucose ≥ 200 mg/dL; fasting plasma glucose ≥ 126 mg/dL; 2-hour plasma glucose ≥ 200 mg/dL during an oral glucose tolerance test; or a hemoglobin A1c ≥ 6.5%. If the patient is asymptomatic, then the test needs to be repeated on a second day to confirm the diagnosis. It is sometimes difficult to determine whether a patient has type 1 or type 2 diabetes because obesity is increasing in all populations in the United States. Because she has a history of obesity, is from a high-risk ethnic population, and has signs of insulin resistance (acanthosis nigricans), she most likely has type 2 diabetes. Regardless of whether she has type 1 or type 2 diabetes, she should be started on insulin injections due to her markedly elevated hemoglobin A1c value of 9.8%. She also has moderate ketones in her urine, which is a sign of insulin deficiency. Due to glucose toxicity and β-cell dysfunction, neither metformin nor a sulfonylurea alone would be effective at this time. The patient has a normal bicarbonate level; therefore, she does not have diabetic ketoacidosis (DKA) and does not need to be started on IV fluids or an insulin drip. Referral to a dietitian would be helpful, but this is not the best initial management to improve her blood sugar control.

(Section 28 – Chapter 537: Diabetes Mellitus, Heading: Treatment of Type 2 Diabetes, Subheading: Insulin)

**Answer 13-43.** E

Type 1 diabetes involves autoimmune destruction of β cells, and diabetic autoantibodies can be assayed as a reflection of β-cell damage. Anti-insulin, islet cell, glutamic acid decarboxylase, and zinc transporter 8 antibodies are commonly present in type 1 diabetes. Diabetic autoantibodies are uncommon in type 2 diabetes (Table 537-4). Blood glucose and hemoglobin A1c will both be elevated in new-onset diabetes and, therefore, are not helpful in differentiating the type of diabetes. Due to glucose toxicity to β cells in type 2 diabetes and β-cell injury in type 1 diabetes, C-peptide and insulin levels may be low in both conditions at diagnosis.

**TABLE 537-4.** Typical Characteristics of Most Frequent Types of Pediatric Diabetes

| | Type 1 Diabetes | Type 2 Diabetes | Maturity-Onset Diabetes of the Young |
|---|---|---|---|
| Age at onset | 6 months to adulthood | More common after puberty | Any |
| Predominant race or ethnicity | White (slight) | Hispanic, African American, American Pacific Islander, American Indian | Any |
| Predominant sex | Males (slight) | Females (slight) | Equal |
| Onset | Acute | Subtle to acute | Subtle |
| Diabetic ketoacidosis at onset | Up to 40% | Possible | Rare |
| Incidental finding | Rare | Common | Common |
| Obesity | As in the population | 90% | As in the population |
| Associated conditions | May have other autoimmune diseases | May have other components of metabolic syndrome | May have diseases associated with specific mutation |
| Islet autoimmunity | Present | Absent | Absent |
| Insulin secretion at onset | Low | Usually elevated | Low-normal |
| Insulin secretion after onset | Noticeable decline over first 1–2 years | Slow decline over many years | No decline |
| Insulin resistance | No | Yes | No |
| Percentage of probands with affected first-degree relative | 5–10% | 80% | 90% |
| Mode of inheritance | Polygenic | Polygenic | Autosomal dominant |
| Diagnostic genetic defect | No | No | Yes |

Mark W. Kline, *Rudolph's Pediatrics*, 23rd Edition. Copyright © McGraw-Hill Education. All rights reserved.

Ketones are a reflection of insulin deficiency and can be present in both conditions as well.

(Section 28 – Chapter 537: Diabetes Mellitus, Heading: Type 1 Diabetes, Subheading: Etiology and Pathogenesis)

**Answer 13-44.** E

The laboratory results in the critical sample are consistent with exogenous insulin administration (or factitious hyperinsulinism). The growth hormone and cortisol levels are appropriately elevated in the setting of hypoglycemia. Patients with sulfonylurea ingestion or an insulinoma would have a detectable C-peptide level since the hypoglycemia results from endogenous insulin release. Prior to decreasing the IV fluid rate, her glucose infusion rate (GIR) was only 1.4 mg/kg/min [(5 × 20 × 0.167)/12 = 1.4 mg/kg/min]. The normal GIR in healthy infants and young children is approximately 6 mg/kg/min. Therefore, her GIR was not elevated before the hypoglycemic events. Children with congenital hyperinsulinism require much higher GIRs to maintain normal blood sugar levels. Because the child is only 2 years old, it is likely that a caregiver is giving her exogenous insulin. A careful history of who in the family has access to insulin and syringes should be solicited.

(Section 28 – Chapter 538: Endocrine Cause of Hypoglycemia, Heading: Factitious Hyperinsulinism [Drug-Induced Hypoglycemia])

**Answer 13-45.** B

This child likely has growth hormone deficiency. On exam, he has midline abnormalities, including a cleft lip and cleft palate, and a micropenis. Children with a cleft lip and palate have a much higher incidence of growth hormone deficiency than children who do not have a cleft lip or palate. In the first few months of life, growth hormone is essential for maintenance of normal blood sugar, and it does not become important for linear growth until about 9 months.

Congenital hyperinsulinism is the most common cause of persistent hypoglycemia in the newborn. Infants with congenital hyperinsulinism are often born large for gestational age. Perinatal stress-induced hyperinsulinism, which occurs in about 10% of small-for-gestational-age infants, is a transient state that can last for a few days or up to a few months or more of life. However, in this case, the infant has an appropriate-for-gestational-age birth weight. Gonadotropins may be deficient in children with midline abnormalities and a micropenis, but this would not be responsible for hypoglycemia. Other pituitary hormone deficiencies that can cause hypoglycemia include adrenocorticotropic hormone (ACTH) deficiency, which results in cortisol deficiency. Infants with Beckwith-Wiedemann syndrome can have hypoglycemia from transient hyperinsulinism, but they do not have a cleft lip, cleft palate, or micropenis.

(Section 28 – Chapter 538: Endocrine Cause of Hypoglycemia, Heading: Growth Hormone Deficiency)

**Answer 13-46.** C

With the infant's history of hypoglycemia and maternal history of eclampsia and hypertension, the infant most likely has a transient form of hyperinsulinism due to perinatal stress. Infants with glucose infusion rates of > 10 mg/kg/min likely have either hyperinsulinism or hypopituitarism. In hyperinsulinism, glycogenolysis is suppressed and glycogen stores are inappropriately not depleted in the setting of hypoglycemia. In this patient, a rise in the plasma glucose of > 30 mg/dL after administration of glucagon indicates inappropriate stores of glycogen at the time of hypoglycemia and is diagnostic of hyperinsulinism. Diazoxide inhibits insulin secretion by activating the opening of the $K_{ATP}$ channel in the β cell (Figure 538-4) and is the initial treatment of choice in infants with hyperinsulinism. Adverse effects of diazoxide include fluid retention and hypertrichosis. Octreotide is a long-acting analog of somatostatin that inhibits insulin release from β cells, but this medication is used only if diazoxide is ineffective. Nifedipine is a calcium channel blocker that has been used in infants with hyperinsulinism but is generally not effective. Growth hormone and hydrocortisone would be indicated if the child has hypopituitarism.

(Section 28 – Chapter 538: Endocrine Cause of Hypoglycemia, Heading: Perinatal Stress-Induced Hyperinsulinism)

**Answer 13-47.** C

The most concerning symptom is that the child is waking up from sleep to drink and urinate. Psychogenic polydipsia is a behavioral problem that leads to compulsive water drinking. Behavioral problems of increased drinking manifest during the daytime when the child is awake but not during the night. Normal children can have primary polydipsia where they drink large volumes of fluid during the day, leading to volume overload and increased urination. Young children may use drinking as a way to get their parent's attention, and they will be upset if the fluids are restricted. However, waking up at night to drink and urinate points to a more pathologic condition, such as diabetes insipidus or diabetes mellitus.

(Section 28 – Chapter 518: Primary Disturbances in Water Homeostasis, Heading: Diagnosis of Diabetes Insipidus)

**Answer 13-48.** B

The differential diagnosis of polyuria and polydipsia includes diabetes mellitus, diabetes insipidus, psychogenic, hypercalcemia, hypokalemia, and hyperthyroidism. Initial screening labs were unremarkable except for a low urine specific gravity. After a water deprivation test, the patient was able to appropriately concentrate her urine, and her serum sodium and osmolality were normal. These labs are most consistent with psychogenic polydipsia or compulsive water drinking.

The SIADH would present with decreased urine output and hyponatremia. After a prolonged fast, patients with

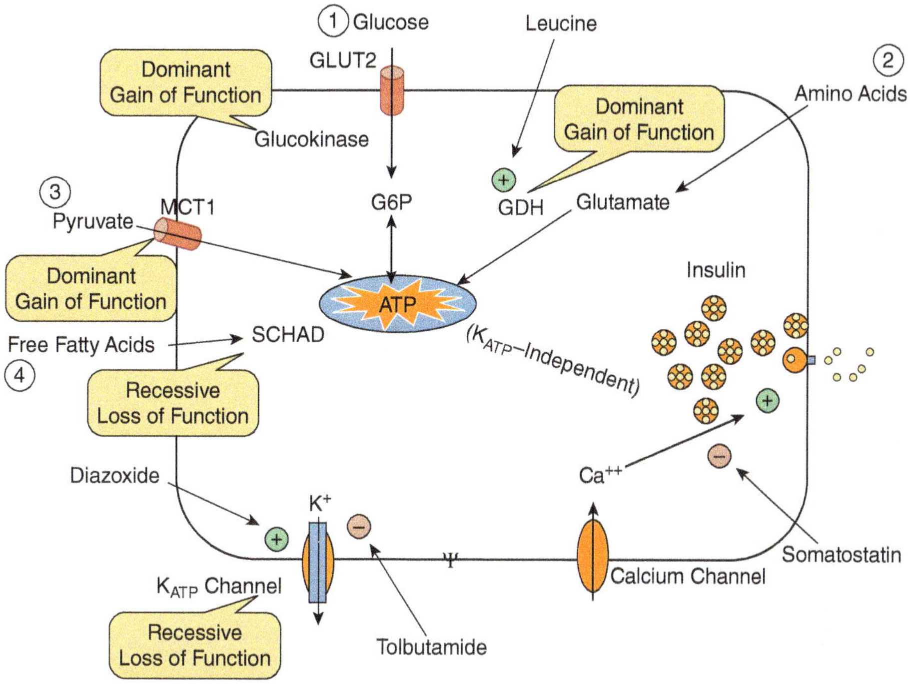


**FIGURE 538-4.** Diagram of insulin secretion and sites of defects leading to congenital hyperinsulinism. Glucose enters the β-cell via GLUT-1 and GLUT-2 transporters and is phosphorylated by glucokinase, the glucosensor of the β-cell. Further metabolism leads to an increase in the ATP-to-ADP ratio, closure of the $K_{ATP}$ channel, β-cell membrane depolarization, opening of voltage-dependent calcium channels, calcium influx, and ultimately insulin secretion. This process is referred to as the $K_{ATP}$ channel-dependent pathway. Amino acids also stimulate insulin secretion through the $K_{ATP}$ channel-dependent pathway via glutamic dehydrogenase (GDH). This process occurs through oxidation of the amino acid, glutamate, by GDH which is allosterically activated by the amino acid leucine. Free fatty acids do not act as direct fuels for insulin secretion. Pyruvate is not normally a fuel-stimulant for insulin secretion. A $K_{ATP}$ channel-independent pathway for insulin secretion also exists. Glucokinase, the $K_{ATP}$ channel, GDH, SCHAD, and monocarboxylate transporter 1 (MCT1, a pyruvate transporter not normally present on the β-cell) are all sites of defects responsible for congenital hyperinsulinism. Sulfonylureas, such as tolbutamide or glyburide, enhance insulin secretion by inhibiting the $K_{ATP}$ channel, whereas diazoxide, a drug used to treat hyperinsulinism, suppresses insulin secretion by activating the $K_{ATP}$ channel. Somatostatin suppresses insulin secretion downstream of calcium entry. (Mark W. Kline, *Rudolph's Pediatrics*, 23rd Edition. Copyright © McGraw-Hill Education. All rights reserved.)

either nephrogenic or central diabetes insipidus would have hypernatremia, hyperosmolality, and an inability to concentrate their urine. Patients with cerebral salt wasting have increased urine output and hyponatremia.

(Section 28 – Chapter 518: Primary Disturbances in Water Homeostasis, Heading: Primary Polydipsia and Hyponatremia without Elevated Vasopressin Secretion)

## Answer 13-49. A

The patient is currently in the second phase of the triphasic response, which commonly occurs after neurosurgery or trauma. The first phase is a transient diabetes insipidus state due to loss of regulation of vasopressin release after neuronal damage. This phase can last for 12 hours or up to several days. The second phase is due to uncontrolled vasopressin release by dying neurons that produce vasopressin, which creates the syndrome of inappropriate antidiuretic hormone (SIADH). This phase can last for a couple of days or up to a couple of weeks. The third phase is due to complete vasopressin deficiency from neuronal death, which results in permanent diabetes insipidus. SIADH is best treated with fluid restriction. Therefore, the best initial management in this patient is to decrease the IV fluid rate.

Hypertonic saline is not part of the initial management of SIADH, and it is only indicated if the patient has acute neurologic symptoms (eg, seizures). Furosemide is also not used in the initial treatment of SIADH. A vasopressin drip would be indicated in a patient with diabetes insipidus and not SIADH. Oral salt supplementation is used in patients with cerebral salt wasting and not SIADH. Cerebral salt wasting and SIADH are sometimes difficult to differentiate as both have hyponatremia. However, in cerebral salt wasting, urine output is increased and urine sodium is more elevated (> 100 mEq/L) than in SIADH.

(Section 28 – Chapter 518: Primary Disturbances in Water Homeostasis, Heading: Treatment of Inappropriate Antidiuretic Hormone Secretion)

## Answer 13-50. B

Unlike other pituitary hormones, prolactin secretion is tonically inhibited by dopamine. With any disruption in the pituitary stalk, prolactin levels will be elevated. The pituitary

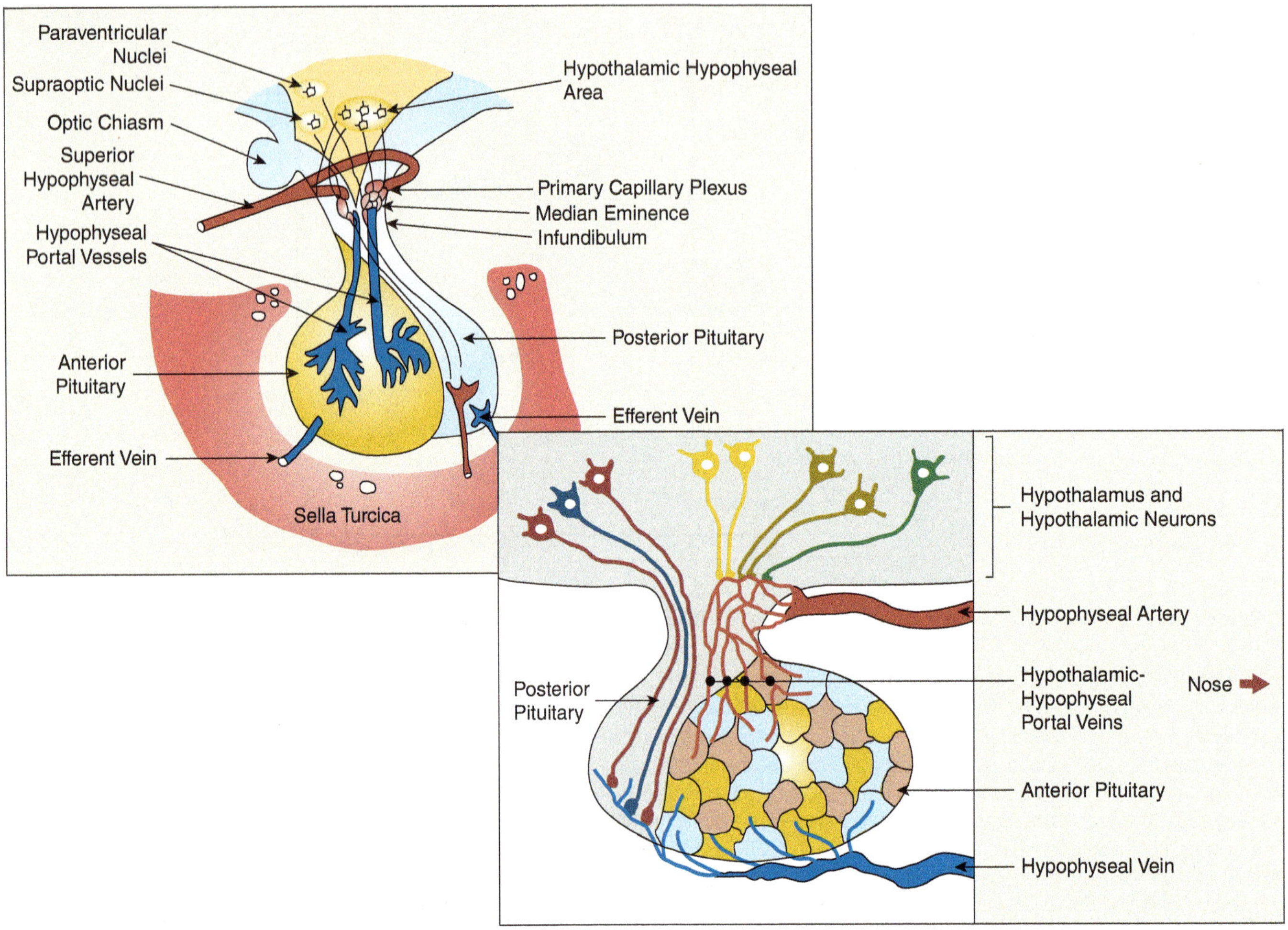


**FIGURE 514-2.** Anatomy of the fully developed pituitary gland with its anterior and posterior parts and the intricate neural and vascular network connecting it to the hypothalamus. (Mark W. Kline, Rudolph's Pediatrics, 23rd Edition. Copyright © McGraw-Hill Education. All rights reserved.)

is connected by a stalk to the hypothalamus (Figure 514-2). Disruption of the stalk results in a decrease in communication between the hypothalamus and pituitary gland. Therefore, growth hormone will be decreased, leading to decreased IGF-1 production; thyroid-stimulating hormone (TSH) will be decreased, leading to decreased free $T_4$ production; and luteinizing hormone (LH) will be decreased, leading to decreased testosterone production. Cortisol may initially be increased due to stress and illness, but it may also be decreased from adrenocorticotropic hormone (ACTH) deficiency.

(Section 28 – Chapter 514: The Anterior Pituitary Gland, Heading: Prolactin)

**Answer 13-51. B**

Constitutional delay is a common variation of normal growth. These patients are often labeled "late bloomers" as the timing of puberty starts at a later age than average. Although the etiology is not completely understood, there appears to be a genetic component, as one or more family members may have a similar history. Growth parameters at birth are typically normal. Between the ages of 6 months and approximately 3 years, growth velocity decreases with crossing of height percentiles downward, after which time affected children grow at a normal growth velocity along this new percentile. Because these patients often have pubertal delay, they grow for a longer period of time than their peers, typically achieving a normal height, although at the lower end of their genetic height potential. Constitutional delay is clinically more common in boys than girls, but this may be due to referral bias.

Growth hormone deficiency and hypothyroidism are endocrine causes of short stature and often present with a delayed bone age, but linear growth velocity is below normal. Children with familial short stature have normal bone ages and normal timing of puberty and achieve a final height consistent with their mid-parental height. Idiopathic short stature is a diagnosis of exclusion in an otherwise healthy child who has a height > 2.25 standard deviations below the mean for age and sex with normal growth velocity, skeletal maturity, timing of puberty, and a predicted height below mid-parental height.

(Section 28 – Chapter 515: Growth and Growth Impairment, Heading: The Case of the Child with Constitutional Delay)

**Answer 13-52.** C

Craniopharyngiomas are derived from squamous rest cell remnants of Rathke's pouch. They are the most common tumor found in the sellar region in children, accounting for 80% to 90% of sellar tumors. They are also the most common tumor causing hypopituitarism in children. Although craniopharyngiomas are benign and slow growing, by the time symptoms arise, they have often invaded local structures including the suprasellar region and sometimes the hypothalamus. The majority of affected patients have pituitary hormone deficiencies at diagnosis and are at risk for additional deficiencies as the result of further damage to the pituitary from treatment, including surgery and/or radiation. For the patient in the vignette, her symptoms are concerning for possible diabetes insipidus, growth hormone deficiency, and/or central hypothyroidism.

Germinomas are most commonly found in the pineal region, although they may also occur in the suprasellar location. Gliomas involve the optic nerve, chiasm, or hypothalamus. Meningiomas can arise in the suprasellar region, but they are more commonly found in other locations and are rare in children. Rathke's cleft cysts are benign and also arise from remnants of Rathke's pouch. The vast majority are found incidentally and do not cause symptoms, but if large, they can cause pituitary dysfunction, visual disturbance from chiasmal compression, or headaches.

(Section 28 – Chapter 516: Endocrine Abnormalities Causing Growth Impairment, Heading: Craniopharyngioma)

**Answer 13-53.** D

This girl most likely has constitutional tall stature because both of her parents are tall. Children with constitutional tall stature grow at normal height velocities at the upper range of normal or sometimes above the 97th percentile, have normal bone ages, and achieve final heights within the range of their mid-parental height. Her mid-parental height is 175 cm (or 69 inches), which is consistent with a final female height at the 97th percentile.

Exogenous obesity is a cause of growth velocity acceleration, and bone ages are often advanced. The patient's BMI is in the normal range, and she is not obese. Hyperthyroidism can cause an increase in growth velocity, but this patient has no hyperthyroid symptoms. Precocious puberty can lead to growth velocity acceleration, and bone ages are usually advanced. Final height in untreated children with precocious puberty is often short and below their genetic height potential due to premature epiphyseal fusion. Marfan syndrome is an autosomal dominant disorder with findings of tall stature, arachnodactyly, joint laxity, ectopia lentis, and aortic root dilatation. Other causes of tall stature include growth hormone excess, homocystinuria, Klinefelter syndrome, and Sotos syndrome. A complete list of causes for tall stature is shown in Table 517-1.

(Section 28 – Chapter 517: Tall Stature, Heading: Constitutional Tall Stature)

**TABLE 517-1.** Differential Diagnosis of Statural Overgrowth

| |
|---|
| Fetal overgrowth |
| Maternal diabetes mellitus |
| Cerebral gigantism (Sotos syndrome) |
| Weaver syndrome |
| Beckwith-Wiedemann syndrome |
| Other IGF-2 excess syndromes |
| Postnatal overgrowth leading to childhood tall stature |
| Familial (constitutional) tall stature |
| Exogenous obesity |
| Excess GH secretion (pituitary gigantism) |
| McCune-Albright syndrome or MEN associated with excess GH secretion |
| Precocious puberty |
| Marfan syndrome |
| Klinefelter syndrome (XXY) |
| Weaver syndrome |
| Fragile X syndrome |
| Homocystinuria |
| XYY syndrome |
| Hyperthyroidism |
| Postnatal overgrowth leading to adult tall stature |
| Androgen or estrogen deficiency/estrogen resistance (in males) |
| Testicular feminization |

GH, growth hormone; IGF-2, insulin-like growth factor-2; MEN, multiple endocrine neoplasia.

Mark W. Kline, *Rudolph's Pediatrics*, 23rd Edition. Copyright © McGraw-Hill Education. All rights reserved.

**Answer 13-54.** D

The next best step is to order a brain MRI once the diagnosis of central diabetes insipidus (CDI) is confirmed. A posterior pituitary bright spot is normally seen on an unenhanced T1-weighted MRI image. This imaging finding is thought to represent stored vasopressin, which creates a hyperintensity on MRI. Absence of the pituitary bright spot is often seen in patients with CDI. A brain MRI can identify serious underlying causes of CDI, which include brain tumors, histiocytosis, septo-optic dysplasia, and other midline defects. A list of causes of CDI is shown in Table 518-1.

An antidiuretic hormone (ADH) level is helpful prior to administering vasopressin during a water deprivation test, but not afterward. It is important to be aware that ADH levels can be misleading, as commercially available assays have poor sensitivity and there is high preanalytical instability. Patients with CDI and an intact thirst should have free access to water

**TABLE 518-1.** Causes of Central Diabetes Insipidus

| |
|---|
| **Congenital** |
| Optic nerve hypoplasia (septo-optic dysplasia) |
| Holoprosencephaly |
| Ectopic or absent pituitary |
| Other midline craniofacial defects |
| **Familial** |
| Autosomal dominant |
| Autosomal recessive |
| Wolfram syndrome (DIDMOAD)—autosomal recessive |
| **Acquired** |
| Postoperative (with triple-phase response) |
| Neoplasms |
| Craniopharyngioma |
| Germinoma |
| Pinealoma |
| Optic glioma |
| Metastatic tumors: leukemias |
| Infiltrative/autoimmune |
| Langerhans cell histiocytosis |
| Lymphocytic hypophysitis |
| Sarcoidosis |
| Trauma: transection of the stalk |
| Drugs: ethanol, phenytoin, opiate antagonists, α-adrenergics |
| Septic shock (infarction) |
| Sheehan syndrome (postpartum hemorrhage) |
| Hypoxic brain injury |
| Infectious (basal meningitis/encephalitis) |
| Aneurysm and cysts |
| Idiopathic |
| Pregnancy: increased vasopressinase |

DIDMOAD, diabetes insipidus, diabetes mellitus, optic atrophy, deafness.

Mark W. Kline, *Rudolph's Pediatrics*, 23rd Edition. Copyright © McGraw-Hill Education. All rights reserved.

because their thirst drive helps to maintain normal sodium levels. A renal ultrasound is not part of the workup for CDI, but it would be indicated in cases of nephrogenic diabetes insipidus.

(Section 28 – Chapter 518: Primary Disturbances in Water Homeostasis, Heading: Diagnosis of Central Diabetes Insipidus)

**Answer 13-55.** E

The most likely diagnosis is hypothyroidism, specifically central hypothyroidism resulting from deficient thyroid-stimulating hormone (TSH) production from the pituitary gland. A normal newborn screen does not rule out central hypothyroidism, which can be missed when TSH is used as the only newborn screening method. However, even newborn screening programs that use both TSH and thyroxine ($T_4$) can miss cases of central hypothyroidism. Thyroid hormone deficiency can result in profound growth failure after birth because thyroid hormone is essential for normal linear growth and neurodevelopment. Unrecognized and untreated hypothyroidism can result in significant developmental delay and intellectual disability. This child may have septo-optic dysplasia, which is a constellation of optic nerve hypoplasia (often seen with nystagmus), pituitary gland dysfunction, and midline brain abnormalities, such as an absent septum pellucidum or agenesis of the corpus callosum.

Growth hormone is essential for normal linear growth starting at the age of about 9 months. Because growth hormone is a counterregulatory hormone to insulin, growth hormone deficiency causes hypoglycemia during infancy. Hyperthyroidism can cause failure to thrive, but it also presents with tachycardia, hypertension, irritability, moist skin, stare, tremor, or goiter. Celiac disease and inadequate caloric intake are also possibilities, but they are less likely given the classic features of central hypothyroidism for the patient in the vignette, as well as his normal weight gain.

(Section 28 – Chapter 520: Hypothyroidism in the Infant, Heading: Central Hypothyroidism)

**Answer 13-56.** A

TBG excess is characterized by a normal TSH and an elevated total $T_4$. Estrogen glycosylates TBG, decreasing its clearance, which leads to elevated levels of TBG. Total $T_4$ circulates in the bloodstream mostly bound to TBG. Total $T_4$ measures both bound and free $T_4$. Most $T_4$ is bound, with only 0.03% circulating in the free form. Because oral contraceptive pills contain estrogen, TBG levels in this patient are elevated, leading to subsequent elevation of bound $T_4$ as well. The free $T_4$ level in this patient would be normal, and free $T_4$ is the biologically active form of $T_4$. Patients with TBG excess are euthyroid and do not have hyperthyroidism. Subclinical hyperthyroidism will have a low TSH with a normal $T_4$ level, and hypothyroidism will have a high TSH and a low $T_4$ level.

(Section 28 – Chapter 520: Hypothyroidism in the Infant, Heading: Thyroxine-Binding Globulin Excess)

**Answer 13-57.** C

Consumptive hypothyroidism can occur with large hepatic hemangiomas or hepatic hemangioendotheliomas due to ectopic production of type 3 iodothyronine deiodinase. This enzyme converts active thyroxine ($T_4$) and triiodothyronine ($T_3$) to inactive metabolites, one of which is reverse $T_3$. This infant will have a very elevated thyroid-stimulating hormone

(TSH), low $T_4$, low $T_3$, and increased reverse $T_3$. Management includes thyroid hormone replacement and treatment of the underlying vascular tumor, which is often associated with increased morbidity and mortality. Very high doses of thyroid hormone replacement are needed to return thyroid hormone levels to a normal range.

(Section 28 – Chapter 521: Acquired Hypothyroidism, Heading: Consumptive Hypothyroidism)

**Answer 13-58.** B

Hashimoto thyroiditis is the most common cause of acquired hypothyroidism in children. Nearly 5% to 10% of patients will present with an initial phase of thyrotoxicosis, termed hashitoxicosis. Inflammation and damage to the thyroid gland cause release of preformed thyroid hormone during hashitoxicosis, which typically lasts a few weeks or months. Laboratory evaluation in this phase will reveal a low TSH, normal or elevated total or free $T_4$, and normal or elevated triiodothyronine ($T_3$) levels. Both Graves' disease and Hashimoto thyroiditis can have positive thyroid peroxidase and antithyroglobulin antibodies, but TSH receptor antibody is typically negative in Hashimoto thyroiditis and positive in Graves' disease.

Subacute thyroiditis is rare in children and often preceded by an upper respiratory infection. Patients present with a painful thyroid gland with viral symptoms, such as fever, malaise, and sore throat. Inflammation from this process may cause a transient hyperthyroid phase. As this phase gradually resolves, hypothyroidism can occur, but the condition is ultimately self-limited. Acute suppurative thyroiditis occurs due to an acute bacterial infection of the thyroid gland. Patients have an acutely painful, warm, and tender thyroid accompanied by dysphagia and dysphonia. Usually patients are euthyroid, but transient thyrotoxicosis can occur. A thyroglossal duct cyst presents in the midline of the neck, and it is the result of cystic expansion of a congenital remnant from the thyroglossal tract. Patients with a thyroglossal duct cyst usually have a normally developed thyroid gland in the correct location.

(Section 28 – Chapter 522: Hyperthyroidism, Heading: Thyroiditis)

**Answer 13-59.** A

Maternal Graves' disease is the most common cause of neonatal hyperthyroidism. It is not common as there is a low incidence of thyrotoxicosis in pregnancy at 1 to 2 cases per 1000 pregnancies. Neonatal Graves' disease occurs in only about 1 in 70 of these pregnancies. Most cases occur due to high maternal titers of thyroid-stimulating immunoglobulins, which are immunoglobulin G (IgG) antibodies that readily cross the placenta from the mother to the fetus. The mother may be euthyroid due to treatment with antithyroid drugs, prior thyroidectomy, or radioactive iodine ablation.

In an infant with a known positive TSH receptor antibody or if the history of maternal Graves' disease comes to attention after birth, it is recommended to check a TSH and free $T_4$ at 3 to 5 days of life and again at 10 to 14 days of life. If thyroid function tests are normal at these times, then additional testing is not needed unless clinical symptoms of hyperthyroidism develop. Symptoms such as irritability, flushing, tachycardia, hypertension, poor weight gain, weight loss, goiter, and exophthalmos can be present at birth, but if the mother is on an antithyroid drug, symptoms may not arise until around 8 to 9 days of life. Once the diagnosis is confirmed, treatment should start quickly in a symptomatic infant. Neonatal Graves' typically resolves around 3 to 12 weeks of age as the maternal antibodies clear from the infant.

(Section 28 – Chapter 522: Hyperthyroidism, Heading: Neonatal Hyperthyroidism)

**Answer 13-60.** C

The most common cause of a pediatric thyroid nodule is a benign follicular adenoma. In children, there is a higher risk (~25%) for malignant thyroid nodules than in adults (5%). The most common thyroid malignancy in children is papillary thyroid carcinoma. When a nodule is palpated on exam, a thyroid ultrasound should be performed to provide detail on the size and characteristics of the nodule. Concerning ultrasound features include solid nodules, hypoechogenicity, microcalcifications, irregular margins, central vascularity, extrathyroidal extension, and abnormal cervical lymph nodes.

If the TSH is decreased, a thyroid uptake scan can be obtained to evaluate for a hyperfunctioning nodule. Suspicious thyroid nodules warrant FNA as the next best step in management. Results of the FNA will dictate further management (ie, whether close surveillance versus surgery is indicated). MRI or computed tomography (CT) may be helpful for identifying suspicious lymph nodes as part of the preoperative planning for thyroid surgery and lymph node dissection.

There is conflicting evidence about the use of levothyroxine suppression therapy for benign thyroid nodules in children in an attempt to reduce nodule size. However, this option is usually not recommended and contraindicated in children.

(Section 28 – Chapter 523: Other Disorders of the Thyroid, Heading: Thyroid Nodules in Children)

**Answer 13-61.** D

Initial testing for Cushing syndrome can be performed with either a low-dose dexamethasone suppression test, at least 2 measurements of 24-hour urine free cortisol, or at least 2 measurements of late-night salivary cortisol. A low-dose dexamethasone suppression test is a simple test that can be done in the outpatient setting; the patient takes 1 mg of dexamethasone orally between 11:00 PM and midnight, and a morning serum cortisol is drawn the following morning at 8:00 AM. A cortisol value of ≤ 1.8 μg/dL is a negative test and rules out Cushing syndrome.

High-dose dexamethasone suppression test is not an initial screening test, but it can be done later to determine the location of cortisol excess. Cortisol levels after a high-dose dexamethasone suppression test will be suppressed in those with Cushing disease, which is caused by excess ACTH production from the pituitary gland, but elevated in those with ectopic ACTH production from a malignant tumor. Cortisol levels after a low-dose dexamethasone suppression test will be elevated in both clinical scenarios. A random ACTH level is not recommended as an initial screen for Cushing syndrome but is obtained once the diagnosis is confirmed to determine if the cause is ACTH dependent or independent. ACTH stimulation tests are performed in the evaluation of adrenal insufficiency, but not Cushing syndrome.

(Section 28 – Chapter 525: Evaluation of Adrenal Function, Heading: Dexamethasone Suppression Test)

### Answer 13-62. C

CAH refers to a group of disorders caused by variable deficiency in one of the enzymes in the adrenal steroidogenesis pathway (Figure 524-1). The most common form of CAH is due to 21-hydroxylase deficiency, which accounts for > 90% of cases. There are different forms of 21-hydroxylase deficiency (classic salt wasting, classic simple virilizing, and nonclassic) depending on the type of mutation in the *CYP21A2* gene and degree of enzyme deficiency. 21-Hydroxylase is important for the production of cortisol and aldosterone, and those with the classic salt-wasting form need replacement of both of these hormones. A male neonate with CAH will have a normal physical exam. However, the spectrum of physical exam findings in an affected female infant with classic CAH is quite broad, ranging from clitoromegaly to a complete phenotypic male appearance. Because male infants appear normal at birth, detection of CAH on the newborn screen is crucial to prevent a salt-wasting adrenal crisis, morbidity, and death.

(Section 28 – Chapter 526: Genetic Lesions in Steroidogenesis, Heading: 21-Hydroxylase Deficiency, Subheading: Pathophysiology, Genetics, and Epidemiology)

### Answer 13-63. E

Pheochromocytoma is a catecholamine-secreting neuroendocrine tumor that most frequently arises in the adrenal medulla. Patients with MEN2A, MEN2B, neurofibromatosis type 1, and Von Hippel-Lindau disease have an increased risk for pheochromocytomas. Measurements of plasma free metanephrines or urinary fractionated metanephrines are the best initial screening tests for a pheochromocytoma, as the sensitivity is nearly 100%.

Urine homovanillic and vanillymandelic acids are metabolites of catecholamines and have inferior sensitivity compared to measurements of plasma free or urinary fractionated metanephrines. Twenty-four-hour urinary creatinine should be obtained when measuring 24-hour excretion of urinary fractionated metanephrines to verify an adequate sample collection. Chromogranin A is elevated in pheochromocytomas, but it can also be detected in carcinoid tumors, insulinomas, neuroblastomas, medullary thyroid cancer, and other neuroendocrine tumors. Although it is not an initial screening test, chromogranin A can be used to support the diagnosis in patients with an initial positive screen. Chromogranin A is a nonspecific tumor marker, and it is a useful tool in monitoring treatment efficacy and to look for disease recurrence of neuroendocrine and carcinoid tumors.

(Section 28 – Chapter 530: Endocrine Neoplasia Syndromes, Heading: Pheochromocytoma, Subheading: Diagnosis)

### Answer 13-64. D

Conditions such as celiac disease, inflammatory bowel disease, cystic fibrosis, short gut syndrome, and gastric bypass surgery can have malabsorption leading to vitamin D deficiency. The best test to screen for vitamin D deficiency is 25-hydroxyvitamin D, which is the storage and main form found in the circulation. It is produced in the liver from ergocalciferol (vitamin $D_2$) or cholecalciferol (vitamin $D_3$) by the enzyme 25-hydroxylase. 25-Hydroxyvitamin D is converted in the kidney by the enzyme 1-α-hydroxylase to 1,25-dihyroxyvitamin D (calcitriol), the active form of vitamin D. Parathyroid hormone stimulates 1-α-hydroxylase enzyme activity.

A 1,25-dihydroxyvitamin D level is difficult to measure since this form is present at very low concentrations in the circulation and has a short half-life, and it does not reflect vitamin D stores in the body. Calcium and phosphorus may be low in vitamin D deficiency because 1,25-dihydroxyvitamin D is necessary for the absorption of these minerals from the intestine. However, in less severe forms of deficiency, these values can be normal or low. Parathyroid hormone is typically elevated in vitamin D deficiency, but there are other reasons that a patient may have an elevated parathyroid hormone level.

(Section 28 – Chapter 536: Disorders of Bone Formation, Heading: Vitamin D Deficiency or Insufficiency)

### Answer 13-65. A

This child has a classic history for ketotic hypoglycemia, which typically occurs in children aged 1 to 5 years. After a period of prolonged fasting, symptomatic hypoglycemia can occur. Ketotic hypoglycemia typically presents in the morning after sleeping in with a delayed morning meal. Affected children commonly have a preceding viral illness and may have skipped or not eaten much at supper the previous evening. This condition is self-limited and typically resolves around age 8 to 9 years. It is a diagnosis of exclusion, so a critical sample should be obtained to rule out other causes. A critical sample includes laboratory specimens obtained at the time of hypoglycemia in order to assist in determining an underlying etiology. Biochemically, children with ketotic hypoglycemia will have positive ketones, so checking the urine for ketones is a diagnostic clue. This child's critical sample would have elevated serum ketones (β-hydroxybutyrate), elevated free fatty acids, and an appropriately suppressed insulin level.

Other causes of hypoglycemia include hyperinsulinism, which can be congenital or transient such as in cases of perinatal stress, small for gestational age, infants of diabetic mothers, or Beckwith-Wiedemann syndrome. Hormonal causes of hypoglycemia include growth hormone deficiency and cortisol deficiency. Hypoglycemia can occur due to late dumping syndrome in patients with prior gastric surgery, including Nissen fundoplication. Metabolic disorders, such as fatty acid oxidation defects, disorders of amino acid metabolism, disorders of glycogenolysis or gluconeogenesis, and galactosemia can also cause hypoglycemia. Thyroid disease is not a cause of hypoglycemia in children.

To diagnose hypoglycemia, it is important to satisfy Whipple's triad: (1) positive symptoms of hypoglycemia, (2) documentation of a low plasma blood glucose in the lab at the time of symptoms, and (3) administration of glucose with subsequent resolution of symptoms once the blood glucose level returns to normal.

(Section 28 – Chapter 538: Endocrine Causes of Hypoglycemia, Heading: The Critical Sample and Fasting Test)

# CHAPTER 14 | Orthopedics and Sports Medicine

Rebecca L. Carl, Sarah B. Kinsella, Natalie C. Stork, Sigrid F. Wolf, and Cynthia R. LaBella

**14-1.** Which of the following statements regarding bone development and postnatal growth is correct?

**A.** The major long bones of the upper limbs generally have 1 physis.

**B.** Endochondral ossification is characterized by the replacement of osteoblasts by chondroblasts.

**C.** Traction or distraction may decrease physeal growth.

**D.** The clavicle forms by intramembranous ossification.

**E.** The resting (germinal) zone is the weakest physeal zone.

**14-2.** A 10-month-old female infant who was recently placed in foster care presents for a well-child visit. The foster mother expresses some concern with regard to her development. She has not previously provided foster care for infants and is not sure what to expect. She reports that the child is rolling and can sit with assistance; however, the child seems wobbly. In addition, she is concerned that she is not crawling consistently yet. Which developmental motor skill is paired correctly with the average age of achievement?

**A.** Sitting independently – 5 months

**B.** Crawling – 10 months

**C.** Rolling back to front – 5 months

**D.** Pulling to a stance – 11 months

**E.** Walking independently – 12 months

**14-3.** A 2-month-old male infant presents for his well-child check. He was born at 38 weeks of gestational age to a G1P1 mother via vaginal delivery. Mom reports the pediatrician noticed his right foot was curved inward during the exam in the newborn nursery and mentioned that the infant may need further treatment to straighten the foot out. Mom is concerned because the right foot is still curved and she does not think it has changed since birth. She has been reading and is concerned her son may have other, additional abnormalities that she has not noticed yet.

On exam, the patient is well appearing and actively moving all the extremities. You notice a curved border on the lateral aspect of the right foot, whereas the left foot has a straight border. The curved appearance of the foot appears to improve as the patient stretches. Ankle motion appears symmetric. The remainder of the exam is normal. Given the patient's exam and mom's concerns, what is the next best course of action?

**A.** Order a dynamic screening hip ultrasound

**B.** Provide reassurance and plan follow-up for 4-month visit

**C.** Refer to orthopedics for stretching casts

**D.** Order a cervical spine radiograph

**E.** Provide a prescription for straight last shoes

**14-4.** An 18-month-old girl presents for concerns with her gait. Mom reports she began walking around 11 months of age and has always been very pigeon toed. Mom is concerned now because her daughter is starting to run and she feels like she trips and falls frequently. She was born at term and has otherwise been healthy. Pregnancy and delivery were uncomplicated. She has been meeting all of her milestones. On exam, you notice that her toes point inward when she is walking or standing, left more than right. You notice a negative thigh–foot angle on exam (Figure 209-2). She demonstrates normal range of motion through her hips and knees and is actively climbing through the exam room. Which of the following statements is true regarding the patient's in-toeing diagnosis?

**A.** There is an increased risk for osteoarthritis.

**B.** Genu varum is commonly appreciated on exam.

**C.** Referral to orthopedics is recommended if any deformity persists after 5 years of age.

**D.** Patients often demonstrate excessive internal rotation of the hips relative to external rotation.

**E.** Some patients may benefit from treatment with a brace.

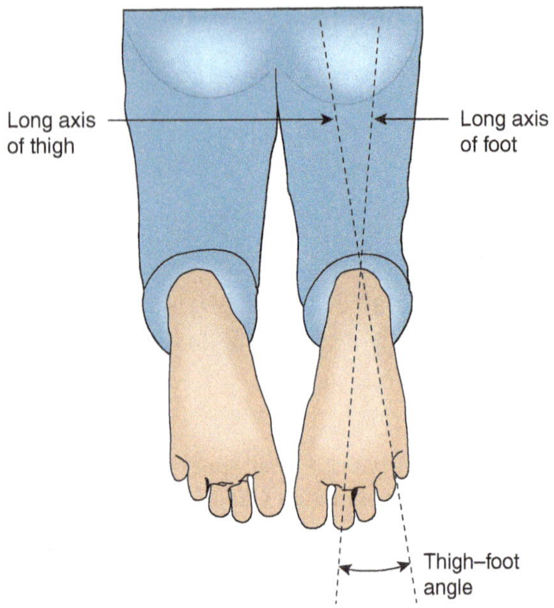


**FIGURE 209-2.** Determination of the thigh–foot angle in the prone position. (Mark W. Kline, *Rudolph's Pediatrics*, 23rd Edition. Copyright © McGraw-Hill Education. All rights reserved.)

**14-5.** A 30-month-old African-American boy presents due to concern for persistent bow-legged appearance. The child was born at term and experienced no complications during the pregnancy or delivery. Family reports they recently moved from northern Minnesota. He was exclusively breastfed until about 7 months of age. He eats whatever the family eats now, which includes a variety of fruits, vegetables, and meat. Mom is not aware of any family history of bow-leggedness.

On exam, he demonstrates marked genu varum bilaterally. As he walks in the exam room, you notice almost a shift or thrust at the knee as he stands on either side. He is active and appears overall well nourished. There is normal range of motion through bilateral hips and knees. Exam is otherwise normal. Radiographs demonstrate a beaked appearance of the medial tibial metaphysis. Which of the following is a known risk factor for the patient's disease process?

**A.** Metatarsus adductus

**B.** Breech positioning

**C.** Delayed walking

**D.** Family history

**E.** Increased body mass index (BMI)

**14-6.** A 2-week-old girl presents for her well-child check after discharge from the hospital. The patient was born at term via normal spontaneous vaginal delivery. There were no complications with the pregnancy or delivery. After delivery, however, the family reports her right lower extremity appeared deformed. The right foot was bent toward the shin. No other abnormalities were appreciated on exam. Mom and dad are healthy, without any medical diagnoses at this time. Due to the clinical appearance, a radiograph of the right leg and foot was obtained and demonstrates consistency with posterior medial bowing of the tibia. Which statement is true regarding posterior medial bowing of the tibia?

**A.** Precursor to pseudoarthrosis

**B.** May require an amputation

**C.** Can be managed in a brace

**D.** Increased risk of a leg length difference

**E.** Often corrects by 5 years of age

**14-7.** An 11-year-old girl presents today for evaluation of scoliosis. Mom reports she noticed that her shoulder blades appeared uneven when she was watching her at a swim meet recently. Mom is concerned because the patient's uncle had surgery for scoliosis. The patient underwent menarche about 6 months ago. She is active in swimming and has no limitations or concerns with her back when swimming. She does report back pain that comes and goes a few times a week. She notices the pain if she is seated in class for a long time. In addition, she thinks this pain has been occurring for about a year.

On exam, you notice the right shoulder blade sits higher relative to the left. In addition, the right iliac crest is about 5 mm higher relative to the left. She has a prominence of the right rib cage when bending forward. Neurologic exam is normal. Radiographs demonstrate findings of Risser 1, a thoracic curve, apex facing the right, with a Cobb angle of 20 degrees, and a lumbar curve with a Cobb angle of 18 degrees. Which of the following is a risk factor of curve progression?

**A.** Early age of menarche

**B.** Leg length discrepancy

**C.** Left thoracic curve

**D.** Female sex

**E.** Associated back pain

**14-8.** A 14-year-old boy presents with chronic back pain. He reports this pain started about a year ago. He denies any history of injury. His pain is located over the thoracic spine. He denies radicular symptoms and reports no change in his bowel or bladder function. His mom thinks his pain is related to his poor posture and heavy backpack.

On exam, he demonstrates normal range of motion through the spine. He has a rounded appearance to his shoulders and increased kyphosis appreciated through the thoracic spine that is more prominent when he bends forward. This does not fully correct with hyperextension. The rest of the exam is normal. Radiographs of his total spine demonstrate similar findings, with increased kyphosis appreciated through the thoracic spine and normal vertebral body size, shape, and alignment. There is also comment of associated Schmorl nodes. Which of the following statements is false regarding the patient's diagnosis?

**A.** Treatment often includes physical therapy.

**B.** Pain is common and commonly located over the apex of the curve.

**C.** Radiographs demonstrate 5 consecutive vertebrae with > 3 degrees of anterior wedging.

**D.** Curve progression commonly can occur during periods of rapid growth.

**E.** The condition is not commonly associated with neurologic symptoms.

**14-9.** A 3-year-old boy presents to clinic due to complaints of back pain. His mom reports that she does not remember any specific injury. He woke up a few days ago complaining of back pain. She states he has not been as active. In addition, she feels as though he is walking differently. He prefers to lie on the couch. Mom reports that on the way to the appointment the patient was quite uncomfortable. However, his car seat was recently updated and replaced. The patient has recently begun toilet training, and mom reports no concerns.

On exam, the patient is overall well appearing; however, he is not interested in cooperating. He becomes irritated when asked to sit. He demonstrates limited motion when asked to bend forward or twist. Neurologic exam is normal. Radiographs of the spine are normal. A magnetic resonance imaging (MRI) scan of the spine demonstrates consistency with diskitis and vertebral body osteomyelitis. Which of the following statements is true regarding the patient's diagnosis?

**A.** *Staphylococcus aureus* is the most common pathogen identified.

**B.** Laboratory values commonly demonstrate elevated white blood cell (WBC) count, erythrocyte sedimentation rate (ESR), and C-reactive protein (CRP).

**C.** Systemic symptoms are common and help differentiate from other back pain causes.

**D.** Injury is often a precursor to the diagnosis.

**E.** The thoracic spine is the most commonly affected area.

**14-10.** A 2-month-old boy presents for a well-child check. On exam, the patient demonstrates social smile and appears to track objects well. You notice, however, that the patient seems to tilt his head to the left and point his chin to the right. In addition, he demonstrates decreased lateral rotation to the left. There does appear to be a small prominence palpable over the left side of the neck. His spine appears straight, but he does have some flattening of the right occiput. The remaining exam is otherwise normal. Mom had not noticed this much but now becomes very concerned that something is wrong. What is the next best course of action?

**A.** Order urgent magnetic resonance imaging (MRI) of the neck due to palpable mass

**B.** Refer to physical therapy and counsel mom on strategic positioning for sleeping and feeding

**C.** Refer to orthopedics for further workup and management

**D.** Order ultrasound of the neck and refer to physical therapy

**E.** Refer to pediatric ophthalmology to evaluate vision

**14-11.** A 14-year-old boy presents to your office for evaluation of a "lump" over the inner aspect of his lower leg near the knee. He denies pain at the site of the lesion. There is no history of fever, and patient has experienced no changes in activity level and no changes in appetite. He is otherwise healthy. The boy and his parents deny family history of bony deformities or tumors.

On exam, you palpate a 2-cm fixed nodular swelling over the medial aspect of the proximal tibia. There are no other lesions. You obtain knee radiographs following the clinic visit; the boy's radiograph is shown in the following figure. Of the following, what is the most appropriate next step in evaluation and management?

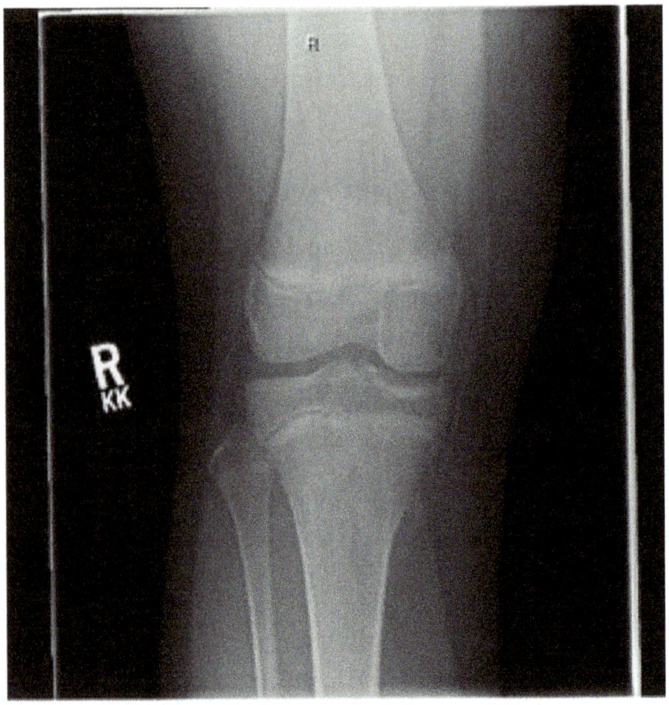


**A.** Obtain a skeletal survey to look for additional lesions

**B.** Obtain magnetic resonance imaging (MRI) of the knee

**C.** Reassure the family about the benign nature of the radiographic finding

**D.** Refer for computed tomography (CT)-guided biopsy of the lesion

**E.** Refer for orthopedic surgery consultation for mass removal

**14-12.** A 12-year-old girl presents to your office for evaluation following a knee injury 3 days ago. The girl tripped over a stair and fell onto the anterior surface of her right knee. She was seen in an urgent care clinic and had radiographs performed. The girl and her mother report that the knee pain has resolved. However, the family is very concerned because the urgent care physician mentioned that the radiographs showed a "bone cyst" and recommended follow-up. The girl denies fever or constitutional symptoms. Physical examination of the knee is normal. The girl's radiograph is shown in Figure 216-2. Of the following, what is the most accurate statement to include in your discussion with the girl and her mother?

**A.** Her radiographic finding indicates the need for advanced imaging of the knee.

**B.** Her radiographic finding is due to infection of the tibia.

**C.** Her radiographic finding is likely a benign neoplasm.

**D.** Her radiographic finding resulted from her fall onto the knee.

**E.** Her radiographic finding will likely resolve without treatment.

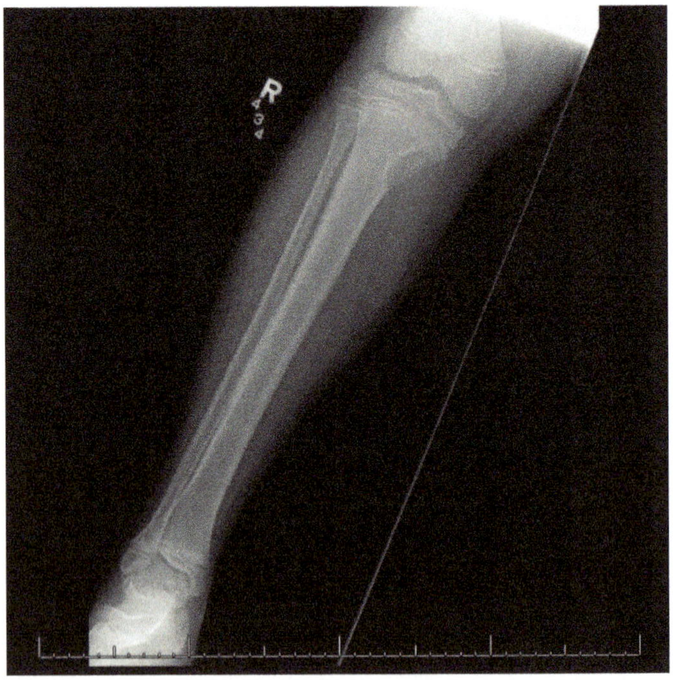


**FIGURE 216-2.** Nonossifying fibroma of the left proximal tibia with typical features: eccentric, radiolucent lesion with well-defined sclerotic margins. (Mark W. Kline, *Rudolph's Pediatrics*, 23rd Edition. Copyright © McGraw-Hill Education. All rights reserved.)

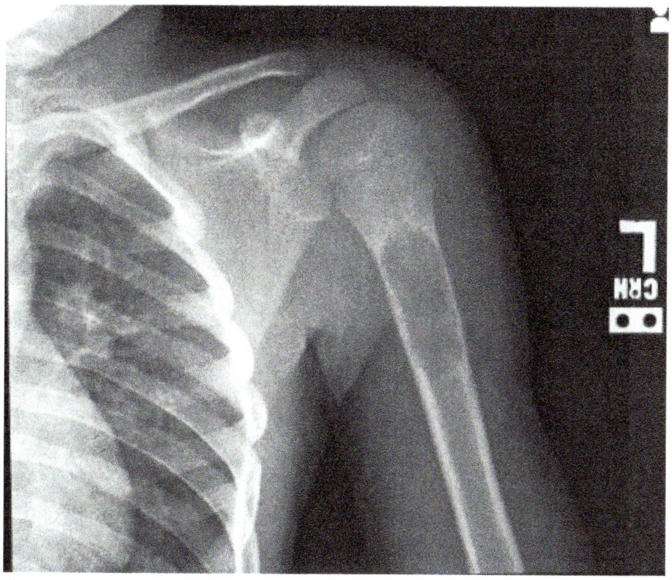

A

**FIGURE 216-3A.** Unicameral bone cyst of the left humerus associated with pain and multiple pathologic fractures. (Mark W. Kline, *Rudolph's Pediatrics*, 23rd Edition. Copyright © McGraw-Hill Education. All rights reserved.)

**14-13.** A 9-year-old girl presents to your clinic to discuss her history of arm pain and injury. About 2 months ago, the girl fell on the left arm and had severe pain in the upper arm near the shoulder. Because she was traveling with her family, they did not seek medical care. After 2 or 3 weeks, the pain improved but her arm still feels a little sore. The girl had a similar, milder episode of pain about 9 months prior. The girl's radiograph is shown in Figure 216-3A. Of the following, what is the next best step in evaluation and management?

**A.** Admit the girl for intravenous (IV) antibiotic treatment

**B.** Obtain magnetic resonance imaging (MRI) of the arm

**C.** Reassure the family that the lesion will resolve without treatment

**D.** Refer to interventional radiology for computed tomography (CT)-guided biopsy

**E.** Refer to orthopedic surgery for operative management

**14-14.** A 7-year-old girl presents to your clinic for evaluation of right anterior mid-thigh pain that has been present for 3 months. You perform a thorough history and physical examination and subsequently obtain radiographs of the hips and femur. Based on the results of your examination, you suspect the girl has an osteoid osteoma. Of the following, which finding is most consistent with your suspected diagnosis?

**A.** Erythema overlying the lesion

**B.** Pain that is worse upon waking in the morning

**C.** Pronounced tenderness at the location of her pain

**D.** Significant relief with ibuprofen

**E.** A 3-cm radiolucent lesion seen on radiographs

**14-15.** You are reviewing radiographs from your teaching file with a group of residents. You present the case of a 5-year-old boy who presents with swelling and pain over the skull associated with a fever. Radiographs of the skull showed a single, round, 1.5-cm "punched out" radiolucent lesion affecting the parietal region. The history and radiographic findings are most consistent with which of the following conditions?

**A.** Aneurysmal bone cyst

**B.** Enchondroma

**C.** Eosinophilic granuloma

**D.** Osteoid osteoma

**E.** Fibrous dysplasia

**14-16.** During a health supervision visit for a 6-year-old child with mild left hemiplegia, you discuss the girl's need for braces, and the girl's father mentions that his daughter "needs a new AFO." Following the appointment, the medical student working with you asks you about the nomenclature for braces. What are these devices typically named after?

**A.** The condition that the brace is typically used to treat

**B.** The material the brace is typically made from

**C.** The muscles stretched by the brace

**D.** The joints crossed by the brace

**E.** The physicians who initially described each type of brace

**14-17.** A newborn with myelodysplasia and a complex medical history including a prolonged neonatal intensive care unit stay is scheduled to begin care with your practice. Prior to her health supervision visit, you initiate a review of her medical records. Of the following, which condition is most likely to be associated with her history of myelodysplasia?

**A.** Anal atresia

**B.** Chiari malformation type I

**C.** Clubfoot

**D.** Horseshoe kidney

**E.** Ventricular septal defect

**14-18.** You are seeing a 3-year-old girl for a follow-up visit in your clinic. The girl is a former premature infant born at 30 weeks gestation. She has been followed by a pediatric neurologist and was recently diagnosed with cerebral palsy (CP) and has mild left hemiplegia. Her family is understandably very upset about the diagnosis and would like to discuss what it means for their child. What is the most accurate statement to include in the discussion with the girl's parents?

**A.** Ataxia is common in children with CP.

**B.** Children with hemiplegic CP typically have only lower extremity involvement.

**C.** Her degree of cognitive dysfunction relates to the degree of physical disability.

**D.** Her hemiplegia is nonprogressive and is not expected to worsen over time.

**E.** Spasticity must be present to make the diagnosis of CP.

**14-19.** You are evaluating a 1-day-old male infant in the newborn nursery. The infant was delivered at term by spontaneous vaginal delivery. On physical examination of the lower extremities, you note that the infant has bilateral talipes equinovarus (clubfoot), bilateral knee contractures with knees held in extension, and limited hip motion. Evaluation of the upper extremities reveals elbow extension contractures, internally rotated shoulders, and wrist flexion contractures. The limbs appear thin with poor muscle definition, whereas the trunk, head, and neck are normal. Of the following, which finding is most likely to be associated with this infant's condition?

**A.** Cognitive disability

**B.** Family history of joint contractures

**C.** History of oligohydramnios

**D.** Maternal history of seizures

**E.** Vertebral anomalies

**14-20.** A 4-year-old boy presents to your clinic for evaluation of abnormal gait and clumsiness. The boy's parents report that he began walking at age 16 months. Initially, they had no concerns about his walking. However, about 1 year ago, he began walking on his "tip toes" at times, and this seems to be increasing in frequency. On exam, the boy has well-developed calf muscles and limited dorsiflexion of his ankles. He uses his hands to push along his thighs in order to rise from a seated position on the floor and consistently toe-walks during the clinic visit. Of the following, which laboratory finding would be most consistent with your suspected diagnosis?

**A.** Decreased aldolase

**B.** Decreased aspartate transaminase

**C.** Increased alkaline phosphatase

**D.** Increased uric acid

**E.** Increased creatine kinase

**14-21.** A 14-year-old girl presents to your office with 3 months of gradual-onset bilateral knee pain. The pain occurs all around her knee caps, and she denies any knee swelling or locking. She has never injured her knees or dislocated her knee caps. The pain is worse with climbing stairs and squatting. She recently increased her hours of volleyball, playing on both her school team and a club team. On exam, both patellae move laterally when the knees are fully extended, and she feels uncomfortable when you move her patellae. There is no focal tenderness, and her exam is otherwise unremarkable. What is the most appropriate initial treatment?

**A.** Intra-articular steroid injection

**B.** Physical therapy

**C.** Patellar strap

**D.** Surgery correction of patellar alignment

**E.** Knee immobilizer

**14-22.** An 11-year-old boy presents to clinic for 2 years of a popping sensation over the lateral aspect of his right knee. The popping occurs with bending and straightening the knee. The popping has increased in frequency and become more painful since he joined his school's running club this year. For the past few weeks, he occasionally has a catching sensation with straightening his knee and reports that the knee will sometimes "give out" when he is walking. His exam is significant for a clicking over the lateral joint on McMurray test. Knee radiographs show a widened lateral joint space. Which further knee imaging would you order to confirm your suspected diagnosis?

**A.** Dual-energy x-ray absorptiometry (DEXA) scan

**B.** Ultrasound

**C.** Magnetic resonance imaging (MRI)

**D.** Computed tomography (CT) scan

**E.** Bone scan

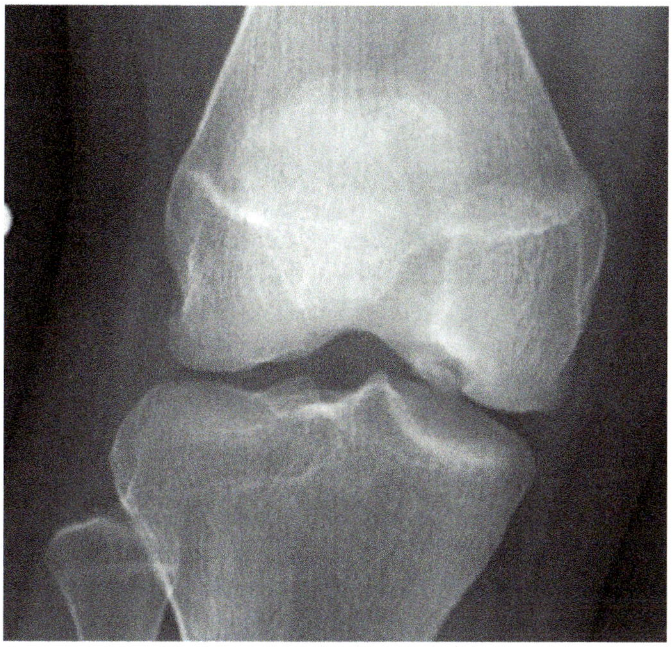

A

**FIGURE 211-2A.** Anteroposterior radiograph of the left knee. (Mark W. Kline, *Rudolph's Pediatrics*, 23rd Edition. Copyright © McGraw-Hill Education. All rights reserved.)

**14-23.** A previously healthy 14-year-old boy presents to your office with 1 year of left knee pain and swelling. The pain and swelling have come and gone over the past year but have recently worsened. He now frequently feels a painful popping and "catching" sensation in his knee and is no longer able to run due to the pain. He denies knee injury, other joint pain, or fevers. On exam, he has a moderate effusion and is tender over the medial femoral condyle. Anteroposterior (AP) radiograph is shown in Figure 211-2A. What is the most likely diagnosis?

**A.** Osgood-Schlatter disease

**B.** Tibial spine fracture

**C.** Meniscus tear

**D.** Salter-Harris III fracture

**E.** Osteochondritis dissecans

**14-24.** A 13-year-old girl presents with bilateral anterior knee pain for 4 months. She is on her school's basketball team and reports that the pain is worse at the end of each practice. She reports that jumping, squatting, and climbing stairs are especially painful. Her parents note that she seems to have grown a lot in the past year. Her physical exam is significant for prominent and tender tibial tubercles bilaterally. Which of the following is the best advice to give her about her condition?

**A.** This pain almost always resolves at skeletal maturity, but it may wax and wane until then.

**B.** She will continue to have pain for the rest of her life unless she has surgery to correct the condition.

**C.** She should not continue to participate in sports because this is the cause of her condition.

**D.** She should wear a patellar stabilization brace to treat the condition.

**E.** This condition usually occurs in elementary school-age children and is rare in teenagers.

**14-25.** A 10-year-old boy presents with bilateral anterior knee pain. The pain began insidiously 2 months ago and has been worsening since the family purchased a trampoline a few weeks ago. The pain primarily occurs with running, climbing stairs, and jumping on the trampoline. The boy denies popping, locking, or the sensation of the knees giving out. The pain improves with ice and rest. On exam, he is very tender and has mild swelling over the inferior poles of both patellae. His knee exam is otherwise normal. What is the best next step in management?

**A.** Magnetic resonance imaging (MRI) of both knees

**B.** Anteroposterior (AP), lateral, and oblique radiographs of both knees

**C.** Bilateral joint aspiration and synovial fluid analysis

**D.** Avoidance of painful activities and supportive care with ice and patellar strap

**E.** Referral to orthopedic surgery to discuss surgical repair

**14-26.** A healthy 5-year-old girl presents to your office with a swelling over her left posterior knee. Her mother noticed the fullness a few days ago when the family was at the beach. There was no known knee injury, and the girl has been participating in all of her normal activities without pain. On exam, the girl is afebrile and well appearing. When the girl is prone with her knees extended, you feel a firm mass over the posteromedial aspect of her left knee. The mass transilluminates and decreases in size with knee flexion. What is the most likely diagnosis?

**A.** Discoid meniscus

**B.** Anterior cruciate ligament injury

**C.** Osteochondroma

**D.** Popliteal (Baker) cyst

**E.** Osgood-Schlatter disease

**14-27.** A mother brings her 4-month-old infant to your office to establish care. The mother states that she was diagnosed with developmental dysplasia of the hip (DDH) when she was a child and is concerned that her child may also have DDH. Which of the following is a risk factor for DDH?

**A.** Male sex

**B.** Breech presentation

**C.** Loose lower extremity swaddling

**D.** History of polyhydramnios

**E.** Prematurity

**14-28.** A father brings his 9-month-old daughter for her well-child check. She was born at term and has no known medical problems. On supine exam, you notice that her left leg is slightly shorter than the right, and her left knee appears shorter when both hips are flexed to 90 degrees. You also find that the left hip abducts less than the right. There is no bruising, swelling, or tenderness. What is the most likely diagnosis?

**A.** Legg-Calvé-Perthes disease

**B.** Slipped capital femoral epiphysis

**C.** Transient synovitis of the hip

**D.** Internal tibial torsion

**E.** Developmental dysplasia of the hip (DDH)

**14-29.** A 6-year-old boy with no known medical problems is brought to clinic for evaluation after his teacher noticed him limping on the playground. He denies pain. He has been well with no recent fevers or illnesses. On exam, he has an antalgic gait and limited internal and external rotation of the left hip. His knee exam is normal. What is your next step in management?

**A.** Standing anteroposterior (AP) and frog-leg radiographs of both hips

**B.** Reassurance

**C.** Referral for emergent surgical intervention

**D.** Fast-acting oral opiate

**E.** Pavlik harness

**14-30.** A 14-year-old boy with a history of acanthosis nigricans, dyslipidemia, and body mass index (BMI) in the 98th percentile is brought to your office by his father. His father is concerned because the boy has been intermittently limping and complaining of right knee pain during soccer practice for the past 2 months. You find no abnormalities on examination of both knees, but you notice that the boy sits with the right leg externally rotated compared to the left leg. What is your next step in management?

**A.** Knee radiographs

**B.** Reassurance

**C.** Hip examination

**D.** Patellar strap

**E.** Physical therapy

**14-31.** Which patient is most likely to be diagnosed with developmental dysplasia of the hip (DDH)?

**A.** A 13-year-old boy who plays lacrosse and has been intermittently limping and complaining of unilateral knee pain for 2 months

**B.** A 5-year-old boy with sickle cell disease and an insidious-onset, painless limp and limited unilateral hip range of motion

**C.** An afebrile 3-year-old girl with acute-onset left hip pain and limp with no known injuries who had a viral upper respiratory tract infection last week

**D.** A 4-month-old girl who was delivered by cesarean section for breech presentation and has limited left hip abduction

**E.** A 14-year-old girl with sudden onset of severe pain directly over the right anterior inferior iliac spine

**14-32.** An immunized, 4-year-old Filipino American girl is brought to an urgent care center after she started complaining of right leg pain and limping at preschool that day. There was no known injury. Her parents report that she is usually healthy, but she had a bad cold last week. On exam, she is afebrile and nontoxic appearing. She cries when you attempt to check her right hip range of motion, and she grimaces and limps when walking across the exam room. Labs show a C-reactive protein (CRP) of 0.6 mg/dL, erythrocyte sedimentation rate (ESR) of 2 mm/h, and white blood cell (WBC) count of 5500 cells/mL. Hip radiographs are unremarkable. Ultrasound of the right hip shows no evidence of joint effusion. What is the next appropriate step in management?

**A.** Admit for right hip arthroscopy and washout

**B.** Admit for surgical stabilization of the capital femoral epiphysis

**C.** Discharge home with Pavlik harness

**D.** Discharge home with nonsteroidal antiinflammatory drug (NSAID) for 3 to 5 days

**E.** Discharge home with physical therapy prescription

**14-33.** A 10-year-old overweight boy with a history of hypothyroidism presents to your office with insidious onset of right knee pain. He denies any injuries and reports that his pain and limp have progressed over the past couple days. The family denies any recent illnesses, fevers, or chills.

On exam, he is well appearing with a normal temperature. His gait is antalgic. He has no tenderness to palpation around the left knee. He has normal knee range of motion without swelling or effusion. He has asymmetric hip range of motion. What test would you order next for this patient?

**A.** Anteroposterior (AP), lateral, and sunrise view radiographs of both knees

**B.** Complete blood count (CBC)

**C.** Knee magnetic resonance imaging (MRI)

**D.** Inflammatory markers (erythrocyte sedimentation rate [ESR] and C-reactive protein [CRP])

**E.** AP and lateral radiographs of both hips

**14-34.** A 12-year-old girl presents with a right ankle injury. She describes "rolling her ankle" at soccer practice. She was unable to continue playing and is now limping. On exam, she is afebrile and well appearing with an antalgic gait. She has right ankle swelling, mostly over the lateral ankle, and point tenderness at her distal fibular physis. Her ankle range of motion is slightly decreased compared to the opposite side. Anteroposterior (AP), lateral, and mortise radiographs of the ankle are unremarkable. What is the most appropriate next step in treatment?

**A.** Reassurance

**B.** Ace wrap of ankle

**C.** Immobilization of ankle (with walking boot or splint)

**D.** Ankle magnetic resonance imaging (MRI)

**E.** Lab evaluation with complete blood count (CBC), erythrocyte sedimentation rate (ESR), and C-reactive protein (CRP)

**14-35.** A 6-year-old boy presents with a limp. He states that his left leg and thigh are painful; however, he denies any injury. He had a cold and 1 day of fever last week. The patient currently has no fever, chills, or rash.

On exam, the patient is afebrile, and his gait is antalgic. His left hip has slightly decreased motion compared to the right, and he complains of pain with left hip motion. Anteroposterior (AP) pelvis and frog-leg lateral views of both hips are unremarkable. Lab evaluation, including complete blood count (CBC), erythrocyte sedimentation rate (ESR), and C-reactive protein (CRP), is also unremarkable. What is the most likely diagnosis?

**A.** Septic hip arthritis

**B.** Legg-Calvé-Perthes disease

**C.** Transient synovitis of the hip

**D.** Occult hip fracture

**E.** Slipped capital femoral epiphysis (SCFE)

**14-36.** A 3-year-old girl presents refusing to walk. Her parents state that she will not bear weight on the left leg. She has been febrile for the past couple days without other symptoms.

On exam, she appears very tired. Her temperature is 38.5°C, and she has resting tachycardia. Her left hip is flexed and externally rotated, and she cries with any attempt to move the hip. She has no tenderness in her femur, knee, tibia, or ankle. Anteroposterior (AP) pelvis and bilateral frog-leg lateral radiographs of the pelvis are normal. Complete blood count (CBC) shows an elevated white blood cell (WBC) count along with an elevated C-reactive protein (CRP) and an elevated erythrocyte sedimentation rate (ESR). What is your next step in management?

**A.** Outpatient follow-up

**B.** Subspecialty consultation

**C.** Immobilization in a long leg splint or cast

**D.** Reassurance

**E.** Radiographs of the knee

**14-37.** Which of the following scenarios increases your clinical suspicion for malignancy?

**A.** A 2 years old with a twisting injury at the park and left leg limp

**B.** A 15 years old obese male with insidious-onset right leg limp

**C.** A 14 years old ice hockey player with a left-sided limp after being checked into the boards

**D.** A 17 years old with a limp and knee effusion after a twisting injury during basketball

**E.** A 10 years old with an insidious-onset limp, various other bone pains, and slightly elevated erythrocyte sedimentation rate (ESR) and C-reactive protein (CRP)

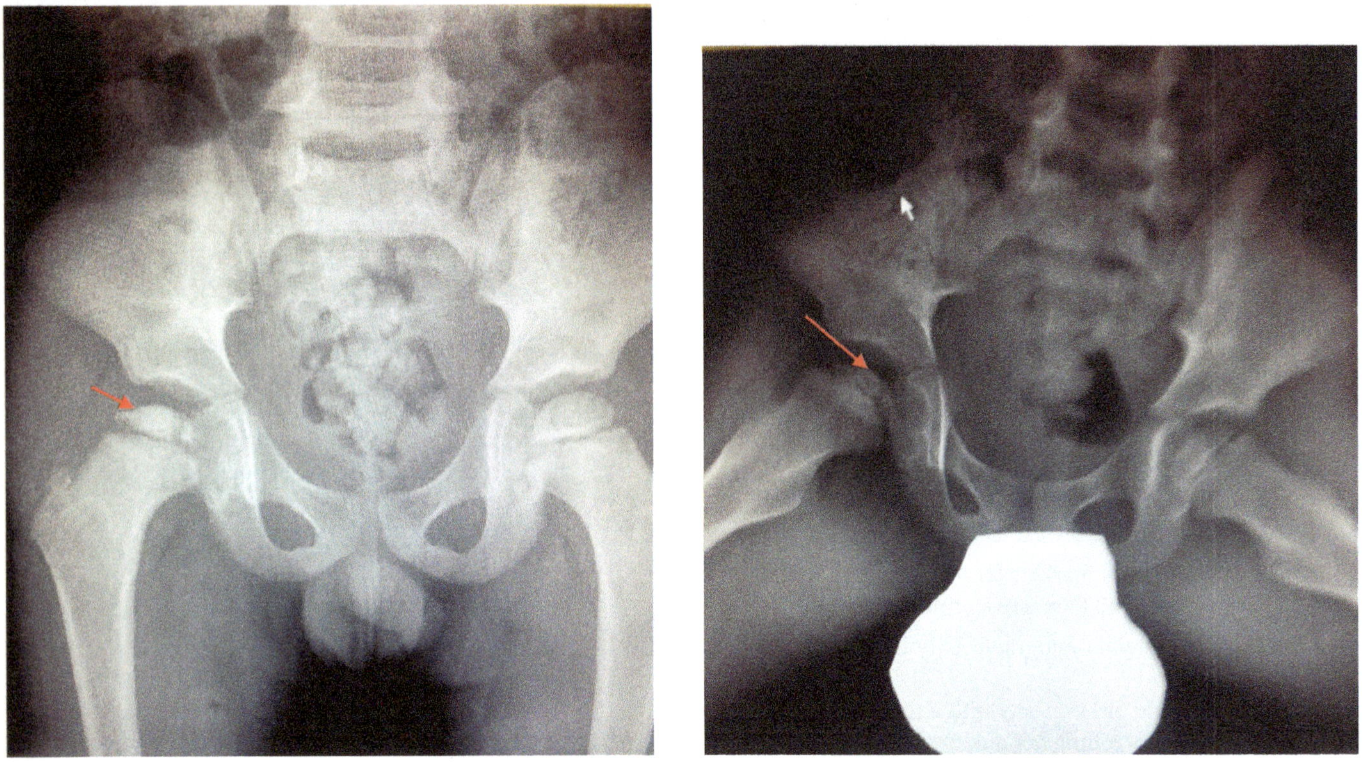

A B

**FIGURE 208-3.** A and B: Anteroposterior pelvis and bilateral frog-leg lateral views of the hip. (Mark W. Kline, *Rudolph's Pediatrics*, 23rd Edition. Copyright © McGraw-Hill Education. All rights reserved.)

**14-38.** A 10-year-old boy presents with an insidious-onset limp. He describes vague upper leg and right hip pain. He denies any injury. On exam, he is well appearing and afebrile. His gait is antalgic. His right hip range of motion is decreased compared to the left side. His knee and ankle exam are unremarkable. You obtain the following radiographs (Figure 208-3, A and B). What is the most likely diagnosis?

**A.** Slipped capital femoral epiphysis (SCFE)
**B.** Septic arthritis
**C.** Transient synovitis
**D.** Legg-Calvé-Perthes disease
**E.** Hip fracture

**14-39.** A 6-year-old girl presents after a fall off a trampoline. She reports elbow pain and swelling with decreased range of motion. On exam, she is well appearing and afebrile. There is no gross deformity, her elbow is held in flexion, and there is swelling. She is tender around all bony prominences. You obtain the following lateral radiograph (Figure 215-1C), which is read as elbow effusion, no fracture identified. What is the next step in treatment?

**A.** Immobilization in a long arm splint
**B.** Reassurance to parents
**C.** Ace wrap applied to the elbow
**D.** A reduction maneuver where the elbow is flexed and supinated
**E.** Ultrasound of the elbow

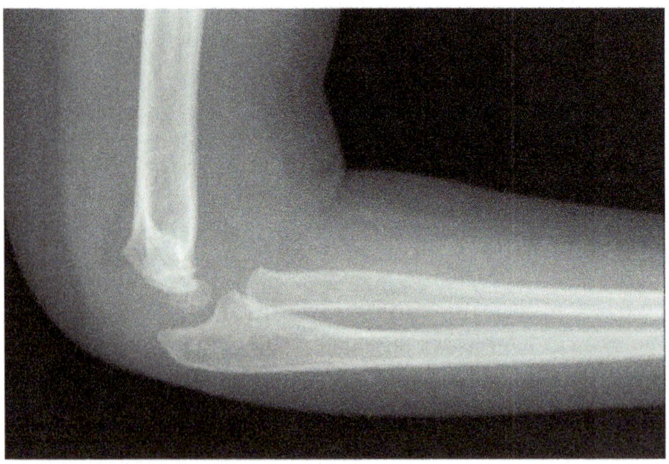

C

**FIGURE 215-1C.** Radiograph with anterior and posterior fat pad signs. (Mark W. Kline, *Rudolph's Pediatrics*, 23rd Edition. Copyright © McGraw-Hill Education. All rights reserved.)

**14-40.** Which of the following fractures should prompt a suspicion of nonaccidental trauma and thus a skeletal survey?

**A.** A greenstick fracture of the distal radius and ulna in a 3 years old

**B.** A posterior rib fracture in a 12 months old

**C.** A spiral fracture of the distal tibia in a 2 years old

**D.** A buckle fracture of the distal radius in a 5 years old

**E.** A Salter-Harris II fracture of the lateral malleolus in a 6 years old

**14-41.** A 16-year-old girl reports a knee injury during soccer. She twisted her knee when running and felt a pop and shift in her knee. On exam, she is afebrile with normal vital signs. She has an antalgic gait. She has a knee effusion and can only flex her knee to 90 degrees. She has diffuse tenderness throughout her knee including her kneecap and is guarding with exam. She has a positive anterior drawer test. Three-view radiographs of the knee are negative. What is your next step in management?

**A.** Hip x-ray

**B.** Knee computed tomography (CT) scan

**C.** Lab evaluation including complete blood count (CBC), erythrocyte sedimentation rate (ESR), and C-reactive protein (CRP)

**D.** Knee magnetic resonance imaging (MRI)

**E.** Repeat x-ray in 7 to 10 days

**14-42.** A 2-year-old boy presents with a limp. There was no clear injury; however, there were a few falls at the playground earlier in the day including a twist on a slide. On exam, he is afebrile with an antalgic gait. There is no appreciable swelling. He has normal hip and knee range of motion. You note that he pulls away with palpation of his left tibia. Two radiographic views of the left tibia and fibula are normal. What is your next step in workup or management?

**A.** Long leg splint with close follow-up in 7 to 10 days

**B.** Lab evaluation including complete blood count (CBC), erythrocyte sedimentation rate (ESR), and C-reactive protein (CRP)

**C.** Ace wrap and reassurance

**D.** Skeletal survey

**E.** Hip radiograph

**14-43.** A 17-year-old girl presents with right ankle pain. She describes an inversion injury while playing lacrosse. She was unable to continue playing and is now unable to bear weight on her leg. On exam, she is afebrile. She has significant lateral ankle swelling. She is tender over her anterior talofibular ligament and around the lateral malleolus. Her ankle has decreased range of motion. There is no laxity when compared to the other ankle. Three-view radiographs of the right ankle are unremarkable. What is the best next step in management?

**A.** Reassurance

**B.** Rest, ice, compression, elevation, and early range-of-motion exercises

**C.** Cast immobilization for 4 to 6 weeks

**D.** Lab evaluation including complete blood count (CBC), erythrocyte sedimentation rate (ESR), and C-reactive protein (CRP)

**E.** Ankle magnetic resonance imaging (MRI)

**14-44.** A 15-year-old boy presents to your office with insidious onset of right shoulder pain for the past 3 months. He is right-handed and denies any injury; however, he does play baseball. He plays pitcher on 2 teams, and sometimes he plays catcher as well. On exam, he has no shoulder asymmetry and mild tenderness of the proximal humerus. He has normal range of motion and strength. You obtain the radiograph as shown in Figure 215-10A. What is the most likely diagnosis?

**A.** Rotator cuff tear

**B.** Shoulder strain

**C.** Epiphysitis

**D.** Clavicle fracture

**E.** Growing pains

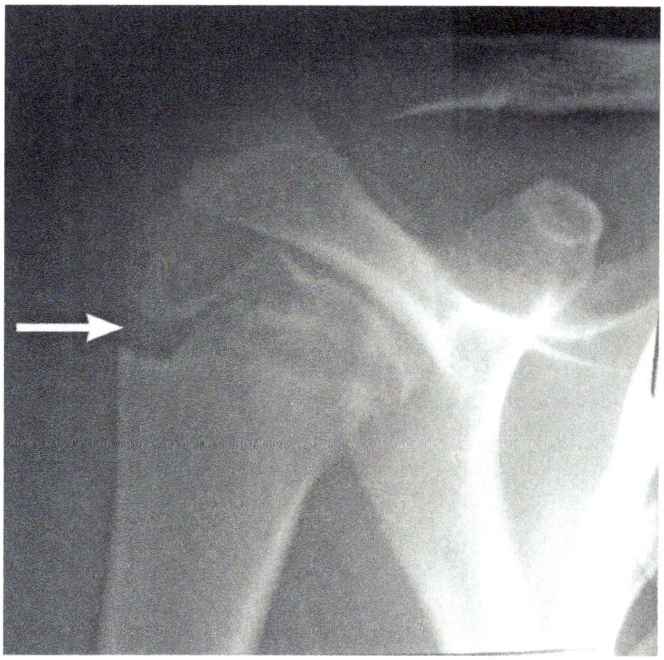

A

**FIGURE 215-10A.** Radiograph of the right shoulder. (Mark W. Kline, *Rudolph's Pediatrics*, 23rd Edition. Copyright © McGraw-Hill Education. All rights reserved.)

**14-45.** A trainee points out an incidental finding of a nonossifying fibroma on a set of knee radiographs. As a part of the discussion about this finding with a group of medical students and residents, you review radiographic features that help physicians distinguish benign bone lesions from malignant ones. During your review, you explain that which of the following types of lesion would be most consistent with a malignant tumor?

**A.** A mixed lytic and sclerotic lesion with extensive periosteal reaction

**B.** A radiolucent nidus with a surrounding rim of sclerosis

**C.** A multiloculated radiolucent lesion with a thin sclerotic rim

**D.** A well-defined lesion with a "ground glass" appearance

**E.** A thin stalk of bone with a large cap arising from the metaphysis

**14-46.** A 4-year-old girl presents for evaluation of "bumps" involving the fingers of the right hand. On physical examination, she has 4 palpable firm nodules over the right hand phalanges of her index, middle, and ring fingers. Radiographs show expansive, lytic lesions of the phalanges with thinning of the overlying cortex. What is the most likely diagnosis?

**A.** Beckwith-Wiedemann syndrome

**B.** Li-Fraumeni syndrome

**C.** Maffucci syndrome

**D.** Multiple hereditary exostosis

**E.** Ollier disease

## ANSWERS

**Answer 14-1.** D

The clavicle and the flat bones of the skull are formed by intramembranous ossification. The major long bones of the upper limbs (ie, the humerus, radius, and ulna) have a physis at either end of the bone, unlike the metacarpals and phalanges, which typically have only 1 physis (Figure 207-2). Endochondral ossification is characterized by the replacement of chondroblasts by osteoblasts. Generally, excessive compression of the physis may result in decreased growth, whereas traction or distraction may accelerate growth. The germinal zone is characterized by a large amount of extracellular matrix, whereas the zone of hypertrophy and provisional calcification are more cellular and generally the weakest of the 4 zones (Figure 207-4).

(Chapter 207: Growth and Development)

**Answer 14-2.** E

On average, infants begin walking independently around 12 months of age. Infants are usually sitting independently by 7 months of age and crawling by 8 months old. Infants achieve the milestone of rolling over by 5 and 6 months of age. On average, infants begin rolling front to back around 5 months of age and back to front by 6 months of age. Pulling to a stance is typically achieved by 9 months of age (Table 207-2).

(Chapter 207: Growth and Development)

**Answer 14-3.** B

The history and exam are consistent with mild metatarsus adductus, the most frequent reason for in-toeing in the first year of life. Metatarsus adductus occurs when there is inward torsion of the mid- or forefoot with the hindfoot in normal position or slight valgus.

The severity of metatarsus adductus is determined by the amount of flexibility of the forefoot and is graded 1 to 3, with 3 being the most severe. A foot that neutralizes itself spontaneously with tickling of the lateral border is termed mild or grade 1. A moderate, or grade 2, foot is passively correctable but does not actively correct itself to neutral. A severe, or grade 3, foot cannot be completely corrected with stretching.

Although there is not a defined standard of treatment, generally the mild deformities will improve with growth and the natural history is generally benign. Infants with moderate, severe, and/or rigid metatarsus adductus benefit from referral to orthopedics. These deformities may benefit from further treatment with straight last shoes and/or serial casting. Although the true etiology of metatarsus adductus is not known, positioning in utero is thought to contribute.

Hip dysplasia has been reported in up to 10% of patients with metatarsus adductus, and thus, a thorough hip exam is recommended. Further imaging of the hips should be considered depending on exam and other associated risk factors. Congenital scoliosis is not commonly associated with metatarsus adductus; however, careful musculoskeletal exam including examining the spine and sacral area is recommended.

(Chapter 209: Torsional and Angular Deformities)

**Answer 14-4.** B

The patient demonstrates an exam consistent with internal tibial torsion, the most common cause of in-toeing in patients between 1 and 3 years old. Genu varum is commonly seen in patients with internal tibial torsion as well. Internal tibial torsion generally has a rather benign natural history. It often improves up until about age 5 years. Persistence of deformity in an otherwise typically developing child does not commonly

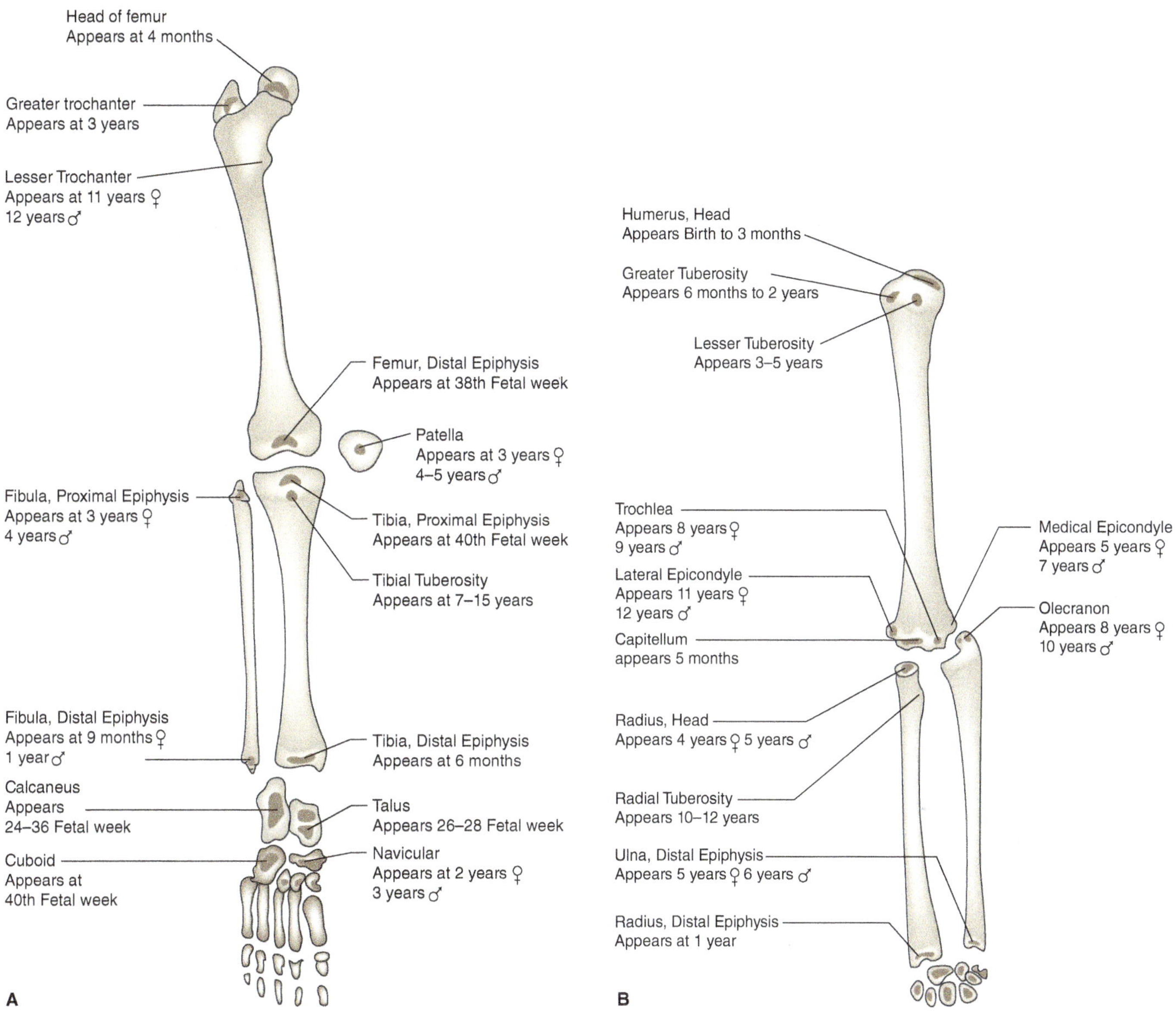


**FIGURE 207-2.** Age of radiographic appearance of the secondary ossific centers of long-bone epiphyses: (**A**) upper extremity and (**B**) lower extremity. These appearances can be used to estimate a child's skeletal age and identify skeletal growth abnormalities and need to be differentiated from fractures. (Mark W. Kline, *Rudolph's Pediatrics*, 23rd Edition. Copyright © McGraw-Hill Education. All rights reserved.)

cause any functional limitations or pain, and thus, orthopedic referral is usually not necessary even if mild deformity persists. Orthopedic referral may be considered if severe deformity persists after 5 years of age and/or if patient has significant functional limitations secondary to the deformity.

The "W" sitting pattern is commonly observed with excessive femoral anteversion, not internal tibial torsion. This pattern correlates with increased internal rotation of the hips relative to external rotation. Bracing and orthotics have not demonstrated any efficacy in the treatment of either increased femoral anteversion or internal tibial torsion in the otherwise typically developing child. Some studies suggest that increased femoral anteversion, another common cause of in-toeing, may correlate with an increased risk of osteoarthritis in the hip. However, other studies suggest a benign natural history associated with femoral anteversion.

(Chapter 209: Torsional and Angular Deformities)

**Answer 14-5.** E

This patient demonstrates an exam and radiographs consistent with infantile Blount disease. Increased BMI or obesity is a common risk factor both for infantile and adolescent Blount disease. In addition, a history of early walking, before 1 year of age, is another known risk factor for infantile Blount disease. Metatarsus adductus, breech positioning, and family history are not known risk factors for infantile Blount disease at this time.

(Chapter 209: Torsional and Angular Deformities)

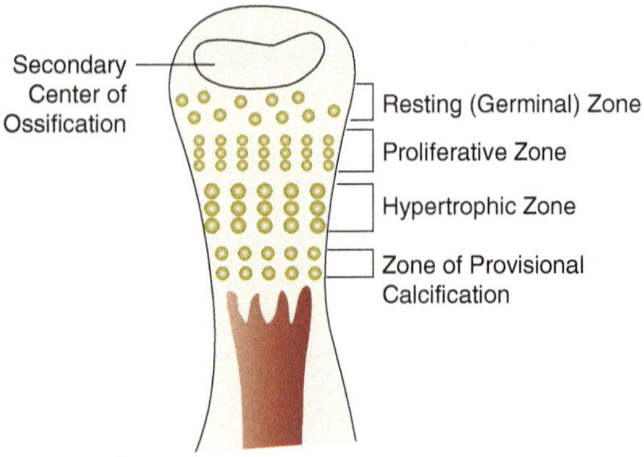


**FIGURE 207-4.** Scheme of the microscopic organization of the physis or growth plate. Traditionally, the physis is separated into 4 contiguous layers from epiphysis to metaphysis: resting (or germinal), proliferative, hypertrophic, and zone of provisional calcification. (Mark W. Kline, *Rudolph's Pediatrics*, 23rd Edition. Copyright © McGraw-Hill Education. All rights reserved.)

### Answer 14-6. D

Posterior medial bowing of the tibia is a congenital deformity of the tibia that is relatively benign in nature despite the obvious abnormality at birth. Patients may develop a leg length discrepancy on the affected side and should be followed through skeletal maturity. Aside from the associated leg length discrepancy, the majority of the deformity will spontaneously correct by about 2 years of age. Unlike anterior lateral bowing of the tibia, which is associated with neurofibromatosis type I, posterior medial bowing of the tibia is not a precursor for pseudoarthrosis and does not require bracing or amputation.

(Chapter 209: Torsional and Angular Deformities)

**TABLE 207-2.** Age of Appearance of Certain Gross Motor Milestones[a]

| Milestone | Age (Months, Average) |
|---|---|
| Rolls over (front to back) | 5 |
| Rolls over (back to front) | 6 |
| Sits independently | 7 |
| Crawls | 8 |
| Pulls to stand | 9 |
| Cruises (walks holding on) | 11 |
| Walks independently | 12 |
| Runs well | 24 |

[a]Note that achievement of these milestones requires development of the neurologic and musculoskeletal systems.

Mark W. Kline, *Rudolph's Pediatrics*, 23rd Edition. Copyright © McGraw-Hill Education. All rights reserved.

### Answer 14-7. D

The patient demonstrates findings consistent with scoliosis. Adolescent idiopathic scoliosis is the most common type of scoliosis and is more common in females. Females also have a higher risk of progression relative to males.

The severity of the curve at presentation may affect risk of progression. For example, a larger curve in a younger patient has a much higher risk of progression than a smaller curve in an older child. Age of menarche is an indicator of how much predicted growth may remain. Menarche happens after the peak growth phase. Thus, the risk of progression in a postmenarchal female, even at an early age, is generally less than the risk of a premenarchal female. A leg length discrepancy may cause a nonstructural scoliosis; however, it is not a separate risk factor for curve progression. Although back pain is common among adolescents, it is not a known risk factor for progression in the setting of idiopathic scoliosis. Severe back pain that limits or affects activity participation or is associated with neurologic findings is not common in idiopathic scoliosis, and if present, further workup may be necessary. A left thoracic curve is commonly referred to as an "atypical" curve. Some authors have demonstrated an increased risk of intraspinal pathology with atypical curve patterns.

(Chapter 213: Disorders of the Neck and Spine)

### Answer 14-8. C

A normal thoracic kyphosis has a 20- to 45-degree Cobb angle from T5 to T12. Increased kyphosis may be postural; however, this patient has Scheuermann's kyphosis. This condition is characterized by a structural (not postural) kyphosis on physical exam, with at least 3 consecutive vertebral bodies demonstrating ≥ 5 degrees of anterior endplate wedging appreciated on plain radiographs. Pain is not uncommon and is often located over the apex of the curve clinically.

Similar to idiopathic scoliosis, the risk of progression is highest among individuals who have significant growth remaining. Associated neurologic symptoms in Scheuermann's kyphosis are rare. Nonoperative treatment of Scheuermann's kyphosis includes physical therapy, core strengthening, and bracing. Surgical treatment for Scheuermann's kyphosis usually is reserved for patients who have demonstrated continued progression of the kyphosis despite skeletal maturity or prolonged pain refractory to conservative treatment.

(Chapter 213: Disorders of the Neck and Spine)

### Answer 14-9. A

The patient presents with acute diskitis, a rare inflammatory disease that can affect the disk or vertebral endplate in children. Children can present with history of back pain and decreased range of motion through the spine and may also have an abnormal gait. *S aureus* is the most common pathogen; however, many authors recommend use of empiric antibiotics to cover both *Kingella kingae* and *S aureus*. Laboratory values, including complete blood count (CBC) and blood cultures, are

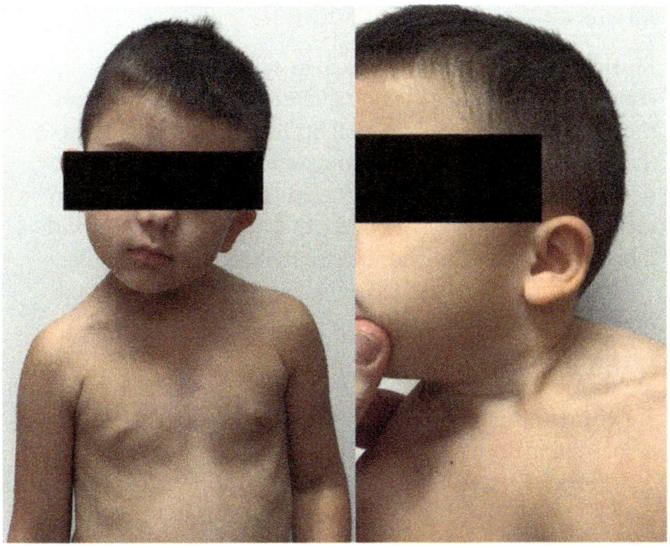

**FIGURE 213-1.** Congenital muscular torticollis in a young boy. The tight left sternocleidomastoid causes the left head tilt and chin rotation to the right. The tight left sternocleidomastoid muscle is evident. (Mark W. Kline, *Rudolph's Pediatrics*, 23rd Edition. Copyright © McGraw-Hill Education. All rights reserved.)

often normal; however, inflammatory markers such as CRP and ESR are usually elevated. Systemic symptoms are not common. The lumbar spine is most commonly affected; however, cases of diskitis affecting the cervical and thoracic spine have been reported. Injury is not a common precursor to onset of diskitis.

(Chapter 213: Disorders of the Neck and Spine)

### Answer 14-10. B

This patient has congenital muscular torticollis. This can be characterized by normal range of motion with postural preference or may also demonstrate limited range of motion secondary to a tight sternocleidomastoid (SCM) muscle. In the presence of a tight SCM, the patient will often demonstrate a tilt of the head (toward the side of the tight SCM) and rotation of the chin toward the opposite side (Figure 213-1). In some cases, a palpable mass can be appreciated in the muscle belly of the affected SCM. Palpation of the mass is typically painless. The mass is located within the mid-substance of the muscle belly and generally does not require further imaging. Referral to orthopedics is generally not necessary unless there is clinical concern for congenital scoliosis and/or the condition is refractory to physical therapy. The patient appears to be demonstrating appropriate vision for his age at this time, and thus, referral to ophthalmology is not indicated.

(Chapter 213: Disorders of the Neck and Spine)

### Answer 14-11. C

The history, examination, and radiographic findings for this child are consistent with an osteochondroma. An osteochondroma, or exostosis, is a common benign bone tumor. Because the boy in the vignette has a solitary osteochondroma, he does not require biopsy or additional imaging.

Indications for surgical removal of an osteochondroma include pain or functional disturbance, which this boy does not have. Therefore, providing reassurance to the boy and his parents is appropriate. The family should also be informed that osteochondromas often increase in size during childhood and adolescence. Osteochondromas consist of a bony base with a cartilage cap. Because the cartilaginous portion is not visible on radiographs, these tumors appear to be smaller on radiographs than on clinical examination. Growth of an osteochondroma in a skeletally mature individual is concerning for malignant transformation, an extremely rare complication of a solitary lesion.

(Chapter 216: Tumors)

### Answer 14-12. E

The radiograph shows a nonossifying fibroma, or fibrous cortical defect. Nonossifying fibromas are areas of bone filled with fibrous tissue and are not true neoplasms. Approximately one-third of children have a nonossifying fibroma, and these lesions are typically discovered as an incidental finding on radiographs. Children with an incidentally discovered nonossifying fibroma do not require additional imaging or treatment. These bony defects typically resolve without treatment. Infection and trauma do not appear to have any connection to the presence of a nonossifying fibroma.

(Chapter 216: Tumors)

### Answer 14-13. E

The girl's radiographs show a unicameral bone cyst (UBC). A UBC, or simple bone cyst, is a benign, serous fluid–filled cyst. Her history of episodic arm pain suggests that she has experienced multiple pathologic fractures. Pathologic fractures are a known complication of UBCs and an indication for surgical treatment. Historically, UBCs have been treated with corticosteroid injection or compounds that fill the bone. However, operative treatment with curettage, decompression, and packing of the cyst is now favored due to improved outcomes with lower risk of recurrence.

Because a UBC is not an infectious condition, the girl does not require antibiotics. Advanced imaging and biopsy are not required for a child with clear evidence of UBC on radiographs. Observation can be an appropriate treatment for a child with a UBC. However, with a history of pathologic fracture, operative treatment is favored. UBCs rarely resolve spontaneously, so counseling the family that the lesion will heal with no treatment would not be appropriate.

(p. 1029, Chapter 216: Tumors)

### Answer 14-14. D

Osteoid osteomas are small, benign bone tumors. These tumors secrete prostaglandin. Therefore, prostaglandin inhibitors, such as nonsteroidal anti-inflammatory drugs (NSAIDs), often provide dramatic relief of the pain associated with these lesions. Osteoid osteomas can occur in any bone but are most common in the tibia and femur. Children and teens are most commonly affected. Affected individuals typically report that pain occurs at night. Swelling, redness, and tenderness are not usually associated with osteoid osteoma. Classic radiographic findings include a radiolucent nidus (typically smaller than 1 cm in size) surrounded by a ring of sclerosis. Computed tomography (CT) is the gold standard for imaging osteoid osteomas.

Symptomatic treatment with NSAIDs may be tried. However, CT-guided radiofrequency or surgical excision is recommended for patients who have persistent pain despite medical management.

(Chapter 216: Tumors)

### Answer 14-15. C

Eosinophilic granuloma refers to a single Langerhans cell histiocytosis (LCH) lesion. School-aged children are most commonly affected. LCH can present at any age, from birth to old age. The incidence in children has been estimated at 3 to 4 per million, with a 2:1 male-to-female ratio. The mildest, most favorable form of histiocytosis X is an eosinophilic granuloma that is confined to a single bone, or occasionally to several bones, without extraskeletal involvement.

LCH is a rare condition; the skull and femur are the bones most frequently affected. The majority of children with LCH have a solitary lesion. Low-grade fever, soft tissue swelling, and pain at the site of the lesion are common associated findings. On radiographs, an eosinophilic granuloma appears as a well-demarcated, "punched out" lucency.

Aneurysmal bone cysts typically occur in the long bones and are not associated with fever. Enchondromas are clusters of atypical cartilage cells that are present in the metaphyses and diaphyses of the long bones. Enchondromas usually occur in the phalanges of the hands and feet. Osteoid osteomas are not associated with swelling or fever. Radiographically, osteoid osteomas appear as a central lucent nidus with surrounding sclerosis. Individuals with monostotic (single lesion) fibrous dysplasia often present in their teens. Fibrous dysplasia can affect the skull. On radiographs, lesions have a "ground glass" appearance with scalloped edges.

(Chapter 216: Tumors)

### Answer 14-16. D

An orthosis, or orthotic, is a brace or device used to support or position the skeleton. Rigid or stiff orthoses are used to position the spine or extremities. Functional orthoses allow some motion of the joints while still providing stability. Orthoses are typically named for the joints or body parts they cross. For example, HKAFO stands for hip-knee-ankle-foot orthosis. Shoe inserts are also referred to as FOs (foot orthoses).

(Chapter 217: Neuromuscular Disorders)

### Answer 14-17. C

Myelodysplasia, often referred to as spina bifida, is a group of congenital conditions including closed neural tube defects, meningocele, and myelomeningocele. Spina bifida occurs when the neural tube fails to close completely during embryonic development. The incidence of spina bifida has declined in recent years due to the discovery that supplementation with folate during pregnancy decreases the risk of this disorder.

Spina bifida is associated with conditions that affect the brain, spine, extremities, and kidneys. Clubfoot, talipes equinovarus deformity, is often present at birth. Chiari malformation type II and hydrocephalus are frequently present. Patients with spina bifida are often followed by urology for associated hydronephrosis.

Ventricular septal defects, horseshoe kidney, and anal atresia may be part of the VACTERL (**v**ertebral defects, **a**nal **atresia**, **c**ardiac defects, **t**racheo-**e**sophageal fistula, **r**enal anomalies, and **l**imb abnormalities) association; individuals with spina bifida are not at risk for these conditions.

(p. 1032, Chapter 217: Neuromuscular Disorders)

### Answer 14-18. D

CP is defined as static encephalopathy due to brain injury. With CP, the injury occurs before brain development is complete. In premature infants, encephalopathy is often caused by intracranial hemorrhage; however, infection and trauma can also cause CP. In children with CP, the brain injury occurs prenatally or early in life, and the geographic classification and extent of disability are typically observable by 2 to 3 years of age. By definition, the encephalopathy with CP is nonprogressive. Children may have some fluctuation in flexibility during periods of rapid growth, but the girl's hemiplegia would not be expected to worsen over time.

The most common type of motor dysfunction with CP is spasticity, which is present in 80% of affected children; ataxia is the least common type. Children affected by hemiplegia have upper extremity and lower extremity dysfunction on the involved side. Cognitive dysfunction is not related to the degree of physical disability.

(p. 1034, Chapter 217: Neuromuscular Disorders)

### Answer 14-19. C

The infant in the vignette has amyoplasia, a form of arthrogryposis. The term *arthrogryposis* is an umbrella term used to describe a variety of disorders that involve contractures of multiple joints. Children with amyoplasia typically have symmetric involvement of the proximal and distal joints of the upper and lower extremities. Individuals with distal arthrogryposis usually have contractures of the hands and feet. Although many forms of distal arthrogryposis appear to be genetic, amyoplasia generally occurs sporadically. Conditions that impede fetal movement, such as bicornate uterus and oligohydramnios, increase the risk of amyoplasia. Children with amyoplasia usually have normal intelligence. Vertebral anomalies and a maternal history of seizures are not associated with amyoplasia.

(Chapter 217: Neuromuscular Disorders)

### Answer 14-20. E

Toe-walking gait is a common variant in young children and is not alarming when it begins around the time children learn to walk. However, the child in the vignette has developed toe-walking and increased clumsiness over the past year. Additionally, his physical examination findings suggest muscle weakness. His combination of history and physical findings raises concerns for the presence of muscular dystrophy. Duchenne muscular dystrophy (DMD) is the most likely type given this child's age, gender, and clinical presentation. Children with DMD tend to have elevated serum creatine kinase, aldolase, aspartate transaminase, and alanine transaminase. Creatine kinase is usually elevated before clinical signs appear, early in the course of the disease. As the disease progresses and as muscle is increasingly replaced with fibrotic tissue, creatine kinase declines. Increases in alkaline phosphatase and uric acid are not typically seen with DMD.

(Chapter 217: Neuromuscular Disorders)

### Answer 14-21. B

The patient in this vignette most likely has patellofemoral pain syndrome. This is a common diagnosis in adolescents with nonspecific anterior knee pain. The pain generally occurs diffusely around the patellae, and there is usually no inciting injury. Many patients with patellofemoral pain also have patellar subluxations. Common physical exam findings include the "J sign," which occurs when the patella moves laterally when the knee is fully extended, and the patellar apprehension sign, which occurs when the patient feels uncomfortable when the examiner pushes the patellae.

Physical therapy is the best treatment for decreasing pain long term. Physical therapy focuses on strengthening the quadriceps and hip muscles and stretching of the iliotibial band and hamstrings. Patellar stabilization braces can alleviate symptoms while patients are undergoing physical therapy.

Intra-articular steroid injection is not indicated for patellofemoral pain in adolescents and would not provide long-term relief. Patellar straps are commonly used for Osgood-Schlatter and Sinding-Larsen-Johansson disease and are not helpful for patellofemoral pain. Surgical correction of patellar alignment is only indicated in cases of recurrent patellofemoral dislocation. Knee immobilizers are generally helpful in the short period immediately after an acute knee injury and would not treat chronic patellofemoral pain syndrome.

(Chapter 211: Disorders of the Knee)

### Answer 14-22. C

Less than 5% of children are born with a thickened, abnormally shaped meniscus known as a lateral discoid meniscus. Discoid menisci can present at any age with popping, catching, and sometimes pain over the lateral knee with flexion and extension. They are more prone to tearing and can limit knee function over time. On exam, the McMurray test, or McMurray circumduction maneuver, can be used to detect internal tears in the knee joint. During the maneuver, any pain or click suggests a meniscal tear.

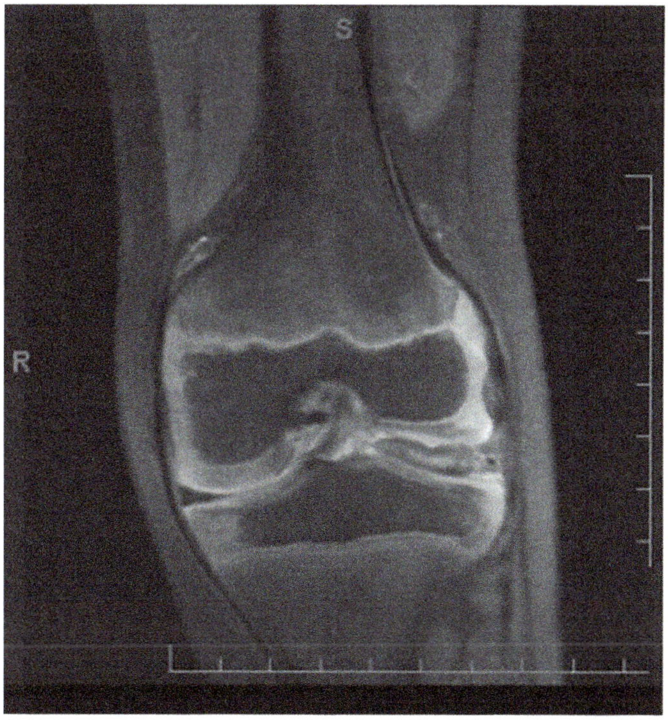


A

**FIGURE 211-1A.** Coronal magnetic resonance imaging of a 7-year-old patient with painful left knee popping due to large, unstable discoid meniscus. (Mark W. Kline, *Rudolph's Pediatrics*, 23rd Edition. Copyright © McGraw-Hill Education. All rights reserved.)

Children with symptomatic discoid menisci often require arthroscopic reconstruction to correct the shape of the meniscus and repair any tears. MRI is the best imaging to evaluate for soft tissue abnormalities and can aid in surgical planning (Figure 211-1A).

DEXA scans are used to evaluate bone density and would not provide any information about the cartilaginous meniscus. Ultrasound will not provide sufficient imaging of the meniscus to fully evaluate its shape and potential tears. CT scans are most helpful when evaluating abnormalities of the bone and would not provide sufficient detail of the soft tissue structures in the knee. A bone scan is a nuclear medicine study used to determine the metabolic activity of bone and is primarily used for evaluating stress fractures.

(Chapter 211: Disorders of the Knee)

### Answer 14-23. E

Osteochondritis dissecans is a lesion of subchondral bone necrosis, shown on the medial femoral condyle in the

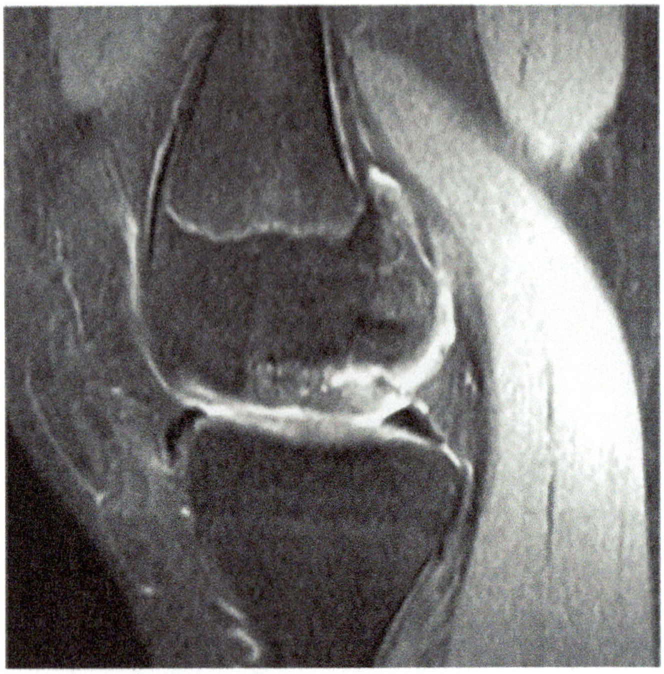

B

**FIGURE 211-2B.** Sagittal magnetic resonance imaging showing fragment instability. (Mark W. Kline, *Rudolph's Pediatrics*, 23rd Edition. Copyright © McGraw-Hill Education. All rights reserved.)

radiograph (Figure 211-2A and B). The cause is unknown, but repetitive microtrauma and low blood supply to the area are thought to contribute. These most commonly occur in the medial femoral condyle but can develop in any joint. The lesion and its overlying cartilage can separate from the rest of the bone and become an intra-articular loose body. Patients may complain of pain, swelling, and mechanical symptoms such as catching or popping.

Patients with Osgood-Schlatter disease have pain over the tibial tubercle and do not have mechanical symptoms. There is no tibial spine fracture on the radiograph. Meniscal tears can present with mechanical symptoms and swelling but would not have the bone lesion shown on the radiograph. There is no fracture on the radiograph. Salter-Harris III fractures extend from the physis (growth plate) to the epiphysis.

(Chapter 211: Disorders of the Knee)

## Answer 14-24. A

Osgood-Schlatter disease is a frequent condition in adolescents in which the tibial tubercle apophysis (growth plate) becomes irritated and inflamed. The patellar tendon inserts into this apophysis, so tight quadriceps and hamstring muscles can aggravate the condition by increasing tension on the patellar tendon and its apophysis. Osgood-Schlatter disease often occurs during the teenage growth spurt when muscles have less flexibility. Pain is worse with repetitive activities such as jumping and running, and the tibial tubercles are tender and can appear prominent on exam. This condition resolves completely at skeletal maturity when the growth plates close, although occasionally, patients may have prominent and tender tibial tubercles into adulthood.

Surgery is not necessary to treat Osgood-Schlatter disease, and the pain resolves at skeletal maturity. Patients with Osgood-Schlatter may continue to participate in sports as long as the pain is not so severe that it causes limping or distraction because this may lead to other injuries. Patellar stabilization braces are used to treat patellar subluxations or dislocation. Patellar straps alleviate symptoms of Osgood-Schlatter by off-loading pressure from the physis. Stretching and ice can also help alleviate symptoms. Sinding-Larsen-Johansson disease (irritation of the apophysis of the inferior pole of the patella) is more common in the preteen years, before the pubertal growth spurt, whereas Osgood-Schlatter usually occurs in the early teen years.

(p. 1002: Chapter 211: Disorders of the Knee)

## Answer 14-25. D

Sinding-Larsen-Johansson disease (SLJ) is an apophysitis, or growth center irritation, of the distal pole of the patella where the patellar tendon originates. SLJ can be unilateral or bilateral. It usually occurs in children aged 10 to 13 years just before the pubertal growth spurt. There is tenderness and sometimes swelling over the inferior pole of the patella. Pain is usually worse with activities that load the knee, such as running, jumping, and squatting, and improves with rest. Other helpful treatments include ice and using a patellar strap to change the directional pull of the patellar tendon. Radiographs are not necessary if there are no other abnormalities on exam.

Imaging with MRI is usually recommended to evaluate soft tissue injuries such as ligament or meniscal tears and is not necessary for SLJ. The swelling seen in SLJ is usually focal over the inferior patellar poles; there is no joint effusion or fevers to suggest septic arthritis, so synovial fluid analysis is not necessary. SLJ resolves naturally with time, so surgical treatment is not necessary.

(Chapter 211: Disorders of the Knee)

## Answer 14-26. D

Popliteal (Baker) cysts generally occur in children aged 4 to 7 years. They arise from the gastrocnemius-semimembranosus bursa and do not communicate with the joint. These generally arise spontaneously and are often nonpainful. On exam, there is a firm, fluid-filled mass in the posterior medial fossa that decreases in size when the knee is flexed. The mass is best appreciated with the patient prone and the knee fully extended. With the knee flexed, there is some mobility to the mass, but it remains firm. In a dark room, the mass will transilluminate. Childhood popliteal cysts resolve without treatment. In contrast, popliteal cysts in adults are associated with underlying joint disease and usually communicate with the joint.

A child with a discoid meniscus presents with popping, mechanical symptoms, and sometimes pain over the lateral knee. Anterior cruciate ligament injuries are rare in young children, and exam usually reveals a joint effusion as well as positive Lachman and anterior drawer signs. Osteochondromas are firm masses that do not change size with positioning and would not transilluminate. Osgood-Schlatter disease is an apophysitis of the tibial tubercle that occurs in adolescents.

(Chapter 211: Disorders of the Knee)

### Answer 14-27. B

Breech positioning, especially frank breech presentation in which the hips are flexed and knees are extended, is an important risk factor for DDH. Other important risk factors include family history of DDH, history of tight lower extremity swaddling with the hips in an extended position, and female sex. Regardless of sex and exam findings, imaging of the hips should be considered in infants with history of breech positioning or family history of DDH. This imaging can consist of a hip ultrasound between 6 weeks and 6 months of age or a radiograph of the pelvis once the femoral heads have sufficiently ossified at 4 to 6 months of age.

Male sex, loose swaddling, polyhydramnios, and prematurity are not risk factors for DDH.

(Chapter 212: Developmental Conditions of the Hip)

### Answer 14-28. E

The most important exam finding in DDH in a child > 3 months of age is limited hip abduction. Other possible exam findings include positive Galeazzi sign, a positive Klisic test, leg length discrepancy, abnormal gait, and asymmetric thigh or gluteal folds. Ortolani and Barlow tests are useful in younger infants but are less sensitive after 3 months of age.

Legg-Calvé-Perthes disease is most prevalent between 4 and 12 years of age and generally presents with a painless limp. On exam, there is limitation in hip abduction and internal rotation, but there is no leg length discrepancy or Galeazzi sign. Slipped capital femoral epiphysis usually occurs during adolescence. These patients can have pain and a limp, and exam is significant for painful, limited internal rotation. Transient synovitis usually occurs between 3 and 8 years of age. Children may have sudden onset of hip pain, limping, and limited range of motion. Internal tibial torsion causes in-toeing in toddlers and resolves with time. Hip exam would be normal in children with internal tibial torsion.

(Chapter 212: Developmental Conditions of the Hip)

### Answer 14-29. A

Legg-Calvé-Perthes disease is idiopathic avascular necrosis of the femoral head. It most commonly occurs between 4 and 12 years of age and is more prevalent in boys. Although the exact etiology is unknown, systemic conditions such as sickle cell disease and hypothyroidism, as well as steroid medications, can increase risk. Standing AP and frog-leg radiographs of both hips are the best initial imaging. If positive, the radiographs will show fragmentation and/or remodeling of the femoral head.

It would be inappropriate to provide reassurance before obtaining imaging. Surgical treatment of Legg-Calvé-Perthes disease is uncommon, and initial imaging should be performed before referral to orthopedic surgery. Treatment is usually conservative: rest, decreased weight bearing on the affected hip, and restoration of hip strength and range of motion. Fast-acting opiates are not necessary for Legg-Calvé-Perthes disease, especially because this child does not currently have any pain. Fast-acting opiates would be more appropriate for a child presenting with sickle cell crisis. Pavlik harnesses are used for treating developmental dysplasia of the hip (DDH) in infants younger than 6 months.

(Chapter 212: Developmental Conditions of the Hip)

### Answer 14-30. C

Chronic, stable slipped capital femoral epiphysis (SCFE) often presents with insidious-onset pain and a limp. It is more common in obese adolescent males, but girls and adolescents with normal weight can also develop SCFE. Because the pain can be referred to the knee, it is important to examine the hips in all adolescents with knee, thigh, or groin pain. A positive exam will reveal increased external rotation at rest and pain with flexion and internal rotation of the affected hip (Figure 212-8). Anteroposterior (AP) and frog-leg radiographs of the hips are diagnostic.

Hip pain is frequently referred to the knee. As a result, providers should examine the hips of children and adolescents with knee pain, especially in the setting of a normal knee exam. Reassurance would be inappropriate in this case because stable, chronic SCFE can progress to acute, unstable SCFE, which has a significant risk of avascular necrosis. Patellar straps are a helpful treatment for adolescents suffering from Osgood-Schlatter disease. Physical therapy is not an effective treatment for SCFE.

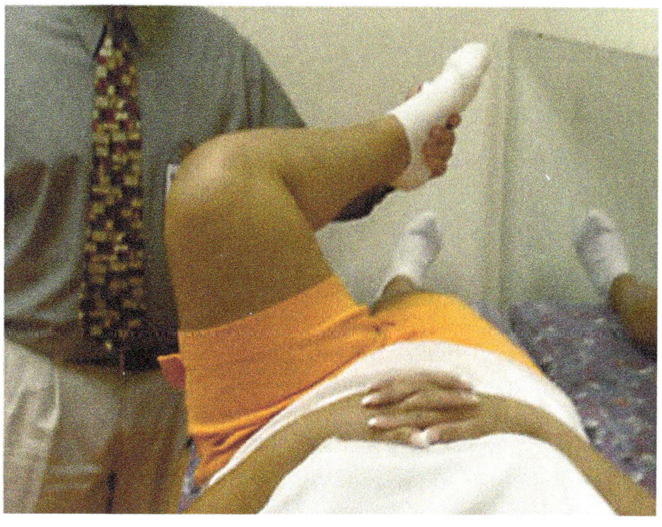

**FIGURE 212-8.** Clinical examination of a patient with stable slipped capital femoral epiphysis. Hip flexion and external rotation are limited. With flexion of the affected hip, the limb rotates externally. (Reproduced with permission from Herring JA. *Tachdjian's Pediatric Orthopaedics*, 4th ed. Philadelphia: Elsevier; 2007.)

Patients with SCFE should be made non–weight bearing and transported to the hospital for urgent surgical repair to stabilize the capital femoral epiphysis and prevent further displacement.

(Chapter 212: Developmental Conditions of the Hip)

**Answer 14-31.** D

The most important risk factors for DDH are breech positioning, family history of DDH, female sex, and history of tight lower extremity swaddling with the hips in an extended position. The most important exam finding in DDH in a child > 3 months of age is limited hip abduction.

Answer choice A describes an adolescent with chronic, stable slipped capital femoral epiphysis (SCFE). SCFE often presents with insidious onset of knee, thigh, or groin pain along with a limp. It is more common in obese adolescent males, but girls and adolescents with a normal body mass index (BMI) can also develop SCFE. Because the pain can be referred to the knee, it is important to examine the hips in all adolescents with knee pain. Answer choice B describes a child with Legg-Calvé-Perthes disease, an avascular necrosis of the femoral head. This condition is most prevalent between 4 and 12 years of age and generally presents with a painless limp. Certain systemic conditions such as sickle cell disease and hypothyroidism, as well as systemic steroids, can increase the risk of developing the condition. Answer choice C describes a child with transient synovitis of the hip. Transient synovitis usually occurs between 3 and 8 years of age and usually presents with sudden onset of hip pain, limping, and limited range of motion. These children often have had a recent illness. Answer choice E describes an adolescent who likely has an avulsion fracture of the anterior inferior iliac spine. Adolescents have an apophysis (minor growth plate) at the anterior inferior iliac spine where the rectus femoris muscle originates. The quadriceps muscle can contract so hard during intense physical activity that the anterior inferior iliac spine apophysis can be pulled away from the pelvis, resulting in an avulsion fracture.

(Chapter 212: Developmental Conditions of the Hip)

**Answer 14-32.** D

The patient in this vignette has transient synovitis of the hip. This diagnosis is a relatively common cause of hip pain, limited range of motion, and limping in children aged 3 to 8 years old. Although the exact cause of transient synovitis is unknown, nearly half of children with transient synovitis have had a recent viral upper respiratory tract infection. The symptoms last an average of 10 days, and conservative treatment with scheduled NSAIDs for the first 3 to 5 days helps alleviate symptoms.

The Kocher criteria help distinguish transient synovitis from septic arthritis and include non–weight bearing, temperature > 38.5°C, ESR > 40 mm/h, and WBC > 12,000 cells/mL. The patient in this vignette has none of these criteria and no effusion on imaging, so septic arthritis is unlikely and surgical washout is not necessary. Slipped capital femoral epiphysis (SCFE) usually occurs in obese adolescent males. In addition, SCFE is usually apparent on radiographs. Pavlik harness is a treatment for infants with developmental dysplasia of the hip (DDH). Physical therapy is not necessary for most patients with transient synovitis because it usually resolves quickly with conservative management.

(Chapter 212: Developmental Conditions of the Hip)

**Answer 14-33.** E

Based on the history and exam, this patient most likely has slipped capital femoral epiphysis (SCFE), a fracture in the proximal femoral growth plate. SCFE is an urgent orthopedic condition that is best diagnosed on AP and lateral radiographs. Imaging of both hips is preferred for comparison to the contralateral side and because SCFE can be bilateral in some cases (Figure 208-4, A and B).

AP pelvis and frog-leg lateral views of the right hip show SCFE, which is best seen on the lateral view. If diagnosed, orthopedic consultation should be obtained urgently for surgical stabilization and the patient should be made non–weight bearing on crutches. Children and adolescents are at risk for SCFE if they are overweight or have endocrine abnormalities. If a patient complains of knee pain, the hip should also be evaluated for possible referred pain. Patients with SCFE often present with external rotation with hip flexion on exam. Lab tests such as CBC and inflammatory markers would be helpful if the patient appeared ill or if a septic joint or transient synovitis was suspected. Knee imaging such as x-rays or MRI would be appropriate to evaluate for knee pathology.

(Chapter 208: The Limping Child)

**Answer 14-34.** C

In this patient, even with unremarkable radiographs, the presence of tenderness directly over the growth plate (physis) suggests a growth plate injury. These injuries should be protected like a fracture with immobilization. A walking boot or splint are options for immobilization. Because the growth plate is susceptible to injury, occult fracture is more likely than sprain in this age group.

Reassurance and/or using an ace wrap would not be appropriate for a possible fracture. A growth plate injury can be suspected based on physical exam alone. As a result, an ankle MRI is not necessarily required. You should consider lab evaluation when there is suspicion for an infection or malignancy. This approach would be less likely in a case with a clear injury and otherwise well-appearing child.

(Chapter 208: The Limping Child)

**Answer 14-35.** C

Transient synovitis is also called irritable hip. It is benign and self-limiting; however, it is challenging to distinguish this diagnosis from septic arthritis. In an afebrile patient with normal labs, transient synovitis is more likely than septic arthritis. Septic arthritis is more likely to present with an

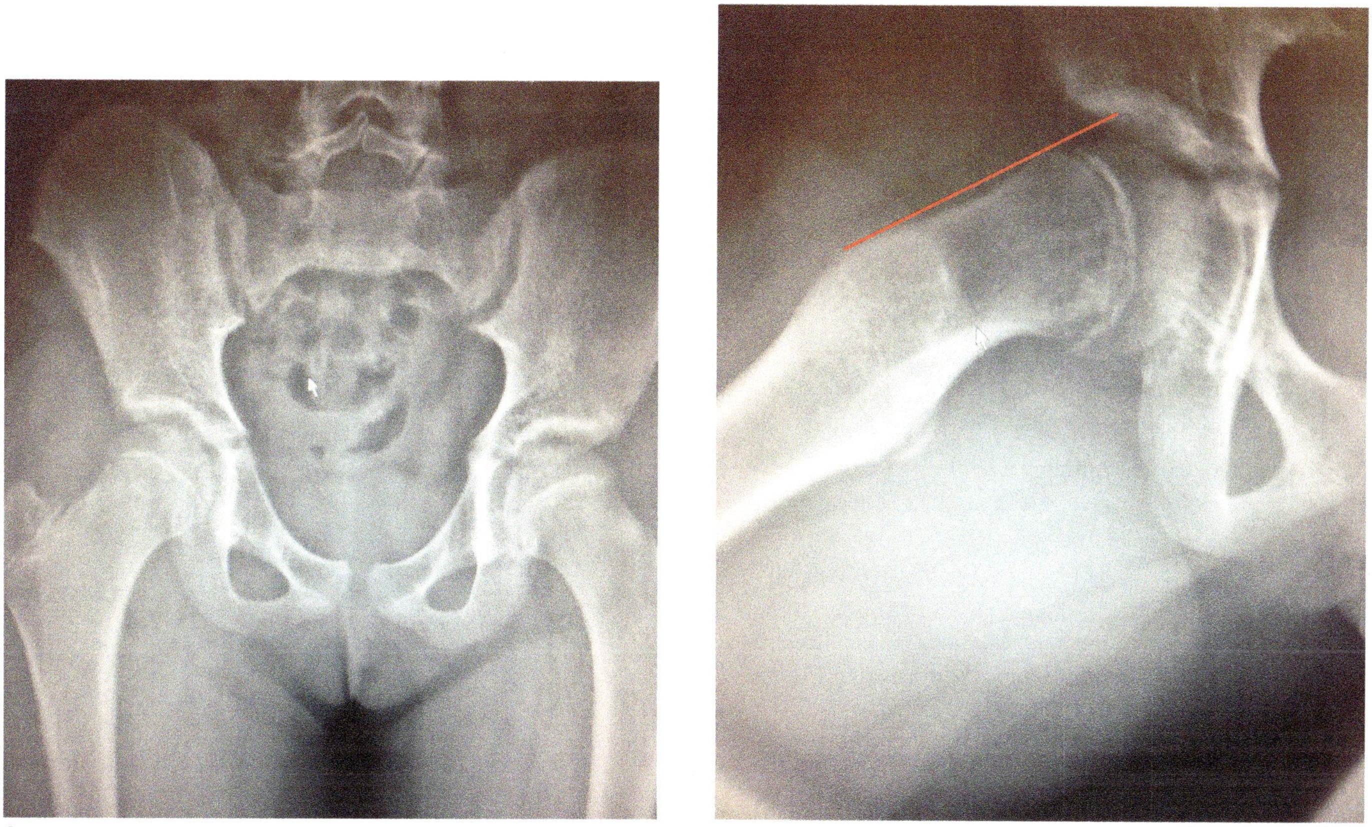


**FIGURE 208-4.** A and B: Anteroposterior pelvis and frog-leg lateral views of the right hip show a slipped capital femoral epiphysis, best demonstrated on the lateral view. It was missed on initial evaluation. (Mark W. Kline, *Rudolph's Pediatrics*, 23rd Edition. Copyright © McGraw-Hill Education. All rights reserved.)

ill-appearing and febrile child who has an elevated white blood cell (WBC) count along with elevated inflammatory markers such as ESR and CRP. Both transient synovitis and septic arthritis are more likely to occur in the hip than other joints.

Legg-Calvé-Perthes disease is a less common cause of hip pain. Radiographs typically show an abnormality of the proximal femoral epiphysis. A hip fracture would be more likely with a history of injury and likely be apparent on radiograph. SCFE would also likely be suggested on radiograph and is more common in adolescents. SCFE should be suspected in an overweight adolescent with insidious onset of hip or leg pain.

(Chapter 208: The Limping Child)

### Answer 14-36. B

This patient likely has a hip effusion given she is presenting with her hip held in flexion and external rotation. A hip effusion with an ill-appearing child, high WBC count, and elevated CRP and ESR is suspicious for septic arthritis. Subspecialty consultation is warranted for likely further imaging (ultrasound or magnetic resonance imaging [MRI]) and possible aspiration or drainage.

Reassurance or outpatient follow-up would not be appropriate for suspected septic arthritis. A leg fracture would be immobilized in a long leg splint, although there would more likely be a history of injury and an abnormal radiograph. Knee radiographs would be appropriate if there was a knee injury, effusion, or tenderness around the knee on exam.

(p. 986, Chapter 208: The Limping Child)

### Answer 14-37. E

Malignancy is an extremely rare cause of childhood limp; however, it should be considered in certain situations. A child without clear injury, various other bone pains, and elevated inflammatory markers should raise suspicion for malignancy. Radiographs should be inspected for changes such as periosteal elevation or lucency. When concerned, a manual differential should be requested because blast cells may be mistakenly identified as atypical lymphocytes on automated differential. A 2 years old with a twisting injury is suspicious for a toddler's fracture. A 15-year-old obese male with insidious-onset right leg limp is more suspicious for slipped capital femoral epiphysis (SCFE). A 14-year-old ice hockey player and a 17-year-old basketball player with injuries are more suspicious for bone or soft tissue injuries given the history.

(Chapter 208: The Limping Child)

**Answer 14-38.** D

The anteroposterior (AP) pelvis and bilateral frog-leg lateral radiograph views show sclerosis and fragmentation of the proximal femoral epiphysis or Legg-Calvé-Perthes disease. Legg-Calvé-Perthes disease is a rare, idiopathic cause of hip pain in children aged 4 to 10 years old.

SCFE is an urgent growth plate fracture that can occur in children aged 9 to 14 years. Children who are overweight or have endocrine abnormalities are at increased risk. A patient with septic arthritis would appear more ill and, along with transient synovitis, is likely to have normal radiographs. Hip fracture would be suspected in a patient with trauma and would likely be visible on radiograph.

(p. 987, Chapter 208: The Limping Child)

**Answer 14-39.** A

An elbow effusion is detected on lateral radiograph with fat pad signs (Figure 215-1, A–C). If there is an elbow effusion, occult fracture is suspected, and the joint should be immobilized with close follow-up and repeat radiographs performed in 7 to 10 days.

Reassurance and ace wrap would not be appropriate for a suspected fracture. A nursemaid's elbow is reduced by flexing the elbow to 90 degrees with supination; however, this injury is typically caused by traction or pulling on the extended arm of a child and is most common under the age of 5 years. An ultrasound may be appropriate if you were concerned about a joint infection; however, this is less likely with a known injury.

(Chapter 215: Injuries)

**Answer 14-40.** B

There are a few fractures that are pathognomonic for signs of abuse, including metaphyseal corner fractures, posterior rib fractures, and several fractures in various stages of healing. Any fracture in a nonambulatory child < 12 months of age should be evaluated carefully for possible nonaccidental trauma, especially femur and elbow fractures.

The other scenarios illustrate common pediatric fractures. Greenstick and buckle fractures of the forearm can occur after a fall. A spiral tibial or "toddler's" fracture is common for a child in the first 2 to 3 years after ambulation. A lateral malleolus fracture can occur after an inversion ankle injury. The Salter-Harris classification defines where the fracture is located in the growth plate.

(p. 1024, Section 215: Injuries)

**Answer 14-41.** D

An injury with a knee effusion and negative radiographs should prompt evaluation for an underlying ligamentous or cartilage injury. As a result, a knee MRI is an appropriate next step. An anterior cruciate ligament tear would be highest on the differential for a twisting injury with an effusion and positive anterior drawer test noted on exam.

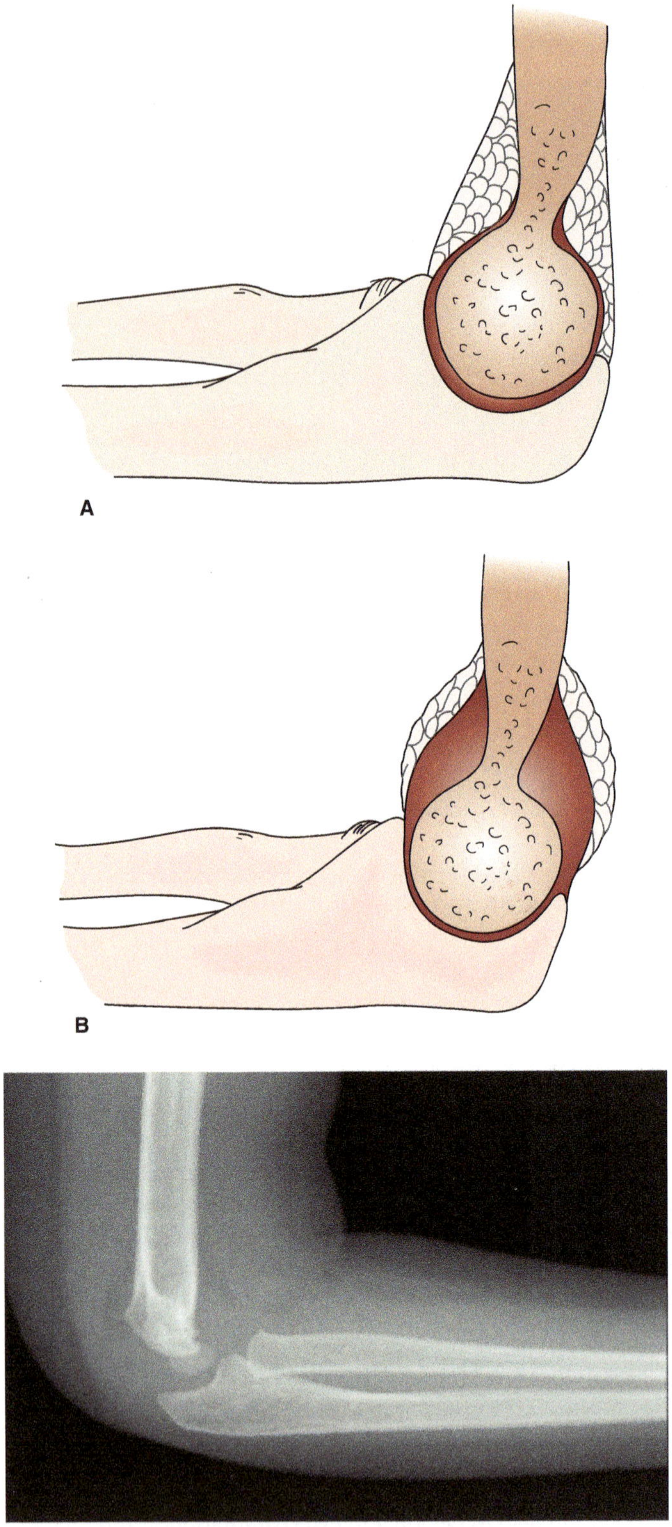

A

B

C

**FIGURE 215-1.** A: Anterior and posterior fat pad positions in a normal elbow. B: Elevation of fat pads secondary to elbow effusion as seen in occult fractures. C: Radiograph with anterior and posterior fat pad signs. (Mark W. Kline, *Rudolph's Pediatrics*, 23rd Edition. Copyright © McGraw-Hill Education. All rights reserved.)

Meniscal tears and patellar dislocations can also cause knee effusions. You may recommend repeat radiographs in 7 to 10 days or a CT scan for a possible fracture. Hip pathologies such as slipped capital femoral epiphysis (SCFE) or Legg-Calvé-Perthes disease would be evaluated with hip radiographs and can present with knee pain; however, they would not typically present with a knee effusion and specific injury. Labs would be warranted if concerned about an infection; however, this is less likely with a clear mechanism of injury.

(Chapter 215: Injuries)

**Answer 14-42.** A

This presentation is consistent with a toddler's fracture, a nondisplaced or occult spiral fracture of the tibia. It typically occurs during the first 2 to 3 years of ambulation and should be treated with immobilization for 3 to 4 weeks. Even with negative radiographs, if there is a history of injury and tibial tenderness, an occult fracture should be treated with immobilization rather than reassurance.

You would consider further lab evaluation if you were concerned for an infection. This diagnosis would more likely present without an injury and be accompanied by an ill-appearing febrile child with joint swelling or loss of hip range of motion. A skeletal survey would be considered to evaluate for nonaccidental trauma if the fracture was suspicious. For example, you might consider a skeletal survey for a child who is less than a year old or nonambulatory. A hip radiograph would be appropriate if the hip exam was abnormal.

(Chapter 215: Injuries)

**Answer 14-43.** B

The patient has a lateral ankle sprain, which is diagnosed clinically by an inversion mechanism of injection, tenderness over the lateral ankle ligaments instead of over bony prominences, and negative radiographs. Ankle sprains are best treated with RICE (rest, ice, compression, elevation) along with early range of motion and weight bearing as tolerated. These active treatments are better than reassurance for this type of injury.

A cast would be appropriate if there was concern for a fracture. Lab evaluation would be appropriate if there was concern for infection, which is less likely in the ankle and with a clear injury mechanism. Advanced imaging such as MRI is rarely needed for the initial management of ankle sprains.

(Chapter 215: Injuries)

**Answer 14-44.** C

A high volume of repetitive activity can stress tissue, including the growth plate in a growing adolescent. The radiograph shows widening of the proximal humeral physis, which is consistent with epiphysitis, or bone edema and growth plate injury. Epiphysitis can also be found at the medial epicondyle of the elbow in baseball pitchers. Radiographs can be normal, so a history of high levels of repetitive activities and activity-related pain should raise suspicion for growth plate stress injury. Treatment is rest from painful activities including throwing. Adhering to pitch count recommendations and rules is an important part of preventing these injuries.

Rotator cuff tears are more common in adults and cannot be diagnosed based on radiographs. Shoulder strain or clavicle fracture would more likely present with an acute injury, and clavicle fracture would be evident on radiographs. Growing pains are a diagnosis of exclusion and more common in the lower extremity.

(Chapter 215: Injuries)

**Answer 14-45.** A

Malignant bony lesions cause damage to surrounding bone. On radiographs, malignant tumors are associated with periosteal reaction and destruction of the cortex. A mixed lytic and sclerotic lesion with extensive periosteal reaction should raise concern for malignancy, specifically osteosarcoma. With osteosarcoma, there is often soft tissue involvement as well; this would be seen with magnetic resonance imaging (MRI).

A surrounding rim of sclerosis suggests a stable, nonprogressive lesion. An osteoid osteoma appears as a radiolucent nidus with a surrounding rim of sclerosis on radiographs. A nonossifying fibroma can appear multiloculated with a thin sclerotic rim. The "ground glass" appearance of a bony lesion is a classic descriptor for fibrous dysplasia. Osteochondromas (or exostoses) are osseous growths that demonstrate continuity with the bony cortex. They usually arise from the metaphyseal region and can be either sessile (having a broad base with a smaller cap) or pedunculated (having a narrow base and a large cap).

(Chapter 216: Tumors)

**Answer 14-46.** E

The description of expansile, lytic lesions involving the phalanges suggests enchondromas. Multiple enchondromatosis can be seen with both Ollier disease and Maffucci syndrome.

Maffucci syndrome is less common than Ollier disease. Individuals with Maffucci syndrome have multiple hemangiomas with associated calcifications seen on radiographs. Osteochondromas (or exostoses) are outgrowths of the bone that demonstrate continuity with the bony cortex. People with Li-Fraumeni syndrome have an increased risk of breast and adrenal cancer, leukemia, and sarcomas. Children with Beckwith-Wiedemann syndrome exhibit hemihypertrophy and have an increased risk of Wilms tumor and hepatocellular carcinoma but do not have benign bony lesions.

(Chapter 216: Tumors)

# CHAPTER 15 Rheumatology

Aimee O. Hersh, Karen E. James, Sara M. Stern, Erin M. Treemarcki, Christi J. Inman, and John F. Bohnsack

**15-1.** A 7-year-old girl is suspected of being infected with *Mycobacterium tuberculosis*. She develops a positive skin test reaction to intradermal injection with purified protein derivative (PPD). Which of the following best describes the mechanism underlying the reaction to the PPD injection?

**A.** Immunoglobulin E (IgE) bound to mast cells triggers mast cell activation after the IgE binds PPD.

**B.** Immunoglobulin G (IgG) binds to PPD, initiating an influx of neutrophils and macrophages.

**C.** Immune complex formation in the walls of blood vessels triggers complement activation and blood vessel damage.

**D.** Antigen-presenting cells ingest PPD and present antigen to T cells, thereby triggering T-cell activation to induce an influx of macrophages and other inflammatory cells.

**E.** Direct activation of complement by PPD results in C5a production and influx of neutrophils.

**15-2.** A 10-year-old boy is being treated for a hypocalcemic seizure and is found to have hypoparathyroidism. He has suffered from chronic thrush and onychomycosis due to *Candida albicans* since he was 1 year of age. In addition, he has had episodes of a recurrent maculopapular rash described as nonpruritic urticaria since 2 years of age. His younger sister also has chronic mucocutaneous candidiasis. His parents are not affected by any of these disorders. Genetic testing of the siblings reveals that they both have biallelic mutations in the *AIRE* gene, which are known to cause loss of function in the protein product of this gene. A diagnosis of autoimmune regulator and autoimmune polyendocrinopathy-candidiasis-ectodermal dystrophy (APECED) is made. What is the underlying mechanism of this disease?

**A.** Lack of development of B-cell tolerance during B-cell development

**B.** Lack of development of T-cell tolerance during T-cell development

**C.** Overproduction of IL-1 and IL-18 by caspase 1

**D.** Lack of expression of major histocompatibility complex (MHC) class I

**E.** Lack of expression of MHC class II

**15-3.** A 7-month-old male infant is admitted to the hospital for education regarding recent-onset diabetes mellitus. He is found to have hypothyroidism during the hospitalization. He has had severe eczema since shortly after birth and was diagnosed as having enteropathy with villous atrophy at 4 months of age. A genetic test reveals a mutation in the *FOXP3* gene. Which of the following is the underlying pathogenic mechanism for his clinical presentation?

**A.** Lack of B-cell tolerance to self-antigens

**B.** Lack of development of T regulatory (Treg) cells

**C.** Overproduction of IL-1 and IL-18 by caspase

**D.** Lack of expression of major histocompatibility complex (MHC) class I

**E.** Lack of expression of MHC class II

**15-4.** A 12-year-old girl with juvenile idiopathic arthritis (JIA) is being treated with rituximab, a monoclonal antibody directed against B cells that is used to treat arthritis. Rituximab is a chimeric antibody, meaning that part of it is derived from a mouse antibody and acts as a foreign antigen in humans. Seven days after her third dose of rituximab, she develops fever, arthritis, proteinuria, and a hive-like rash that subsequently becomes petechial and ecchymotic. She recovers after several days of treatment with a systemic corticosteroid. Which of the following best describes the underlying mechanism of her reaction to rituximab?

**A.** She has developed immunoglobulin E (IgE) antibodies against murine antigens in rituximab, which activate her mast cells.

**B.** Rituximab lyses B cells, resulting in release of intracellular cytokines.

**C.** She has developed immunoglobulin G (IgG) antibodies against murine antigens in rituximab, and immune complexes consisting of rituximab and antirituximab deposit in skin, kidney, and joints, triggering complement activation and blood vessel damage.

**D.** Rituximab depletes B cells, allowing T helper cells directed against self-antigens to proliferate and attack the affected tissues.

**E.** Rituximab depletes Treg cells, leading to an autoimmune reaction against skin, kidney, and joint antigens.

**15-5.** A 7-year-old boy is brought in for evaluation of joint pain. His mother reports that this has been an ongoing concern for the past month, but she initially thought it was just growing pains. What element of the history is most concerning for an inflammatory arthritis?

**A.** Waking up with pain at night

**B.** Being unable to button his shirt in the morning

**C.** Limping after soccer practice

**D.** A maternal history of rheumatoid arthritis

**E.** Having pain since falling off his scooter

**15-6.** A 5-year-old boy is brought in for evaluation of joint pain. Pain has been gradually worsening over the past month. He tells his mother that his legs hurt on a daily basis. You are concerned he may have juvenile idiopathic arthritis (JIA). What pattern of pain is most consistent with JIA?

**A.** Worse in morning, improves with activity

**B.** Worse in morning, worse with activity

**C.** Persistent all day, no change with activity

**D.** Worse in afternoon, improves with activity

**E.** Worse in afternoon, worse with activity

**15-7.** A 6-year-old boy is brought in for evaluation of knee pain and swelling. His mother states that he refused to walk this morning, at which time she noticed that his right knee was swollen. Which physical exam finding would be most suggestive of septic arthritis?

**A.** Limited flexion of the knee

**B.** Warmth of the knee

**C.** Erythema overlying the knee

**D.** Boggy effusion of the knee

**E.** Raised purpura distal to the knee

**15-8.** A 14-year-old girl has complained of fatigue and diffuse musculoskeletal pain for 4 months. She has missed school and is falling behind on her school work. Her complete review of symptoms is otherwise unremarkable. She is tired appearing with a somewhat flat affect. She has no objective findings of arthritis, and her exam is otherwise normal. Her complete blood count (CBC), comprehensive metabolic panel, and urinalysis are normal, but her antinuclear antibody (ANA) is positive at a titer of 1:80. Which of the following is the next best step in her evaluation and management?

**A.** Order a panel of specific, autoimmune disease–associated antibodies, such as anti–double-stranded DNA or anti-Smith antibodies

**B.** Consider causes for her symptoms other than systemic lupus erythematosus (SLE)

**C.** Refer her to a pediatric rheumatologist because she has SLE

**D.** Tell her family that she has juvenile idiopathic arthritis (JIA) and that the presence of a low-positive ANA indicates that she is at increased risk of developing uveitis

**E.** Order a serum C3 and C4

**15-9.** A 15-year-old girl has a 3-month history of morning stiffness lasting 2 hours in her wrists and fingers. Her exam reveals mild swelling in her wrists, metacarpophalangeal joints, and proximal interphalangeal joints of her hands. She has pain on passive range of motion in these joints and cannot completely make a fist. Her rheumatoid factor is 123 IU/mL, with a normal value being < 15 IU/mL. Which of the following statements is true?

**A.** Rheumatoid factors are more likely to be false positive in adolescents than in adults.

**B.** Measuring rheumatoid factors is not useful in juvenile idiopathic arthritis (JIA).

**C.** Persistently positive high titer rheumatoid factors indicate an increased risk of more aggressive arthritis in children.

**D.** Positive anti–cyclic citrullinated peptide (CCP) antibodies are less specific for childhood-onset rheumatoid arthritis than are rheumatoid factors.

**E.** High titer rheumatoid factors in childhood are only seen in seropositive JIA.

**15-10.** A 15-year-old boy is hospitalized with hemoptysis. He has a 3-month history of malaise, epistaxis, and arthralgias. Examination of his nose reveals a nasal septal perforation. A chest radiograph shows bilateral alveolar infiltrates. A serum anti–proteinase 3 (PR3) antibody is positive, and antinuclear antibody (ANA) is negative. Which of the following is the most likely diagnosis?

**A.** Granulomatosis with polyangiitis (GPA)

**B.** Microscopic polyangiitis

**C.** Systemic lupus erythematosus (SLE)

**D.** Antiphospholipid syndrome

**E.** Evans syndrome

**15-11.** A 14-year-old boy presents to the emergency department (ED) with shortness of breath and a nonproductive cough. He has a history of recurrent sinus infections, nosebleeds, and joint pain. On physical exam, he looks unwell. He is afebrile with tachycardia and tachypnea. His oxygen saturation is 90% on room air. There are bilateral nasal septal ulcerations, a saddle nose deformity, and a swollen left ankle. There are coarse breath sounds bilaterally but no wheeze or rales. He does not have a rash. A complete blood count (CBC) demonstrates a hemoglobin of 8.9 g/dL, a creatinine of 1.8 mg/dL, and an erythrocyte sedimentation rate (ESR) of 90 mm/h. A chest radiograph is performed and shows nonspecific perihilar and basilar opacities; there is no radiographic evidence for pneumonia. What is the next most appropriate diagnostic test for this patient?

**A.** Computed tomography (CT) angiogram of the chest, abdomen, and pelvis

**B.** Renal biopsy

**C.** Antineutrophil cytoplasmic antibodies (ANCA) testing with proteinase 3 (PR3) and myeloperoxidase (MPO) antibodies

**D.** High-resolution pulmonary CT scan

**E.** Magnetic resonance imaging (MRI) with contrast of ankle

**15-12.** A 5-year-old girl presents to your office for evaluation of foot pain. She has also been having pain in both wrists for 2 months. She experienced an ice skating injury where she fell on her right hand prior to the onset of pain. She says that her wrists hurt more in the morning but cannot describe if there is morning stiffness. The family states that she no longer wants to play on the monkey bars; however, she tells you it is because she does not like them. She is hesitant to let you examine her and cries when you move her wrists. Based on her limited physical exam, you are unable to determine if there is swelling. There are no obvious deformities of her wrists, and she has pain with range of motion and limits her range of motion by guarding of both her wrists. Previous plain radiograph of her right wrist performed the week after the injury was read as normal. Which diagnostic test is most likely to aid you in a definitive diagnosis of arthritis when physical exam and history are unclear?

**A.** Magnetic resonance imaging (MRI) with gadolinium of the right wrist

**B.** Antinuclear antibody (ANA)

**C.** Repeat a plain radiograph of the right wrist

**D.** Rheumatoid factor testing

**E.** Computed tomography (CT) of the right wrist

**15-13.** The parents of a child newly diagnosed with juvenile idiopathic arthritis (JIA) are worried that their daughter will develop uveitis. You talk to them about her risk factors as well as the screening guidelines. Which of the following patients is in the highest risk category of developing uveitis?

**A.** A 12-year-old girl with antinuclear antibody (ANA)-positive, rheumatoid factor–positive polyarticular JIA diagnosed 7 years ago

**B.** A 6-year-old boy with systemic JIA complicated by pericarditis diagnosed 1 month ago

**C.** A 6-year-old boy with ANA-negative oligoarticular JIA diagnosed 5 years ago

**D.** A 2-year-old girl with ANA-positive oligoarticular JIA diagnosed 6 months ago

**E.** A 3-year-old boy with ANA-negative, rheumatoid factor–negative polyarticular JIA diagnosed 2 years ago

**15-14.** A 7-year-old boy has had spiking fevers for the past 2 weeks. When he has the fever, he develops a pink rash that comes and goes. He also has joint and muscle pain. Recently, he developed mild joint swelling in his knees. Based on his clinical symptoms and physical examination findings, he was diagnosed with systemic-onset juvenile idiopathic arthritis (JIA). Despite starting appropriate treatment, the patient experiences clinical worsening of his condition and is ill appearing. There is concern that he has developed macrophage activation syndrome. What laboratory test change is seen with macrophage activation syndrome?

**A.** Increase in erythrocyte sedimentation rate (ESR)

**B.** Rheumatoid factor testing goes from negative to positive

**C.** Prolonged prothrombin time and partial thromboplastin time

**D.** Decreased ferritin level

**E.** Significant leukocytosis and thrombocytosis

**15-15.** A 5-year-old girl is diagnosed with rheumatoid factor–negative polyarticular juvenile idiopathic arthritis (JIA). She has arthritis in multiple joints and complains about daily joint pain and morning stiffness lasting for 45 minutes. Her recent radiographs show that she has erosions in both of her wrists. Which of the following will increase the likelihood of a sustained remission for this patient?

**A.** Using nonsteroidal anti-inflammatory drugs (NSAIDs) as the mainstay of treatment

**B.** Treatment with systemic corticosteroids for months to years

**C.** Starting methotrexate as early as possible

**D.** Clinical follow-up for active JIA every 6 months

**E.** Avoiding anticytokine agents because they are less effective in controlling arthritis

**15-16.** A mother brings in her child who has been complaining of joint pain and stiffness for the past 2 months, and you note that he has active arthritis. Which of the following characteristics is most suggestive of the enthesitis-related arthritis/spondyloarthropathy subtype of juvenile idiopathic arthritis (JIA)?

**A.** Chronic upper back pain in a 15-year-old girl

**B.** A swollen right knee in a 4-year-old boy

**C.** Presence of HLA-B27 antigen

**D.** Presence of rheumatoid factor

**E.** Family history including an aunt with psoriasis

**15-17.** A 14-year-old girl is brought in by her mother with 2 months of joint pain. Physical exam reveals a thin female with warmth, swelling, and tenderness of her bilateral knees. Vital signs are notable for a body mass index (BMI) in the 15th percentile for age, which is decreased from the 40th percentile at her last well-child check. She states that she has not been eating well because a lot of foods upset her stomach. You send some preliminary labs. Which of the following labs will be most helpful in making a diagnosis?

**A.** Albumin

**B.** Complete blood count (CBC)

**C.** Erythrocyte sedimentation rate (ESR)

**D.** Fecal calprotectin

**E.** Urinalysis

**15-18.** A 16-year-old boy presents to the emergency department (ED) with 4 days of diffuse arthralgias. He states that he has not been entirely well for the past 3 weeks, since he got "food poisoning" during a camping trip. Vital signs are stable with a temperature of 37.0°C. On physical exam, you note warmth, swelling, and tenderness of the left knee and right ankle. Radiographs demonstrate moderate joint effusions of the knee and ankle. What is the most appropriate initial treatment for this patient?

**A.** A 10-day course of doxycycline

**B.** A 2-week course of nonsteroidal antiinflammatory drugs (NSAIDs)

**C.** A 3-day course of high-dose glucocorticoids

**D.** Weekly subcutaneous methotrexate

**E.** A 14-day course of amoxicillin

**15-19.** A 6-year-old boy presents to your office with a chief complaint of rash. His parents also report he has been complaining of abdominal pain on and off for the past 4 days. Yesterday, he developed a rash around his ankles that seemed to spread over his legs. He has been otherwise well, without fevers. On exam, you note that he is generally well appearing and has raised, nonblanching purpuric lesions scattered over his legs with coalescing areas over his buttocks (Figure 200-1). What monitoring test should you order for this patient?

**A.** Stool guaiac

**B.** Urinalysis

**C.** Hemoglobin

**D.** Serum creatinine

**E.** Liver function tests

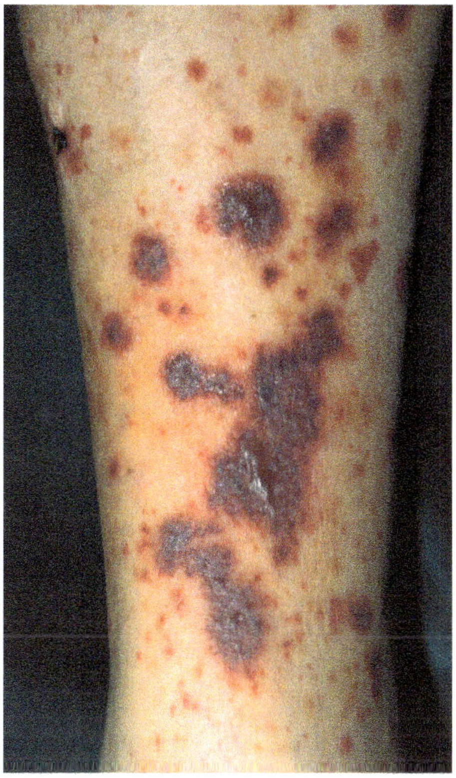

**FIGURE 200-1.** Classic palpable purpura on the lower legs of a patient with Henoch-Schönlein purpura. (Reproduced with permission from Wolff K, Johnson RA. *Fitzpatrick's Color Atlas & Synopsis of Clinical Dermatology*, 6th ed. New York: McGraw-Hill; 2009.)

**15-20.** A 15-year-old boy comes in to your office complaining of a cough. He has also noticed that his urine has been very dark lately. He was seen in your office a week ago for joint pain and malaise. You review his chart and notice he has been seen in your office 5 times in the past 4 months for sinus infections. He is hypertensive. You check a urine dipstick in the office that shows 3+ blood and protein. A chest radiograph shows several pulmonary nodules, one of which is cavitating. You suspect that he has granulomatosis with polyangiitis (GPA). What test would help confirm this diagnosis?

**A.** Rheumatoid factor
**B.** Antinuclear antibody (ANA)
**C.** Anti–double-stranded DNA (dsDNA)
**D.** Anti-Sjögren's-syndrome-related antigen A (anti-SSA)
**E.** Antineutrophil cytoplasmic antibodies (ANCA)

**15-21.** A 9-year-old girl comes into your office complaining of fevers, rash, and myalgias. One week ago, she developed a lacy purplish rash all over her legs, and the following day, she began to develop painful nodules scattered on her lower legs. Her calf muscles started to hurt, and the pain is so severe that she cannot put her heels down. She has had fevers up to 102°F on and off for the past week. You are suspicious that she has polyarteritis nodosa (PAN). What common childhood infection can be a trigger for PAN?

**A.** Influenza
**B.** Group A *Streptococcus*
**C.** Staphylococcal skin infections
**D.** Rhinovirus
**E.** Coxsackievirus

**15-22.** A 15-year-old girl presents to your clinic, and you suspect she might have systemic lupus erythematosus (SLE) based on the presence of 1 month of fevers, ulcerations on the hard palate, swelling of the proximal interphalangeal joints of her fingers, and a urinalysis concerning for nephritis with hematuria and proteinuria. Which of the following test results would be most specific to confirm a diagnosis of SLE?

**A.** Elevated erythrocyte sedimentation rate (ESR)
**B.** Elevated aspartate aminotransferase
**C.** Positive double stranded DNA (dsDNA) antibody
**D.** Elevated C-reactive protein (CRP)
**E.** Mild anemia

**15-23.** You see a patient in your clinic with suspected systemic lupus erythematosus (SLE). Which of the following clinical manifestations is most specific for SLE?

**A.** Malar rash
**B.** Joint pain
**C.** Fatigue
**D.** Chest pain
**E.** Headache

**15-24.** A 13-year-old girl presents with Raynaud phenomenon, diffusely swollen fingers, and weakness. You are concerned that she might have an overlap syndrome such as mixed connective tissue disease (MCTD). Which of the following test results would help confirm a diagnosis of MCTD?

**A.** Increased erythrocyte sedimentation rate (ESR)
**B.** Low complement levels
**C.** Anemia
**D.** Positive U1 ribonucleoprotein (RNP) antibody
**E.** Urinalysis with proteinuria

**15-25.** A mother brings her 4-year-old daughter in for a facial rash. At first, she thought that the rash might be a sunburn because it started after a trip to the water park. After several weeks, the rash has not faded. It seems to get worse every time she goes out in the sun, but still does not go away even if she avoids the sun. On exam, you notice a red rash on the cheeks crossing over the bridge of the nose but sparing the nasolabial folds, consistent with a malar rash. Besides cutaneous lupus and systemic lupus erythematosus (SLE), what other diagnosis should you consider?

**A.** Juvenile idiopathic arthritis (JIA)
**B.** Behçet disease
**C.** Juvenile dermatomyositis (JDM)
**D.** Polyarteritis nodosa (PAN)
**E.** Psoriasis

**15-26.** An 8-year-old boy in your clinic was recently diagnosed with juvenile dermatomyositis (JDM) after he developed a heliotrope rash and muscle weakness. He had an magnetic resonance imaging (MRI) performed of his thighs that showed edema of the muscle. On exam, he has 2 hard nodules on his forearms and effusions of both his knees. There is a violaceous discoloration of his eyelids. Looking under magnification with an ophthalmoscope and lubricating jelly, you are able to see dilated, tortuous nailfold capillaries. Which of the following is a poor prognostic factor?

**A.** Presence of heliotrope rash
**B.** Presence of muscle edema on MRI
**C.** Presence of calcinosis
**D.** Presence of arthritis
**E.** Presence of nailfold capillary changes

**15-27.** Which of the following is not considered evidence of muscle inflammation according to the Bohan and Peter criteria for the diagnosis of dermatomyositis and polymyositis?

**A.** Symmetric proximal and axial weakness
**B.** Evidence of chronic inflammation on muscle biopsy
**C.** Elevation of lactate dehydrogenase
**D.** Characteristic electromyographic changes
**E.** Muscle edema on short T1 inversion recovery (STIR) sequences of magnetic resonance imaging (MRI)

**15-28.** You see a 10-year-old girl for a well-child examination. You note that she has some tightening of the skin around her mouth, and you suspect that she has systemic sclerosis. Which of the following is the most common early clinical manifestation included in the classification criteria for systemic sclerosis, apart from skin hardening?

**A.** Raynaud phenomenon
**B.** Arthritis
**C.** Cough
**D.** Nephritis
**E.** Fatigue

**15-29.** An otherwise healthy, 8-year-old girl presents to your office for an urgent visit. She and her mother have noticed that over the past several months she has developed a skin lesion with hyperpigmentation extending from her right thigh down to her ankle. You note that the associated skin has a somewhat waxy texture and she is developing a flexion contracture of her right knee (Figure 203-5). The remainder of her skin exam is unremarkable. You suspect she has a form of morphea. What form of morphea is this child most likely to have?

**A.** Generalized morphea
**B.** Linear scleroderma
**C.** Circumscribed morphea
**D.** Systemic sclerosis
**E.** Pansclerotic morphea

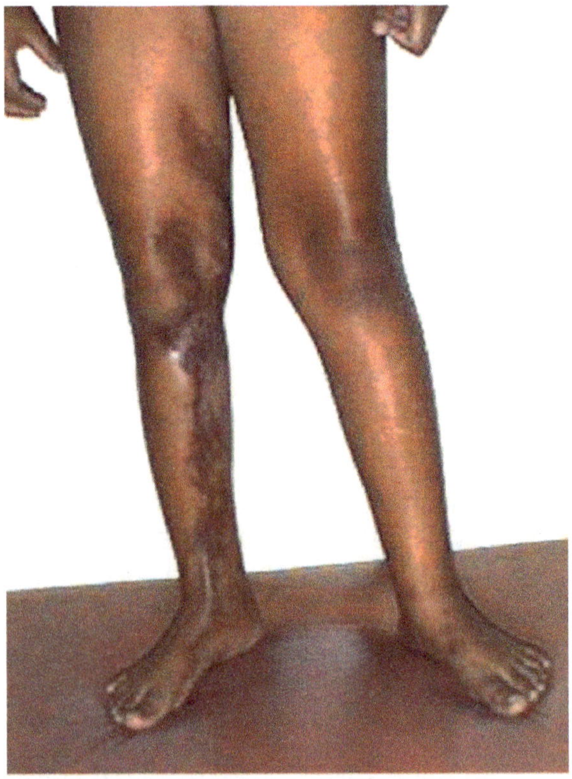

**FIGURE 203-5.** Hyperpigmentation of the right leg. (Mark W. Kline, *Rudolph's Pediatrics*, 23rd Edition. Copyright © McGraw-Hill Education. All rights reserved.)

**15-30.** A 4-year-old boy is brought in for his well-child check. His mother states that he has been waking up in the middle of the night screaming that his legs hurt. This has been occurring on and off for the past few months. He seems fine during the day, although he sometimes has pain in his legs at bedtime. Vitals are stable. Exam reveals an active healthy boy without joint pain, joint swelling, or limitations in range of motion. What would be the most appropriate next step for this child with a diagnosis of growing pains?

**A.** Reassure parents that this will resolve without long-term consequences

**B.** Order radiographs of both lower extremities

**C.** Order complete blood count (CBC)

**D.** Order antinuclear antibody (ANA)

**E.** Referral to psychiatry

**15-31.** A 10-year-old girl presents with 4 months of pain in her wrists, elbows, and knees. Her mother notes that she is a competitive gymnast. The pain has started to limit her participation. Exam demonstrates hyperextension of the elbows and knees in addition to the ability to place her palms on the floor with her knees straight. Which of the following would prompt further evaluation in this patient?

**A.** History of 4 ankle sprains

**B.** Family history of "double-jointed" father

**C.** Chronic back pain

**D.** Increased skin elasticity

**E.** Height in the 15th percentile for age

**15-32.** A 10-year-old girl presents with refusal to bear weight on her right foot for the past month since she sprained it during gymnastics. Exam is notable for significant tenderness to palpation over the ankle and dorsum of the foot and limitation of the right ankle in all planes of passive motion due to pain. What additional finding would suggest complex regional pain syndrome?

**A.** Focal, reproducible tenderness inferior to the medial malleolus

**B.** Cool right foot with a blue discoloration

**C.** Bone radiographs demonstrating periarticular osteopenia

**D.** Elevated erythrocyte sedimentation rate (ESR)

**E.** Daily fevers for the past week

**15-33.** A 16-year-old girl presents with 3 months of worsening joint pain, joint swelling, and morning stiffness. Pain is present in her hands, wrists, neck, back, hips, knees, and feet. She states that she stopped running cross country because the pain got so bad. Now, she barely has the energy to get out of bed because she hurts so much. She admits to poor appetite because her stomach hurts whenever she eats. She has worsening "migraines" and gets dizzy when she stands up too quickly. Her mother states that her daughter is becoming increasingly anxious because her school absences are starting to affect her grades. Vital signs are stable. Exam demonstrates diffuse abdominal tenderness and tenderness of her joints without limitation, warmth, erythema, or swelling. What is the next best step?

**A.** Order radiographs of the sacroiliac joints

**B.** Check antinuclear antibodies (ANA)

**C.** Check thyroid studies

**D.** Reassure family that with treatment her symptoms will improve

**E.** Refer to neurology

**15-34.** A teenage boy in your practice is diagnosed with chronic fatigue syndrome after presenting with 4 months of fatigue that was precipitated by a viral illness and is not relieved by rest. He also has difficulty falling and staying asleep, generalized muscle pain, and difficulty maintaining focus in school. Which of the following would be an appropriate laboratory test to evaluate for an underlying condition as a cause of these symptoms?

**A.** Antinuclear antibody (ANA)

**B.** Double-stranded DNA (dsDNA)

**C.** Thyroid studies

**D.** Rheumatoid factor

**E.** Human leukocyte antigen B27 (HLA-B27)

**15-35.** A 3-year-old boy presents to your office with a history of recurrent fevers. His fevers have been occurring for 2 years. His parents are worried that he could have an autoinflammatory syndrome. Which of the following is an important aspect of the history to consider during your evaluation of an autoinflammatory syndrome?

**A.** He gets fevers every 4 weeks.

**B.** He has 4 brothers.

**C.** One of his brothers has juvenile idiopathic arthritis (JIA).

**D.** He has a positive antinuclear antibody (ANA) with a value of 1:1280.

**E.** He has celiac disease.

**15-36.** A patient presents to your office with recurrent fever. There is a high suspicion for an autoinflammatory syndrome. Which scenario has the highest risk of the patient developing amyloidosis?

**A.** A 4-year-old boy with periodic fever, aphthous stomatitis, pharyngitis, adenitis (PFAPA) who has fever episodes every 3 weeks

**B.** A 7-year-old Armenian boy with familial Mediterranean fever (FMF) and an M694V mutation in the *MEFV* gene

**C.** A 1-year-old girl with familial cold autoinflammatory syndrome (FCAS) who develops urticarial rash when exposed to cold weather

**D.** A 10-year-old Dutch girl with hyperimmunoglobulin D syndrome (HIDS) who develops a morbilliform rash and severe abdominal pain with her fever episodes

**E.** A 9-year-old girl with systemic juvenile idiopathic arthritis (JIA) for the past 8 years with uncontrolled disease

**15-37.** A 10-year-old boy with inflammatory bowel disease (IBD) presents with bone pain for the past 6 months in his chest, back, and legs. Recently, he developed swelling and pain in his right clavicle. A magnetic resonance imaging (MRI) of his chest showed areas of bone marrow edema in his left second rib, right clavicle, and fifth thoracic vertebrae. He has a bone biopsy that reveals chronic inflammation. The bacterial culture from the bone biopsy was negative for bacteria or other infectious etiology. What is a possible common complication of ineffective treatment of this disease?

**A.** Respiratory distress with pneumonitis

**B.** Progressive lipodystrophy

**C.** Stroke

**D.** Sensorineural hearing loss

**E.** Leg length inequality

**15-38.** A 4-year-old boy presents to clinic with a history of recurrent fevers. He has had recurrent fevers for the past 2 years. His parents have taken him to the pediatrician for most of his fever episodes and have been unable to find a source for his fevers. He has had numerous throat cultures and urine cultures, which have all been negative. His blood work shows a mildly elevated white blood cell (WBC) count, erythrocyte sedimentation rate (ESR), and C-reactive protein (CRP). His parents are worried that he could have periodic fever, aphthous stomatitis, pharyngitis, adenitis (PFAPA). Which symptom would be most consistent with a diagnosis of PFAPA?

**A.** The most common symptoms are rash and abdominal pain.

**B.** The attacks occur every 21 days and last 5 days in duration.

**C.** Prednisone does not stop the fever episode.

**D.** Fifteen years later, he continues to have recurrent fevers.

**E.** His inflammatory markers continue to be elevated when he is not febrile.

## ANSWERS

**Answer 15-1. D**

The PPD test is based on type IV hypersensitivity in which resident antigen-presenting cells (eg, macrophages and dendritic cells) internalize, process, and present the PPD antigenic epitopes in the surface class II major histocompatibility complex (MHC) molecule to T cells. T cells that have been previously sensitized by exposure to *M tuberculosis* during infection recognize the antigen in the MHC molecule and are activated, releasing cytokines that further activate macrophages. The activated macrophages release cytokines, such as tumor necrosis factor (TNF) and interleukin (IL)-1, that upregulate molecules on the endothelium, such as the selectins, and induce increased blood flow and vascular leak in the area. The selectins traffic inflammatory cells into the site of the injection. These inflammatory cells and the edema resulting from vascular leak cause the characteristic induration and erythema at 24 to 72 hours after the injection.

Answer choices A, B, and C are descriptions of type I, II, and III hypersensitivity, respectively, whereas answer choice D is a description of type IV hypersensitivity. Some substances and bacteria activate complement directly, but PPD does not.

(Chapter 195: Pathogenesis of Inflammatory and Autoimmune Disorders [pp. 914–915])

**Answer 15-2. B**

APECED is a rare monogenic disease caused by mutations in the *AIRE* gene. AIRE is a transcription factor that induces the expression of 500 to 1200 genes in the thymus that encode self-antigens that would otherwise only be produced by other tissues. T-cell precursors that recognize these self-antigens in the thymus during T-cell development are deleted by undergoing apoptosis. Thus, the major pathogenic mechanism in APECED is lack of development of T-cell tolerance because these genes are not expressed in the absence of a functional *AIRE* gene product, and autoreactive T cells are allowed to continue development.

Development of B-cell tolerance involves different mechanisms that negatively select autoreactive B cells during immunoglobulin gene rearrangement, although some potentially autoreactive B cells survive B-cell development. In APECED, the development of autoreactive T helper cells apparently triggers autoreactive B cells, leading to the production of antibodies that recognize self-antigens, which contribute to the disease manifestations. Despite the contribution of autoantibodies to the disease process, APECED is a disease caused by lack of T-cell tolerance.

Overproduction of IL-1 and IL-18 by caspase 1 results from genetic mutations in the gene encoding NLRP3, which results in a variety of autoinflammatory diseases including neonatal-onset multisystem inflammatory disease, Muckle-Wells syndrome, and cold-induced urticaria. These syndromes are not felt to have an autoimmune component but rather are disorders of the innate immune system.

Lack of expression of MHC class I and MHC class II is found in rare diseases associated with both lack of immune response to foreign antigens and autoimmune manifestations, but none of these diseases are caused by defects in the *AIRE* gene.

(Chapter 195: Pathogenesis of Inflammatory and Autoimmune Disorders [pp. 913–915])

## Answer 15-3. B

This patient has immune dysregulation, polyendocrinopathy, enteropathy, X-linked (IPEX) syndrome. This is an X-linked disorder caused by mutations in *FOXP3*, a transcription factor critical for the development of Treg cells. These cells are important for limiting activation of T cells by self-antigen. In the absence of Treg cells, T cells infiltrate and damage a variety of organs, particularly the gut, thyroid, and islet cells of the pancreas.

Development of B-cell tolerance involves different mechanisms that negatively select autoreactive B cells during immunoglobulin gene rearrangement, although some potentially autoreactive B cells survive B-cell development.

Overproduction of IL-1 and IL-18 by caspase 1 results from genetic mutations in the gene encoding NLRP3, which results in a variety of autoinflammatory diseases including neonatal-onset multisystem inflammatory disease, Muckle-Wells syndrome, and cold-induced urticaria.

Lack of expression of MHC class I and MHC class II is found in rare diseases associated with both lack of immune response to foreign antigens and autoimmune manifestations, but none of these diseases are caused by defects in the *AIRE* gene.

(Chapter 195: Pathogenesis of Inflammatory and Autoimmune Disorders [p. 916])

## Answer 15-4. C

This is an example of a serum sickness–like reaction resulting from an infusion of a foreign protein (rituximab). This was originally observed in patients receiving infusions of horse diphtheria toxin antiserum but has also been described in patients receiving antithymocyte globulin. This reaction is classified as type III hypersensitivity. It is self-limited after the inciting antigen is eliminated. The offending antigen should not be reintroduced.

IgE antibodies generally incite type I immediate hypersensitivity, which manifests as urticaria, angioedema, and anaphylaxis. Rituximab does lyse and deplete B cells, but this effect does not play a role in serum sickness. Rituximab is not known to deplete Treg cells.

(Chapter 195: Pathogenesis of Inflammatory and Autoimmune Disorders [p. 914])

## Answer 15-5. B

A characteristic feature of inflammatory arthritis is morning stiffness, and difficulties with morning activities of daily living, such as buttoning a shirt, can indicate morning stiffness. Stiffness may also be seen following periods of prolonged inactivity, such as long car rides or sitting in classes in school. This is known as the "gel effect." Joint stiffness is often relieved with warmth or activity, both of which raise the temperature within the joint and allow synovial fluid to return to a liquid state.

Children with inflammatory arthritis might not experience pain. If there is pain, it should not wake a child from sleep. Nighttime pain should raise suspicion of an alternate diagnosis, such as malignancy or growing pains. For children with inflammatory arthritis and joint pain, their pain is generally improved by activity. A child may limp first thing in the morning and then be able to exercise vigorously later in the day. Pain exacerbated by activity is more typical of mechanical pain. Having a family member with inflammatory arthritis does not increase the risk that the child will have the same disease, although it increases the risk of having a rheumatologic disorder. Pain following an injury would necessitate ruling out other causes of joint pain before considering inflammatory arthritis. An injury may reflect a traumatic injury or may unmask preexisting pathology, such as osteogenic sarcoma.

(Chapter 196: History and Physical Examination in Rheumatology [p. 918])

## Answer 15-6. A

When obtaining a rheumatology history, one should elicit the following details:

- Nature of onset (acute vs chronic)
- Timing of symptoms
- The number of affected sites
- Exacerbating and remitting factors (eg, activity, medications, heat, ice)
- Associated symptoms

Children with inflammatory pain, such as those with JIA, typically have pain that is worst right after waking and improves throughout the day (Table 196-1). Pain tends to improve with activity. Mechanical pain is the opposite of inflammatory pain,

**TABLE 196-1.** Categories of Musculoskeletal Pain Based on Timing of Symptoms

| | AM | PM | Night | Effect of Activity on Symptoms |
|---|---|---|---|---|
| Inflammatory (eg, arthritis) | +++ | + | – | Improves |
| Mechanical (eg, overuse syndromes) | ± | ++ | ± | Worsens |
| Bony (eg, tumors) | ++ | ++ | ++ | No consistent change |
| Neuropathic (eg, radiculopathy) | + | ++ | +++ | No consistent change |
| Functional | +++ | +++ | +++ | No physiologic pattern |

Mark W. Kline, *Rudolph's Pediatrics*, 23rd Edition. Copyright © McGraw-Hill Education. All rights reserved.

such that pain gets worse during the day and with activity. Bony pain can occur with infection, trauma, or tumors. This pain is not affected by time of day or activity. Neuropathic pain tends to be worse at bedtime because the child is no longer distracted by activity.

(Chapter 196: History and Physical Examination in Rheumatology [pp. 918–919])

**Answer 15-7.** C

Clinical findings are important in making a rheumatologic diagnosis; therefore, a thorough physical exam is warranted in a child presenting for evaluation of joint pain and/or joint swelling. Warmth, swelling, and limitations in range of motion are characteristic of arthritis and do not differentiate between causes of arthritis. Overlying erythema would be suggestive of septic arthritis. Children with juvenile idiopathic arthritis (JIA) generally do not have color changes to the joint, although there is sometimes some mild pink discoloration. However, patients with septic arthritis can have bright pink or red discoloration to the skin overlying their joint. A boggy effusion would be more suggestive of synovial proliferation, which is seen in chronic JIA. Palpable purpura is suggestive of Henoch-Schönlein purpura (HSP/IgA vasculitis). The arthritis seen in HSP is typically oligoarticular (1–4 joints) and nondeforming. Arthritis may be transient or migratory, and it may precede the appearance of purpura by 1 to 2 days. See Table 196-3 for common causes of arthritis.

(Chapter 196: History and Physical Examination in Rheumatology [p. 920])

**Answer 15-8.** B

Patients with SLE rarely have ANA titers that are ≤ 1:160. This patient's only clinical manifestations that are consistent with SLE are fatigue and diffuse musculoskeletal pain, and she does not have any other laboratory evidence of SLE. Thus, there is no rationale for ordering specific autoimmune disease–associated antibodies or for referring her to a pediatric rheumatologist. Patients who have JIA and have a low titer positive ANA are at an increased risk of developing uveitis compared to patients

**TABLE 196-3.** Common Causes of Arthritis

| |
|---|
| **Monoarticular** |
| *Acute Onset* |
| Septic arthritis |
| Reactive arthritis |
| Trauma |
| Hemophilia |
| Lyme disease |
| *Chronic* |
| Juvenile idiopathic arthritis |
| Lyme disease |
| Tuberculosis (rare without pulmonary disease) |
| Tumor (eg, pigmented villonodular synovitis) (rare) |
| **Polyarticular** |
| Juvenile rheumatoid arthritis |
| Spondyloarthropathies |
| Systemic autoimmune diseases |
| Systemic lupus erythematosus |
| Vasculitis |
| Sarcoidosis |
| Arthritis associated with inflammatory bowel disease |
| Viral arthritis |
| Reactive arthritis |
| Serum sickness |
| Rheumatic fever (migratory arthritis) |
| Malignancies |
| Periodic fever syndromes |

Mark W. Kline, *Rudolph's Pediatrics*, 23rd Edition. Copyright © McGraw-Hill Education. All rights reserved.

with JIA and a negative ANA, but this patient does not have any evidence of arthritis on exam. Serum C3 and C4 levels correlate inversely with some aspects of disease activity in SLE because immune complexes consume complement, but C3 and C4 are not screening tests for SLE.

(Chapter 197: Diagnostic Testing in Rheumatology [pp. 923–924])

**Answer 15-9.** C

This young woman likely has childhood-onset rheumatoid arthritis, also known as rheumatoid factor–positive polyarticular JIA. The diagnosis becomes more secure if the rheumatoid factor is persistently elevated over the course of 2 to 3 months and her symptoms and clinical findings of arthritis also persist. Rheumatoid factors are *less* likely to be false positive in adolescents than in adults, although false-positive rheumatoid factors, usually of low titer, are sometimes found in the pediatric population.

Measuring rheumatoid factors in JIA is useful because persistently elevated titers indicate a more aggressive arthritis. Positive anti-CCP antibodies are rarely false positives and are thus more specific than rheumatoid factors for rheumatoid factor–positive polyarticular JIA. High titer rheumatoid factors can be seen in other disorders besides seropositive JIA, and their detection should lead the clinician to consider other diagnoses associated with positive rheumatoid factors, such as cryoglobulinemia, Sjögren syndrome, and systemic lupus erythematosus (SLE).

(Chapter 197: Diagnostic Testing in Rheumatology [p. 923])

**Answer 15-10.** A

This young man has GPA. This is a form of vasculitis characterized by necrotizing granulomas in the upper and lower airways and, frequently, by rapidly progressive glomerulonephritis. The presence of anti-PR3 antibodies in the setting of these clinical findings is largely diagnostic of this disorder. Anti-PR3 antibodies are correlated closely with the cytoplasmic pattern of antineutrophil cytoplasmic antibodies (ANCA), and hence, this disease is a form of ANCA-associated vasculitis. Microscopic polyangiitis is a related disorder more closely associated with anti-myeloperoxidase (MPO) antibodies, which correlate with the presence of the perinuclear pattern of ANCA, and does not generally have destructive upper airway disease. Positive anti-PR3 antibodies are sometimes found in patients with SLE, but the clinical findings and negative ANA make SLE less likely. Anti-PR3 antibodies are not useful in antiphospholipid syndrome or in Evans syndrome, which refers to autoimmune hemolytic anemia together with autoimmune thrombocytopenia.

(Chapter 197: Diagnostic Testing in Rheumatology [p. 923])

**Answer 15-11.** D

The clinical presentation is most consistent with granulomatosis with polyangiitis (GPA). The anemia and shortness of breath are concerning for pulmonary hemorrhage. A high-resolution CT scan would be able to evaluate for bleeding in the lungs. Chest radiograph is not sensitive enough to delineate intra-alveolar blood from atelectasis and cannot rule out pulmonary hemorrhage. The high-resolution CT would be better to evaluate for pulmonary hemorrhage, which is a life-threatening complication of GPA. A CT angiogram is unlikely to show evidence of vasculitis because GPA is a small- to medium-size vasculitis in which the arteries are too small to be seen by CT angiogram. Additionally, contrast is required to perform a CT angiogram and would be contraindicated in a patient with chronic renal disease due to the risk of additional renal injury from contrast. The elevated creatinine is concerning for GPA nephritis, and a renal biopsy will be valuable in confirming a diagnosis assessing potential renal damage. However, the results will not be available in a timely manner or address the immediate life-threatening condition of pulmonary hemorrhage. ANCA testing with PR3 and MPO antibodies is indicated in this scenario; however, they will not be available in a timely manner. An MRI of the ankle can confirm the presence of clinically suspected arthritis in this patient. The urgent condition in this adolescent is pulmonary hemorrhage and confirming arthritis would not change clinical management in this acute setting.

(Chapter 197: Diagnostic Testing in Rheumatology [p. 923])

**Answer 15-12.** A

MRI with gadolinium is the definitive diagnostic test for arthritis when the clinical picture is unclear. The addition of gadolinium allows for evaluation of inflammation in the synovium (synovitis), which would be consistent with a diagnosis of inflammatory arthritis. An MRI can also detect joint effusions, which can be difficult to assess in a small child who is reticent to undergo a physical exam. Plain radiographs are limited in their ability to detect joint effusions. Plain radiographs are useful in ruling out other causes on the differential diagnosis of joint pain such as a fracture or a tumor. In this clinical scenario, the patient has pain in the bilateral wrists and fell only on her right wrist with a previous normal radiograph. Repeating the plain radiograph is unlikely to give a definitive diagnosis of arthritis. A CT of the right wrist would give more precise imaging of the bones if there is a high suspicion for a fracture. A CT would not be able to evaluate for synovial enhancement. Laboratory evaluation does not confirm a diagnosis of juvenile idiopathic arthritis (JIA). An ANA is a marker of future risk of uveitis associated with JIA and guides the frequency of screening eye exams. A positive rheumatoid factor cannot definitively diagnose arthritis, and a negative rheumatoid factor does not rule out a diagnosis of JIA.

(Chapter 197: Diagnostic Testing in Rheumatology [p. 925])

**Answer 15-13.** D

Based on the guidelines for ophthalmology examinations for JIA, the patient with the highest risk for developing uveitis

**TABLE 198-3.** Guidelines for Ophthalmologic Examinations

| | Arthritis Onset ≤ Age 6 | | | Arthritis Onset > Age 6 | |
|---|---|---|---|---|---|
| **JRA Subtype at Onset** | **First 4 years after onset, exam every:** | **Next 3 years after onset, exam every:** | **After 7 years from onset, exam every:** | **First 4 years after onset, exam every:** | **After 4 years from onset, exam every:** |
| Pauci-ANA + | 3 mo | 6 mo | 12 mo | 6 mo | 12 mo |
| Pauci-ANA – | 6 mo | 6 mo | 12 mo | 6 mo | 12 mo |
| Poly-ANA + | 3 mo | 6 mo | 12 mo | 6 mo | 12 mo |
| Poly-ANA – | 6 mo | 6 mo | 12 mo | 6 mo | 12 mo |
| Systemic | 12 mo | 12 mo | 12 mo | 12 mo | 12 mo |

Abbreviations: ANA, antinuclear antibodies; JRA, juvenile rheumatoid arthritis.

Data from American Academy of Pediatrics Section on Rheumatology and Section on Ophthalmology: Guidelines for ophthalmologic examinations in children with juvenile rheumatoid arthritis, *Pediatrics*. 1993 Aug;92(2):295-296; Cassidy J, Kivlin J, Lindsley C, et al: Ophthalmologic examinations in children with juvenile rheumatoid arthritis, *Pediatrics*. 2006 May;117(5):1843-1845.

is the patient in answer choice D, a 2-year-old girl with ANA-positive oligoarticular JIA diagnosed 6 months ago. The screening guidelines are shown in Table 198-3. These guidelines were developed using the American College of Rheumatology (ACR) criteria for defining JIA instead of the newer International League of Associations for Rheumatology (ILAR) criteria (Table 198-1). The most important aspects determining risk are ANA positivity and younger age of onset (< 7 years old). Additionally, pauciarticular juvenile arthritis (known as oligoarticular JIA in the ILAR criteria) and polyarticular JIA have higher rates of uveitis than systemic-onset JIA. Finally, ophthalmology screening for uveitis is recommended to be done frequently earlier in the disease course and then spaced out to 3, 4, or 7 years after making the diagnosis, depending on risk. In these guidelines, high-risk patients see ophthalmology every 3 months, moderate-risk patients every 6 months, and low-risk patients every 12 months.

Uveitis is defined as inflammation of the uveal tract, which includes the iris, ciliary body, and choroid. At each ophthalmology visit, a slit-lamp examination is completed to look for inflammation in the uveal tract (uveitis). Asymptomatic uveitis is a common extra-articular complication in JIA. Twenty percent of patients with oligoarticular JIA will develop uveitis, and 80% of those patients are ANA positive. Uveitis can lead to multiple complications including vision loss, glaucoma, and cataracts.

(Chapter 198: Juvenile Idiopathic Arthritis [p. 930])

**TABLE 198-1.** Comparison of Classification System Nomenclature of Chronic Arthritis in Children

| ACR | EULAR | ILAR |
|---|---|---|
| Juvenile Rheumatoid Arthritis | Juvenile Chronic Arthritis | Juvenile Idiopathic Arthritis |
| • Systemic onset | • Systemic onset | • Systemic arthritis |
| • Polyarticular onset | • Polyarticular onset | • Persistent oligoarthritis |
| • Pauciarticular onset | • Oligoarticular onset | • Extended oligoarthritis |
| | • Juvenile rheumatoid arthritis | • RF-negative polyarthritis |
| | • Juvenile psoriatic arthritis | • RF-positive polyarthritis |
| | • Juvenile ankylosing spondylitis | • Psoriatic arthritis |
| | | • Enthesitis-related arthritis |
| | | • Undifferentiated arthritis |

NOTE. Terminologies apply to children less than age 16 years.

ACR, American College of Rheumatology; EULAR, European League against Rheumatism; ILAR, International League of Associations for Rheumatology; RF, rheumatoid factor.

Mark W. Kline, *Rudolph's Pediatrics*, 23rd Edition. Copyright © McGraw-Hill Education. All rights reserved.

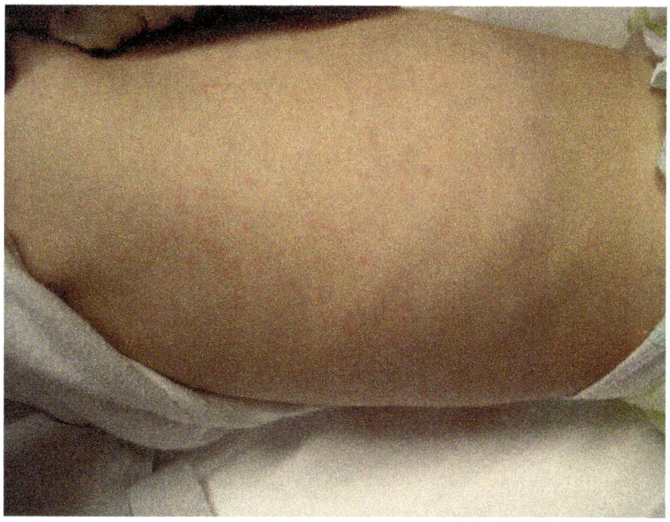

**FIGURE 198-1.** Salmon-pink rash in systemic-onset juvenile idiopathic arthritis. (Mark W. Kline, *Rudolph's Pediatrics*, 23rd Edition. Copyright © McGraw-Hill Education. All rights reserved.)

**Answer 15-14.** C

Systemic-onset JIA is a type of JIA that consists of arthritis with systemic disease manifestations including a high spiking fever (quotidian pattern), salmon-colored evanescent rash (Figure 198-1), lymphadenopathy, hepatosplenomegaly, and serositis (Table 198-2). With systemic JIA, typical laboratory abnormalities include leukocytosis, thrombocytosis, and elevated inflammatory markers. Elevated transaminases, a mild/moderate anemia, and low serum albumin levels can also be seen. A urinalysis is typically normal, and a rheumatoid factor is rarely positive.

When a patient with systemic-onset JIA develops macrophage activation syndrome, there are distinct trends in the laboratory findings. First, in contrast to a patient with systemic JIA who has leukocytosis or thrombocytosis, patients with macrophage activation syndrome typically develop leukopenia and/or thrombocytopenia. A profound anemia can also occur. Because macrophage activation syndrome can cause disseminated intravascular coagulation, hypofibrinogenemia is seen. Because fibrinogen is a key protein in the ESR assay, a patient's ESR can drop precipitously and the prothrombin

**TABLE 198-2.** International League of Associations for Rheumatology Classification System for Juvenile Idiopathic Arthritis (JIA)

| |
|---|
| JIA is arthritis of unknown etiology that begins before the 16th birthday and persists for at least 6 weeks; other known conditions including infections, neoplasms, orthopedic disorders, chronic inflammatory or autoimmune conditions, or metabolic inherited and endocrine diseases. |
| **Systemic Arthritis** |
| Arthritis in 1 or more joints with or preceded by fever of at least 2 weeks in duration that is documented to be daily ("quotidian") for at least 3 days, and accompanied by 1 or more of the following:<br>1. Evanescent (nonfixed) erythematous rash<br>2. Generalized lymph node enlargement<br>3. Hepatomegaly and/or splenomegaly<br>4. Serositis<br>*Exclusions:* a, b, c, d |
| **Oligoarthritis** |
| Arthritis affecting 1–4 joints during the first 6 months of disease. Two subcategories are recognized:<br>1. Persistent oligoarthritis: Affecting not more than 4 joints throughout the disease course<br>2. Extended oligoarthritis: Affecting a total of more than 4 joints after the first 6 months of disease<br>*Exclusions:* a, b, c, d, e |
| **Polyarthritis (Rheumatoid Factor [RF] Negative)** |
| Arthritis affecting 5 or more joints during the first 6 months of disease; a test for RF is negative.<br>*Exclusions:* a, b, c, d, e |
| **Polyarthritis (RF Positive)** |
| Arthritis affecting 5 or more joints during the first 6 months of disease; 2 or more tests for RF at least 3 months apart during the first 6 months of disease are positive.<br>*Exclusions:* a, b, c, e |

(*Continued*)

**TABLE 198-2.** International League of Associations for Rheumatology Classification System for Juvenile Idiopathic Arthritis (JIA) (*Continued*)

| |
|---|
| **Psoriatic Arthritis** |
| Arthritis and psoriasis, or arthritis and at least 2 of the following:<br>1. Dactylitis<br>2. Nail pitting or onycholysis<br>3. Psoriasis in a first-degree relative<br>*Exclusions:* b, c, d, e |
| **Enthesitis-Related Arthritis** |
| Arthritis and enthesitis, or arthritis or enthesitis with at least 2 of the following:<br>1. The presence of or a history of sacroiliac joint tenderness and/or inflammatory lumbosacral pain<br>2. The presence of HLA-B27 antigen<br>3. Onset of arthritis in a male over 6 years of age<br>4. Acute (symptomatic) anterior uveitis<br>5. History of ankylosing spondylitis, enthesitis-related arthritis, sacroiliitis with inflammatory bowel disease, Reiter syndrome, or acute anterior uveitis in a first-degree relative<br>*Exclusions:* a, d, e |
| **Undifferentiated Arthritis** |
| Arthritis that fulfills criteria in no category or in 2 or more of the above categories. |
| **Exclusions** |
| (a) Psoriasis or a history of psoriasis in the patient or first-degree relative. (b) Arthritis in an HLA-B27–positive male beginning after the 6th birthday. (c) Ankylosing spondylitis, enthesitis-related arthritis, sacroiliitis with inflammatory bowel disease, Reiter syndrome, or acute anterior uveitis, or a history of one of these disorders in a first-degree relative. (d) The presence of IgM rheumatoid factor on at least 2 occasions at least 3 months apart. (e) The presence of systemic JIA in the patient. |
| **Definitions of Terms** |
| *Dactylitis:* Swelling of 1 or more digits, usually in an asymmetric distribution, which extends beyond the joint margin. *Enthesitis:* Tenderness at the insertion of a tendon, ligament, joint capsule, or fascia to bone. *Inflammatory lumbosacral pain:* Lumbosacral spinal pain at rest with morning stiffness that improves on movement. *Nail pitting:* A minimum of 2 pits on 1 or more nails at any time. *Positive test for RF:* At least 2 positive results (as routinely defined in an accredited laboratory), at least 3 months apart, during the first 6 months of disease. *Quotidian fever:* Fever that rises to ≥ 39°C once a day and returns to ≤ 37°C between fever peaks. *Serositis:* Pericarditis and/or pleuritis and/or peritonitis. *Sacroiliac joint arthritis:* Presence of tenderness on direct compression over the sacroiliac joints. *Spondyloarthropathy:* Inflammation of entheses and joints of the lumbosacral spine. *Uveitis:* Chronic anterior uveitis as diagnosed by an ophthalmologist. |

Data from Petty RE, Southwood TR, Manners P, et al: International League of Associations for Rheumatology classification of juvenile idiopathic arthritis: second revision, Edmonton, 2001, *J Rheumatol.* 2004 Feb;31(2):390-392.

and partial thromboplastin times can become prolonged. D-dimer and ferritin also typically increase. Over time, serum transaminases increase dramatically, and a bone marrow biopsy may demonstrate hemophagocytosis. The rheumatoid factor continues to be negative. If the diagnosis or management of macrophage activation syndrome is delayed, then there is a 10% to 20% mortality rate.

(Chapter 198: Juvenile Idiopathic Arthritis [pp. 930–931])

**Answer 15-15.** C

Earlier and aggressive medication management is the cornerstone of JIA treatment. Therefore, methotrexate should be started as early as possible in patients with polyarthritis or persistent or extended oligoarthritis, such as the patient in this scenario. Methotrexate is a disease-modifying antirheumatic drug frequently used in the treatment of JIA.

NSAIDs are no longer the mainstay of treatment in JIA. They are used for pain control as well as a daily anti-inflammatory medication. Systemic corticosteroids are used to treat the systemic manifestations seen with systemic-onset JIA, which this patient does not have. Short courses of systemic corticosteroids are also given to JIA patients to manage disease flares or while awaiting the maximal effectiveness of other treatments. Anticytokine agents have been shown to be *more* effective in controlling arthritis and preventing long-term damage. Anticytokine agents include anti-tumor necrosis factor (TNF) therapy (eg, etanercept, infliximab, adalimumab, golimumab) and co-stimulatory blocking agents (abatacept). Anti–IL-1 (eg, anakinra, rilonacept, canakinumab) and anti–IL-6 (tocilizumab) agents have shown efficacy and tolerability for the treatment of systemic JIA.

Medication management requires close follow-up to evaluate for side effects and medication efficacy every 1 to 3 months. Regular testing is required to evaluate for medication toxicity. Cytopenias and liver function abnormality are the most common laboratory abnormalities seen.

(Chapter 198: Juvenile Idiopathic Arthritis [p. 932])

**Answer 15-16.** C

The term *spondyloarthropathy* refers to a set of conditions characterized by axial joint involvement, presence of HLA-B27 haplotype, absence of rheumatoid factor, and a positive family history of these diseases. These conditions include ankylosing spondylitis, psoriatic arthritis, the arthropathy of inflammatory bowel disease (IBD), and reactive arthritis.

Traditional ankylosing spondylitis is not common in childhood. Under the International League of Associations for Rheumatology (ILAR) classification, children with arthritis and/or enthesitis primarily affecting the lower extremities who may go on to develop disease in the spine or sacroiliac joints are considered to have enthesitis-related arthritis. Those who ultimately develop ankylosing spondylitis typically present with peripheral arthritis in addition to enthesitis, onset in late childhood, a family history of ankylosing spondylitis or related diseases, and presence of HLA-B27 antigen. A child with axial involvement would present with persistent low back pain, not upper back pain.

Psoriatic arthritis is a type of spondyloarthropathy characterized by arthritis and psoriasis. However, not all children classified with juvenile psoriatic arthritis have psoriasis. According to the ILAR criteria, diagnosis of psoriatic arthritis requires arthritis and psoriasis or arthritis and 2 additional criteria including dactylitis, nail pitting, onycholysis, and a family history of psoriasis in a first-degree relative. Psoriasis in an aunt would not meet criteria for diagnosis.

(Chapter 199: Spondyloarthropathies [pp. 933–944])

**Answer 15-17.** D

This patient has inflammatory bowel disease (IBD)-associated arthritis. Inflammatory arthritis occurs in 7% to 20% of patients with IBD. It is associated with active intestinal inflammation and usually resolves as the IBD is treated. However, joint disease may occur at the onset of IBD or even precede the diagnosis of IBD by months to years. Peripheral arthritis is twice as common as axial arthritis in patients with IBD and usually involves the large weight-bearing joints. Those who have axial involvement are often males who are HLA-B27 positive, and that disease tends to be more persistent rather than dependent on bowel inflammation.

Symptoms that should raise suspicion for IBD include fatigue, weight loss, unexplained growth failure, and fevers. Gastrointestinal manifestations include abdominal pain or tenderness, oral ulcers, diarrhea, and hematochezia. Extraintestinal manifestations of IBD include erythema nodosum, pyoderma gangrenosum, and clubbing. Other musculoskeletal complaints seen in children with IBD include arthralgias, nonspecific myalgia, deconditioning secondary to illness, glucocorticoid-induced osteopenia, pes planus, and hypertrophic osteoarthropathy.

In a child with IBD-associated arthritis, laboratory studies demonstrate chronic inflammation including anemia, hypoalbuminemia, and elevated ESR. Elevated fecal calprotectin indicates intestinal inflammation, which could be due to IBD. Therefore, although gastrointestinal endoscopy and biopsy are needed for confirmation, measurement of serum and/or fecal calprotectin is a less invasive test to evaluate for possible IBD.

(Chapter 199: Spondyloarthropathies [p. 936])

**Answer 15-18.** B

This patient has reactive arthritis. Reactive arthritis is a type of spondyloarthropathy that typically occurs 1 to 4 weeks after a gastrointestinal or genitourinary infection. Common causative organisms include *Yersinia enterocolitica*, *Yersinia tuberculosis*, *Shigella flexneri*, *Salmonella typhimurium*, *Campylobacter jejuni*, *Chlamydia trachomatis*, and *Ureaplasma urealyticum*. Respiratory infections due to *Mycoplasma pneumoniae* or *Chlamydia pneumoniae* are less common causes of reactive arthritis. The frequency of reactive arthritis varies based on genetic factors and the prevalence of arthritogenic infections in the community. A history of recent infection, infectious contact, or travel should increase suspicion for reactive arthritis. In this case, this patient had a history of a gastrointestinal infection 2 to 3 weeks prior to onset of joint pain and swelling.

Reactive arthritis typically presents with warmth, erythema, tenderness, and pain of 1 or 2 large, weight-bearing joints but may also present as asymmetric involvement of the small and large joints. Additional joint manifestations include dactylitis, enthesitis, tenosynovitis, and bursitis. Associated symptoms may include fever, fatigue, polyarthralgia, and myalgias. Reactive arthritis may be accompanied by conjunctivitis and/or urethritis, but extra-articular manifestations are rare in children. Laboratory investigations may show elevated acute phase reactants. There is no recommendation to search for a causative organism with reactive arthritis if there is clear evidence of a preceding infection, although presence of a causative organism would increase suspicion for reactive arthritis.

The differential for reactive arthritis includes other postinfectious arthritides, such as poststreptococcal, postgonococcal, Lyme, and viral arthritis. Lyme arthritis commonly presents as arthritis in a single joint, typically the knee. Poststreptococcal and postgonococcal arthritis differ in pattern of involvement, course, and prognosis. Acute warmth, swelling, and tenderness in the setting of fever would raise concern for septic arthritis.

In a child with reactive arthritis, short-term treatment with NSAIDs may be effective for symptomatic relief. Although reactive arthritis is triggered by an infection, antibiotic therapy has not been demonstrated to alter the natural history of reactive arthritis. In cases of significant discomfort and inflammation, a short-term course of glucocorticoids may be used, but high-dose steroids would not be appropriate.

Reactive arthritis is usually transient or self-limited with resolution in days to weeks. After 6 months, the patient would be classified as having chronic arthritis, which differs from the juvenile idiopathic arthritis (JIA) criterion of 6 weeks of arthritis. In cases of persistent arthritis, it is often indistinguishable from enthesitis-related arthritis and should be treated as such with disease-modifying drugs such as sulfasalazine. There is an association between reactive arthritis and HLA-B27 positivity, and HLA-B27–positive individuals are more likely to develop persistent arthritis following an infection.

(Chapter 199: Spondyloarthropathies [pp. 936–937])

### Answer 15-19. B

This patient has classic findings suggestive of Henoch-Schönlein purpura (HSP). HSP is a form of small-vessel vasculitis. Essentially all patients will develop rash at some point during the disease course, and the diagnosis is dependent on the classic "palpable purpura" rash. Arthritis is the second most common feature, occurring in 75% of patients, followed by gastrointestinal involvement in 50% to 75% of patients. Gastrointestinal involvement is often colicky in nature, ranging from mild to severe enough to mimic appendicitis, and may lead to intussusception in 1% to 5% of patients. Nephritis is less common, occurring in only 40% to 50% of patients, but has the potential for severe renal involvement and ongoing nephropathy in 1% to 2% of those with renal involvement. About 75% to 90% of patients with nephritis develop urinary abnormalities within 4 weeks, but they may occur up to 3 months after symptom onset.

Urinalysis should be performed on all HSP patients once weekly while disease is active and then monthly for the next 3 months. If at any point there is evidence of nephritis, long-term monitoring of urinalyses, renal function, and blood pressure should continue until urinary abnormalities resolve.

(Chapter 200: Vasculitides [p. 939])

### Answer 15-20. E

GPA is a form of ANCA-associated vasculitis. It is a necrotizing granulomatous vasculitis of small- to medium-sized vessels. Its classic triad of manifestations is upper airway, lower airway, and renal involvement; however, any organ system can be involved, and children may frequently present predominantly with constitutional symptoms and arthralgias/arthritis. A positive test for ANCA can facilitate the diagnosis in the appropriate clinical context; however, confirmatory biopsy of involved tissue is often necessary. GPA is most strongly associated with the cytoplasmic staining of the ANCAs (c-ANCA) on indirect immunofluorescence testing. These antibodies are targeted against PR3, detectable by enzyme-linked immunosorbent assay (ELISA) testing.

Less commonly, GPA may be associated with the perinuclear staining pattern (p-ANCA), targeted against myeloperoxidase (MPO). GPA may also be ANCA negative, particularly in early disease and disease limited to the upper airway. Consequently, ANCA testing can support a diagnosis but is not adequate by itself for diagnosis or necessary for diagnosis.

(Chapter 200: Vasculitides [p. 941])

### Answer 15-21. B

PAN is a necrotizing vasculitis of medium-sized arteries. Most patients present predominantly with constitutional symptoms; however, many have some form of skin rashes (classically livedo reticularis and skin nodules), abdominal pain, musculoskeletal involvement (myalgias and myositis are common), neurologic involvement (mononeuritis multiplex, peripheral neuropathy, stroke), and hypertension from renal vessel aneurysms. Acute phase reactants may be highly elevated.

A subset of PAN patients have cutaneous PAN, which is characterized by livedo reticularis, crops of painful nodules, and sometimes myalgias or arthralgias. Patients with cutaneous PAN do not have constitutional symptoms and generally have normal acute phase reactants. Patients with cutaneous PAN require monitoring for development of systemic involvement and may require immunosuppressive treatment; patients with systemic involvement require immunosuppression. PAN, including cutaneous PAN, has been associated with streptococcal infections. Patients may require prophylaxis with penicillin to prevent recurrences of their PAN if it is felt to be triggered by streptococcal infections.

(Chapter 200: Vasculitides [p. 940])

### Answer 15-22. C

Laboratory abnormalities and, specifically, the presence of autoantibodies are common in patients with SLE. The majority of patients (> 95%) are antinuclear antibody (ANA) positive. A positive dsDNA is present in 50% to 60% of patients. Other autoantibodies commonly seen in SLE include anti-Smith and ribonucleoprotein (RNP) antibodies, as well as antibodies associated with antiphospholipid antibody syndrome (anticardiolipin and anti–$\beta_2$-glycoprotein antibodies). The presence of autoantibodies is part of the classification criteria for SLE. Many patients with SLE have elevated inflammatory markers (ESR is more commonly elevated than the CRP), increased liver function studies, and mild anemia. However, the presence of a positive dsDNA antibody is most specific for SLE.

(Chapter 201: Systemic Lupus Erythematosus, Overlap Connective Tissue Diseases, and Mixed Connective Tissue Disease [pp. 943–948])

**Answer 15-23.** A

The malar rash, which is a fixed (not transient), flat, or raised rash, typically extending from the nose to the cheeks and sparing the nasolabial folds (commonly referred to as a "butterfly rash"), is a very specific clinical finding in SLE. The only other rheumatic disease that causes a malar rash is juvenile dermatomyositis. The malar rash is present in about 40% of patients with SLE and is included in both the American College of Rheumatology (ACR) 1982 criteria for classification of SLE and the more recent Systemic Lupus International Collaborating Clinics (SLICC) classification criteria.

(Chapter 201: Systemic Lupus Erythematosus, Overlap Connective Tissue Diseases, and Mixed Connective Tissue Disease [pp. 943–948])

**Answer 15-24.** D

MCTD is an overlap syndrome that combines clinical features of systemic lupus erythematosus (SLE), polymyositis/dermatomyositis, scleroderma, and juvenile arthritis. The most common features are Raynaud phenomenon, fever, arthritis, rash, finger swelling (sclerodactyly), and myositis. By definition, all patients with MCTD have a high positive antinuclear antibody (ANA) and increased anti-U1RNP antibodies. Given the clinical features, elevated muscle enzymes and a positive rheumatoid factor are common as well.

(Chapter 201: Systemic Lupus Erythematosus, Overlap Connective Tissue Diseases, and Mixed Connective Tissue Disease [pp. 948–950])

**Answer 15-25.** C

The patient described in this question has a classic, photosensitive malar rash. Only 2 diseases are associated with malar rashes: lupus (including cutaneous lupus erythematosus and SLE), and JDM. Malar rashes in both conditions are photosensitive. Based on the young age, cutaneous lupus erythematosus and JDM are more likely than SLE. A patient with JDM might also have other rashes, which point toward the diagnosis. A heliotrope rash appears as a purple to red discoloration over the eyelids, sometimes associated with periorbital edema (Figure 202-1). Gottron papules (Figure 202-2) are erythematous plaques overlying extensor surfaces, most frequently the small joints. Calcinosis—firm, generally painful nodules—can occur from calcium deposits in affected skin and muscle. Ulcerations of the skin may also occur, in addition to erythema of the cuticles. Many patients with JDM, although not all, will have weakness.

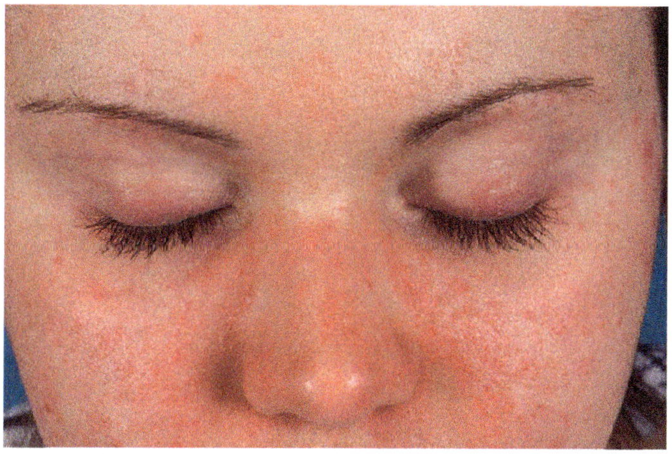

**FIGURE 202-1.** Heliotrope rash, a purplish discoloration over the eyelids with associated periorbital edema, which is characteristic of dermatomyositis. This child also has a malar rash. (Mark W. Kline, Rudolph's Pediatrics, 23rd Edition. Copyright © McGraw-Hill Education. All rights reserved.)

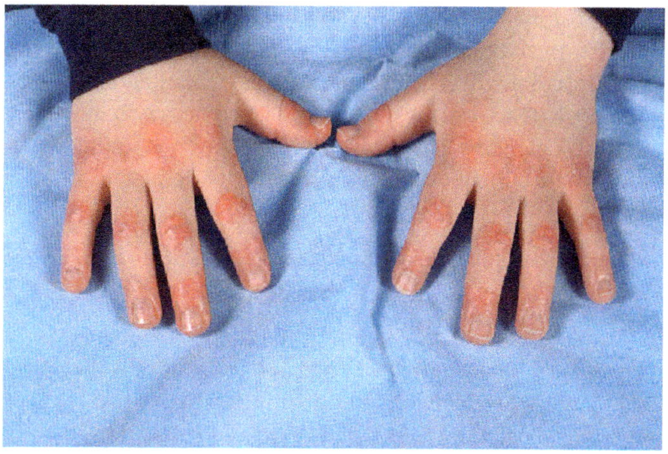

**FIGURE 202-2.** Gottron papules. Raised erythematous plaques over joint extensor surfaces, here over the finger joints, which are generally symmetric and characteristic of dermatomyositis. (Mark W. Kline, *Rudolph's Pediatrics*, 23rd Edition. Copyright © McGraw-Hill Education. All rights reserved.)

(Chapter 202: Juvenile Dermatomyositis [pp. 946, 953])

**Answer 15-26.** C

Risk factors for poor outcome in JDM include severe and/or chronic disease activity, ulcerations, calcifications, severe dysphagia, interstitial lung disease, cardiac involvement, some myositis-specific autoantibodies, some features on muscle biopsy, delay in treatment, and persistent skin disease activity. Heliotrope rash is a common finding in JDM, affecting 66% to 100% of patients. Essentially all children with JDM have some skin findings: a heliotrope rash, malar rash, and/or Gottron papules. Muscle edema demonstrated by MRI is frequently used by rheumatologists in North America as confirmation of the presence of myositis. Arthritis is a less common manifestation, occurring in only 10% to 65% of children with JDM, but does not portend a poor prognosis. Nailfold capillary changes—dilation, dropout, and tortuosity—are seen in > 90% of children diagnosed with dermatomyositis. These changes typically require magnification to see but can lead to reddened inflamed-appearing cuticles to the naked eye.

Calcinosis is dystrophic calcification that occurs in skin, subcutaneous tissue, or muscle, frequently at pressure point sites. There is increased risk for calcinosis with long-standing active disease (including those who have had a delay in diagnosis/initiation of treatment), more severe disease, a chronic or polycyclic course, and cardiopulmonary disease.

Calcinosis typically appears 1 to 3 years after the onset of disease. In addition to being painful, it can also lead to cellulitis, skin breakdown, joint contractures, and ulcerations at the site of calcinosis. Once calcinosis develops, it can be very challenging to treat. Calcinosis can resolve on its own over an unpredictable time frame but typically progresses if active dermatomyositis is inadequately controlled.

(Chapter 202: Juvenile Dermatomyositis [p. 956])

**Answer 15-27.** E

There are 5 Bohan and Peter criteria, one of which is the characteristic rash of dermatomyositis (heliotrope rash or Gottron papules); the other 4 criteria address clinical, laboratory, electromyographic (EMG), or histopathologic evidence of myositis. The latter 4 criteria include symmetric, often progressive proximal and axial weakness, elevation of muscle-associated enzymes (creatine kinase, aldolase, lactate dehydrogenase, and transaminases), a triad of characteristic EMG changes, and biopsy showing evidence of chronic muscle inflammation. The diagnosis of dermatomyositis requires the presence of rash as well as 3 other criteria, whereas the diagnosis of polymyositis requires the absence of rash and the presence of the other 4 criteria.

MRI was not available at the time of the development of these criteria, but many pediatric rheumatologists in North America use STIR sequences (which suppress fat signal) on MRI to detect myositis and frequently forgo biopsy and EMG if the MRI shows muscle edema. Biopsy is strongly recommended in cases of juvenile polymyositis, a disease not associated with a characteristic rash. The presence of muscle edema on MRI is *not* specific for myositis and can occur in other inflammatory myopathies as well as in muscular dystrophy.

(Chapter 202: Juvenile Dermatomyositis [p. 955])

**Answer 15-28.** A

Raynaud phenomenon occurs in up to 70% of patients with systemic sclerosis and may precede other clinical manifestations by several years. Raynaud phenomenon is caused by vasospasm, usually in response to cold or stress. Patients experience a triphasic color change with a white phase due to vasoconstriction, subsequent purplish discoloration, and then a red phase when reperfusion occurs (Figure 203-1). Although Raynaud phenomenon is common, even among otherwise healthy individuals, it is more likely to be part of an underlying autoimmune condition if a patient develops fingertip ulcerations (Figure 203-2) or if nailfold capillary changes are visible by capillaroscopy. The treatment of Raynaud includes rewarming techniques and medication management including calcium channel blockers.

Musculoskeletal findings, including arthritis, arthralgias, and myositis, are a part of the classification criteria for systemic sclerosis, but these manifestations are not as common as Raynaud phenomenon. Pulmonary fibrosis is one of the minor criteria for systemic sclerosis, but a cough would be a late clinical symptom. Nephritis is not a common renal manifestation

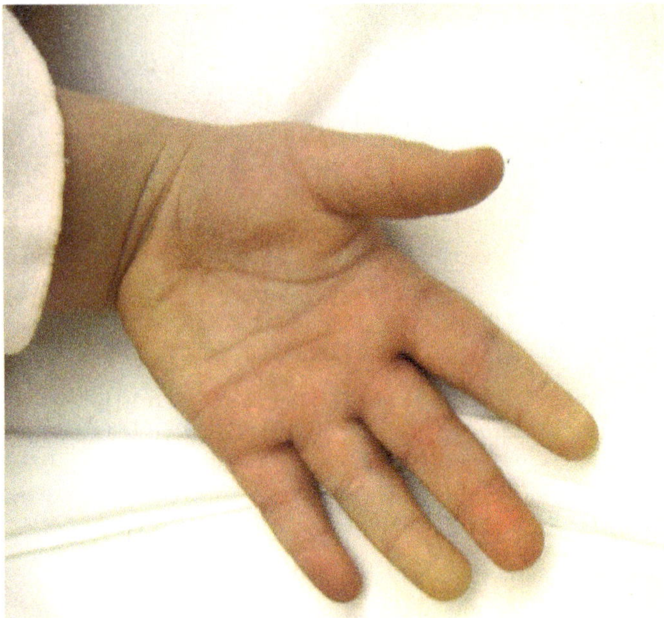

**FIGURE 203-1.** Classic Raynaud phenomenon in a 4-year-old girl. Note the ischemic changes (blanching phase) of the second and fourth fingers and the cyanosis (bluish phase) of the fifth finger. (Mark W. Kline, *Rudolph's Pediatrics*, 23rd Edition. Copyright © McGraw-Hill Education. All rights reserved.)

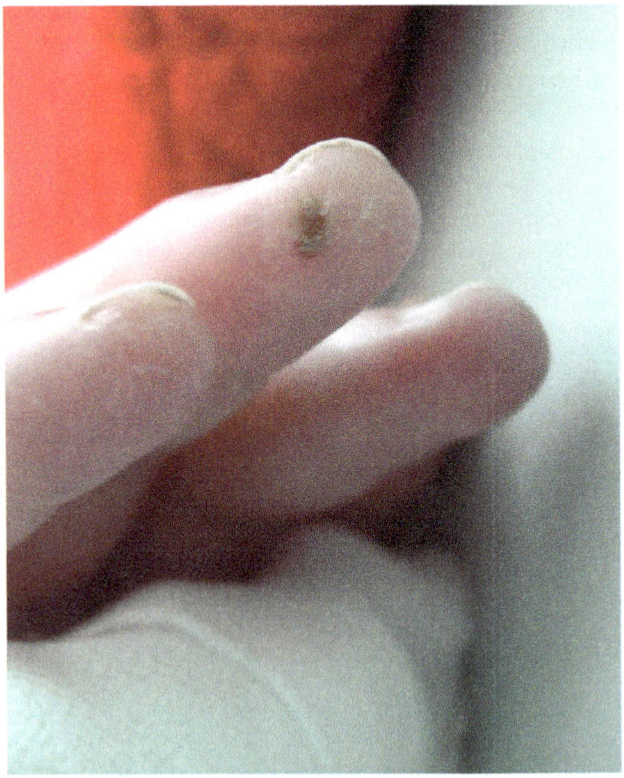

**FIGURE 203-2.** Pitting of the fingertips. Note a small ulceration of the tip of the right third finger and shiny, tightly stretched skin over the fingertips. (Mark W. Kline, *Rudolph's Pediatrics*, 23rd Edition. Copyright © McGraw-Hill Education. All rights reserved.)

of systemic sclerosis. Patients with systemic sclerosis may experience fatigue, but this symptom is not included in the classification criteria for juvenile systemic sclerosis.

(Chapter 203: Juvenile Scleroderma [pp. 959–961])

**Answer 15-29.** B

Linear scleroderma is the most common form of juvenile scleroderma. It is characterized by linear hyperpigmentation of the skin, most commonly on the extremities, which can involve multiple layers of the skin and soft tissue including the dermis, fat, muscle, and bone, leading to joint contractures and other deformities. Linear scleroderma involving the face is called "en coup de sabre" or "strike of the sword." In most cases, patients with linear scleroderma will have an unremarkable laboratory evaluation including normal inflammatory markers. Treatment of all forms of progressive and potentially disabling morphea includes systemic immunosuppressive therapy such as corticosteroids, methotrexate, and mycophenolate mofetil.

(Chapter 203: Juvenile Scleroderma [pp. 961–963])

**Answer 15-30.** A

This is a child whose presentation is consistent with growing pains. Growing pains are the most common cause of recurrent limb pain in childhood and occur in children between the ages of 3 and 12. Growing pains are of unclear etiology and are characterized by intermittent nighttime nonarticular pain, most commonly in the legs. Pain tends to be bilateral and occur in the evening or night. Growing pains are not associated with limping, limitations in mobility, joint swelling, color changes, warmth, or morning stiffness.

If a child presents with a typical picture for growing pains, no additional workup is needed. However, radiographs and laboratory tests may be needed to alleviate parental concern. Laboratory workup typically consists of CBC, erythrocyte sedimentation rate (ESR), and muscle enzymes, which should all be normal in growing pains. An ANA would not be of benefit because it is a nonspecific antibody and is not required for a diagnosis of juvenile idiopathic arthritis (JIA). Additional workup is recommended if a child has a limp, joint pain, an abnormal physical exam, or history of trauma or illness because these would not be consistent with this condition.

Symptomatic treatment for growing pains includes heat, massage, and analgesics. Children tend to outgrow this condition by middle school with no long-term sequelae. Reassurance that this is a benign condition without serious progression is important because growing pains can be disruptive and concerning to parents.

(Chapter 204: Musculoskeletal Pain Syndromes [pp. 963–964])

**Answer 15-31.** D

This patient has benign joint hypermobility syndrome (BJHS) and meets both major Brighton criteria (Table 204-1):

**TABLE 204-1.** 1998 Revised Brighton Criteria for Benign Joint Hypermobility Syndrome

| |
|---|
| **Major Criteria** |
| 1. A Beighton score of 4 out of 9 or greater (either currently or historically) |
| 2. Arthralgia for longer than 3 months in 4 or more joints |
| **Minor Criteria** |
| 1. A Beighton score of 1, 2, or 3 out of 9 |
| 2. Arthralgia (≥ 3 months) in 1–3 joints or back pain (≥ 3 months), spondylosis, spondylolysis/spondylolisthesis |
| 3. Dislocation/subluxation in >1 joint, or in 1 joint on > 1 occasion |
| 4. Soft tissue rheumatism, at least 3 lesions (eg, epicondylitis, tenosynovitis, bursitis) |
| 5. Marfanoid habitus (tall, slim, span/height ratio < 1.03, upper-to-lower segment ratio < 0.89, arachnodactyly [positive Steinberg/wrist signs]) |
| 6. Abnormal skin: striae, hyperextensibility, thin skin, papyraceous scarring |
| 7. Eye signs: drooping eyelids or myopia or antimongoloid slant |
| 8. Varicose veins or hernia or uterine/rectal prolapse |

Mark W. Kline, *Rudolph's Pediatrics*, 23rd Edition. Copyright © McGraw-Hill Education. All rights reserved.

a Beighton score of 4 out of 9 or greater and arthralgia for longer than 3 months in 4 or more joints.

She has a Beighton score of 5 out of 9, which is calculated by awarding 1 point for hypermobility of each of the following sites (Figure 204-1):

1. Extension of the wrist and fifth metacarpophalangeal joint so that the fifth digit is parallel to the dorsum of the forearm
2. Passive apposition of the thumb to the flexor aspect of the forearm
3. Hyperextension of the elbows 10 degrees or more
4. Hyperextension of the knees 10 degrees or more
5. Flexion of the trunk with the knees fully extended so the palms rest on the floor

In a patient with BJHS, one should look for stigmata of heritable connective tissue diseases, such as Marfan syndrome and Ehlers-Danlos syndrome. Stigmata of Marfan syndrome include Marfanoid habitus, arachnodactyly, high-arched palate, and ocular abnormalities such as drooping eyelid or dislocated lens. Ehlers-Danlos syndrome may present with increased elasticity of skin, abnormal papyraceous scars, and velvety texture of the skin. Of the answer choices given, only choice D is a stigmata of heritable connective tissue disease. Patients with a Marfanoid habitus are typically tall with long limbs (answer choice E).

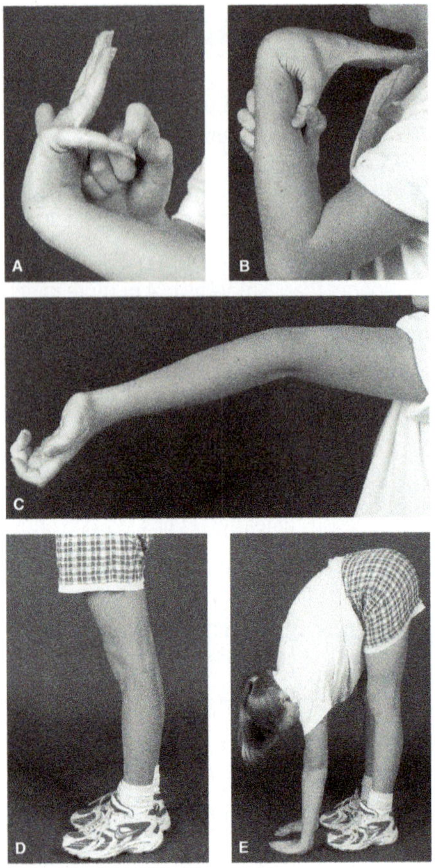


**FIGURE 204-1.** Demonstrations of Beighton score components. **A:** Extension of the wrist and metacarpophalangeal joints so that the fingers are parallel to the dorsum of the forearm. **B:** Passive apposition of the thumb to the flexor aspect of the forearm. **C:** Hyperextension of the elbows 10 degrees or more. **D:** Hyperextension of the knees 10 degrees or more. **E:** Flexion of the trunk with the knees fully extended so the palms rest on the floor. (Mark W. Kline, *Rudolph's Pediatrics*, 23rd Edition. Copyright © McGraw-Hill Education. All rights reserved.)

BJHS tends to be more common in younger patients and females. There is a tendency for BJHS to run in families. BJHS may present with joint and muscle pain, transient joint swelling, subjective stiffness, and pain that is worse with increased physical activity. Up to 20% of children with BJHS have recurrent sprains. Chronic nonspecific back pain may also be secondary to hypermobility.

(Chapter 204: Musculoskeletal Pain Syndromes [pp. 964–965])

**Answer 15-32.** B

Complex regional pain syndrome (CRPS) is characterized by pain, swelling, and disuse of an extremity with associated vasomotor instability. Onset may occur after an antecedent illness or minor trauma, and pain is out of proportion to the severity of the injury. In children, CRPS most commonly affects the legs and feet. Children with CRPS tend to report worsening pain during rest and immobilization after a minor injury.

The Budapest criteria for CRPS in adults requires continuing pain out of proportion to the initial injury in addition to symptoms in the following domains:

- Sensory: allodynia, hyperesthesia
- Vasomotor: skin temperature or color asymmetry
- Sudomotor: asymmetry of sweating or edema
- Motor/trophic: spasticity, dystonia, hair/nail changes

This child demonstrates allodynia with her out-of-proportion tenderness to palpation. Focal pain would suggest an alternative diagnosis. A cool and discolored affected foot would meet the vasomotor criteria for CRPS. Fevers should not be present in CRPS and would raise concern for alternate pathology, such as septic arthritis or other infectious etiology. Bony abnormalities are not common in children with CRPS, but any demineralization would be diffuse rather than focal.

(Chapter 204: Musculoskeletal Pain Syndromes [pp. 965–966])

**Answer 15-33.** D

This young lady has juvenile fibromyalgia. This is a condition of unknown etiology that tends to predominately affect females. Common symptoms include arthralgias, myalgias, fatigue, sleep disturbance, and characteristic tender points. Further associations include irritable bowel syndrome, migraine or tension headaches, paresthesias, Raynaud phenomenon, and dizziness attributed to postural orthostatic tachycardia syndrome or neurocardiogenic orthostatic hypotension. Patients also tend to share certain personality traits and behavior patterns, such as anxiety and depression, compulsion, overwork, and perfectionism.

There are no diagnostic tests for juvenile fibromyalgia. Laboratory studies may be done to exclude other conditions and include complete blood count (CBC), erythrocyte sedimentation rate (ESR), rheumatoid factor, ANA, muscle enzymes, and thyroid function tests. Laboratory studies should be considered when there are abnormalities on exam because juvenile fibromyalgia is characterized by multiple tender points in the absence of other physical findings. At this time, additional laboratory testing or imaging is not indicated based on her history or exam.

The first priority of treatment is to confirm the diagnosis and reassure the family that symptoms are not due to a serious or life-threatening disorder. Nonmedical approaches that have been shown to be effective in children include exercise and cognitive-behavioral therapy. The goals of treatment include pain reduction, return to normal activity, and improved quality of sleep. A structured exercise program, sometimes done in conjunction with physical therapy, has been shown to reduce pain, although patients may initially experience increased pain at the start of treatment.

(Chapter 204: Musculoskeletal Pain Syndromes [pp. 966–967])

**Answer 15-34.** C

Although clear criteria for the diagnosis of chronic fatigue syndrome in children has not been established, it is a diagnosis that should be considered in a child with at least 3 months of fatigue, frequently precipitated by a specific illness or event. Patients with chronic fatigue syndrome frequently have other somatic complaints such as headaches or abdominal pain, as well as widespread musculoskeletal pain. Many patients also have disorganized or disrupted sleep. Because chronic fatigue syndrome is a diagnosis of exclusion, the evaluation for this diagnosis should include an evaluation for an underlying condition that can present with similar symptoms, including thyroid disease.

An ANA, which is a sensitive screening test for systemic lupus erythematosus (SLE) and other systemic autoimmune conditions, is not an appropriate test without more specific manifestations of SLE (eg, malar rash, arthritis, evidence of nephritis). Similarly, a dsDNA is an appropriate test to send in case of suspected SLE. A rheumatoid factor is an appropriate test for a patient with focal joint pain or symptoms and examination findings consistent with arthritis. HLA-B27 testing should be reserved for a patient with a likely HLA-B27–associated disease such as arthritis/sacroiliitis or symptomatic inflammatory eye disease (uveitis/iritis).

(Chapter 201: Chronic Fatigue Syndrome [pp. 968–950])

**Answer 15-35.** A

Carefully asking about key aspects of autoinflammatory syndrome is essential in arriving at the correct diagnosis in a patient with recurrent fevers (Table 206-2). Age of onset, ethnicity, consanguinity, and family history are important distinguishing points for autoinflammatory syndromes because many are due to monogenetic mutations (Table 206-4).

**TABLE 206-2.** Characteristics of the Main Autoinflammatory Syndromes

| Disease | Onset Age | Typical Ethnicity | Common Triggers | Episode Duration | Interval Between Episodes |
|---|---|---|---|---|---|
| Familial Mediterranean fever (FMF) | Mostly first decade (~80%) | Sephardic Jewish, Armenian, Arab Muslim, Turks, Italian | None known, exercise, stress, menstrual period | Hours to 3 days | Variable |
| Mevalonate kinase deficiency (MKD)/hyperimmunoglobulin D syndrome (HIDS) | First year of life | Dutch, western Europe | Vaccines, infections | 3–7 days | 3–6 weeks |
| Tumor necrosis factor (TNF) receptor–associated periodic syndrome (TRAPS) | Mostly first decade<br>Can start in adults (~25%) | Any, mainly Scottish, Irish (Hibernian) | Exercise, stress, minor trauma | Days to 6–8 weeks | Variable, usually > 8 weeks |
| Familial cold autoinflammatory syndrome (FCAS) | First year of life | United States | Cold | < 24 hours | Variable |
| Muckle-Wells syndrome (MWS) | Any age | Western Europe | None known | 1–3 days | Variable |
| Neonatal-onset multisystem inflammatory disorder (NOMID) | Birth, infancy | Any | None known | Continuous | None |
| Pyogenic sterile arthritis, pyoderma gangrenosum, acne (PAPA) syndrome | Mostly first decade | Western Europe | Minor trauma | Variable | Variable |
| Periodic fever, aphthous stomatitis, pharyngitis, adenitis (PFAPA) | Toddler (1–5 years) | Any | None known | 5–7 days | 3–4 weeks, truly periodic |
| Deficiency of interleukin-1 receptor antagonist (DIRA) | Birth, infancy | Puerto Rico, Lebanon, Newfoundland, Netherlands | None known | Continuous | None |
| Deficiency of adenosine deaminase 2 (DADA2) | First year of life, adolescence | Georgian Jewish | None known | Unclear, often episodic | Years |
| Chronic atypical neutrophilic dermatosis with lipodystrophy and elevated temperature (CANDLE) syndrome | Early childhood | Any | None known | Continuous | None |

Mark W. Kline, *Rudolph's Pediatrics*, 23rd Edition. Copyright © McGraw-Hill Education. All rights reserved.

**TABLE 206-4.** Important Historical Points to Consider During Investigations of Autoinflammatory Syndromes

| |
|---|
| Age of onset |
| Ethnicity (eg, Mediterranean) |
| Consanguinity |
| Family history |
| Triggers for attack (eg, infection, cold, vaccines, stress, exercise) |
| Duration of attacks |
| Frequency of attacks (including periodicity) |
| Clinical features (eg, fever, rash, serositis, gastrointestinal, chest, musculoskeletal, eye, neurologic) |
| Response to therapy (colchicine, corticosteroids, tumor necrosis factor and interleukin-1 inhibitors) |

Mark W. Kline, *Rudolph's Pediatrics*, 23rd Edition. Copyright © McGraw-Hill Education. All rights reserved.

Triggers for attacks, duration of attacks, frequency of attacks, clinical features, and response to therapy help to distinguish the most likely disease associated with the patient's symptoms. Clinical features most commonly affect the following organ systems: skin, gastrointestinal tract, joints, eyes, and central nervous system. Asking parents to keep a symptoms and fever journal helps to obtain the essential information.

An autoinflammatory-driven history helps to gain the essential information needed so that the correct diagnosis can be postulated for genetic testing.

The number of siblings, family history of JIA, ANA status, and history of celiac disease are not key components of autoinflammatory syndrome history.

(Chapter 206: Autoinflammatory Disorders [pp. 972–973])

## Answer 15-36. B

Amyloidosis is the feared complication for many autoinflammatory syndromes. Understanding the risk for amyloidosis for each autoinflammatory syndrome is important to understanding the future risk and screening appropriately (Table 206-5). Specific questions about chronic renal failure and amyloidosis in the family history can help elucidate the risk of amyloidosis and can hone down the specific autoinflammatory disease.

FMF has one of the highest rates of amyloidosis (up to 25%). There are several risk factors for the development of amyloidosis in FMF: homozygous for 694 and 680 mutations, family history of amyloidosis, geographic location outside the United States, male gender, serum amyloid A genotype, and poor compliance to colchicine (because colchicine is protective against developing amyloidosis). The 3 syndromes associated with cryopyrin-associated periodic syndromes have different rates of amyloidosis: amyloidosis is rare in FCAS and is somewhat associated with neonatal-onset multisystem inflammatory disorder (NOMID); however, in Muckle-Wells

**TABLE 206-5.** The Risk of Amyloidosis in Untreated Autoinflammatory Syndromes

| Disease | Risk of Amyloidosis | Risk Factors |
|---|---|---|
| Familial Mediterranean fever (FMF) | Yes (up to 25%) | 680, 694 mutations |
| | | Ethnicity (increased in Armenians, Sephardic Jewish, Arab Muslims) |
| | | Geography of patients (decreased in United States, western Europe) |
| | | Family history |
| | | Increased in males |
| | | Serum amyloid A genotype |
| Mevalonate kinase deficiency (MKD)/hyperimmunoglobulin D syndrome (HIDS) | Rare (0%–5%) | |
| Tumor necrosis factor (TNF) receptor–associated periodic syndrome (TRAPS) | Yes (14%–25%) | Cysteine mutations |
| Familial cold autoinflammatory syndrome (FCAS) | Rare | |
| Muckle-Wells syndrome (MWS) | Yes (25%–33%) | Unknown |
| Neonatal-onset multisystem inflammatory disorder (NOMID) | Yes, in survivors | Unknown |
| Pyogenic sterile arthritis, pyoderma gangrenosum, acne (PAPA) syndrome | Unknown | |
| Periodic fever, aphthous stomatitis, pharyngitis, adenitis (PFAPA) | No | |

Mark W. Kline, *Rudolph's Pediatrics*, 23rd Edition. Copyright © McGraw-Hill Education. All rights reserved.

syndrome, it is quite high (25%–33%). Amyloidosis is also rarely associated with mevalonate kinase deficiency (MKD)/HIDS and JIA. Amyloidosis is not associated with PFAPA.

(Chapter 206: Autoinflammatory Disorders [p. 974])

**Answer 15-37.** E

The disease described in this question is chronic recurrent multifocal osteomyelitis (CRMO). The correct answer is answer choice E because a complication of CRMO is leg length inequality, along with chronic bone deformities and disability. CRMO is a chronic inflammatory condition that primarily affects the bones. Unlike infectious osteomyelitis, the bacterial cultures of bone biopsies of CRMO are negative. The inflammatory bone lesions can include osteolytic and sclerotic bone lesions. Lesions preferentially occur in the metaphysis of long bones. Any bone can be affected in CRMO, including areas uncommonly affected in infectious osteomyelitis such as the clavicle, ribs, and vertebrae. Technetium bone scan and MRI are the imaging modalities used to visualize the lesions, and whole-body MRI is the best imaging modality for these patients. Common associated clinical features include synovitis, isolated palmoplantar pustulosis, psoriasis, sacroiliitis, IBD, and pyoderma gangrenosum.

Respiratory distress with pneumonitis, progressive lipodystrophy, stroke, and sensorineural hearing loss are not associated complications of CRMO. Respiratory distress with pneumonitis is a pulmonary manifestation seen in deficiency of the IL-1 receptor antagonist (DIRA). DIRA is an autoinflammatory bone disease that presents in infancy. Progressive lipodystrophy is seen in proteasome-associated autoinflammatory syndromes such as chronic atypical neutrophilic dermatosis with lipodystrophy and elevated temperature (CANDLE) syndrome. Stroke is a complication seen in deficiency of adenosine deaminase 2 (DADA2). Sensorineural hearing loss is seen in Muckle-Wells syndrome. Fifty percent to 70% of patients develop sensorineural hearing loss that affects high-frequency sounds first and typically starts in adolescence.

(Chapter 206: Autoinflammatory Disorders [p. 974])

**Answer 15-38.** B

PFAPA is likely the most common etiology for periodic fever syndromes. Currently, there is no known genetic mutations for PFAPA. The onset of PFAPA is usually in children < 5 years of age. It is the only autoinflammatory syndrome that is truly periodic. The attacks occur every 21 to 28 days, and each fever episode lasts 3 to 7 days. Pharyngitis and cervical adenopathy are the most common symptoms, occurring in 80% to 100% of cases. Aphthous stomatitis occurs in 60% to 70% of cases. Other common symptoms are abdominal pain, nausea/vomiting, arthralgias, and headaches. Patients with PFAPA have elevated inflammatory markers during an attack that normalize between flares. A single dose of prednisone at the onset of symptoms usually aborts the attack, although it can also decrease the interval between fevers. The natural course of PFAPA is benign, and the attacks diminish or completely resolve over time. Amyloidosis is not a complication of PFAPA.

(Chapter 206: Autoinflammatory Disorders [p. 978])

# CHAPTER 16 Neurology

Andres Jimenez-Gomez and Sarah Risen

**16-1.** A 13-year-old girl with acne vulgaris presents with a headache 2 weeks after completing a course of treatment with 2 unspecified medications. Her headache began 1 week ago and is dull in quality, diffuse in location, and constant. It is worse at night and has started to wake her up from sleep. In the past 2 days, she has also developed diplopia. On examination, she is overweight. Neurologic examination is significant for bilateral papilledema and a right sixth nerve palsy. Magnetic resonance imaging (MRI) of the brain, including magnetic resonance venogram, is normal. Opening pressure on lumbar puncture is 30 cm $H_2O$, and cerebrospinal fluid (CSF) composition is normal. Which medication would be most appropriate for her treatment?

**A.** Propranolol

**B.** Acetazolamide

**C.** Ibuprofen

**D.** Cyproheptadine

**E.** Sumatriptan

**16-2.** A 12-year-old boy complains of episodic severe headaches for the past 6 months. The headaches occur once every 2 weeks and last for up to 2 hours. He says it hurts "all over" his head and feels like something is going "boom boom" in his head. His mother notes that he pulls the covers over his head and he asks her to turn off the lights when he has a headache. There are no cranial autonomic symptoms (eg, lacrimation) with the headaches. The mother experiences severe headaches every month before her period that are associated with nausea and vomiting. The child's neurologic examination is normal. What feature would suggest that migraine, rather than other types of headache, is the most likely diagnosis?

**A.** Duration of the headaches

**B.** Throbbing sensation

**C.** Photophobia or phonophobia

**D.** Gender

**E.** Normal neurologic examination

**16-3.** Which of the following would be the most appropriate medication for an adolescent girl with juvenile myoclonic epilepsy?

**A.** Oxcarbazepine

**B.** Divalproex sodium

**C.** Lamotrigine

**D.** Clonazepam

**E.** Diazepam

**16-4.** A 10-year-old girl has migraine headaches once every 2 weeks. Her head pain is severe in intensity, and there is significant associated nausea and vomiting. Her parents have tried giving her ibuprofen; however, she usually vomits the medication within minutes of taking it. Her parents ask if there is anything else she could try for these headaches. Which of the following would be the most appropriate treatment to recommend?

**A.** Sumatriptan nasal spray

**B.** Continue to use ibuprofen

**C.** Ondansetron oral dissolving tablet

**D.** Oxygen at 12 L/min

**E.** Amitriptyline

**16-5.** A 3-day-old term neonate presents to the emergency department (ED) because of tachypnea and poor feeding. He was born to a 25-year-old G1P1 mother by normal spontaneous vaginal delivery after an uncomplicated pregnancy. Apgar scores were 8 and 9. His examinations in the nursery were normal, and he was discharged to home on day of life 2 latching well and taking colostrum, although his mother's milk had not yet come in. In triage, he is noted to have a respiratory rate of 72 breaths/min. His eyes are closed, and he is sluggishly reactive to painful stimuli. Emergent computed tomography (CT) of the head rules out intracranial hemorrhage but suggests diffuse cerebral edema. Which laboratory test is most likely to reveal the reason for his encephalopathy?

**A.** Blood glucose

**B.** Ammonia

**C.** Venous blood gas

**D.** Urine toxicology screen

**E.** Sodium

**16-6.** A term neonate develops recurrent focal motor seizures at 12 hours of life. The seizures were first noted by the mother while she was breastfeeding. She reports the infant's left arm began to jerk rhythmically and then the left side of his face began to jerk as well. This lasted for 1 minute before self-resolving. The infant was brought to the nursery where he had a second event, identical to the first. Review of his history reveals that he was born to a 28-year-old G1P1 mother by vaginal delivery. Labor was complicated by a prolonged second stage; however, his fetal heart tracing remained reassuring and he was delivered spontaneously with Apgar scores of 8 and 9. The infant was vigorous at delivery. His neurologic examination at the time of the evaluation was normal. A bedside head ultrasound was performed and intracranial hemorrhage ruled out. Electrolytes were normal. A lumbar puncture was performed, and cell counts and chemistries were normal. What feature would suggest an arterial ischemic stroke as the most likely cause of this presentation?

**A.** Head ultrasound does not show blood

**B.** Focal onset seizures

**C.** Prolonged labor

**D.** Normal Apgar scores

**E.** Breastfeeding

**16-7.** A 3-year-old boy presents with hypotonia and gross motor delay. He can pull to stand but is not yet walking. He was born at term. His mother recalls decreased fetal movements in utero. The neonatal period was complicated by feeding difficulty. On examination, he has a high-arched palate and a narrow face. There is facial diplegia, and his mouth tends to hang open. His speech is nasal in quality and dysarthric. Muscle bulk is diminished throughout. He has hypotonia and proximal weakness in a limb-girdle distribution. The weakness is not fatigable. Sensation is normal. Deep tendon reflexes are present. What is the localization of his neurologic condition?

**A.** Upper motor neuron disease

**B.** Neuromuscular junction

**C.** Muscle

**D.** Lower motor neuron disease

**E.** Peripheral nerve

**16-8.** A 9-month-old baby girl is evaluated for profound global developmental delay. Examination is notable for coarsened facial features, a gibbous deformity of the thoracolumbar spine, and hepatomegaly. Neurologic examination reveals hypotonia and positional plagiocephaly. Laboratory analysis reveals low β-galactosidase activity. Which of the following would be most likely on ophthalmologic examination?

**A.** Cherry-red spot

**B.** Optic nerve hypoplasia

**C.** Coloboma

**D.** Uveitis

**E.** Congenital cataract

**16-9.** A 12-year-old boy presents to the emergency department (ED) complaining of a severe headache that involves only the right side of his face. He has been having this type of headache on and off for 2 days. The headaches occur twice a day and last for 1 hour each time. There is associated right-sided conjunctival injection, lacrimation, and nasal rhinorrhea during the attacks. His mother notes that he had a similar bout of headaches 6 months ago that lasted for 3 weeks. Of the following, which would be the best first-line therapy?

**A.** Intramuscular ketorolac

**B.** Intravenous (IV) prochlorperazine

**C.** Oxygen via non-rebreather

**D.** Topiramate

**E.** IV sodium valproate

**16-10.** A baby boy was born at term to a 34-year-old G3P2 mother. Pregnancy was complicated by borderline gestational diabetes. Delivery was complicated by shoulder dystocia, although the infant was ultimately able to be delivered vaginally. Apgar scores were 8 and 9. Birth weight was 4700 g. In the delivery room, the pediatrics team noted the infant was not moving his left arm. What symptom would suggest a brachial plexus injury is a likelier diagnosis than a neonatal ischemic stroke?

- **A.** Focal seizures of affected arm
- **B.** Affected leg ipsilaterally
- **C.** Difficulty feeding due to dysphagia
- **D.** Ipsilateral Horner syndrome
- **E.** Disconjugate gaze

**16-11.** A 12-year-old boy presents to the emergency department (ED) complaining of an acute-onset, severe, holocephalic headache that began 12 hours ago. There was no antecedent head trauma. He vomited once at headache onset. He reports this is the worst headache of his life. He is afebrile, and neurologic examination is normal; however, he has some neck stiffness. A computed tomography (CT) scan is negative for intracranial hemorrhage. What is the next most appropriate step in his care?

- **A.** Reassurance that his headache is benign and ibuprofen for pain
- **B.** Lumbar puncture to evaluate for xanthochromia
- **C.** Magnetic resonance imaging (MRI) scan to rule out ischemic stroke
- **D.** Electroencephalogram (EEG) to evaluate for seizure
- **E.** Start antibiotics for presumed meningitis

**16-12.** A 7-year-old Mexican boy comes to see you for "funny movements" for the past 6 weeks. These are happening frequently and involve his head and shoulders mostly. He is attentive, communicates during episodes, seems uncomfortable, and cannot make them go away. They do go away fully when he sleeps. It is also now affecting his gait. Which is an appropriate next step in management?

- **A.** Obtain an electroencephalogram (EEG)
- **B.** Order a magnetic resonance imaging (MRI) of the brain
- **C.** Send a serum ceruloplasmin level
- **D.** Recommend further immunologic evaluation, including antistreptolysin O titers
- **E.** Order a lumbar puncture

**16-13.** You see a 13-year-old girl with a history of migraine headaches that have required abortive treatment on many previous occasions. She reports that her headaches tend to be unilateral, severe, and associated with nausea and photophobia. She reports that, on a prior occasion, she went to the emergency department (ED) where she received intravenous (IV) fluids and prochlorperazine. She improved almost immediately but remembers having a severe reaction where her neck and tongue stiffened for several hours. Given the potential benefit of the medication, what additional medication could be used concomitantly to prevent or diminish the intensity of this reaction?

- **A.** Diphenhydramine
- **B.** Chlorpromazine
- **C.** Phenytoin
- **D.** Acetaminophen
- **E.** Sumatriptan

**16-14.** An 8-year-old boy comes in with 2 days of left-sided facial weakness. He awoke with it in the morning, and it has been stable since. His taste sensation has also changed. On examination, the left side of his face moves significantly less than the right. What aspect of his neurologic examination would suggest Bell palsy is a likelier diagnosis than stroke?

- **A.** Involvement of the lower face
- **B.** Age
- **C.** Forehead involvement
- **D.** Preceding viral infection
- **E.** Hyperacusis

**16-15.** A 15-year-old boy comes to the office complaining of headache for 1 day. The day prior, he had played in a football game and banged his helmet against another player's during a tackle. He did not lose consciousness; however, he felt "dazed" immediately following the event and had to sit out for the rest of the game. The headache began within an hour of the event. He also reports trouble concentrating and sensitivity to light and sound. Neurologic examination is normal. Neuropsychological testing indicates he is currently performing below his preseason baseline. He asks if he can go to football practice later that afternoon. What would be the most appropriate counseling?

- **A.** He can warm up with the team but should not participate in any tackling drills.
- **B.** He can play, but if his headache starts to get worse, he should sit out.
- **C.** He should stay home for now on cognitive and physical rest until symptoms resolve.
- **D.** He should focus on schoolwork and only return to football once he can concentrate on academics again.
- **E.** He can practice as long as his headache improves with ibuprofen.

**16-16.** A 2-month-old baby boy comes into the emergency department (ED) after having a focal convulsive seizure at home. The parents state that he rolled off the bed onto a carpeted floor, hitting his head. On examination, he is lethargic and difficult to arouse; a bruise is seen on the side of his head, and he has several bruises on his extremities. Which combination of tests would be an appropriate next step in the acute care of this patient?

- **A.** Skeletal survey, hearing testing, pre- and post-ductal oxygen saturation tests, neurosurgery evaluation
- **B.** Skeletal survey, neurosurgery evaluation, computed tomography (CT) imaging of the head, ophthalmology evaluation
- **C.** Skeletal survey, hearing testing, neurosurgery evaluation, CT imaging of the head
- **D.** Hearing testing, pre- and post-ductal oxygen saturation tests, CT imaging of the head, ophthalmology evaluation
- **E.** Pre- and post-ductal oxygen saturation tests, ophthalmology evaluation, CT imaging of the head, neurosurgery evaluation

**16-17.** A term infant is born by emergency cesarean section for fetal distress. Intraoperatively, the obstetricians suspect that a placental abruption has caused the fetal distress. Labor had been uneventful until the fetal heart rate dropped suddenly. At delivery, the infant has low tone, a poor suck, and an absent Moro reflex. Apgar scores were 1 and 4 at 3 and 5 minutes, respectively. He is treated with therapeutic hypothermia for presumed hypoxic-ischemic injury. At 18 hours of life, he develops seizures, which are controlled with phenobarbital and stop after 24 hours. His neurologic examination reveals increased sleepiness and higher tone than normal; however, he is opening his eyes and beginning to breastfeed. His electroencephalogram (EEG) background is normalized by 48 hours of life. A magnetic resonance imaging (MRI) scan suggests moderate brain injury. Which of the following is the most accurate way to counsel the family?

- **A.** Therapeutic hypothermia prevented any permanent neurologic injury, and the child will definitely develop normally.
- **B.** The baby now has epilepsy and will need antiepileptic medication for at least 2 years.
- **C.** The baby is at risk for both motor and cognitive disabilities and needs close neurodevelopmental monitoring.
- **D.** An elective cesarean section could have prevented the child's injury.
- **E.** The child is neurologically devastated and will never learn to walk, talk, or feed himself.

**16-18.** A 9-year-old girl with a history of severe birth asphyxia with resultant quadriplegic cerebral palsy comes to clinic. Her mother reports that the child's legs are so stiff that the physical therapists are having difficulty doing range-of-motion exercises with her. On examination, she has severe spasticity in all extremities, particularly the legs. She appears uncomfortable when the examiner tries to range her lower extremities, and she has contractures at the ankles. What medications would be options in treating her spasticity?

- **A.** Baclofen, phenobarbital, botulinum toxin
- **B.** Diazepam, phenobarbital, baclofen, botulinum toxin
- **C.** Baclofen, diazepam, clonazepam, botulinum toxin
- **D.** Baclofen, clonazepam, phenobarbital, botulinum toxin
- **E.** Botulinum toxin only

**16-19.** A 3-year-old girl comes to urgent care because since she woke up that morning she has been "clumsy" and "has been falling much more than usual." She has not vomited. On examination, she is afebrile and well appearing. There is horizontal nystagmus on end-gaze bilaterally. When she reaches for a toy, her accuracy is poor bilaterally. Her gait is wide based, and she tends to veer to the side and prefers to walk along the hallway wall to help her balance. Her mother notes that about 10 days earlier she had a febrile illness with vomiting and diarrhea. What would be the most likely magnetic resonance imaging (MRI) finding?

- **A.** Posterior fossa mass
- **B.** Hydrocephalus
- **C.** Cerebellar edema
- **D.** Cerebellar hemorrhage
- **E.** Midbrain stroke

**16-20.** A 6-year-old boy presents to the emergency department (ED) with fever and altered mental status. On neurologic examination, he is somnolent, pupils are dilated and slow to react to light, and there is nuchal rigidity. The treating physician is concerned about bacterial meningitis. Which of the following correctly describes the optimal timing of when antibiotics should be started?

- **A.** After the computed tomography (CT) scan is done
- **B.** Without any delay
- **C.** Once the lumbar puncture has been performed
- **D.** When the lab calls with the stat Gram stain results
- **E.** After the hearing test

**16-21.** A 16-year-old girl tells you her neurologist started her on a preventive medication for migraine. She can't remember the name of the medication but tells you her neurologist advised her to start on birth control medication concomitantly and check lab work periodically. Which medication was she most likely started on?

**A.** Propranolol

**B.** Topiramate

**C.** Valproate

**D.** Amitriptyline

**E.** Gabapentin

**16-22.** A 16-year-old girl complains of left eye pain and visual blurring in the left eye. Her acuity in that eye is 20/100 compared with 20/20 in the right eye. When the examiner shows her a red object, she states it appears "less red" on the left compared with the right. The fundoscopic examination is normal, and there are no eye movement abnormalities. The remainder of her neurologic examination is normal. What is the neuroanatomic localization of her visual disturbance?

**A.** Retina

**B.** Optic nerve

**C.** Lateral geniculate nucleus

**D.** Visual cortex

**E.** Not localizable (eg, conversion disorder)

**16-23.** A 21-month-old girl is brought to the pediatrician's office for several days of unusual eye movements. Her mother notes that she also has not been sleeping well for the past couple of weeks and has been fussier lately. On examination, she has random, conjugate, chaotic eye movements. She has dysmetria when reaching for objects bilaterally and is unsteady when sitting on the exam table. What condition should she be promptly investigated for?

**A.** Ovarian teratoma

**B.** Limbic encephalitis

**C.** Glucose transporter type 1 (GLUT) deficiency

**D.** Neuroblastoma

**E.** Arterial ischemic infarct

**16-24.** At a well-child check, an astute pediatrician notices that a 6-month-old male infant who was born full term without any complications does not track toys that do not also make noise and also has significantly declined percentiles on the growth curve for height and weight. He blinks to light and fixates on the pediatrician's face briefly but does not track and does not blink to threat. The infant has normal tone in his arms and legs; he is rolling over front to back only and does not yet sit with anterior propping. He is laughing and babbling. Concerned about impaired vision, the pediatrician refers him to an ophthalmologist who sees him the following day and notes bilateral optic nerve hypoplasia. In addition to laboratory tests of pituitary function, the pediatrician orders a brain magnetic resonance imaging (MRI). What is most likely to be seen on brain MRI?

**A.** Hypothalamic hamartoma

**B.** Absence of the septum pellucidum

**C.** Stenosis of the cerebral aqueduct

**D.** Cerebellar-pontine hypoplasia

**E.** Hypoxic-ischemic injury

**16-25.** You have been referred a new 7-year-old patient to your clinic. She has a history of neurofibromatosis type 1 (NF1). What screening examination should young children with NF1 have annually?

**A.** Ophthalmologic examination

**B.** Brain magnetic resonance imaging (MRI)

**C.** Hearing tests

**D.** Cardiac echocardiography

**E.** Wood's lamp examination

**16-26.** A 2-year-old boy presents because the mother is concerned that he is having seizures. She describes that when he gets frustrated or upset, he will cry and then turn purple in the face and lose consciousness. He has a few seconds of jerking movements after losing consciousness. He regains consciousness immediately and does not seem sleepy afterward. He never has a spell without first becoming upset and crying. He is meeting all of his developmental milestones. What is the most likely diagnosis?

**A.** Epilepsy

**B.** Child abuse

**C.** Gastroesophageal reflux

**D.** Cardiac arrhythmia

**E.** Breath-holding spells

**16-27.** A 9-month-old infant has episodes of torticollis every 3 weeks that last between 20 and 30 minutes. He typically does not want to feed during these periods and sometimes looks pale. He is also not as playful as he usually is. Between episodes, he returns completely to normal. His neurologic examination is normal, and he has achieved normal developmental milestones. What condition might he develop later in childhood?

**A.** Epilepsy

**B.** Depression

**C.** Migraine

**D.** Breath-holding spells

**E.** Anxiety

**16-28.** A 12-year-old girl presents complaining of fatigue for the past few weeks. She notes that although she feels normal in the morning, as the day goes on, she gets more tired. She cannot exercise as much as she used to. In the evenings, she sometimes gets double vision while watching TV and needs to rest while eating dinner or she notes that she starts to drool. On examination, she has mild ptosis bilaterally at baseline, although it is more noticeable on the right. On sustained upgaze testing, the ptosis becomes more prominent and she complains of diplopia. What is the localization for her symptoms?

**A.** Muscle

**B.** Nerve

**C.** Neuromuscular junction

**D.** Pons

**E.** Spinal cord

**16-29.** A 2.5-month-old baby boy comes into urgent care for seizures. He has been feeding poorly with minimal weight gain. His mom notes that recently he stopped tracking her face and can no longer lift his head up during tummy time. On exam, he has sagging facial features and lightly pigmented hair with a strange kinky texture and is significantly hypotonic. His prenatal course was unremarkable, and he had a normal newborn screen. What is his most likely diagnosis?

**A.** Phenylketonuria

**B.** Menkes disease

**C.** Biotinidase deficiency

**D.** Urea cycle defect

**E.** GM1 gangliosidosis

**16-30.** You are asked to see a child with Fabry disease. He has bouts of crises that often involve "burning" or "piercing" pains that originate in the hands and feet. What medication can be used to treat the pain crises that often occur in children with Fabry disease?

**A.** Carbamazepine

**B.** Baclofen

**C.** Propranolol

**D.** Diphenhydramine

**E.** Prochlorperazine

**16-31.** A 9-year-old boy is told to follow-up with his pediatrician from the emergency room after he had his first generalized tonic-clonic seizure. His mom reports that 6 months ago he was diagnosed with attention-deficit/hyperactivity disorder (ADHD) by a psychiatrist after he began to have trouble in school. Mom explains his grades declined this school year, and he has seemed overly active despite being on a good dose of methylphenidate. After the seizure, mom feels he is walking funny and he seems to be having more trouble performing motor tasks. He tells you that things look blurrier now. His exam reveals a very hyperactive boy with dysmetria on exam and spasticity in his legs. A magnetic resonance imaging (MRI) of the brain shows abnormalities of the parieto-occipital white matter. Plasma levels of very-long-chain fatty acids are elevated. What is the most likely diagnosis?

**A.** Aicardi-Goutières syndrome

**B.** X-linked adrenoleukodystrophy

**C.** ADHD

**D.** Neuronal ceroid lipofuscinosis

**E.** Juvenile-onset Alexander disease

**16-32.** Where is the port-wine stain characteristic of Sturge-Weber syndrome most commonly found?

**A.** In an upper motor neuron seventh nerve pattern

**B.** In a lower motor neuron seventh nerve pattern

**C.** In the first division of the trigeminal nerve, bilaterally

**D.** In the first division of the trigeminal nerve, unilaterally

**E.** In the distribution of the greater occipital nerve

**16-33.** A 2-day-old, former full-term neonate has seizures that are difficult to control and was recently intubated for respiratory distress and apnea. Her mother reports that in utero the baby had significantly more "hiccups" than her other children did. On examination, the infant is intubated, does not open her eyes, does not move spontaneously, and is very hypotonic. Labor and delivery were uneventful, and the infant had Apgar scores of 8 and 9. What test or intervention would be most useful in identifying the etiology for her seizures?

**A.** Brain magnetic resonance imaging (MRI)

**B.** Electroencephalogram (EEG)

**C.** Lumbar puncture

**D.** Electromyography (EMG)

**E.** Response to therapeutic hypothermia

**16-34.** A 3-year-old boy has been having headaches that wake him up from sleep for the past week. He has vomited several times, and mom feels he is falling more. He says he sees "2 doctors" when he looks at you. On examination, he has end-gaze horizontal nystagmus bilaterally and truncal ataxia. He has limitation of his horizontal eye movements, where he cannot move his left eye past midline when looking left. He is unable to tolerate a funduscopic examination. What is the most likely etiology for his headaches?

A. Migraine
B. Tension-type headache
C. Idiopathic intracranial hypertension
D. Cerebral aneurysm
E. Posterior fossa mass

**16-35.** Which cranial nerve is most likely to be affected by Lyme disease?

A. Optic nerve
B. Oculomotor nerve
C. Trigeminal nerve
D. Facial nerve
E. Hypoglossal nerve

**16-36.** A 12-year-old girl is being evaluated for possible seizures. She has a seizure about once a week. Typically, they occur when she is in a stressful situation or frightened. Her eyes roll up, and she has asynchronous jerking movements of all extremities and pelvic thrusting for about 15 minutes. A routine electroencephalogram (EEG) is normal; however, no events were captured. What is the next best step in her evaluation and management?

A. Start an antiepileptic medication
B. Prescribe benzodiazepines as needed
C. Refer to physical therapy
D. Admit for sedated electromyography (EMG) testing
E. Admit for video EEG monitoring

**16-37.** A 10-year-old boy presents with 10 hours of progressive bilateral lower extremity weakness and urinary retention. He is awake and alert. Cranial nerve function is normal. What is the neuroanatomic localization of his symptoms?

A. Brain stem
B. Spinal cord
C. Muscle
D. Brain
E. Neuromuscular junction

**16-38.** A 5-day-old, 36-week gestational age, male infant in the neonatal intensive care unit (NICU) started having abnormal movements of the left arm and leg. He is not intubated and has been working with therapists on his oral feeding. Electroencephalogram (EEG) confirmed these movements are seizures. The NICU attending orders an initial phenobarbital load and starts maintenance phenobarbital. The phenobarbital level the following morning is 29 μg/mL. He begins to have more frequent seizure and activity, and the NICU team is ordering another loading dose of phenobarbital. What is the most likely side effect the neonatology team should be prepared for?

A. Hyponatremia
B. Respiratory suppression
C. Anaphylaxis
D. Hypertension
E. Dystonic reaction

**16-39.** A 15-month-old girl presents to the emergency department (ED) after a reported generalized convulsion at home that lasted 60 seconds. A rectal temperature on arrival is 39.5°C. She is well appearing and back to her baseline with a normal neurologic examination. She is an otherwise healthy and normally developing girl. Mom had a febrile seizure when she was 2 years old. What are the clinical features that would increase this child's risk of future epilepsy?

A. Family history of febrile seizures in a first-degree relative
B. Age of first febrile seizure < 18 months
C. Level of temperature at first seizure
D. Complex febrile seizure (focal, prolonged, or repeated)
E. Duration of illness before seizure

**16-40.** A 6-month-old normally developing boy presents to pediatric urgent care for episodes of brief arm jerks for the past 5 days. The movements occur in clusters on awakening. The parents report he is quiet during the arm jerks, which last only a few seconds, but he cries after each jerk. You are most concerned about infantile spasms. What is the typical electroencephalogram (EEG) pattern that will confirm the diagnosis?

A. Suppression
B. 3-Hz spike and wave
C. Hypsarrhythmia
D. Trace alternant
E. Asynchronous spindles

**16-41.** A healthy 7-year-old girl presents to your clinic with her mother, who claims she has noticed that her daughter has been "spacing out" many times a day over the past month. On further questioning, mom reports that these episodes last about 10 seconds, during which her daughter is unresponsive with a behavioral arrest. Her teachers have also reported similar episodes at school. The patient endorses feeling that she "loses time" sometimes and was recently hit on the head with a soccer ball during one of these episodes. Her examination is normal. Based on the most likely diagnosis, what is the best next step?

**A.** Obtain blood work, including complete blood count (CBC) and liver function tests
**B.** Schedule a referral to a neurologist and an electroencephalogram (EEG)
**C.** Obtain a brain magnetic resonance imaging (MRI)
**D.** Ask the patient's mother to keep an event diary and schedule follow-up in 1 month
**E.** Schedule a referral to a psychiatrist

**16-42.** Which of the following antiepileptic drugs is most likely to cause an allergic skin reaction?

**A.** Levetiracetam
**B.** Topiramate
**C.** Valproic acid
**D.** Lamotrigine
**E.** Zonisamide

**16-43.** You are taking care of a 5-year-old boy who has had recurrent seizures and was recently diagnosed as having idiopathic epilepsy. What is the most common form of idiopathic epilepsy in children?

**A.** Childhood absence epilepsy
**B.** Juvenile myoclonic epilepsy
**C.** Benign epilepsy with centrotemporal spikes (BECTS)
**D.** Childhood occipital epilepsy, Gastaut type
**E.** Benign occipital epilepsy (Panayiotopoulos syndrome)

**16-44.** A 13-year-old girl with a history of generalized tonic-clonic seizures arrives to the emergency department (ED) by ambulance after having a convulsion lasting 5 minutes at home. In the ED, she is sleepy but arousable without any focal neurologic findings. Vital signs are normal. There is no history of illness or trauma. Her last seizure was 2 years ago. She takes lamotrigine for seizure control. As part of her diagnostic evaluation, what test would be most important in this situation?

**A.** Head computed tomography (CT) scan
**B.** Electroencephalogram (EEG)
**C.** Lamotrigine level
**D.** Complete blood count (CBC) and liver function tests
**E.** Lumbar puncture

**16-45.** A 6-month-old girl with developmental regression and a 1-month history of seizures is seen for a follow-up visit in your clinic. The cause of her developmental regression and new-onset seizures is unknown. Imaging and laboratory tests have not yet been performed. The local neurologist's first available clinic appointment is in 4 weeks. In the interim, which of the following antiepileptic medications should *not* be started in this child?

**A.** Oxcarbazepine
**B.** Valproic acid
**C.** Topiramate
**D.** Levetiracetam
**E.** Zonisamide

**16-46.** A 12-year-old boy presents to the emergency department (ED) after having an episode of unresponsiveness with shaking of all extremities lasting 2 minutes. The event occurred during wakefulness and was witnessed by his mother. When the paramedics arrived, he was sleepy but arousable. His serum glucose was 100 mg/dL. When he arrives to the ED by ambulance, he is well appearing with normal vital signs and is alert with a normal neurologic examination. What is the most appropriate course of action?

**A.** Admit to the hospital for observation
**B.** Perform a lumbar puncture to exclude meningitis
**C.** Diagnose the patient with epilepsy
**D.** Coordinate an outpatient referral to a child neurologist
**E.** Start an antiepileptic medication

**16-47.** An 8-month-old boy with unexplained global developmental delay who recently moved to the area presents in urgent care for worsening spells over the past month. These spells are described as "jackknife" movements in which there is a quick head drop with flexion at the waist and his arms extend out. These episodes have been occurring over the past 3 weeks with increasing frequency, and they tend to cluster on waking up. On examination, he is hypotonic, and 5 hypomelanotic macules are noted. What is the patient's most likely underlying diagnosis?

**A.** Tuberous sclerosis complex
**B.** Dravet syndrome
**C.** Benign myoclonic epilepsy in infancy
**D.** Ohtahara syndrome
**E.** Neurofibromatosis

**16-48.** A healthy 2-year-old girl presents to your clinic for a routine checkup. She is meeting her developmental milestones and has a normal examination, including her neurologic exam. Her mother is concerned about her history of febrile seizures, which includes 4 simple febrile seizures over the past 12 months. She asks you if her risk of future epilepsy is increased due to the number of febrile seizures. How will you counsel this patient?

**A.** If she continues to have frequent febrile seizures past age 2 years, then her risk will increase.

**B.** The number of seizures does not predict risk of future epilepsy, but her age of onset (before 18 months) does increase her risk.

**C.** The number of simple febrile seizures does not correlate with risk of future epilepsy.

**D.** If she has 1 more simple febrile seizure, then her risk of epilepsy increases.

**E.** Her risk of developing future epilepsy is already 15%.

**16-49.** What percentage of children with new-onset epilepsy will eventually be able to discontinue medication and remain seizure-free?

**A.** 10%

**B.** 30%

**C.** 50%

**D.** 70%

**E.** 90%

**16-50.** You are taking care of a 4-year-old girl who has had several generalized tonic-clonic seizures over the past 6 weeks. She has no significant past medical history and has reached all developmental milestones appropriately. You decide to refer her to a neurologist in hopes of pursuing a formal diagnosis. Which of the following is the most important reason for accurate identification of an epilepsy syndrome?

**A.** It may avoid the need to obtain an electroencephalogram (EEG).

**B.** It may avoid the need to check antiepileptic drug levels and drug interactions.

**C.** It may prompt the family to seek school services for learning disabilities.

**D.** It may help with prognosis and choice of antiepileptic therapy.

**E.** It can determine whether prenatal and environmental exposures were associated with symptoms.

**16-51.** A 4-month-old infant is seen in the office for a new patient visit. The patient's mother reports that her daughter had "seizures" involving clonic movements starting at 5 days of life and remitting at 1 month of life spontaneously. Brain magnetic resonance imaging (MRI) and metabolic studies at the time of seizure onset were normal. Her examination and development are normal. There is no family history of seizures. What is the most likely diagnosis?

**A.** Infantile spasms

**B.** Early myoclonic epilepsy

**C.** Benign neonatal convulsions

**D.** Birth trauma–associated convulsions

**E.** Transient hypocalcemia

**16-52.** A 9-month-old infant with a history of seizures is admitted to the pediatric intensive care unit for status epilepticus. The infant has had seizures since several days of life, and the etiology is unclear. In addition to traditional antiepileptic medications, which of the following therapies should be considered in an infant with unexplained intractable epilepsy?

**A.** Folic acid

**B.** Pyridoxine (vitamin $B_6$)

**C.** Vitamin D

**D.** Glucose

**E.** Cobalamin (vitamin $B_{12}$)

**16-53.** A 6-month-old infant presents to the emergency department (ED) after a brief convulsion at home in the setting of fever for 3 days. In the ED, his temperature is 40.0°C, he is lethargic, his anterior fontanelle is bulging and firm, and his pupils are unequal, dilated, and sluggish. Besides antibiotics, what should be an immediate next step in this patient's evaluation?

**A.** Neurosurgical evaluation

**B.** Lumbar puncture

**C.** Antiepileptic medication

**D.** Elevated head of bed

**E.** Head computed tomography (CT)

**16-54.** A 1-year-old boy presents to your clinic for a well-child visit. You notice that his head circumference plots below the third percentile. He additionally appears somewhat delayed in his development and failed a recent audiologic evaluation. Besides his head circumference, his physical examination is unrevealing. You review his birth history, which reveals no abnormal prenatal or perinatal events; he passed his newborn hearing screen. He has a healthy 3-year-old sibling. Which of the following conditions is most likely causative of this patient's presentation?

**A.** Cri-du-chat (5p deletion syndrome)

**B.** Hypoxic-ischemic encephalopathy at birth

**C.** Congenital cytomegalovirus (CMV) infection

**D.** Congenital Zika infection

**E.** Sotos syndrome

**16-55.** You are evaluating an otherwise healthy and normally developing 6-month-old infant with stable macrocephaly. Which part of the history is most helpful in making the diagnosis?

A. Birth history
B. Family history of seizures
C. Parental head circumference scores
D. Pregnancy history
E. Immunization status

**16-56.** A 10-year-old girl with a history of transient left-sided weakness due to a partial transverse myelitis now presents to urgent care with a 3-day history of right arm numbness. Other than these sensory changes, the rest of her neurologic examination is normal. Lumbar puncture reveals normal cell count and normal glucose and protein. Brain magnetic resonance imaging (MRI) with contrast shows multiple periventricular and subcortical white matter lesions, some with enhancement. What is the most likely diagnosis?

A. Acute disseminated encephalomyelitis (ADEM)
B. Clinically isolated syndrome
C. Increased intracranial pressure (ICP)
D. Focal arterial ischemic stroke
E. Multiple sclerosis (MS)

**16-57.** A 12-year-old girl with a history of transverse myelitis now presents to urgent care with a 2-day history of worsening blurry vision of her right eye. On examination, her right eye demonstrates decreased visual acuity and papillitis. What is the best acute treatment for this patient?

A. Antibiotics
B. Plasmapheresis
C. High-dose methylprednisolone
D. Oral steroids
E. Cytoxan

**16-58.** A 10-year-old boy presents with altered mental status and lower extremity weakness. Based on neuroimaging, he is diagnosed with acute disseminated encephalomyelitis (ADEM). What percentage of children who present with ADEM will have only 1 event without recurrence?

A. 10%
B. 20%
C. 40%
D. 60%
E. 80%

**16-59.** An 8-year-old, previously healthy boy develops subacute onset of bilateral leg weakness with bowel and bladder incontinence over 3 days. On examination in the emergency department (ED), he has bilateral leg weakness, increased lower extremity deep tendon reflexes, and absent anal wink reflex. Emergent spinal magnetic resonance imaging (MRI) is indicated to exclude which of the following diagnoses?

A. Multiple sclerosis (MS)
B. Guillain-Barré syndrome
C. Acute arterial ischemic stroke
D. Spinal epidural hematoma
E. Spina bifida

**16-60.** A 12-year-old girl with a recent diagnosis of multiple sclerosis (MS) presents to your clinic with complaints of blurry vision. Which of the following symptoms or signs would support a diagnosis of optic neuritis?

A. Proptosis
B. Color vision deficit
C. Inability to abduct the affected eye
D. Foreign body sensation
E. Eyelid swelling

**16-61.** A 15-year-old girl has a history of multiple episodes of transient neurologic symptoms with associated T2 hyperintense white matter lesions on magnetic resonance imaging (MRI), suggestive of multiple sclerosis (MS). Which of the following diagnostic tests offers further support of a diagnosis of MS?

A. Cerebrospinal fluid (CSF) xanthochromia
B. Serum oligoclonal bands
C. CSF oligoclonal bands
D. Highly elevated CSF protein
E. Conduction block on electromyography (EMG)

**16-62.** A 3-month-old infant is brought to the pediatrician for evaluation of excessive startle response to tactile stimulation and developmental regression over the past month. On examination, there is mild hepatosplenomegaly. He does not make good eye contact, does not vocalize, and has axial hypotonia with appendicular hypertonia and increased reflexes. Ophthalmologic examination performed earlier that day showed a macular cherry red spot. What is the enzyme deficiency in this disease?

A. Phenylalanine hydroxylase deficiency
B. $\beta$-Hexosaminidase $\beta$-subunit
C. Ornithine transcarbamylase
D. Acid $\alpha$-glucosidase
E. $\alpha$-Galactosidase A

**16-63.** Which statement is correct regarding diagnostic tests in Tay-Sachs disease and Sandhoff disease?

**A.** Tay-Sachs is associated with hexosaminidase A deficiency in white blood cells (WBCs), whereas Sandhoff disease is associated with hexosaminidase A and B deficiency.

**B.** Tay-Sachs is associated with hexosaminidase B deficiency in WBCs, whereas Sandhoff disease is associated with hexosaminidase A and B deficiency.

**C.** Tay-Sachs is associated with hexosaminidase A and B deficiency in WBCs, whereas Sandhoff disease is associated with hexosaminidase A deficiency.

**D.** Tay-Sachs is associated with hexosaminidase A and B deficiency in WBCs, whereas Sandhoff disease is associated with hexosaminidase B deficiency.

**E.** Tay-Sachs is associated with hexosaminidase A deficiency in WBCs, whereas Sandhoff disease is associated with hexosaminidase B deficiency.

**16-64.** Gaucher disease displays which type of inheritance pattern?

**A.** Autosomal dominant

**B.** X-linked recessive

**C.** X-linked dominant

**D.** Autosomal recessive

**E.** Mitochondrial

**16-65.** A 2-year-old boy has a history of myoclonic seizures since 9 months of life, slowly progressive ataxia, acquired microcephaly, and recent-onset visual decline. His ophthalmologic examination reveals macular degeneration, retinal degeneration, and optic atrophy. Electroencephalogram (EEG) displays epileptiform discharges in response to low-frequency photic stimulation. What is the most likely diagnosis?

**A.** Dravet syndrome

**B.** Infantile spasms

**C.** Neuronal ceroid lipofuscinosis (NCL)

**D.** Lennox-Gastaut syndrome

**E.** Ohtahara syndrome

**16-66.** What clinical characteristic can be seen in all of the following metabolic disorders: sialidosis type I, Gaucher, Sandhoff, and Niemann-Pick type A?

**A.** Hepatosplenomegaly

**B.** Cherry red spot

**C.** Hyperpigmented skin lesions

**D.** Cognitive impairment

**E.** Early death

**16-67.** You are seeing a 7-year-old boy with new-onset attention-deficit, hyperactivity disorder (ADHD) and cognitive decline. Despite trials of multiple medications by his primary care physician, he presents with worsening cognitive decline. His history is significant for a deceased male sibling. On examination, his skin looks notably tanner than that of his parents. He has brisk reflexes. Given the prior history, and besides a brain magnetic resonance imaging (MRI), what would be an appropriate immediate evaluation for this patient?

**A.** Urine organic acids

**B.** Chromosomal microarray

**C.** Cerebrospinal fluid (CSF) oligoclonal bands

**D.** Serum very-long-chain fatty acids

**E.** Spine MRI

**16-68.** In a child diagnosed with X-linked adrenoleukodystrophy (xALD), what is an important initial assessment?

**A.** Adrenocorticotropic hormone (ACTH) level

**B.** Vitamin $B_{12}$

**C.** Platelets

**D.** Erythrocyte sedimentation rate (ESR)

**E.** Bicarbonate

**16-69.** A 4-month-old girl presents with extreme irritability and developmental regression. On examination, there is diffusely increased tone. Cerebrospinal fluid (CSF) evaluation reveals increased protein. Magnetic resonance imaging (MRI) shows extensive T2 hyperintense lesions involving the brain stem and centrum semiovale and T2 hypointensity of the bilateral thalami. Which laboratory test is diagnostic of this disorder?

**A.** Undetectable galactocerebrosidase level

**B.** Elevated galactocerebrosidase level

**C.** Elevated very-long-chain fatty acids

**D.** Absence of arylsulfatase A activity

**E.** Duplication of *PLP1*

**16-70.** You see a 6-month-old infant with Pelizaeus-Merzbacher disease (PMD) in your office for routine checkup. Which statement about this disease is correct?

**A.** It has a mitochrondial inheritance pattern.

**B.** Typical clinical presentation occurs in boys and girls with equal frequency.

**C.** It is caused by mutations in *ATP7B* gene, which plays an important role in copper transportation and metabolism.

**D.** In the connatal and classic forms of PMD, nystagmus is one of the defining clinical features.

**E.** Surgical removal of the lesion after one year of age is curative in 95% of cases.

**16-71.** Lennox-Gastaut syndrome refers to the triad including which features?

**A.** Abnormal neuroimaging, abnormal development, abnormal electroencephalogram (EEG)

**B.** Abnormal cognition, microcephaly, abnormal EEG

**C.** Abnormal cognition, abnormal EEG, infantile spasms

**D.** Abnormal development, abnormal EEG, multiple seizure types

**E.** Abnormal neuroimaging, abnormal EEG, multiple seizure types

**16-72.** The ketogenic diet would be a reasonable option relatively early in the course of all of the following epilepsies except which one?

**A.** Dravet syndrome

**B.** Lennox-Gastaut syndrome

**C.** Doose syndrome

**D.** Benign rolandic epilepsy

**E.** Infantile spasms

**16-73.** A 17-year-old, otherwise healthy boy presents to the emergency department (ED) 1 hour after experiencing sudden-onset right face and arm weakness along with expressive and receptive aphasia as witnessed and reported by his mother. There were no preceding symptoms. His examination reveals right-sided hemiparesis and global aphasia. What is the first diagnosis to exclude?

**A.** Migraine

**B.** Conversion disorder

**C.** Seizure

**D.** Multiple sclerosis (MS)

**E.** Childhood stroke

**16-74.** A 5-year-old girl with acute bacterial meningitis is comatose in the intensive care unit with an intracranial pressure (ICP) monitor, which shows raised ICP. What measure would help lower the ICP acutely?

**A.** Administer mannitol

**B.** Change the dose of antibiotics

**C.** Hypoventilation

**D.** Perform a neuroimaging study

**E.** Put the patient in Trendelenburg position

**16-75.** A 2-month-old girl with developmental delay, new-onset infantile spasms, and chorioretinal lacunae received a brain magnetic resonance imaging (MRI). What is the most likely finding?

**A.** Normal

**B.** Hypoplastic cerebellum

**C.** Astrocytoma

**D.** Focal stroke

**E.** Absent corpus callosum, partial or complete

## ANSWERS

**Answer 16-1. B**

Idiopathic intracranial hypertension (IIH), previously known as pseudotumor cerebri, is characterized by elevated intracranial pressure (ICP) in the absence of any structural cause or CSF abnormality. The underlying cause is not well understood. Before puberty, girls and boys are equally likely to be affected. After puberty, there is a female predominance. Recent use of certain medications, including isotretinoin and minocycline (both often used for treatment of acne), has been associated with idiopathic intracranial hypertension. Being overweight is also associated, and weight loss is an important component of long-term management in overweight patients.

Elevated ICP should be suspected in a patient who complains of a headache that is worse when lying flat; the patient may describe this as worse when they lie down to go to sleep or that the headache is waking them up from sleep. A fundoscopic examination is essential to evaluate for papilledema, which is swelling of the optic nerve head due to increased pressure. However, early on, this finding can be absent. Neuroimaging, including venous imaging, is necessary to rule out other causes of elevated ICP such as an intracranial mass or venous sinus thrombosis. Following neuroimaging, lumbar puncture with measurement of opening pressure should be performed with the patient in the lateral decubitus position with the legs extended. IIH can be vision threatening, and close monitoring of visual function is needed.

Carbonic anhydrase inhibitors, such as acetazolamide, are first-line therapies because they decrease CSF production. Topiramate also has weak carbonic anhydrase inhibition. Propranolol and cyproheptadine are used as migraine preventives in children; ibuprofen and sumatriptan are acute therapies for migraine.

(p. 2672, Section 29: Disorders of the Nervous System, Chapter 546: Hydrocephalus and Pseudotumor Cerebri)

**Answer 16-2. C**

Primary headache disorders are relatively common in pediatrics. This child meets diagnostic criteria for migraine. Migraineurs may describe a pounding or pulsating quality to their head pain, and children may describe this as "booming" like their heartbeat; however, in pediatric patients, specific quality descriptors may be hard to elicit. Although there is a postpubertal preponderance for migraines in females, both sexes can be affected through life. Accompanying symptoms such as photophobia (light sensitivity) and phonophobia (sound sensitivity) and nausea or vomiting are characteristic of migraines. In this child, photophobia can be inferred from the child's behavior, such as pulling the covers over his head. There is usually a family history of migraine, although it is not uncommon for the family member to think it is "normal" to get frequent headaches. Interviewing family members directly about the features of their headaches can be helpful.

Tension-type headaches are not accompanied by migrainous features such as photophobia or nausea. Idiopathic intracranial hypertension is characterized by head pain that is worse when lying flat, whereas migraineurs typically prefer to lie down when they have severe headache. Cluster headache is a rare headache disorder that is characterized by unilateral headache associated with at least 1 cranial autonomic symptom (eg, ptosis, conjunctival injection, nasal congestion). All of the listed headache disorders may present with a normal physical and neurologic examination. Although headache can occur postictally, isolated ictal headache would be quite rare.

(p. 2706, Section 29: Disorders of the Nervous System, Chapter 557: Migraine and Headache Disorders)

**Answer 16-3.** C

Juvenile myoclonic epilepsy is a specific epilepsy syndrome typically presenting in adolescence and characterized by early morning myoclonic seizures and generalized tonic-clonic seizures, especially associated with sleep deprivation and alcohol use. In addition, patients may present with absence seizures. A characteristic electroencephalogram (EEG) pattern of generalized polyspike and wave with photoparoxysmal response (response to photic stimulation) has been described. Lifelong management with antiepileptic medications is required, mainly those with a broad-spectrum mechanism of action. Traditionally, valproic acid has been used as first-line treatment; however, the inherent risks for neural tube defects, in addition to the required monitoring for potential side effects (liver function testing and bone marrow suppression), make it a suboptimal medication for young females in childbearing age. Lamotrigine is a broad-spectrum antiepileptic with effect over glutamate and sodium channels and has been widely used in juvenile myoclonic epilepsy. Oxcarbazepine, a sodium channel inhibitor, is typically used for focal (partial) seizures and is not recommended as monotherapy in juvenile myoclonic epilepsy. Benzodiazepines, such as clonazepam and diazepam, may aid in the management of generalized and focal seizures; however, their effect duration, significant side effects, and potential for abuse make them undesirable as first-line therapy or monotherapy in juvenile myoclonic epilepsy.

(p. 2696, Section 29: Disorders of the Nervous System, Chapter 554: Epilepsy Treatment: Antiepileptic Drug Therapy)

**Answer 16-4.** A

Sumatriptan nasal spray has been well studied in children for the treatment of acute migraine in children as young as age 6. It is an appropriate choice in children who have severe head pain, particularly those who have difficulty taking oral medication due to nausea and vomiting. Triptans are migraine-specific therapies that treat head pain. Their use is also associated migraine symptoms such as photophobia, phonophobia, nausea, and vomiting. Her attack frequency is low enough that using sumatriptan would not be expected to lead to medication overuse headache.

Ibuprofen is an excellent first-line agent for many children with acute migraine. However, in this patient's case, she cannot tolerate it due to emesis. Ondansetron oral dissolving tablets could be used to treat the nausea but will have no impact on the headache. Oxygen therapy can be useful in cluster headache, another headache disorder, but is not a proven therapy for migraine. Amitriptyline is a preventive migraine agent and not useful in the acute setting.

(p. 2706, Section 29: Disorders of the Nervous System, Chapter 557: Migraine and Headache Disorders)

**Answer 16-5.** B

This is a classic presentation of a hyperammonemic neonate. Although neonatal hyperammonemia can be due to fatty acid oxidation disorders or disorders of amino acid metabolism, the most common cause is a urea cycle defect. There are 6 enzymes in the urea cycle, and a defect in any one of them can lead to hyperammonemia. A neonatal presentation in a male infant would be most suggestive of ornithine transcarbamylase (OTC) deficiency, the only enzyme that has an X-linked inheritance. Breastfed infants with OTC deficiency are asymptomatic until the mother's milk comes in, which is typically on day of life 3, particularly in a primiparous mother. Often the infants have already gone home before they become symptomatic. Although some urea cycle defects can be tested for with routine newborn screening, not all can be detected. Furthermore, results of newborn screening tests usually are not completed by the time infants with OTC deficiency present, requiring clinicians to have a high index of suspicion.

Ammonia levels are often elevated at presentation. Urgent diagnosis is critical because significant prolonged hyperammonemia leads to cerebral edema, neurologic damage, and, potentially, death. Hemodialysis should be rapidly initiated and ammonia-scavenging medications provided. The infant should be transferred to a center that is experienced in the management of inborn errors of metabolism. Hyperammonemia is often accompanied by a respiratory alkalosis. This can be detected via arterial blood gas; a venous sample will not be as helpful.

Methamphetamine or cocaine ingestion, via mother's milk, would only cause an acute encephalopathy by causing an intracranial bleed, and hemorrhage was ruled out by imaging. Hypoglycemia and hyponatremia would not cause tachypnea, and although cerebral edema can result from hyponatremia, breastfed infants are at lower risk for this than formula-fed infants because formula can be prepared incorrectly.

(p. 642, Section 11: Inherited Disorders of Metabolism, Chapter 141: Urea Cycle Disorders)

**Answer 16-6.** B

Focal motor seizures in a neonate are often due to arterial ischemic stroke. Perinatal stroke is significantly more common than previously appreciated. It is usually not possible to pinpoint the exact timing of stroke onset, but it is generally thought to be at or near the time of birth. Neonates do not typically present with a hemiparesis after an ischemic stroke, as an older child or an adult would. Instead, recurrent focal motor seizures in day 1 or 2 of life are the most typical presentation. Some infants with perinatal stroke will be asymptomatic in the nursery and then present later in infancy (~6–9 months) with an early hand preference (eg, being left-handed or right-handed). Head ultrasound is significantly more sensitive for intracerebral hemorrhage than for ischemic stroke; magnetic resonance imaging (MRI) is preferred for evaluating for ischemic stroke.

(p. 2668, Section 29: Disorders of the Nervous System, Chapter 545: Stroke in Neonates and Children)

**Answer 16-7.** C

This child has a congenital myopathy. There are several different forms of congenital myopathies, each with a different pathologic change in muscle on histology. Typical clinical features include feeding or respiratory difficulty in the neonatal period and a high-arched palate at birth. However, the diagnosis may not be made until the child presents with delayed motor milestones. Neurologic examination findings that suggest a muscle localization include diminished bulk, hypotonia, and proximal greater than distal weakness. Upper motor neuron injury presents with hypertonia (spasticity), hyperreflexia, and distal greater than proximal weakness. Weakness in neuromuscular junction disease is fluctuating and fatigable. The bulbar musculature is not commonly involved in peripheral nerve disease. More typical features would be sensory abnormalities and diminished or absent reflexes (depending on severity). Lower motor neuron disease that presents in the neonatal period would be spinal muscular atrophy, which is typically progressive and entirely spares the cranial nerves.

(p. 2728, Section 29: Disorders of the Nervous System, Chapter 563: Myopathies)

**Answer 16-8.** A

This infant has GM1 gangliosidosis, an inborn error of metabolism due to β-galactosidase deficiency. Buildup of GM1 ganglioside in neurons leads to progressive neurologic dysfunction, and buildup of metabolites in the bone, liver, and soft tissues of the face leads to bony malformations, organomegaly, and coarsened facial features. Metabolites also build up in the retina nerve fiber layer; however, the macula is spared because the nerve fiber layer is thinned in this region. This leads to the macula appearing as a bright "cherry-red spot" compared with the surrounding retina. Optic nerve hypoplasia is a congenital anomaly that can be seen in other neurodevelopmental disorders, for example, septo-optic dysplasia, but would not have the other systemic features observed. Congenital cataracts are seen in certain metabolic and genetic disorders such as trisomy 21. They are important to diagnose early, as there is a critical period to early vision development. Uveitis is seen in inflammatory autoimmune disorders such as multiple sclerosis.

(p. 693, Section 11: Inherited Disorders of Metabolism, Chapter 155: Mucopolysaccharidosis, Glycoproteinosis, and Mucolipidosis)

**Answer 16-9.** C

This child suffers from a cluster headache, a primary headache disorder. Cluster headache pain is severe in intensity, lateralized, and associated with at least 1 cranial autonomic symptom. Examples of cranial autonomic symptoms include conjunctival injection, lacrimation, periorbital edema, and nasal congestion or rhinorrhea. The cranial autonomic symptoms lateralize to the side of the headache. High-flow oxygen via non-rebreather mask for 20 minutes is an effective acute therapy in some patients. Both prochlorperazine (a dopamine receptor antagonist) and ketorolac (a nonsteroidal anti-inflammatory drug) are used in the acute treatment of migraine in children in the ED setting, with prochlorperazine being superior. Topiramate is a migraine preventive medication. Sodium valproate is also a preventive migraine medication, although there are several small studies suggesting some efficacy of an IV load of sodium valproate in the treatment of acute migraine.

(p. 2706, Section 29: Disorders of the Nervous System, Chapter 557: Migraine and Headache Disorders)

**Answer 16-10.** D

This baby has brachial plexus injury, most likely due to birth injury. Shoulder dystocia and macrosomia are risk factors for brachial plexus injury. In this infant, the accompanying Horner syndrome helps with the localization as the sympathetic chain runs close to the brachial plexus and its involvement signals this is a severe, proximal injury that will not spontaneously recover. Physical findings of Horner syndrome include ptosis (drooping of eyelid) and miosis (smaller pupil). The pupillary asymmetry is most easily appreciated in a darkened room as the other pupil will dilate. Anhidrosis, or decreased facial sweating on that side, can be part of Horner syndrome but is difficult to appreciate in a neonate. Infants with severe brachial plexus injury at birth should be referred for evaluation for possible surgical reconstruction of the plexus within the first few months of life. Neonates with stroke do not present with a hemiparesis at birth. Focal seizures of the affected arm are concerning for perinatal stroke, but not brachial plexus injury, and may have an associated postictal paralysis (Todd paralysis, which is not moving the limb following focal seizure). Leg weakness is also more concerning for a cortical process, not a brachial plexus injury that innervated the upper extremities. Difficulty feeding or disconjugate gaze may signal abnormalities elsewhere in the brain stem, not the brachial plexus, although a disconjugate gaze may be normal in infancy.

(p. 2718, Section 29: Disorders of the Nervous System, Chapter 561: Peripheral Nerve Disorders and Anterior Horn Cell Diseases)

**Answer 16-11.** B

Acute-onset severe headache is concerning for aneurysmal subarachnoid hemorrhage. Although CT scan is generally highly sensitive for acute intracranial blood, a small bleed can be missed, particularly if several hours have passed since headache onset. When subarachnoid hemorrhage is suspected (acute onset of the worst headache plus neck stiffness), a negative CT scan should be followed up by a lumbar puncture to evaluate for xanthochromia in cerebrospinal fluid (CSF). Xanthochromia is the pigment seen after blood has begun to break down; its presence distinguishes a subarachnoid hemorrhage from a traumatic lumbar puncture. In this patient, his neck stiffness suggests meningeal irritation, which can be from subarachnoid blood. Although a CT scan is not as sensitive as MRI for ischemic stroke, isolated acute headache with no other neurologic symptoms or examination findings would be unusual for stroke. Similarly, isolated, severe, ongoing headache is not suggestive of seizure. An afebrile patient with normal mental status would be relatively unlikely to have an infectious meningitis; however, lumbar puncture should be performed if there is a clinical suspicion for central nervous system (CNS) infection. A benign headache disorder, such as migraine, is a diagnosis of exclusion and should not be made until the evaluation for secondary causes of headache has been completed.

(p. 2668, Section 29: Disorders of the Nervous System, Chapter 545: Stroke in Neonates and Children)

**Answer 16-12.** D

Abnormal movements are not an uncommon phenomenon in this age group, but understanding of the potential etiology is very important. Motor and vocal tics commonly present in this age group, and boys are more likely to be affected. However, patients with tics describe being able to suppress the movements for a few minutes, but the urge to perform them mounts, and when they do them, they typically feel a sense of relief; none of these are described by the patient in the vignette. Tic disorders are generally benign and may require no treatment whatsoever.

This foreign-born patient presents with worsening symptoms of severe, erratic movements affecting face and neck and, ultimately, ambulation. The movements do not impair consciousness and disappear at night. This is highly suggestive of chorea. The most frequent type of chorea in developing countries is Sydenham chorea (SC), which constitutes one of the Jones major criteria for acute rheumatic fever. SC may present months after acute streptococcal infection, which explains why the patient does not recall any preceding illness. Treatment is supportive, but further workup for acute rheumatic fever may require immunologic, cardiologic, and renal evaluations, including erythrocyte sedimentation rate (ESR)/C-reactive protein (CRP), antistreptolysin O titers, electrocardiogram (ECG), and echocardiogram. The fact that there is no impairment of consciousness and no postictal state makes these episodes unlikely to be seizures. Low ceruloplasmin levels can help to diagnose Wilson disease, an inherited condition of copper accumulation that often manifests as a movement disorder. However, the abnormal movements are usually dystonia or chorea rather than tics. There are also neuropsychiatric symptoms that frequently accompany the movement disorder. Examination of cerebrospinal fluid (CSF) would be indicated if there was a question of an inflammatory etiology for a movement disorder, for example, anti-*N* -methyl-D-aspartate (NMDA) receptor encephalitis. However, these patients characteristically have abnormal mental status and sometimes seizures and cardiovascular instability.

(p. 2709, Section 29: Disorders of the Nervous System, Chapter 558: Pediatric Movement Disorders)

**Answer 16-13.** A

Prochlorperazine (Compazine) is a commonly used acute migraine therapy in children in the ED setting. It is a dopamine receptor antagonist and therefore can cause movement-related side effects, most commonly dystonic reactions or akathisia (a sense of needing to move). Diphenhydramine is typically effective in relieving this side effect. Observation is an option; however, the dystonic reaction is typically uncomfortable and so treatment is generally preferred. Chlorpromazine is another dopamine receptor antagonist used to treat migraine and would be expected to worsen the dystonic reaction. Acetaminophen may help with discomfort but would not treat the underlying abnormality. Phenytoin is a seizure medication and would not be expected to have an effect.

(p. 500, Section 8: Acute and Critical Illness, Chapter 114: Toxic Ingestions and Exposures)

**Answer 16-14.** C

This child has a Bell palsy. This results from an abnormality of the seventh cranial nerve on the affected side. Many cases are idiopathic, although some cases are associated with infections such as Lyme disease or herpes simplex virus. Early treatment (within 72 hours of onset) with corticosteroids improves recovery. Some patients with Bell palsy experience hyperacusis due to weakness of the stapedius muscle, an inner ear muscle that is innervated by the seventh nerve and responsible for dampening sound intensity. The seventh nerve also provides taste sensation to the anterior two-thirds of the tongue; hence, many patients with Bell palsy report abnormal taste on the affected side. The seventh nerve also innervates the forehead; therefore, involvement of the forehead denotes a lower motor neuron (peripheral) cause of facial weakness; facial weakness from a central cause (eg, a stroke affecting cortical function) would spare the forehead because there is bilateral cortical innervation to the forehead. The seventh nerve is in the pons, which is below the midbrain in the brain stem. A lesion of the eighth cranial nerve would be expected to cause diminished hearing.

(p. 2718, Section 29: Disorders of the Nervous System, Chapter 561: Peripheral Nerve Disorders and Anterior Horn Cell Diseases)

**Answer 16-15.** C

This young athlete has suffered a concussion, sometimes referred to as mild traumatic brain injury. The majority of concussions are not associated with loss of consciousness. Typically, postconcussive symptoms take 7 to 10 days to resolve, although more recent evidence shows children with concussion take longer to recover (1 month on average). Both cognitive and physical rest are recommended while recovering from a concussion. However, cognitive rest does not mean a child should not return to school until all symptoms resolve. After a few days of rest, the child should return to school with concussion-related accommodations (see the American Academy of Pediatrics "Returning to Learn" guidelines). Athletics, and any contact activities, should remain on hold until symptoms resolve, although the child may participate in daily activities and noncontact activities as tolerated as recovery progresses. Returning to contact play before he has fully recovered (although most often within the first week of injury) puts him at risk for second-impact syndrome, a potentially fatal consequence that can result from suffering a second concussion before the first has resolved. Although ibuprofen or other medications may help his headache, he should not return to athletics until he is symptom free without medications.

(p. 2664, Section 29: Disorders of the Nervous System, Chapter 544: Trauma to the Nervous System)

**Answer 16-16.** B

The clinical story is concerning for nonaccidental head trauma or abusive head trauma. Two-month-old infants do not have the gross motor control to roll over; hence, the parents' story is questionable. Additionally, evidence does not support significant brain injury following a fall from a couch or bed. A skeletal survey to look for bone fractures is indicated, as is an ophthalmologic examination to look for retinal hemorrhages. The seizure was likely provoked by trauma and intracranial blood; hence, immediate intracranial investigation should include tomography (head CT), which quickly evaluates for blood and bone fractures and may help detect late acute to chronic injury. Any findings could warrant immediate neurosurgical intervention. Brain magnetic resonance imaging (MRI) and magnetic resonance venography are likely to be needed as part of the ongoing evaluation, but head CT should be performed emergently for evaluation of bleeding and fracture. A trauma panel looking for other organ injury is also a part of the evaluation. A hearing test is not a part of the standard initial evaluation for abusive head trauma, although hearing testing may be needed prior to discharge depending on the injury severity and clinical symptoms. Assessment of pre- and post-ductal saturations is an screening test for newborn infants in the nursery that is used to screen for critical congenital heart defects (CCHD). It is not part of the standard evaluation for abusive head trauma.

(p. 2664, Section 29: Disorders of the Nervous System, Chapter 544: Trauma to the Nervous System)

**Answer 16-17.** C

This infant suffered hypoxic-ischemic injury. He was appropriately treated with therapeutic hypothermia, and his acute symptomatic seizures were appropriately managed. Although he is at risk for epilepsy, he does not yet meet criteria for diagnosis of epilepsy (as his seizures were provoked in the setting of hypoxic-ischemic encephalopathy). This infant's neurologic examination, EEG background, and brain MRI suggest moderate brain injury. Certainly, normal development cannot be assured; however, it would be equally inappropriate to suggest to the family that the child's developmental prospects are dire. He is at risk for both motor and cognitive disabilities and will need close neurodevelopmental monitoring during early childhood, with early referral for therapies if developmental concerns arise. Elective cesarean section does not eliminate the risk of birth asphyxia and carries higher risks of maternal morbidity and mortality than vaginal delivery.

(p. 2672, Section 29: Disorders of the Nervous System, Chapter 547: Cerebral Palsy and Static Encephalopathies)

**Answer 16-18.** C

Central nervous system (CNS) damage can lead to an imbalance between the afferent excitatory and descending inhibitory pathways, which is associated with muscle hypertonia and involves γ-aminobutyric acid (GABA). Baclofen can be useful in the treatment of spasticity. It is a derivative of GABA and an agonist for GABA receptors. It can be given orally or, in more severe cases, through a continuous intrathecal pump. Some degree of spasticity can actually be helpful in some individuals in making transfers easier or helping with ambulation, so treating spasticity is an individualized decision that often depends on factors such as discomfort or the inability to participate fully in therapies. Benzodiazepines such as clonazepam and diazepam can be used as first- or second-line treatment in tone disturbances associated with brain injury, with or without concomitant use of baclofen; in addition, they may provide some benefit in epilepsy control, if present. Phenobarbital is an antiepileptic and may indirectly mildly lower tone; however, it is not typically used for that purpose and side effects, including cognitive changes, are a concern in vulnerable populations. Botulinum toxin is a commonly used therapy for focal management of tone disturbances and is injected directly to the affected muscle, typically over 3 to 4 months.

(p. 2672, Section 29: Disorders of the Nervous System, Chapter 547: Cerebral Palsy and Static Encephalopathies)

**Answer 16-19.** C

Acute cerebellar ataxia is an infectious or postinfectious process that typically affects preschool-aged children. The course of the illness is typically monophasic. For those in the postinfectious category, there is often a history of a recent febrile or gastrointestinal illness. The MRI may be unremarkable or may show cerebellar edema. It is important to rule out more serious causes of new ataxia in young children, such as a posterior fossa mass or a cerebellar hemorrhage, with brain MRI. However, most children with cerebellar hemorrhage are not well appearing, and the onset of ataxia is quite acute. Ataxia from a posterior fossa mass is usually more insidious in onset, unless there has been bleeding into the mass. Hydrocephalus can cause gait disturbance; however, it would not explain the nystagmus or limb ataxia. Midbrain cerebrovascular accidents typically display a myriad of symptoms beyond ataxia, including cranial nerve compromise and other sensorimotor changes.

(p. 1088, Section 17: Infectious Diseases, Chapter 227: Viral Infections of the Central Nervous System)

**Answer 16-20.** B

This clinical situation is concerning for bacterial meningitis. His neurologic examination suggests elevated intracranial pressure (ICP) given his lethargy and slowly reactive pupils. When there is concern for high ICP, a CT scan should be performed before performing a lumbar puncture as there is the potential to precipitate herniation through the foramen magnum. If necessary, lumbar puncture can be put off even longer until the patient is stable. However, empiric antibiotic coverage at meningitic doses should be started without delay. Concerns about being able to identify the specific organism do not justify a delay in treatment. It may still be possible to identify the infectious organism through blood or urine culture, and if necessary, an empiric course of antibiotics can be completed based on the most likely etiologic agents.

(p. 1077, Section 17: Infectious Diseases, Chapter 226: Bacterial Infections of the Central Nervous System)

**Answer 16-21.** C

All of these medications can be used for migraine prevention. Some of the more frequent side effects of topiramate are cognitive slowing and word-finding difficulties. Propranolol can decrease exercise tolerance. Valproate is a known teratogenic, particularly in relation to neural tube defects. Additionally, it can cause weight gain, hepatic damage, and bone marrow suppression, warranting laboratory monitoring with long-term use. Amitriptyline can cause fatigue and dry mouth. Gabapentin can also cause fatigue.

(p. 2706, Section 29: Disorders of the Nervous System, Chapter 557: Migraine and Headache Disorders)

**Answer 16-22.** B

This girl has an optic neuritis, a disorder of the optic nerve that can be inflammatory or infectious in etiology. Typical symptoms include diminished visual acuity, red desaturation, and sometimes pain with eye movement. Optic neuritis may be an isolated condition or may be an initial presentation of a pediatric demyelinating disorder. Children < 10 years of age are more likely to present with bilateral optic neuritis, whereas older children are more likely to present with unilateral disease. The retina is not involved in optic neuritis. The optic nerve is anterior to the optic chiasm, where inputs from both eyes cross, so all visual information in the optic nerve is coming from a single eye. Once the optic chiasm is reached, visual information is crossing, so manifestations will be apparent in both eyes. This holds true for the lateral geniculate nucleus in the thalamus and the visual cortex as well.

(p. 2676, Section 29: Disorders of the Nervous System, Chapter 548: Immune- and Inflammatory-Mediated Central Nervous System Disorders)

**Answer 16-23.** D

This child has opsoclonus-myoclonus-ataxia syndrome. About half of children with this condition have a detectable neuroblastoma, so a chest radiograph (CXR), abdominal ultrasound, and urine vanillylmandelic and homovanillic acid should be promptly performed. These studies are typically followed by magnetic resonance imaging (MRI) of chest, abdomen, and pelvis and then a metaiodobenzylguanidine (MIBG) scan, which is used to assess for metastases. Not all patients with opsoclonus-myoclonus-ataxia syndrome will have all 3 of these neurologic symptoms, and it is possible for 1 symptom to precede the others. Ovarian teratomas can be associated with the *N*-methyl-D-aspartate (NMDA) receptor antibody syndrome, most often in adolescents and adults, which is typically characterized by seizures, autonomic instability, and mental status or behavioral changes. Limbic encephalitis also typically presents with seizures and behavioral or mental status changes. GLUT-1 deficiency often presents in infancy with seizures, global developmental delays, spasticity and/or dystonia, and acquired microcephaly but may also have associated abnormal eye movements and ataxia. The overall clinical presentation of this patient (lacking developmental delays, seizures, or movement disorder) is more consistent with opsoclonus-myoclonus-ataxia syndrome rather than GLUT-1 deficiency. Arterial ischemic infarcts (strokes) are rare in children. Cerebellar strokes are also rare and present with a variety of cerebellar signs, which may include ataxia and abnormal eye movements. However, strokes typically present abruptly without progression of deficits and do not have opsoclonus eye movements; therefore, this patient does not need urgent head computed tomography (CT)/CT angiography or stroke protocol MRI.

(p. 2676, Section 29: Disorders of the Nervous System, Chapter 548: Immune- and Inflammatory-Mediated Central Nervous System Disorders)

**Answer 16-24.** B

This infant has septo-optic dysplasia (also known as de Morsier syndrome), a condition characterized by optic nerve hypoplasia, absence of the septum pellucidum or dysgenesis of corpus callosum or other cortical malformations, and abnormalities of the hypothalamic-pituitary axis with resultant endocrine dysfunction; however, only approximately 40% of children with septo-optic dysplasia have all 3 features. In most cases, there is no etiology found, although there are now 3 known genes associated with septo-optic dysplasia. Symptoms of septo-optic dysplasia are variable and related to the involved structures. Optic nerve hypoplasia results in poor vision and nystagmus. Neurodevelopmental delays (ranging from mild to severe) are common in children with septo-optic dysplasia. Hypothalamic-pituitary dysfunction presents most often in children < 2 years of age, with central hypothyroidism and growth hormone deficiency being most common, followed by adrenal insufficiency and diabetes insipidus.

Hypothalamic hamartoma is a nonprogressive malformation that may present with 2 distinct phenotypes: (1) central precocious puberty and (2) epilepsy (including the classic gelastic seizures) with neurodevelopmental delays or deterioration and neurobehavioral symptoms. Optic nerve hypoplasia is not associated with hypothalamic hamartomas. The corpus callosum is the white matter tract that connects the 2 hemispheres of the brain. Agenesis of the corpus callosum is the result of abnormal prosencephalic development and can be acquired (intrauterine infections, fetal alcohol exposure) or genetic (autosomal recessive, X-linked, Aicardi syndrome). Although dysgenesis of the corpus callosum may be seen in septo-optic dysplasia, agenesis of the corpus callosum is not the classic finding, and other forms of agenesis of the corpus callosum are not typically associated with optic nerve hypoplasia or endocrine abnormalities. Stenosis of the cerebral aqueduct can be seen in X-linked hydrocephalus and is often diagnosed in utero. Common associated symptoms include seizures, global developmental delays, and spasticity. There are several types of cerebellar-pontine hypoplasia. Infants often have abnormalities of tone or movements, visual impairment, seizures, and global developmental delay. An infant with hypoxic-ischemic injury would have had complications reflecting encephalopathy following birth. Furthermore, visual impairment and pituitary dysfunction are not the expected or most common symptoms of hypoxic-ischemic injury.

(p. 2655, Section 29: Disorders of the Nervous System, Chapter 541: Cranial Developmental Abnormalities)

**Answer 16-25.** A

Children with NF1 are at increased risk for optic pathway gliomas; therefore, annual ophthalmologic screening examinations are recommended for children 10 years of age or younger.

Screening neuroimaging is not recommended and should only be done to evaluate neurologic symptoms including persistent headaches, visual changes, seizures, or rapid increase in head size. Vestibular schwannomas are associated with NF2, not NF1. Patients with NF1 should have blood pressure checked annually because they are at risk for hypertension; however, annual cardiac echocardiography in the absence of symptoms is not necessary. Although revisiting the skin examination annually in a patient with known or suspected NF1 may help satisfy diagnostic criteria and track the number of neurofibromas, a Wood's lamp examination is not necessary. Wood's lamp examination is useful in detecting the hypopigmented lesions sometimes seen in tuberous sclerosis, so-called ash leaf macules, which can be difficult to see in light-skinned individuals.

(p. 836, Section 12: Clinical Genetics and Dysmorphology, Chapter 176: Neurocutaneous Disorders)

**Answer 16-26.** E

This child's history is characteristic for breath-holding spells. Typically, breath-holding spells occur in young children and are an involuntary reflex response triggered by being frightened or upset. The child will cry and then hold their breath in expiration and turn either pale or cyanotic. Loss of consciousness is possible, and convulsive movements are relatively common. Electroencephalogram (EEG) during the spell shows no electrographic seizure. Children with epilepsy typically do not have a reliable trigger for their seizures, except in the rare case of reflex epilepsies. Although it is important to have a low index of suspicion for child abuse, nothing about this child's story is developmentally or medically inconsistent or concerning for abuse. Reflux can cause crying or accompany crying but does not typically lead to loss of consciousness. A cardiac arrhythmia is possible, for example, due to long QT syndrome; however, the age of the patient and the clinical presentation are quite classic for breath-holding spells. Prolonged QTc in children often presents in older children with syncope, seizures, or cardiac arrest often preceded by exercise or other exertion.

(p. 2750, Section 29: Disorders of the Nervous System, Chapter 568: Autonomic Dysfunction)

**Answer 16-27.** C

Benign paroxysmal torticollis of infancy is an episodic disorder characterized by bouts of torticollis that can last from minutes to hours or even several days. Episodes are often accompanied by emesis, pallor, and ataxia. Onset occurs within the first year of life with resolution by 5 years of age. In between bouts, children are completely normal. Although based on small cohorts in the literature, benign paroxysmal torticollis of infancy is reported as a migraine variant as some children go on to develop vertigo and then vestibular migraine. Many of these infants also have a family history of migraine. There is no known association with mood disorders, seizures, or breath-holding spells.

(p. 2711, Section 29: Disorders of the Nervous System, Chapter 558: Pediatric Movement Disorders)

**Answer 16-28.** C

This girl has myasthenia gravis, an autoimmune disorder with antibodies affecting the postsynaptic membrane of the neuromuscular junction, most often the nicotinic acetylcholine receptor in adolescents and adults (note: prepubertal patients are more likely to be seronegative or have other postsynaptic membrane antibodies). Diurnal variation is common, with patients feeling relatively well in the morning but becoming more symptomatic as the day goes on. Rest can often improve symptoms. Exercise and sustained muscle use precipitates the weakness, which is why prolonged upgaze is a useful clinical measure when there is concern for myasthenia gravis. Predominance of ocular and bulbar symptoms is common in myasthenia gravis. Weakness from a muscle cause typically does not have such marked diurnal fluctuation. There are no sensory symptoms to suggest sensory nerve involvement, and motor involvement at the nerve level is not fluctuating. Symptoms from a pontine lesion would typically be persistent and would not be associated with her more diffuse muscular weakness that worsens throughout the day. Additionally, the nucleus for innervation of the levator palpebrae muscle is in the midbrain, not the pons. Ocular and bulbar symptoms exclude a spinal cord localization.

(p. 2723, Section 29: Disorders of the Nervous System, Chapter 562: Diseases of the Neuromuscular Junction)

**Answer 16-29.** B

This baby's presentation is consistent with Menkes disease, a lethal neurodegenerative disorder of copper transport due to mutation in the X-linked *ATP7A* gene that results in copper deficiency and dysfunction of copper-dependent enzymes. As an X-linked disorder, Menkes predominantly affects males. Infants present within the first few weeks or months of life with systemic signs and evidence of neurologic dysfunction including hypotonia, developmental regression, and seizures. Connective tissue dysfunction leads to lax ("sagging") skin, and the hair is typically twisted ("kinky") and lightly pigmented ("silvery"). Bones and blood vessels are also affected. Phenylketonuria is detected on the newborn screening tests in all states. Biotinidase deficiency also has neurologic, skin, and hair findings. In biotinidase deficiency, infants have hypotonia, seizures, developmental delay with vision and hearing loss, and a more diffuse "eczematous" rash and alopecia. Many urea cycle defects present in early infancy but do not have the associated skin and hair findings observed in this child. GM1 gangliosidosis is a neurodegenerative storage disease, and the infantile form typically presents within 6 months with developmental regression and an exaggerated startle. The progression of GM1 gangliosidoses includes coarsened facial features, seizures, hepatosplenomegaly, cardiomyopathy, visual loss with corneal clouding, and a cherry red spot noted on retinal exam.

(p. 766, Section 11: Inherited Disorders of Metabolism, Chapter 164: Disorders of Metal Metabolism)

**Answer 16-30.** A

Fabry disease is an X-linked lysosomal disorder that results in accumulation of glycosphingolipids throughout the body. It is caused by a deficiency of the enzyme α-galactosidase A. The incidence is estimated to be 1 in 55,000 male births. It is probably underdiagnosed because individuals with milder phenotypes may go undiagnosed. Patients may also complain of numbness and paresthesias of the hands and feet (acroparesthesia). Another classic manifestation of the disease is bouts of painful crises that often involve burning or lancinating (eg, cutting or piercing) pains that originate in the hands and feet. Carbamazepine and gabapentin can be useful therapeutically as neuropathic pain management. Children with Fabry disease may also have associated gastrointestinal dysfunction, angiokeratomas, and corneal dystrophy. Renal and cardiac involvement typically occurs in adolescence or adulthood. Baclofen is a treatment for spasticity. Propranolol is used as an antihypertensive or migraine preventive. Diphenhydramine is an antihistamine useful in treating dystonic reactions that sometimes arise from use of dopamine receptor antagonists such as prochlorperazine, but neither medication is used as treatment in Fabry disease.

(p. 2733, Section 29: Disorders of the Nervous System, Chapter 564: Batten Diseases and Lipidoses)

**Answer 16-31.** B

The cerebral form of X-linked adrenoleukodystrophy is a degenerative disorder secondary to a mutation in the *ABCD1* gene on the X chromosome, leading to impaired peroxisomal β-oxidation of very-long-chain fatty acids. The childhood cerebral X-linked adrenoleukodystrophy is the most severe and rapidly progressive form and presents between 4 and 10 years of age. New behavioral disturbances, often concerning for ADHD, are often the first symptom. However, other symptoms such as visual impairment, difficulty understanding language, seizures, and spasticity then follow. Brain MRI most typically shows white matter changes in the parieto-occipital cortex involving the visual cortex. The condition is caused by a mutation in the gene that codes for the adrenoleukodystrophy protein, which plays a role in β-oxidation of very-long-chain fatty acids. Disruption in this protein's function leads to accumulation of very-long-chain fatty acids. Aicardi-Goutières syndrome is a leukoencephalopathy that presents in infancy with global developmental delay or developmental regression, hepatosplenomegaly and thrombocytopenia, sterile pyrexia, irritability, and eventually chilblain skin lesions. Neuronal ceroid lipofuscinosis is a group of disorders characterized by neuronal dysfunction due to accumulation of autofluorescent material in the lysosomes. The juvenile form can present at a similar age and is also characterized by visual and behavioral problems; however, there is no male predominance, and the typical imaging and lab findings are different. Juvenile-onset Alexander disease is another leukoencephalopathy that can present in this age group; however, the presenting symptoms are spasticity and bulbar dysfunction, and the MRI findings typically have a frontal predominance to the white matter changes.

(p. 2736, Section 29: Disorders of the Nervous System, Chapter 566: Leukodystrophies)

**Answer 16-32.** D

Sturge-Weber syndrome is caused by a mutation in the *GNAQ* gene that affects the development of certain areas of blood vessels, skin, and brain. Sturge-Weber is characterized by a port-wine stain skin lesion, leptomeningeal angioma, and seizures. Glaucoma is common, and diffuse choroid hemangioma can lead to visual loss. Migraines and hemiparesis may develop as well. The port-wine stain is usually unilateral and most often involves the first (ophthalmic) division of the trigeminal nerve (along the forehead, around the eye and nasal bridge), although lower divisions can also be involved (Figure 359-11).

The seventh cranial nerve, the facial nerve, innervates the muscles of facial expression. The forehead receives bilateral innervation and so an upper motor neuron lesion, such as a stroke, will result in unilateral facial weakness that spares the forehead. Lower motor neuron facial weakness, such as that from a Bell palsy, involves the forehead. The greater occipital nerves provide sensation over the back of the head, with innervation from the upper cervical cord.

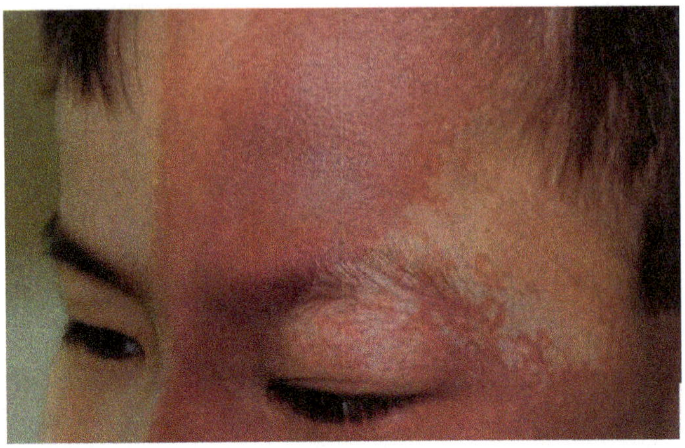

**FIGURE 359-11.** Child with a capillary malformation in the V1 distribution and associated with Sturge-Weber syndrome. (Mark W. Kline, *Rudolph's Pediatrics*, 23rd Edition. Copyright © McGraw-Hill Education. All rights reserved.)

(p. 2743, Section 29: Disorders of the Nervous System, Chapter 567: Neurocutaneous Disorders)

**Answer 16-33.** C

Glycine encephalopathy (nonketotic hyperglycinemia) classically presents in the neonatal period with apnea and difficult-to-control seizures in an encephalopathic (lethargic), hypotonic infant. Some infants will have experienced seizures in utero, which the mother may report as frequent "hiccups." A high cerebrospinal fluid (CSF) to plasma glycine ratio, and therefore lumbar puncture with measurement of serum and CSF glycine (obtained in serum and CSF amino acids), is essential in making the diagnosis. A glycine peak may be seen on magnetic resonance spectroscopy, but brain imaging is not the primary diagnostic tool. EEG will show frequent seizures and often a burst suppression pattern but will not be specific to etiology. EMG is used to evaluate for peripheral nerve, neuromuscular junction, or muscle pathology (which are not affected in glycine encephalopathy). Neonates who have experienced hypoxic-ischemic brain injury at birth may suffer seizures and benefit from therapeutic hypothermia; however, this infant had an uncomplicated delivery with good Apgar scores; furthermore, the apnea and in utero hiccups are classic for glycine encephalopathy and not hypoxic-ischemic injury.

(p. 622, Section 11: Inherited Disorders of Metabolism, Chapter 134: Disorders of Glycine Metabolism)

**Answer 16-34.** E

This patient's clinical picture is concerning for increased intracranial pressure (ICP) given that his headaches wake him from sleep and he has a left sixth nerve palsy (presenting as diplopia). In addition, he has nystagmus and ataxia, which suggest a cerebellar localization. He may have papilledema, but it can be difficult to get a good funduscopic examination in young children. Taken together, this clinical situation is concerning for a posterior fossa mass. Children with a primary headache disorder such as migraine or tension-type headache should have a normal neurologic examination. Idiopathic intracranial hypertension is rare in this age group and does not have cerebellar examination findings. Cerebral aneurysms typically do not cause pain unless they rupture and cause subarachnoid hemorrhage with acute onset of severe ("thunderclap-onset") headache.

(p. 2651, Section 29: Disorders of the Nervous System, Chapter 540: Clinical Approach to Neurologic Disease)

**Answer 16-35.** D

Neurologic complications of Lyme disease include cranial nerve palsies and meningitis. The facial nerve is most likely to be affected, and Lyme disease is an important consideration in evaluating a child with a Bell palsy. In idiopathic Bell palsy, early treatment (within 72 hours of onset) with corticosteroids improves recovery, but for Lyme disease facial nerve palsy, antibiotics are the primary treatment (and steroid use may be associated with worse outcome in Lyme disease facial palsy). Some patients with facial nerve palsy experience hyperacusis due to weakness of the stapedius muscle, an inner ear muscle that is innervated by the seventh nerve and responsible for dampening sound intensity. The seventh nerve also provides taste sensation to the anterior two-thirds of the tongue; hence, many patients report abnormal taste on the affected side.

(p. 1227, Section 17: Infectious Diseases, Chapter 262: Lyme Disease)

**Answer 16-36.** E

This girl's events are suspicious for psychogenic nonepileptic seizures, a form of conversion disorder. The asynchronous jerking of the limbs and pelvic thrusting are common manifestations of psychogenic nonepileptic seizures. However, many patients with nonepileptic seizures also have epilepsy, so an admission for video EEG monitoring to capture events is essential in clarifying the diagnosis. Starting a medication typically should be delayed until the diagnosis is clear, particularly as the goal of the admission is to record events. If the diagnosis is ultimately shown to be psychogenic nonepileptic seizures, then referral for behavioral therapy or counseling would be recommended. Physical therapy is not indicated, and an EMG is not appropriate in this patient, in whom there is no concern for a muscular or neuropathic process.

(p. 2709, Section 29: Disorders of the Nervous System, Chapter 558: Pediatric Movement Disorders)

**Answer 16-37.** B

Bowel or bladder symptoms, along with lower extremity weakness, point to the spinal cord as the localization. His clinical picture is that of a transverse myelitis, for which there are a number of infectious and inflammatory etiologies. Hydrocephalus can cause bladder and gait dysfunction; however, with rapid onset of hydrocephalus over just a few hours, he would have more diffuse or additional symptoms such as impaired mental status and visual changes. Therefore, brain is an unlikely etiology. Absence of cranial nerve involvement rules out a brain stem localization. Neuromuscular junction pathology usually causes fluctuating weakness without bowel or bladder symptoms. Similarly, muscle diseases, such as muscular dystrophy, do not have bowel or bladder symptoms.

(p. 2676, Section 29: Disorders of the Nervous System, Chapter 548: Immune- and Inflammatory-Mediated Central Nervous System Syndromes)

**Answer 16-38.** B

Multiple loading doses of phenobarbital can sometimes be required to control neonatal seizures. Respiratory suppression is common, and infants may need respiratory support, particularly with escalating phenobarbital levels. Phenobarbital-induced electrolyte disturbances are not expected. Allergic reactions are rare. Hypotension is more likely than hypertension. Dystonic reactions are associated with dopamine receptor antagonists, not barbiturates.

(p. 2696, Section 29: Disorders of the Nervous System, Chapter 554: Epilepsy Treatment: Antiepileptic Drug Therapy)

**Answer 16-39.** D

Several studies have shown that the factors associated with a complex febrile seizure are risk factors for subsequent epilepsy after a first febrile seizure. These factors include a focal seizure, prolonged seizure, and/or repeated seizures within a single febrile illness. Developmental delay, abnormal neurologic examination, and a family history of epilepsy (note: not a family history of only febrile seizures) are also associated with an increased risk of future epilepsy. Children with a history of febrile seizures with no risk factors for epilepsy have a 2% chance of developing epilepsy. A single risk factor increases the risk of epilepsy to 5%, and 2 or more risk factors increase the risk to 15%. Even so, the majority of all children with febrile seizures will not develop epilepsy. The other choices listed are risk factors for having a recurrent febrile seizure after a first febrile seizure. Positive family history and younger age of first febrile seizure are most predictive, but low temperature and shorter duration of illness at first seizure are also risk factors.

(p. 2689, Section 29: Disorders of the Nervous System, Chapter 551: Febrile Seizures)

**Answer 16-40.** C

Infantile spasm is an epileptic encephalopathy marked by epileptic spasms and a characteristic interictal EEG pattern called hypsarrhythmia (large-amplitude, chaotic wave pattern). The spasms are classically characterized by a sudden flexion contraction of the trunk with bilateral extension of the extremities; however, spasms may have other presentations such as unilateral flexion, an extension-predominant movement, or brief head jerks. Spasms occur in clusters, often shortly after waking. Infants may have irritability or crying with or after spasms. Emergent EEG should be obtained for infants with suspicion for infantile spasms because earlier treatment is associated with improved developmental outcome. Accurate diagnosis of infantile spasms is important because traditional first-line antiepileptic medications are ineffective in this disorder. Instead, high-dose steroids, adrenocorticotropic hormone (ACTH), and vigabatrin are the initial treatment options (selection varies based on etiology, institute preference, medication availability, insurance approval, and other factors).

(p. 2683, Section 29: Disorders of the Nervous System, Chapter 549: Seizures and Epilepsy: Epidemiology and Seizure Classification)

**Answer 16-41.** B

The patient's age and clinical description of her spells are most consistent with childhood absence epilepsy, and therefore, she should be evaluated by a neurologist as soon as possible given her presumed frequent seizures. The EEG shows a typical pattern of 3-Hz generalized spike and wave during the absence seizures, which are easily provoked by hyperventilation. Childhood absence epilepsy is an age-related idiopathic generalized epilepsy that occurs in otherwise typically developing children, more frequently in girls. There is a strong genetic predisposition. Treatment is most often with ethosuximide, although lamotrigine and valproate are also effective. Remission usually occurs before the age of 12 years, but approximately 10% to 15% of patients may develop other seizure types in adolescence. Brain imaging is normal and therefore unnecessary in children with childhood absence epilepsy. Similarly, laboratory evaluations are not required for diagnosis. Because this is a typical story for absence seizures and they are occurring many times per day and affecting her school and sports, planning to see the patient back in a month is inappropriate. Neurologic diagnoses should be excluded prior to concluding that these symptoms are a psychiatric or behavioral issue.

(p. 2683, Section 29: Disorders of the Nervous System, Chapter 549: Seizures and Epilepsy: Epidemiology and Seizure Classification)

**Answer 16-42.** D

The overall risk of a skin reaction with lamotrigine is approximately 5%. Phenytoin and carbamazepine also carry roughly similar risks of an allergic skin reaction. The risk of an antiepileptic drug skin reaction is increased if there is a history of prior antiepileptic drug skin reaction. The other choices have reported rates of rash that are < 1%.

(p. 2696, Section 29: Disorders of the Nervous System, Chapter 554: Epilepsy Treatment: Antiepileptic Drug Therapy)

**Answer 16-43.** C

BECTS is the most common form of idiopathic epilepsy in children, accounting for up to nearly 25% of epilepsies in children < 16 years of age. BECTS is a genetic epilepsy characterized by childhood onset of partial motor seizures occurring mostly but not exclusively during sleep. Children are typically developing, and the seizures do not affect ongoing intelligence. The characteristic electroencephalogram (EEG) has centrotemporal spikes. Except for benign occipital epilepsy (Gastaut type), the other epilepsy syndromes listed are still quite common, with Panayiotopoulos syndrome occurring most often in younger children (3–6 years of age) and juvenile myoclonic epilepsy occurring in older children (12–18 years of age).

(p. 2683, Section 29: Disorders of the Nervous System, Chapter 549: Seizures and Epilepsy: Epidemiology and Seizure Classification)

**Answer 16-44.** C

It is important to check a lamotrigine level to determine whether the patient is taking the medication, as this will affect the management plan going forward. Nonadherence is a significant problem in patients with epilepsy. The patient has known epilepsy without recent trauma, no fever, and a nonfocal neurologic examination; therefore, lumbar puncture, routine blood work, and head CT scan are unnecessary. An EEG is also unnecessary at this time because she has known epilepsy and is waking (and therefore at low risk of ongoing subclinical seizures).

(p. 2696, Section 29: Disorders of the Nervous System, Chapter 554: Epilepsy Treatment: Antiepileptic Drug Therapy)

**Answer 16-45.** B

The risk of valproic acid–associated fatal hepatotoxicity is highest in young children, with the risk reaching 1 in 600 in children < 3 years of age receiving valproic acid as polytherapy. Developmental delay and coincident metabolic disorders are also risk factors for valproic acid–associated hepatotoxicity. Valproic acid should not be started in any young child with abnormal neurodevelopment of unknown cause prior to performing basic laboratory studies to screen for a metabolic disorder. Valproic acid is known to inhibit mitochondrial β-oxidation, and therefore, particular attention to excluding an underlying mitochondrial disorder is important. The other antiepileptic drugs listed are often used in young children.

(p. 2696, Section 29: Disorders of the Nervous System, Chapter 554: Epilepsy Treatment: Antiepileptic Drug Therapy)

**Answer 16-46.** D

After a first-time afebrile seizure, a child should be evaluated by a neurologist. As in this case, if a child quickly returns to baseline and the history and examination are not concerning for an acute medical or neurologic process, then the evaluation, including electroencephalogram (EEG), can be done as an outpatient. Given that the child is otherwise well and has a normal neurologic examination in the ED, an admission to the hospital and lumbar puncture are unnecessary. Epilepsy is defined by 2 or more unprovoked seizures; therefore, this patient does not meet criteria for a diagnosis of epilepsy. Without other risk factors, the standard of care is to wait to start a daily antiepileptic medication until the second seizure.

(p. 2692, Section 29: Disorders of the Nervous System, Chapter 552: New-Onset Seizures)

**Answer 16-47.** A

This infant has infantile spasms. The history of developmental delay and hypomelanotic macules, or ash leaf spots, seen on exam raise high suspicion for tuberous sclerosis. Tuberous sclerosis is a neurocutaneous genetic disorder that causes hamartomatous lesions primarily affecting the skin, central nervous system (CNS), eye, kidney, heart, and lung. Clinically, there are defined major and minor criteria used in diagnosis, and then genetic testing is sent to confirm clinical suspicion. Cortical tubers are common in patients with tuberous sclerosis, occurring in up to 95% of patients, although tubers or other cortical malformations may not be visible on initial brain imaging. Infantile spasms develop in approximately one-third of individuals with tuberous sclerosis. Dravet syndrome, benign myoclonic epilepsy in infancy, and Ohtahara syndrome are epilepsy syndromes that present in infancy, but none have the characteristic ash leaf spots. Neurofibromatosis is another neurocutaneous disorder with associated café-au-lait spots, not ash leaf spots.

(p. 2687, Section 29: Disorders of the Nervous System, Chapter 550: Etiologies of Epilepsy)

**Answer 16-48.** C

Children with simple febrile seizures have a 2% chance of developing subsequent epilepsy (compared with the 1% prevalence of epilepsy in children). The number of febrile seizures does not increase this risk. Complex febrile seizures and abnormal neurodevelopment or an abnormal neurologic examination increase the risk of future epilepsy. The other options are incorrect. Earlier age of onset (< 18 months) increases the risk of recurrent febrile seizures but not epilepsy. The risk of developing subsequent epilepsy in a child with 2 or more risk factors (eg, focal febrile seizures and abnormal neurodevelopment) is up to 15%.

(p. 2689, Section 29: Disorders of the Nervous System, Chapter 551: Febrile Seizures)

**Answer 16-49.** C

About 50% of all children with new-onset epilepsy will ultimately outgrow their epilepsy and no longer require medication. Response to medication is a positive predictor, with about 65% of children who are seizure-free for 2 years on medication remaining seizure-free after weaning medication.

(p. 2696, Section 29: Disorders of the Nervous System, Chapter 554: Epilepsy Treatment: Antiepileptic Drug Therapy)

**Answer 16-50.** D

It is important to correctly identify epilepsy syndromes because some idiopathic epilepsy syndromes of childhood such as childhood absence epilepsy and benign rolandic epilepsy are not associated with structural brain disorders and, therefore, neuroimaging is not necessary. Furthermore, prognosis is greatly impacted by the epilepsy syndrome. Finally, seizures may respond better to particular medications depending on the syndrome. A key part of the diagnostic evaluation in all children with a first-time seizure or epilepsy is an EEG. In fact, an EEG is required to diagnose many epilepsy syndromes. The EEG should never be deferred because it can identify abnormalities that place an individual at risk of recurrent seizures and it can help confirm epilepsy syndromes.

(p. 2683, Section 29: Disorders of the Nervous System, Chapter 549: Seizures and Epilepsy: Epidemiology and Seizure Classification)

**Answer 16-51.** C

Benign neonatal convulsions, also known as fifth-day fits, are marked by seizure onset between 4 and 6 days of life in otherwise healthy newborns. Diagnostic evaluation for an underlying cause is negative. The seizures remit by 2 months of life. The diagnosis is made retrospectively, after the seizures remit and development remains normal. Infantile spasms present around 6 months of age and are generally associated with poor developmental outcomes. Similarly, early myoclonic epilepsy is associated with poor developmental outcomes, and the early-onset myoclonic seizures tend to be refractory to treatment. Birth trauma can produce small subdural hematomas (most often in the posterior fossa) that rarely lead to seizures, and therefore, this is not the most likely cause for this patient's clinical presentation. Transient neonatal hypocalcemia may occur predominantly in breastfeeding Latino patients, but typically presents during the second week of life.

(p. 2683, Section 29: Disorders of the Nervous System, Chapter 549: Seizures and Epilepsy: Epidemiology and Seizure Classification)

**Answer 16-52.** B

Pyridoxine-dependent (vitamin $B_6$-dependent) epilepsy is a rare metabolic disorder manifesting as unexplained medically refractory seizures usually in the neonatal period that rapidly respond to a trial of intravenous (IV) pyridoxine (although sometimes the response can occur over a longer period, so oral pyridoxine is often continued following the IV pyridoxine trial until genetic testing results are received). The underlying genetic abnormality is a deficiency in α-aminoadipic semialdehyde dehydrogenase (antiquitin). Importantly, folinic acid–dependent seizures have been found to be allelic with pyridoxine dependency, and therefore, a trial of folinic acid should also be considered. The other choices do not abort intractable seizures.

(p. 585, Section 11: Inherited Disorders of Metabolism, Chapter 129: Principles of Inborn Errors of Metabolism)

**Answer 16-53.** E

The patient described in this vignette additionally presents signs and symptoms suggestive of increased intracranial pressure (ICP), including a tense bulging fontanelle, pupillary anisocoria, and pupils that are large and sluggishly reactive. Given the history, this is likely in the setting of meningitis; therefore, a lumbar puncture will be needed, but if there is concern for increased ICP, it is important to obtain a head

CT first to assure there is not impending herniation. In this context, management of potentially elevated ICP should include neurosurgical consultation, prompt imaging to determine the potential cause, and supportive measures including an elevated head of bed. Antiepileptics are included in the armamentarium for management of seizures, including potential nonconvulsive (subclinical) seizures in this patient. Lumbar puncture, albeit important, as mentioned earlier, should be deferred due to the hypothetical risk of brain herniation with elevated ICP.

(p. 1077, Section 17: Infectious Diseases, Chapter 226: Bacterial Infections of the Central Nervous System)

**Answer 16-54.** C

This patient presents with a history of delay, microcephaly, and hearing loss. There are no described risk factors for hypoxic-ischemic encephalopathy, which may result in either normocephaly or microcephaly if the injury was significant enough to cause poor brain growth. Multiple genetic conditions can lead to microcephaly and developmental delay, including cri-du-chat (5p deletion); however, characteristic dysmorphisms such as hypertelorism, a rounded face, and low-set ears are not present. Contrary to this, other genetic syndromes such as Sotos syndrome present with macrocephaly and frontal bossing. Congenital viral infections are also a potential culprit. In this patient's presentation, the presence of a possible asymptomatic primary CMV infection in the mother during pregnancy is likely, particularly when preschool siblings are present in the household. Sensorineural hearing loss may or may not be present at birth, explaining our patient's evolution. Although recently popularized, an association between Zika virus infection and congenital microcephaly is much less likely than CMV, and the vignette provides no history of recent travel to Zika-endemic areas.

(p. 2663, Section 29: Disorders of the Nervous System, Chapter 543: Microcephaly and Macrocephaly)

**Answer 16-55.** C

Increased head size with an autosomal dominant inheritance pattern, known as familial macrocephaly, is the most common type of anatomic macrocephaly. The other choices would not contribute to making the diagnosis in this case of a normally developing child with a normal neurologic examination. It is important to establish the diagnosis to avoid unnecessary testing.

(p. 2663, Section 29: Disorders of the Nervous System, Chapter 543: Microcephaly and Macrocephaly)

**Answer 16-56.** E

MS is a chronic demyelinating disorder affecting the brain and spinal cord. The diagnosis is suspected clinically and confirmed radiographically. The first demyelinating attack of the central nervous system (CNS) is termed a clinically isolated syndrome. The new clinical symptoms and new imaging findings, some of which are "active" (enhancing), confirm the diagnosis of multiple sclerosis through the dissemination of both time and space. ADEM is typically monophasic and presents with encephalopathy and multifocal symptoms, with MRI showing demyelinating lesions affecting the brain and sometimes spinal cord. Increased ICP can present with bilateral papilledema rather than unilateral papillitis. Focal ischemic arterial stroke presents with an acute-onset neurologic deficit rather than subacute onset, and imaging shows an infarct in an arterial vascular territory.

(p. 2676, Section 29: Disorders of the Nervous System, Chapter 548: Immune- and Inflammatory-Mediated Central Nervous System Disorders)

**Answer 16-57.** C

The first-line therapy for an acute demyelinating central nervous system (CNS) attack is a course of high-dose intravenous steroids. Although it does not appear that this treatment alters long-term disability, it does hasten functional recovery. Oral steroids are not recommended as initial treatment, although she will be started on an oral steroid taper following the course of IV steroids. As second-line therapy, plasmapheresis is also used. Cytoxan can be considered, but due to the adverse side effect profile, it is reserved for cases in which other treatments have failed. With lack of systemic symptoms, antibiotics are not indicated in this case.

(p. 2676, Section 29: Disorders of the Nervous System, Chapter 548: Immune- and Inflammatory-Mediated Central Nervous System Disorders)

**Answer 16-58.** E

About 80% of children who present with ADEM will only have a single event. The remaining 20% of children will have a recurrent event, usually within the first 3 months. Those who have a recurrence after 3 months of the initial event can be classified as having recurrent ADEM (if the symptoms are the same as the initial event) or multiphasic ADEM (if the symptoms are different). Even if there is clear encephalopathy with the recurrence in multiphasic ADEM, the classification of this group remains controversial. More recently, ADEM recurrence has been linked to the presence of the myelin oligodendrocyte glycoprotein (MOG) antibody. Overall, about 10% of children who are initially diagnosed with ADEM will go on to be diagnosed with multiple sclerosis.

(p. 2676, Section 29: Disorders of the Nervous System, Chapter 548: Immune- and Inflammatory-Mediated Central Nervous System Disorders)

**Answer 16-59.** D

Emergent neuroimaging is indicated in this case to exclude a compressive spinal lesion, such as an epidural hematoma or abscess, which would require an emergent neurosurgical procedure to prevent severe neurologic disability. Although an acute stroke does require emergent neuroimaging, this child has been symptomatic for 3 days, and therefore, acute therapy would not be indicated; furthermore, the clinical history of subacute-onset weakness is not consistent with acute stroke. This is the first clinical event, excluding a diagnosis of MS. Guillain-Barré could also present with these symptoms, although the reflexes would be decreased or absent. Spina bifida is a congenital spinal malformation and would not present in an 8-year-old boy.

(p. 2676, Section 29: Disorders of the Nervous System, Chapter 548: Immune- and Inflammatory-Mediated Central Nervous System Disorders)

**Answer 16-60.** B

Color vision deficit can be seen in optic neuritis. The major presenting symptom of optic neuritis is vision loss, which typically affects the central visual field more than the periphery. In children, vision loss is usually severe, with acuity of 20/200 or worse. Bilateral involvement occurs in about 50% of patients. The inability to abduct the affected eye, which implies a cranial nerve VI palsy, would not be seen in isolated optic neuritis, which involves cranial nerve II exclusively. Proptosis, foreign body sensation, and eyelid swelling would also not be expected with optic neuritis.

(p. 2676, Section 29: Disorders of the Nervous System, Chapter 548: Immune- and Inflammatory-Mediated Central Nervous System Disorders)

**Answer 16-61.** C

Oligoclonal band testing involves a comparison of immunoglobulin patterns in the CSF to the serum. The presence of bands in the CSF but not the serum indicates abnormal synthesis of immunoglobulin in the CSF, and the presence of 2 or more of such bands is considered a positive result and supports the diagnosis of MS. The presence of bands in the serum is suggestive of a systemic process, rather than an isolated central nervous system (CNS) process. Xanthochromia is typically a marker of red blood cell breakdown in the spinal fluid, as is the case in subarachnoid hemorrhage. Highly elevated CSF protein, especially in the absence of cells (cytoalbuminologic dissociation), is a marker for Guillain-Barré syndrome. Equally so, conduction block abnormalities in EMG studies suggest acute demyelination, as is the case in Guillain-Barré syndrome.

(p. 2676, Section 29: Disorders of the Nervous System, Chapter 548: Immune- and Inflammatory-Mediated Central Nervous System Disorders)

**Answer 16-62.** B

β-Hexosaminidase β-subunit deficiency causes Sandhoff disease, which differs clinically from β-hexosaminidase α-subunit deficiency (Tay-Sachs) only by the occasional presence of hepatosplenomegaly. The age of onset, duration, neurologic symptoms, and ophthalmologic signs in patients with Sandhoff disease are otherwise identical to Tay-Sachs disease. Symptoms can include excessive startle response, motor delay and loss of motor skills, loss of verbal skills, and loss of awareness of environment. Physical findings common to both disorders include macular cherry red spot and macrocephaly. Affected children can also develop seizures. Answer choices A, C, D, and E are other enzymes involved in metabolic disorders (phenylketonuria, urea cycle disorder, Pompe disease, and Fabry disease).

(p. 2733, Section 29: Disorders of the Nervous System, Chapter 564: Batten Diseases and Lipidoses)

**Answer 16-63.** A

The clinical presentations of Tay-Sachs and Sandhoff diseases are often indistinguishable, and therefore, the diagnosis is confirmed with evaluation of hexosaminidase A and B in the WBCs, with both being deficient in Sandhoff disease and only hexosaminidase A being deficient in Tay-Sachs disease. The age of onset, duration, neurologic symptoms, and ophthalmologic signs in patients with Sandhoff disease are identical to those in patients with Tay-Sachs disease, with the exception of occasional mild hepatosplenomegaly in Sandhoff disease. Symptoms can include excessive startle response, motor delay and loss of motor skills, loss of verbal skills, and loss of awareness of environment. Physical findings common to both disorders include macular cherry red spot and macrocephaly. Affected children can also develop seizures.

(p. 2733, Section 29: Disorders of the Nervous System, Chapter 564: Batten Diseases and Lipidoses)

**Answer 16-64.** D

Gaucher disease is an autosomal recessive disorder that results from deficiency of the lysosomal enzyme glucocerebrosidase and is inherited in an autosomal recessive pattern. This leads to accumulation of glycolipid in the macrophage–monocyte system throughout the body. Three major clinical types are determined by presence or absence of central nervous system (CNS) involvement: type 1, nonneuronopathic; type 2, infantile onset, acute neuronopathic; and type 3, chronic neuronopathic.

(p. 2733, Section 29: Disorders of the Nervous System, Chapter 564: Batten Diseases and Lipidoses)

**Answer 16-65.** C

NCLs are a group of progressive hereditary neurodegenerative disorders characterized by the accumulation of an autofluorescent material rich in lipid, protein, and carbohydrate in the lysosomes. Although all tissues have this accumulation, only neurons are affected. NCLs are characterized by progressive neurodegeneration, with cognitive and motor dysfunction, seizures, and vision loss. Progressive visual decline is a hallmark of NCL and usually occurs as the initial symptom in juvenile-onset NCL. The other choices, although associated with seizures and developmental delay or regression, are not associated with progressive visual loss.

(p. 2733, Section 29: Disorders of the Nervous System, Chapter 564: Batten Diseases and Lipidoses)

**Answer 16-66.** B

Cherry red macula can be seen in all of these disorders. Hepatosplenomegaly is not seen in sialidosis type I. Hyperpigmented skin lesions, or café-au-lait spots, are not seen in any of these disorders. Sialidosis type I is not associated with cognitive decline or premature death.

(p. 2733, Section 29: Disorders of the Nervous System, Chapter 564: Batten Diseases and Lipidoses)

**Answer 16-67.** D

X-linked adrenoleukodystrophy (xALD; cerebral form) is marked by onset of ADHD symptoms in a previously healthy childhood-age boy, followed by progressive cognitive decline, visual abnormalities, ataxia, and spasticity. Adrenal dysfunction may be present, and signs such as excessive skin tanning may be present (Addison disease). The diagnosis is confirmed by elevated very-long-chain fatty acids in the serum but can be evidenced by genetic testing as well. Prognosis is poor, with mean time from onset to a vegetative state of approximately 2 years. The spinal form, adrenomyeloneuropathy, represents a later onset phenotype with slower progression but similar final prognosis. Urine organic acids are useful in the diagnosis of developmental delays, regression, and seizures in infants, but lend no clue to xALD. Genetically, xALD is caused by mutations in the *ABCD1* gene and is detectable by exome sequencing; conventional chromosomal microarray would not detect these changes. CSF oligoclonal bands help in the diagnosis of multiple sclerosis.

(p. 2736, Section 29: Disorders of the Nervous System, Chapter 566: Leukodystrophies)

**Answer 16-68.** A

The majority of symptomatic boys with xALD (cerebral form) have abnormal adrenal function, and therefore, adrenal assessment through plasma ACTH level or cortical response in an ACTH stimulation test is important. The other choices do not have abnormal values in xALD.

(p. 2736, Section 29: Disorders of the Nervous System, Chapter 566: Leukodystrophies)

**Answer 16-69.** A

This clinical presentation is suggestive of Krabbe disease, which is a leukodystrophy due to a mutation of the *GALC* gene on chromosome 14q31 encoding the lysosomal enzyme galactocerebrosidase. The mutation results in an undetectable or extremely low activity level, not an elevated level. Answer choices C, D, and E are abnormalities found in other leukodystrophies.

(p. 2736, Section 29: Disorders of the Nervous System, Chapter 566: Leukodystrophies)

**Answer 16-70.** D

PMD is inherited in an X-linked autosomal recessive pattern, with males being affected and females being carriers who are either mildly affected or asymptomatic. *PLP1* gene abnormalities are identified in the majority of cases (80%–95%). Children presenting with the early-onset forms (connatal and classic) have abnormal eye movements (nystagmus) and hypotonia early in the course and then develop progressive spasticity, ataxia, and cognitive impairment. Spastic paraplegia type 2 presents at an older age, typically between 2 and 5 years, with lower extremity spasticity and bladder dysfunction, although nystagmus can be seen in some of these cases as well. At this time, there is no treatment other than supportive care. Wilson disease, not PMD, is caused by mutations in *ATP7B* gene, which plays an important role in copper transportation and metabolism.

(p. 2736, Section 29: Disorders of the Nervous System, Chapter 566: Leukodystrophies)

**Answer 16-71.** D

Lennox-Gastaut syndrome refers to the triad of multiple seizure types (most frequently tonic seizures), abnormal cognition, and a particular abnormal EEG (slow spike and wave, 2 Hz). It often is the end point of evolution of other epileptic encephalopathies such as West syndrome (infantile spasms, abnormal development, and hypsarrhythmia on EEG). Abnormal imaging and microcephaly are not characteristic of Lennox-Gastaut syndrome.

(p. 2683, Section 29: Disorders of the Nervous System, Chapter 549: Seizures and Epilepsy: Epidemiology and Seizure Classification)

**Answer 16-72.** D

Studies have shown that the ketogenic diet can be quite effective for seizure control in some epileptic encephalopathies such as those listed in answer choices A, B, C, and E. The ketogenic diet requires significant parental dedication and can be very difficult to administer effectively, and therefore, it is typically reserved for severe epilepsies that do not respond to typical antiepileptic medications. Benign rolandic epilepsy is an age-dependent epilepsy associated with spontaneous seizure cessation and normal developmental outcomes, and medication is rarely necessary. Therefore, the ketogenic diet would not be an optimal therapeutic choice.

(p. 2701, Section 29: Disorders of the Nervous System, Chapter 555: Epilepsy Treatment: Ketogenic Diet and Neurostimulation)

**Answer 16-73.** E

Childhood stroke is the most likely diagnosis in this case, and it is the first diagnosis to exclude because emergent therapies/interventions (eg, thrombectomy) may be an option in the first several hours (up to 24 hours) following the stroke. Migraine can present with transient unilateral weakness, but there are no typical migrainous features to suggest this diagnosis, and it also is a diagnosis of exclusion. Conversion disorder is a diagnosis of exclusion and should never be diagnosed prior to excluding other treatable neurologic conditions. Unlike the sudden onset of maximum neurologic deficit in this case, demyelinating episodes such as those in MS evolve in severity over the course of the attack. Seizure itself is typically not associated with unilateral weakness, but postictal hemiparesis is common and suggests a focal seizure onset.

(p. 2668, Section 29: Disorders of the Nervous System, Chapter 545: Stroke in Neonates and Children)

**Answer 16-74.** A

As an osmotic diuretic, mannitol increases water and sodium excretion and therefore decreases extracellular fluid volume, which then lowers ICP. Hypoventilation raises ICP by causing cerebral vasodilatation and increased cerebral blood volume, whereas hyperventilation lowers ICP by causing cerebral vasoconstriction and decreased cerebral blood volume. Putting the patient in Trendelenburg position with the head below the feet will increase cerebral blood volume and therefore raise ICP. The dosing of antibiotics and neuroimaging studies do not change the patient's ICP.

(p. 459, Section 8: Acute and Critical Illness, Chapter 105: Management of Acute Brain Injury; p. 2668, Section 29: Disorders of the Nervous System, Chapter 545: Stroke in Neonates and Children)

**Answer 16-75.** E

This patient has Aicardi syndrome, which is an X-linked dominant disorder with lethality, but no gene or region on the X chromosome has been identified. The classic triad consists of chorioretinal lacunae identified on ophthalmologic examination, infantile spasms, and agenesis of or dysplastic corpus callosum. The brain MRI is seldom normal. Hypoplastic cerebellum is not a feature of this disorder, although other cerebral malformations such as polymicrogyria can be seen. Astrocytomas and strokes are not associated with this syndrome.

(p. 2655, Section 29: Disorders of the Nervous System, Chapter 541: Cranial Development Abnormalities)

# CHAPTER 17 Ear, Eye, Nose, and Throat

Charu J. Sehgal, Anna Rueda, Elisha Acosta, Jennifer Benjamin, Lynda Chima Aririguzo, Judy Kim, Elton Lambert, Wallis Molchen, Andria Tatem, Margaret Wood, and Scott D. Burge

**17-1.** You are counseling the mother of a 3-month-old baby. The mother is concerned because the infant has noisy breathing on inspiration, especially when agitated. You identify the sound as high-pitched stridor, consistent with laryngomalacia. What is the most accurate statement regarding laryngomalacia?

**A.** The condition will require surgery.

**B.** Most children outgrow laryngomalacia around 12 to 18 months of age.

**C.** The noise is worse when the child is prone or upright and better when supine.

**D.** The condition is commonly associated with failure to thrive.

**E.** The condition has a bimodal age distribution and also commonly presents during adolescence.

**17-2.** Late one evening, the mother of a 3-year-old boy calls the after-hours provider on call and states that she saw her son put something in his left nostril 30 minutes ago. He was recently playing with a battery-operated toy, and the mother suspects that he most likely put a small round battery in his nose. He has left-sided rhinorrhea, no bleeding, no respiratory distress, and no fever or pain. She tried to remove the item with a cotton-tip applicator but was unsuccessful. What do you advise the mother to do?

**A.** Come to the outpatient clinic for the first appointment tomorrow morning to remove the nasal foreign body.

**B.** Go to the emergency department (ED) within the next 12 hours to remove the nasal foreign body.

**C.** Provide reassurance that the nasal foreign body will fall out on its own within 24 hours.

**D.** Go to the ED immediately for removal of the nasal foreign body.

**E.** Arrange an ear, nose, and throat (ENT) appointment for tomorrow to remove the nasal foreign body.

**17-3.** Which of the following statements is true about laryngotracheobronchitis (croup)?

**A.** Intubation is rarely necessary, and if it is required, the presence of an underlying congenital lesion such as subglottic stenosis or vascular ring should be considered.

**B.** For mild croup, the first-line treatment at home is a β-agonist given every 4 hours via a metered-dose inhaler or nebulizer.

**C.** Prospective, randomized studies show that treatment with dexamethasone makes no difference in severity or length of treatment.

**D.** Respiratory syncytial virus (RSV) accounts for most cases of croup in young children. Croup occurs more commonly in girls than in boys.

**E.** Stridor is more common on expiration because the negative expiratory pressure tends to collapse the already partially narrowed intrathoracic structures.

**17-4.** A mother brings her 2-year-old daughter to the clinic with a 1-day history of fever, pain with swallowing, and drooling. Her mother reports that she has been drinking oral rehydration solution and having normal wet diapers. On exam, she has moist mucous membranes and vesicular lesions on her soft palate; the remainder of her oropharynx is clear. Her vital signs and skin exam are normal. What is the best treatment for this child?

**A.** Acyclovir 15 mg/kg 5 times per day for 7 days

**B.** Amoxicillin 90 mg/kg twice a day for 7 days

**C.** Acetaminophen as needed and oral hydration at home

**D.** Hospitalization for intravenous (IV) fluids

**E.** Benzocaine gel applied to the lesions

**17-5.** A 16-year-old boy presents with concern for a foul-smelling otorrhea from his left ear for the past 2 weeks. Over the past 2 days, he has also noted decreased hearing in this ear. He denies pain, fever, or trauma to his ear. He has no history of frequent ear infections or tympanostomy tubes. On exam, the tympanic membrane is intact and mobile on otoscopy. A white mass is seen behind the tympanic membrane, and there is yellow-colored squamous debris on the superior aspect of the tympanic membrane at the pars flaccida. He fails his hearing screen on the left side and passes on the right. What is the next best step in management for this patient?

**A.** Treat him with high-dose amoxicillin for 10 days

**B.** Refer him to otolaryngology for surgical intervention

**C.** Treat him with ciprofloxacin/dexamethasone otic drops for 10 days

**D.** Perform a tympanometry test

**E.** Observation and follow-up for repeat hearing screen in 12 weeks

**17-6.** A previously healthy and normally developing 3-year-old boy is brought to the emergency department (ED) by his grandmother for fever to 103°F, pain with swallowing, and drooling that started 2 hours ago. Since onset, he has had worsening of symptoms, and the grandmother is concerned because he has become more tired appearing. Vitals on presentation are temperature of 101.6°F, heart rate of 120 bpm, respiratory rate of 35 breaths/min, blood pressure of 94/56 mm Hg, and oxygen saturation of 85% on room air. On initial exam, he is sitting on his grandmother's lap leaning forward with his chin extended, and he appears in severe distress with audible stridor at rest and perioral cyanosis. What is the next best step in management of this patient's condition?

**A.** Emergent intubation in the ED

**B.** Have both ED medical assistants work simultaneously to establish intravenous (IV) access and obtain a baseline arterial blood gas

**C.** Have the grandmother gently provide supplemental oxygen to this child while you contact the anesthesiology or otolaryngology team to ready an operating room for intubation under controlled conditions

**D.** Give nebulized β-agonist while you order a chest radiograph and ask the radiologist to rule out a foreign body

**E.** Give intramuscular dose of dexamethasone, observe for 4 hours, and then discharge home

**17-7.** A 10-year-old boy comes in to your office with abdominal pain for about 6 months, on and off. You note from the chart that he has lost some weight. He also has been having some knee pain that his mother attributes to "growing pains," and mom also is concerned about his color; she feels that he looks pale. The patient has also had some eye redness of the sclera for the past month, which improved with the antibiotic drops that you prescribed for him but keeps coming back. He says his eyes feel uncomfortable most of the time, even painful at times. There is no discharge today. In the chart, you note a family history of inflammatory bowel disease (IBD). Given the symptoms that the patient has, what is the most likely eye finding presented here?

**A.** Episcleritis

**B.** Viral conjunctivitis

**C.** Hyphema

**D.** Trachoma

**E.** Bacterial conjunctivitis

**17-8.** In December, a 10-year-old boy comes to the office after the school nurse sent him home with possible pink eye. He had symptoms including right sclera redness about 3 days ago, but since then, the redness has moved to the other eye. He states his eyes are itchy and watery, but he has no discharge during the day. In the morning, he wakes up with dried white residue in the corners of his eyes. His review of systems is negative for ear pain, vomiting, diarrhea, or headache, but positive for rhinorrhea and mild sore throat. There is no reported trauma to the eyes. This is not a repeated occurrence; he has never had red eyes before, and there is no noted trigger for it.

On exam, he is afebrile. He does have some nasal congestion and mucus in his nose, and his throat looks mildly erythematous but without enlarged tonsils. His tympanic membranes are clear. He has preauricular lymphadenopathy on the right side. Both sclerae are erythematous and watery without mucopurulent discharge. Conjunctiva are not inflamed, and eyelids do not appear to be swollen. You ran out of fluorescein strips and are unable to assess further. What should be the treatment for the eye redness?

**A.** Antibacterial ophthalmic drops

**B.** Observation with possible referral to ophthalmologist

**C.** Steroid drops

**D.** Topical anesthetic ophthalmic drops

**E.** $H_1$ antagonist/mast cell inhibitor ophthalmic drops

**17-9.** You are attending a delivery of a 35-week-gestation infant. He is born in acute respiratory distress. On the warmer, you note a cyanotic infant who has improved color when he cries. He is tachypneic with increased work of breathing and retractions, but strangely, he has no nasal flaring. He has clear lung fields and no murmur, and with a quick physical exam, you note a small ear on the right and a nonexistent ear on the left. There appears to be a cleft palate and possible sacral deformity that looks like a meningocele. You attempt to pass a suction catheter in the nostrils, and it does not pass on either side. You then put in an oral airway. The baby's oxygen saturations drop to 85% and do not improve on oxygen. The heart rate drops to 60 bpm, so you start bag-mask ventilation. What is the best next step in management of the airway of this child?

**A.** Tracheotomy

**B.** Observation

**C.** Intubation

**D.** Non-rebreather mask

**E.** Start gavage feedings

**17-10.** A 5-year-old girl presents to your clinic. Her chief complaint is halitosis. Her father had not noticed it before because he travels overseas for work, but he received a call from her school teacher regarding this issue. The child is often ostracized due to her breath, and this is affecting her emotionally. There is no history of cough, congestion, sore throat, ear pain, vomiting, or reflux. She eats healthy food and not a lot of sugar. The child loves to brush her teeth, and even lets her parents floss her teeth. She recently visited the dentist for the same issue, but her teeth and oral mucosa looked healthy. Her father notes one strange detail; she seems to have thick nasal mucus but only in the right nostril. What is the most likely diagnosis?

**A.** Adenoidal hypertrophy

**B.** Gastroesophageal reflux disease (GERD)

**C.** Sinusitis

**D.** Nasal foreign body

**E.** Dental caries

**17-11.** An 8-year-old girl came to clinic for ear pain. She is on the swim team and has been practicing 3 days a week for an upcoming meet. She has been using swimmer's ear drops and cotton-tipped swabs to clean her ears at night. However, her right ear has been hurting since this morning, so much so that she cannot sleep on it or put her phone to it. She has no cough, congestion, sore throat, or fever. Upon exam, she starts crying when you pull the pinna. The ear canal appears swollen and red. You note a lack of cerumen on the outside of the ear but cannot visualize the tympanic membrane well because the ear canal is edematous. There is some yellowish clear discharge on the otoscope tip when you take it out. You prescribe ciprofloxacin otic drops for treatment. However, she comes back 2 weeks later with similar symptoms. What is the next logical treatment?

**A.** Ofloxacin otic drops

**B.** Acetic acid/alcohol drops

**C.** Oral amoxicillin-clavulanic acid

**D.** Stop swimming

**E.** Antifungal otic drops

**17-12.** Which of the following patients would *not* be at risk for ototoxicity?

**A.** A 7-year-old boy with cystic fibrosis who takes daily inhaled tobramycin

**B.** A 4-year-old boy with ruptured otitis media on fluoroquinolone otic drops

**C.** A 15-year-old girl who purposely overdosed on aspirin

**D.** A 10-year-old girl receiving cisplatin for chemotherapy

**E.** A 2-year-old girl who is a former 29-week premature infant treated with gentamicin in the past

**17-13.** A 3-year-old boy presents for a well-child check-up. He is well appearing without craniofacial abnormalities and uses 3-word sentences. He denies ear pain or pressure. He does not have a history of ear infections. He had an upper respiratory infection 1 week ago but is afebrile today. He has mild congestion that is improving. His head and neck examination is normal except for the left otoscopic examination noted in Figure 238-1B. What is the next best step?

**A.** Start amoxicillin

**B.** Start amoxicillin-clavulanic acid

**C.** Observation

**D.** Consultation for placement of bilateral myringotomy tube

**E.** Refer to child protective services for suspected child abuse

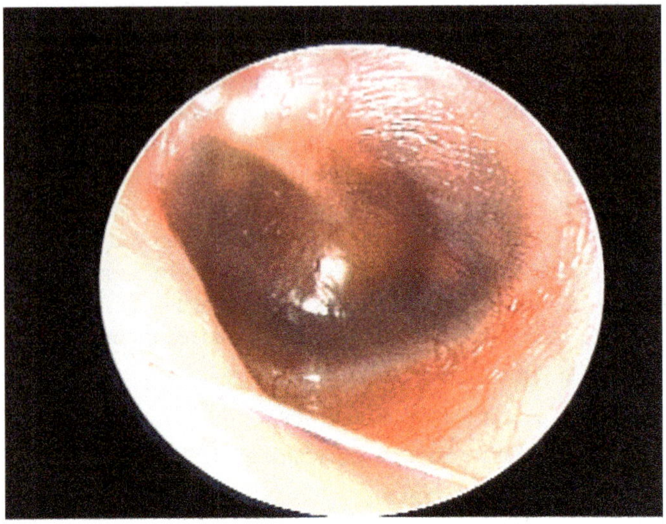

B

**FIGURE 238-1B.** (Used with permission from David P. McCormick, MD.)

**17-14.** A 6-year-old girl presents with a 10-day history of intermittent fever to 102°F, nasal congestion, and greenish rhinorrhea. Her rhinorrhea was clear about 5 days ago, but the fever and rhinorrhea have worsened over the past 2 to 3 days. Today, her parents noted acute onset of left-sided eye swelling. What is the next best step?

**A.** Nasal steroid spray

**B.** Amoxicillin-clavulanic acid

**C.** Amoxicillin-clavulanic acid and nasal decongestant

**D.** Computed tomography (CT) scan with intravenous (IV) contrast

**E.** Observation

**17-15.** A 2-year-old boy presents to the emergency department (ED) after a witnessed choking episode. The child is tachypneic, diaphoretic, and fussy and has a wet cough. Auscultation reveals decreased breath sounds and wheezing at the right lung bases. What is the next step?

**A.** Inspiratory and expiratory chest radiographs (CXR)

**B.** Consultation for bronchoscopy and foreign body removal

**C.** Nebulized bronchodilators

**D.** Intravenous (IV) steroids

**E.** Chest computed tomography (CT) scan

**17-16.** A 12-year-old girl presents with a 1-year history of a slowly enlarging neck mass. It is painless and fluctuates with sicknesses. Upon examination, it is a fluctuant, nontender midline neck mass and moves when she sticks out her tongue. A photograph of the mass is shown in Figure 367-4. What is the underlying pathophysiology of this mass?

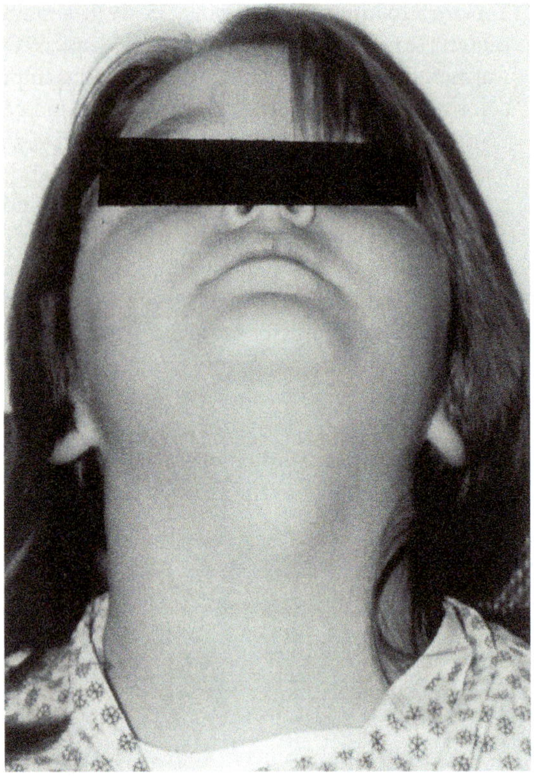

**FIGURE 367-4.** Midline neck mass in an adolescent girl. (Reproduced with permission from Tintinalli JE, Kelen GD, Stapczynski JS. *Emergency Medicine: A Comprehensive Study Guide*, 6th ed. New York: McGraw-Hill; 2004.)

**A.** Aberration in the normal descent of the thyroid gland

**B.** Blockage of the submandibular duct with secondary infection of the submandibular gland

**C.** Anomaly in the development of the branchial arches

**D.** Inflammation due to bacterial suppuration of a cervical lymph node

**E.** Insufficient iodine consumption

**17-17.** A 12-year-old girl comes to the office for left-sided ear drainage. This has been present off and on for 3 months. There have been at least 5 separate episodes during this time. She has been on courses of topical antibiotics, including ofloxacin and ciprofloxacin-dexamethasone. She denies ear pain, but there is some fullness and decreased hearing. On exam, you notice thick drainage and edema of the ear canal, but the tympanic membrane while thickened shows no erythema, and there is no middle ear effusion. The auricle is normal, and there is no postauricular tenderness. What is the best next step?

**A.** Start amoxicillin

**B.** Send a culture of the ear drainage

**C.** Request a consultation for myringotomy tube insertion

**D.** Computed tomography (CT) scan with intravenous (IV) contrast

**E.** IV ampicillin

**17-18.** A 2-year-old boy presents with a 1-day history of nasal congestion, rhinorrhea, low-grade fever, and a barky cough. Upon examination, he has biphasic stridor and has mild subcostal retractions. This child would most likely have pathology in which anatomic region?

**A.** Subglottis

**B.** Posterior choanae

**C.** Bronchioles

**D.** Tonsils

**E.** Anterior choanae

**17-19.** A 2-year-old boy presents for a well-child check-up. The parents notice that he only says about 2 to 3 words, and he is hard to understand. He passed a newborn hearing screening. He has not had any ear infections. He has no motor delays. Upon examination, he is well appearing, both ear canals and tympanic membranes are normal and show good mobility, and there are no middle ear effusions. His intranasal examination is normal, and he has 1+ tonsils, no ankyloglossia, and no palatal abnormalities. What is the next most appropriate step?

**A.** Consultation for myringotomy tube placement

**B.** Observation and anticipatory guidance

**C.** Consultation for cochlear implantation

**D.** Audiogram

**E.** Speech therapy referral

**17-20.** A 14-year-old girl presents to the emergency department (ED) with a 4-day history of progressive fever, sore throat, left ear pain, muffled voice, and decreased oral intake. She is alert but uncomfortable and has full neck range of motion. Ear examination is normal. Her oral exam shows medial displacement of the left tonsil, left soft palate erythema and fullness, deviation of the uvula, and deviation of the soft palate to the right. What is the underlying pathophysiology of this condition?

**A.** Necrosis and abscess formation of a retropharyngeal lymph node

**B.** Epstein-Barr virus (EBV) infection

**C.** Abnormal persistence of a branchial pouch derivative

**D.** Spread of infection to the peritonsillar space

**E.** Spread of infection to the mastoid process

**17-21.** You are called to resuscitation involving a 38-week-gestation female infant who was born a few minutes ago. The child is intermittently cyanotic, which is relieved by crying. There is nasal flaring with severe suprasternal and subcostal retractions. The child is tachypneic and is grunting but has no stridor. Breath sounds are normal. An 8-French catheter cannot be advanced through nasal cavity. What is the next best step?

**A.** Obtain a computed tomography (CT) scan of the face

**B.** Insert an oral airway

**C.** Proceed with endotracheal intubation

**D.** Start a nasal decongestant

**E.** Observation for improvement over time

**17-22.** A 3-year-old boy presents with a 1-year history of snoring. He has associated mouth breathing and nasal obstruction. He has no apneic events. Parents deny rhinorrhea, itchy eyes, and itchy nose. There is no seasonal variability with his symptoms. On exam, the ear canal and tympanic membranes are clear. His intranasal exam reveals pink and healthy-appearing inferior turbinates, no rhinorrhea, and no nasal airway obstruction. His tonsils are 1+, and you notice open-mouth breathing. His lungs are clear. What is the next step?

**A.** Begin an oral antihistamine

**B.** Request a consultation for tonsillectomy

**C.** Order a lateral neck radiograph (CXR)

**D.** Start a bronchodilator

**E.** Refer for allergy testing

**17-23.** A 2-month-old female infant presents for a routine well-child exam. Her father is concerned that her right eye consistently produces more tears than her left eye. She also has been blinking more over the past week. He denies cough, rhinorrhea, fever, or sick contacts. She has otherwise been doing well. On exam, you note a well-nourished infant with clear conjunctivae, white sclera, increased right eye lacrimation, blepharospasms, and a slightly asymmetric red reflex. What would be the most appropriate next step in management?

**A.** Offer reassurance and follow up at next well-child visit

**B.** Lacrimal massage at home with a clean, warm cloth

**C.** Arrange prompt referral to pediatric ophthalmology

**D.** Prescribe dexamethasone ophthalmic drops for 5 days

**E.** Prescribe trimethoprim ophthalmic drops for 7 days

**17-24.** A 4-year-old boy with a past history of frequent ear infections presents for a well-child examination. He is at the 60th percentile for weight and 45th percentile for height. He has been meeting developmental milestones and is preparing to enter preschool. His ear exam is notable for a left tympanic membrane with retraction pockets and a pearly white mass superior to the short process of the malleolus. His father reports that the child occasionally has ear discharge but has not experienced fever, cough, or rhinorrhea recently. What would be the most appropriate management of this child's condition?

**A.** Referral to infectious disease for evaluation and assistance with recurrent infection

**B.** Referral to otolaryngology for evaluation and surgical treatment

**C.** Counsel on ear wicking technique and avoidance of swimming

**D.** Prescribe amoxicillin-clavulanic acid and follow up in 3 months

**E.** Offer reassurance and return precautions, with follow-up as needed

**17-25.** A 5-week-old, former full-term female infant is brought to your office for noisy breathing for the past 2 weeks. According to her parents, her breathing becomes noisier when she cries and occasionally when she feeds. They notice that laying her on her back when she is upset also makes the breathing louder. She is otherwise eating well and developing normally. On exam, you note a sleeping, well-developed infant in no acute distress with lungs clear to auscultation bilaterally. Her neurologic exam is unremarkable. As she awakens, she begins to cry, and you note mild stridor that decreases when she is placed on her side and increases in the supine position. Her oxygen saturation at this time remains at 98% on room air. Given the mild nature of her condition, you offer reassurance, close observation with return precautions, and the expected course of this condition. Her condition should resolve by what age?

**A.** 3–9 months of age

**B.** 9–12 months of age

**C.** 12–18 months of age

**D.** 18–24 months of age

**E.** 24–36 months of age

**17-26.** A 9-year-old girl presents to your office for a well-child visit. Her father expresses concern that she seems to be congested all the time. She snores frequently but denies itchy nose or eyes. Nasal saline washes and oral antihistamines do not seem to improve her congestion. She has no known allergies to food or medication. There is no family history of atopic dermatitis, allergic rhinitis, or asthma. She is at the third percentile for height and fifth percentile for weight. Her frontal and maxillary sinuses are nontender to palpation. Inspection of the nasal cavity reveals grayish, gelatinous, grape-like masses near the turbinates of both nares. Given her presentation, which of the following tests would be most important for making a definitive diagnosis?

**A.** Skin prick test

**B.** Hemoglobin electrophoresis

**C.** Head and neck radiographs

**D.** Sweat chloride test

**E.** Rapid influenza antigen assay

**17-27.** A 5-year-old boy is brought to clinic for evaluation of recurrent swelling on his neck. His father reports that this is the third time the child has had swelling at the front of his neck. Swelling typically is associated with erythema and soreness to the area and usually occurs during or shortly after he has a cold. This current episode of swelling is slightly larger than the previous episode, which prompted the family to seek medical attention. He has not experienced fever, difficulty breathing, or decreased oral intake. His examination is significant for an erythematous, mildly tender mass along his left lateral neck at the border of the sternomastoid. Which of the following is the definitive treatment for the boy's condition?

**A.** Oral antibiotic therapy

**B.** Intravenous (IV) antibiotic therapy

**C.** Incision and drainage

**D.** Complete excision

**E.** Chemotherapy

**17-28.** You come on service in the neonatal intensive care unit (NICU) and take over the care of a term 2-day-old male infant who frequently has cyanotic episodes. He is on high-flow nasal cannula, but his breathing at rest is still labored with significant subcostal retractions. His lungs are otherwise clear on auscultation. He had routine prenatal care and had a normal echocardiogram yesterday. When he cries, both his color and oxygen saturations significantly improve. A 5-French catheter is unable to be passed completely through either side of the nose. What is the best next step in the management of this child?

**A.** Obtain a computed tomography (CT) maxillofacial scan

**B.** Consult ear, nose, and throat (ENT) surgery

**C.** Obtain a magnetic resonance imaging (MRI) skull base scan

**D.** Intubate to secure the airway

**E.** Carefully dilate the nasal passages starting with a smaller catheter

**17-29.** A 4-year-old girl presents to your clinic with a 1-cm mass under the skin of the nasal bridge. This was first noticed 1 month ago while she was crying after her younger brother stole her favorite toy. There has been no trauma to the area and no pain, erythema, or drainage. She has also been afebrile. The child denies nasal obstruction and nosebleeds. When you compress her jugular veins on exam, the mass expands and then goes back down to baseline upon release. She has normal extraocular movements on exam. What is the best next step in management?

- **A.** Consult ear, nose, and throat (ENT) surgery to biopsy the mass
- **B.** Perform a magnetic resonance imaging (MRI) of the skull base with and without contrast
- **C.** Perform an ultrasound with Doppler signal of the nasal region
- **D.** Perform a computed tomography (CT) of the neck with and without contrast
- **E.** Obtain an ophthalmology consultation

**17-30.** Which of the following is most characteristic of a juvenile nasopharyngeal angiofibroma?

- **A.** They most commonly occur in prepubescent males and are benign tumors.
- **B.** They most commonly occur in prepubescent females and are malignant tumors.
- **C.** They most commonly occur in adolescent males and are benign tumors.
- **D.** They most commonly occur in neonatal females and are malignant tumors.
- **E.** They most commonly occur in adolescent females and are benign tumors.

**17-31.** A 7-year-old boy presents to your clinic with otorrhea from his left ear and associated pain when pulling on the ear to perform otoscopy. The otorrhea started 5 days ago, and he remembers going swimming a lot while on vacation with his family last week. He has been afebrile, and your exam reveals no postauricular swelling or erythema. You note white debris within the left ear canal as well as moderate ear canal swelling, which limits complete visualization of the tympanic membrane. What should be done along with antibiotic otic drops to treat this condition?

- **A.** Tell the patient to use cotton-tipped swabs twice a day to help remove the otorrhea so that the ear can heal
- **B.** Get a computed tomography (CT) temporal bone scan to see if the infection has extended into the mastoid cavity
- **C.** Avoid getting pool or shower water in the ears as this will allow the infection to persist
- **D.** Avoid placing a wick as this will only contribute to keeping the infected drainage in place
- **E.** Obtain a culture from both ears to compare what is likely normal flora with what is causing infection in the affected ear

**17-32.** You suspect that a 3-year-old girl has Jervell and Lange-Nielsen syndrome based on your history and an audiogram. Which of the following should be considered next?

- **A.** Obtain a renal ultrasound
- **B.** Obtain an electrocardiogram (ECG)
- **C.** Obtain a magnetic resonance imaging (MRI) of the brain with and without contrast
- **D.** Obtain a thyroid ultrasound
- **E.** Obtain a urinalysis

**17-33.** A 10-year-old boy comes to see you in clinic because his mom has noticed a slight odor to the right ear over the past 3 months. He has not been on any ear drops or oral antibiotics, but he also states that the ear does not hurt. He has a history of needing several sets of ear tubes due to "chronic ear issues." He has subjectively noticed some decreased hearing on the right side. On exam, you confirm the odor from the right ear and see a white mass and debris in a retracted portion of the eardrum in the posterior-superior quadrant. How should this condition be treated?

- **A.** Irrigate the ear and use a loop curette to see if the debris can be completely cleared from the retraction pocket
- **B.** Have the patient return in 3 to 6 months to see if the debris clears on its own because it will be difficult to clear all of the debris in clinic
- **C.** Prescribe oral antibiotics because otic drops alone will not penetrate the infection to resolve it
- **D.** Refer to child protective services for concern for neglect since this has been going on for at least 3 months
- **E.** Surgical excision with tympanoplasty and mastoidectomy will be needed to remove all of the squamous debris

**17-34.** An 8-year old girl presents to clinic with a 4-day history of a midline neck mass. She does not have any respiratory distress or concerns with swallowing. You notice that the mass is erythematous and swollen, and you treat her with antibiotics. At the 1-week follow-up, the mass is decreased in size and significantly less erythematous. It is still palpable at 1 cm in size. It also moves vertically when she swallows. What is the best next step?

**A.** Obtain a head and neck ultrasound and refer for surgical excision
**B.** Refer to interventional radiology to perform a fine-needle aspiration biopsy of the mass
**C.** Observe and follow up in 3 months as it should resolve by then
**D.** Prescribe a macrolide antibiotic as this is likely an atypical mycobacterial infection
**E.** Obtain a computed tomography (CT) of the chest to make sure that there are no other midline masses

**17-35.** A 7-year-old boy with cerebral palsy, spastic paraplegia, and global developmental delay is admitted to your service with his third case of aspiration pneumonia in the past year. He was started on antibiotics and has been improving in his oxygen requirements. He is fed via gastric tube and is nonverbal, but his mom is concerned about the amount of drooling that he has and wonders if this is contributing to his recurrent pneumonias. He was started on an anticholinergic medication, which has been increased to the maximum dose as of 4 months ago. He also received onabotulinumtoxinA (Botox®) injections to the major salivary glands 3 months ago. His sialorrhea is still a significant issue. Which of the following statements is true regarding this child's management?

**A.** Tracheostomy should not be considered because it will not address the issue of the increased saliva production.
**B.** Surgical excision of the submandibular glands and parotid duct ligations should be considered.
**C.** You should add another anticholinergic medication to help control his symptoms.
**D.** You should recommend continued observation because there has not been enough time for the onabotulinumtoxinA to work.
**E.** You should not recommend administering another dose of onabotulinumtoxinA due to concerns that it will cause toxicity.

**17-36.** A 16-year-old boy presents to the emergency department (ED) after running into a door while holding a pencil in his mouth. On arrival he has no mental status changes and no signs of Horner syndrome. He has good neck range of motion and is afebrile. You are able to adequately visualize a full-thickness penetrating trauma to the soft palate, which is located < 1 cm to the right of midline. What is the best next step in the management of this child?

**A.** Order a computed tomography (CT) neck angiogram to rule out an internal carotid injury
**B.** Repair the laceration under sedation to prevent a palatal fistula
**C.** Order a carotid duplex scan of the neck to better evaluate the carotid arteries
**D.** Observe overnight to rule out a delayed embolic event
**E.** Consult neurology for a full neurologic exam to evaluate for sequelae of the injury

**17-37.** A 13-year-old girl presents to the emergency department (ED) after being "clothes-lined" during a soccer game 1 hour ago. She attempts to tell you the story but has difficulty due to the pain in her neck and the hoarseness of her voice. You see bruising on the anterior neck and suspect a laryngeal fracture injury. You also notice that she is becoming more anxious. What is the best next step in her management?

**A.** Give her a dose of a benzodiazepine such as lorazepam to help her calm down so she can breathe more easily
**B.** Obtain a computed tomography (CT) neck angiogram to better evaluate the injury to the larynx and major vessels
**C.** Start cardiopulmonary resuscitation (CPR) to make sure that she is getting enough oxygen perfusion to the body
**D.** Place her on oxygen and monitors, administer steroids and racemic epinephrine, and consult the in-house ear, nose, and throat (ENT) surgeon or general surgeon for possible intervention
**E.** Perform intubation in the ED to secure the airway

**17-38.** A 13-year-old boy presents after injury to his auricle following soccer yesterday. He complains of pain at the swollen site, which he did not notice before. What is the next best step in management?

**A.** Provide adequate pain control with a nonsteroidal anti-inflammatory drug (NSAID)
**B.** Closely follow up in 2 days to monitor for complications
**C.** Perform an incision and drainage and apply compression dressing to prevent reaccumulation
**D.** Provide reassurance and apply cold compress to improve swelling
**E.** Start topical antibiotics to avoid secondary infection

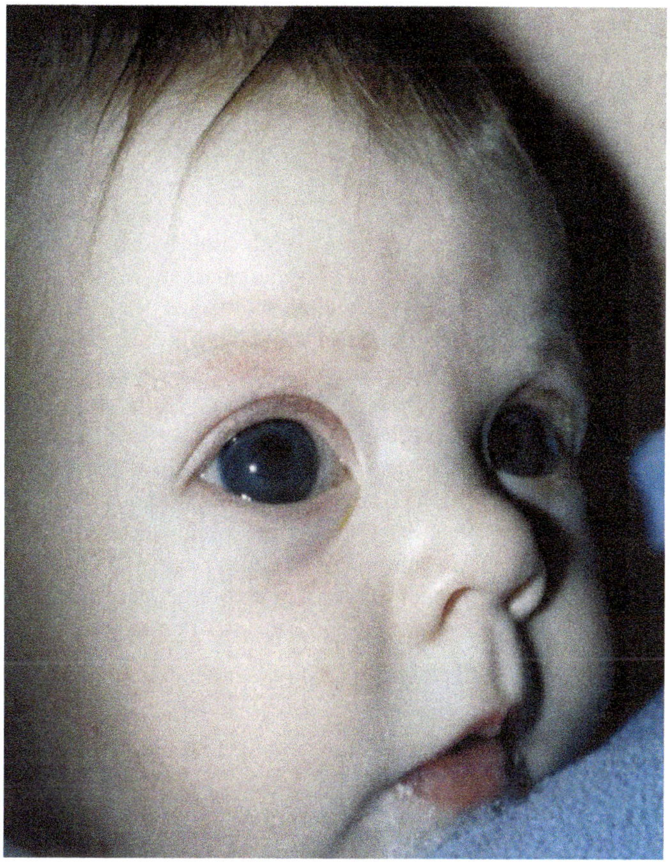

**FIGURE 580-1.** (Mark W. Kline, *Rudolph's Pediatrics*, 23rd Edition. Copyright © McGraw-Hill Education. All rights reserved.)

**17-39.** A 2-month-old female infant who was born by normal delivery presents for her well-child check. She is breastfeeding and is attempting to roll over. Her mother reports that she has noticed that her daughter has increased blinking and tearing for the past few days. There is no history of trauma to her eye. Her eye examination is shown in Figure 580-1. What is the next best step in her management?

**A.** Apply topical antibiotic eye drops
**B.** Explain appropriate clearing of secretions from the medial aspect of each eye using clean cotton wool
**C.** Follow up in 2 weeks to monitor symptoms
**D.** Treat with moisturizing eye drops
**E.** Place urgent referral to ophthalmology

**17-40.** You are seeing a 1-week-old newborn female child born to a 20-year-old primigravida female who had poor antenatal care. She was discharged 2 days after birth. The mother's main concern today is sticky eyes. The secretions first started as thin and watery and have recently been noticed to be more purulent and thicker. You notice swelling of eyelids and greenish secretions from both eyes. You send for cultures and Gram stain. What is the next best step in treatment?

**A.** Topical erythromycin ointment and antibiotic eye drops for 7 days
**B.** Topical erythromycin ointment and oral azithromycin for 1 day
**C.** Topical silver nitrate
**D.** Topical rinse with normal saline and topical antibiotics
**E.** Oral erythromycin for 14 days

**17-41.** Which of the following statements is true of neonatal conjunctivitis?

**A.** *Chlamydia trachomatis* is the most common cause of neonatal conjunctivitis.
**B.** Gonococcal conjunctivitis usually presents 2 to 3 weeks after birth.
**C.** Routine prophylaxis with erythromycin ointment has proven to reduce the rate of infections.
**D.** *C trachomatis* is associated with corneal perforation.
**E.** Penicillin derivatives are usually effective in management.

**17-42.** What is the most common cause of infectious conjunctivitis in children?

**A.** Bacterial conjunctivitis caused by *Chlamydia trachomatis*
**B.** Bacterial conjunctivitis caused by *Streptococcus pneumoniae*
**C.** Bacterial conjunctivitis caused by *Moraxella*
**D.** Viral conjunctivitis caused by adenovirus
**E.** Viral conjunctivitis caused by herpes virus

**17-43.** An 8-year-old girl presents to you, her primary care physician, for evaluation of persistent rhinitis for > 1 year despite daily second-generation antihistamine and steroid nasal spray use. What initial diagnostic test may help direct further treatment?

**A.** Nasal swabs for bacterial and viral etiologies
**B.** Allergy testing (skin prick or allergen-specific antibody test)
**C.** Computed tomography (CT) of sinuses
**D.** Complete blood count (CBC)
**E.** C-reactive protein (CRP)

**17-44.** A 5-year-old boy moves to a new city and presents to his pediatrician to establish care. The boy and his parents deny any acute concerns. They report a past medical history of congenital heart disease with spontaneous resolution. Initial exam by the pediatrician is normal except the boy has limited mobility of his cervical spine associated with a short neck with a webbed appearance and a low posterior hairline. A radiograph of the cervical spine is ordered. What finding is expected on the plain film of the cervical spine?

**A.** Fusion of single or multiple levels of the cervical spine
**B.** Atlantoaxial instability
**C.** Absence of C5
**D.** Cervical kyphosis
**E.** Squaring of the vertebral bodies ("bamboo spine")

**17-45.** What is the most common cause of cheilitis?

**A.** Atopic dermatitis
**B.** Nutritional deficiencies
**C.** Bacterial infections
**D.** Licking the lips or perioral skin
**E.** Fungal infection

**17-46.** An 8-month-old child is brought to her pediatrician by her parents who are concerned by their daughter's frequent tearing and blinking. The parents report that increasingly since birth their child has experienced frequent eye tearing not associated with irritability or crying. The tearing happens throughout the day and does not necessarily seem related to light, although the baby does appear to prefer dark rooms. On exam, a well-developed 8-month-old baby girl is noted to have prominent eyes with cloudy corneas. There is no icterus or injection, and pupils are equal and reactive to light, with equal red reflex. What is the most likely cause of this patient's symptoms?

**A.** Lacrimal duct stenosis
**B.** Primary congenital glaucoma
**C.** Infantile cataract
**D.** Glaucoma secondary to Soto syndrome
**E.** Sclerocornea

**17-47.** An 18-year-old woman presents to your office with a history of ear swelling, erythema, and pain. She underwent piercing of her helix last week, after which she developed progressive pain and redness in her ear. On exam, the upper two-thirds of her auricle are diffusely swollen, erythematous, and exquisitely tender to touch. Antibiotics for this patient should ensure coverage for which organism(s)?

**A.** *Staphylococcus aureus*
**B.** *Streptococcus pyogenes* (group A *Streptococcus*)
**C.** *Pseudomonas aeruginosa*
**D.** *S aureus* and *S pyogenes*
**E.** *P aeruginosa* and *S aureus*

**17-48.** A 7-year-old boy presents to your clinic with his mom, who is concerned about chronic, persistent rhinorrhea for the past year. The patient's rhinorrhea persists throughout the year and at times is triggered by strong odors such as perfumes and soaps. The patient has not had any recent illness and has had a recent negative skin prick test. The patient denies nasal congestion, throat pain, ear pain, or eye redness/irritation. He reports that he overall feels well, and medical history and review of systems are otherwise negative. Family history is negative for asthma, allergies, and eczema. Which of the following treatments should be recommended?

**A.** Oral second-generation antihistamine
**B.** Intranasal glucocorticoid (eg, fluticasone propionate or beclomethasone)
**C.** Intranasal topical anticholinergic (eg, ipratropium bromide nasal spray)
**D.** Intranasal topical antihistamine (eg, azelastine)
**E.** Intranasal glucocorticoid (eg, fluticasone propionate or beclomethasone) plus intranasal topical antihistamine (eg, azelastine)

**17-49.** Congenital anomalies of the third or fourth branchial arches are most likely to present as which of the following?

**A.** Painless sinus tract near the ear noted at birth
**B.** Draining sinus in the lateral neck at the anterior border of the sternocleidomastoid
**C.** Enlarging mass near the parotid gland
**D.** Recurrent left neck abscesses or suppurative thyroiditis
**E.** Mobile, painless, midline neck mass

**17-50.** A 14-year-old boy presents to the emergency department (ED) with an anterior lip laceration sustained after falling from his bike. On exam, he has a through-and-through lip laceration of the skin through the oral mucosa. After suturing the laceration, antibiotics should be prescribed for this patient to cover which of the following organisms?

**A.** Staphylococcal species
**B.** Streptococcal species
**C.** *Actinomyces* species
**D.** *Corynebacterium* species
**E.** *Prevotella* species

**17-51.** A mother brings her 7-year-old son to your office with concern for a "growth" along his mid-maxillary gumline. On exam, both maxillary central incisors are missing, and in this region appears a soft, bluish, dome-shaped swelling that is minimally tender to palpation with a tongue depressor. The surrounding gingiva appears healthy without evidence of inflammation. Which of the following is the most appropriate next step?

**A.** Urgent referral to pediatric dentist for further evaluation

**B.** Referral to an emergency department (ED) with dental providers for incision and drainage

**C.** Reassurance that this typically resolves spontaneously

**D.** Antibiotic prescription for probable gingival abscess

**E.** Referral to ear, nose, and throat (ENT) for surgical removal

**17-52.** A 10-year-old girl presents to the clinic for evaluation of right eye pain. She was flying a kite with her father at the beach when the pain started. On examination, she is unable to open her eye, and there is profuse clear tearing. Using a Wood's lamp, fluorescein dye reveals an area of epithelial cell loss. What is the most appropriate next step?

**A.** Refer to an ophthalmologist

**B.** Prescribe an oral antibiotic

**C.** Apply a pressure patch to the eye

**D.** Prescribe a topical antibiotic ointment

**E.** Wash the eye out with water

**17-53.** A child is referred to you after failing his hearing test at school. His mother noticed foul-smelling drainage on his pillow this morning and is concerned he has an ear infection. Using an otoscope, you examine his left ear and see squamous debris within a retraction pocket most consistent with the diagnosis of a cholesteatoma. The mother asks you about treatment options. You refer the child to a specialist and order which of the following?

**A.** Magnetic resonance imaging (MRI) of brain

**B.** Ultrasound of the neck

**C.** Computed tomography (CT) scan of temporal bone

**D.** Bilateral ultrasound of the kidneys

**E.** Chest radiograph

**17-54.** A 3-year-old boy presents to the emergency department with rhinorrhea and an erythematous lump on the left side of his neck. The mother is unsure if he has a fever but believes he is warm to touch. She also offers that this is the third time he has had this same bump on his neck. She asks you why her son keeps getting the same infection. Which of the following statements concerning branchial anomalies is correct?

**A.** Treatment is complete excision of the cyst and/or sinus tract.

**B.** They do not form fistulas or sinus tracts.

**C.** Anomalies of the third and fourth branchial arches are most common.

**D.** They usually present as recurrent neck abscesses almost exclusively on the right side of the neck.

**E.** Amoxicillin is the antibiotic of choice.

**17-55.** You are the physician on call in the emergency department when the trauma pager goes off. A 12-year-old boy is brought in by emergency medical services following an unwitnessed skateboarding accident. The boy arrives intubated with a C-collar in place. As you walk into the trauma room, you notice a broken tree branch emerging from the anterior part of his neck. You also see fluid draining from the area and are concerned about an esophageal injury. What is the most appropriate next step in the management of this patient?

**A.** Magnetic resonance imaging (MRI) with contrast of the neck

**B.** Perform a secondary survey

**C.** Consult the ear, nose, and throat (ENT) specialist

**D.** Remove the foreign body

**E.** Contrast barium esophagram

**17-56.** A 4-year-old girl presents with her mother to the pediatrician's office for evaluation of a mass on her neck that has been worsening for the past 5 days. You send the eager medical student in to perform a history and physical. He reports that the patient has had fever, poor appetite, and fatigue. Mother denies recent travel, animal exposure, and weight loss. On exam, temperature is 101°F, and the patient is fussy with a mobile, tender to palpation, 4-cm erythematous mass on the right side of her neck. No other skin lesions are observed. Exam is negative for hepatosplenomegaly. Which of the following imaging modalities is the most appropriate in the initial evaluation of this patient's neck mass?

**A.** Computed tomography (CT) scan without contrast

**B.** Complete blood count (CBC)

**C.** CT scan with contrast

**D.** Ultrasound

**E.** Magnetic resonance imaging (MRI) with and without contrast

**17-57.** A 14-year-old boy with a history of asthma, allergic rhinitis, and atopic dermatitis presents with 2 days of "pink eye." Symptoms include itchy and watery eyes and runny nose. Physical exam reveals hyperemia to the tarsal and bulbar conjunctive with mild edema of the upper and lower eyelids with clear watery discharge. There is no pain with eye movement. He's been rubbing his eyes constantly because of the itching. He recently started conditioning for spring soccer. What is the most likely cause for this patient's "pink eye"?

**A.** Preseptal cellulitis

**B.** Allergic conjunctivitis

**C.** Subconjunctival hemorrhage

**D.** Bacterial conjunctivitis

**E.** Viral conjunctivitis

**17-58.** A 5-year-old boy presents with subjective hearing loss and ringing in his ear for the past month. He was recently discharged from a prolonged hospitalization for a bacterial infection. His mother read that some of the medications that were used for his treatment could cause these symptoms. You agree with her. Which of the following antibiotics is ototoxic?

**A.** Gentamicin

**B.** Ampicillin

**C.** Ciprofloxacin

**D.** Ceftriaxone

**E.** Metronidazole

**17-59.** A 3-year-old girl presents with a foreign body in her nose. Her mother reports that she was playing with an old watch and she noticed that the back was off of the watch and the battery was missing. You suspect the child placed the battery in her nose. What treatment plan do you recommend to the mother?

**A.** Wait for it to fall out on its own

**B.** See an ear, nose, and throat (ENT) specialist within the next 48 hours

**C.** Go for emergent removal of the battery

**D.** Treat with nasal rinses with saline

**E.** Treat with nasal rinses with oxymetazoline

**17-60.** During a routine well-child examination, a mother asks if her child could have a referral to ear, nose, and throat (ENT) for a preventive tonsillectomy. She read on a blog that this would prevent her child from getting sick in the future. You counsel her regarding the appropriate indications for tonsillectomy. Which of the following scenarios is an indication for a tonsillectomy?

**A.** A single episode of acute tonsillitis

**B.** Recurrent, acute tonsillitis, with 3 episodes per year for 2 years

**C.** Enlarged tonsils without obstruction or tonsillitis

**D.** Recurrent, acute tonsillitis, with > 7 episodes in 1 year

**E.** Family history of tonsillectomy

**17-61.** A 3-year-old girl presents with a lump on her neck. She was seen by her pediatrician 3 weeks ago and was diagnosed with a viral upper respiratory infection. One week ago, her mother noticed the lump on her neck getting bigger. On physical exam, she has a temperature of 101.5°F. There is a 5-cm swollen lymph node on the right side of her neck. The area is red, warm to touch, and tender to palpation. The lesion is also described as fluctuant. Diagnosis is confirmed with ultrasound. What is the most appropriate treatment for this condition?

**A.** Incision and drainage and antibiotic therapy

**B.** Reassurance

**C.** Nonsteroidal anti-inflammatory drugs (NSAIDs)

**D.** Surgical excision

**E.** Neck radiograph

## ANSWERS

**Answer 17-1. B**

Laryngomalacia is the most common cause of stridor in newborns. Its exact pathogenesis is unknown. Laryngoscopy demonstrates an omega shape of the epiglottis, and the aryepiglottic folds and false vocal cords are drawn into the laryngeal lumen. The resulting narrowing leads to high-pitched stridor, which is worse when the infant is agitated, feeding, or in the supine position. The stridor often worsens with severity over time.

In the majority of cases, laryngomalacia is benign and resolves around 12 to 18 months of age. More severe cases of laryngomalacia can result in poor growth and/or cyanotic or apneic events. In those rarer patients, supraglottoplasty (surgical trimming of the aryepiglottic folds) is recommended.

(Section 19: Disorders of the Ear, Nose, and Throat, Chapter 366: The Pharynx and Upper Airway)

**Answer 17-2. D**

This patient has a retained nasal foreign body, most likely a button battery from a toy, and should be advised to go to the ED for immediate removal.

Children often place foreign bodies in their noses without parental knowledge. This results in delayed diagnosis and classically presents with unilateral rhinorrhea and foul odor. Many intranasal foreign bodies may be removed in the office setting with appropriate preparation and equipment. However, some may require general anesthesia. Unlike other foreign bodies, button batteries are more hazardous and should be removed immediately. Local nasal damage can occur within the first hour after lodgment in the nose, and nasal septum perforation can occur within 7 hours. Nasal septum perforation has associated symptoms of foul-smelling discharge, epistaxis, and saddle nose deformity. Button batteries can be found in household items such as toys, clothing, watches, and greeting cards. Parents should be advised to keep these batteries out of reach of children.

(Section 19: Disorders of the Ear, Nose, and Throat, Chapter 365: Nose and Sinus)

**Answer 17-3.** A

Human parainfluenza virus types I and II account for most cases of croup in young children. Other causes of croup include other types of human parainfluenza virus, influenza A and B, RSV, measles, or other viruses. With an RSV infection, croup is the least common clinical manifestation. The barking cough and stridor that are associated with croup are caused by edema of the subglottic airway, specifically at the level of the cricoid cartilage where the airway is narrowest. Stridor is most common on inspiration because the negative inspiratory pressure tends to collapse already partially narrowed extrathoracic structures. Stridor on inspiration and expiration occurs only if the subglottis is extremely narrowed. The first-line treatment for croup is cool mist. At home, a cool mist vaporizer, a bathroom filled with steam from a shower, or taking the child outside in the cool night air can improve symptoms. In the hospital, treatment consists of hydration, cool mist with or without supplemental oxygen, and steroids. Prospective, randomized studies have demonstrated that steroid therapy decreases the length and severity of respiratory symptoms associated with croup. Racemic epinephrine is used in only severe cases. Most children improve in 2 to 3 days without further treatment, but some require intervention for impending respiratory failure.

(Section 19: Disorders of the Ear, Nose, and Throat, Chapter 366: The Pharynx and Upper Airway)

**Answer 17-4.** C

The child in this vignette has herpangina. Herpangina is typically caused by coxsackievirus or an echovirus, and it presents with vesicular lesions solely on the soft palate. This illness is associated with headache and quick-onset fever and usually lasts from 1 to 4 days. The best treatment is supportive care with hydration and acetaminophen for any fever or pain. The lesions usually resolve in 7 to 10 days. Because this illness is caused by a virus, amoxicillin would not be effective. Acyclovir would be a good treatment if the patient was in the prodromal period of an infection with herpetic gingivostomatitis. Herpetic lesions typically present in clusters on the gingival tissue, lips, tongue, buccal mucosa, and soft palate. This patient is well hydrated and able to tolerate oral fluids well; therefore, she would not require hospitalization for IV fluids.

(Section 20: Disorders of the Oral Cavity, Chapter 373: Oral Pathology)

**Answer 17-5.** B

This patient has a cholesteatoma and should be referred to otolaryngology for surgical excision. A cholesteatoma is an expanding epithelial-lined sac containing squamous debris, often infected with purulent discharge. It can be congenital or acquired and presents as a pearly white keratin mass seen behind an intact tympanic membrane. The most likely etiology is the embryologic retention of an epithelial cell rest, whereas acquired cholesteatomas can be the result of perforation or severe retraction of the tympanic membrane or occur at the site of insertion of a tympanostomy tube. The acquired types cause inhibition of natural epithelia migration of desquamated debris. This debris can become wet and infected, producing malodorous discharge and a mass lesion of squamous debris. Treatment involves surgical removal of the retained epithelium in the middle ear and mastoid. Oral or antibiotic treatment is not appropriate treatment because this is not a bacterial infection. He will have an abnormal tympanometry test, but this will not aid in the diagnosis. This patient warrants timely referral and treatment and will not benefit from observation or repeat hearing screening.

(Section 19: Disorders of the Ear, Nose, and Throat, Chapter 364: The Ear)

**Answer 17-6.** C

This patient's presentation is consistent with epiglottitis. Epiglottitis is caused by an infection of the epiglottis and/or its associated structures such as the supraglottis, leading to edema and inflammation. It is classically caused by *Haemophilus influenzae* type B (HIB), but due to the HIB vaccine the incidence of *H influenzae*–related epiglottitis has declined. Some other etiologic agents include *Streptococcus*, *Staphylococcus*, and *Pseudomonas* species.

The first step in management would be to administer supplemental oxygen while awaiting definitive airway management. Manipulation of the oropharynx in this child could be unsafe, potentially leading to more severe respiratory compromise and respiratory failure. Intubation should occur under controlled conditions, preferably in the operating room with skilled anesthesiologists and otolaryngologists. After the airway is secure, it would be appropriate to establish IV access, collect blood cultures, and provide IV parenteral antibiotics. Early intubation and IV antibiotics have been shown to reduce mortality significantly. A nebulized β-agonist and intramuscular steroids would not improve the patient's symptoms or improve his outcome.

(Section 8: Acute and Critical Illness, Chapter 118: Acute Upper Airway Obstruction)

**Answer 17-7.** A

Episcleritis is one of the extraintestinal findings of IBD, namely Crohn disease. Episcleritis is a self-limiting disorder, with attacks lasting up to a month and often recurring. There is a circumscribed area of redness deep to the conjunctiva, which can become elevated or nodular. No cause is usually found in children, but some children may have this disorder in combination with autoimmune systemic disease. Often in Crohn disease, episcleritis may be the only or early finding of IBD. The boy in the question stem had several nondescript symptoms that contributed to diagnosis of autoimmune disease and IBD, including episcleritis.

Viral conjunctivitis presents acutely, is often associated with upper respiratory infection, may present with preauricular or submandibular adenopathy, lymphadenopathy, conjunctival edema, discomfort, mild photophobia, or small subconjunctival hemorrhages. Our patient did not have upper respiratory infection symptoms or lymph nodes mentioned in the clinical stem, and the fact that it seems recurrent also does not go along with viral conjunctivitis.

Hyphema results from blunt trauma to the globe and surrounding tissues; injury to the globe may vary from periorbital ecchymosis to rupture of the globe. There was no history of trauma to the eye in the clinical vignette, so hyphema is less likely the correct diagnosis.

Trachoma is responsible for about 3% of cases of blindness worldwide, with approximately 1.3 million people worldwide blind from trachoma. Eighty-four million people have active trachoma infection. Trachoma is caused by *C trachomatis* serovars A, B, and C, which spread through contact with eye discharge from the infected person (eg, on towels, handkerchiefs, fingers) and through transmission by eye-seeking flies. It is associated with poverty and unsanitary living conditions. There is no history of contagious infections of the eye the patient may have been exposed to or flies that could have transmitted infection.

Bacterial conjunctivitis is caused by many bacteria, including *Staphylococcus aureus, Moraxella,* streptococci, *Clostridium diphtheriae,* and *Haemophilus,* among others. It often will result in mucopurulent discharge that will pass from eye to eye. The patient in the clinical question did not have eye discharge, itchiness, or other findings of bacterial conjunctivitis. In addition, the fact that his symptoms did not clear completely with antibiotic drops suggests the conjunctivitis is not infectious.

(Section 21: Disorders of the Gastrointestinal System, Chapter 405: Inflammatory Bowel Disease)

**Answer 17-8.** B

Antibacterial eye drops for confirmed mucopurulent bacterial conjunctivitis would be appropriate, but not in the clinical diagnosis of viral conjunctivitis. Bacterial conjunctivitis is typically more purulent than viral conjunctivitis and becomes bilateral within a very short period. It is a common disorder in young children, and typical organisms include *Streptococcus pneumoniae, Moraxella,* and nontypeable *Haemophilus influenzae.* Our patient's eye symptoms took 3 days to move to the other eye; in bacterial conjunctivitis, it likely would have taken hours to 1 day to move to the other eye. Bacterial conjunctivitis usually does not have the associated symptoms of cough, upper respiratory symptoms, or lymphadenopathy.

The most common infectious cause of conjunctivitis is viral, most often due to adenoviruses. There may be an associated upper respiratory tract infection. Viral conjunctivitis is highly contagious and spreads by eye-to-hand contact. Parents are advised to use a separate hand towel for their child and to wash their hands after touching the child's eye, hands, or secretions. The cornea may be affected, initially with a fine, diffusely spread, punctate epithelial disturbance, followed by subepithelial infiltrates. Both can produce photophobia. Viral conjunctivitis is typically self-limited and can last from a few days to 4 weeks or more. If the course is prolonged, the condition is most likely epidemic keratoconjunctivitis, due to adenovirus serotypes. Viral conjunctivitis often begins with unilateral involvement and becomes bilateral after a few days. There is often a swollen preauricular or submandibular lymph node. Other viruses that can cause conjunctivitis include coxsackieviruses, echoviruses, and even herpes simplex virus. It may be appropriate to seek ophthalmology consultation, because photophobia with corneal pathology may require specialized treatment. With the other symptoms listed (preauricular lymphadenopathy, upper respiratory symptoms, and timing), the most likely diagnosis is viral conjunctivitis. Therefore, the patient's condition does not warrant treatment at this time, other than observation to see if it will be self-limiting.

Steroid eye drops are not indicated, except in the most severe cases, and then only under the care of an ophthalmologist, who must exclude herpes simplex keratitis and monitor for steroid-induced side effects. The ophthalmologist would perform a slit-lamp exam to monitor for side effects of steroids once treatment was started and would be able to visualize a corneal ulcer upon exam and determine the correct treatment. Prescribing steroids without being able to monitor side effects would not be clinical standard of care for a pediatric patient.

Topical anesthetic drops would be helpful only in displacing a foreign body that may have gotten into the eye. Our patient did not have a listed history of trauma to the eye in recent days; in addition, the eye redness moved to the other eye. Thus, topical anesthetic drops would not be the right answer.

$H_1$ antagonist/mast cell inhibitor drops are prescribed for allergic conjunctivitis. Allergic conjunctivitis is common and typically seasonal, being worse in spring and summer. It is often accompanied by nasal congestion (rhinoconjunctivitis). It is also known as "hay fever" conjunctivitis and represents a type I hypersensitivity response to a seasonal allergen. The itching is usually far more conspicuous than in infectious conjunctivitis. The patient in the clinical question has itchy eyes, but the sclerae are red instead of the conjunctiva; his eyelids are not reported as swollen. He has lymphadenopathy, which is not typically present in allergic conjunctivitis. Finally, his symptoms occurred in winter, which is not associated with seasonal allergy time, and are not repeatedly occurring.

(Section 30: Disorders of the Eyes, Chapter 578: Red Eye)

**Answer 17-9.** C

Choanal atresia occurs when the posterior nasal cavity fails to communicate with the nasopharynx. It may be unilateral or bilateral, most commonly occurs on the right side, and usually is a mixed bony and membranous atresia. Infants born with complete bilateral choanal atresia present with respiratory distress. Cyclic cyanotic events broken by crying are common occurrences. Acute management includes opening the mouth using an oral airway. Gavage feedings may be necessary due to feeding difficulties because the infant is unable to coordinate breathing, sucking, and swallowing without an adequate nasal airway. Some infants will require intubation until the atresia is surgically repaired. Unilateral choanal atresia is twice as common as bilateral choanal atresia, but symptoms are less obvious; therefore, diagnosis may be delayed. Traditionally, an attempt is made to pass an 8-French catheter through both nasal cavities at birth; passage of the catheter rules out complete choanal atresia but does not guarantee adequate nasal airflow. Nasal obstruction warrants further evaluation, including endoscopy and, in cases of complete obstruction, a computed tomography (CT) scan. Bilateral choanal atresia is associated with other congenital abnormalities in 50% of patients. It is most frequently associated with CHARGE syndrome (coloboma, heart disease, atresia choanae, retarded development of the nervous system, genital hypoplasia, and ear anomalies or deafness), although it is also seen with polydactyly, Crouzon syndrome, craniosynostosis, microencephaly, meningocele, facial asymmetry, cleft palate, hypertelorism, and nasal and auricular deformities.

Tracheotomy may very well be warranted in the future, but doing so emergently leaves a lot of room for error. Often, this is done to allow the facial bones to grow in preparation of choanal atresia repair as patients would have to have an artificial airway for a long time. Many of these children may just require repair of the choanal atresia without having to intubate. Observation in a code situation would not help this infant who is currently desaturating and has a low heart rate. Intubation would be the correct intervention in this situation to stabilize the airway and help the infant oxygenate. If an oropharyngeal airway is placed and the oxygen saturations are not increasing, then a non-rebreather will not work due to structural defects. Gavage feeding may very well be needed (in this case, orally) in the future, but the airway needs to be stabilized first.

(Section 19: Disorders of the Ear, Nose, and Throat, Chapter 365: Nose and Sinus)

**Answer 17-10.** D

The adenoids are located behind the nasal cavity in the roof and posterior wall of the nasopharynx, just above and behind the uvula. Due to their location, they are difficult to examine. Adenoid hypertrophy or chronic adenoiditis may contribute to sinonasal disease. Adenoids consist of lymphoid tissue and are present early in life, with growth continuing until about 4 to 10 years of age, followed by regression in size by adolescence. Adenoid hypertrophy can be evaluated with a lateral neck radiograph or by endoscopy, whereas chronic adenoiditis is diagnosed based on symptoms and may occur without adenoid enlargement. Nasal obstruction, mouth breathing, and persistent nasal congestion or discharge in the child who "always seems to have a cold" may indicate chronic adenoiditis. Adenoidectomy is indicated for chronic adenoiditis, adenoid hypertrophy with upper airway obstruction, and, selectively, chronic middle ear disease and chronic sinusitis. There is no mention of mouth breathing or the fact that she has recurrent upper respiratory infections in the child presented in the vignette.

GERD is unlikely because this patient eats a healthy diet and would not have any clinical reason to have GERD. In addition, no other GERD symptoms are mentioned such as spitting up, vomiting, abdominal pain, or intolerance of food. No evidence of enamel breakdown on teeth per dental exam is mentioned as well.

Sinusitis may be in the differential, but the history of one nostril with drainage and no recurrence or other symptoms mentioned makes it less of a possibility. Sinusitis would usually present with fever and mucopurulent drainage. In addition, due to anatomic differences in children versus adults, sinusitis would not usually present in a 5-year-old child because their sinuses are still developing.

A nasal foreign body in this case is the most likely diagnosis. With the unilateral nasal drainage, her halitosis is most likely caused by postnasal drip from inflammation surrounding the foreign body. Upon exam, if it can be seen (eg, if it is the father's ear plugs for when he is on an airplane for work), it can be taken out with nasal forceps. Assistance from otolaryngology may be warranted in this case.

Dental caries are usually found by a good dental exam. Radiographs may be needed to detect small caries. Still, good dental hygiene and flossing often prevent halitosis. The child in the question actually does have appropriate oral hygiene measures in place; thus, dental caries are less likely to be the cause of halitosis.

(Section 19: Disorders of the Ear, Nose, and Throat, Chapter 365: Nose and Sinus)

**Answer 17-11.** E

Ofloxacin otic drops belong to the fluoroquinolone class of drops, as do ciprofloxacin drops, so a drug from the same class may not make much progress in treatment of the otitis externa described in the clinical vignette. Acetic acid/alcohol drops are available in a pharmacy to help prevent otitis externa. The alcohol dries the ear of remnants of pool water, and the acetic acid returns the ear environment back to a neutral pH; the chlorine in the swimming pool makes the pH too basic. However, when there is already an active infection, these drops would not make much of a difference. Oral antibiotics would not typically be active against the usual bacteria and fungi responsible for otitis externa; these bacteria and fungi include *Staphylococcus aureus*, *Pseudomonas aeruginosa*, and *Candida albicans*. However, amoxicillin-clavulanic acid is often effective against otitis media, which is usually caused by *Streptococcus pneumoniae, Haemophilus influenzae,* or *Moraxella catarrhalis.* Stopping swimming may lessen future infections, but it is a lifestyle choice and is more advisable to find a way to continue doing the patient's activity because it is important for personal development. However, the patient may need to stop inserting cotton-tipped applicators so deeply and to just clean the outer ear. Because fluoroquinolone drops were not effective, the other thought is that this may be a fungal infection or candidiasis of the outer ear; thus, trying antifungal treatment would be appropriate.

(Section 19: Disorders of the Ear, Nose, and Throat, Chapter 364: The Ear)

**Answer 17-12. B**

Ototoxicity is defined as damage to the inner ear. The manifestations of ototoxicity can include hearing loss, tinnitus, and vestibulopathy, with different drugs causing one or more of these symptoms depending on the pharmacologic properties of the particular drug. For many drugs, ototoxicity is a well-known risk, and the benefits of treatment must be weighed against the risks of their use to the inner ear.

A child taking regular doses of an aminoglycoside, such as tobramycin or gentamicin, can definitely be at high risk for hearing loss due to ototoxicity. Otic drops such as fluoroquinolone drops to treat otitis media that has ruptured or otitis externa would not increase the risk of hearing loss due to the medication's effect on the inner ear. Aspirin is a salicylate that can cause ototoxicity that is reversible if caught early; signs are tinnitus, hearing loss, and disequilibrium. Cisplatin can affect the cochlear hair cells and can cause high-frequency hearing loss. Premature infants who spent time in the neonatal intensive care unit (NICU) often were treated with antibiotics routinely for suspected sepsis, meningitis, or pneumonias; many of these antibiotics are ototoxic. All of the patients described should have routine hearing screening due to their history.

(Section 19: Disorders of the Ear, Nose, and Throat, Chapter 364: The Ear)

**Answer 17-13. C**

The otoscopic exam shows a unilateral serous middle ear effusion. Antibiotic therapy is not indicated. The serous effusion could have been caused by the recent upper respiratory infection. A hemotympanum is the presence of blood in the tympanic cavity of the middle ear. A hemotympanum, not a serous effusion, is associated with trauma. The child is afebrile, has good speech, and has not had recurrent ear infections. Myringotomy tube insertion is not indicated.

(Section 19: Disorders of the Ear, Nose, and Throat, Chapter 364: The Ear)

**Answer 17-14. D**

Acute bacterial rhinosinusitis should be suspected with the history of worsening symptoms of fever, nasal congestion, and rhinorrhea. With acute-onset eye swelling, an orbital complication should be suspected. CT scan with IV contrast of the orbit/sinus/maxillofacial tissues is the next step.

(Section 19: Disorders of the Ear, Nose, and Throat, Chapter 365: Nose and Sinus)

**Answer 17-15. B**

The patient has a history consistent with foreign body aspiration. Typically, a CXR can be ordered to assist in the diagnosis, and bronchodilators can be initiated with a history of asthma. However, the patient is in respiratory distress, so foreign body removal should be done without delay.

(Section 19: Disorders of the Ear, Nose, and Throat, Chapter 366: The Pharynx and Upper Airway)

**Answer 17-16. A**

The midline neck mass represents a thyroglossal duct cyst, which forms as a result of the interruption of the normal descent of the thyroid gland, with persistence of the thyroglossal duct. A goiter is an abnormal enlargement of the thyroid gland. Lack of iodine is a common cause of goiter worldwide. In the United States, the more common causes of childhood goiter are chronic autoimmune thyroiditis (Hashimoto thyroiditis) and colloid goiter.

(Section 19: Disorders of the Ear, Nose, and Throat, Chapter 368: Head and Neck Masses)

**Answer 17-17. B**

The patient has a history consistent with recurrent/persistent acute otitis externa (AOE). She has failed appropriate topical otic drops, and so an ear culture is the next appropriate step. Oral or IV antibiotics are not typically needed for uncomplicated AOE, unless there is associated cellulitis of the auricle or postauricular area. Amoxicillin is less likely to cover the organisms most associated with AOE (*Pseudomonas* species). Myringotomy tubes are indicated for recurrent acute otitis media or persistent middle ear effusion. A CT scan would be indicated if there are concerns for tympanic and intracranial complications. Referral for aural suctioning would also be considered.

(Section 19: Disorders of the Ear, Nose, and Throat, Chapter 364: The Ear)

**Answer 17-18. A**

This child has a history consistent with viral laryngotracheobronchitis or croup. Of the choices, airway narrowing will occur at the level of the subglottis. Biphasic stridor is characteristic of severe fixed subglottic narrowing.

(Section 19: Disorders of the Ear, Nose, and Throat, Chapter 366: The Pharynx and Upper Airway)

**Answer 17-19.** D

Speech delay can be one of the first signs of hearing loss. An assessment of hearing is the best choice. At 2 years old, the child should have a broader vocabulary and should be using 2-word sentences, so observation is not appropriate. There is no history of ear infections and no fluid behind the ears, so myringotomy tube placement is not warranted. A child should have an audiogram showing severe to profound hearing loss and a trial of hearing aids prior to consideration of cochlear implant.

(Section 19: Disorders of the Ear, Nose, and Throat, Chapter 364: The Ear)

**Answer 17-20.** D

The patient has a classic presentation of a peritonsillar abscess. She has full neck range of motion and peritonsillar swelling, so a retropharyngeal abscess is less likely. EBV infection usually results in bilateral tonsillar swelling with gray exudates. The tonsillar fossa is a second branchial pouch derivative, but the presentation represents a peritonsillar abscess and not a branchial cleft cyst. Mastoiditis occurs when a middle ear infection spreads to the area of the skull behind the ear, specifically the mastoid process in the temporal bone. Mastoiditis is unlikely with a normal ear examination and no ear symptoms.

(Section 19: Disorders of the Ear, Nose, and Throat, Chapter 366: The Pharynx and Upper Airway)

**Answer 17-21.** B

Newborn infants are obligate nasal breathers, so nasal obstruction can cause significant airway distress. The inability to pass an 8-French catheter is suspicious for a bilateral choanal atresia, although other forms of nasal obstruction can be associated with this finding. Observation is not appropriate, as the condition will not improve over time. In a patient who has respiratory distress and suspected nasal obstruction, the next best step is to insert an oral airway. Insertion of an oral airway should precede endotracheal intubation. A nasal decongestant can be a temporizing measure but is less appropriate in a patient with respiratory distress.

(Section 19: Disorders of the Ear, Nose, and Throat, Chapter 365: Nose and Sinus)

**Answer 17-22.** C

This child has a history of mouth breathing and nasal obstruction. The history and physical examination are not consistent with allergic rhinitis. With the anterior nasal airway appearing clear, consideration should be given to adenoid hypertrophy. A lateral neck CXR can be diagnostic. Without an obvious history of apneic events and due to the small tonsils, a tonsillectomy would not be appropriate.

(Section 19: Disorders of the Ear, Nose, and Throat, Chapter 366: The Pharynx and Upper Airway)

**Answer 17-23.** C

This 2-month-old presents with signs concerning for primary (isolated) congenital glaucoma. Early clinical manifestations of congenital glaucoma include tearing, blepharospasms (frequent blinking), light sensitivity, corneal clouding, and corneal enlargement. The eyeball can become enlarged due to increased intraocular pressure. Eighty percent of those with primary congenital glaucoma are diagnosed within the first year of life, with 10% diagnosed at birth. Congenital glaucoma causes 2% to 15% of blindness in children. Vision prognosis is directly linked to early diagnosis and treatment, which often entails prompt surgical treatment. Therefore, any child with an abnormal reflex or concerns for glaucoma requires prompt evaluation by an ophthalmologist. The other answer choices can lead to delayed ophthalmologic evaluation. Lacrimal duct stenosis (answer choice B) and conjunctivitis (answer choice E) are not associated with an abnormal red reflex. Steroid ophthalmic drops (answer choice D) can potentially increase intraocular pressure, which would worsen this child's glaucoma.

(Section 30: Disorders of the Eyes, Chapter 580: Anterior Segment Disorders)

**Answer 17-24.** B

This child has signs concerning for a cholesteatoma. A cholesteatoma is an expanding, epithelial-lined sac of squamous debris that forms behind an intact membrane. They can be congenital or acquired. Acquired cholesteatomas can form after chronic negative middle ear pressure causes an area of the tympanic membrane to weaken and retract, often in the attic region superior to the short process of the malleolus. Patients may have a history of chronic otorrhea. Cholesteatomas expand and can cause erosion of the ossicles and/or labyrinth, leading to hearing loss and disequilibrium. Treatment involves surgical removal of the cholesteatoma. Given the natural progression, risk of complications, and need for surgery, prompt referral to an otolaryngologist is warranted. Therefore, the most appropriate answer is referral to otolaryngology for evaluation and surgical treatment.

(Section 19: Disorders of the Ear, Nose, and Throat, Chapter 364: The Ear)

**Answer 17-25.** C

The most likely cause of this infant's stridor is laryngomalacia. Laryngomalacia is the most common cause of stridor in the neonate. Infantile laryngeal cartilage is very flexible and allows the lumen of the larynx to narrow during inspiration. The stridor often occurs several weeks after birth and increases in severity, although the stridor is sometimes present at birth. Stridor can worsen with agitation, during feeds, and in the supine position and can improve or resolve in prone or side-lying position and when the child is relaxed. Other causes of stridor must be ruled out. Laryngomalacia typically self-resolves by 12 to 18 months when the laryngeal cartilage has become stiffer. In rare cases, severe laryngomalacia can cause oxygen desaturation during sleep or failure to thrive and may need surgical management.

(Section 19: Disorders of the Ear, Nose, and Throat, Chapter 366: The Pharynx and Upper Airway)

**Answer 17-26.** D

This child presents with nasal polyps. She has chronic congestion and airway obstruction by history, and symptoms have not improved with treatments used to alleviate allergic rhinitis, another possible cause of chronic nasal congestion. Furthermore, her exam reveals grayish, gelatinous masses characteristic of nasal polyps. Polyps typically are seen extending from the middle meatus. Nasal polyps generally are a rare finding prior to adolescence; the exception is in children with cystic fibrosis (CF). Approximately 15% to 20% of patients with CF can have nasal polyps, which can present at the end of the first or during the second decade of life and can be the first sign of CF. Not only does this child have nasal polyps, but she also falls within low anthropometric percentiles, further raising suspicion for malabsorption disorder as seen in CF-related pancreatic insufficiency. She should undergo a sweat chloride test, which is the primary diagnostic test for CF.

(Section 19: Disorders of the Ear, Nose, and Throat, Chapter 365: Nose and Sinus, Section 27: Disorders of the Respiratory System, Chapter 507: Cystic Fibrosis)

**Answer 17-27.** D

This child has signs and symptoms of a second branchial cleft anomaly. Branchial cleft anomalies sometimes present at birth as an asymptomatic sinus, fistula opening, or cyst along the anterolateral aspect of the neck. Other times, they are not noticed until they become secondarily infected later on (as seen with this patient). Infection and painful enlargement of cysts are often associated with an upper respiratory infection. Of all the branchial cleft anomalies, second branchial anomalies are the most common; they typically are located on the lateral neck along the border of the sternomastoid muscle. Although this patient may benefit from antibiotics while the cyst is secondarily infected, definitive treatment of branchial cleft anomalies involves complete excision of the cyst and/or sinus tract.

(Section 19: Disorders of the Ear, Nose, and Throat, Chapter 367: The Head, Face, and Neck)

**Answer 17-28.** D

Based on the history and physical exam, this child likely has bilateral choanal atresia/stenosis. The fact that his oxygen saturations improve when he cries speaks to his ability to breathe better orally, whereas neonates are otherwise obligate nasal breathers. However, he is still in respiratory distress, and high-flow nasal cannula oxygen will likely not provide adequate oxygen supplementation because he has nasal obstruction. Although an 8-French catheter may rule out choanal atresia in a neonate, an adequate nasal airway is no smaller than the size of a 5- or 6-French catheter. Therefore, because he is unable to have a 5-French catheter completely pass through either side of the nose and due to his other findings, we can assume that his nasal obstruction is his major issue.

The first step in the management of patients with airway obstruction is to secure the airway by bypassing the obstruction. In this case, because choanal atresia/stenosis is highly suspected, he should be intubated. Further evaluation with imaging or endoscopy by ENT should only occur secondary to stabilization of the patient. Because this child was born at term and otherwise had routine prenatal care, we can assume that he does not need anesthesia or ENT assistance for intubation. Finally, any attempts at serial dilation should be reserved for the operating room because bedside intervention could lead to bleeding or trauma from the catheter and further complications.

(Section 19: Disorders of the Ear, Nose, and Throat, Chapter 365: Nose and Sinus)

**Answer 17-29.** B

Based on the history and the positive Furstenberg sign (compression of the jugular veins or crying that results in temporary swelling of the nasal mass), this child likely has an encephalocele. The best way to diagnose an intracranial connection from the mass through the foramen cecum is with an MRI skull base scan. It would not be wise to biopsy the mass without first ruling out the intracranial connection, as this could lead to the introduction of bacteria into the cerebrospinal fluid (CSF) or even damage to the brain contents. Ultrasound with or without evaluating blood flow through the mass will not be sufficient to diagnose an intracranial connection. Although a CT scan of the skull base (with 1-mm slices) could give information about the bony structure in this area, a CT neck scan will not be helpful in this case. Finally, there is no indication as of yet to involve ophthalmology based on the history, but imaging may give you more information once performed.

(Section 19: Disorders of the Ear, Nose, and Throat, Chapter 365: Nose and Sinus)

**Answer 17-30.** C

Juvenile nasopharyngeal angiofibromas are aggressive but benign masses that most commonly occur in the nasopharynx of adolescent males. These typically present with unilateral epistaxis and nasal obstruction in this group of children, but symptoms of facial edema, proptosis, and cerebrospinal fluid (CSF) rhinorrhea can signify more extensive disease. If visualized on physical exam, these masses should not be biopsied due to their high vascularity and risk of significant bleeding. Management often includes preoperative embolization followed by surgical excision; however, significant or unresectable disease is sometimes managed with radiotherapy to try to limit further growth of the mass.

(Section 19: Disorders of the Ear, Nose, and Throat, Chapter 365: Nose and Sinus)

**Answer 17-31.** C

Based on the clinical vignette, the child appears to have a left otitis externa. When treating otitis externa, there are 3 main strategies for treatment. The first is to remove the infected debris but only if this can be done safely and effectively. The second is to treat the infection with antibiotics, making sure that the otic drops can reach the site of infection. Third, the patient should avoid getting water in the affected ear as this could promote further infection.

In this scenario, cotton-tipped swabs should be avoided as they are not an effective tool for removing otorrhea and they may also cause more trauma to the ear canal skin, which would only propagate the infection. Instead, it is sometimes required that the debris be suctioned out under microscopic visualization because this is a safer alternative. In regard to answer choice B, mastoiditis is a clinical diagnosis and can be ruled out based on the lack of findings on history and exam. Therefore, a CT temporal bone scan is not needed at this time. Contrary to answer choice D, a wick may actually be helpful for this patient to ensure that the otic drops are effectively reaching the infected tissue since ear canal edema can often be a barrier to adequate treatment. Finally, a culture of the infected otorrhea can be helpful (especially in resistant infections), but a contralateral culture is not needed for comparison.

(Section 19: Disorders of the Ear, Nose, and Throat, Chapter 364: The Ear)

**Answer 17-32.** B

Jervell and Lange-Nielsen syndrome is an autosomal recessive condition associated with profound bilateral sensorineural hearing loss and cardiac arrhythmias. These children may present with syncopal episodes due to the QT prolongation often seen on ECG.

Branchio-oto-renal syndrome is an autosomal dominant condition associated with several characteristics for which the syndrome is named. These children may present with branchial anomalies seen as bilateral preauricular pits or skin tags as well as branchial anomalies in the neck. They will often have associated conductive, sensorineural, or mixed hearing loss. Finally, developmental abnormalities of the kidneys are often seen, and a renal ultrasound is warranted in the workup.

An MRI of the brain may be appropriate when a child is suspected to have a neurologic deficit, and an MRI temporal bone scan can be appropriate in children with asymmetrical sensorineural hearing loss to rule out a tumor compressing the cochlear nerve. However, a child with Jervell and Lange-Nielsen syndrome does not generally need an MRI of the brain on initial evaluation.

Pendred syndrome is an autosomal recessive condition commonly associated with severe to profound sensorineural hearing loss and the development of a thyroid goiter, which is an enlargement in the thyroid gland. A thyroid ultrasound is helpful to identify and monitor the size of these goiters as the patient grows.

Urinalysis would not be helpful in confirming the diagnosis of Jervell and Lange-Nielsen syndrome during the initial workup.

(Section 19: Disorders of the Ear, Nose, and Throat, Chapter 364: The Ear)

**Answer 17-33.** E

Based on the history and exam in this scenario, this child appears to have a cholesteatoma. A cholesteatoma is a benign mass that develops in the ear due to an accumulation of desquamated epithelium. This squamous debris often becomes infected and propagates inflammation. Some by-products of this process, such as inflammatory cytokines and proteinases, can have a destructive effect on surrounding structures, leading to erosion of the ossicles or dehiscence of the tegmen tympani (skull base).

There are 3 types of middle ear cholesteatomas that arise by different mechanisms but can be equally destructive. Congenital cholesteatomas are thought to arise during embryologic development as an epithelial rest of cells becomes trapped within the middle ear. These often present in preschool- or elementary-age children. Primary cholesteatomas commonly occur after trauma to the eardrum or even multiple ear tube surgeries as the epithelium is thought to heal in a way that it affects the normal migration of epithelium. Finally, a third type of cholesteatoma is the secondary cholesteatoma, which is likely what this child has. These tend to occur in the pars flaccida (posterior-superior region of the tympanic membrane) where the eardrum is weakest. Chronic negative pressure from eustachian tube dysfunction leads to the development of a deep retraction pocket. This becomes a site for accumulation of moisture and desquamated epithelial debris, which by definition is a cholesteatoma.

In the situation presented in this vignette, attempts at completely clearing the debris from the retraction pocket are not advised because removal of debris could accidentally dislocate the ossicles because these masses are often intimately involved with the surrounding structures. However, observation is also not advised because this will only allow more time for the disease process to progress. Treatment with oral antibiotics and/or otic drops may temporarily resolve the otorrhea, but the infection is likely to persist, and this would only delay definitive treatment. Unfortunately, cholesteatomas often go a long time before being diagnosed, so it is not uncommon that these children will present after several months of otherwise benign-appearing symptoms. Therefore, a referral to child protective services in this case is not necessary. Instead, definitive treatment requires surgical excision with a tympanoplasty and mastoidectomy whereby all of the epithelium is removed from the middle ear space, after which time the hearing reconstruction can then be performed.

(Section 19: Disorders of the Ear, Nose, and Throat, Chapter 364: The Ear)

**Answer 17-34.** A

Based on this clinical vignette, there is a high suspicion that this child has a thyroglossal duct cyst. The workup of a midline neck mass is often different than that of a lateral neck mass in children. Thyroglossal duct cysts make up the large majority of midline neck masses in children, and the finding on exam that the mass moves vertically with swallowing is significant.

During embryologic development, the thyroid gland descends from the base of the tongue (at the foramen cecum) to its normal location in the neck. The sac that contains the glandular tissue should obliterate by the second trimester but sometimes does not. In this case, when a tract persists, it can often become symptomatic later in childhood, leading to infection with swelling and pain in the midline neck. Answer choice A is the next best step in this scenario because this will help identify that the mass is in fact a cyst and it will also confirm the presence of normal thyroid tissue so that accidental surgical excision of an ectopic thyroid does not lead to hypothyroidism. Definitive treatment includes surgical excision. Because these masses are cysts, the likelihood that they will resolve on their own after any amount of time is low. In regard to answer choice D, the scenario does not likely represent an atypical mycobacterial infection given the location and presenting symptoms. Finally, although a thyroglossal duct cyst is a congenital midline mass, it is not necessary to explore the chest anatomy unless there is separate concern for a mediastinal process.

(Section 19: Disorders of the Ear, Nose, and Throat, Chapter 368: Head and Neck Masses)

**Answer 17-35.** B

Sialorrhea (or ptyalism) is a condition that can significantly affect neurologically impaired children because they often do not have the coordination to effectively control their salivary secretions. This can lead to significant social and health problems like recurrent aspiration pneumonias, such as in this patient. Anticholinergic medications are a first-line therapy because they tend to be a conservative option. However, they can also have side effects, and increasing this class of drugs beyond the maximum dosage can be dangerous.

A slightly more invasive approach is the injection of onabotulinumtoxinA into the major salivary glands. This can usually be done at the bedside under moderate sedation or in the operating room. The onabotulinumtoxinA will generally start working within a couple of days until reaching a peak after a couple of weeks. The effects tend to wear off by 3 months, which is why repeat injections are often performed at 3-month intervals. However, there are generally no major concerns with repeat injections at 3-month intervals.

The next more invasive treatment of sialorrhea in these children involves surgically excising the submandibular glands and ligating the parotid ducts. This will effectively decrease the salivary production but not stop it completely. Therefore, answer choice B is the best option in this question; however, tracheostomy should be considered as well in these children to provide the function of "pulmonary toilet" whereby continued aspiration is more easily managed and the secretions can be suctioned to prevent recurrent pneumonias.

(Section 19: Disorders of the Ear, Nose, and Throat, Chapter 366: The Pharynx and Upper Airway)

**Answer 17-36.** B

Based on the clinical vignette, this child has a penetrating trauma to the soft palate of the oropharynx that is fairly midline. You should complete your own neurologic exam including evaluation of the cranial nerves and gross motor function. However, further imaging with a CT neck angiogram or a carotid duplex scan is not necessary (nor is a neurology consult at this time) because the injury was not lateral within the tonsillar bed and there are no neurologic deficits. Answer choice B is correct because improper healing of this injury could lead to a palatal fistula, resulting in oronasal reflux during swallowing and speech disarticulation issues. The risk of a delayed embolic event is more likely when the injury is lateral within the oropharynx, but even observation overnight may not identify such an event because these can occur up to 3 days after the injury.

(Section 19: Disorders of the Ear, Nose, and Throat, Chapter 366: The Pharynx and Upper Airway)

**Answer 17-37.** D

This child likely has a laryngeal fracture, which can present in several ways. Depending on the initial injury, the laryngeal airway may only have mild edema or may have complete tracheal separation. The rapid progression in this child is worrisome because she already has edema or a hematoma contributing to her hoarseness. However, the onset of anxiety is generally a sign of carbon dioxide retention due to poor ventilation from airway obstruction. Medications such as benzodiazepines in this scenario are contraindicated due to their effect of respiratory depression. Furthermore, it would not be wise to send her to the CT scanner when she is unstable like this because she will be more isolated from access to immediate care if the situation worsens. She is not in cardiac arrest at this time, so CPR is not warranted. The best next step is to provide her with medical therapy such as oxygen, steroids, and racemic epinephrine until surgical evaluation for a possible tracheostomy can be completed. Intubation in a patient with a laryngeal injury is often not advised because this can lead to further laryngotracheal injury or accidental wrong placement of the endotracheal tube.

(Section 19: Disorders of the Ear, Nose, and Throat, Chapter 367: The Head, Face, and Neck)

**Answer 17-38.** C

Blunt trauma to the auricle is a common injury sustained during athletic activities and routine childhood play. These injuries are best prevented with the routine use of bike helmets and sports-specific head protection. Because of the thin skin covering and delicate perichondrium, hematomas and seromas of the auricle are frequent findings. When undiagnosed or untreated, these injuries can result in auricular cartilage damage and auricular deformity. Appropriate treatment consists of drainage of the fluid collection and subsequent application of a pressure dressing to prevent reaccumulation of fluid. The child should be reevaluated at close intervals for signs of perichondritis.

(Section 19: Disorders of the Ear, Nose, and Throat, Chapter 364: The Ear)

**Answer 17-39.** E

Childhood glaucoma is an uncommon eye disease but an important cause of blindness. Primary congenital glaucoma is caused by abnormal development of the aqueous humor drainage system. It occurs in about 1 in 10,000 births in the United States and is the most common form of glaucoma in infants. Secondary glaucoma results from other disorders of the eye and may or may not be genetic; these include cataract surgery, trauma, and uveitis. Both types may be associated with other medical conditions. Ten percent of primary congenital glaucoma is present at birth, and 80% is diagnosed during the first year of life. The first signs of glaucoma include clouding or enlargement of the cornea. The elevated intraocular pressure can cause the eyeball to enlarge, with injury to the inner layers of the cornea (Haab striae). Important early symptoms of glaucoma in infants and children are blepharospasm (frequent blinking), light sensitivity, and tearing. The prognosis for vision is directly related to early recognition and treatment and to the severity at presentation.

Many patients will require surgery, with the goal of reducing pressure either by increasing the outflow of fluid from the eye or decreasing the production of fluid within the eye. Goniotomy and trabeculotomy are important surgical procedures that open the natural drainage mechanism (the trabecular meshwork) of the eye.

(Section 30: Disorders of the Eye, Chapter 580: Anterior Segment Disorders)

**Answer 17-40.** E

Topical treatment of neonatal conjunctivitis is not recommended because local eye treatment does not prevent or clear nasopharyngeal carriage and thus results in further risk of developing pneumonia or repeated episodes of conjunctivitis. Therefore, treatment with oral erythromycin for 14 days is appropriate.

(Section 30: Disorders of the Eye, Chapter 578: Red Eye)

**Answer 17-41.** A

*C trachomatis* is the most common cause of neonatal conjunctivitis. Acute purulent chlamydial conjunctivitis in the newborn has an incubation period from 5 to 12 days. There is a watery discharge from the eyes that becomes progressively more purulent, with swelling of the eyelids if left untreated. Patients can develop membranous conjunctivitis that can last up to months. The conjunctivitis should be distinguished from other bacterial infections (*Neisseria gonorrhoeae* and *Staphylococcus aureus*) and from chemical conjunctivitis resulting from silver nitrate prophylaxis. Gonococcal conjunctivitis typically occurs in the first 2 to 5 days after birth, whereas chlamydia conjunctivitis occurs later, but it may be difficult to distinguish between the two clinically.

(Section 30: Disorders of the Eye, Chapter 578: Red Eye)

**Answer 17-42.** D

Infectious conjunctivitis with all of the organisms listed is possible, but viral conjunctivitis is the most common infectious conjunctivitis in children, with adenovirus occurring the most often. Viral conjunctivitis is highly contagious, usually starts as unilateral involvement with spread to bilateral involvement after a few days, and can last from a few days to a few weeks. Bacterial conjunctivitis is typically more purulent than viral conjunctivitis and becomes bilateral quickly. Conjunctivitis caused by *Chlamydia* is a more common cause of conjunctivitis in newborns.

(Section 30: Disorders of the Eye, Chapter 578: Red Eye)

**Answer 17-43.** B

Nonallergic rhinitis and allergic rhinitis can have similar presentations, and although they often coexist, allergy testing can help provide further information on a possible trigger for this patient's symptoms that should be avoided. Although viral upper respiratory infection is the most common case of rhinorrhea in children, the length of symptoms (> 1 year) makes bacterial or viral pathogens an unlikely cause of all of this patient's symptoms. CT of the sinuses may be necessary but is not the most appropriate initial test. CBC and CRP would provide nonspecific information in this case.

(Section 19: Disorders of the Ear, Nose, and Throat, Chapter 365: Nose and Sinus)

**Answer 17-44.** A

This patient has the classic triad of Klippel-Feil syndrome: short webbed neck, low posterior hairline, and limited mobility of the cervical spine. Klippel-Feil syndrome is a spectrum of abnormalities secondary to congenital fusion of the cervical spine. The classic triad only occurs in 40% to 50% of patients. Klippel-Feil syndrome has also been associated with an elevated scapula (in ~30% of patients), congenital scoliosis (in ~60%), cardiac abnormalities (ventricular septal defect most commonly), hearing impairment, neural axis abnormalities (eg, Chiari malformations or tethered cord), and urologic abnormalities. Atlantoaxial instability is a concern for patients with Down syndrome, but this patient does not present with other phenotypic features consistent with Down syndrome.

Absence of C5 would not fully explain the patient's clinical presentation. Cervical kyphosis may be present in conjunction with congenital cervical spine fusion but would not explain all of the patient's anomalies. Squaring of the vertebral bodies is a radiologic finding on plain film of patients with spondyloarthritis, which is not consistent with this clinical presentation.

(Section 16: The Musculoskeletal System, Chapter 213: Disorders of the Neck and Spine)

**Answer 17-45.** D

Cheilitis is a common inflammatory condition in children characterized by erythema, mild edema, and a thin layer of scaling of the lips or perioral areas. It is commonly caused by the chronic habit of licking the lips or the skin surrounding the lips. It is less frequently caused by bacterial or fungal (usually candidal) infections, nutritional deficiencies, or atopic dermatitis. Allergic cheilitis can also occur; it occurs more frequently in women using lipstick or lip balm, although spearmint oil in toothpaste has also been identified as an allergen.

(Section 20: Disorders of the Oral Cavity, Chapter 373: Oral Pathology)

**Answer 17-46.** B

Primary congenital glaucoma occurs in about 1 in 10,000 births in the United States and is a result of abnormal development of the aqueous humor drainage system. Approximately 10% of primary congenital glaucoma is present at birth, and 80% is diagnosed within the first year of life. Congenital or infantile glaucoma presents initially with clouding and enlargement of the cornea. Early symptoms also include blepharospasm (blinking), tearing, and light sensitivity. Lacrimal duct stenosis presents with exudative drainage and swelling in the area of the medial canthus on the affected side. Lens opacification would be seen on exam in the case of infantile cataract. The child has no other signs of Soto syndrome, making glaucoma secondary to this etiology less likely. Sclerocornea presents with cloudiness of the cornea but not excessive tearing or light sensitivity.

(Section 30: Disorders of the Eyes, Chapter 580: Anterior Segment Disorders)

**Answer 17-47.** E

This patient likely has perichondritis, an infection of the perichondrium (tissue surrounding the cartilage) of the auricular cartilage. Perichondritis usually occurs in the setting of recent local trauma (eg, piercings, laceration, or burns) and can lead to chondritis—infection of the cartilage. The most common infective organisms are *P aeruginosa* and *S aureus*, and systemic antibiotics should be given that are active against both organisms. Typical antibiotic regimens are an antipseudomonal penicillin or a combination of antipseudomonal quinolone plus penicillinase-resistant penicillin. Incision and drainage can be considered for obtaining culture and may help with resolution of infection, which can take weeks.

(Section 19: Disorders of the Ear, Nose, and Throat, Chapter 364: The Ear)

**Answer 17-48.** C

This patient likely has nonallergic rhinitis (NAR) given his negative skin prick testing and negative allergen-specific antibody tests. Symptoms of NAR are typically long lasting and can be triggered by strong odors (eg, perfumes, smoke, soaps, paint, fumes), foods, or changes in temperature or weather. Treatment includes avoiding environmental triggers. Azelastine (topical antihistamine) and intranasal fluticasone propionate and beclomethasone are approved by the US Food and Drug Administration for treatment of NAR. However, when rhinorrhea is the predominant symptom, as it is with this patient, intranasal ipratropium (topical anticholinergic) is recommended. Oral second-generation antihistamines are generally not as effective in treatment of NAR as when used to treat allergic rhinitis. First-generation oral antihistamines may be somewhat effective due to their anticholinergic properties.

(Section 19: Disorders of the Ear, Nose, and Throat, Chapter 365: Nose and Sinus)

**Answer 17-49.** D

Branchial arch anomalies often present as lesions of the anterolateral neck and may present as sinuses, fistulas, or cysts. Anomalies of the first branchial arch can present as sinus tracts or masses close to the ear or parotid gland (answer choices A and C) and at times may involve the ear canal and facial nerve. Second branchial arch anomalies are the most common and usually present as enlarging masses or draining sinuses along the lateral neck along the border of the sternocleidomastoid (answer choice B). Anomalies of the third or fourth branchial arches are relatively rare, and they typically present as recurrent left-sided neck abscesses or suppurative thyroiditis. Midline neck masses are most commonly of thyroid origin, such as thyroglossal duct cysts (answer choice E) or ectopic cervical thyroids.

(Section 19: Disorders of the Ear, Nose, and Throat, Chapter 367: The Head, Face, and Neck)

**Answer 17-50.** A

Lip lacerations commonly occur in the setting of trauma; thus, examination requires a thorough oral exam and possible radiograph to assess for fractured teeth or possible foreign body. Suturing of lip lacerations requires careful attention to ensure aesthetic closure, especially if the vermillion border is involved. Through-and-through lip lacerations involve communication between the skin and oral environment and, therefore, are often contaminated. The intraoral lesion should be sutured before the skin lesion, and antibiotics should be

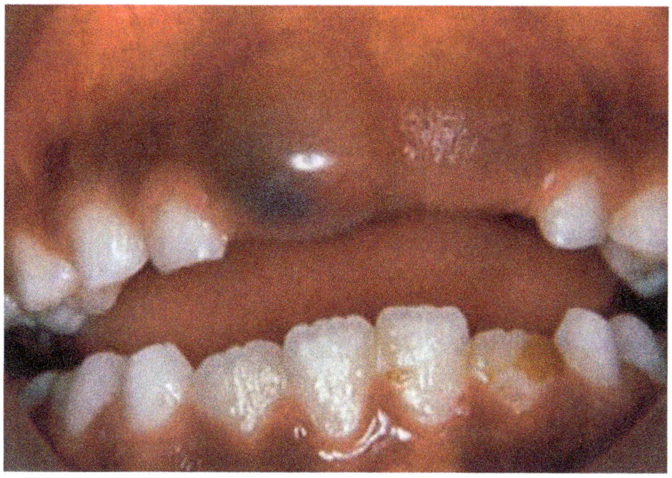

**FIGURE 373-4.** Eruption hematoma. Often associated with an erupting primary tooth, these benign lesions are the result of hemorrhage into the cystic cavity surrounding the crown of the involved tooth. (Mark W. Kline, *Rudolph's Pediatrics*, 23rd Edition. Copyright © McGraw-Hill Education. All rights reserved.)

prescribed that provide coverage against staphylococcal species.

(Section 20: Disorders of the Oral Cavity, Chapter 370: Dental Emergency Care)

**Answer 17-51.** C

This patient most likely has an eruption hematoma, a dentigerous cyst that often forms around the crown of an erupting primary or permanent tooth (Figure 373-4). These lesions are benign and are formed from hemorrhage into the cyst surrounding the crown of the emerging tooth. Eruption hematomas usually self-resolve with emergence of the erupting tooth. Excision is rarely needed.

(Section 20: Disorders of the Oral Cavity, Chapter 373: Oral Pathology)

**Answer 17-52.** D

Corneal abrasion is one of the most frequent ocular injuries of childhood. The abrasion results from mechanical removal of the superficial epithelial layers of the cornea. This can cause intense pain, protective spasm closure of the lids, tearing, and photophobia, although some children may be surprisingly asymptomatic. Examination is facilitated by a drop of topical anesthetic followed by fluorescein dye. The fluorescein will define the extent of epithelial cell loss when examined with cobalt blue illumination.

Use of a cycloplegic agent and topical antibiotic ointment will provide comfort and prevent infection. The placement of a pressure patch to close the eyelid and promote healing of the epithelium was traditional care for children and adults, but more recent studies indicate that the patch may not increase the rate of healing or comfort. Younger children may resist or remove the patch. Normal eye closure during sleep will usually be enough to promote a rapid recovery. Corneal abrasions typically are healed within 1 to 2 days.

(Section 30: Disorders of the Eye, Chapter 573: Eye Emergencies and Trauma)

**Answer 17-53.** C

In a patient with a history of chronic otorrhea, pneumatic otoscopy can help differentiate whether the affected portion of the tympanic membrane is a perforation or a retraction pocket. It may also be possible to observe squamous debris or granulation tissue within a perforation or a retraction pocket. This finding is suggestive of cholesteatoma. Squamous epithelium desquamating from a cholesteatoma has an appearance resembling cheese. This diagnosis is best made with otomicroscopy using an operating microscope and suction debridement. If a cholesteatoma is suspected, CT scanning of the temporal bone may provide information on the size of the mass and whether surrounding landmarks are involved.

The treatment of a cholesteatoma involves surgical removal of squamous epithelium in the middle ear and mastoid. Although several different surgical approaches are used, almost all of them involve a mastoidectomy. Surgical removal of the cholesteatoma is performed initially. It is followed by a second procedure allowing confirmation of squamous epithelial removal and subsequent reconstruction of the ossicles if necessary. This second stage of treatment is performed approximately 6 to 12 months after the initial procedure.

(Section 19: Disorders of the Ear, Nose, and Throat, Chapter 364: The Ear, Cholesteatoma)

**Answer 17-54.** A

Lesions of the anterolateral neck often are of branchial system origin. Each of the 4 mesodermal branchial arches was separated from one another by an external cleft of ectodermal origin and by an internal pouch of endodermal origin with a thin epithelial plate separating cleft and pouch. The likely arch of origin classifies branchial cleft anomalies, with second branchial anomalies being most common. They form sinuses, fistulas, or cysts. A sinus tract with either an external or internal opening represents a vestigial cleft or pouch. Branchial cleft sinuses with external openings to the skin typically are associated with the first and second arches. Second branchial anomalies can present as enlarging neck masses or as small draining sinuses in the lateral neck at the border of the sternomastoid muscle. Anomalies of the third and fourth branchial arches, sometimes referred to as *piriform fistulas*, are quite rare. They usually present as recurrent neck abscesses or suppurative thyroiditis, almost exclusively on the left side. Although excision of these piriform fistulas and the associated mass/tract is curative, recent reports have indicated at least short-term benefits from cautery of endoscopically demonstrated fistula tracts in the piriform sinus. Recurrence of branchial anomalies after surgical excision is more common after multiple infections, so early removal of these lesions usually is recommended. Treatment is complete excision of the cyst and/or sinus tract.

(Section 19: Disorders of the Ear, Nose, and Throat, Chapter 367: The Head, Face, and Neck, Congenital Anomalies of the Head and Neck)

**Answer 17-55. B**

The evaluation of a patient with penetrating neck trauma always should start with advanced trauma life support (ATLS), a paradigm that begins with a directed primary survey emphasizing airway, breathing, and circulation (ABC). Once the patient is stabilized, a secondary survey that includes a complete history and thorough physical examination should be performed. In few other regions of the body are so many vital structures located in so small an area. The sternocleidomastoid muscle delineates the posterior and anterior regions of the neck. Most of the vital structures are located in the anterior or lateral regions. Penetrating injuries are those that violate the platysma muscle. Such injuries and those that cross the midline have the greatest potential for damage.

Tracheobronchial and esophageal injuries resulting from penetrating trauma may have a mortality rate as high as 20%. Traumatic cervical esophageal injuries can result in devastating complications. Leakage of saliva and gastroesophageal fluid contents can produce early suppurative infection and an intense necrotizing inflammatory response in the neck and mediastinum. The overall mortality rate increases when esophageal injuries are not diagnosed within 12 hours. Diagnostic testing needed to ascertain the level and degree of injury includes direct hypopharyngoscopy and esophagoscopy, computed tomography (CT), and contrast barium esophagram.

(Section 19: Disorders of the Ear, Nose, and Throat, Chapter 367: The Head, Face, and Neck, Head and Neck Trauma, Neck and Laryngotracheal Trauma)

**Answer 17-56. D**

A thorough history and physical examination are key to determining the correct diagnosis of neck masses in children. They help determine which labs and/or imaging, if any, are needed for further evaluation. Key historical information that should be obtained includes duration and changes in size of the neck mass, recent illnesses or travel, animal exposure, and exposure to tuberculosis, human immunodeficiency virus (HIV), or radiation. Systemic symptoms such as fever, weight loss, decreased appetite, fatigue, night sweats, or cough also should be questioned. Physical examination findings should include mass location, size, tenderness, mobility, overlying skin changes, and characteristics of the mass on palpation.

When clinically indicated, laboratory tests should be directed based on the history and physical examination findings. When acute inflammation is suspected, a complete blood cell count and C-reactive protein may be useful for confirmation. Serologic testing for various suspected infections is available: *Bartonella henselae* for cat-scratch disease and antibody titers for Epstein-Barr virus, toxoplasmosis, cytomegalovirus, and HIV. Intradermal skin testing and QuantiFERON tuberculosis blood testing are available if mycobacterial infection is suspected.

Ultrasound is often the initial imaging study of choice for pediatric head and neck masses. It is relatively low cost, there is no need for anesthesia, and results are obtained quickly. Ultrasound may be helpful in characterizing superficial lesions, obtaining information about vascularity of a mass, identifying cystic versus solid masses, and identifying superficial neck abscesses. CT of the neck with intravenous (IV) contrast may be necessary to determine anatomic details in deeper neck masses or deep neck space infections/abscesses. It involves ionizing radiation exposure, which has long-term risks in pediatric patients. MRI with and without IV contrast is helpful for identifying further soft-tissue characteristics, as well as masses that are suspected to be vascular anomalies or masses that may extend into areas of the central nervous system. MRIs are not associated with ionizing radiation. The main concern about obtaining MRIs in young children is that, due to the length of examination, anesthesia may be required, which has its own potential long-term risks in pediatric patients.

(Section 19: Disorders of the Ear, Nose, and Throat, Chapter 368: Head and Neck Masses, Diagnostic Evaluation)

**Answer 17-57. B**

Given the patient's history and symptoms, this patient has allergic conjunctivitis. This is typically worse in the spring and summer and accompanied by nasal congestion. Symptoms include watery discharge and itching. The itching is what differentiates this from infectious causes of conjunctivitis.

Preseptal cellulitis is an infectious process involving the tissue anterior to the orbital septum. Physical exam shows eyelids that are edematous, erythematous, and warm to touch. This is commonly caused by trauma or severe underlying conjunctivitis. Subconjunctival hemorrhage is spontaneous or traumatic bleeding of a conjunctival blood vessel. Physical exam shows redness that looks like blood; eyes are painless, and the patient may report the sensation of a foreign body. Bacterial and viral conjunctivitis are infectious causes of a red eye. Bacterial conjunctivitis is usually caused by *Staphylococcus aureus*, *Moraxella*, streptococci, and other bacteria. Symptoms are usually bilateral with mucopurulent discharge and eye swelling. Viral conjunctivitis is usually caused by adenovirus, coxsackieviruses, and rarely, enterovirus. Symptoms are usually associated with upper respiratory infections and adenopathy. Patient may complain of discomfort and mild photophobia.

(Section 30: Disorders of the Eye, Chapter 578: Red Eye)

**Answer 17-58.** A

Many commonly used medications can cause ototoxicity. Clinical symptoms associated with ototoxicity can include hearing loss, tinnitus, and vestibulopathy. Of the antibiotics listed, gentamicin is the only one known to have ototoxicity. Use of drugs known to cause ototoxicity is beneficial in certain clinical cases. However, the benefits of treatment must be weighed against the risk of ototoxicity.

(Section 19: Disorders of the Ear, Nose, and Throat, Chapter 364: The Ear)

**Answer 17-59.** C

A button battery as a nasal foreign body is very hazardous and should be removed emergently. Local damage to the nasal passage may occur within 1 hour of placement, and nasal septum perforation has been reported within 7 hours of a battery placement.

Most nasal foreign bodies do not fall out on their own and should be removed by a medical professional. Foreign bodies left in the nasal canal without parent knowledge usually result in unilateral rhinorrhea with a foul odor. For most patients with nasal foreign bodies, a referral to an ENT is not necessary. Most pediatric emergency physicians can remove the foreign body successfully. Nasal rinses are not typical methods for removal of nasal foreign bodies. However, oxymetazoline can be used with topical anesthetic prior to foreign body removal.

(Section 19: Disorders of the Ear, Nose, and Throat, Chapter 365: Nose and Sinus)

**Answer 17-60.** D

The appropriate indication for tonsillectomy due to recurrent acute tonsillitis is more than 7 episodes in 1 year, 5 episodes per year for 2 years, or 3 episodes per year for 3 years.

A single episode of acute tonsillitis is not an indication for tonsillectomy. Asymmetric growth or tonsillar lesion suspicious for neoplasm is an indication for tonsillectomy but not asymptomatic enlarged tonsils. Family history of tonsillectomy is not an approved indication for a tonsillectomy.

(Section 19: Disorders of the Ear, Nose, and Throat, Chapter 366: The Pharynx and Upper Airway)

**Answer 17-61.** A

The most likely diagnosis for this patient is acute bacterial lymphadenitis concerning for abscess formation. This is commonly seen in young children. Clinical presentation includes a swollen lymph node that is warm to touch, red, and tender with fluctuance or induration. Diagnosis is suspected clinically and confirmed with ultrasound or computed tomography (CT) scan. Treatment includes incision and drainage and antibiotic therapy.

Reassurance is not recommended when abscess formation is suspected. The abscess must be drained for appropriate treatment. NSAIDs can be used for supportive management but are not the mainstay treatment. Surgical excision is not typical treatment for uncomplicated abscess. A neck radiograph is not necessary. The best methods for confirmation are ultrasound and CT.

(Section 19: Disorders of the Ear, Nose, and Throat, Chapter 368: Head and Neck Masses)

# CHAPTER 18 Disorders of the Heart

Antonio G. Cabrera and S. Yukiko Asaki

**18-1.** A 2 years old presents with an atrial septal defect (ASD). Her mother also had an ASD that was closed with device closure. Her grandfather also had an ASD and has a pacemaker due to complete atrioventricular (AV) block. Of the following, which pathogenic mutation is most likely associated with this finding?

**A.** *NOTCH1*

**B.** *NKX2.5*

**C.** *NF1*

**D.** *TBX5*

**E.** *JAG1*

**18-2.** A newborn has hypotonia, dysmorphic features (see following figure), and a murmur. What chromosomal abnormality and form of congenital heart disease best fits these exam findings?

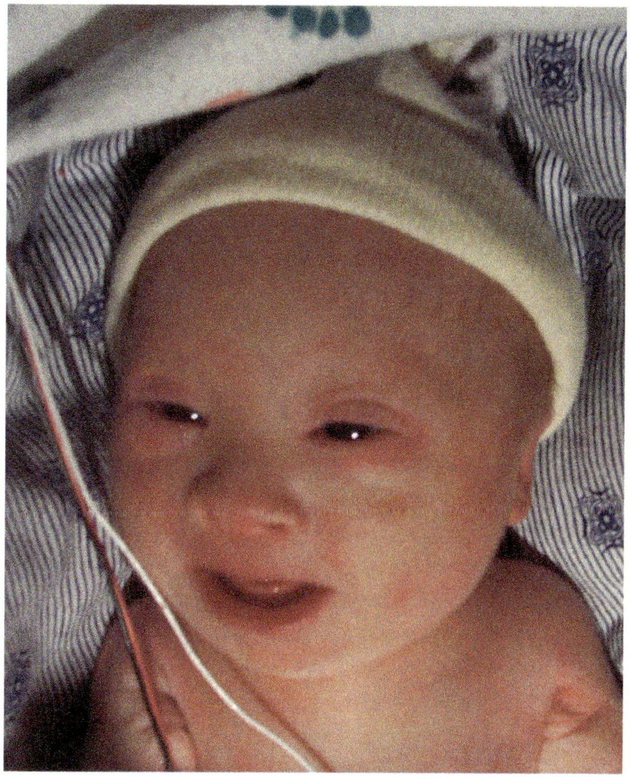

(Reproduced, with permission, from Rudolph CD, Rudolph AM, Lister GE, First LR, Gershon AA. *Rudolph's Pediatrics*. 22nd ed. New York: McGraw-Hill, 2011.)

**A.** Trisomy 13: ventricular septal defect (VSD)

**B.** Trisomy 21: complete atrioventricular (AV) canal defect

**C.** Microdeletion 7q11: supravalvular aortic stenosis

**D.** Microdeletion 22q11: tetralogy of Fallot

**E.** Trisomy 18: VSD

**18-3.** A 12-year-old girl presents with lack of pubertal development, short stature, and broad chest. What is the best next step to evaluate this patient?

**A.** Genetic testing of the genes implicated in Noonan syndrome

**B.** Genetic testing of the genes implicated in Alagille syndrome

**C.** Echocardiogram and blood pressure measurement in all 4 extremities

**D.** Cardiac magnetic resonance imaging (MRI)

**E.** Cardiac catheterization

**18-4.** A 2.2-kg term infant is admitted to the neonatal intensive care unit (NICU) after birth with cleft palate, small chin, and a murmur. An echocardiogram demonstrates truncus arteriosus, with no visible thymus seen. What is the most likely underlying genetic abnormality?

**A.** Deletion of 22q11.2

**B.** *PTPN11* mutation in the RAS/MAP pathway

**C.** *JAG1* mutation

**D.** A mutation in *NKX2.5*

**E.** A deletion of 7q11

**18-5.** A 6-year-old girl in your clinic has widely spaced eyes, a broad forehead, and low-set ears on physical exam (see following figure). She has normal first and second heart sounds and a grade 3–4/6 systolic ejection murmur without any ejection clicks. You obtain an echocardiogram, which demonstrates asymmetric septal hypertrophy with no left ventricular outflow tract gradient and a 40-mm peak gradient across her pulmonary valve. What is the most likely underlying genetic abnormality?

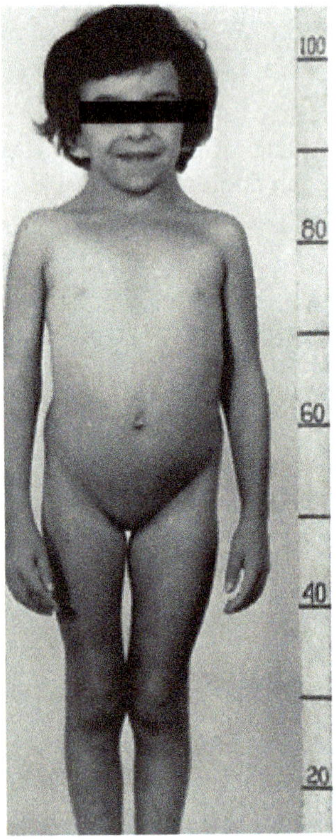


(Reproduced, with permission, from Rudolph CD, Rudolph AM, Lister GE, First LR, Gershon AA. *Rudolph's Pediatrics*. 22nd ed. New York: McGraw-Hill, 2011.)

**A.** Deletion of 22q11.2

**B.** *PTPN11* mutation in the RAS/MAP pathway

**C.** *JAG1* mutation

**D.** A mutation in the β-myosin heavy gene 14q 11.2-3

**E.** A deletion of 7q11

**18-6.** A 3-year-old boy with jaundice, cholestasis, and a murmur is referred to clinic for evaluation. He has a history of mild developmental delay and unusual facial features (broad forehead, deep-set eyes, pointed chin). The chest radiograph (CXR) shows a normal cardiac silhouette but butterfly-shaped vertebrae. He has a normal $S_1$ and $S_2$, no clicks, and peripheral pulmonic stenosis (PS) murmurs bilaterally. What gene defect should you test for?

**A.** Deletion of 22q11.2

**B.** *PTPN11* mutation in the RAS/MAP pathway

**C.** *JAG1* mutation

**D.** A mutation in the β-myosin heavy gene 14q 11.2-3

**E.** A deletion of 7q11

**18-7.** The mother of a patient with a large ventricular septal defect is pregnant with her second child and wants to know if she should have a fetal echocardiogram. Which of the following is the most appropriate response?

**A.** There are no maternal medication exposures or prepregnancy maternal conditions that would be an indication for fetal echocardiogram.

**B.** A fetal echocardiogram is indicated only if a routine obstetric ultrasound shows an extracardiac abnormality.

**C.** The majority of pregnancies with fetal heart disease have known risk factors for congenital heart disease, such as family history.

**D.** Fetal echocardiograms are only indicated for certain forms of congenital heart disease, such as left-sided obstructive lesions.

**E.** A family history of congenital heart disease, which includes any first-degree relative, is an indication for fetal echocardiogram.

**18-8.** A term baby is born to a 32-year-old G1P0 woman with no significant past medical history. The pregnancy was complicated by fetal bradycardia without evidence of hydrops and was followed by the maternal-fetal high-risk obstetrician. The baby is able to maintain spontaneous respirations, is warm and well perfused with good pulses, and is admitted to the neonatal intensive care unit (NICU) where the electrocardiogram (ECG) shown in the figure below was obtained. What does this ECG show, and what is the best next workup for this kind of bradycardia?

**A.** This ECG is consistent with L-looped ventricles and associated complete heart block. Obtain echocardiogram to delineate cardiac anatomy and function.

**B.** This ECG is consistent with sinus bradycardia. Begin workup for sepsis and start antibiotics.

**C.** This ECG is consistent with first-degree atrioventricular (AV) block and a superior axis. Obtain echocardiogram to evaluate for endocardial cushion defect.

**D.** This ECG is consistent with complete heart block. Send mother's blood for autoantibodies anti-SSA-Ro and anti-SSB-La to evaluate for neonatal lupus erythematosus, and obtain an echocardiogram on the baby to evaluate for myocardial depression and presence of congenital heart disease.

**E.** This ECG is consistent with complete heart block. Send the neonate's blood for the *NKX2.5* mutation, and obtain an echocardiogram to evaluate for associated atrial septal defect (ASD).

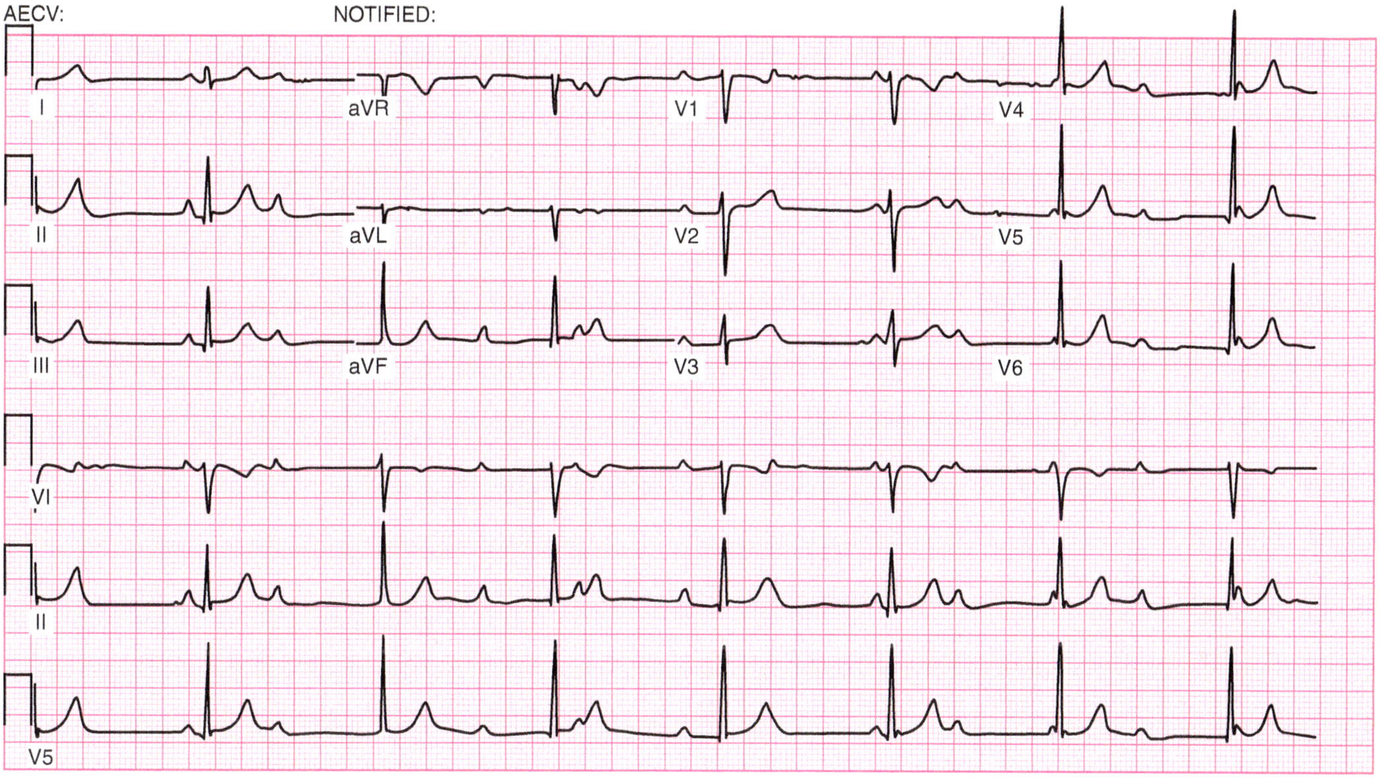


**18-9.** A full-term baby girl in the well-baby nursery is found to have an early systolic click and harsh 3/6 systolic ejection murmur heard best at the second left intercostal space. $S_1$ is normal, and $S_2$ has normal physiologic split. She is comfortable with respiratory rate at 40 breaths/min and heart rate of 140 bpm. On pulse oximetry, she is desaturated at 82%. Several hours later, after transfer to the neonatal intensive care unit, her saturations are 73%. After prostaglandins are given, the saturation increases again to the low 80s. There is no pre- or postductal split in saturations. What is the most likely diagnosis?

**A.** Transposition of the great arteries

**B.** Critical pulmonary stenosis (PS)

**C.** Tricuspid atresia with transposed great vessels

**D.** Truncus arteriosus with truncal valve stenosis

**E.** Large ventricular septal defect (VSD)

**18-10.** A 10-day-old neonate presents with "heavy breathing" and difficulty breastfeeding that developed over the past day following an uncomplicated pregnancy and delivery and an unremarkable 2-day stay in the well-baby nursery. His vital signs are as follows: heart rate is 170 bpm, respiratory rate is 65 breaths/min and labored, and it is difficult to obtain blood pressure in the leg. On exam, there is a strong pulse in the right brachial artery but very weak pulses at both femoral arteries. On pulse oximetry, saturation in the right hand is 99% and in the left foot is 82%. What condition does this infant most likely have?

**A.** Critical coarctation of the aorta

**B.** Left ventricular dysfunction due to cardiomyopathy

**C.** Critical pulmonary stenosis (PS)

**D.** Total anomalous pulmonary venous return (TAPVR) with obstruction

**E.** Tricuspid atresia with normally related great vessels

**18-11.** A 4-month-old child born at full term presents with decreased feeding for the past several days. He was taking up to 3 oz, but over the past few weeks, he only takes 1.5 to 2 oz and gets tired by the end of feeding. His birth weight was 3.3 kg; current weight is 5.1 kg. He has had minimal weight gain since his well-child visit at 4 months. A pulse oximeter reads 85%. There is a soft 1–2/6 systolic murmur and widely split $S_2$, which are new cardiac findings. A chest radiograph (CXR) shows moderate cardiomegaly and mild pulmonary edema. What is the most likely cardiac lesion?

**A.** Tetralogy of Fallot

**B.** Total anomalous pulmonary venous return without obstruction (TAPVR)

**C.** Truncus arteriosus

**D.** Transposition of the great arteries

**E.** Ventricular septal defect (VSD)

**18-12.** A 2-day old, full-term infant presents with tachypnea (respiratory rate, 80 breaths/min), cyanosis, sinus tachycardia (heart rate, 170 bpm), hepatomegaly (5 cm below the costal margin), and a palpable spleen tip. He has a hyperdynamic precordium, normal $S_1$, prominent $S_2$, an $S_3$, and bounding pulses. A chest radiograph (CXR) shows cardiomegaly, increased pulmonary vascular markings, and a dilated mediastinum. Auscultation for which of the following additional physical findings will help you identify the malformation causing cyanosis and congestive heart failure?

**A.** Cranial bruit

**B.** Continuous murmur at left upper sternal border

**C.** Harsh, late-peaking systolic ejection murmur at right upper sternal border

**D.** Pericardial rub

**E.** Holosystolic murmur at left lower sternal border with low-pitched diastolic rumble

**18-13.** A 6-month-old child with a doubly committed subarterial ventricular septal defect (VSD) presents with a new decrescendo diastolic murmur. On past visits, the murmur has been a holosystolic murmur without a diastolic component. What is the most likely cause for this new murmur?

**A.** Aortic regurgitation due to prolapse of the aortic valve cusp into the defect

**B.** Relative mitral stenosis due to increased flow across the valve

**C.** Flow across an atrial septal defect (ASD) due to increased pulmonary venous return in the left atrium

**D.** Pulmonary regurgitation from pulmonary hypertension

**E.** Endocarditis of the tricuspid valve related to turbulence near the VSD, which has caused a left ventricle to right atrium shunt

**18-14.** A 26-month-old boy with a small ventricular septal defect (VSD) was noted to have a louder systolic murmur than at the past several visits. On examination today, he has a grade 4–5/6 systolic ejection-type murmur at the high to mid left sternal border and a grade 1/4 high-frequency diastolic decrescendo murmur at the lower left sternal border. There are no ejection clicks, and the rest of the exam is normal.

His electrocardiogram (ECG) shows right ventricular hypertrophy. His echocardiogram demonstrates a small perimembranous ventricular septal defect (VSD) with partial aneurysmal closure, a fibrous subaortic ridge with an estimated peak left ventricular outflow gradient of 20 mm Hg, and trivial to mild aortic regurgitation. What other cardiac lesion would also likely be shown on this echocardiogram?

**A.** Coarctation of the aorta

**B.** Patent ductus arteriosus

**C.** Mitral valve prolapse

**D.** Prominent right ventricular muscle bundles

**E.** Left superior vena cava to the coronary sinus

**18-15.** A 3-month-old boy with tetralogy of Fallot presents with fever, diarrhea, and poor feeding over the past 24 hours. On physical examination, you note cyanosis of the extremities and perioral area, tachypnea, hyperpnea, and a heart rate of 180 bpm. At the last visit, you recall a harsh 3/6 systolic ejection murmur; today, you do not hear a murmur. Of the following, what is the most appropriate next management strategy?

**A.** Administer antipyretics for fever

**B.** Reassure his mother because the murmur is gone

**C.** Order echocardiogram to evaluate the pulmonary valve

**D.** Encourage oral intake of fluids

**E.** Place him in the knee-chest position with oxygen

**18-16.** A 4-year-old child has an ejection click and a 3/6 harsh systolic murmur that increases with squatting on exam. What is the most likely lesion, and what is the best treatment?

**A.** Congenital aortic stenosis; balloon valvuloplasty

**B.** Subaortic stenosis due to hypertrophic cardiomyopathy; septal myectomy

**C.** Bicuspid aortic valve and coarctation; coarctation repair

**D.** Pulmonary stenosis (PS); balloon valvuloplasty

**E.** Ventricular septal defect (VSD); surgical repair

**18-17.** A 7-month-old infant has had noisy breathing since birth that his mother notes worsened when he began eating solid foods. The arch vessel sequence on echocardiogram from proximal to distal is: left common carotid, right common carotid, right subclavian, and left subclavian arteries. There are patent vessels anterior to, to the right of, and posterior to the trachea but not to the left. There is a bulge in the proximal portion of the left subclavian artery. Which of the following statements is correct?

**A.** This may be a vascular ring, but angiography is needed to confirm the diagnosis.

**B.** This is a right arch with retroesophageal subclavian artery that does not form a true ring.

**C.** This may be a vascular ring, but the child needs a barium swallow to confirm the diagnosis.

**D.** This is a vascular ring, and the patient should have surgical division based on this imaging test alone.

**E.** This is a left pulmonary artery sling, and the left pulmonary artery should be reimplanted surgically to relieve the symptoms.

**18-18.** A 9-week-old infant presents with a holosystolic blowing murmur best heard at the apex. An electrocardiogram (ECG) shows S-segment changes and Q waves in leads I and aVL. Echocardiography shows a dilated left ventricle with an ejection fraction of 20%. The right coronary artery appears dilated. What is the most likely cause of the cardiomyopathy?

**A.** Anomalous left coronary artery from the pulmonary artery

**B.** Intramural left coronary artery from the right sinus

**C.** Dilated cardiomyopathy

**D.** Myocarditis

**E.** Kawasaki disease

**18-19.** A 6-year-old girl is admitted for appendectomy. After noting an irregular heart rate on preoperative examination, the nurse hands you this rhythm strip (Figure 480-11). What is the next most appropriate step?

**A.** Reassurance—this is sinus arrhythmia

**B.** Reassurance—this is second-degree Mobitz type I/ Wenckebach atrioventicular (AV) block, a normal variant

**C.** Consult cardiology—this is second-degree Mobitz type II AV block and could deteriorate to complete heart block

**D.** Consult cardiology—this is type III/complete heart block and may be very problematic for safe anesthesia

**E.** Check electrolytes—this is a junctional escape rhythm with a narrow QRS complex

**18-20.** A 13-year-old boy presents to the emergency department (ED) with palpitations and tachycardia. He has had two 20- to 30-minute episodes over the past week, but he only told his mother about it this morning when he felt it for the third time after drinking an energy drink. He does not complain of chest pain or dizziness, and other vital signs are normal for age. He has never had syncope. The rhythm strip is shown in Figure 480-14. The echocardiogram displays normal structure and function. What is the next most appropriate step in his evaluation and management?

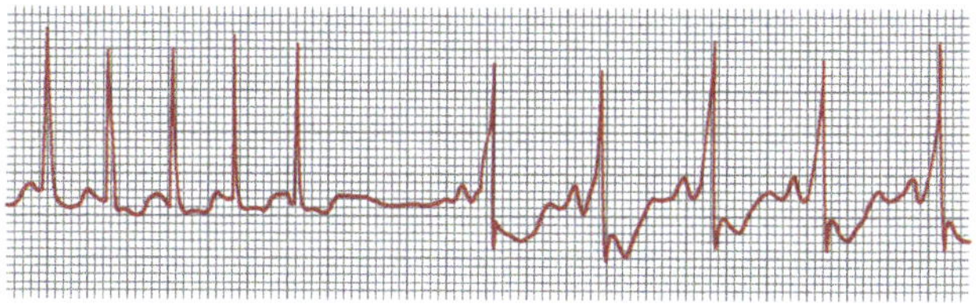

**FIGURE 480-14.** (Mark W. Kline, *Rudolph's Pediatrics*, 23rd Edition. Copyright © McGraw-Hill Education. All rights reserved.)

**A.** Refer to cardiology clinic and discharge from ED with prescription for verapamil

**B.** Refer to cardiology clinic and discharge from ED with prescription for atenolol

**C.** Refer to cardiology clinic and discharge from ED with prescription for digoxin

**D.** Admit to the cardiology ward for close monitoring and an urgent electrophysiology test with ablation of the accessory pathway

**E.** Discharge from ED with instructions to cut back on caffeine intake and to follow up if the palpitations reoccur

**18-21.** A 15-year-old boy whose father recently drowned while swimming presents for evaluation. Upon further inquiry, his father had lost consciousness while running a few months ago but had attributed this to dehydration. Your patient admits that he has had some episodes of dizziness and palpitations during track practice, for which he took breaks, but he has never fainted or had any chest pain. He has a normal cardiovascular examination. What changes on his electrocardiogram (ECG) would be most worrisome?

**A.** Mobitz type I second-degree atrioventricular (AV) block

**B.** Possible right ventricular hypertrophy

**C.** Prolonged QTc interval

**D.** Upright T wave in $V_1$

**E.** Premature ventricular contractions

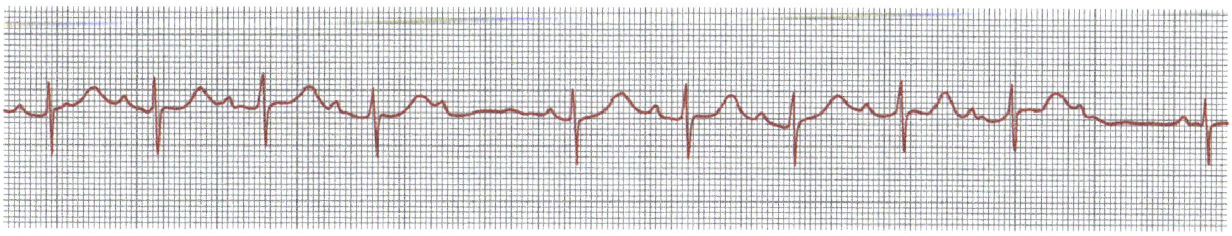

**FIGURE 480-11.** (Mark W. Kline, *Rudolph's Pediatrics*, 23rd Edition. Copyright © McGraw-Hill Education. All rights reserved.)

**18-22.** A 9-year-old boy with a history of syncope has a prolonged QTc interval on electrocardiogram (ECG). What would be the most appropriate therapy?

**A.** Implant an intracardiac defibrillator
**B.** Initiate β-blocker therapy
**C.** Start digoxin
**D.** Start amiodarone
**E.** Perform left cardiac sympathetic denervation

**18-23.** A 2-year-old patient with DiGeorge syndrome presents with hypocalcemia, seizure, and the following rhythm strip (see following figure). Which of the following choices is the most likely cause of this rhythm?

**A.** Ventricular fibrillation
**B.** Ventricular flutter
**C.** Atrial fibrillation
**D.** Movement artifact
**E.** Supraventricular tachycardia

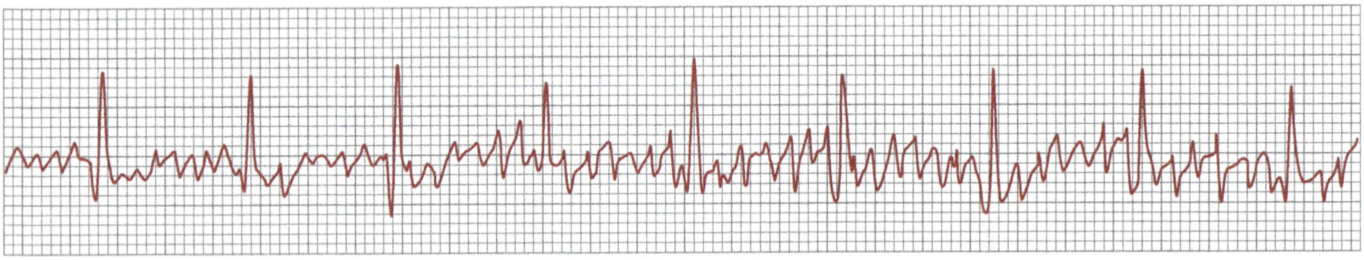

**18-24.** A 14-year-old boy presents with a rash (see following figure), nonspecific joint pain, and the electrocardiogram (ECG) shown in Figure 480-10. What disease process most appropriately explains these findings?

**A.** Rheumatic fever
**B.** Lyme disease
**C.** Myocarditis
**D.** Kawasaki disease
**E.** Juvenile rheumatoid arthritis

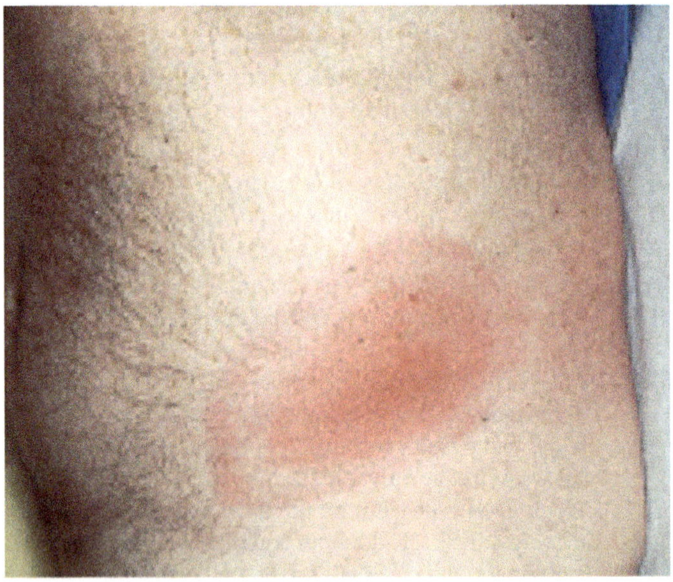

(Reproduced, with permission, from Weinberg S, Prose NS, Kristal L. *Color Atlas of Pediatric Dermatology*. 4th ed. New York: McGraw-Hill, 2007.)

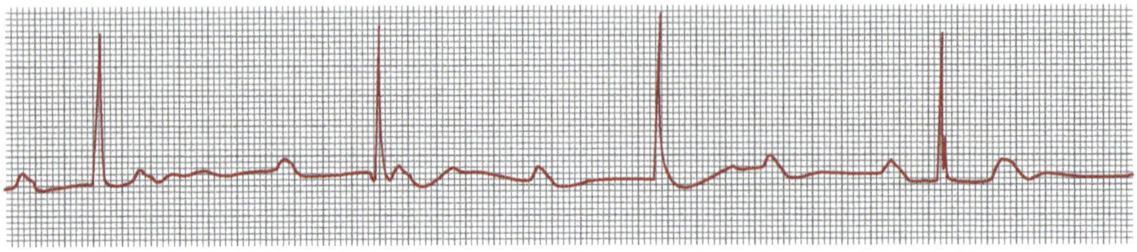

**FIGURE 480-10.** (Mark W. Kline, *Rudolph's Pediatrics*, 23rd Edition. Copyright © McGraw-Hill Education. All rights reserved.)

**18-25.** A newborn develops tachycardia on day of life 1. She is feeding with good pulses and a blood pressure of 65/45 mm Hg. An electrocardiogram (ECG) is obtained and shown here (see following figure). Which of the following is the most appropriate therapy?

**A.** Discharge for home with a Holter monitor

**B.** Intravenous (IV) adenosine to convert orthodromic reciprocating tachycardia

**C.** Synchronized direct-current (DC) cardioversion

**D.** Defibrillation

**E.** Vagal maneuvers to convert atrioventricular (AV) node reentry tachycardia

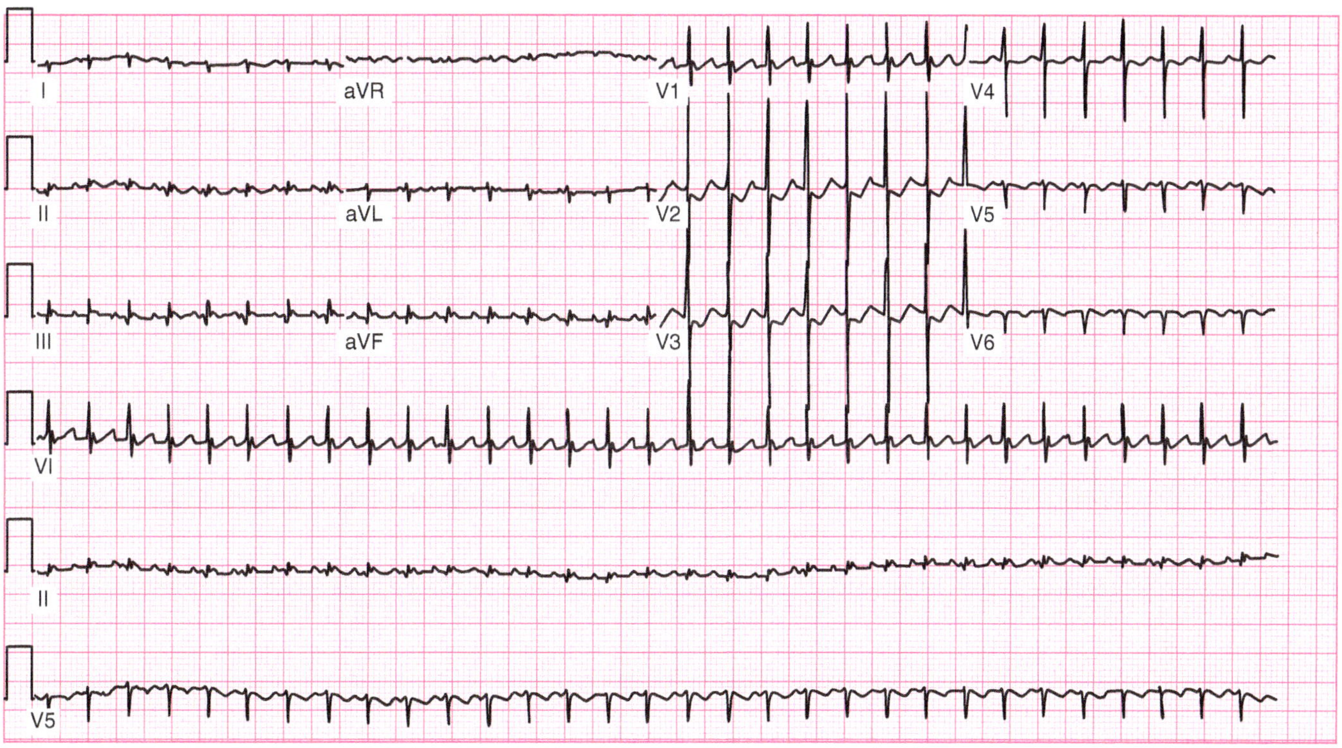


**18-26.** A healthy 4-year-old girl has a murmur on exam at her annual health supervision visit. Further exam findings include clear breath sounds, strong distal pulses, and a quiet precordium. Your partner noted a murmur at last year's visit. Of the following, which description is *most* consistent with the diagnosis of an innocent murmur?

**A.** A continuous machine-like murmur under the left clavicle

**B.** A harsh systolic murmur at the right upper sternal border

**C.** A high-pitched systolic murmur in the back between the scapulae

**D.** A low-pitched, long, diastolic murmur at the left sternal border

**E.** A low-pitched, vibratory systolic murmur at the left sternal border

**18-27.** A healthy 3-year-old boy is referred for evaluation of a murmur. His peripheral pulses are normal. The first and second heart sounds are normal. There is a grade 2/6 low- to mid-frequency vibratory murmur along the left sternal border. One would expect this murmur to increase in intensity at what point?

**A.** When going from sitting to standing position

**B.** With handgrip maneuver

**C.** With deep inhalation

**D.** During the Valsalva maneuver

**E.** When moving from sitting to supine position

**18-28.** A 2-year-old boy who was recently adopted internationally presents for evaluation of exertional dyspnea. His parents note that he squats down and breathes heavily with vigorous play. On examination, he has room air saturations of 80%, a right ventricular heave, and a harsh systolic ejection murmur at the left upper sternal border that radiates to the lung fields. There is no hepatomegaly. Pulses are equal in all extremities. His upper and lower extremity blood pressures are normal for age. Which congenital cardiac lesion do you suspect?

**A.** Coarctation of the aorta

**B.** Double outlet right ventricle with transposed great arteries

**C.** Tetralogy of Fallot

**D.** Atrioventricular septal defect (AVSD)

**E.** Ventricular septal defect (VSD)

**18-29.** A healthy 10-year-old boy has a loud first heart sound and a widely split second heart sound that does not vary with respiration. He has a right ventricular lift and a soft systolic flow murmur at the left upper sternal border. Pulses are normal. He is a good soccer player and has been healthy. What lesion is most likely to explain these findings?

**A.** Atrial septal defect (ASD)

**B.** Ventricular septal defect (VSD)

**C.** Coarctation of the aorta

**D.** Aortic stenosis

**E.** Pulmonic valve stenosis

**18-30.** A 16-year-old soccer player comes to the clinic complaining of left-sided chest pain for the past week. She has no history of chest trauma, fever, recent illness, palpitations, dizziness, or syncope. The pain is worse when she breathes deeply. Her cardiovascular and pulmonary examinations are normal. She has tenderness to palpation along the left sternal border. Of the following, which is the most likely diagnosis?

**A.** Anomalous coronary origin

**B.** Costochondritis

**C.** Infective endocarditis

**D.** Myocarditis

**E.** Pericarditis

**18-31.** A 13-year-old boy presents with a history of multiple syncopal episodes during church services. He describes the episodes to you: after standing quietly for 5 to 10 minutes, he feels warm, his vision darkens from the periphery, he feels sweaty, and his heart races. He feels dizzy and loses consciousness. He has never injured himself during fainting episodes and returns to his usual baseline shortly afterward. He drinks plenty of water every day. His mother recalls that she had similar episodes in adolescence. His physical examination in clinic is normal. His electrocardiogram (ECG) shows normal axes, normal conduction, and normal QRS and QT intervals for his age. What is the most likely etiology of his syncope?

**A.** Long QT syndrome

**B.** Premature atrial contractions

**C.** Supraventricular tachycardia (SVT)

**D.** Vasovagal syncope

**E.** Hypertrophic cardiomyopathy

**18-32.** A 6-year-old obese boy has a right arm blood pressure of 145/60 mm Hg and a left arm blood pressure of 143/59 mm Hg using an appropriately sized blood pressure cuff. There is a family history of systemic hypertension. He has an aortic valve click on examination. You do not hear a murmur. He has good radial pulses, but you have difficulty identifying lower extremity pulses. His electrocardiogram (ECG) has voltage criteria for left ventricular hypertrophy. What is the best next step?

**A.** Check a lower extremity blood pressure

**B.** Order a fasting lipid profile

**C.** Obtain a urinalysis to evaluate for proteinuria

**D.** Recommend portion control with a low-fat and low-salt diet

**E.** Check chemistries with blood urea nitrogen and creatinine

**18-33.** A 13-year-old girl has a blood pressure in the right arm of 152/96 mm Hg. Her heart rate is 75 bpm, her body mass index is 23, and her exam is otherwise normal. Her past medical history is significant for urinary tract infections in early childhood. She also had a high fever and rash at age 5 that responded after treatment with amoxicillin. She has had normal growth and development. Her family history is notable for a father with hypertension. What is the most likely cause of her hypertension?

**A.** Coarctation of the aorta

**B.** Renal artery stenosis

**C.** Poststreptococcal glomerulonephritis

**D.** Atrophic pyelonephritis

**E.** Pheochromocytoma

**18-34.** Of the following patients, who is at *highest* risk for bacterial endocarditis?

**A.** A child with tetralogy of Fallot with a Blalock-Taussig shunt

**B.** A toddler with transposition of the great arteries following an arterial switch operation at age 1 week

**C.** A child who had a cardiac transplantation 4 years ago

**D.** An infant with unrepaired total anomalous pulmonary venous connection

**E.** A child with mild mitral stenosis

**18-35.** A 4-year-old girl with tuberous sclerosis and seizures is most likely to have which of the following intracardiac masses?

**A.** Hamartoma

**B.** Rhabdomyoma

**C.** Myxoma

**D.** Teratoma

**E.** Hemangioma

**18-36.** A 5-year-old boy presents with irritability and 5 days of persistent high fever (39–40°C) despite multiple doses of antipyretics. He has a bright red tongue, cracked red lips, conjunctivitis without eye discharge, and a diffuse erythematous rash. His joints are not tender or swollen, but his hands and feet are edematous. His palms and soles are erythematous. What is the most likely diagnosis?

**A.** Kawasaki disease

**B.** Streptococcal infection

**C.** Stevens-Johnson syndrome

**D.** *Staphylococcus* scaled skin syndrome

**E.** Rheumatic fever

**18-37.** A 5-year-old boy has had a fever for 5 days, a bright red tongue, cracked red lips, conjunctivitis, a large cervical lymph node, and a diffuse erythematous rash. His erythrocyte sedimentation rate (ESR) is 120 mm/h. What is the next best step to treat this patient?

**A.** Perform a blood culture and start broad-spectrum antibiotics

**B.** Admit tonight for intravenous immunoglobulin (IVIG) and high-dose aspirin; order an echocardiogram for tomorrow

**C.** Discharge from the emergency department (ED) with follow-up if fever persists another 48 hours

**D.** Prescribe amoxicillin and follow up in primary care clinic tomorrow

**E.** Perform a lumbar puncture and start broad-spectrum antibiotics due to concern for meningitis

**18-38.** Two weeks after having a nonspecific upper respiratory tract infection, a previously healthy 4-year-old boy has a gallop and a 1/6 blowing systolic murmur at the apex. He has moderate hepatomegaly. Of the following, what is the most likely diagnosis?

**A.** Acute rheumatic fever (ARF)

**B.** Infective endocarditis (IE)

**C.** Viral myocarditis

**D.** Paroxysmal atrial tachycardia

**E.** Pericarditis

**18-39.** A 6-year-old boy with no previous cardiac history is admitted to the pediatric intensive care unit in congestive heart failure. Upon questioning his parents, he had a fever and culture-proven strep throat 3 weeks ago, but the family could not fill the antibiotic prescription. Your differential diagnosis includes acute rheumatic fever (ARF). Carditis is a major criterion. What other major criterion do you need to confirm to make this diagnosis?

**A.** Arthritis

**B.** Elevated erythrocyte sedimentation rate (ESR)

**C.** Elevated C-reactive protein (CRP)

**D.** Anemia and elevated white blood cell count

**E.** Prolonged PR interval on electrocardiogram (ECG)

**18-40.** A 7-year-old boy has documented antecedent streptococcal infection, positive antistreptolysin O (ASO), and evidence of carditis on echocardiography. How many additional minor criteria are required to make the diagnosis of acute rheumatic fever (ARF)?

**A.** 1

**B.** 2

**C.** 3

**D.** 4

**E.** 5

**18-41.** A previously healthy 10-year-old girl has a 4-week history of low-grade fever, malaise, decreased appetite, weight loss, myalgia, and headaches. On examination, she has a new diastolic murmur, petechiae, and a palpable spleen tip. What is the most likely diagnosis?

**A.** Infective endocarditis (IE)

**B.** Tuberculosis

**C.** Kawasaki disease

**D.** Rheumatic fever

**E.** Scarlet fever

**18-42.** An otherwise healthy, 14-year-old girl complains of chest pain that is particularly severe over the left precordium when she is lying supine. She has begun sleeping upright due to chest pain. She has had a mild viral respiratory infection and intermittent, low-grade fever (< 38.5°C) for the past 2 weeks. Physical examination is remarkable only for mild jugular venous distention and distant heart sounds. The chest radiograph (CXR) shows a moderately enlarged cardiac silhouette, and the electrocardiogram (ECG) shows low-voltage QRS and diffuse ST elevation. Of the following, which is the most likely diagnosis?

**A.** Acute rheumatic fever (ARF)

**B.** Costochondritis

**C.** Infective endocarditis (IE)

**D.** Myocarditis

**E.** Pericarditis

**18-43.** A 15-year-old boy with recently diagnosed systemic lupus erythematosus and a normal echocardiogram last month has developed progressive chest discomfort with inspiration, shortness of breath, and dyspnea on exertion over the past week. He is ill appearing although afebrile, is tachycardic with a heart rate in the 130s, and has cold, clammy extremities. His electrocardiogram (ECG) shows sinus tachycardia and diffusely decreased QRS voltages. His chest radiograph (CXR) shows an enlarged cardiac silhouette without infiltrates, pulmonary edema, or pleural effusions. What physical examination finding would help you make a diagnosis of tamponade at the bedside?

**A.** Comparison of upper and lower extremity blood pressures

**B.** Absent femoral pulses

**C.** Conjunctival injection and strawberry tongue

**D.** Splinter hemorrhages and Janeway lesion

**E.** Blood pressure assessment with deep inspiration

**18-44.** A previously healthy 4-year-old girl presents with a witnessed syncopal episode. She had been running on the playground and lost consciousness for < 1 minute. Her mother thinks she "looked a bit blue" during the episode. There was no incontinence or seizure activity. On examination, she had a prominent left hemithorax and marked right ventricular impulse. She has a regular rate and rhythm, normal $S_1$, and a loud, single $S_2$ that is palpable. There are no murmurs. Her abdominal examination is normal. She has full, equal pulses in all extremities and no blood pressure gradient between the arms and legs. There is no digital clubbing. Her room air saturations are 98%. Chest radiograph (CXR) shows enlarged right ventricle and main pulmonary artery silhouettes. The electrocardiogram (ECG) shows sinus rhythm, right axis deviation, and significantly increased right ventricular voltages. What is your leading diagnosis based on the exam, ECG, and CXR?

**A.** Tetralogy of Fallot with severe subvalvular outflow obstruction

**B.** Severe pulmonary arterial hypertension

**C.** Pulmonary valve stenosis

**D.** Coarctation of the aorta

**E.** Hypertrophic obstructive cardiomyopathy

**18-45.** A 12-year-old child with Williams syndrome and supravalvar aortic stenosis has an echocardiogram that measured the velocity of flow just above the aortic valve at 4.5 m/s by spectral Doppler. What is the estimated pressure gradient across the stenotic area?

**A.** 91 mm Hg

**B.** 18 mm Hg

**C.** 45 mm Hg

**D.** 20 mm Hg

**E.** 81 mm Hg

**18-46.** Which of the following is a normal pulmonary vascular resistance (PVR) range in children and adults (in indexed Woods units)?

**A.** 1–3 units/m$^2$

**B.** 4–6 units/m$^2$

**C.** 7–10 units/m$^2$

**D.** 10–15 units/m$^2$

**E.** > 15 units/m$^2$

**18-47.** A cardiac catheterization was performed in room air ($FiO_2$ = 0.21) on a 6-month-old child with a right arm blood pressure of 70/40 mm Hg. Based on the catheterization data in the following table, what congenital heart defect does this infant have?

| Chamber | Saturation (%) | Pressure (mm Hg) |
|---|---|---|
| Superior vena cava | 60 | |
| Right atrium | 60 | 5 |
| Left atrium | 99 | 8 |
| Right ventricle | 85 | 70/5 |
| Left ventricle | 85 | 70/8 |
| Pulmonary artery | 85 | 10/5 |
| Ascending aorta | 85 | 70/40 |
| Descending aorta | 85 | 75/40 |

**A.** Moderate membranous ventricular septal defect (VSD)

**B.** Tetralogy of Fallot

**C.** Large secundum atrial septal defect (ASD)

**D.** Aortic valve stenosis

**E.** Coarctation of the aorta

**18-48.** A cardiac catheterization was performed in room air ($FiO_2$ = 0.21) on a 16-year-old child with a right arm blood pressure of 160/70 mm Hg. Based on the catheterization data in the following table, what congenital heart defect does this adolescent have?

| Chamber | Saturation (%) | Pressure (mm Hg) |
|---|---|---|
| Superior vena cava | 75 | |
| Right atrium | 75 | 8 |
| Left atrium | 100 | 10 |
| Right ventricle | 75 | 25/8 |
| Left ventricle | 100 | 160/10 |
| Pulmonary artery | 75 | 10/5 |
| Ascending aorta | 100 | 160/70 |
| Descending aorta | 100 | 100/80 |

**A.** Moderate membranous ventricular septal defect (VSD)

**B.** Tetralogy of Fallot

**C.** Large secundum atrial septal defect (ASD)

**D.** Aortic valve stenosis

**E.** Coarctation of the aorta

**18-49.** A 4-month-old infant breathes quickly and becomes sweaty with feeds, which take longer to finish. He has not gained much weight in the past month. He has little subcutaneous tissue, resting tachypnea, hepatomegaly, and a murmur on examination. Which lesion is *not* likely to cause this clinical picture?

**A.** Large patent ductus arteriosus

**B.** Large ventricular septal defect (VSD)

**C.** Truncus arteriosus

**D.** Complete common AV canal

**E.** Secundum atrial septal defect (ASD)

**18-50.** A patient with low cardiac output due to myocarditis is started on milrinone. How does this medication work?

**A.** This medication is a calcium-sensitizing agent with inotropic and afterload-reducing effects. It binds to troponin C and improves the efficiency of the contractile apparatus.

**B.** This medication acts by stimulating myocardial surface β-adrenergic receptors, leading to increased adenylate cyclase and intracellular cyclic adenosine monophosphate.

**C.** This medication inhibits phosphodiesterase type III and lowers filling pressures, systemic and pulmonary artery pressures, and systemic and pulmonary vascular resistances, while improving the cardiac index.

**D.** This medication is a sodium-potassium ATPase inhibitor with positive inotropy, negative chronotropy, and inhibition of neurohormonal activation.

**E.** This medication is a recombinant B-type natriuretic peptide and causes natriuresis, diuresis, vasodilatation, increased renal blood flow, and increased cardiac output and urine output.

**18-51.** Which of the following is *not* a cardiac lesion with a single-ventricle physiology?

**A.** Pulmonary atresia with intact ventricular septum

**B.** Hypoplastic left heart syndrome

**C.** Tricuspid atresia with normally related great vessels and a restrictive bulboventricular foramen

**D.** Unbalanced atrioventricular septal defect (AVSD) with straddling AV valve chordae

**E.** Tetralogy of Fallot with subpulmonary stenosis

**18-52.** A 4-day-old infant presents with decreased oral intake and decreased activity. Birth history was unremarkable, and he was discharged home on day 2 of life. Physical exam reveals a cool, mottled infant with decreased pulses. No significant murmur is audible. Which is the most likely congenital heart defect?

**A.** Tetralogy of Fallot

**B.** Transposition of the great arteries

**C.** Ebstein anomaly

**D.** Hypoplastic left heart syndrome

**E.** Ventricular septal defect (VSD)

**18-53.** A newborn born full term at a community hospital with Apgar scores of 8 and 8 is noted to be cyanotic at 9 hours of life. Oxygen is given by facemask at 10 L/min, but pulse oximetry readings in the right hand remain in the low 70s. An umbilical arterial line is placed, and the first blood gas shows pH of 7.23, $PCO_2$ of 38 mm Hg, and $PaO_2$ of 33 mm Hg. Her lungs are clear, and her breathing is unlabored with mild tachypnea and no retractions. She has full pulses at femoral and brachial areas and is well perfused. What intervention should be done while transport is arranged?

**A.** Infusion of indomethacin

**B.** Infusion of prostaglandin $E_1$

**C.** Bolus of digoxin

**D.** Infusion of adenosine

**E.** Bolus of saline

**18-54.** A 14-year-old child presents for a presports physical examination. A patient with which of these conditions may compete in school athletics without restrictions?

**A.** Unrepaired tetralogy of Fallot

**B.** Congenital atrioventricular block with transvenous pacemaker

**C.** D-transposition of the great arteries, status post arterial switch operation

**D.** Moderate aortic valve stenosis

**E.** Moderate pulmonary valve stenosis

**18-55.** A 10-year-old boy with hypoplastic left heart syndrome has been stable for several years after his Fontan procedure. His family is considering a ski trip to Colorado and seeks your advice. Which of the following statements is most appropriate?

**A.** Given his repair and Fontan physiology, he should have no problem at elevation.

**B.** The patient will not be able to tolerate the airline flight.

**C.** The patient will develop symptoms of respiratory distress and cyanosis within hours.

**D.** The patient may tolerate the high elevation, but his exercise tolerance will be affected.

**E.** The patient should not travel above 500 ft above sea level.

**18-56.** A healthy 16-year-old boy presents for preparticipation sports screening. The boy states that his older brother was diagnosed with a seizure disorder and died suddenly during high school track practice. He also has a younger sister who has a history of syncope. Before approving him for sports participation, which of the following tests must be performed?

**A.** Magnetic resonance imaging (MRI) of the head

**B.** Electrocardiogram (ECG)

**C.** Electroencephalography

**D.** Twenty-four-hour Holter monitor

**E.** Tilt-table test

**18-57.** Which of the following is the most common cause of sudden death during competitive exercise?

**A.** Postoperative congenital heart disease

**B.** Hypertrophic cardiomyopathy

**C.** Marfan syndrome

**D.** Anomalous coronary arteries

**E.** Long QT syndrome

**18-58.** A 2-week-old full-term baby presents to the emergency department (ED) after 2 days of poor feeding and increasing respiratory distress. An electrocardiogram (ECG) is obtained on presentation and shown in the figure. Following successful termination of tachycardia, what is the appropriate management strategy for this patient?

**A.** Admit for sepsis evaluation

**B.** Reassurance and discharge from ED without follow-up

**C.** Obtain echocardiogram and admit to initiate antiarrhythmic

**D.** Admit for observation without antiarrhythmics

**E.** Give first dose of antiarrhythmic in the ED, then discharge home on an antiarrhythmic regimen

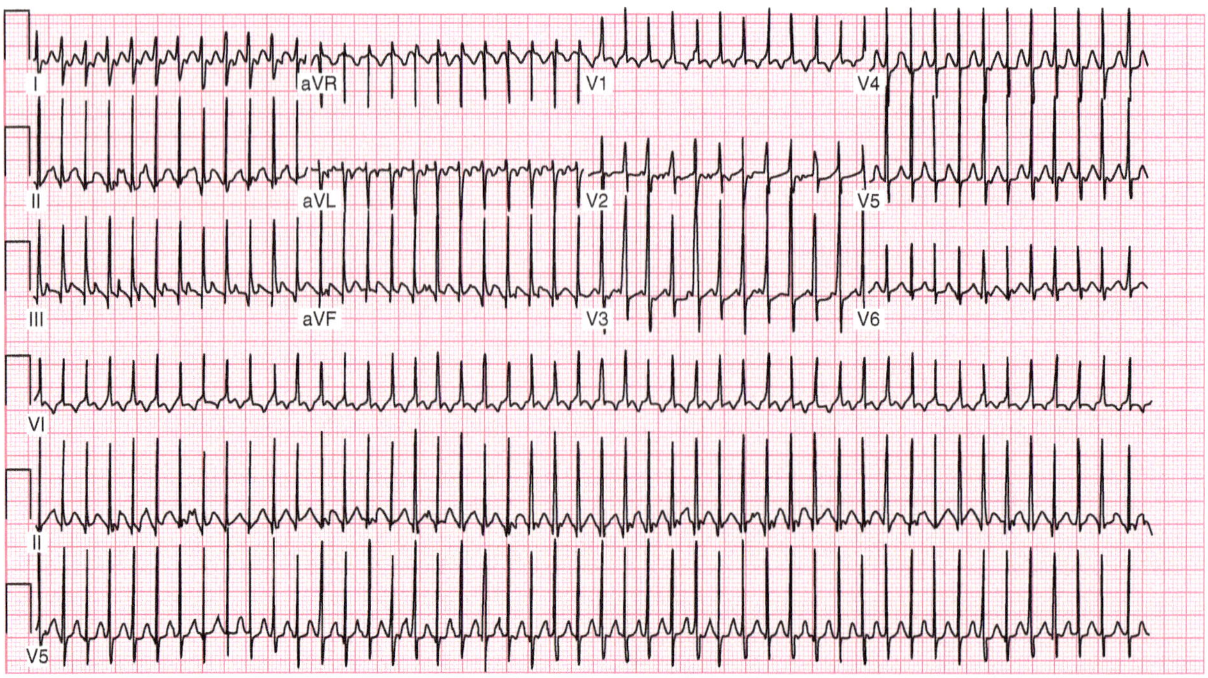

**18-59.** An otherwise healthy, full-term newborn baby has profound bradycardia, and an electrocardiogram (ECG) is obtained (see following figure). What is the most appropriate management strategy for this patient?

**A.** Obtain echocardiogram to evaluate for congenital heart disease

**B.** Perform sepsis evaluation

**C.** Initiate caffeine

**D.** Transfer to the neonatal intensive care unit (NICU) for close monitoring and initiation of propranolol

**E.** Place an epicardial pacemaker

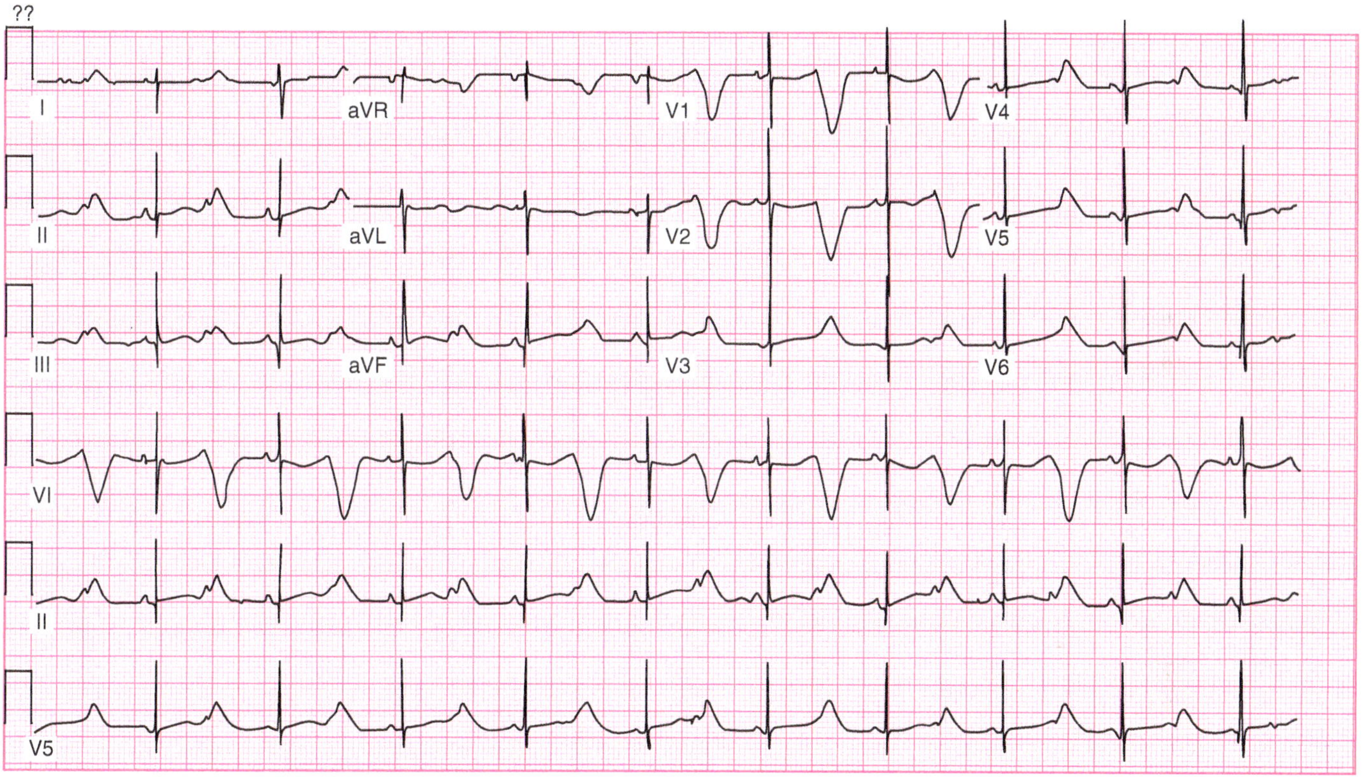


**18-60.** An 11-year-old boy with a history of Kawasaki disease at age 5 has coronary artery Z-score measurements of 4.5 on echocardiogram this year. He undergoes routine fasting lipid screening at his pediatrician's office and is found to have a low-density lipoprotein (LDL) level of 150 mg/dL, which is confirmed on appropriate follow-up testing. What is the most appropriate course of treatment?

**A.** No intervention because this LDL level is normal for age

**B.** Lifestyle modification with diet and exercise

**C.** Lifestyle modification, with intention to start statin therapy in 6 months if no improvement in LDL level

**D.** Lifestyle modification, with intention to start statin therapy in 3 months if no improvement in LDL level

**E.** Lifestyle modification and initiation of statin therapy now

**18-61.** A 26-year-old man with repaired coarctation of the aorta presents for his first visit with the adults with congenital heart disease team. He has no significant residual gradient across his aortic arch, and his upper extremity blood pressure in both arms is not elevated. What condition is he at higher risk for developing compared to the general adult population?

**A.** Deep vein thrombosis

**B.** Hepatocellular carcinoma

**C.** Type 2 diabetes mellitus

**D.** Intracranial aneurysms

**E.** Pulmonary arterial hypertension

## ANSWERS

### Answer 18-1. B

Mutations in *NKX2.5* are associated with ASDs and progressively disrupt electrical conduction and can progress to complete heart block. Over time, the specialized conduction cells in the AV node are lost and replaced by fibrotic tissue, resulting in progressive defects in electrical conduction. This patient should be monitored for AV block in the long term due to the strong family history of both ASD and conduction abnormalities.

*NOTCH1* mutations in humans cause bicuspid aortic valves. Neurofibromatosis is associated with thickened valves and is caused by mutation of the *NF1* gene. *TBX5* is associated with Holt-Oram syndrome. Although patients with the Holt-Oram syndrome can have ASDs, progressive conduction problems would be unexpected. *JAG1*, a NOTCH ligand, can cause outflow tract defects associated with the autosomal dominant disease Alagille syndrome.

(Section 26: Disorders of the Cardiovascular System)

### Answer 18-2. B

This child's features are most consistent with Down syndrome, or trisomy 21. The prevalence of congenital heart defect (CHD) in this population is approximately 40% to 50%. Complete AV septal defect (AVSD; also termed endocardial cushion defect or AV canal defect) accounts for 40% of all CHDs in Down syndrome patients, and this figure increases to almost 60% when partial AVSD (primum ASD and inlet or canal-type VSD) is included.

The American Academy of Pediatrics recommends routine echocardiographic screening of neonates with Down syndrome to facilitate early diagnosis of CHD and intervention because of the increased risk of pulmonary vascular disease in this population.

(Section 26: Disorders of the Cardiovascular System)

### Answer 18-3. C

The features presented here most likely represent those of Turner syndrome, or monosomy X. Approximately 25% to 30% of patients have associated congenital heart disease, predominately left-sided obstructive lesions. Coarctation of the aorta is present in 10% to 20% of patients; therefore, screening for coarctation is indicated at 5-year intervals. Major intracardiac anomalies are not commonly found with isolated coarctation of the aorta, although there is a high association of this lesion with bicuspid aortic valve.

Genetic testing of the genes involved in Noonan syndrome would not be indicated unless Turner syndrome is ruled out. There can be overlap of the features between Noonan and Turner syndromes. Genetic testing for Alagille syndrome is not indicated. Although cardiac MRI and cardiac catheterization may offer additional clinical information, they are not indicated as first-line tests.

(Section 26: Disorders of the Cardiovascular System)

### Answer 18-4. A

The physical characteristics of the infant described in this vignette are classically associated with DiGeorge syndrome (22q11 microdeletion deletion syndrome). This includes neonatal hypocalcemia, micrognathia, thymic hypoplasia, immunodeficiency, feeding and speech disorders, behavioral and psychiatric disorders, renal anomalies, and congenital heart disease. Approximately 75% of affected individuals have congenital heart disease, most commonly conotruncal and aortic arch anomalies, including interrupted aortic arch, truncus arteriosus, and tetralogy of Fallot.

Consider microarray testing for the 22q11 deletion in all infants with the following cardiac lesions: type B interrupted arch, ventricular septal defect with aortic arch anomaly, truncus arteriosus, isolated aortic arch anomaly, and tetralogy of Fallot, especially when associated with absent pulmonary valve, aortic arch or pulmonary artery anomalies, or aortopulmonary collaterals.

*PTPN11* mutation in the RAS/MAP pathway is one of the genetic abnormalities associated with Noonan syndrome. A *JAG1* mutation is seen in Alagille syndrome. Mutation in the β-myosin heavy gene 14q 11.2-3 is the genetic abnormality that is frequently seen in hypertrophic cardiomyopathy. A deletion of 7q11 is associated with William syndrome. None of these are associated with conotruncal cardiac abnormalities and cleft palate.

(Section 26: Disorders of the Cardiovascular System)

### Answer 18-5. B

The patient most likely has Noonan syndrome. Noonan syndrome is an autosomal dominant disorder that presents with hypertelorism, ptosis, epicanthal folds, low-set posteriorly rotated ears, short stature, and congenital heart defects (CHDs). CHDs occur in 80% to 90% of patients with Noonan syndrome, most often valvular pulmonic stenosis (PS) and hypertrophic cardiomyopathy. This patient's cardiac exam and echocardiogram are consistent with a dysplastic pulmonary valve and hypertrophic cardiomyopathy. *PTPN11* mutation in the RAS/MAP pathway is one of the genetic abnormalities associated with Noonan syndrome.

Deletion of 22q11 is the genetic anomaly seen with DiGeorge syndrome. A *JAG1* mutation is seen in Alagille syndrome. Mutation in the β-myosin heavy gene 14q 11.2-3 is the genetic abnormality that is frequently seen in hypertrophic cardiomyopathy. Although the patient in this vignette shows evidence of hypertrophic cardiomyopathy, the physical exam consistent with a dysplastic pulmonary valve and the classic facial features are diagnostic of Noonan syndrome. A deletion of 7q11 is associated with Williams syndrome.

(Section 26: Disorders of the Cardiovascular System)

**Answer 18-6.** C

The constellation of symptoms and facial features is most consistent with Alagille syndrome. Alagille syndrome is caused by mutations in *JAG1*, which encodes a cell surface protein that acts as a ligand in the NOTCH signaling pathway. Alagille syndrome is characterized by a paucity of bile ducts, cholestasis, and jaundice. Some patients need liver transplantation. Alagille patients have distinctive facial features and vertebral anomalies. The cardiac defects usually involve stenosis in the peripheral pulmonary arteries. Rare patients will have tetralogy of Fallot.

Deletion of 22q11.2 is the genetic abnormality associated with DiGeorge syndrome, which does not have associated hepatic disease or skeletal involvement. *PTPN11* mutation in the RAS/MAP pathway is one of the genetic abnormalities associated with Noonan syndrome. Noonan patients usually have dysplastic pulmonary valves and can also develop hypertrophic cardiomyopathy. Skeletal and hepatic abnormalities are not associated with Noonan syndrome. The genetic abnormality in the β-myosin heavy gene is frequently seen in hypertrophic cardiomyopathy. A defect in the elastin gene with deletion of 7q11 is the abnormality associated with Williams syndrome. It causes an arterial vasculopathy and can cause supravalvar aortic stenosis, supravalvar pulmonary stenosis, and branch pulmonary artery stenosis, as well as aortic hypoplasia and renal artery stenosis.

(Section 26: Disorders of the Cardiovascular System)

**Answer 18-7.** E

Fetal echocardiograms are used to evaluate structural, functional, and rhythm-related defects. A family history of congenital heart defects (CHDs) in the fetus's mother, father, or siblings is an indication for fetal screening. Additionally, a family history of a syndrome associated with CHD is also an indication. Maternal indications include associated diseases such as diabetes, phenylketonuria, or autoimmune disorders. Fetal indications include suspected cardiac abnormalities on routine ultrasound, suspected extracardiac abnormalities, and abnormal fetal rhythms. Importantly, the majority of positive referrals come from a low-risk population without known risk factors who were referred because of suspicion for CHD on routine ultrasound.

(Section 26: Disorders of the Cardiovascular System)

**Answer 18-8.** D

This ECG shows complete heart block with complete atrial (P wave) and ventricular (QRS complex) dissociation. The ventricular rate is in the 60s, and although this is much slower than the typical neonatal heart rate, the child is compensating with larger stroke volume and has adequate cardiac output. The QRS complexes are narrow and normal, indicating that the escape focus generating the ventricular rhythm is high in the conducting system. The block often occurs in utero, and at times, cesarean section is done due to concern for fetal distress suspected to be from the slow heart rate. A nonhydropic fetus should not be considered for early delivery to avoid the comorbidities of prematurity. The autoantibodies anti-SSA-Ro and anti-SSB-La are observed in maternal systemic lupus erythematosus or mixed connective tissue disease, but also occur in the absence of clinical autoimmune disease. It is important to evaluate the neonate's myocardial function because 15% to 20% of fetuses with maternal autoimmune-mediated AV block can develop more diffuse myocardial disease. The presence of congenital heart disease is important to establish because the guidelines for pacemaker implantation in the neonatal period have different heart rate cutoffs in neonates with structurally normal hearts versus congenital heart defects.

This ECG does not have the features of L-looped ventricles. Although complete heart block is associated with this form of congenital heart disease, it is much less common than neonatal lupus and often presents at an older age with progressive AV block. Although the most common form of fetal bradycardia is sinus bradycardia, this ECG shows complete AV dissociation and is not consistent with sinus bradycardia. The ECG is not consistent with first-degree AV block (when there is prolongation of the PR interval, but otherwise preserved conduction) or a superior axis (with a frontal plane QRS axis of −90 to −180 degrees [or 0 to +270 degrees]) seen in atrioventricular septal defects. *NKX2.5* is also associated with ASDs. Although complete heart block is associated with this genetic mutation, it is much less common than neonatal lupus.

(Section 26: Disorders of the Cardiovascular System)

**Answer 18-9.** B

This vignette describes a neonate with inadequate pulmonary blood flow. This patient's exam and clinical course are most consistent with severe PS, which presents in the immediate postnatal period with severe cyanosis and cardiac collapse as the ductus arteriosus closes. Once the ductus closes, pulmonary blood flow decreases substantially. In this patient, at the time of the first exam, the ductus was still patent; several hours later, it was more restrictive, and saturations improved with prostaglandins. Although the ductus is patent, there is left to right flow across it from the aorta to the pulmonary artery, increasing pulmonary blood flow. In infants with PS, there will be right ventricular hypertrophy and right axis deviation, with the degree depending on the severity of the stenosis. Apart from the systolic ejection murmur, there is typically a loud variable ejection click. The electrocardiogram (ECG) shows the right atrial hypertrophy with peaked P waves. The right precordial leads show tall R waves, and with severe stenosis, they may also show T-wave inversion and ST-segment depression.

Transposition of the great arteries would present with neonatal cyanosis due to the parallel systemic and pulmonary circulations and may present with reverse differential cyanosis (ie, higher saturation in lower extremities than upper extremities) in the immediate period after birth while the pulmonary vascular resistance is high. Further, in the absence of a VSD or outflow tract obstruction, there is typically not a harsh systolic ejection murmur, as described in the vignette.

Although patients with tricuspid atresia with transposed great vessels are cyanotic, they typically have unrestricted pulmonary blood flow and are at risk for decreased systemic blood flow as the VSD/bulboventricular foramen becomes restrictive. A patient with truncus arteriosus with truncal valve stenosis would be cyanotic with a harsh systolic ejection murmur but would not have a split $S_2$ because there are not separate aortic and pulmonary valve components and would typically have excess pulmonary blood flow. A VSD results in a left-to-right shunt and does not cause cyanosis.

(Section 26: Disorders of the Cardiovascular System)

**Answer 18-10.** A

The child in this vignette most likely has a critical coarctation of the aorta. The coarctation usually occurs in the region of the aorta across from the ductus arteriosus, at the distal end of the aortic isthmus. Children will present with increasing respiratory distress secondary to pulmonary venous hypertension and shock secondary to inadequate cardiac output. Workup should include pulses and upper and lower blood pressures. Systolic, not mean, pressures should be compared because blood flows through the aortic arch in systole.

Although patients with left ventricular dysfunction present with respiratory distress due to a similar mechanism as described in the vignette, we would expect equally diminished pulses in upper and lower extremities in the presence of cardiogenic shock and would not expect differential cyanosis. Both PS and tricuspid atresia with normally related great vessels present with decreased pulmonary blood flow. This physiology would not lead to differential saturations, differential pulses, or respiratory distress. Obstructed TAPVR presents with profound cyanosis and respiratory distress with low cardiac output, often in the first hours of life, but would not present with differential saturations and pulses.

(Section 26: Disorders of the Cardiovascular System)

**Answer 18-11.** B

TAPVR without obstruction often presents as failure to thrive because the respiratory distress is so subtle and these children often do not have a significant heart murmur on exam unless they develop tricuspid regurgitation or turbulent blood flow across the pulmonary valve secondary to increased flow. Cardiac findings include a widely split second heart sound in the setting of markedly increased pulmonary blood flow and a right ventricular heave. Cyanosis becomes more significant as congestive heart failure progresses.

In tetralogy of Fallot, the murmur would have a harsh quality and ejection type. CXR shows darker lung fields, indicating decreased pulmonary blood flow. In truncus arteriosus, there is no split $S_2$ because there is only 1 semilunar valve and there is usually a systolic ejection click. Truncus arteriosus commonly presents with tachypnea and modest desaturations. In transposition of the great arteries, there is a single loud $S_2$ because the aorta is anterior. In ventricular septal defect, there should not be desaturation or a widely split $S_2$.

(Section 26: Disorders of the Cardiovascular System)

**Answer 18-12.** A

A cranial bruit may be present in the vein of Galen malformation, a type of intracranial arteriovenous fistula. These arteriovenous fistulas usually produce immediate, severe hemodynamic changes in neonates. They involve vessels of large caliber, and the left-to-right shunt is often large, causing severe high-output congestive heart failure in the first days after birth. Clinically, they have continuous murmurs over either side of the skull, bounding carotid pulses, and distended jugular veins. The superior vena cava is generally markedly dilated on CXR, and there is significant right and left ventricular volume overload.

A large ductal shunt and a large ventricular septal defect (VSD) will not cause congestive heart failure until the pulmonary vascular resistance drops in the first weeks of life, and this will present with symptoms of pulmonary overcirculation. A pericardial rub caused by a pericardial effusion is not associated with congestive heart failure. Critical valvar aortic stenosis would present with cardiogenic shock and decreased systemic perfusion rather than high-output failure.

(Section 26: Disorders of the Cardiovascular System)

**Answer 18-13.** A

The murmur in the vignette is characteristic of aortic regurgitation: a high-pitched, early diastolic murmur that starts at the aortic component of the second heart sound. This occurs due to prolapse of the aortic valve cusp into the subpulmonic or doubly committed subarterial defect. With a VSD adjacent to the aortic annulus, the support of the adjacent aortic cusp is weakened. The cusp tends to sag into the left ventricle, and the left-to-right shunt through the VSD exerts force on the cusp through the defect. Repair of the defect may buttress the aortic cusp sufficiently to reduce the aortic regurgitation and prevent surgery on the aortic valve.

The murmur described does not correlate with mitral stenosis or ASDs. Pulmonary regurgitation is not associated with VSDs. Infective endocarditis (IE) is a rare problem, and this clinical vignette is not consistent with endocarditis or a Gerbode defect.

(Section 26: Disorders of the Cardiovascular System)

**Answer 18-14.** D

There is a strong association between VSD, anomalous right ventricular muscle bundles, and subpulmonic stenosis. This is known as double-chambered right ventricle. This double-chambered right ventricle is caused by large, aberrant muscular bands that divide the right ventricular cavity into 2 separate chambers and obstruct flow through the subpulmonic infundibular area.

Although VSD, subaortic stenosis, and coarctation of the aorta are frequently related, this is not the best answer based on the ECG and physical exam (with normal distal pulses). The physical exam does not suggest mitral valve prolapse or a patent ductus arteriosus, and these lesions are not associated with a VSD and subpulmonic stenosis. A patent ductus arteriosus in a toddler would most likely be heard as the classic machinery-type continuous murmur. Left superior vena cava to the coronary sinus is not associated with VSD and subpulmonic stenosis.

(Section 26: Disorders of the Cardiovascular System)

**Answer 18-15.** E

Placing the patient in the knee-chest position with supplemental oxygen is one of the ways to help abort a tet spell. Tet spells are hypercyanotic episodes with paroxysmal hyperpnea that occur spontaneously, after early morning feedings, prolonged crying, or fever. The attacks may last only a few moments and have no sequelae; they may cause obtundation, limpness, deep exhaustion, or sleep; rarely, they may end in unconsciousness, convulsions, or even death. Administering antipyretics or oral hydration is not correct because the patient's hypoxia is the most acute concern. The absence of murmur is not reassuring; it is one of the signs of a tet spell and represents lack of blood flow across the pulmonary valve, and steps to correct the hypoxia are the most important. An echocardiogram would not help with management because the diagnosis has already been made and would delay care.

(Section 26: Disorders of the Cardiovascular System)

**Answer 18-16.** A

The heart murmur described in the question is most consistent with aortic stenosis. This is a loud crescendo-decrescendo systolic murmur, often grade 4 to 5 in intensity and associated with a suprasternal notch thrill. Additionally, a prominent apical third sound is frequently heard. Balloon valvoplasty has become the treatment of choice (see Chapter 479 for more information about balloon valvoplasties).

Although a bicuspid valve may also cause an ejection click, the coarctation would result in a blood pressure and pulse intensity differential not noted in the vignette. In subaortic stenosis due to hypertrophic cardiomyopathy, when the patient squats, this increases venous return, and this increase in preload can overcome dynamic outflow obstruction, which results in a softer murmur. The murmur of PS is an ejection systolic murmur of the crescendo-decrescendo type best heard at the upper left sternal border, with radiation to the left infraclavicular area. A PS murmur does not change with squatting, although it does decrease with Valsalva. The murmur of a moderate-sized VSD would be holosystolic and should not appreciably change with Valsalva.

(Section 26: Disorders of the Cardiovascular System)

**Answer 18-17.** D

The vignette is most consistent with either a right aortic arch with aberrant left subclavian causing a ring or a double arch with an atretic left arch. Elective surgery should be done, and no other imaging is necessary. Infants with severe obstructions are very ill with vomiting, choking, and often dysphagia, which often lead to feeding difficulties and poor weight gain. Wheezing and stridor, usually inspiratory, are often symptoms and are made worse by feeding. These infants frequently will hyperextend their heads to reduce tracheal compression. The most common malformation is the double aortic arch, which can result from failure of absorption of any part of the embryonic fourth arches. The subclavian artery is not causing the patient's noisy breathing. The large proximal left subclavian bulge is known as a diverticulum of Kommerell. This indicates that there is a ring with either a ligamentum arteriosum or an atretic left arch (or both). Although a left pulmonary artery sling can cause symptoms similar to those in the vignette, dysphagia is rare. The echocardiogram would show that the left pulmonary artery arises from the right pulmonary artery and passes between the esophagus and trachea, compressing the trachea and the right main bronchus.

(Section 26: Disorders of the Cardiovascular System)

**Answer 18-18.** A

Patients with an anomalous left coronary artery arising from pulmonary artery (ALCAPA) present with myocardial failure from ischemia or even a myocardial infarct between 2 weeks and 6 months of age. Episodes of restlessness and crying associated with pallor and sweating have been described in infants, along with poor feeding, tachypnea, and respiratory symptoms related to left ventricular failure. Other findings include severe cardiomegaly with the murmur of mitral regurgitation secondary to infarction of the papillary muscles, the presence of a gallop rhythm, and ECG findings consistent with an anterolateral infarct pattern.

A primary dilated cardiomyopathy could present with similarly depressed systolic function, but the ECG changes and dilated right coronary artery seen on the ECG would not be expected. Although intramural left coronary artery from the right sinus can be associated with sudden death, especially after exercise, this does not present as cardiomyopathy in infancy. Although ECG changes and poor ventricular function are common findings in myocarditis, the mitral regurgitation and specific ischemic changes on the ECG make ALCAPA more likely. Kawasaki disease can affect infants and could explain the dilation of the right coronary artery; however, it is unusual to present this young with these ischemic findings without other preceding Kawasaki symptoms.

(Section 26: Disorders of the Cardiovascular System)

**Answer 18-19.** B

This figure shows second-degree, Mobitz type I/Wenckebach AV block. The tracing shows 2 Wenckebach cycles with progressive lengthening of the PR interval until the atrial beat is not conducted to the ventricles. The first atrial impulse of a group of beats is conducted normally, but the next atrial impulse reaches the AV node while it is still partly refractory and thus is conducted more slowly, resulting in a longer PR interval. The next atrial impulse arrives even earlier in the AV nodal relative refractory period, resulting in an even longer PR interval. Eventually, the atrial impulse reaches the AV node in its absolute refractory period and is blocked so that no QRS complex follows. Mobitz type I second-degree AV block may occur in healthy people, particularly athletes. In this setting, it occurs at night and is caused by increased vagal tone. If it is asymptomatic in someone with no structural or functional heart disease, it does not require aggressive evaluation or treatment.

In contrast, Mobitz type II second-degree AV block occurs when a QRS complex drops out without prior lengthening of the PR intervals. It is less common but more serious than type I second-degree AV block and is more likely to lead to complete AV block. It usually results from disease in the His-Purkinje system below the level of the compact AV node and always requires careful evaluation; therefore, reassurance would be incorrect. Third-degree AV block occurs if no atrial beats are conducted and ventricular contraction is stimulated by a junctional or ventricular escape focus. There are normal P waves at one rate and QRS complexes at a slower rate, with no fixed relationship between P waves and QRS complexes (AV dissociation). Phasic sinus arrhythmia is a normal variant in which the sinus rate varies with increases with inspiration and slows with expiration secondary to changing right heart filling with negative intrathoracic pressure with inspiration. During expiration, the sinus rate may be sufficiently slowed to allow escape beats from an atrial or junctional pacemaker. An escape beat is recognized by its late appearance (R-R interval longer than normal) and evidence of a nonsinus focus (abnormal P-wave axis and morphology for an atrial ectopic focus, or no P wave, very short PR, or retrograde P wave for junctional focus).

(Section 26: Disorders of the Cardiovascular System)

**Answer 18-20. B**

This patient has Wolff-Parkinson-White (WPW) syndrome. Supraventricular tachycardia (SVT; the orthodromic reciprocating form of atrioventricular [AV] reentrant tachycardia) terminates suddenly to preexcited sinus rhythm. Note the short PR interval and the delta wave (slurred initial QRS deflection) resulting in a wide-complex QRS in preexcited sinus rhythm. It is important to document an echocardiogram because WPW is associated with Ebstein anomaly, congenitally corrected transposition of the great arteries, left ventricular noncompaction cardiomyopathy, and hypertrophic cardiomyopathy. A β-blocker, such as atenolol, is the treatment of choice to prevent recurrences of tachycardia. This child would also be referred for elective radiofrequency ablation as definitive treatment since he has been symptomatic with SVT due to the WPW. Radiofrequency ablation of the accessory pathway is the treatment of choice for patients with WPW syndrome, with a > 90% cure rate. However, this patient has not had episodes suggestive of preexcited atrial fibrillation or aborted sudden cardiac death, and it can be done on an elective basis.

AV nodal blocking agents, including verapamil and digoxin, are contraindicated in WPW due to the potential for enhancing anterograde conduction down the accessory pathway. Although caffeine can increase automaticity and may cause increased frequency of SVT due to a premature atrial or ventricular beat initiating reentry, premature atrial and ventricular contractions are common in the absence of caffeine, and cutting back will not always prevent further episodes. Additionally, any symptomatic child should be referred for definitive treatment with radiofrequency ablation.

(Section 26: Disorders of the Cardiovascular System)

**Answer 18-21. C**

This clinical history is concerning for a cardiac cause for syncope (with his family history of sudden death and his exertional syncope). A referral to a pediatric cardiologist is warranted.

Long QT syndrome is a cause of ventricular arrhythmias and sudden death and would be the most worrisome of these findings. Sudden death while swimming in particular raises the concern for type 1 long QT syndrome. All first-degree relatives of a child with a long QTc interval should be screened by a cardiologist. Mobitz type I/Wenckebach second-degree AV block is often a normal finding in healthy adolescents and does not raise the concern for higher-grade AV block. Possible right ventricular hypertrophy on ECG is often poorly correlated with true right ventricular hypertrophy on echocardiogram and is likely a false-positive finding in the absence of physical exam findings suggestive of pathologic processes that would result in a volume or pressure overload to the right ventricle. An upright T wave in $V_1$ is normal in adolescents and adults. Frequent premature ventricular contractions can cause a premature ventricular contraction cardiomyopathy due to mechanical dyssynchrony, but typically, these are not inherited findings, and his and his father's clinical symptoms are not consistent with this.

(Section 26: Disorders of the Cardiovascular System)

**Answer 18-22. B**

β-Blockers are the primary treatment for long QT syndrome. β-Blockers are useful for minimizing the adrenergic stimulation that increases early and late afterdepolarizations and increase the ventricular fibrillation threshold in the setting of increased dispersion of repolarization across the myocardium. The afterdepolarizations are thought to be the inciting events for torsades de pointes. Intracardiac defibrillator or sympathetic denervation may be needed in cases of frequent ventricular tachycardia or ventricular fibrillation arrest despite optimal β-blocker therapy; however, they are not a substitute for β-blockers, which remain the primary treatment for long QT syndrome. Digoxin increases atrial and ventricular ectopy, and amiodarone is a class III antiarrhythmic that further prolongs the QTc; thus, these are contraindicated.

(Section 26: Disorders of the Cardiovascular System)

**Answer 18-23.** D

Children with DiGeorge syndrome and hypocalcemia are prone to having seizures from hypocalcemia. A rhythm strip during the seizure may have muscle or motion artifact that may be confused with supraventricular or ventricular tachycardia. Careful marching of the R waves will show an underlying sinus rhythm. This is important to distinguish from true arrhythmias, as a patient with severe hypocalcemia is at risk for QTc prolongation and malignant ventricular arrhythmias.

(Section 26: Disorders of the Cardiovascular System)

**Answer 18-24.** B

The ECG and rash depicted above are consistent with Lyme disease. The incidence of cardiac involvement in Lyme disease has been estimated to be 8% and usually occurs within a few weeks of the onset of the illness. The most common feature of Lyme carditis is atrioventricular (AV) block, as shown here. The AV block usually resolves gradually with normalization of the PR interval in 1 to 2 weeks. Persistence of AV block requiring a pacemaker is unusual.

Although first-degree AV block (PR prolongation) is a minor criterion in acute rheumatic fever (ARF), higher-grade AV block is not seen. Typical ECG findings in pericarditis are diffuse ST elevation and reciprocal PR depression, but not of the AV block. Although Kawasaki disease may affect the coronary arteries, it does not affect AV conduction unless there is involvement of the AV nodal branch, typically off the right coronary artery. Juvenile rheumatoid arthritis is not associated with AV block.

(Section 26: Disorders of the Cardiovascular System)

**Answer 18-25.** C

The rhythm strip shows a regular and rapid atrial rate, consistent with atrial flutter. Atrial flutter is characterized by intra-atrial reentry at rapid atrial rates of about 300 per minute in older children and adolescents and as high as 450 to 500 bpm in newborns. The ECG strip below (see following figure) shows a marking at each flutter wave at an atrial rate of 375 bpm and a ventricular rate of 188 bpm, representing 2:1 AV conduction. Atrial flutter can sometimes occur transiently in otherwise normal newborn infants. Synchronized DC cardioversion is an effective treatment to terminate intra-atrial reentry.

The patient should be treated before discharge. The patient described is stable and does not require emergent DC cardioversion. This rhythm strip is not consistent with AV node reentry tachycardia or orthodromic reciprocating tachycardia. Vagal maneuvers and adenosine will not convert atrial flutter to sinus rhythm. They can, however, slow the ventricular rate so that the sawtooth pattern is more easily seen for diagnostic purposes.

(Section 26: Disorders of the Cardiovascular System)

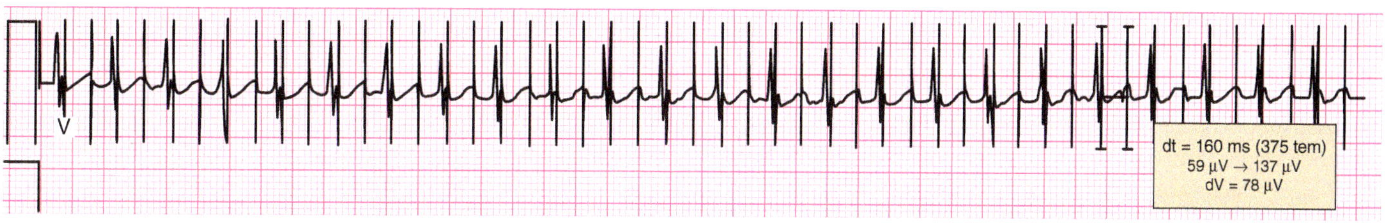


**Answer 18-26.** E

The classic functional murmur, Still's murmur, is a low-pitched, vibratory systolic murmur best heard between the left sternal border and apex. Typically, this murmur decreases in intensity as the patient moves from supine to sitting position. These innocent murmurs are frequently heard after age 3 years, when the child is quietly cooperative with the physical exam.

A continuous machine-like murmur under the left clavicle describes a patent ductus arteriosus. The harsh systolic ejection murmur of valvar aortic stenosis is best heard at the right upper sternal border and radiates to the carotid arteries in the neck. It often is associated with a suprasternal notch thrill. The murmur of an aortic coarctation is best heard in the interscapular area, which is closest to the aortic narrowing. Diastolic murmurs are always pathologic.

(Section 26: Disorders of the Cardiovascular System)

**Answer 18-27.** E

Functional (innocent) murmurs increase in intensity when the child moves from sitting to supine position. It is flow dependent and should change in intensity during postural change that increases venous return and preload to the heart. Moving from sitting to standing, deep inspiration, and the Valsalva maneuver decrease preload on the heart and, therefore, would cause the murmur to decrease in intensity. The handgrip maneuver causes an increase in afterload, which will not change a functional murmur.

(Section 26: Disorders of the Cardiovascular System)

**Answer 18-28.** C

Given his examination and low baseline oxygen saturations, this child likely has tetralogy of Fallot: right ventricular hypertrophy, pulmonary stenosis, overriding aorta, and a VSD. This is the most common form of cyanotic heart disease. He is having hypercyanotic (tet) spells, which are caused by an acute reduction in pulmonary blood flow during exertion. Squatting increases the systemic vascular resistance, decreases the volume of right-to-left shunting across the VSD, and thereby increases pulmonary blood flow. Double outlet right ventricle with transposition of the great arteries would have cyanosis but would not be at risk for dynamic outflow obstruction. VSD and AVSD would shunt from left to right and therefore would not be associated with cyanosis in a toddler, although patients with unrepaired VSDs are at risk for Eisenmenger syndrome when older. Normal blood pressures and pulses make coarctation unlikely in this cyanotic patient.

(Section 26: Disorders of the Cardiovascular System)

**Answer 18-29.** A

An ASD shunt increases the volume of flow across the pulmonic valve, causing the fixed split $S_2$ and the flow murmur in the main pulmonary artery. Most children with an ASD are asymptomatic, and the lesion is detected on routine examinations. There is minimal pressure difference between the atria, so the murmur is due to increased flow volume across the pulmonic valve.

Aortic stenosis, pulmonic valve stenosis, and VSD murmurs are generally detected early in infancy/childhood with prominent murmurs due to high pressure gradients. The pulses are normal, so aortic coarctation is unlikely.

(Section 26: Disorders of the Cardiovascular System)

**Answer 18-30.** B

Reproducible chest wall tenderness at the costochondral border supports the diagnosis of costochondritis. Adolescents often develop nonspecific inflammation of the costochondral cartilage, which is relieved by nonsteroidal anti-inflammatory medications. Rheumatic fever, endocarditis, myocarditis, and pericarditis are all more likely to present with fever and other systemic signs of infection. The pain associated with pericarditis is not associated with tenderness.

(Section 26: Disorders of the Cardiovascular System)

**Answer 18-31.** D

His description of the episodes, the normal exam, and ECG are characteristic of vasovagal syncope. It is a benign condition and can be avoided by increasing fluid and salt intake and by avoiding situations that promote venous blood pooling in the lower extremities and reduce systemic venous return, such as standing for prolonged periods of time. Once the patient faints, and thereby lies flat, the systemic venous return increases and the relative cerebral blood flow increases, thus reestablishing consciousness.

Long QT syndrome, hypertrophic cardiomyopathy, and SVT have distinct ECG patterns. Premature atrial contractions are benign. Syncopal episodes due to long QT syndrome are often associated with increased emotion or exercise.

(Section 26: Disorders of the Cardiovascular System)

**Answer 18-32.** A

Having documented elevated arm blood pressures with a proper-sized cuff, it is important to rule out an aortic coarctation. His distal pulses are difficult to feel. With an aortic click on exam, he likely has a bicuspid aortic valve; however, there is no evidence of aortic stenosis on exam. There is left ventricular hypertrophy on ECG. If his lower extremity blood pressure is lower than his arms, he is likely to have an aortic coarctation. He needs a cardiology evaluation and an echocardiogram.

Once a coarctation has been ruled out, then you should investigate other etiologies of systemic hypertension, including renal disease, familial hypercholesterolemia, and essential hypertension.

(Section 26: Disorders of the Cardiovascular System)

**Answer 18-33.** D

Atrophic pyelonephritis is the most likely cause for her hypertension. The key is the history of urinary tract infections causing scar over time.

Coarctation is unlikely since her diastolic blood pressure is also high; most children with coarctation have isolated systolic hypertension. You would also expect an abnormal physical exam such as a murmur in the back and weak femoral pulses. Although renal artery stenosis could cause this degree of blood pressure elevation, you might expect to hear an abdominal bruit. The history of high fever and rash may represent a streptococcal infection. However, an elevated blood pressure at age 13, 8 years after this episode, is more consistent with glomerular scarring rather than glomerulonephritis. Pheochromocytoma is unlikely since she is not tachycardic and does not have other historical features consistent with this diagnosis. Additionally, pheochromocytoma is a rare diagnosis.

(Section 26: Disorders of the Cardiovascular System)

**Answer 18-34.** A

Patients with prosthetic material used during palliative or corrective surgery are at the highest risk for bacterial endocarditis. In the current 2007 American Heart Association guidelines, patients with aortopulmonary shunts continue to be in the small subset of patients for whom antibiotic prophylaxis is recommended. The other patients in this vignette would not warrant prophylaxis unless they had a history of prior bacterial endocarditis (or if there is valve disease in the transplantation patient). Prophylaxis would have been recommended for the child with transposition and transplantation for the first 6 months after the operation. The child with unrepaired total anomalous pulmonary veins and the child with mitral stenosis have not had surgical or cardiac interventional procedures.

(Section 26: Disorders of the Cardiovascular System)

**Answer 18-35.** B

Rhabdomyomas are the most common cardiac tumor of childhood, and approximately half are associated with tuberous sclerosis. Most are asymptomatic, and many regress; however, they may cause arrhythmias, heart block, or even death by obstructing blood flow. Mortality is highest among children < 5 years old. Hamartomas are a type of fibroma that can occur in the ventricular wall. Myxomas are benign and usually arise from the atrial septum. Teratomas are rare and usually occur in infants at the base of the heart. Hemangiomas are usually in the atrial wall and spontaneously resolve. Any of these lesions may present with similar symptoms of arrhythmia or obstruction but are not associated with tuberous sclerosis.

(Section 26: Disorders of the Cardiovascular System)

**Answer 18-36.** A

This patient meets the clinical criteria for Kawasaki disease. The persistent high fever, conjunctival injection, changes in the extremities, red lips, and strawberry tongue are diagnostic features of Kawasaki disease. Cervical lymphadenopathy (node > 1.5 cm) is the fifth principal feature (Table 482-1). To meet the classical definition, the patient must have at least 5 days of fever and 4 of the 5 principal features. His presentation is not as consistent with streptococcal infection, which usually presents with a pharyngeal exudate and without mucosal involvement. Children with Stevens-Johnson syndrome and staphylococcal scaled skin syndrome typically have a more toxic appearance. Rheumatic fever classically has a history of joint swelling, pain, or erythema.

(Section 26: Disorders of the Cardiovascular System)

**TABLE 482-1.** Clinical and Laboratory Features of Kawasaki Disease

| | |
|---|---|
| **Epidemiologic Case Definition (Classic Clinical Criteria)** | • Central nervous system |
| • Fever of at least 5 days in duration | Extreme irritability |
| • Presence of at least 4 of the following principal features: | Aseptic meningitis |
| Changes in extremities | Peripheral facial nerve palsy |
| Polymorphous exanthem | Sensorineural hearing loss |
| Bilateral conjunctival injection | • Genitourinary system |
| Changes in the lips and oral cavity | Urethritis/meatitis |
| Cervical lymphadenopathy | Testicular swelling |
| • Exclusion of other diseases with similar findings | • Other findings |
| **Other Clinical and Laboratory Findings** | Erythema and induration at bacillus Calmette-Guérin (BCG) inoculation site |
| • Cardiovascular findings | Anterior uveitis |
| Congestive heart failure, myocarditis, pericarditis, or valvular regurgitation | Desquamating rash in groin |
| Coronary artery abnormalities | • Laboratory findings in acute Kawasaki disease |
| Aneurysms of medium-sized noncoronary arteries | Neutrophilia with immature forms |
| Raynaud phenomenon | Elevated erythrocyte sedimentation rate |
| Peripheral gangrene | Elevated C-reactive protein |
| • Musculoskeletal system | Elevated serum $\alpha_1$ antitrypsin |
| Arthritis, arthralgia | Anemia |
| • Gastrointestinal tract | Abnormal plasma lipids |
| Diarrhea, vomiting, abdominal pain | Hypoalbuminemia |
| Hepatic dysfunction | Thrombocytosis after first week |
| Hydrops of the gallbladder | Sterile pyuria |
| • Respiratory tract | Elevated serum transaminases |
| Pulmonary nodules and interstitial infiltrates | Pleocytosis of cerebrospinal fluid |
| Pleural effusion | Leukocytosis in synovial fluid |

Reproduced with permission from Newburger JW, Takahashi M, Gerber MA, et al: Diagnosis, treatment, and long-term management of Kawasaki disease: a statement for health professionals from the Committee on Rheumatic Fever, Endocarditis and Kawasaki Disease, Council on Cardiovascular Disease in the Young, American Heart Association, *Circulation*. 2004 Oct 26;110(17):2747-2771.

**Answer 18-37. B**

If the patient meets the clinical criteria for diagnosis of Kawasaki disease, the treatment of choice is IVIG and high-dose aspirin to reduce inflammatory response and decrease the risk of coronary aneurysm formation. There is a limited window of time in which one can give IVIG to help prevent coronary aneurysm formation (< 10 days after the onset of fever).

Blood cultures and antibiotics or a lumbar puncture and antibiotics are appropriate if sepsis and meningitis are primary concerns; however, the patient meets diagnostic criteria for Kawasaki disease, and antibiotics have no role in its treatment. To discharge the patient and follow up the next day in clinic would delay diagnosis and treatment of the Kawasaki disease and may increase the risk of coronary involvement.

(Section 26: Disorders of the Cardiovascular System)

**Answer 18-38. C**

This patient most likely has acute myocarditis. Its course ranges from very mild to fulminant, with death in a few days or weeks. Often there is a history of a recent upper respiratory tract infection, and viruses are usually the causative agents. Viral myocarditis is commonly associated with ventricular dysrhythmias and conduction abnormalities. The murmur is most likely from mitral regurgitation.

Although ARF can cause myocarditis, there are no other signs of the disease such as prior infection with *Streptococcus*, arthritis, or rash. IE is unlikely in a previously healthy patient, and he has not had persistent fevers or other signs of IE. Paroxysmal atrial tachycardia would not cause this degree of illness with hepatomegaly and would not explain the murmur or gallop. Pericarditis can follow a viral upper respiratory infection, but typically would cause chest pain and not cause a gallop.

(Section 26: Disorders of the Cardiovascular System)

**Answer 18-39. A**

To diagnose ARF, a patient must have 2 major criteria or 1 major and 2 minor criteria. The 5 major criteria include (1) migratory polyarthritis, (2) carditis, (3) subcutaneous nodules, (4) erythema marginatum, and (5) Sydenham chorea. Minor criteria include fever, arthralgia, increased ESR or CRP, leukocytosis, ECG changes showing features of heart block, evidence of streptococcal infection such as elevated DNAse or antistreptolysin O (ASO), and previous history of rheumatic fever. Rheumatic myocarditis can occur early in ARF and almost always causes mitral or aortic valve regurgitation.

(Section 26: Disorders of the Cardiovascular System)

**Answer 18-40. A**

This patient has 1 major criterion of ARF: carditis. He also has 1 minor criterion: documented evidence of recent streptococcal infection with a positive antistreptolysin O. He needs 1 additional minor criterion to meet diagnostic criteria for ARF. Minor criteria include elevated erythrocyte sedimentation rate, positive C-reactive protein, anemia, leukocytosis, electrocardiogram changes of PR and QT prolongation, and arthralgia.

(Section 26: Disorders of the Cardiovascular System)

**Answer 18-41. A**

IE is an infection of the endocardium, typically involving the cardiac valves. The presentation of endocarditis can be variable. Presentation can be slow onset or subacute with intermittent fevers and few other symptoms. Other cases may present with fever, fulminant symptoms of heart failure, and embolic complications. IE can occur in children with or without underlying cardiac disease. The diagnosis is primarily dependent on clinical features (Table 484-1 for revised Duke clinical diagnostic criteria). Importantly, identifying the causative organism through multiple blood cultures is imperative *before* starting an antibiotic. Treatment usually lasts for 4 to 6 weeks. Echocardiography is a secondary diagnostic modality; it can identify the valve involved and the potential risk of embolic events.

Tuberculosis can present with intermittent fevers and a pericardial friction rub, but generally does not directly involve the heart or the valves. Kawasaki disease has a 4- to 5-day course of high fever, irritability, conjunctivitis, and rash. Acute rheumatic fever (ARF) can present with carditis; however, this presentation does not fit the major or minor criteria of ARF. Scarlet fever has a more self-limited course (< 1 week) and is associated with pharyngitis and a rash.

(Section 26: Disorders of the Cardiovascular System)

**Answer 18-42. E**

Given this history, examination, and CXR, this patient most likely has acute pericarditis with a pericardial effusion. Symptoms of acute pericarditis include sharp precordial chest pain that is improved by sitting up, an intermittent pericardial friction rub, and fever. Pericardial effusions alone may have no symptoms; however, they can present as in this vignette, with muffled heart sounds, enlarged cardiac silhouette on CXR, and low voltages on ECG. Importantly, pulsus paradoxus should be checked. She should have an echocardiogram to assess the size of the effusion. She may need pericardiocentesis to drain the effusion.

The patient in the vignette does not have an antecedent streptococcal infection or other physical findings to support ARF. There is no chest wall tenderness consistent with costochondritis. IE is a possibility with the history of intermittent fevers, but the viral respiratory infection history and cardiomegaly on CXR make pericardial effusion more likely. Myocarditis is possible with the history of viral illness, but her need to sleep upright, dyspnea, ECG, and CXR are more consistent with pericarditis.

(Section 26: Disorders of the Cardiovascular System)

**TABLE 484-1.** Definitions of Terms Used in Modified Duke Criteria for Diagnosis of Infective Endocarditis (IE)

| |
|---|
| **Major Criteria** |
| 1. Positive blood culture for infective endocarditis |
| A. Typical microorganism consistent with IE from ≥ 2 blood cultures, as noted below: |
| (i) Viridans streptococci,[a] *Streptococcus bovis*, or HACEK group OR |
| (ii) Community-acquired *Staphylococcus aureus* or enterococci, in the absence of a primary focus |
| B. Microorganisms consistent with IE from persistently positive blood cultures, defined as: |
| (i) ≥ 2 Positive cultures of blood samples drawn > 12 h apart OR |
| (ii) All of 3 or a majority of ≥ 4 blood cultures, irrespective of the timing OR |
| (iii) 1 Positive blood culture for *Coxiella burnetii* or antiphase-I immunoglobulin G antibody titer > 1:800 |
| 2. Evidence of endocardial involvement |
| A. Positive echocardiogram (transesophageal echocardiography recommended in prosthetic valves, rated at least possible IE by clinical criteria, or the first test in other patients) for IE, defined as: |
| (i) Oscillating intracardiac mass on valve or supporting structures, in the path of regurgitant jets, or on implanted material or in the absence of an alternative anatomic explanation OR |
| (ii) Abscess OR |
| (iii) New partial dehiscence of prosthetic valve |
| 3. New valvar regurgitation (worsening or changing of preexisting murmur not sufficient) |
| **Minor Criteria** |
| 1. Predisposition: predisposing heart condition or intravenous drug use |
| 2. Fever: temperature ≥ 38.0°C |
| 3. Vascular phenomena: major arterial emboli, septic pulmonary infarcts, mycotic aneurysm, intracranial hemorrhage, conjunctival hemorrhages, and Janeway lesions |
| 4. Immunologic phenomena: glomerulonephritis, Osler nodes, Roth spots, and rheumatoid factor |
| 5. Microbiologic evidence: positive blood culture but does not meet a major criterion as noted above or serologic evidence of active infection with organism consistent with IE |

[a]Includes nutritionally variant strains (*Abiotrophia* species). Excludes single positive cultures for coagulase-negative staphylococci and organisms that do not cause endocarditis.

Reproduced with permission from Durack DT, Lukes AS, Bright DK: New criteria for diagnosis of infective endocarditis: utilization of specific echocardiographic findings. Duke Endocarditis Service, *Am J Med.* 1994 Mar;96(3):200-209.

**Answer 18-43.** E

Pulsus paradoxus is the single most important bedside test for tamponade. To measure pulsus paradoxus, blood pressure is measured with the patient breathing normally and then with deep inspiration. In tamponade, the systolic blood pressure with inspiration will be > 10 mm Hg lower than the resting blood pressure. This is due to the inability of the right heart to fill during diastole when there is a constricting effusion. This effect profoundly compromises systemic cardiac output.

An upper extremity systolic blood pressure that is > 15 mm Hg more than the lower extremity blood pressure and absent femoral pulses are signs of aortic coarctation. Nonpurulent conjunctival injection and strawberry tongue are seen in Kawasaki disease. Splinter hemorrhages and Janeway lesions are findings in infective endocarditis.

(Section 26: Disorders of the Cardiovascular System)

**Answer 18-44.** B

Pulmonary arterial hypertension has multiple etiologies but a common pathophysiology. The small pulmonary arteries (the lung does not have arterioles) are muscularized, which elevates the pulmonary vascular resistance and pulmonary arterial pressures. The right ventricle dilates and hypertrophies in response. During exercise, when the right heart is unable to maintain cardiac output through the hypertensive pulmonary vascular bed, syncope occurs. It is an ominous sign in late-stage pulmonary hypertension. Both tetralogy of Fallot and pulmonary stenosis would have right ventricular hypertrophy on ECG, but on examination, patients with these cardiac defects should present with a murmur. Coarctation is unlikely given the normal pulses and blood pressures. Both coarctation and hypertrophic cardiomyopathy would have increased left ventricular voltages on ECG.

(Section 26: Disorders of the Cardiovascular System)

**Answer 18-45.** E

The quantitative assessment of flow events in the heart and great vessels is performed using spectral Doppler velocity measurement of flow velocities. In many situations, the blood velocity can be used to predict a pressure drop across the area of flow. Using the modified Bernoulli equation, the pressure drop is 4*v*2, where *v* is the velocity in meters per second. Thus, a peak jet velocity of 4.5 m/s predicts a peak pressure drop of 4 × 4.52, or 81 mm Hg. This gradient can be used to predict a chamber or vessel pressure or may be used to assess stenosis severity. A gradient of 81 mm Hg denotes severe left ventricular outflow tract obstruction, and surgical correction would be warranted.

(Section 26: Disorders of the Cardiovascular System)

**Answer 18-46.** A

The normal PVR is < 3 units/m$^2$. Although high at birth, the PVR drops to adult levels by 4 weeks of age. If the patient has mild-moderate pulmonary vascular disease, the PVR will be in the 4 to 12 units/m$^2$ range. Severe pulmonary vascular disease is characterized by high PVR (> 15 units/m$^2$). By testing the responsiveness of the pulmonary vasculature to vasodilators (oxygen, nitric oxide, and iloprost), cardiologists can assess the patient's suitability for various medications or lung transplant.

(Section 26: Disorders of the Cardiovascular System)

### Answer 18-47. B

There is a 60-mm Hg pressure drop from the right ventricle and pulmonary artery, indicating severe right ventricular outflow obstruction. There are equal pressures in the right and left ventricles due to the associated large VSD. Because there is right-to-left shunting at the VSD level, the saturation in the left ventricle and aorta are lower than normal. These data describe a child with tetralogy of Fallot.

A moderate VSD would cause mildly elevated right ventricle and pulmonary artery pressures but would be expected to have only left-to-right shunting and no desaturation in the left ventricle or aorta. There is no left-to-right shunting at the atrial level, as indicated by the fact that there is no increase in saturations from the superior vena cava to the right atrium. The left atrial saturation is normal. There is no pressure gradient from the left ventricle to the ascending aorta, ruling out aortic valve stenosis. And there is no pressure gradient between the ascending and descending aorta, excluding coarctation of the aorta. The mildly increased descending aortic systolic pressure is normal. This elevation is caused by the standing wave effect of the blood rushing down the abdominal aorta.

(Section 26: Disorders of the Cardiovascular System)

### Answer 18-48. E

There is a 60-mm Hg pressure gradient between the ascending and descending aorta, indicating the presence of a severe aortic coarctation.

A moderate VSD would cause mildly elevated right ventricular and pulmonary artery pressures but would be expected to have only left-to-right shunting and no desaturation in the left ventricle or aorta. These data show normal pressures and saturations in the right ventricle and pulmonary artery, excluding right ventricular outflow obstruction as in tetralogy of Fallot. There is no shunting at the atrial level, with no increase in saturations from the superior vena cava to the right atrium. There is no pressure gradient from the left ventricle to the ascending aorta, ruling out aortic valve stenosis.

(Section 26: Disorders of the Cardiovascular System)

### Answer 18-49. E

This patient is presenting with heart failure. Infants and young children present with poor feeding, failure to thrive, respiratory distress, diaphoresis, and pallor. Patients with a large patent ductus arteriosus, large VSD, truncus arteriosus, and complete common AV canal all develop high-pressure/high-volume left-to-right shunts after the pulmonary vascular resistance drops. This subsequently causes an increase in pulmonary blood flow relative to systemic blood flow (increased Qp:Qs), which results in symptoms of congestive heart failure. These patients may also have decreased systemic blood flow. Even large ASDs will not cause congestive heart failure at this age.

(Section 26: Disorders of the Cardiovascular System)

### Answer 18-50. C

Milrinone is a nonglycoside, noncatecholamine inotropic agent with additional vasodilatory and lusitropic properties. It inhibits phosphodiesterase type 3, increasing intracellular cyclic adenosine monophosphate (AMP) and intracellular calcium, thus enhancing myocardial contractility. It also enhances diastolic relaxation of the myocardium by increasing the rate of reuptake of calcium after systole. It may also act synergistically with a β-adrenergic agonist such as dopamine and has fewer side effects. Milrinone lowers filling pressures, systemic and pulmonary artery pressures, and systemic and pulmonary vascular resistances, while improving the cardiac index. Milrinone is usually initiated at 0.25 μg/kg/min and can be titrated gradually to 1 μg/kg/min based on the clinical response.

Levosimendan is a calcium-sensitizing agent with inotropic and afterload-reducing effects. It binds to troponin C and improves the efficiency of the contractile apparatus. Catecholamines, either endogenous (eg, dopamine or epinephrine) or synthetic (eg, dobutamine), act by stimulating myocardial surface β-adrenergic receptors, leading to increased adenylate cyclase and intracellular cyclic AMP. Digoxin is a sodium-potassium ATPase inhibitor with positive inotropy, negative chronotropy, and inhibition of neurohormonal activation. Nesiritide causes natriuresis, diuresis, vasodilatation, and increased renal blood flow, and increased cardiac output and urine output.

(Section 26: Disorders of the Cardiovascular System)

### Answer 18-51. E

Patients with single-ventricle physiology have complete mixing of the pulmonary and systemic circulation. The balance between systemic and pulmonary blood flow depends on anatomic obstruction and resistance.

In patients with tricuspid atresia with normally related great vessels and pulmonary atresia with an intact ventricular septum, the right ventricle cannot pump blood to the lungs, and therefore, pulmonary blood flow is dependent on left to right flow through the patent ductus arteriosus. In the hypoplastic left heart syndrome, the left ventricle and left ventricular outflow tract are hypoplastic, and therefore, the right ventricle provides pulmonary blood flow and systemic blood flow through the patent ductus arteriosus. An unbalanced AVSD may have a right- or left-dominant ventricle. In tetralogy of Fallot with subpulmonary stenosis, the pulmonary blood flow primarily is supplied by the right ventricle and is not a complete mixing lesion and thus is not an example of single-ventricle physiology.

(Section 26: Disorders of the Cardiovascular System)

**Answer 18-52.** D

This infant is in cardiac shock and is presenting due to closure of the ductus arteriosus, which supports the systemic output. Most infants with hypoplastic left heart complex are acutely ill, with signs of congestive heart failure within the first days or weeks after birth. There are signs and symptoms of severe right-sided and left-sided heart failure: cyanosis of varying degree and often a characteristic grayish pallor and poor peripheral pulses, which contrast with hyperdynamic cardiac pulsations. Murmurs are not prominent, but a short soft midsystolic murmur and middiastolic rumble may be present. The second heart sound is single, heard loudest at the upper left sternal border, and is accentuated until clinical deterioration with gross right heart failure is advanced.

Tetralogy of Fallot is not expected to cause cardiac shock and is most commonly associated with systolic ejection murmurs due to pulmonary stenosis and varying degrees of cyanosis without respiratory distress. Although transposition of the great arteries also would likely not cause a murmur, the more typical presentation is a cyanotic infant without cardiac shock. If there is restriction to mixing, such as with restrictive atrial septal communication, the cyanosis can be profound, and there can be signs of decreased systemic output. Ebstein anomaly, when severe enough to cause symptoms in the neonate, typically is immediate in onset. Although large VSDs at 4 days of age may not cause a murmur, they also would not cause cardiac shock.

(Section 26: Disorders of the Cardiovascular System)

**Answer 18-53.** B

This infant's presentation is very concerning for ductal-dependent cyanotic congenital heart disease, in this case pulmonary atresia with intact ventricular septum. She failed to increase saturations and had a low $PaO_2$ after oxygen was administered. To reopen and keep the ductus arteriosus patent, prostaglandin $E_1$ should be given as soon as ductal-dependent heart disease is suspected. Because this medication can cause hypoventilation, the transport team should be prepared to intubate and mechanically ventilate.

Indomethacin is used to promote closure of patent ductus arteriosus. Digoxin is not useful in this scenario. Adenosine is used to treat supraventricular tachycardia. This child has adequate perfusion and pulses, and a saline bolus is not warranted.

(Section 26: Disorders of the Cardiovascular System)

**Answer 18-54.** E

Mild-to-moderate pulmonary valve stenosis is very well tolerated. As long as the right ventricular pressures are less than one-half systemic and the right ventricular function is normal, patients should not have any restrictions. Patients who are dependent on pacemakers should not participate in contact sports. The pacemaker leads and generators are at risk for damage during contact sports. Tetralogy of Fallot patients should not compete in any sports until after they are repaired because of the risks of ventricular arrhythmias, hypercyanosis, and thromboembolic events associated with right-to-left shunting. D-transposition patients, who have had arterial switch repairs, have had their coronary arteries moved as part of the operation. They are potentially at risk for coronary ischemia and sudden death. They should all have appropriate coronary artery imaging prior to approval for competitive sports. Additional sequelae that may affect their ability to participate are supravalvar PS or supravalvar aortic stenosis and dilation of the neoaortic root.

Asymptomatic patients with moderate aortic stenosis (defined as a catheterization gradient of 30–50 mm Hg or a mean gradient of 25–40 mm Hg on echocardiogram) may participate in some sports, but they will need an echocardiogram/exercise testing prior to approval. Because all forms of subvalvar, valvar, and supravalvar aortic stenosis tend to progress with time, these patients will need serial follow-up every 1 to 2 years with the possibility of a change in recommendations.

(Section 26: Disorders of the Cardiovascular System)

**Answer 18-55.** D

At higher altitudes, the partial pressure of oxygen ($PO_2$) is reduced, which decreases the alveolar oxygen ($PaO_2$). In individuals with normal cardiopulmonary function, this only becomes significant at high elevation when the $PO_2$ is $< 60$ mm Hg. This is due to the S-shaped oxygen dissociation curve. However, as the $PaO_2$ falls, the pulmonary vascular resistance will increase due to hypoxia-induced vasoconstriction. In individuals with heart lesions that do not tolerate pulmonary vasoconstriction, such as single ventricles with Fontan circulation, this will cause cyanosis and respiratory distress. Most of these individuals are able to visit or live at moderate elevations (5000–10,000 ft) or tolerate air travel. The longer they stay and the higher the elevation, the more likely they are to develop symptoms. Even if they are not symptomatic at rest, their exercise tolerance will be affected. Ski trips should include contingency plans that allow the individual to return to a lower altitude quickly, and supplemental oxygen can be helpful.

(Section 26: Disorders of the Cardiovascular System)

**Answer 18-56.** B

According to the 2007 American Heart Association guidelines for sports screening, a positive family history includes sudden death, syncope, chest pain, arrhythmias, or heart disease. It is particularly likely in hypertrophic cardiomyopathy, right ventricular dysplasia, long QT syndrome, premature atherosclerosis, and Marfan syndrome. This patient has a very strong family history of syncope and sudden death, and an ECG would help evaluate for long QT syndrome and possibly hypertrophic cardiomyopathy.

A brain MRI and electroencephalography can be useful in diagnosing seizure disorders. This patient has no history of seizures, and most likely, his brother, with his history of exertion-related sudden death, was having postsyncopal seizures and not primary seizures. A 24-hour Holter monitor would be useful in diagnosing an arrhythmia; however, an ECG would be the first step in this workup. A tilt-table test is done to evaluate vasovagal causes of syncope.

(Section 26: Disorders of the Cardiovascular System)

### Answer 18-57. B

There are approximately 3000 to 5000 sudden death episodes per year in children and adolescents in the United States. The majority, approximately 40% to 50% of sudden deaths, are caused by hypertrophic cardiomyopathy. Between 10% and 20% will be caused by coronary abnormalities—usually the left or right coronary artery arising from the wrong sinus origin or a single coronary artery origin. The remaining 30% will be caused by such lesions as myocarditis, dilated cardiomyopathy including noncompaction, ion channelopathies (long QT) syndrome, Brugada syndrome, catecholaminergic polymorphic ventricular tachycardia, arrhythmogenic right ventricular dysplasia, Wolff-Parkinson-White (WPW) syndrome, previous Kawasaki disease with undiagnosed coronary involvement, commotio cordis, and connective tissue disorders with dilated aortic roots (eg, Marfan).

(Section 26: Disorders of the Cardiovascular System)

### Answer 18-58. C

This ECG shows the orthodromic reciprocating form of atrioventricular reciprocating tachycardia, a form of reentrant supraventricular tachycardia (SVT) using a retrograde conducting accessory pathway. Based on the history of several days of poor feeding and respiratory distress, it is likely he was in SVT for several days and has developed tachycardia-induced cardiomyopathy (TIC). The most appropriate management strategy would be to obtain an echocardiogram to evaluate for ventricular systolic function and the presence of congenital heart disease and admit to initiate an antiarrhythmic. The most appropriate choice of antiarrhythmic depends on the degree of ventricular dysfunction seen because many antiarrhythmics are negative inotropes.

This rhythm is not sinus tachycardia, and the patient's presenting symptoms are less consistent with sepsis than with TIC following sustained SVT. Reassurance would not be appropriate in the setting of suspected TIC. Observation without antiarrhythmics would leave the baby at risk for future episodes of SVT. Although a high percentage of babies with accessory pathways outgrow these pathways in the first year of life, it is most appropriate to minimize the chance of recurrent SVT with an antiarrhythmic during this time that the substrate to sustain SVT remains. Not only would it be inappropriate to discharge a patient with suspected TIC, but also there are currently no antiarrhythmics that are considered safe to initiate as an outpatient in the infant population.

(Section 26: Disorders of the Cardiovascular System)

### Answer 18-59. D

This ECG shows profound QTc prolongation (> 630 ms) and 2:1 atrioventricular (AV) conduction with an atrial rate of 125 bpm and a ventricular rate of 63 bpm. Although there is not 1:1 conduction of every P wave, this is not due to AV nodal block—rather, the ventricular myocardium repolarizes too slowly and is still refractory at the time a sinus beat is conducted through the AV node and His-Purkinje system. This patient has long QT syndrome, and neonatal 2:1 AV conduction is a very-high-risk population to develop torsades de pointes, which may degenerate into ventricular fibrillation. This patient should be transferred to the NICU for telemetry monitoring and initiation of propranolol. Although it may seem counterintuitive to start a β-blocker to treat bradycardia, a β-blocker will decrease the likelihood that this patient will go into torsades de pointes or ventricular fibrillation by decreasing sympathetic tone and ventricular ectopy that may initiate torsades de pointes, possibly shortening the QTc, and raising the ventricular fibrillation threshold.

Long QT syndrome is not associated with congenital heart defect, and thus, an echocardiogram would not contribute to this patient's diagnosis or management. Although sinus bradycardia can be a sign of neonatal sepsis, this patient's sinus rate is normal at 125 bpm. Caffeine treats transient sinus bradycardia that often follows episodes of apnea of prematurity, but this patient is full term and is not having apneic episodes, and this rhythm is not sinus bradycardia. An epicardial pacemaker is not indicated because the patient's AV nodal conduction is intact, and pacing a refractory myocardium in the setting of the patient's markedly prolonged QTc would result in pacemaker noncapture and would not increase the patient's ventricular rate.

(Section 26: Disorders of the Cardiovascular System)

### Answer 18-60. E

Hypercholesterolemia is defined as a fasting LDL level ≥ 130 mg/dL or total cholesterol ≥ 200 mg/dL measured on initial screening and confirmed on repeat testing 2 weeks to 3 months later. Kawasaki disease with persistent coronary artery aneurysms is a high-risk condition for early cardiovascular disease and warrants lifestyle modification and pharmacologic therapy at the time of diagnosis for patients age ≥ 10 years. Additional high-risk conditions and risk factors include homozygous familial hypercholesterolemia, type 1 or 2 diabetes mellitus, end-stage kidney disease, solid organ transplant vasculopathy, childhood cancer survivor following stem cell transplantation, and multiple comorbidities (moderate-risk condition plus ≥ 2 additional moderate- or at-risk conditions or factors). The LDL treatment target for high-risk patients is < 100 mg/dL. Children < 10 years of age with a high-risk condition may benefit from and should be considered for early statin therapy in addition to lifestyle changes.

For all non–high-risk patients with hypercholesterolemia, initial treatment includes lifestyle modification with a heart-healthy diet, exercise, optimal management of comorbidities (eg, hypertension, obesity), and avoidance of nicotine exposure. This is the mainstay of therapy for non–high-risk patients < 10 years of age. Statin therapy should be initiated for moderate-risk patients ≥ 10 years old if the LDL remains ≥ 160 mg/dL after 3 months of lifestyle changes and after 6 months for at-risk patients. Patients with isolated hypercholesterolemia and no cardiovascular disease risk factors should be considered for statin therapy if their LDL remains ≥ 190 mg/dL after 6 months of lifestyle modification. The treatment target for all non–high-risk patients is < 130 mg/dL.

(Section 26: Disorders of the Cardiovascular System)

**Answer 18-61. D**

Patients with coarctation of the aorta have approximately 10% incidence of intracranial aneurysms, which is 5-fold that of the general population. Coarctation is not associated with increased risk of venous thrombosis, hepatocellular carcinoma, diabetes, or pulmonary hypertension.

(Section 26: Disorders of the Cardiovascular System)

# CHAPTER 19 Pulmonary and Sleep Disorders

Amy G. Filbrun and Fauziya Hassan

**19-1.** A 7-year-old boy presents with an 8-month history of inconsolable screaming 3 to 4 times per week. The father states that after falling asleep his son will typically awaken 1 to 2 hours later screaming at the top of his lungs and sweating. He is inconsolable and terrified. He does not remember what happens the following morning. What do you tell dad?

- **A.** The symptoms are consistent with sleep terrors.
- **B.** The symptoms are consistent with nightmares.
- **C.** The symptoms are concerning for seizure disorder.
- **D.** The child needs to be evaluated by a mental health professional.
- **E.** The child needs to be evaluated by a neurologist.

**19-2.** A 10-year-old girl presents with an inability to stop fidgeting for the past 6 months. Her mother states that both she and her teachers are complaining that the girl "cannot sit still." The nonrhythmic movement occurs when she is awake prior to bedtime. Her physical exam is unremarkable. The girl states that she feels as if "bugs are crawling up her legs," and she only feels better when she moves her legs as if trying to squash them. What is the most likely diagnosis?

- **A.** Essential tremor
- **B.** Periodic limb movement disorder
- **C.** Physiologic myoclonus
- **D.** Restless legs syndrome (RLS)
- **E.** Tourette syndrome

**19-3.** A 6-year-old girl presents with an 8-month history of being unable to fall asleep at night. The mother reports that just as she starts to fall asleep, her daughter starts crying and rubbing her legs. The mother states that she also suffered from similar discomfort when she was pregnant. The mother's symptoms resolved after her doctor did a test and started her on daily pills. The mother cannot remember the name of the pills but recalls that they left a bad taste in her mouth. What is the most likely test that the mother's doctor ordered?

- **A.** Thyroid-stimulating hormone
- **B.** Complete metabolic panel
- **C.** Purified protein derivative
- **D.** Complete blood count (CBC) and serum ferritin level
- **E.** Serum copper level

**19-4.** A 16-year-old boy presents to clinic for excessive daytime sleepiness (EDS) for the past year. Per mom, his teachers state that he is falling asleep in class. He feels a little better on the weekends but gets worse again during the school week. There is no history of snoring or mouth breathing. What is the most likely cause of EDS in this patient?

- **A.** Apnea
- **B.** Obstructive sleep apnea (OSA)
- **C.** Insufficient sleep
- **D.** Narcolepsy
- **E.** Alcohol abuse

**19-5.** A father brings his 13-year-old daughter in because she refuses to go to bed at 8:00 PM. Dad states that 8:00 PM had been her nightly bedtime since she was a toddler. She tells you that she just does not feel sleepy at 8:00 PM. What physiologic change during adolescence occurs that may be affecting her ability to fall asleep at 8:00 PM?

- **A.** Phase advance
- **B.** Phase delay
- **C.** Growing pains
- **D.** Menarche
- **E.** Gastroesophageal reflux disease (GERD)

**19-6.** A 28-month-old girl presents to your office for a second opinion for persistent irritability. Mom states that her previous pediatrician said she was fine. Her physical exam is normal. Mom brings in laboratory tests (complete blood count and thyroid), which are normal. What screening tool may be helpful in determining the cause of her persistent irritability?

**A.** BEARS

**B.** DREAMS

**C.** CAGE

**D.** SALSA

**E.** HEEADSSS

**19-7.** A 10-week-old, former 32-week premature male infant comes to clinic today. He was recently discharged from the neonatal intensive care unit, and they are now establishing care at your practice. During the visit, the parents state that they are worried that because he was a premature infant that his lungs will not grow. What do you tell them?

**A.** The lungs stop growing at birth.

**B.** The lung tubes or conducting airways continue to grow in number after birth.

**C.** The lung sacs or alveoli continue to grow in number after birth.

**D.** The lung tubes and sacs continue to grow in number throughout life.

**E.** The lung tubes and sacs continue to remodel throughout life.

**19-8.** A 2-week-old boy presents to clinic for observed pauses in his sleep by his parents. His mother says that she now places the child on her own stomach to make sure he is breathing. What test would be most helpful is assessing his breathing pattern while he sleeps?

**A.** Spirometry

**B.** Polysomnogram

**C.** Chest radiograph (CXR)

**D.** Arterial blood gas (ABG)

**E.** Electroencephalogram (EEG)

**19-9.** An 8-year-old boy comes to clinic with complaint of persistent cough and wheeze with respiratory infections. His parents state that he has no problems when he is well. The parents state that he was given a "breathing medication" but that they do not know what it is for. What test in your office clinic could be done to assess his lung function?

**A.** Spirometry

**B.** Chest radiograph (CXR)

**C.** Arterial blood gas (ABG)

**D.** Plethysmography

**E.** Peak flow meter

**19-10.** A 12-year-old boy with a history of mild persistent asthma presents for his annual well-child visit. He is currently on a daily controller medication. His typical triggers include seasonal allergies, smoke exposure, and mold. He has been hospitalized 3 times, with the most recent hospitalization 2 years ago. Which of the following statements is correct regarding this patient's asthma control?

**A.** For this patient, asthma control should be assessed at a visit at least every 6 months.

**B.** It is not possible to assess asthma control for this patient because he has already been started on a daily controller medication.

**C.** The patient's asthma control is optimal because he has had no hospitalizations or emergency department (ED) visits in the past year.

**D.** Asthma control describes the patient's intrinsic intensity of disease, whereas his asthma severity is based on the intensity of disease and the appropriateness of asthma management.

**E.** There are no validated questionnaires to help measure asthma control for children.

**19-11.** A 2-year-old boy comes to the emergency department with sudden onset of cough and respiratory distress. His father was watching football on television and eating popcorn when he noted his son coughing on the floor. On exam, you hear wheezing in the left lung. What is the most appropriate study to order?

**A.** Computed tomography (CT) scan of the chest

**B.** Bronchoscopy

**C.** Complete blood count (CBC)

**D.** Chest radiograph (CXR)

**E.** Spirometry

**19-12.** A 13-year-old girl with a history of asthma presents for her annual well-child visit. She has mild, intermittent asthma. She has recently been seen by an allergist who has confirmed that she is sensitive to house dust mite allergen. House dust mite allergen seems to be a trigger for her asthma exacerbations. Which of the following allergen avoidance strategies would be *inappropriate* for this patient?

**A.** Use of a warm mist humidifier at night in the child's bedroom

**B.** Removal of wall-to-wall carpeting in the bedroom

**C.** Weekly washing of all the sheets and bedding in hot water at a temperature > 130°F

**D.** Use of encasings for the child's bedroom mattresses

**E.** Use of encasings for the child's bedroom pillows

**19-13.** A 1-month-old boy comes to the emergency department with stridor and respiratory distress. His parents state that he developed a runny nose and then a harsh barky cough. From the following choices, which would be the most appropriate test to order?

**A.** Computed tomography (CT) scan

**B.** Frontal and lateral neck radiographs

**C.** Chest radiograph (CXR)

**D.** Ultrasound

**E.** Complete blood count (CBC)

**19-14.** A 2-year-old girl comes to the emergency department with sudden onset of wheezing. The patient's mother says she heard the wheezing right after the family opened up their holiday gifts. The patient's mother states that the girl's older brother received a large set of miniature action figures. What is the most appropriate test to order?

**A.** Inspiratory and expiratory films

**B.** Decubitus films

**C.** Ultrasound

**D.** Computed tomography (CT) scan

**E.** Magnetic resonance imaging (MRI)

**19-15.** A 16-year-old girl presents to the emergency department with sudden onset of chest pain. She just came off a 16-hour flight from Europe. On exam, you note that she is in a cast because she broke her leg a week ago skiing. What is the most appropriate test to order to rule out a pulmonary embolism?

**A.** Ultrasound of the lower extremities

**B.** Computed tomography (CT) angiography

**C.** Ventilation/perfusion scan

**D.** Magnetic resonance imaging (MRI)

**E.** Chest radiograph (CXR)

**19-16.** A 3-month-old infant is brought to your office by her parents for evaluation of "noisy breathing." The parents have noticed that as she has gotten more active, her breathing has become noisier. Her breathing is louder when she gets active or excited and was much louder when she had a recent cold. Her breathing is quiet when she sleeps. They deny cough, fever, feeding intolerance, or cyanosis. On your exam, the baby is thriving, with normal vital signs and excellent growth. As she gets excited, you note inspiratory stridor and mild chest wall retractions. Of the following, what is the most appropriate next step?

**A.** Order a chest radiograph (CXR) of the neck looking for a steeple sign

**B.** Refer the child for surgical correction

**C.** Reassure the family that this will improve with time

**D.** Initiate therapy with bronchodilators

**E.** Order an upper gastrointestinal series

**19-17.** Primary ciliary dyskinesia (PCD) is a rare condition. An appropriate index of suspicion in the primary care setting is important for timely referral, early diagnosis, and appropriate management of the condition. You are seeing a 2-year-old child in the primary care clinic. Which of the following findings would most likely be present in a 2-year-old child with PCD that has not yet been diagnosed?

**A.** Prominent digital clubbing

**B.** Bronchiectasis

**C.** Situs inversus

**D.** Rhinosinusitis since birth

**E.** Nasal polyps

**19-18.** A 16-year-old girl who is a competitive cheerleader presents for evaluation of chest tightness and dyspnea during a cheerleading competition. She notices symptoms within a few minutes of activity. Upon further questioning, you learn that she feels she cannot catch her breath and has more difficulty breathing in. She has felt lightheaded at times and once thought she was going to faint. If she stops and rests and takes a drink of water, she feels better in a few minutes and can return to activity. She denies symptoms at other times and has no sleep-related symptoms. She has a history of allergic rhinitis and eczema but feels these have been well controlled. Pulmonary function testing shows flattened inspiratory loops. Which of the following diagnoses is most likely?

**A.** Exercise-induced asthma

**B.** Vocal cord dysfunction

**C.** Restrictive lung disease

**D.** Cystic fibrosis

**E.** Gastroesophageal reflux disease (GERD)

**19-19.** Which of the following statements about tracheobronchomalacia (TBM) is correct?

**A.** TBM is usually an isolated abnormality.

**B.** Chest radiography and neck films are usually diagnostic.

**C.** Rigid bronchoscopy should be used for direct visualization of the airways.

**D.** TBM will generally improve by 1 year of age.

**E.** Chest physiotherapy can be helpful to clear retained secretions.

**19-20.** A 4-year-old, previously healthy boy presents with a fever of 102.5°F, sore throat, irritability, and refusal to eat or drink. Symptoms began that morning and have progressed over the past few hours. You note the child to be ill appearing, leaning forward, and drooling. There are no ill contacts, and the child has received all immunizations. You keep the child comfortable with his mother and immediately contact anesthesia and otolaryngology to assist with further management. If neck films are ordered, what is the most likely finding?

**A.** Thumbprint sign
**B.** No acute abnormality
**C.** Steeple sign
**D.** Reverse spine sign
**E.** Irregularity of the tracheal air column

**19-21.** The chest radiograph of a 12-hour-old, full-term baby boy with respiratory distress shows a uniformly dense left upper lobe and a shift of the mediastinum from left to right. On repetition of the study at 72 hours of age, the left upper lobe is more lucent than the rest of the lung, but mediastinal shift persists. Of the following, which is the most likely diagnosis?

**A.** Respiratory distress syndrome
**B.** Meconium aspiration syndrome
**C.** Congenital small lung
**D.** Congenital large hyperlucent lobe
**E.** Congenital thoracic malformation

**19-22.** Which of the following statements is true regarding antenatal diagnosis of fetal lung lesions?

**A.** If a fetal lesion demonstrates an aortic blood supply, pulmonary sequestration may be definitively diagnosed.
**B.** All abnormalities should be detectable on second-trimester scans.
**C.** Oligohydramnios is often associated with congenital cystic lesions and confers poorer prognosis.
**D.** All neonates prenatally diagnosed with a fetal lung lesion require a chest computed tomography (CT) scan prior to discharge.
**E.** Congenital thoracic malformations peak in size at 25 weeks and then regress.

**19-23.** You follow a baby diagnosed with primary ciliary dyskinesia who was found to have a bilateral right lung (right isomerism). The parents are reluctant to provide routine immunizations but are willing to provide those that you feel are most critical. Which of the following vaccines do you recommend is most important for your patient to receive?

**A.** DTaP (diphtheria, tetanus, and pertussis) vaccine
**B.** MMR (measles-mumps-rubella) vaccine
**C.** Hepatitis B vaccine
**D.** Pneumococcal vaccine
**E.** Respiratory syncytial virus (RSV) prophylaxis

**19-24.** A 14-year-old boy followed in your practice comes in with his third episode of pneumonia in the past 8 months. He was previously healthy with no symptoms between episodes. His symptoms started with nasal congestion, postnasal drainage, cough, and low-grade fever. On exam, you note a temperature of 38°C, respiratory rate of 16 breaths/min, and oxygen saturation of 97% on room air. He does have cloudy nasal drainage. Lung exam reveals slightly coarse breath sounds bilaterally without focal wheezing or crackles. The remainder of exam is within normal limits. Chest radiograph (CXR) reveals a round infiltrate in the same area in the left lower lobe as seen previously. You order a follow-up CXR 6 weeks after treatment with antibiotics. Despite complete resolution of clinical symptoms, the same appearance is noted on repeat imaging. You suspect this may be a congenital anomaly. Which of the following is most likely?

**A.** Pulmonary arteriovenous malformation
**B.** Pulmonary sequestration
**C.** Bronchogenic cyst
**D.** Tracheomalacia
**E.** Congenital cystic adenomatoid malformation

**19-25.** Which of the following statements about swallowing dysfunction is correct?

**A.** The inflammatory response is characterized by eosinophilic infiltration.
**B.** Acute-onset, large-volume aspiration is a common complication.
**C.** Neurologically intact children are more likely to have silent aspiration.
**D.** The larynx must lower during the pharyngeal phase in order for a food bolus to pass into the esophagus.
**E.** If left untreated, chronic dysphagia can lead to bronchiectasis as well as chronic hypoxia and dyspnea.

**19-26.** Which of the following statements about diagnostic tests for gastroesophageal reflux is true?

**A.** An upper gastrointestinal (GI) series (or barium swallow study) is considered the gold standard for diagnosing gastroesophageal reflux.

**B.** Multichannel intraluminal impedance with pH monitoring can detect both acid and nonacid reflux.

**C.** Bronchoscopy with bronchoalveolar lavage can definitively diagnose gastroesophageal reflux.

**D.** Twenty-four-hour esophageal pH probe monitoring can determine aspiration.

**E.** Gastroesophageal scintigraphy, or "milk scan," has a high sensitivity for aspiration in children.

**19-27.** You are seeing a 14-year-old boy with exercise-induced bronchoconstriction. As you counsel him regarding his condition, which of the following factors can potentially increase the likelihood of an episode of exercise-induced bronchospasm?

**A.** Recent use of a bronchodilator 10 to 20 minutes before exercise

**B.** Implementing a warm-up period prior to exercise

**C.** Participation in sports associated with cold weather (eg, skiing, speed skating) versus a warm, moist air environment (eg, swimming)

**D.** Wearing a mask to cover the nose and mouth during exercise when the weather is cold

**E.** Exercising indoors during days with high pollen counts or high levels of pollution

**19-28.** A 7-year-old girl presents to your office for evaluation of chronic cough and wheeze. By history, you determine that triggers for her symptoms include upper respiratory infections, weather change, exercise, and laughter. She was seen in the emergency department once and received an oral corticosteroid burst and was sent home with bronchodilator therapy. She reports that any time she is active, she will use bronchodilators often to relieve her symptoms. Her mother reports that the girl has nighttime cough at least once a week. You diagnose her with asthma and classify the severity as which of the following?

**A.** Exercise-induced bronchospasm

**B.** Mild intermittent asthma

**C.** Mild persistent asthma

**D.** Moderate persistent asthma

**E.** Severe persistent asthma

**19-29.** An 8-year-old obese boy comes to see you for follow-up of his asthma. His mother reports that he has been having more difficulties with exacerbations and that they note an increase in nighttime cough. He has not had symptoms of acute upper respiratory infection and has no fevers. His allergic symptoms seem to be controlled without nasal congestion, itching, or rhinorrhea. There is no abdominal pain, emesis, or heartburn. His mother describes a decline in his energy level, and he has been using more rescue medication recently, which does help some of his symptoms. They both report that he is taking his combination high-dose inhaled corticosteroid–long-acting bronchodilator well, with rare missed doses. He is also taking his leukotriene modifier every day. What is your next step in managing his asthma?

**A.** Order a chest radiograph to evaluate for pneumonia

**B.** Make no changes to the current regimen

**C.** Order a polysomnogram to evaluate for obstructive sleep apnea (OSA)

**D.** Order a methacholine challenge test to assess airway reactivity

**E.** Order a sinus computed tomography (CT) to evaluate for acute sinusitis

**19-30.** A 15-year-old boy has recently transferred his care to your office. He and his parents report that he was recently diagnosed with exercise-induced asthma. He began noticing symptoms when he started participating on the high school cross-country team. Prior to this, he had not had difficulty with exercise. He has no history of prolonged upper respiratory infections or pneumonia. He denies frequent sinus infections or otitis media. He does have a history of peanut allergy and carries an epinephrine autoinjector.

He denies chronic rhinorrhea, sneezing, or other signs of environmental allergy. There is no history of eczema. He reports that he eats well and denies abdominal discomfort, heartburn, or emesis. Generally, his symptoms begin within the first 5 minutes of exercise, and he feels a tightness in his throat and upper chest. He generally stops and rests for a few minutes and then can return to running again. He has tried an inhaler but did not feel it helped as much as a brief rest. What is the most definitive diagnostic test you can order?

**A.** Upper gastrointestinal (GI) series

**B.** Methacholine challenge

**C.** Spirometry

**D.** Flexible laryngoscopy

**E.** Nasal ciliary biopsy

**19-31.** A 14-year-old boy with cystic fibrosis (CF) has a low-grade fever, sore throat, fatigue, and increased urinary frequency. Since his last visit 2 months ago, he has a 4.0-kg weight loss, essentially unchanged findings on chest examination, and only minimally decreased pulmonary function (3% decrease in forced expiratory volume in 1 second [$FEV_1$] and 8% decrease in forced expiratory flow at 25%–75%). Which of the following is the most likely diagnosis?

**A.** Urinary tract infection

**B.** Diabetes mellitus

**C.** Distal intestinal obstruction syndrome

**D.** Pulmonary exacerbation

**E.** Allergic bronchopulmonary aspergillosis

**19-32.** Which of the following descriptions meets accepted criteria for the diagnosis of cystic fibrosis (CF)?

**A.** Positive newborn screen and sweat chloride value of 65 mEq/L with adequate sweat volume

**B.** Four-year-old with failure to thrive and steatorrhea and sweat chloride value of 45 mEq/L with adequate sweat volume

**C.** Positive newborn screen that identifies 1 disease causing CF mutations on the state's newborn screen DNA testing

**D.** Positive newborn screen in an infant with a sibling with CF

**E.** Twelve-year-old with recurrent sinusitis and nasal polyps with 1 known CF mutation identified on DNA testing

**19-33.** A 12-year-old girl with cystic fibrosis returns to your office after a second course of oral and inhaled antibiotics for a pulmonary exacerbation. She reports she has been doing extra airway clearance. She continues to have an increased cough. In addition, her lung function has not yet returned to her usual baseline. She has lost almost 1 kg since her last visit and continues to have fatigue. What is the most appropriate next step?

**A.** Begin an appetite stimulant to improve appetite and encourage weight gain

**B.** Begin treatment for allergic bronchopulmonary aspergillosis

**C.** Admit her for initiation of intravenous (IV) antibiotics for a 10- to 14-day course

**D.** Perform outpatient bronchoscopy to clear mucus and continue increased airway clearance

**E.** Assume this is her new baseline and continue routine therapies

**19-34.** Which class of cystic fibrosis transmembrane conductance regulator (CFTR) mutation is most commonly associated with pancreatic sufficiency and milder lung disease?

**A.** Class I

**B.** Class II

**C.** Class IIa

**D.** Class III

**E.** Class IV

**19-35.** A 16-year-old football player with cystic fibrosis (CF) presents with complaints of diffuse crampy abdominal pain. Football season began 2 weeks ago, and he is practicing 3 days per week, with games on weekends. He reports that he has not had a regular formed bowel movement in the past 3 days. He has had some loose stool the morning of his appointment. He usually has 2 formed stools per day. He reports feeling well between pain episodes. He denies any blood or mucus in his stools. He denies vomiting, heartburn, or epigastric pain. He has been eating less in the past day but does not note worsening after eating. What is the most likely diagnosis?

**A.** Gallstones

**B.** Gastroesophageal reflux

**C.** Intussusception

**D.** Distal intestinal obstruction syndrome

**E.** Fibrosing colonopathy

**19-36.** A 15-year-old girl is found to have anemia, cough, and bibasilar infiltrates on chest radiograph. Bronchoalveolar lavage is performed and confirms pulmonary hemorrhage. Video-assisted thoracoscopic lung biopsy is performed, and there is evidence on pathology of small- and medium-vessel neutrophilic inflammation. Which of the following can be eliminated from the differential diagnosis?

**A.** Granulomatosis with polyangiitis

**B.** Eosinophilic granulomatosis with polyangiitis

**C.** Microscopic polyangiitis

**D.** Polyarteritis nodosa

**E.** Takayasu arteritis

**19-37.** A 13-year-old girl presents with sinusitis and epistaxis. She is admitted to the hospital for nasal cautery and is found to have proteinuria and renal insufficiency with increasing creatinine levels. On further review of her history, she was found to have pneumonia 2 years ago, which was associated with microcytic anemia and bilateral pulmonary infiltrates. What is the most likely diagnosis?

**A.** Eosinophilic granulomatosis with polyangiitis
**B.** Polyarteritis nodosa
**C.** Behçet disease
**D.** Granulomatosis with polyangiitis
**E.** Sarcoidosis

**19-38.** A 15-year-old boy with a history of epistaxis, proteinuria, and hemoptysis presents with hypoxemia, respiratory distress, and acute worsening hemoptysis. His vital signs include a respiratory rate of 45 breaths/min, heart rate of 120 bpm, blood pressure of 100/60 mm Hg, oxygen saturation of 88% on room air, continued hemoptysis, and severe suprasternal and subcostal retractions. What is the most appropriate next step in treatment?

**A.** Administer intravenous (IV) corticosteroids
**B.** Intubate using 100% oxygen
**C.** Administer IV cyclophosphamide
**D.** Give a blood transfusion
**E.** Start chest compressions

**19-39.** A 12-year-old girl presents with hemoptysis. Her evaluation has thus far included a complete blood count showing microcytic anemia, chest radiograph with bilateral opacities, and chest computed tomography (CT) scan also with bilateral opacities and a right upper lobe cavitary lesion. Flexible bronchoscopy with bronchoalveolar lavage demonstrates the presence of hemosiderin-laden macrophages, and video-assisted thoracoscopic lung biopsy demonstrates small- to medium-vessel vasculitis. What test would help confirm the diagnosis?

**A.** C-reactive protein
**B.** Angiotensin-converting enzyme level
**C.** Antiribonucleoprotein antibody
**D.** Antiphospholipid antibody profile
**E.** Antineutrophil cytoplasmic antibodies

**19-40.** Which of the following statements is true about pulmonary surfactant?

**A.** It decreases alveolar surface tension, thereby preventing alveolar collapse.
**B.** It is composed primarily of proteins (90%) and also of lipids (10%).
**C.** It is secreted into alveoli by type I alveolar epithelial cells.
**D.** Surfactant protein B deficiencies are reported to occur in 1 in 1000 births.
**E.** Surfactant protein C deficiencies are associated with alveolar lung disease and *Escherichia coli* infections.

**19-41.** A 1-year-old boy develops cough and increased work of breathing. He has a thorough evaluation including lung biopsy. This demonstrates well-preserved alveolar wall architecture, but filling of the alveoli with surfactant. The diagnosis in this case is most likely which of the following?

**A.** ABCA3 dysfunction
**B.** Surfactant protein B deficiency
**C.** Surfactant protein C dysfunction
**D.** NKTF-1 (thyroid transcription factor) dysfunction
**E.** Granulocyte-macrophage colony-stimulating factor receptor α chain dysfunction

**19-42.** A 5-year-old girl develops cough and hypoxemia. She has a thorough evaluation including chest computed tomography (CT) scan, which shows diffuse ground-glass opacities in both lungs. Which of the following diagnostic tests should be performed next?

**A.** Thoracoscopic lung biopsy
**B.** Bronchoalveolar lavage for surfactant levels
**C.** Genetic testing for lysinuric protein intolerance
**D.** Genetic testing for *ABCA3* mutations
**E.** Genetic testing for granulocyte-macrophage colony-stimulating factor receptor α chain mutations

**19-43.** A 5-year-old girl develops cough and hypoxemia. She has a thorough evaluation including chest computed tomography (CT) scan, which shows diffuse ground-glass opacities in both lungs. Genetic testing confirms the presence of 2 mutations in the *ABCA3* gene. What is the next step in treatment of this disorder?

**A.** Surfactant administration
**B.** Whole-lung lavage
**C.** Supplemental oxygen
**D.** Chronic systemic steroids
**E.** Lung transplantation

**19-44.** Which of the following is true regarding the pulmonary physiology of an infant?

**A.** Compliance of the chest wall is less than in the adult.

**B.** Laryngeal braking helps maintain functional residual capacity.

**C.** As an infant ages, less of the diaphragm is in direct contact with the inner thoracic cavity.

**D.** The chest wall of an infant is less likely to collapse inward.

**E.** Prolonged expiration helps to maintain functional residual capacity.

**19-45.** Which of the following muscles helps to increase the intrathoracic volume by a "bucket handle" mechanism?

**A.** Scalenes

**B.** Serratus anterior

**C.** Diaphragm

**D.** Sternocleidomastoids

**E.** External intercostals

**19-46.** A 10-year-old boy is being evaluated for Duchenne muscular dystrophy. His spirometry suggests decreased forced vital capacity compared to the standards for his age and height. Which of the following abnormalities is most likely to be found on testing?

**A.** Elevated total lung capacity (TLC)

**B.** Increased residual volume to total lung capacity (RV/TLC) ratio

**C.** Increased maximum expiratory pressure

**D.** Decreased end-tidal carbon dioxide

**E.** Increased oxyhemoglobin saturation

**19-47.** A 16-year-old female athlete is being evaluated for exercise-induced asthma with an exercise test. During her run on the treadmill, which of the following is true regarding her pulmonary physiology?

**A.** Contraction of the internal intercostal muscles may aid in expiration.

**B.** Contraction of the abdominal muscles may aid in inspiration.

**C.** Expiration is passive and dependent on the elastic recoil of the lung and chest wall.

**D.** Contraction of the sternocleidomastoids may aid in expiration.

**E.** Contraction of the serratus anterior may aid in expiration.

**19-48.** A 4-month-old infant presents with choking when taking his bottles, tongue fasciculation, and profound hypotonia. Which of the following would you tell the parents?

**A.** Without assisted ventilation, median age of death is 12 years.

**B.** Their child will likely be able to sit but not walk.

**C.** The chest wall may increase in diameter over time due to weakness of the intercostal muscles.

**D.** Tracheostomy is the only option for survival.

**E.** Cough is impaired, and use of an airway clearance device is recommended.

**19-49.** A term newborn whose mother did not have prenatal care presents with short-limb dwarfism; a small, narrow, bell-shaped rib cage with shortened ribs; hypoxemia; respiratory distress; and renal insufficiency. Which of the following is true regarding this patient and disorder?

**A.** It is inherited in an autosomal dominant fashion.

**B.** It results in obstructive lung disease.

**C.** Vertically expandable prosthetic titanium rib placement is a treatment option.

**D.** Recurrent pneumonia is unlikely.

**E.** It is known as achondroplasia.

**19-50.** A 15-year-old girl with chronic cough productive of sputum and poor growth is found to have enlargement of the terminal segments of her fingers and toes. No other family members have this finding. Which of the following is true regarding this finding?

**A.** It is likely to be idiopathic and does not need further evaluation.

**B.** The depth of the finger at the proximal nail fold is less than the depth of the distal interphalangeal joint.

**C.** It is likely to be painful and recognized by the patient.

**D.** The nail bed shows increased numbers of blood vessels and primitive fibroblasts.

**E.** When this finding is present, Schamroth sign should disappear.

**19-51.** A 10-month-old infant presents to her pediatrician's office with a respiratory rate of 70 breaths/min, diffuse crackles on auscultation of all lung fields, and an oxygen saturation of 88% on room air. Her symptoms continue for months and do not respond to inhaled bronchodilators. She is kept on supplemental oxygen. Chest computed tomography (CT) scan reveals ground-glass opacities most prominent in the right middle lobe and lingula. Lung biopsy demonstrates normal lung histology but increased cells that stain positive for bombesin. Which of the following is correct regarding this diagnosis?

**A.** It most commonly occurs following adenovirus infection.

**B.** Treatment with corticosteroids is usually effective.

**C.** The most common cause in children is exposure to avian antigens.

**D.** Supplemental oxygen may be required for a period of years.

**E.** Lung transplantation is ultimately required for the majority of cases.

**19-52.** A 3-year-old girl presents to the hospital with tachypnea, hypoxemia, and bilateral diffuse infiltrates on chest radiograph (CXR). She becomes more comfortable on 2-L nasal cannula oxygen, and her respiratory rate is 30 breaths/min. The patient is found to be anemic. What is the next step you would take in the management of this patient?

**A.** Request lung biopsy using video-assisted thoracoscopy

**B.** Perform bronchoscopy with bronchoalveolar lavage

**C.** Prescribe high-dose intravenous corticosteroids

**D.** Order high-resolution computed tomography (CT) of the chest

**E.** Order genetic testing for mutations in surfactant proteins B and C

**19-53.** An 18-year-old man with cystic fibrosis (CF) underwent lung transplantation 1 year ago due to severe airway obstruction and progressive disease. He had been doing well but has noticed over the past 2 months that he has been increasingly short of breath with exercise and is also coughing more. His spirometry suggests increased airway obstruction compared to baseline. High-resolution computed tomography (CT) of the chest shows mosaic perfusion and central bronchiectasis. What recommendations would you give to the patient and his family regarding his most likely diagnosis?

**A.** Reassure the family that the symptoms are unlikely to be progressive, and therefore, no treatment is necessary

**B.** Explain to the family that steroids have been proven in multiple studies to prevent airway fibrosis

**C.** Counsel the family that anti–tumor necrosis factor (TNF) has been used successfully for treatment and can be started immediately

**D.** Recommend bronchoscopy with bronchoalveolar lavage to help make a definitive diagnosis

**E.** Suggest treatment with systemic corticosteroids and consideration of lung biopsy if symptoms continue

**19-54.** A 4-year-old child with snoring is found to have obstructive sleep apnea (OSA) on a polysomnogram. Which of the following is true regarding the upper airway physiology in this patient?

**A.** Decreased inspiratory effort results in collapse of the upper airway.

**B.** Impaired arousal responses to obstructive events result in obstructive alveolar hypoventilation.

**C.** Increased growth rate of lymphadenoid tissue compared to other upper airway structures contributes to upper airway obstruction.

**D.** Pharyngeal airway neuromotor responses are increased compared to normal children.

**E.** Hypoxia and hypercapnic ventilatory drive are impaired compared to normal children.

**19-55.** An infant is found to have obstructive sleep apnea (OSA). Which of the following is true regarding this condition in the first year of life?

**A.** A child with trisomy 21 and laryngomalacia is at increased risk.

**B.** It is more common in females than males.

**C.** The upper airway is most likely obstructing in the retroglossal region.

**D.** It is not commonly associated with hypoxemia.

**E.** The laryngeal chemoreflex is less likely to play a role in OSA in an infant compared to an older child.

**19-56.** A full-term infant is born to a G1P0 mother without prenatal complications by vaginal delivery. The infant weighs 2.74 kg and is vigorous at birth but develops respiratory failure and cyanosis during sleep. Arterial blood gas reveals $PCO_2$ of 80 mm Hg. The infant is intubated and mechanically ventilated. After thorough evaluation in the neonatal intensive care unit, genetic testing reveals the presence of a heterozygous mutation in the paired-like homeobox 2B (*PHOX2B*) gene with a 20/27 polyalanine expansion, consistent with congenital central hypoventilation syndrome (CCHS). What can you tell the parents regarding CCHS?

**A.** It is inherited in an autosomal recessive fashion.

**B.** Their child is likely to outgrow the disorder as maturation of the autonomic nervous system occurs.

**C.** Hirschsprung disease is associated with this condition.

**D.** Their child's mutation is *not* the most common to cause this disorder.

**E.** Ventilation is most affected during rapid eye movement (REM) sleep.

**19-57.** A 12-month-old girl with normal birth history and normal development until 6 months of age is found to have developmental delay, loss of ability to babble, and flapping hand movements. The girl also develops breath-holding spells and rapid shallow breathing during sleep. These events lead to oxygen desaturations during sleep. Which of the following is also consistent with this condition?

**A.** Mutation in the gene encoding methyl-CpG-binding protein 2 (MECP2)

**B.** Absence of the paternally inherited genes on the proximal long arm of chromosome 15

**C.** Autosomal dominant inheritance

**D.** Cerebellar aplasia with thickened superior cerebellar peduncles ("molar tooth sign")

**E.** Abnormal development and survival of unmyelinated sensory and autonomic neurons

**19-58.** An infant born at 33 weeks of gestation to a mother without prenatal problems is admitted to the neonatal intensive care unit. At several hours of life, the baby is found to have pauses in his breathing of 15 to 25 seconds in duration associated with bradycardia (heart rate to the 60 bpms). The events occur 1 to 2 times per hour, and the infant does require stimulation by the nurse to stop the episodes. The infant has a temperature of 38°C, heart rate of 140 bpm, respiratory rate of 36 to 48 breaths/min, and pulse oximetry of 99% on room air and does not appear in distress in between these episodes. Arterial blood gas shows a normal pH, $PCO_2$, $PO_2$, and bicarbonate. Electrolytes and serum glucose are within normal limits. What is your next step in the management of this infant?

**A.** Start caffeine citrate

**B.** Start nasal continuous positive airway pressure (CPAP)

**C.** Order a pH probe

**D.** Order a head ultrasound

**E.** Order a blood culture and complete blood count

**19-59.** A 10-year-old boy with normal growth and development is being evaluated by his pediatrician for obstructive sleep apnea (OSA) due to parental complaint that the boy snores loudly every night. Which of the following is true regarding assessment for OSA?

**A.** The predictive value of clinical history is increased when the patient is referred to a sleep specialist, often obviating the need for a polysomnogram.

**B.** Diagnosis can be made with an overnight pulse oximetry study or with an overnight polysomnogram.

**C.** Less than 20% of children with OSA report excessive daytime sleepiness (EDS).

**D.** Transcutaneous carbon dioxide tension measurements are recommended in addition to end-tidal capnography.

**E.** Children are more likely to manifest electroencephalographic arousals after obstructive apneas.

**19-60.** A 12-week-old, former 27-week preterm infant presents to your clinic to establish care after discharge from the neonatal intensive care unit 4 days ago. The infant was on continuous positive airway pressure (CPAP) for 3 weeks, followed by transition to nasal cannula oxygen. He was discharged home on 1/4 L oxygen by nasal cannula. At what stage of lung development was this infant's lung growth disrupted?

**A.** Alveolar

**B.** Canalicular

**C.** Embryonic

**D.** Pseudoglandular

**E.** Saccular

**19-61.** You are seeing a 2-month-old infant for inspiratory stridor. The parents report the infant has had noisy breathing since birth, but it has become louder over time. The baby is loudest when upset or excited and quieter during sleep. She is feeding and growing well without respiratory distress. What is the most likely cause of the infant's inspiratory stridor?

**A.** Adenotonsillar hypertrophy

**B.** Asthma

**C.** Bronchomalacia

**D.** Laryngomalacia

**E.** Right lower lobe pneumonia

**19-62.** You are evaluating a term newborn with respiratory distress. As part of the evaluation, a chest radiograph (CXR) is obtained (see following figure). At what stage of lung development did this defect likely occur?

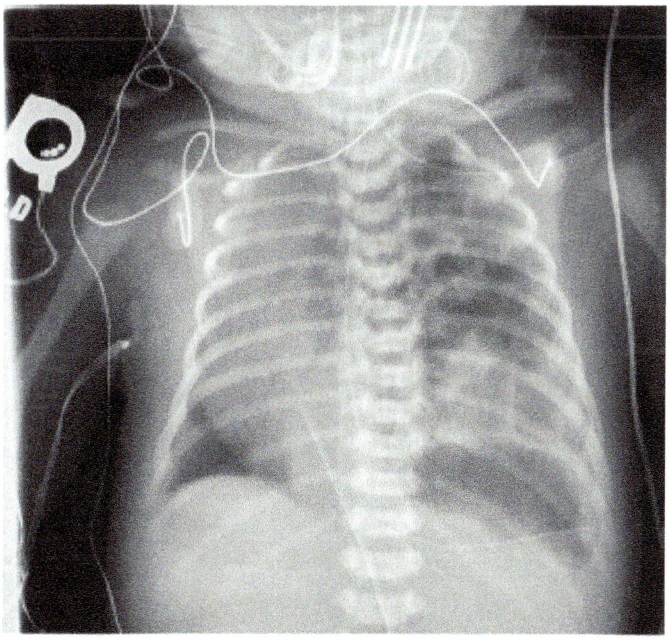

**A.** Alveolar

**B.** Canalicular

**C.** Embryonic

**D.** Pseudoglandular

**E.** Saccular

**19-63.** You are following a 3-year-old boy with a history of recurrent wheeze. He was hospitalized at 6 months of age with respiratory distress in the setting of a respiratory syncytial virus infection. He has since wheezed with upper respiratory infections as well as when he is more active. He has nighttime cough 2 to 3 nights per week, even when well. He has albuterol, which he uses for acute symptoms with a good response. What is the most appropriate course of treatment for this child?

**A.** Daily low-dose inhaled corticosteroid

**B.** Bronchodilator twice a day

**C.** Combination inhaled corticosteroid and long-acting bronchodilator daily

**D.** Inhaled epinephrine as needed

**E.** Low-dose amoxicillin daily

**19-64.** You measure functional residual capacity (FRC) by gas dilution and plethysmography in your patients. Of the following, which patient is most likely to have a lower FRC measured by gas dilution compared to plethysmography?

**A.** An 8 years old with Duchenne muscular dystrophy

**B.** A 9 years old with pectus excavatum

**C.** A 12 years old with rheumatoid arthritis

**D.** A 14 years old with mild idiopathic scoliosis

**E.** A 16 years old with cystic fibrosis (CF)

**19-65.** You are seeing a 2-year-old boy who has had a cough for 6 weeks. The cough is described as wet, and he has intermittent wheeze with chest rattling. The child has otherwise been healthy and thriving. He eats well without symptoms of acid reflux. He has no distress and no chronic rhinorrhea or eczema. What is the most appropriate course of treatment for this child?

**A.** Daily low-dose inhaled corticosteroid

**B.** Bronchodilator twice a day

**C.** A 5-day course of azithromycin

**D.** A 4-week course of amoxicillin/clavulanate

**E.** Low-dose amoxicillin daily

**19-66.** Your 12-year-old patient with well-controlled moderate persistent asthma performs spirometry with good technique. Forced vital capacity (FVC) is 74% predicted, forced expiratory volume in 1 second ($FEV_1$) is 73% predicted, and $FEV_1$/FVC is 86%. You decide to order a complete lung function test to confirm your suspicion regarding your patient's lung function. Of the following, which is the most likely finding when lung volume measurements are completed?

**A.** Residual volume (RV) 130% predicted

**B.** Total lung capacity (TLC) 74% predicted

**C.** RV/TLC 75%

**D.** Airways resistance 62% predicted

**E.** Diffusing capacity 65% predicted

**19-67.** You are caring for a 2-year-old patient who is recovering from pneumonia that required intubation in the intensive care unit (ICU). The patient is now completing an antibiotic course and weaning off oxygen. Of the following, which factor is most likely contributing to this child's increased risk of severe disease?

**A.** Child's age
**B.** Child's human immunodeficiency virus (HIV)-positive status
**C.** Father smokes outside of the home
**D.** Child is breastfed
**E.** Strong family history of asthma

**19-68.** A 7-year-old child presents with a 5-week history of cough that started after an upper respiratory tract infection. The cough is persistent and wet sounding. The parents do not report weight loss but do report reduced activity levels and, on rare occasions, chest pain. They did not note significant sick contacts at home or at school that they are aware of. What would be your next step in management?

**A.** Watchful waiting since the cough has not been persistent
**B.** Broad-spectrum antibiotics for suspected infection
**C.** Chest radiograph (CXR) to assess for underlying pathology
**D.** Oral corticosteroids for treatment of asthma
**E.** Referral to a pulmonologist

**19-69.** You are seeing a 12-month-old child for the first time with the diagnosis of spinal muscular atrophy (SMA; type I), or Werdnig-Hoffmann disease. Parents report that they have not seen the child cough or choke with feedings, and the child is drinking milk and eating some table foods. The only symptom they may have noted is that the child may tire prior to the end of feeding. Based on your evaluation in clinic today, what would be the next likely step in management?

**A.** Ask the parents to feed smaller volumes and monitor the child
**B.** Order a video fluoroscopic swallow study
**C.** Order an upper gastrointestinal (GI) series
**D.** Order a fiberoptic endoscopic evaluation of swallowing/sensory testing (FEES)
**E.** Continue to monitor because there is nothing concerning

**19-70.** Which of the following is a factor that contributes to immune protection of the lower respiratory tract, especially in the youngest children?

**A.** Alveolar macrophages located within air spaces providing innate immunity
**B.** Endothelial cells lining the respiratory surface
**C.** Dendritic cells providing innate immune responses
**D.** Antibiotics
**E.** Breastfeeding and nutrition

**19-71.** Among the diagnoses considered for lung transplantation, which is the most common diagnosis?

**A.** Interstitial lung disease
**B.** Pulmonary hypertension
**C.** Cystic fibrosis (CF)
**D.** Bronchopulmonary dysplasia
**E.** Bronchiolitis obliterans

**19-72.** What is the primary graft dysfunction manifestation of early post–lung transplantation complications?

**A.** Ischemia-reperfusion injury
**B.** Bacteremia
**C.** Bronchiolitis obliterans (BO)
**D.** Renal insufficiency
**E.** Seizures

**19-73.** You are seeing a 3-day-old neonate who was born at 35 weeks' gestation for an abnormal respiratory pattern. Upon observation, you note that the infant will take 3 to 4 quick breaths alternating with brief pauses of < 10 seconds. With which of the following is this respiratory pattern most consistent?

**A.** Central apnea
**B.** Cheyne-Stokes breathing
**C.** Hypopnea
**D.** Kussmaul breathing
**E.** Periodic breathing

**19-74.** A 7-year-old child with cerebral palsy and a history of recurrent aspiration pneumonia presents with respiratory failure. He has a gastrostomy tube and is not orally fed. Mother reports that he had a Nissen fundoplication, and she has not noted emesis or spit ups prior to the episodes of aspiration pneumonia. The child also has significant upper airway secretions and prominent stertor. What would be the next radiographic test that you would like to proceed with to ascertain the cause behind the chronic aspiration?

**A.** Upper gastrointestinal (GI) series
**B.** Radionuclide salivagram
**C.** Esophageal pressure monitoring
**D.** Computed tomography (CT) scan of the chest
**E.** Chest radiograph

## ANSWERS

**Answer 19-1.** A

A sleep terror is a parasomnia characterized by nighttime awakening in an agitated state from non–rapid eye movement (REM) sleep. The events correspond to prominent slow-wave sleep. Sleep terrors are associated with intense autonomic nervous system manifestations such as dilated pupils, diaphoresis, tachypnea, and tachycardia. After the event, the child is not consolable but returns to sleep after a few minutes. In the morning, the child has *no* recollection of the event. It is estimated that up to 6.5% of children experience night terrors, which are most common between 2 and 6 years of age. Sleep terrors can be precipitated by stress, sleep deprivation, anxiety, and environmental noises.

In contrast, a nightmare is a frightening dream that awakes a child. Nightmares occur during REM sleep. The child is consolable after the event and may also have a recollection of the event in the morning. Although night terrors occur in younger children, nightmares are more common in school-age children and adolescents. The occurrence is normal, and management is counseling and reassurance.

Night terrors and nightmares do not require referral to a mental health professional or a neurologist. There is no reported association with seizure disorders.

(Section 27: Disorders of the Respiratory System, Chapter 502: Sleep Disorders)

**Answer 19-2.** D

Based on the history and physical examination, this patient most likely has RLS. RLS is a clinical diagnosis characterized by uncomfortable leg sensations that usually occur *prior* to sleep onset. Periodic limb movements during sleep can be associated with obstructive sleep apnea or RLS. Periodic limb movement disorder (PLMD) is less common and is characterized by periodic limb movements *during* sleep, as noted on polysomnography, and can be associated with symptoms of insomnia or excessive daytime sleepiness.

Both RLS and PLMD are common in adults, with a prevalence of up to 10%. Approximately one-third of adult patients report the onset of symptoms before the age of 20 years. Nonspecific symptoms, such as growing pains, restless sleep, and hyperactivity, may accompany RLS or PLMD. A family history of RLS and PLMD is common.

The etiology of RLS and PLMD is not known. Pregnancy, uremia, iron deficiency, and anemia are associated with increased risk of RLS and PLMD (secondary RLS). Treatment of RLS and PLMD includes iron studies, avoidance of caffeine, and sleep hygiene. There is currently no US Food and Drug Administration–approved medication available to treat RLS and PLMD in children.

A tremor is defined as an involuntary oscillating movement with a fixed frequency. The most common cause of tremor in children is essential (familial) tremor, which is transmitted in autosomal dominant trait. In this case, the child does not have a movement with fixed frequency. Myoclonus is characterized by sudden, brief, shock-like movements, which can be rhythmic or nonrhythmic, focal, multifocal, or generalized. Myoclonic movement can be activated by another movement or sensory stimulation. Physiologic myoclonus can occur as nocturnal myoclonus during sleep or as myoclonus induced by anxiety. Tourette syndrome is part of the spectrum of tic disorders. In this case, the child does not have a tic, which is an involuntary, sudden, rapid, repetitive, nonrhythmic, stereotyped movement.

(Section 27: Disorders of the Respiratory System, Chapter 502: Sleep Disorders)

**Answer 19-3.** D

Based on the history and physical examination, this patient most likely has restless legs syndrome (RLS), which is a clinical diagnosis characterized by uncomfortable leg sensations that usually occur *prior* to sleep onset. Other nonspecific symptoms include growing pains, restless sleep, and hyperactivity. The prevalence of RLS is estimated to be approximately 2% in children 8 to 17 years of age.

Many children with RLS have low iron storage, as evidenced by low serum ferritin and/or iron. Because iron deficiency and anemia are associated with RLS, it is important to screen for this condition. The mother's physician most likely ordered a CBC to screen for anemia and iron deficiency. Based on the mother's history, she was most likely treated with iron supplementation.

Although the etiology of RLS is not known, studies suggest that genetic predisposition, dopamine dysfunction, and low iron stores are related to the pathophysiology of RLS. Thyroid disease, electrolyte anomalies, urinary tract disease, and copper metabolism have not been linked to RLS. As a result, it is unlikely that any of the other tests were previously ordered.

(Section 27: Disorders of the Respiratory System, Chapter 502: Sleep Disorders)

**Answer 19-4.** C

Although adolescents need on average 9 hours of sleep a night, most sleep only 7 to 7.5 hours each night, with irregular sleep patterns as well. This "sleep debt" can lead to significant issues in adolescents, such as daytime sleepiness, as in this case. Other associated problems are changes in mood, memory, behavior, and decreased academic performance.

During puberty, physiologic changes and a shift in melatonin secretion and circadian sleep phase occur. These changes lead to a phase delay and a greater likelihood of later onset of sleep as well as a later wake-up time. In addition, changes in academic demands and social activities during adolescence increase the likelihood of sleep deprivation and sleeping longer during the weekend, which can make the phase delay worse.

OSA is defined as partial or complete upper airway obstruction during sleep, resulting in disruption of normal gas exchange and sleep patterns. Although one of the symptoms of OSA is daytime sleepiness, other daytime symptoms include morning headaches, mouth breathing, difficulty in waking up, moodiness, nasal obstruction, and cognitive problems. Severe OSA is associated with cor pulmonale. The prevalence is 2% to 3% of children. No other symptoms of OSA are present, which makes OSA less likely in this case.

Narcolepsy is unlikely in this case due to the history, symptoms, and epidemiology of the condition. Although narcolepsy is also associated with EDS, it is also associated with cataplexy (sudden loss of muscle tone), hypnagogic hallucinations, and sleep paralysis, which were not reported in this case. Normally, rapid eye movement (REM) sleep occurs after deep sleep; however, patients with narcolepsy enter REM sleep immediately in the sleep cycle. The prevalence of narcolepsy is approximately 1 in 1000 to 1 in 10,000 in the United States. The diagnosis of narcolepsy is based on clinical history and sleep study.

Although anemia can cause fatigue, the patient does not have any risk factors associated with anemia. A complete social history is always helpful; however, based on the information provided, there is no specific reason to suspect alcohol abuse in this case.

(Section 27: Disorders of the Respiratory System, Chapter 502: Sleep Disorders, pp. 2409–2413)

### Answer 19-5. B

The major change in sleep patterns during adolescence is a shift in melatonin secretion and circadian sleep phase. These changes lead to phase delay with propensity to later onset of sleep and later wake-up time.

"Growing pains" most commonly occur between the ages of 3 and 12 years and can sometimes be confused with restless legs syndrome (RLS), which is an uncomfortable sensation in the legs occurring prior to sleep onset. Growing pains, unlike RLS, mainly occur during the day. Similarly, although symptoms of GERD can be worse in a supine or prone position, GERD is not directly associated with difficulty falling asleep. Phase advance is not a standard term. Menarche is generally not a risk factor for sleep disturbances.

(Section 27: Disorders of the Respiratory System, Chapter 502: Sleep Disorders, p. 2412)

### Answer 19-6. A

The BEARS (**B**edtime, **E**xcessive daytime sleepiness, **A**wakenings, **R**egularity, **S**noring) instrument provides a screening tool to assess for the common sleep disorders. The instrument can be used for children 2 to 18 years of age. Five basic sleep domains are incorporated and thought to represent the most common presenting sleep complaints in children. They are **b**edtime problems, **e**xcessive daytime sleepiness, **a**wakenings during the night, **r**egularity and duration of sleep, and **s**noring. Because parents may not be aware of sleep problems in their children, it is important to ask both children and their parents about these issues. Developmentally appropriate trigger questions are made from each domain, with the intent of promoting further discussion after any affirmative responses.

The CAGE questionnaire is used for alcoholism. The HEEADSSS (**H**ome, **E**ducation [or **E**mployment], **E**ating, **A**ctivities, **D**rugs, **S**exuality, **S**uicidality, **S**trengths) exam is a psychosocial interview tool to address adolescent health and risk behaviors. SALSA is a depression screening mnemonic (**s**leep disturbance, **a**nhedonia, **l**ow self-esteem, **a**ppetite decreased). DREAMS is not a standard screening tool.

(Section 27: Disorders of the Respiratory System, Chapter 502: Sleep Disorders)

### Answer 19-7. C

Lung development (Figure 495-1) begins in embryonic life with outpouching of the tracheal primordium from foregut endoderm. There are 5 characteristic periods, including the embryonic period, pseudoglandular period, the canalicular period, the terminal saccular period, and the alveolar period. Normal development of the lung during postnatal development in infancy and childhood is dominated by formation and differentiation of alveoli during the first years of life.

The formation of functional units of gas exchange occurs during the alveolar period. This is accomplished by the secondary formation of septae, which partitions saccules into alveolar ducts and alveoli and facilitates formation of the alveolar-capillary membrane. The alveolar stage begins at 36 weeks after conception and continues postnatally. The bulk of alveolar formation occurs in the first 2 years of life, with the remainder being completed at approximately 8 to 10 years. However, recent data suggest that alveoli can continue to be formed even in adulthood.

(Section 27: Disorders of the Respiratory System, Chapter 495: Lung Growth in Infancy and Childhood)

### Answer 19-8. B

Assessing the function of the respiratory control centers is not straightforward. Polysomnography measures a wide variety of physiologic variables during sleep, including nasal and oral airflow, chest and abdominal wall motion, oxygen saturation ($SpO_2$), end-tidal (exhaled) $PCO_2$, and electrocardiogram (Table 501-6). Sleep state is monitored by EEG, electro-oculogram, and electromyogram. Abnormalities of respiratory drive (especially central apneas and periodic breathing) can be detected with this testing.

Spirometry is the measurement of pulmonary airflow during a maximally forced exhalation. CXR, ABG, and EEG would not be helpful for assessing breathing patterns.

(Section 27: Disorders of the Respiratory System, Chapter 501: Disorders of Respiratory Control and Sleep-Disordered Breathing)

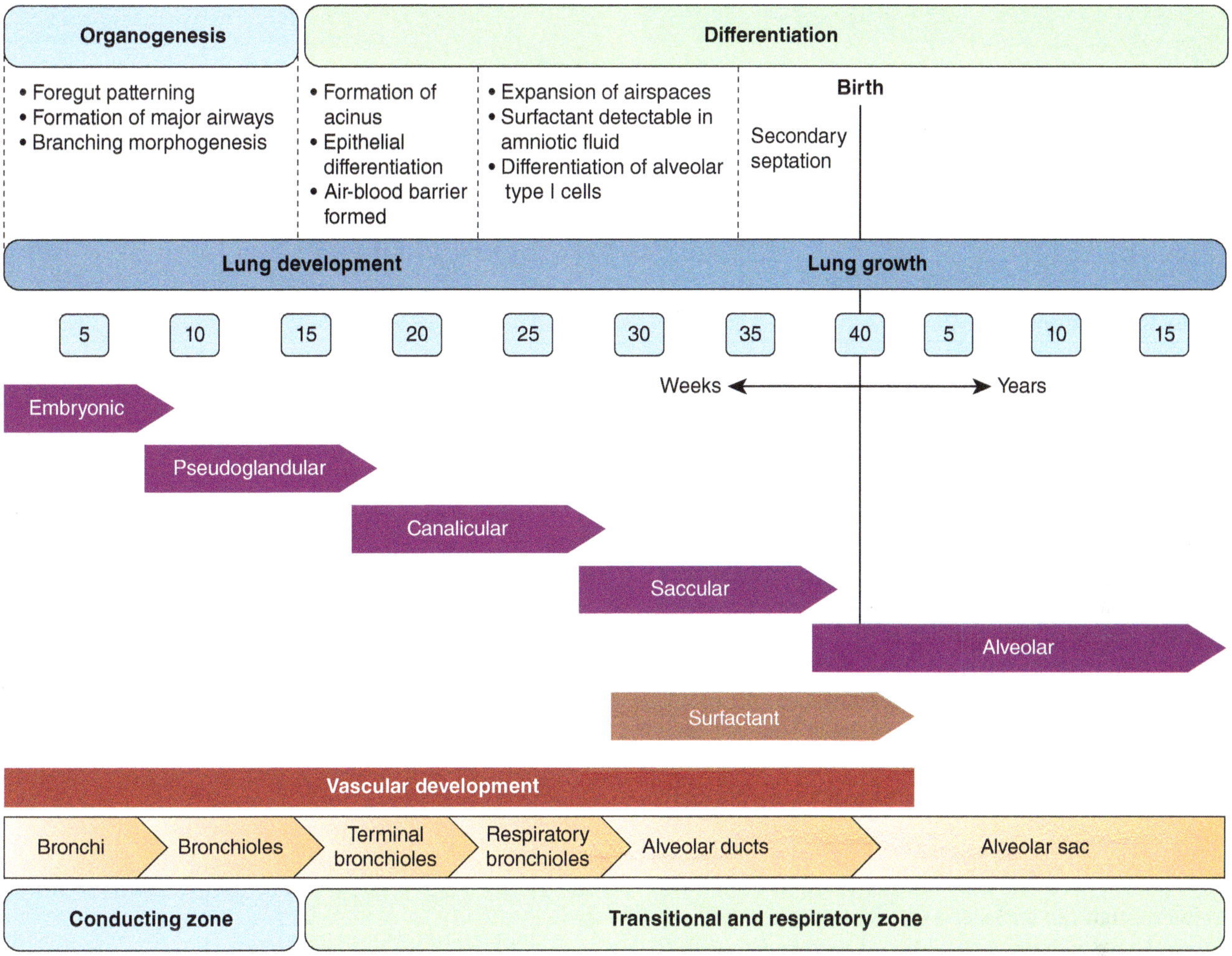


**FIGURE 495-1.** Stages of lung development. (Mark W. Kline, *Rudolph's Pediatrics*, 23rd Edition. Copyright © McGraw-Hill Education. All rights reserved.)

**Answer 19-9. A**

Spirometry is the measurement of airflow during a maximally forced exhalation. Many common pediatric lung diseases (asthma and cystic fibrosis) are obstructive in nature and are characterized by reduced airflows based on the shape of the flow-volume curve. Furthermore, in the smaller airways, minimal effort is needed to achieve a maximal flow rate. The tests are reproducible within subjects, making them useful for assessing response to treatment over time.

Peak flow meter readings are useful for characterizing large airway disease; however, there is less information about small airway obstruction. Plethysmography is useful for measuring airway resistance. CXR and an ABG are not directly useful for assessing lung function.

(Section 27: Disorders of the Respiratory System, Chapter 496: Physiologic Basis of Pulmonary Function)

**Answer 19-10. A**

According to the National Institutes of Health Expert Panel Report 3, even if a patient reports good asthma control, it is important to assess asthma control every 6 months. Asthma control is the degree to which the manifestations of asthma (symptoms, impairments, and risk) are minimized and the goals of therapy are met. Asthma control can help guide decisions to maintain or adjust asthma therapy for this patient.

Although asthma severity describes the patient's intrinsic intensity of disease, asthma control is based on the intensity of disease and the appropriateness of asthma management. Thus, it is possible that a patient with very severe asthma can still have well-controlled asthma. Likewise, a patient with very mild asthma can still have very poorly controlled asthma. Because asthma severity describes the intrinsic intensity of disease, it is not possible to assess asthma severity for this patient because he has already been started on a daily controller medication. However, it is possible to assess asthma control for this patient.

Asthma control is not only based on recent hospitalizations (Table 505-2). Components of asthma control include the level of impairment (frequency of symptoms, nighttime awakenings, interference with normal activity, use of short-acting β-agonists, forced expiratory volume in 1 second [$FEV_1$], and the results from validated questionnaires) and risk (exacerbations in the past year, loss of lung function, and treatment-related adverse events). There are several validated

**TABLE 501-6.** Usual Polysomnographic Montage in Children Evaluated for Suspected Sleep-Disordered Breathing

| |
|---|
| Electroencephalogram: minimum 2 channels (central and occipital leads); recommended 4–8 channels |
| Chin electromyogram |
| Anterior tibial electromyogram: left and right limbs |
| Electro-oculogram: left and right |
| Electrocardiogram |
| Pulse oximeter and pulse waveform |
| Oronasal airflow thermistor |
| Nasal pressure catheter |
| End-tidal capnography and waveform |
| Chest and abdominal respiratory inductance plethysmography |
| Body position sensor |
| Tracheal sound sensor or microphone |
| Time-synchronized video |

Note: In younger children, transcutaneous carbon dioxide tension measurements should be included.

Mark W. Kline, *Rudolph's Pediatrics*, 23rd Edition. Copyright © McGraw-Hill Education. All rights reserved.

questionnaires that can be used to assess asthma control in children. These include the Childhood Asthma Control Test (C-ACT) for children 4 to 11 years of age, as well as the Asthma Therapy Assessment Questionnaire (ATAQ), Asthma Control Questionnaire (ACQ), and Asthma Control Test (ACT) for children 12 years and older.

ED, emergency department; $FEV_1$, forced expiratory volume in 1 second; GERD, gastroesophageal reflux disease; ICS, inhaled corticosteroids; ICU, intensive care unit; SABA, short-acting β-agonist.

(Section 27: Disorders of the Respiratory System, Chapter 505: Childhood Asthma)

**Answer 19-11.** D

Plain radiographs of frontal and lateral views of the chest remain the mainstay of screening imaging for any child with a suspected abnormality within the chest. In this case, it would be the most appropriate initial study for suspected foreign body aspiration (FBA). Plain films may be normal with FBA, but certain findings may be present and strongly support the diagnosis in the context of this clinical history. If the object causes lower airway obstruction and air trapping, local hyperinflation of the lung can be seen. Partial obstruction can lead to atelectasis. If the aspiration is more remote, later developments that can be seen include pneumonia, lung abscess, and bronchiectasis.

**TABLE 505-2.** Approach to Assessment of Asthma Control in Children

Assess Asthma Control

- Determine symptom control over the last 4 weeks
  - Daytime asthma symptoms (including wheezing, cough, chest tightness, or shortness of breath)
  - Nocturnal awakening as a result of asthma symptoms
  - Frequency of use of SABA for relief of symptoms
  - Inability or difficulty performing normal activities (including exercise) because of asthma
- Assess treatment issues
  - Document the patient's current treatment step level
  - Assess inhaler technique
  - Assess adherence
- Measure lung function at diagnosis/start of treatment and then 3–6 months after starting or adjusting controller treatment; spirometry is recommended at least every 1–2 years to assess the maintenance of airway function, as well as during any progressive or prolonged increase in asthma symptoms
  - A reduction in $FEV_1$ at an annual visit is associated with increases in the risk of an attack of wheezing and shortness of breath over the next 12 or 36 months
- Identify risk factors for exacerbations
  - Severe airflow limitation; determined by spirometry[a]
  - Uncontrolled asthma symptoms
  - High SABA use
  - Inadequate treatment
  - Poor adherence[a]
  - Poor inhaler technique
  - Exposures: smoking, traffic pollution, fungal
  - Ever intubated[a]
  - ICU admission for asthma[a]
  - 1 or more prior severe exacerbation(s) in last 12 months (2 or more ED visits or hospitalization in the last year[a])
- Risk factors for medication side effects
  - Systemic: frequent oral corticosteroids; long-term, high-dose ICS
  - Local: high-dose or potent ICS; poor inhaler technique
- Assess comorbidities
  - Rhinitis
  - Sinusitis
  - GERD
  - Obesity
  - Obstructive sleep apnea
  - Internalization disorders: depression, anxiety[a]

[a]Risk factors for asthma-related death.

Mark W. Kline, *Rudolph's Pediatrics*, 23rd Edition. Copyright © McGrawHill Education. All rights reserved.

CT involves a much larger dose of ionizing radiation, and this would not be the first study to pursue. Bronchoscopy may be appropriate upon further workup, but a CXR should be done prior to bronchoscopy. CBC and spirometry have no utility in this scenario.

(Section 27: Disorders of the Respiratory System, Chapter 499: Tools for Diagnosis and Management of Respiratory Disease, pp. 2377–2378)

**Answer 19-12.** A

House dust mites (HDMs; *Dermatophagoides pteronyssinus* and *Dermatophagoides farinae*) feed on human skin flakes, which are shed onto and into mattresses, pillows, carpets, stuffed toys, and upholstered furniture. HDMs also prefer a humid environment. As a result, the use of a warm mist humidifier at night could potentially improve the environment for HDMs.

The feces of HDMs contain allergens (*Der p1* and *Der f1*), which can trigger asthma symptoms for some sensitized children. Removal of wall-to-wall carpeting in the bedroom, weekly washing of all the sheets and bedding in hot water at a temperature > 130°F, and the use of encasings for the child's bedroom mattresses and pillows can all help eradicate HDMs and exposure to HDM feces.

(Section 27: Disorders of the Respiratory System, Chapter 505: Childhood Asthma)

**Answer 19-13.** B

This child is presenting with stridor and barky cough and shows signs of upper airway obstruction. In such cases, radiographs of the neck with frontal and lateral projections can be helpful in distinguishing whether the obstruction is due to an intrinsic or extrinsic mass, foreign body, or inflammation such as croup or epiglottitis. Masses that may be seen include abscesses, cysts, or abnormal vessels. Croup is classically associated with a "steeple sign" due to subglottic narrowing. Epiglottitis is associated with a "thumb sign" from an enlarged epiglottis.

CT scan and ultrasound would not be appropriate first-line tests to order but may be needed for further evaluation of neck masses causing obstruction. CXR would not be as helpful in this child with signs of upper airway obstruction. CBC would not be indicated.

(Section 27: Disorders of the Respiratory System, Chapter 499: Tools for Diagnosis and Management of Respiratory Disease)

**Answer 19-14.** B

This child's history is suspicious for foreign body aspiration (FBA). Plain films may be normal with FBA, but certain findings may be present that strongly support the diagnosis. If children are old enough to cooperate with breath-holding, obtaining inspiratory and expiratory radiographs increases the sensitivity of identifying air trapping and local hyperinflation from foreign body obstruction.

Decubitus views of the chest do not require cooperation for inspiratory and expiratory breath-holding and are more useful for infants and young children. With FBA, the expected deflation of the dependent lung is not seen due to the foreign body causing air trapping. Ultrasound, CT scan, and MRI would not be the first-line tests in this scenario.

(Section 27: Disorders of the Respiratory System, Chapter 499: Tools for Diagnosis and Management of Respiratory Disease, pp. 2378–2379)

**Answer 19-15.** B

CT angiography to evaluate pulmonary embolism (PE) is faster and more sensitive than nuclear medicine ventilation/perfusion scanning.

When the probability of PE is high, CT angiography is the preferred method for confirming this diagnosis. When the probability of PE is low, D-dimer may be used to help rule out the diagnosis. Ultrasound of the lower extremity can support the diagnosis of PE if a deep vein thrombosis is found but cannot rule out PE. CXR and MRI are not used in the diagnosis of PE.

(Section 27: Disorders of the Respiratory System, Chapter 499: Tools for Diagnosis and Management of Respiratory Disease)

**Answer 19-16.** C

The symptoms are most consistent with laryngomalacia. Laryngomalacia commonly presents as stridor that worsens with activity and crying. It may improve when the infant is placed in the prone position. Diagnosis is usually based on the history and physical examination. The lack of fever or other signs of upper respiratory infection make croup less likely. In more severe cases, surgery (supraglottoplasty) may be necessary; however, this infant is thriving. Bronchodilators would more likely provide relief of wheezing, such as in asthma. Gastroesophageal reflux disease (GERD), has been linked to laryngomalacia, and the possibility of concurrent GERD should be considered if suggested by history.

(Section 27: Disorders of the Respiratory System, Chapter 503: Disorders Causing Airway Obstruction, p. 2414)

**Answer 19-17.** D

PCD is a rare condition with an estimated prevalence of 1 in 15,000 to 30,000. Nasal congestion is a nonspecific symptom of PCD that can occur in all individuals; however, in the child who has nasal congestion from birth, PCD should be considered. In PCD, the cilia demonstrate abnormal or no motility. As a result, there is stasis of secretions, which can lead to upper and lower respiratory tract infections.

Other factors that would alert the clinician to the diagnosis of PCD are chronic wet cough, wheeze, and particularly severe recurrent sinusitis and otitis media. Situs inversus is seen in 50% of people with PCD. Bronchiectasis is generally a later finding. Digital clubbing and nasal polyposis, often seen in cystic fibrosis, are not often present in PCD.

(Section 27: Disorders of the Respiratory System, Chapter 503: Disorders Causing Airway Obstruction)

**Answer 19-18.** B

Vocal cord dysfunction, also known as paradoxical vocal fold motion, has gained recognition recently as a cause of upper airway obstruction as a result of paradoxical closure of the true vocal folds during inspiration. It is most commonly seen in females and usually presents in early adolescence. Vocal cord dysfunction may be confused with a diagnosis of asthma, and patients are placed on unnecessary medications such as corticosteroids. Spirometry may reveal attenuation of inspiratory flow with flattened inspiratory loops, indicating extrathoracic airway obstruction. Reductions in expiratory flows, reduced forced expiratory volume in 1 second ($FEV_1$)/forced vital capacity (FVC) ratio, and air trapping suggested by elevated residual volume (RV)/total lung capacity (TLC) ratio are consistent with intrathoracic airway obstruction commonly seen with asthma. Restrictive lung disease with reduced TLC would not be expected. GERD and asthma may be comorbidities associated with vocal cord dysfunction.

(Section 27: Disorders of the Respiratory System, Chapter 503: Disorders Causing Airway Obstruction)

**Answer 19-19.** E

Secretions are often trapped by collapsible airways, and airway clearance devices can be used to facilitate removal of retained secretions in children with TBM. Most infants and children with TBM have an underlying or associated problem. Cardiovascular anomalies may occur in up to 60% of the cases, and half of infants with TBM have bronchopulmonary dysplasia and/or gastroesophageal reflux. Because it does not "stent" open collapsible airways, flexible bronchoscopy is a better alternative to rigid bronchoscopy when evaluating TBM. Bronchoscopy not only identifies the area of TBM but can determine the etiology. Plain radiographs of the neck and chest are not helpful for evaluating TBM. Fluoroscopy of the neck and chest provides a cinegraphic view of the airway, allowing the observer to determine if there is dynamic collapse of the airway. TBM will improve by 2 to 3 years of age, although those with tracheoesophageal fistula may have significant problems into adult years.

(Section 27: Disorders of the Respiratory System, Chapter 503: Disorders Causing Airway Obstruction)

**Answer 19-20.** A

Acute epiglottitis can progress quickly to becoming a life-threatening emergency. Children affected are usually between 2 and 8 years old. It presents quite suddenly (over 6–24 hours) with high fever, irritability, throat pain, stridor, and what is known as a "hot potato" or muffled voice. Unlike croup, there is usually no preceding viral prodrome or cough. A "thumbprint sign," which describes a round and thickened epiglottis, can be seen on the neck radiograph (Figure 258-2).

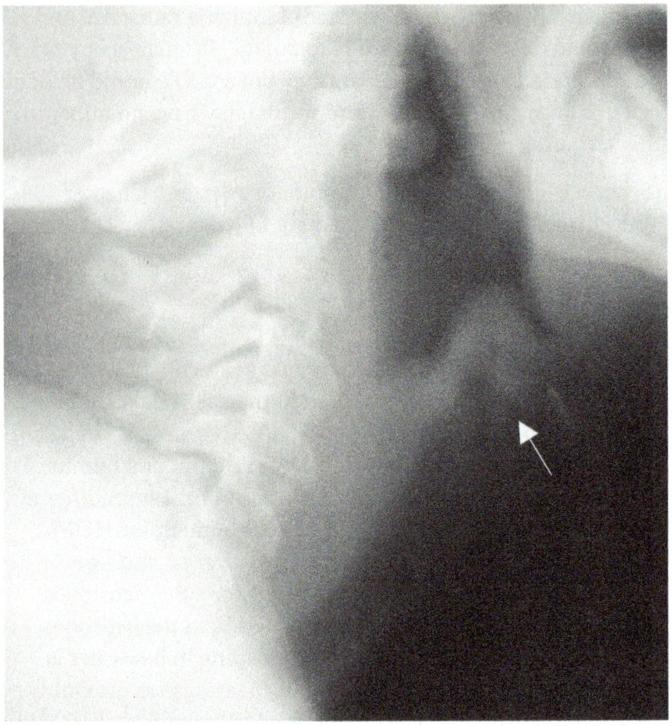

**FIGURE 258-2.** Lateral soft tissue radiograph of the neck demonstrating thickening of aryepiglottic folds and thumbprint sign of epiglottis (*arrow*). (Used with permission from Richard M. Ruddy, MD.)

In croup, a "steeple sign," which is the tapering of the subglottic airway, may be seen, but many patients will also have normal radiographs. Reverse curve of the thoracic spine signifies an enlarged retropharyngeal space seen with retropharyngeal abscess. Irregularity of the tracheal air column (indicating sloughing of pseudomembranous material from the tracheal wall) is most consistent with bacterial tracheitis.

(Section 27: Disorders of the Respiratory System, Chapter 503: Disorders Causing Airway Obstruction, p. 2415)

**Answer 19-21.** D

Congenital large hyperlucent lobe (previously known as congenital lobar emphysema; see Table 500-1) is a rare condition that affects the left upper (42%), right middle (35%), right upper (21%), and lower lobes (2%). The affected lobe is overdistended and displaces adjacent structures. There is resulting respiratory distress from compression and collapse of the adjacent lung, ipsilateral depression of the diaphragm, and mediastinal shift.

Respiratory distress syndrome typically has a "ground-glass" appearance. Congenital thoracic malformations include bronchogenic cysts, which are most often located near the carina and are distinguished by cartilage in the wall. Congenital thoracic malformations can include pulmonary sequestration, which occurs most often in the left lower lobe, and symptoms in neonates are uncommon. In addition, congenital cystic adenomatoid malformations usually present as either larger (> 2 cm) cysts or multiple smaller cysts. Rarely, there is a fully adenomatous lesion that appears solid. A chest radiograph

**TABLE 500-1.** Comparison of Present and Past Terms Used to Describe Clinical Appearances of Congenital Lung Malformations

| New Nomenclature | Old Terms Superseded |
|---|---|
| Congenital large hyperlucent lobe (CLHL) | Congenital lobar emphysema |
| | Polyalveolar lobe |
| Congenital thoracic malformation (CTM) | Cystic adenomatoid malformation (type 0–4 pathologically) |
| | Sequestration (intra- and extrapulmonary) |
| | Bronchogenic cyst |
| | Reduplication cyst |
| | Foregut cyst |
| Congenital small lung (CSL) | Pulmonary hypoplasia |
| Absent lung, absent trachea | Agenesis of lung, tracheal aplasia |
| Absent bronchus | Bronchial atresia |

Mark W. Kline, *Rudolph's Pediatrics*, 23rd Edition. Copyright © McGraw-Hill Education. All rights reserved.

suggestive of meconium aspiration syndrome generally shows patchy atelectasis and hyperinflation.

(Section 27: Disorders of the Respiratory System, Chapter 500: Congenital Disorders of the Lower Airways and Mediastinum)

**Answer 19-22.** E

The prognosis for a fetus with a congenital thoracic malformation is good because the lesions often regress in the third trimester. Pulmonary sequestrations are not the only malformations with an aortic blood supply, because congenital cystic adenomatoid malformation may also have an aortic blood supply. While most abnormalities are detectable after 20 weeks, diaphragmatic hernia and pleural effusion may not be detected until later in the third trimester. Congenital cystic lesions are often associated with hydrops or polyhydramnios, which may indicate poor prognosis and has led to consideration of fetal interventions. Although chest CT is the gold standard for congenital thoracic malformations, because many fetal lung lesions may regress prior to birth, chest radiograph is the recommended initial screening test, particularly for asymptomatic neonates.

(Section 27: Disorders of the Respiratory System, Chapter 500: Congenital Disorders of the Lower Airways and Mediastinum)

**Answer 19-23.** D

Nearly 80% of children with bilateral right lung have asplenia and are thus at risk of overwhelming pneumococcal sepsis. They are therefore particularly at risk from polysaccharide encapsulated bacteria, including pneumococcus, *Haemophilus influenzae*, and meningococcus. Bilateral left lung is associated with polysplenia in nearly 80% of patients. Other associated abnormalities with both right and left isomerism include midline liver, malrotation of the gut, and cardiac abnormalities.

(Section 27: Disorders of the Respiratory System, Chapter 500: Congenital Disorders of the Lower Airways and Mediastinum)

**Answer 19-24.** B

Pulmonary sequestration is often diagnosed after adolescence, and symptoms are uncommon in infants. Intralobar sequestration is more common than extralobar, and treatment is surgical excision. The vascular supply must be carefully delineated preoperatively.

Pulmonary arteriovenous malformation is characterized by dyspnea, cyanosis, and possibly hemoptysis, and clubbing is generally seen on exam. Bronchogenic cyst is most often located near the carina, and when infected, it will usually have an air-fluid level. Tracheomalacia would present with wheeze and/or stridor and would not present with left lower lobe infiltrate. Congenital cystic adenomatoid malformations are generally multicystic abnormalities rather than a single round infiltrate.

(Section 27: Disorders of the Respiratory System, Chapter 500: Congenital Disorders of the Lower Airways and Mediastinum, p. 2390)

**Answer 19-25.** E

Chronic aspiration from swallowing dysfunction leads to increased levels of interleukin-8 and tumor necrosis factor-α, and there is a significant neutrophilic migration to the site of aspiration with subsequent activation and sequestration of the neutrophils. Generally, swallowing dysfunction leads to chronic small-volume aspiration with typical symptoms including cough, wheeze, choking, and gagging that are temporally related to the intake of food.

Children with neuromuscular disorders are among those who are at higher risk for chronic aspiration, and those with neurologic compromise in particular are more likely to have silent aspiration of food. There are 3 phases of swallowing: the oral phase, the pharyngeal phase, and the esophageal phase. During the pharyngeal phase, the larynx elevates and the glottis closes to prevent aspiration into the airway and to allow relaxation of the upper esophageal sphincter so the bolus may pass into the esophagus. If left untreated, children can develop progressive irreversible lung disease that may progress to respiratory failure and death.

(Section 27: Disorders of the Respiratory System, Chapter 504: Aspiration Syndromes, p. 2421)

**Answer 19-26.** B

Multichannel intraluminal impedance with pH monitoring has some advantages over standard pH probe monitoring. It can track the movement of a bolus along the length of the esophagus and detects both acid and nonacid liquid boluses. It can tell how high in the esophagus a bolus goes, so it is better able to detect pharyngeal level reflux. However, it is not yet widely available.

Standard 24-hour pH probe monitoring remains the gold standard for the diagnosis of gastroesophageal reflux but does not differentiate acid from above (aspiration) versus below (reflux). An upper GI series can be used to diagnose reflux but captures gastroesophageal reflux only if it happens to occur during the test. Bronchoalveolar lavage can detect the presence of lipid in the lower airways but cannot distinguish between gastroesophageal reflux and aspiration.

(Section 27: Disorders of the Respiratory System, Chapter 504: Aspiration Syndromes)

**Answer 19-27.** C

Asthma should not limit physical activity. For patients with exercise-induced asthma or bronchoconstriction, the airways are sensitive to changes in humidity and temperature. During exercise or vigorous physical activity, the body temperature increases and the respiratory rate increases quickly, leading to a loss of airway moisture. For some patients, these changes trigger bronchoconstriction.

Methods to address this issue include a gradual warm-up period prior to planned exercise or activity. In addition, the use of a bronchodilator prior to exercise can also help relax the airways. Sports in low-humidity and cold conditions (eg, skiing, speed skating) are a greater risk for exercise-induced bronchoconstriction compared to sports in more humid settings (eg, swimming, diving). It may be helpful to avoid exercise outdoors during high pollen counts or during days with high levels of pollution. Also, it may be helpful to wear a mask to cover the nose and mouth during exercise when the weather is cold.

(Section 27: Disorders of the Respiratory System, Chapter 505: Asthma, p. 2430)

**Answer 19-28.** D

According to the Expert Panel Report 3, this child would have moderate persistent asthma based on having nighttime symptoms at least once per week and likely daily symptoms given the activity-related symptoms described (Figure 505-3).

**Classification of Asthma Severity in Children**

**(Children ≥ 5 years of age)**

| | Intermittent | Mild Persistent | Moderate Persistent | Severe |
|---|---|---|---|---|
| | Step 1 | Step 2 | Step 3/Step 4 | Step 5/Step 6 |
| Symptoms | ≤ 2 days/week | > 2 days/week but not daily | Daily | Throughout the day |
| Nighttime symptoms | ≤ 2x/month | 3–4x/month | > 1x/week but not nightly | Often 7x/week |
| Short-acting beta2-agonist use for symptom control | ≤ 2 days/week | ≤ 2 days/week but not daily | Daily | Several times per day |
| Interference with normal activity | None | Minor limitation | Some limitation | Extremely limited |
| Lung function | Normal $FEV_1$ between exacerbations<br>$FEV_1$ > 80% predicted<br>$FEV_1$/FVC normal | $FEV_1$ ≥ 80%<br>$FEV_1$/FVC normal | $FEV_1$ ≤ 60% but < 80% predicted<br>$FEV_1$/FVC reduced 5% | $FEV_1$ ≤ 60% predicted<br>$FEV_1$/FVC reduced 5% |
| Exacerbations requiring oral systemic corticosteroids | 0–1/year | ≥ 2/year | | |

Classification of Severity of Asthma by Clinical Features Before Treatment according to the Guidelines for the Diagnosis and Management of Asthma, Highlights of the Expert Panel Report 3.
An individual should be assigned to the most servere grade in which any feature occurs.
An individual's classification may change over time.
Patients at any level of severity can have mild, moderate, or severe exacerbations.
Key: $FEV_1$ = forced expiratory volume in 1 second; FVC = forced vital capacity

**FIGURE 505-3.** Classification of asthma severity in children. Asthma severity is classified as intermittent (step 1) or persistent, which is further broken down into step 2, steps 3/4, and steps 5/6 based on the frequency of symptoms, use of quick-relief medications, interference with normal activity, exacerbations, and lung function. (Mark W. Kline, *Rudolph's Pediatrics*, 23rd Edition. Copyright © McGraw-Hill Education. All rights reserved.)

Given her age, she would need to have nighttime symptoms every night to be classified as having severe persistent asthma or only have symptoms 3 to 4 times per month to classify as having mild persistent asthma. Spirometry would also be useful in classifying her asthma severity. She clearly has too many symptoms for her asthma to be considered mild intermittent. Keep in mind that an individual should be assigned to the most severe category in which any feature occurs.

(Section 27: Disorders of the Respiratory System, Chapter 505: Childhood Asthma, p. 2432)

**Answer 19-29.** C

OSA and nocturnal asthma can present with similar symptoms. According to the National Guidelines Expert Panel Report 3, evaluation for OSA is recommended in patients with unstable, poorly controlled asthma, particularly those who are overweight or obese. Without daytime cough, fever, or acute respiratory symptoms, pneumonia or acute sinusitis is less likely. A methacholine challenge is unlikely to be helpful in this scenario, as it will likely be positive given the patient's history. Given the increase in asthma flares and use of rescue medications, continuing current care without further investigation is not optimal.

(Section 27: Disorders of the Respiratory System, Chapter 505: Asthma, p. 2429)

**Answer 19-30.** D

This young man's symptoms are most consistent with vocal cord dysfunction. It is most definitively diagnosed via flexible laryngoscopy with direct observation of paradoxical vocal cord movement. Spirometry can show flattened inspiratory loops, but it is not a definitive diagnostic test and is often highly variable. A methacholine challenge may be negative in the absence of asthma, but that will not make the diagnosis of vocal cord dysfunction. An upper GI series would likely show normal anatomy and, given the lack of abdominal symptoms, would not likely show frank reflux leading to the respiratory symptoms. However, gastroesophageal reflux can be a contributing factor to the development of vocal cord dysfunction. A nasal ciliary biopsy would be used to diagnose ciliary dyskinesia, which is not consistent with this history.

(Section 27: Disorders of the Respiratory System, Chapter 503: Disorders Causing Airway Obstruction, Chapter 505: Childhood Asthma, pp. 2414, 2431)

**Answer 19-31.** B

There are many complications associated with CF (Table 507-5). The constellation of features in this case is most suggestive of CF-related diabetes mellitus. This complication becomes more common with age. Annual screening is recommended for early diagnosis and timely management. Insulin remains the standard therapy at this time.

A pulmonary exacerbation or allergic bronchopulmonary aspergillosis would generally show a significant decline in lung function, with more respiratory symptoms. Distal intestinal obstruction syndrome generally presents with abdominal pain and change in bowel habits. Minimally decreased pulmonary function makes a pulmonary exacerbation less likely.

**TABLE 507-5.** Clinical Manifestations of Cystic Fibrosis

| System | Primary CFTR-Related Manifestations | Secondary Complications |
|---|---|---|
| Airway | Inflammation<br>Infections<br>Bronchiectasis<br>Chronic sinusitis<br>Nasal polyps | Pneumothorax<br>Hemoptysis<br>Allergic bronchopulmonary aspergillosis<br>Respiratory failure |
| Gastrointestinal tract | Meconium ileus<br>Constipation<br>Distal intestinal obstruction syndrome<br>Appendiceal abscess<br>Intussusception | Gastroesophageal reflux disease<br>Fibrosing colonopathy<br>Rectal prolapse<br>Intestinal dysbiosis<br>Intestinal inflammation |
| Pancreas | Pancreatic insufficiency<br>Pancreatitis<br>Cystic fibrosis related diabetes | |
| Hepatobiliary tract | Biliary cirrhosis<br>Gallbladder and biliary tract disease | Portal hypertension<br>Extrinsic compression of common bile duct |
| Nutrition | | Growth failure<br>Protein calorie malnutrition<br>Micronutrient deficiency |
| Musculoskeletal | | Osteoporosis<br>Arthropathy/arthritis<br>Clubbing<br>Hypertrophic osteoarthropathy |

Mark W. Kline, *Rudolph's Pediatrics*, 23rd Edition. Copyright © McGraw-Hill Education. All rights reserved.

(Section 27: Disorders of the Respiratory System, Chapter 507: Cystic Fibrosis)

**Answer 19-32.** A

The accepted criteria for the diagnosis of CF are listed in Table 507-2. Diagnosis is based on a combination of clinical history and laboratory test results.

**TABLE 507-2.** According to Consensus Guidelines, a Diagnosis of Cystic Fibrosis (CF) Can be Made According to the Criteria Listed Below

| Diagnostic Criteria |
|---|
| At least 1 characteristic phenotypic feature (chronic obstructive pulmonary disease, exocrine pancreatic insufficiency, sweat salt loss syndrome, male infertility) |
| OR |
| Family history of cystic fibrosis (sibling) |
| OR |
| Positive newborn screening test |
| AND |
| Sweat chloride concentration > 60 mEq/L |
| OR |
| Identification of 2 CF-causing mutations |

Mark W. Kline, *Rudolph's Pediatrics*, 23rd Edition. Copyright © McGraw-Hill Education. All rights reserved.

(Section 27: Disorders of the Respiratory System, Chapter 507: Cystic Fibrosis)

### Answer 19-33. C

This patient has evidence of ongoing pulmonary exacerbation that has not responded to outpatient antibiotics. In addition, the patient has continued to lose weight and has fatigue, which may impair the ability to complete all the treatments necessary in the home. An IV antibiotic course is indicated in this scenario and may be completed in the hospital or in the home setting based on individual scenario.

An appetite stimulant may be useful but would not treat the pulmonary exacerbation, which is likely contributing to the weight loss. Allergic bronchopulmonary aspergillosis may be considered, but treatment should not be initiated until a diagnosis is confirmed. Bronchoscopy may be helpful in identifying other organisms to target with therapy, but generally in this situation, bronchoscopy without further treatment would not adequately treat the exacerbation. It would be early to make an assumption that this patient could not recover lung function, and aggressive treatment should be implemented before this conclusion is made.

(Section 27: Disorders of the Respiratory System, Chapter 507: Cystic Fibrosis)

### Answer 19-34. E

Class I to III mutations result in more severe disease, whereas class IV to VI mutations are thought to be milder mutations.

Class IV mutations are those of altered conductance, with CFTR that reaches the membrane but does not activate properly (Figure 507-1). These are commonly associated with pancreatic sufficiency. Delta F508 is the most common CFTR mutation and is a class II mutation, a block in processing.

The understanding of the different molecular mechanisms of CFTR dysfunction has led to the development of novel therapies that target the basic underlying defect and improve CFTR functioning.

(Section 27: Disorders of the Respiratory System, Chapter 507: Cystic Fibrosis)

Class of mutation

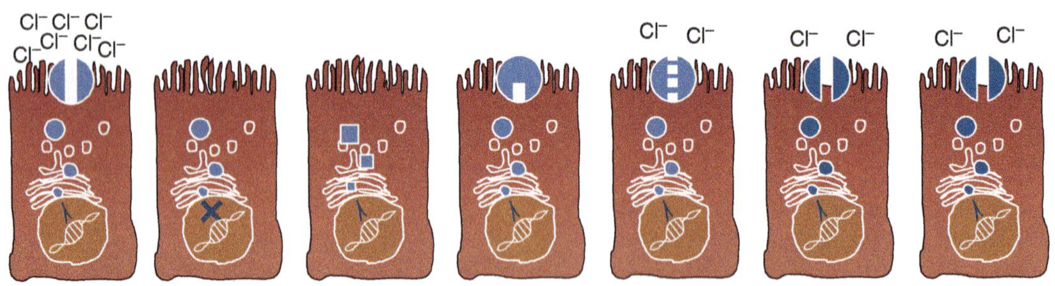


| Normal | I | II | III | IV | V | VI |
|---|---|---|---|---|---|---|
| Molecular defect | No synthesis | Block in processing | Block in regulation | Reduced conductance | Reduced synthesis | Reduced half-life |
| Functional abnormality | Protein is not synthesized | Folding defect | Channel opening defect | Ion transport defect | Decreased protein synthesis | Decreased half-life of the protein |
| Main mutations | Gly542X<br>Tip128X<br>Arg553X<br>621+1G→T | Phe508del<br>Asn1303Lys<br>lie507del<br>Arg560Thr | Gly551Asp<br>Gly178Arg<br>Gly551Ser<br>Ser549Asn | Arg117His<br>Arg347Pro<br>Arg117Cys<br>Arg334Trp | 3849+10kbC→T<br>2789+5G→A<br>3120+1G→A<br>5T | 4326delTC<br>Gln1412X<br>4279insA |

**FIGURE 507-1.** Functional classification of cystic fibrosis transmembrane conductance regulator (CFTR) mutations. (Reproduced with permission from Wat D. *Cystic Fibrosis in the Light of New Research*. London: InTech; 2015.)

**Answer 19-35.** D

There are many complications associated with CF (Table 507-5). Distal intestinal obstruction syndrome is often triggered in warmer months when patients become dehydrated more easily. The condition generally begins with constipation and progresses to obstruction if not treated promptly. Symptoms include crampy abdominal pain with decreased stooling, with or without bilious emesis. It is usually treated with bowel cleanout. Enzyme therapy should be reviewed and optimized.

The symptoms described are not classic for gastroesophageal reflux disease or gallstones. Intussusception can present with similar symptoms but may also include currant jelly stools and is less common than distal intestinal obstruction syndrome. Fibrosing colonopathy is uncommon and generally is seen when high doses of enzymes are being used. Fibrosing colonopathy generally presents with signs of obstruction and bloody stools.

(Section 27: Disorders of the Respiratory System, Chapter 507: Cystic Fibrosis, p. 2451)

**TABLE 507-5.** Clinical Manifestations of Cystic Fibrosis

| System | Primary CFTR-Related Manifestations | Secondary Complications |
|---|---|---|
| Airway | Inflammation<br>Infections<br>Bronchiectasis<br>Chronic sinusitis<br>Nasal polyps | Pneumothorax<br>Hemoptysis<br>Allergic bronchopulmonary aspergillosis<br>Respiratory failure |
| Gastrointestinal tract | Meconium ileus<br>Constipation<br>Distal intestinal obstruction syndrome<br>Appendiceal abscess<br>Intussusception | Gastroesophageal reflux disease<br>Fibrosing colonopathy<br>Rectal prolapse<br>Intestinal dysbiosis<br>Intestinal inflammation |
| Pancreas | Pancreatic insufficiency<br>Pancreatitis<br>Cystic fibrosis related diabetes | |
| Hepatobiliary tract | Biliary cirrhosis<br>Gallbladder and biliary tract disease | Portal hypertension<br>Extrinsic compression of common bile duct |
| Nutrition | | Growth failure<br>Protein calorie malnutrition<br>Micronutrient deficiency |
| Musculoskeletal | | Osteoporosis<br>Arthropathy/arthritis<br>Clubbing<br>Hypertrophic osteoarthropathy |

Mark W. Kline, *Rudolph's Pediatrics*, 23rd Edition. Copyright © McGraw-Hill Education. All rights reserved.

**Answer 19-36.** E

There are many different types of pulmonary vasculitis syndromes (Table 510-1). The girl described in the vignette has

**TABLE 510-1.** Pulmonary Vasculitis Syndromes

| | |
|---|---|
| **Primary Vasculitides** | |
| Small-vessel vasculitides | Granulomatosis with polyangiitis (GPA) |
| | Microscopic polyangiitis (MPA) |
| | Eosinophilic granulomatosis with polyangiitis (EGPA) |
| | Henoch-Schönlein purpura |
| Medium-vessel vasculitides | Kawasaki disease |
| | Polyarteritis nodosa (PAN) |
| Large-vessel vasculitides | Takayasu arteritis |
| Other vasculitides | Behçet syndrome |
| | Cogan syndrome |
| **Secondary Vasculitides** | |
| Connective tissue diseases | Systemic lupus erythematosus (SLE) |
| | Systemic sclerosis (SSc) |
| | Juvenile dermatomyositis (JDM) |
| Autoinflammatory diseases | Familial Mediterranean fever (FMF) |
| | Tumor necrosis factor receptor–associated periodic syndrome (TRAPS) |
| | Hyperimmunoglobulinemia D and periodic fever syndrome (HIDS) |
| | Cryopyrin associated periodic syndromes (CAPS) |
| | NOD2-associated pediatric granulomatous arthritides (Blau syndrome and early-onset sarcoidosis) |
| | STING-associated vasculopathy with onset in infancy (SAVI) |
| Other | Anti–glomerular basement membrane (GBM) disease |

Mark W. Kline, *Rudolph's Pediatrics*, 23rd Edition. Copyright © McGraw-Hill Education. All rights reserved.

a small- to medium-vessel vasculitis with inflammation of these vessels on lung pathology.

Answer choices A through D all fit into this category of small- to medium-vessel vasculitis. Only Takayasu arteritis (answer choice E) is incorrect because this is a large-vessel vasculitis.

(Section 27: Disorders of the Respiratory System, Chapter 510: Pulmonary Vasculitis Syndromes)

**Answer 19-37.** D

The girl described in the vignette is most likely to have granulomatosis with polyangiitis (formerly known as Wegener granulomatosis), based on the triad of involvement of the upper respiratory tract with sinusitis and epistaxis, the lower respiratory tract with history of pneumonia and likely pulmonary hemorrhage, and the kidney with proteinuria and renal insufficiency.

Eosinophilic granulomatosis with polyangiitis (formerly known as Churg-Strauss syndrome) is more likely to be associated with asthma and eosinophilia and is very rare in the pediatric population. Polyarteritis nodosa is not usually associated with upper respiratory findings, but instead may involve fever, weight loss, arthritis, skin lesions, and central nervous system disease. Behçet disease is a large-vessel vasculitis more likely associated with oral and genital ulcers and iritis rather than upper and lower respiratory and kidney findings. Sarcoidosis is a multisystem granulomatous disease, typically with multiple organ involvement, but respiratory symptoms are more likely to include cough and dyspnea rather than pulmonary hemorrhage.

(Section 27: Disorders of the Respiratory System; Chapter 510: Pulmonary Vasculitis Syndromes)

**Answer 19-38.** B

The patient described in the vignette has severe respiratory distress with continuing hemoptysis, and his airway needs to be protected. Following basic cardiopulmonary resuscitation measures, attention to airway, breathing, and circulation should ensue before other interventions. Therefore, intubation is the correct next step in treatment. The patient may need a blood transfusion, but this would occur after initial assessment and stabilization. The patient does not yet require chest compressions because he has an adequate heart rate and blood pressure.

The patient also likely has granulomatosis with polyangiitis (formerly known as Wegener granulomatosis) and may at some point require IV corticosteroids or IV cyclophosphamide as part of chronic therapy, but these would not be the next step in acute management of his hemoptysis and respiratory distress.

(Section 27: Disorders of the Respiratory System, Chapter 510: Pulmonary Vasculitis Syndromes)

**Answer 19-39.** E

The most likely diagnoses for the patient in the vignette include granulomatosis with polyangiitis (formerly known as Wegener granulomatosis) and microscopic polyangiitis, both of which are antineutrophil cytoplasmic antibody (ANCA)-associated vasculitides.

C-reactive protein is likely to be elevated with pulmonary vasculitides but is not specific so will not help confirm the diagnosis. Angiotensin-converting enzyme level would likely be elevated with sarcoidosis rather than with granulomatosis with polyangiitis or microscopic polyangiitis, which are the 2 diagnoses under consideration based on the clinical vignette. Antiribonucleoprotein antibody would be elevated in mixed connective tissue disease. Antiphospholipid antibody profile would be ordered to give an assessment of autoimmune-related thrombosis risk rather than confirm the diagnosis of either granulomatosis with polyangiitis or microscopic polyangiitis.

(Section 27: Disorders of the Respiratory System, Chapter 510: Pulmonary Vasculitis Syndromes)

**Answer 19-40.** A

The function of pulmonary surfactant is to *reduce* surface tension, which prevents alveolar collapse. Surfactant is composed primarily of lipids (90%) and also of proteins (10%). Surfactant is secreted by type II alveolar epithelial cells, not type I cells. Surfactant protein B deficiencies occur in an estimated 1 in 1 to 1.5 million births. Surfactant protein C deficiencies are autosomal dominant or sporadic and are associated with interstitial lung disease.

(Section 27: Disorders of the Respiratory System, Chapter 511: Pulmonary Surfactant and Pulmonary Alveolar Proteinosis)

**Answer 19-41.** E

Lung histopathology in primary alveolar proteinosis, which is caused by granulocyte-macrophage colony-stimulating factor receptor α chain dysfunction, is most consistent with that described in the vignette. Namely, there is preserved alveolar wall architecture but filling of the alveoli with surfactant. All of the other answer choices are associated with surfactant metabolic dysfunction disorders, the pathologic findings of which include fibrosis, alveolar wall thickening, and significant parenchymal lung distortion.

(Section 27: Disorders of the Respiratory System, Chapter 511: Pulmonary Surfactant and Pulmonary Alveolar Proteinosis)

**Answer 19-42.** D

The child described in the vignette is most likely to have *ABCA3* mutations leading to surfactant dysfunction, especially given the ground-glass appearance throughout both lungs on chest CT scan, as opposed to primary alveolar proteinosis, in which there are normal-appearing secondary pulmonary lobules adjacent to highly abnormal secondary lobules. Therefore, genetic testing for surfactant mutations should be performed before lung biopsy because this approach is less invasive, as long as the patient is stable enough to do so.

Bronchoalveolar lavage for surfactant levels is performed on a research basis only and is not routinely recommended for clinical decision-making. If genetic testing for surfactant mutations is negative, then genetic testing for lysinuric protein intolerance should be considered. Lung biopsy plays a more important role in diagnosing primary alveolar proteinosis, rather than genetic testing for granulocyte-macrophage colony-stimulating factor receptor α chain mutations. Based on the clinical and radiologic appearance, the patient described in this question is more likely to have *ABCA3* dysfunction rather than primary alveolar proteinosis.

(Section 27: Disorders of the Respiratory System, Chapter 511: Pulmonary Surfactant and Pulmonary Alveolar Proteinosis)

**Answer 19-43.** C

Treatment for pulmonary surfactant dysfunction disorders typically includes supportive care first, including oxygen supplementation and nutritional support. Therefore, treatment should begin with supplemental oxygen. In older children, surfactant administration does not result in improvement in clinical condition. Whole-lung lavage is technically challenging and of uncertain efficacy for surfactant dysfunction disorders but is the treatment of choice for autoimmune pulmonary alveolar proteinosis. Chronic systemic steroid use has been reported, but there are no controlled studies supporting its clinical utility. Lung transplantation should be considered in severe and progressive disease from *ABCA3* mutations but not before supportive care such as supplemental oxygen is given.

(Section 27: Disorders of the Respiratory System, Chapter 511: Pulmonary Surfactant and Pulmonary Alveolar Proteinosis, p. 2476)

**Answer 19-44.** B

Laryngeal braking helps to maintain an adequate volume of air in the thorax, thus helping to maintain functional residual capacity.

The chest wall of the newborn infant is very compliant, much more so than the chest wall of an adult. Due to the increased compliance of an infant's chest wall, there is an increased likelihood of collapse inward. As an infant ages, *more* of the diaphragm is actually in direct contact with the inner surface of the thoracic cavity. Premature termination of the expiratory phase, rather than prolonged expiration, helps to maintain functional residual capacity.

(Section 27: Disorders of the Respiratory System, Chapter 512: Chest Wall and Respiratory Muscle Disorders)

**Answer 19-45.** D

The sternocleidomastoids help to lift the sternum and increase intrathoracic volume by a "bucket handle" mechanism. Although the scalenes and serratus anterior are accessory muscles of inspiration, their mechanisms of action do not involve the "bucket handle" movement. The function of the diaphragm is to act like a piston and increase intrathoracic volume by displacing abdominal contents downward.

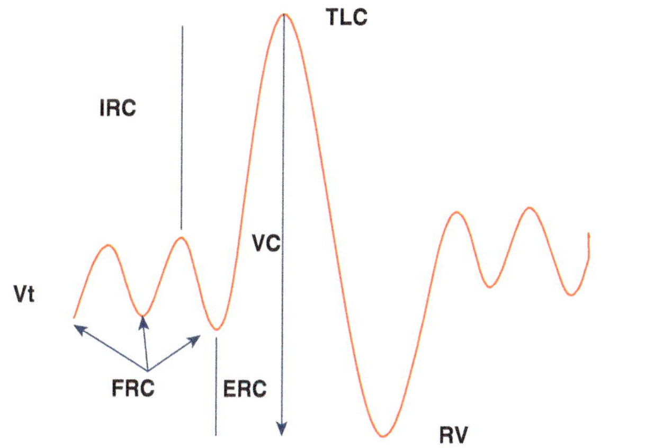


**FIGURE 496-1.** Subdivisions of lung volumes. ERC, expiratory reserve capacity; FRC, functional residual capacity; IRC, inspiratory reserve capacity; RV, residual volume; TLC, total lung capacity; VC, vital capacity; Vt, tidal volume. (Mark W. Kline, *Rudolph's Pediatrics*, 23rd Edition. Copyright © McGraw-Hill Education. All rights reserved.)

The external intercostals act to increase the anteroposterior diameter of the thorax.

(Section 27: Disorders of the Respiratory System, Chapter 512: Chest Wall and Respiratory Muscle Disorders)

**Answer 19-46.** B

With neuromuscular weakness as in Duchenne muscular dystrophy, there are decreases in lung volumes, consistent with the restrictive nature of the lung disease, and the TLC should be low, not elevated. The RV/TLC ratio is increased. This is secondary to weaker muscles of expiration compared to inspiration. These patients are unable to actively expire to lung volumes below functional residual capacity (FRC). The relationships of the different lung volumes are shown in Figure 496-1.

With neuromuscular weakness, there should also be reduced muscle pressures, including maximum expiratory pressure. End-tidal carbon dioxide is more likely to be elevated, rather than decreased, as neuromuscular weakness progresses. These patients should have normal or potentially low oxyhemoglobin saturations over time.

(Section 27: Disorders of the Respiratory System, Chapter 512: Chest Wall and Respiratory Muscle Disorders)

**Answer 19-47.** A

The internal intercostal muscles are accessory muscles of expiration that may be used during exercise. Contraction decreases the anteroposterior diameter of the thorax, aiding in expiration.

The abdominal muscles are also accessory muscles of expiration, not inspiration. Expiration is passive only during normal tidal breathing, not during exercise, coughing, sneezing, or speaking. Both the sternocleidomastoids and serratus anterior muscles are accessory muscles of inspiration rather than expiration.

(Section 27: Disorders of the Respiratory System, Chapter 512: Chest Wall and Respiratory Muscle Disorders)

### Answer 19-48. E

The infant described in the vignette has spinal muscular atrophy (SMA) type I (Werdnig-Hoffmann disease or severe infantile SMA). Clinical features of SMA include hypotonia; muscle weakness, including extensive involvement of the intercostal muscles; muscle atrophy; and fasciculations. Cough is expected to be impaired, and the use of a cough assist device (mechanical in-exsufflator) will help to clear secretions. Without assisted ventilation, children with SMA type I usually die within the first 2 years of life. With SMA type II, the median age of survival is 12 years without assisted ventilation. Children with SMA type I are unlikely to be able to sit or walk. The chest wall may start to become bell-shaped and also tends to draw inward due to the weakness of the intercostal muscles. Although assisted ventilation will be necessary to prolong survival, noninvasive ventilation may also be presented as an option in addition to invasive ventilation via tracheostomy.

(Section 27: Disorders of the Respiratory System, Chapter 512: Chest Wall and Respiratory Muscle Disorders)

### Answer 19-49. C

The newborn described in the clinical vignette has asphyxiating thoracic dystrophy (Jeune syndrome), which is an autosomal recessive disorder known to be part of the ciliopathy spectrum, related to intraflagellar transport genes. The disorder results in fixed chest wall size with restrictive (not obstructive) lung disease due to the mechanical limitations of the chest. These patients are at risk for development of recurrent atelectasis, pneumonia, and impaired lung growth. Vertically expandable prosthetic titanium rib placement has been used for treating children with thoracic dystrophy.

Achondroplasia is an autosomal dominant condition associated with dwarfism but not with the characteristic features of the narrow bell-shaped chest with shortened ribs as described in this case for Jeune syndrome.

(Section 27: Disorders of the Respiratory System, Chapter 512: Chest Wall and Respiratory Muscle Disorders)

### Answer 19-50. D

The girl described in the vignette has digital clubbing of the fingers and toes. Clubbing is associated with increased caliber and number of blood vessels, as well as primitive fibroblasts and an increased number of lymphocytes and eosinophils.

In a girl with chronic productive cough and poor growth, clubbing is likely a sign of respiratory disease, such as bronchiectasis due to cystic fibrosis (CF) or other causes, chronic lung infection, or pulmonary abscess. With clubbing, the depth of the finger at the proximal nail fold exceeds the depth of the distal interphalangeal joint. Clubbing is usually painless and *not* recognized by the patient. When clubbing is present, Schamroth sign is present (Figure 498-2); that is, there is an obliteration of the normal rhombus that is seen when the dorsal surfaces of corresponding fingers on the right and left hand are placed against each other.

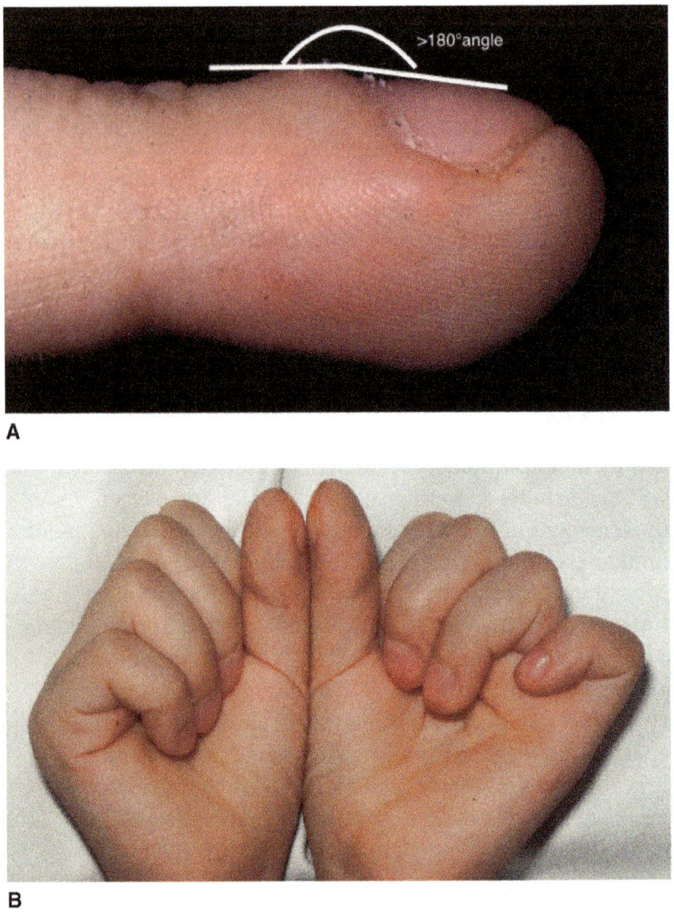


**FIGURE 498-2.** A: The upper image shows the changed hyponychial angle. B: The lower image demonstrates Schamroth sign, with the obliterated diamond-shaped gap between the nails of the opposed thumbs. (Mark W. Kline, *Rudolph's Pediatrics*, 23rd Edition. Copyright © McGraw-Hill Education. All rights reserved.)

(Section 27: Disorders of the Respiratory System, Chapter 498: The Clinical Presentation of Respiratory Illness)

### Answer 19-51. D

The description in the case is consistent with neuroendocrine cell hyperplasia of infancy (NEHI), which is associated with prolonged supplemental oxygen requirements in many cases. The cause of NEHI is largely unknown, and patients do not usually respond to corticosteroids. Fortunately, the majority of patients with NEHI do improve over time and do not need to undergo lung transplantation. Adenovirus infection most commonly leads to bronchiolitis obliterans and is not involved in the pathophysiology of NEHI. Exposure to avian antigens is the most common cause of hypersensitivity pneumonitis in children.

(Section 27: Disorders of the Respiratory System, Chapter 508: Interstitial Lung Disease)

### Answer 19-52. B

The patient described in the question has hypoxemia, bilateral diffuse infiltrates on CXR, and anemia and most likely has diffuse alveolar hemorrhage. The next step in management would be to confirm pulmonary hemorrhage by looking for hemosiderin-stained macrophages in the bronchoalveolar lavage fluid. Lung biopsy would be performed to look for pulmonary capillaritis, but due to the invasiveness of the procedure, one would perform bronchoalveolar lavage to confirm pulmonary hemorrhage first and then perform serologic tests to rule out immune-mediated lung disease, cardiac evaluation, and lung biopsy.

High-dose IV corticosteroids are used for idiopathic pulmonary hemosiderosis and other causes of pulmonary hemorrhage but are not indicated for immediate management unless the diffuse alveolar hemorrhage is life threatening. High-resolution CT of the chest would not be performed next in the management of this patient because it may not provide much additional information and would expose the patient to unnecessary radiation. Surfactant protein B and C mutations cause surfactant dysfunction and can be associated with respiratory distress but are not characteristically associated with anemia in combination with infiltrates on CXR.

(Section 27: Disorders of the Respiratory System, Chapter 508: Interstitial Lung Disease, pp. 2359–2360)

**Answer 19-53.** E

The patient described in the clinical vignette has bronchiolitis obliterans (BO) after lung transplantation for CF. BO affects small- to medium-sized airways and causes obstruction during exhalation. Chronic rejection can also manifest as BO. Median time to diagnosis of BO after transplantation is 16 to 20 months.

Lung biopsy may not be necessary for diagnosis if clinical signs and symptoms and radiography are consistent with the diagnosis. Still, treatment should be initiated with corticosteroids, and consideration of lung biopsy should occur if there is no improvement with therapy. Unfortunately, BO after lung transplantation usually follows a progressive course, so treatment is indicated. Although steroids are often given and have been somewhat helpful in the treatment of BO, the studies behind this practice are lacking. Anti-TNF has been used in BO related to bone marrow transplantation, but not related to lung transplantation. Lung biopsy would help confirm the diagnosis, but bronchoscopy with bronchoalveolar lavage would not by itself help make the diagnosis.

(Section 27: Disorders of the Respiratory System, Chapter 508: Interstitial Lung Disease, p. 2459)

**Answer 19-54.** B

Children with OSA do have impaired arousal responses to obstructive events. The upper airway behaves as a collapsible tube; therefore, *increased* inspiratory effort (rather than decreased inspiratory effort) may only result in more collapse of the airway rather than increased flow.

Contrary to popular belief, the growth rate of lymphadenoid tissue is proportional to other tissues within the upper airway in children aged 2 to 8 years. Pharyngeal airway neuromotor responses are impaired in children with OSA compared to normal children. Hypoxic and hypercapnic ventilatory drive appears to be normal in children with OSA; however, centrally mediated augmentation of upper airway neuromotor function is abnormal.

(Section 27: Disorders of the Respiratory System, Chapter 501: Disorders of Respiratory Control and Sleep-Disordered Breathing)

**Answer 19-55.** A

OSA in infants is more common in children with chromosomal disorders such as trisomy 21, with craniofacial abnormalities, or with any disease leading to soft tissue infiltration, such as inflammation or laryngomalacia. OSA is also more likely in premature infants and in males, which may be attributable to sex-related differences in anatomy or to a protective role of female hormones.

Magnetic resonance imaging (MRI) and manometry studies have shown that infants with clinically significant OSA are more likely to have upper airway obstruction in the retropalatal region (80%) compared with the retroglossal region (20%). In infants, OSA *is* commonly associated with hypoxemia. This finding is likely due to the higher chest wall compliance in infants and the need for dynamically active maintenance of functional residual capacity (FRC). Therefore, in sleep, when FRC is reduced, infants are more likely to desaturate, even in the absence of apnea. The laryngeal chemoreflex is more likely to play a role in an infant than in an older child because the reflex is reduced with maturation. The reflex is more prominent in premature infants as well, such that episodes of gastroesophageal reflux can lead to apnea and bradycardia.

(Section 27: Disorders of the Respiratory System, Chapter 501: Disorders of Respiratory Control and Sleep-Disordered Breathing)

**Answer 19-56.** C

CCHS is inherited in an autosomal dominant fashion, rather than in an autosomal recessive manner. There are also de novo mutations described. CCHS is a lifelong disorder, and patients usually require up to 24 hours per day of assisted ventilation. Hirschsprung disease is found in 20% of CCHS patients, whereas autonomic neural crest tumors such as neuroblastoma are found in 5% to 10% of CCHS patients.

The most common mutations causing CCHS are those in the *PHOX2B* gene, which plays essential roles in the embryogenesis of the autonomic nervous system. Ventilation is most affected during quiet or non-REM sleep, a time when autonomic control is most prominent.

(Section 27: Disorders of the Respiratory System, Chapter 501: Disorders of Respiratory Control and Sleep-Disordered Breathing)

**Answer 19-57.** A

This question describes a young girl with Rett syndrome, who is likely to have abnormal cardiorespiratory patterns and can have hyperventilation, apnea, breath holding, and rapid shallow breathing during wakefulness and sleep. This disorder is caused by a mutation in the *MECP2* gene. Rett syndrome is X-linked. Most cases are sporadic, not inherited.

Prader-Willi syndrome is due to a microdeletion defect on chromosome 15 and is a disorder that can lead to excessive daytime sleepiness or disturbances in circadian rhythms. Obesity and hypotonia may also lead to obstructive sleep apnea in Prader-Willi syndrome. The inheritance for Joubert syndrome is associated with cerebellar abnormalities. The respiratory manifestations of Joubert syndrome include marked hyperpnea with severe alveolar hypoventilation. Finally, abnormal development and survival of unmyelinated sensory and autonomic neurons is characteristic of familial dysautonomia (Riley-Day syndrome), in which abnormalities in the autonomic nervous system lead to inappropriate cardiovascular or catecholamine responses to physical stress, exercise, or position change. Patients can have breath-holding episodes with emotional outbursts, as well as periodic breathing and central apnea during sleep.

(Section 27: Disorders of the Respiratory System, Chapter 501: Disorders of Respiratory Control and Sleep-Disordered Breathing)

**Answer 19-58.** E

Based on the clinical information, the infant was born prematurely and may be more at risk for apnea of prematurity, which is defined as pauses in breathing of > 20 seconds or an apneic event of < 20 seconds but associated with bradycardia or cyanosis. However, because the baby has a low-grade temperature of 38°C in addition to the apneic pauses, it is prudent to rule out underlying sepsis or infection as a cause of apnea first.

Central nervous system problems should also be ruled out, and a head ultrasound would be indicated after a thorough evaluation looking for infection. pH probe could be done to look for gastroesophageal reflux; however, infection and intracranial abnormalities would take precedence over this evaluation. In addition, there is no clear evidence that treating gastroesophageal reflux, if present, will lead to a decrease in the frequency or severity of apnea of prematurity in preterm infants.

Treatment for apnea of prematurity with caffeine citrate should not be initiated until sepsis, seizure disorders, and severe gastroesophageal reflux disease (GERD) have been ruled out because caffeine can lower the seizure threshold and decrease muscle tone in the esophageal sphincter. Treatment of apnea of prematurity with CPAP may also be considered if apnea is frequent or severe; however, evaluation for other etiologies should be undertaken first, as described earlier.

(Section 27: Disorders of the Respiratory System, Chapter 501: Disorders of Respiratory Control and Sleep-Disordered Breathing)

**Answer 19-59.** C

The assessment of OSA involves clinical history and examination and then polysomnogram. Only 7% of children with OSA present with EDS. When sleepiness was measured objectively using multiple sleep latency testing, 13% to 20% of children were noted to have increased sleepiness, with obese children having more prominent symptoms.

In young children, the measurement of transcutaneous carbon dioxide tension is recommended in addition to end-tidal capnography to increase the sensitivity of the test, and it is typically performed when respiratory rate is high, in infants, or if prominent mouth breathing is noted. This assessment is needed because, in children, complete obstructive events are less likely due to the resistance of the pediatric upper airway to collapse. The clinical history, even when performed by a sleep medicine specialist, does not have high predictive accuracy for OSA. At this time, the gold standard for diagnosis is only the overnight polysomnogram and not overnight pulse oximetry. Other methods for making the diagnosis are being evaluated, such as video monitoring and overnight pulse oximetry. Finally, children are less likely to have electroencephalographic arousals after obstructive events, and sleep architecture is more likely preserved in children.

(Section 27: Disorders of the Respiratory System, Chapter 501: Disorders of Respiratory Control and Sleep-Disordered Breathing)

**Answer 19-60.** E

The infant in the vignette has bronchopulmonary dysplasia. Preterm birth occurred at 27 weeks of gestation, which falls in the saccular stage of lung development. During the saccular stage (26–36 weeks), true alveolar units form. Terminal alveolar saccules form from dilated acinar tubules, and differentiation of alveolar type 1 cells leads to an increase in gas exchange surface area. Type 2 alveolar cells also mature, and there is an increase in lamellar bodies, which store surfactant. However, surfactant levels are still low during this time, leading to respiratory distress syndrome and often the development of bronchopulmonary dysplasia in preterm infants born during this stage of lung development.

(Section 27: Disorders of the Respiratory System, Chapter 495: Lung Growth in Infancy and Childhood, p. 2360)

**Answer 19-61.** D

The infant in the vignette most likely has laryngomalacia. Laryngomalacia is the most common cause of noninfectious persistent stridor in infants and is due to prolapse of laryngeal structures (usually epiglottis or arytenoid cartilage) into the airway during inspiration. Stridor is generally a musical, high-pitched sound that is often audible without a stethoscope. Inspiratory stridor is an indication of narrowing of the extrathoracic airways.

Asthma and bronchomalacia are more likely to cause wheeze, which is usually an expiratory sound, indicating partial obstruction in the intrathoracic airways. Adenotonsillar hypertrophy is a cause of snoring, which is generally an inspiratory sound that is due to oropharyngeal obstruction. Crackles are the abnormal respiratory sound often associated with pneumonia. Crackles are usually nonmusical inspiratory sounds that can be fine or coarse. Fine crackles are thought to be due to the sudden opening of small airways, whereas coarse crackles are attributed to the movement of secretions within the lower airways.

(Section 27: Disorders of the Respiratory System, Chapter 498: The Clinical Presentation of Respiratory Illness)

**Answer 19-62.** D

The newborn in the vignette has a left-sided congenital diaphragmatic hernia. The diaphragm is formed during weeks 4 to 12 of embryogenesis. Approximately 90% of congenital diaphragmatic hernias are posterior (Bochdalek) hernias. This occurs due to a failure of the pleuroperitoneal folds to fuse with the transverse septum and intercostal muscles. When the pleuroperitoneal cavity does not close properly, abdominal contents herniate into the chest (intestine is seen in the left side of the chest in the CXR), which leads to pulmonary hypoplasia. Development of the diaphragm coincides with the pseudoglandular stage of lung development (weeks 6–16). During this stage, the conducting airways are formed through branching morphogenesis.

(Section 27: Disorders of the Respiratory System, Chapter 495: Lung Growth in Infancy and Childhood)

**Answer 19-63.** A

The preschool boy in the vignette has wheezing with acute exacerbation and symptoms between episodes. Daily maintenance with inhaled corticosteroids in the lowest dose possible to control symptoms has been shown to reduce exacerbations, symptoms, and bronchodilator use.

Bronchodilators should be used as needed for acute symptoms and are not generally recommended for daily maintenance. Selective $\beta_2$-agonists are preferred because they have less cardiac effects. As such, inhaled epinephrine would not be recommended. Combination inhalers with inhaled corticosteroid and long-acting β-agonist are used for management of asthma, but this medication class would not be recommended as first-line treatment for preschool wheezing. Antibiotic prophylaxis is not indicated for preschool wheezing.

(Section 27: Disorders of the Respiratory System, Chapter 506: Preschool Wheeze: Diagnosis and Management)

**Answer 19-64.** E

Lung volumes, specifically FRC, can be measured by 2 different techniques: gas dilution and whole-body plethysmography. Plethysmography measures all the gas contained in the chest, whereas gas dilution measures only the gas that is able to communicate with the airway opening. Therefore, patients with airflow obstruction, such as asthma or CF, are more likely to have lower volumes when measured by gas dilution techniques. In these cases, some of the airways are not patent and not freely communicating.

In healthy lungs or in patients with diseases that are likely to cause restriction, the 2 techniques should yield very similar results. The remaining examples would all likely be either normal or demonstrate restrictive changes.

(Section 27: Disorders of the Respiratory System, Chapter 496: Physiologic Basis of Pulmonary Function, pp. 2367–2368)

**Answer 19-65.** D

The patient in the vignette has symptoms consistent with protracted bacterial bronchitis (PBB). PBB is characterized by persistent wet cough for at least 4 weeks, usually with wheezing and rattily breathing. Other causes of chronic suppurative lung disease such as cystic fibrosis or bronchiectasis should be ruled out. Children with PBB who undergo bronchoscopy are more likely to have a lower respiratory tract infection based on culture results than controls. Treatment is a prolonged course of a broad-spectrum oral antibiotic. Duration ranges from 2 to 6 weeks, with a recommendation to start with 2 weeks and assess response to determine if continuation is warranted.

(Section 27: Disorders of the Respiratory System, Chapter 506: Preschool Wheeze: Diagnosis and Management)

**Answer 19-66.** A

Asthma is an obstructive lung disease, usually leading to an obstructive pattern on spirometry. However, asthma is also characterized by air trapping. At times, a restrictive pattern is noted on spirometry, confounding the picture. In this situation, air trapping should be suspected and can be confirmed with lung volume measurement. Air trapping is suggested when total lung capacity is normal but RV is elevated, leading to an elevated RV/TLC. Understanding the relationship of the lung volumes is important when interpreting results of lung function testing (Figure 496-1).

(Section 27: Disorders of the Respiratory System, Chapter 496: Physiologic Basis of Pulmonary Function)

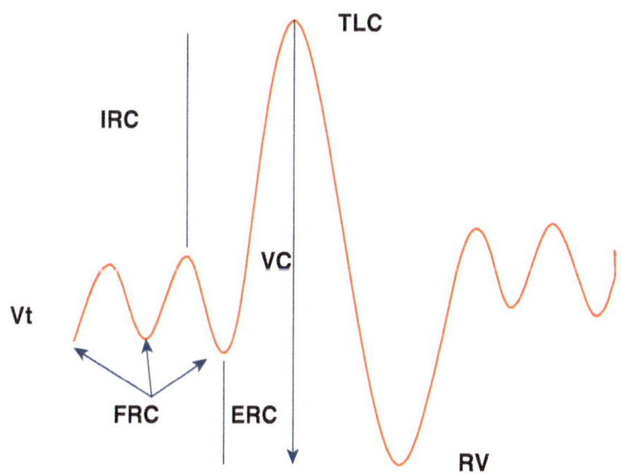


**FIGURE 496-1.** Subdivisions of lung volumes. ERC, expiratory reserve capacity; FRC, functional residual capacity; IRC, inspiratory reserve capacity; RV, residual volume; TLC, total lung capacity; VC, vital capacity; Vt, tidal volume. (Mark W. Kline, *Rudolph's Pediatrics*, 23rd Edition. Copyright © McGraw-Hill Education. All rights reserved.)

**Answer 19-67.** B

This child is recovering from a severe pneumonia. The incidence and severity of pneumonia are highest in the first year of life, particularly in the first 6 months. HIV infection is a significant risk factor for pneumonia, with a 6-fold higher risk of developing severe pneumonia compared to uninfected children and a 6-fold higher risk of death. Ninety percent of HIV-infected children reside in sub-Saharan Africa, and childhood deaths outside the neonatal period are disproportionately high in this region. Smoke exposure is a risk factor for severe pneumonia, but the father smoking outside the home is less likely to be the main contributor to this child's risk compared to the risk with HIV infection. Other risk factors include lack of breastfeeding, low socioeconomic status, crowded housing conditions, prematurity or low birth weight, and chronic underlying disease. A family history of asthma may certainly increase this child's risk for asthma; however, asthma is not likely the main contributor to risk for severe pneumonia.

(Section 27: Disorders of the Respiratory System, Chapter 497: The Global Burden of Lower Respiratory Tract Infections and Mucosal Immunology of the Lower Respiratory Tract in Children)

**Answer 19-68.** C

Cough that has been persistent for 4 weeks or more is considered as chronic cough and warrants further evaluation. Hence, answer choice A is incorrect. CXR is the most appropriate next step, along with a thorough history and examination, for further evaluation because chronic cough (Figure 498-3) can be a symptom of a more significant underlying lung pathology.

Antibiotics would be incorrect because prescribing antibiotics without ascertaining the underlying etiology of chronic cough may potentially lead to missed diagnosis of significant underlying respiratory illness such as primary ciliary dyskinesia (PCD) or cystic fibrosis (Table 498-3).

Oral corticosteroids would be an option if this was dry cough or there was a possibility of asthma, but given that it has been a wet-sounding cough, this is less likely. A referral to a pulmonologist can be done after the initial workup but would not be the likely next step.

(Section 27: Disorders of the Respiratory System, Chapter 498: The Clinical Presentation of Respiratory Illness, pp. 2376–2377)

**Answer 19-69.** B

Patients with neuromuscular disorders such as SMA, muscular dystrophy, and cerebral palsy are at high risk of chronic primary aspiration, which is likely to be of small volume and often silent. The current recommendation per the latest SMA guideline published in 2018 is to evaluate for swallowing abnormalities shortly after diagnosis and when any clinical signs suggestive of dysphagia occur by a video fluoroscopic swallow study. This is the gold standard in evaluating all stages of swallowing function and can distinguish issues with different consistencies of food and liquids. A fiberoptic evaluation of swallowing (FEES) study is a flexible laryngoscope examination done by a physician with a speech therapist; it allows direct visualization of the larynx with regard to swallowing mechanism and can be done with and without feedings. It is helpful in assessment of aspiration of oral secretions as well as feedings, which is not the primary challenge in this child.

Feeding in small volumes or continuing to monitor would not be optimal because even small-volume feeds can cause silent aspiration. An upper GI series would evaluate for aspiration secondary to gastroesophageal reflux disease, but it would not be helpful in evaluation of aspiration secondary to dysphagia.

(Section 27: Disorders of the Respiratory System, Chapter 504: Aspiration Syndromes)

**Answer 19-70.** A

Epithelial cells lining the respiratory surface can be stimulated by microbes or macrophage cytokines to stimulate the production of a distinct set of cytokines to stimulate local neutrophil recruitment and activation. Dendritic cells provide adaptive immune responses, and alveolar macrophages participate in innate immune responses and are located within the air spaces.

Although promoting breastfeeding and nutrition is essential in promoting immunity, the benefits of breastfeeding are not specific to immunity of the lower respiratory tract. Antibiotic use is useful in treating bacterial infection; however, antibiotics do not confer immune protection.

(Section 27: Disorders of the Respiratory System, Chapter 497: The Global Burden of Lower Respiratory Tract Infections and Mucosal Immunology of the Lower Respiratory Tract in Children)

**Answer 19-71.** C

The first lung transplant was performed in 1963, and since then, only 9 free-standing pediatric lung transplant centers exist in the Unites States. CF is the leading indication for lung transplantation among adolescents (> 60%) and among children aged 6 to 11 years. Among children younger than 5 years of age, rare diffuse lung diseases, bronchopulmonary dysplasia, pulmonary and hypertension with or without congenital heart disease are the leading indications for lung transplantation.

(Section 27: Disorders of the Respiratory System, Chapter 509: Pediatric Lung Transplantation)

**Answer 19-72.** A

Ischemia-reperfusion injury to the lung presents with symptoms similar to adult respiratory distress syndrome. It is the cause of 11% to 25% of all postsurgical lung transplant complications. Prolonged ventilator support with high positive end-expiratory pressure would be recommended for recovery.

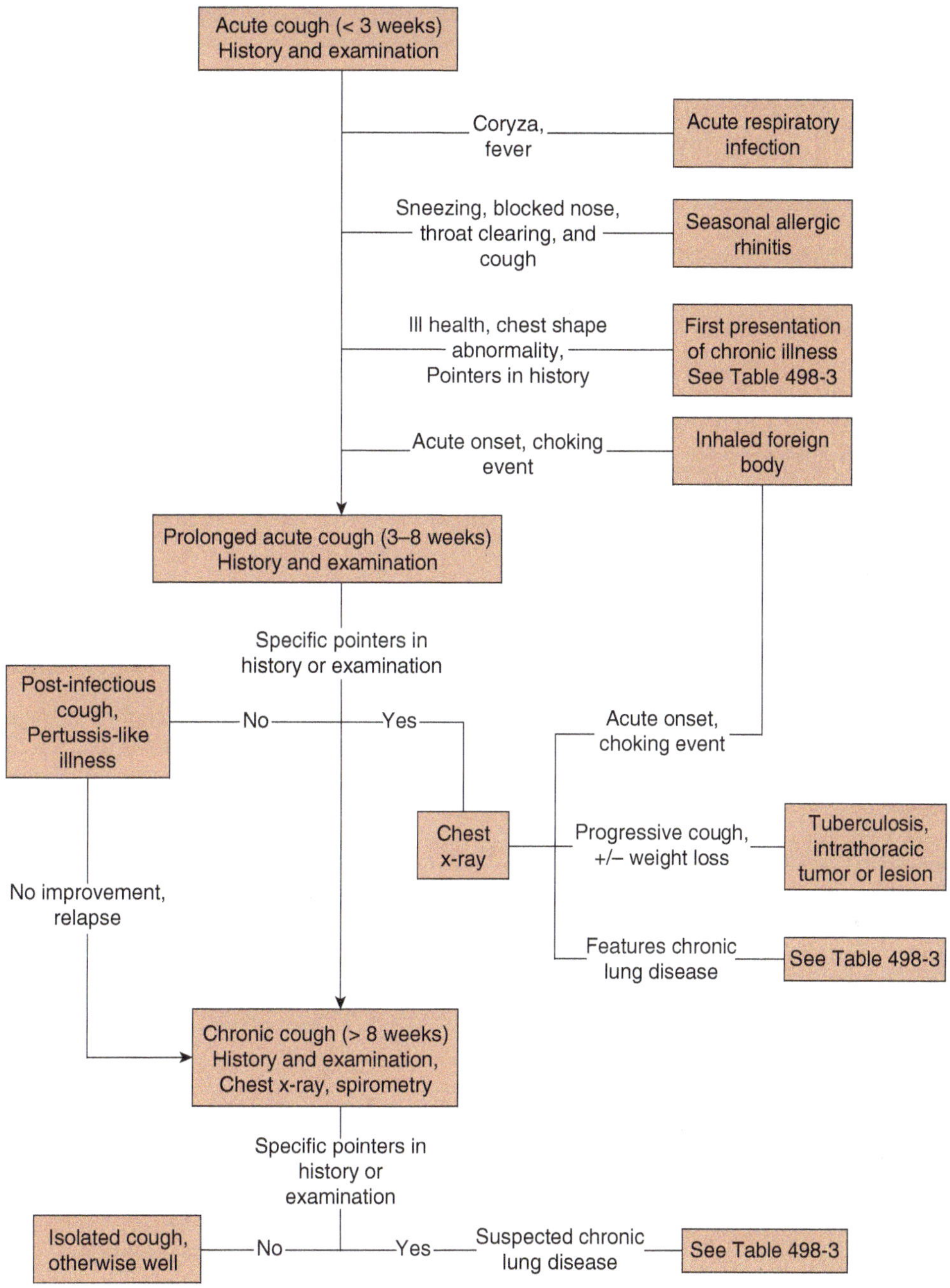


**FIGURE 498-3.** Assessment of acute and chronic cough. (Mark W. Kline, *Rudolph's Pediatrics*, 23rd Edition. Copyright © McGraw-Hill Education. All rights reserved.)

Primary graft dysfunction is the most common cause of early mortality from lung transplant.

Bacteremia is more likely among patients with cystic fibrosis after lung transplant. Seizures can occur in about 10% to 20% of lung transplant patients within the first month after transplant and are secondary to use of medications such as tacrolimus and cyclosporine. Renal insufficiency is noted after lung transplantation, but it is likely transient and mild, secondary to hypotension from surgery or cardiopulmonary bypass. Chronic lung allograft dysfunction manifests as BO, which is a sustained 20% drop in forced expiratory volume in 1 second ($FEV_1$). This condition affects about 50% of survivors of lung transplant.

(Section 27: Disorders of the Respiratory System, Chapter 509: Pediatric Lung Transplantation)

**Answer 19-73.** E

The respiratory pattern described in the vignette is most consistent with periodic breathing. Periodic breathing is frequently seen in neonates, especially those born preterm, and is described as clusters of breaths interrupted by apneas lasting

**TABLE 498-3.** Pathologies Associated with Chronic Cough

| Diagnosis | Further Clues to Diagnosis |
|---|---|
| **Reversible Airway Obstruction** | |
| Asthma | Cough elicited by exercise and associated with wheeze |
| **Chronic Infection** | |
| Cystic fibrosis (CF) | Chronic productive cough, chronic sinusitis, growth failure, clubbing, steatorrhea |
| Primary ciliary dyskinesia | Chronic rhinorrhea, chronic otitis media/sinusitis, situs inversus, neonatal respiratory distress |
| Immunodeficiency | Frequent/prolonged/unusual infections, growth failure, lymphadenopathy |
| Isolated bronchiectasis | Wet cough, history of infection, missed foreign body, chronic aspiration |
| **Aspiration** | |
| Swallowing difficulties (eg, in neuromuscular diseases), laryngeal clefts, H-type tracheoesophageal fistula, vocal cord paralysis | Choking and cough associated with drinking liquids, poor response to asthma or reflux therapy, patchy infiltrates on chest radiograph |
| Gastroesophageal reflux disease | Frequent wet burps, cough associated with meals, postprandial cough, patchy infiltrates on chest radiograph |
| Foreign body inhalation | Acute onset of choking, asymmetric breath sounds or wheezing |
| **Interstitial Lung Disease** | |
| Eosinophilic pneumonitis, hypersensitivity pneumonitis | Dyspnea, exposure to potential inhalant hazards, dry cough, normal lung sounds or fine crackles |
| **Airway Abnormalities** | |
| Tracheobronchomalacia | Wheeze, stridor, harsh barking cough, unilateral changes to breath sounds |
| Extrinsic bronchial compression | |
| **Cardiac Causes** | |
| Pulmonary hypertension | Signs and symptoms of cardiac failure |
| Pulmonary edema | |
| **Others** | |
| Recurrent rhinosinusitis with "postnasal" drip | Cough occurring after lying down, purulent nasal discharge, face pain, morning posttussive emesis |
| Tuberculosis | Exposure history, positive Mantoux test, weight loss, night sweats, abnormal chest radiograph |
| Allergic bronchopulmonary aspergillosis | Eosinophilia, high IgE levels, patchy infiltrates on chest radiograph and associated wheeze |
| Primary and secondary lung tumors, mediastinal tumors | Chest pain, hemoptysis, dyspnea, tachypnea, wheeze, symptoms of vascular compression (superior vena cava syndrome) |
| **Isolated Cough** | |
| Persistent bacterial bronchitis | Protracted isolated wet cough in otherwise healthy children |
| Pertussis/*Mycoplasma*/postviral | Persistent, mostly dry cough after respiratory tract infection |
| Somatic cough syndrome/tic | Harsh or honking in nature; disappears during sleep |

Mark W. Kline, *Rudolph's Pediatrics*, 23rd Edition. Copyright © McGraw-Hill Education. All rights reserved.

as long as 10 seconds. It generally resolves with time, in the first few weeks of life.

Central apnea is a complete cessation of breathing without respiratory effort. Cheyne-Stokes breathing is a repetitive pattern of increasing then decreasing tidal volumes followed by an apnea and is a respiratory pattern suggestive of brain injury. Hypopneas are shallow breaths. Kussmaul breathing is indicative of metabolic acidosis and is characterized by deep and labored breaths.

(Section 27: Disorders of the Respiratory System, Chapter 498: The Clinical Presentation of Respiratory Illness, p. 2372)

**Answer 19-74.** B

Radionuclide salivagram is the gold standard for detection of salivary aspiration by detection of the radiotracer in the lower airways or lungs. This is helpful in confirming the diagnosis of aspiration of oral secretions. Radionuclide salivagram is a noninvasive test, and if negative, fiberoptic endoscopic evaluation of swallowing can be considered as the next step.

Upper GI series and esophageal pressure monitoring (pH probe) are used to test for gastroesophageal reflux disease. In this case, the child is not orally fed. If the Nissen fundoplication is intact, then secondary aspiration is less likely. Upper GI series would not be helpful in a child who is fed via gastrostomy tube. CT scan of the chest and chest radiograph would only be useful to assess for any sequelae of aspiration.

(Section 27: Disorders of the Respiratory System, Chapter 504: Aspiration Syndromes, p. 2422)

# CHAPTER 20 Gastroenterology

Eric Chiou and Kristin Whitfield Van Buren

**20-1.** Vomiting is a common presenting symptom in general pediatrics. In addition, cyclic vomiting syndrome (CVS) has an estimated prevalence of 2%. Which of the following scenarios is consistent with a child with the diagnosis of CVS?

**A.** A 5-year-old boy with recurrent episodes of nonbilious vomiting that occur after he sleeps in during the weekend or after a high-protein meal

**B.** A 6-year-old girl with recurrent episodes of fast-paced vomiting (up to 4 emeses per hour) every 3 weeks that begin in the morning and last about 24 hours

**C.** A 6-month-old girl with recurrent episodes of bilious vomiting and abdominal pain every 4 to 6 hours

**D.** A 5-year-old girl with recurrent episodes of nonbilious vomiting every 4 hours, occipital headache, and mild ataxia

**E.** A 6-week-old girl with recurrent episodes of nonbilious vomiting after every feed

**20-2.** A 7-year-old girl presents to the emergency department (ED) after vomiting 15 times over the past 8 hours. The vomiting began suddenly upon awakening that morning. After examining her medical record, you note that she has had similar 24-hour episodes of vomiting approximately every 4 weeks for the past 3 months. All the episodes required intravenous (IV) fluid rehydration. Aside from the 24-hour vomiting episodes, she has been otherwise healthy.

She has a heart rate of 130 bpm, has a blood pressure of 105/76 mm Hg, and appears listless, but is able to answer your questions appropriately. She has urinated once earlier today. Physical examination reveals tacky mucous membranes. There are no focal neurologic findings or symptoms. She takes sips of water in the ED, but 10 minutes later, she has an episode of nonbloody, nonbilious emesis. You suspect cyclic vomiting syndrome (CVS). What would be the next appropriate step in management of this patient?

**A.** Administer IV fluid rehydration

**B.** Send blood for electrolytes, glucose, blood urea nitrogen (BUN), and creatinine

**C.** Order an abdominal radiograph

**D.** Administer an IV proton pump inhibitor

**E.** Order head computed tomography (CT)

**20-3.** A 10-year-old girl has acute pancreatitis. She was hospitalized yesterday and has been given intravenous (IV) fluids for 24 hours. The girl is feeling better, and her mother would like to know when the girl can begin eating again. Of the following, which is the most appropriate response to give to the patient's mother?

**A.** She can begin clear liquids after 24 hours with no pain.

**B.** She can eat when her lipase levels have normalized.

**C.** She should be able to start eating within the next 24 hours.

**D.** You will order parenteral nutrition before she eats by mouth.

**E.** You will request nasojejunal tube feedings today.

**20-4.** A 12-year-old girl is admitted to the hospital with elevated lipase and suspected pancreatitis based on initial evaluation completed in the emergency department. She is tearful and complaining of pain in her lower neck and shoulders. What is the reason for the location of her pain?

**A.** Inflammation of the pancreas in direct contact with pleural surface

**B.** Direct activation of the visceral efferent nervous system

**C.** Irritation of the parietal peritoneum surrounding the inflamed pancreas

**D.** Convergence of activated visceral afferent nerves with somatic afferent nerves in the spinal cord

**E.** Unreliable reporting of symptoms due to patient distress

**20-5.** A 32-month-old girl presents to clinic for evaluation of constipation. Which of the following findings in the child's medical history suggests an organic cause of constipation rather than functional cause?

**A.** Daily fecal soiling in undergarments
**B.** Two urinary tract infections within the past 6 months
**C.** Large-caliber stools that sometimes clog the toilet
**D.** Small-caliber, thin-appearing stools
**E.** Episodes of posturing during which the child crosses legs and screams

**20-6.** A 4-month-old breastfed infant is seen in clinic for a well-child exam. His mother describes him as a generally happy baby, but expresses concern that he is constipated because he only passes stool every 3 to 5 days. She explains that when he does have a bowel movement, he will briefly become red in the face and fuss and then pass a large soft yellow stool that sometimes spills out of his diaper. His physical exam is unremarkable, and his weight gain and growth have been excellent. What is the most appropriate response to this mother's concern about the infant's stooling pattern?

**A.** The infant is constipated, and she should offer 2 oz. of diluted apple juice daily.
**B.** The infant is constipated, and she should give lactulose 1 mL/kg/d divided twice per day.
**C.** The infant is constipated and should undergo barium enema to evaluate for possible Hirschsprung disease.
**D.** The infant is not constipated, and this may be a normal stooling pattern for a healthy breastfed baby.
**E.** The infant is not constipated and is displaying behavior consistent with colic.

**20-7.** A 7-year-old boy has had 3 episodes of acute pancreatitis. This boy's father and paternal grandmother also have a history of recurrent pancreatitis. The boy's grandmother had pancreatic cancer and is deceased. The boy's father takes pain medication daily for chronic pancreatitis (CP). On further testing, what is the study most likely to elucidate the etiology of this boy's pancreatitis?

**A.** Cystic fibrosis transmembrane conductance regulator (CFTR) mutation testing
**B.** Endoscopic retrograde cholangiopancreatography
**C.** Magnetic resonance cholangiopancreatography
**D.** Cationic trypsinogen (*PRSS-1*) mutation testing
**E.** Serine protease inhibitor Kazal type 1 mutation testing

**20-8.** A 14-year-old female adolescent who has severe juvenile rheumatoid arthritis presents to your office with epigastric abdominal pain. Six weeks earlier, she began taking a nonsteroidal anti-inflammatory drug (NSAID) because of worsening joint complaints. The most appropriate *initial* management of her symptoms would be which of the following?

**A.** Administration of an antibiotic effective against *Helicobacter pylori*
**B.** Administration of a proton pump inhibitor
**C.** Dietary modification
**D.** Substitution of salicylate for NSAID
**E.** Upper endoscopy and gastric biopsy for gastric adenocarcinoma

**20-9.** A 17-year-old boy presents with a several-week history of progressive abdominal pain, nausea, and 1 episode of coffee-ground emesis. He localizes the pain primarily to the epigastrium and describes the pain as "burning" in character. The pain occurs 2 to 3 hours after meals and is relieved by antacids. He denies taking any nonsteroidal anti-inflammatory drugs (NSAIDs) but is noted to have a mild iron deficiency anemia on laboratory testing. Of the following, what is the most appropriate *initial* step in the evaluation and management of suspected *Helicobacter pylori* infection?

**A.** Begin an empiric 2-week course of amoxicillin therapy
**B.** Begin a trial of omeprazole therapy
**C.** Refer for urea breath testing
**D.** Obtain blood sample for *H pylori* antibody testing
**E.** Refer for endoscopy and gastric biopsy for *H pylori* culture

**20-10.** A 2-day-old term infant presents with feeding intolerance and bilious emesis in the newborn nursery. The abdominal exam is notable for distension and a "doughy" character on palpation. The infant has not yet passed meconium. The rectal exam reveals a small amount of white mucus in the vault but is otherwise normal without explosive passage of stool. A plain abdominal radiograph shows multiple fluid-filled loops of bowel, which have a "ground glass" appearance. An upper gastrointestinal tract contrast study is normal, without evidence of malrotation. Retrograde contrast enema is then performed and is significant for a small-caliber colon, or microcolon, but normal length. Contrast fills the colon and is refluxed into the terminal ileum, which appears to be filled with pellet-like masses. A 24-hour postevacuation radiograph is obtained and shows complete clearance of contrast. These findings are *most* consistent with which of the following?

**A.** Hirschsprung disease

**B.** Cystic fibrosis (CF)

**C.** Cow's milk protein allergy

**D.** Duodenal atresia

**E.** Congenital anal stenosis

**20-11.** A 16-year-old boy with a history of cystic fibrosis (CF) presents to the emergency department with complaint of acute-onset, crampy, right lower quadrant abdominal pain, abdominal distension, vomiting, and no bowel movements for the past 3 days. A plain abdominal film is obtained and shows a large amount of stool in the distal ileum. After the patient is admitted, a nasogastric tube is placed for decompression. The patient receives several retrograde enemas with water-soluble contrast as well as oral osmotic laxatives and is successfully disimpacted. Of the following, which would be the *most* important in preventing a recurrence of this patient's symptoms?

**A.** Increased dietary fiber intake

**B.** Daily use of high-dose stimulant laxatives

**C.** Daily use of rectal glycerin suppository

**D.** Optimization of fat-soluble vitamin supplementation

**E.** Optimization of pancreatic enzyme supplementation

**20-12.** Which of the following scenarios would be *most* concerning for a diagnosis of infantile hypertrophic pyloric stenosis (IHPS)?

**A.** A 4-month-old baby boy with postprandial vomiting and weight maintained at the 50th percentile for age

**B.** A 3-week-old baby girl with recurrent regurgitation, frequent gagging while feeding, and lack of interest in feeding

**C.** A 3-day-old baby boy with trisomy 21 and postprandial, bilious emesis

**D.** A 6-week-old baby boy with jaundice and hypochloremic hypokalemic alkalosis but who appears hungry and eager to feed

**E.** A 3-month-old baby girl with 3 days of severe vomiting, now with profuse diarrhea, and found to have hypernatremic, metabolic acidosis

**20-13.** A 6-week-old male infant presents with a history of progressive, postprandial vomiting. The infant's parents report forceful, projectile vomiting after every feeding. On exam, the patient appears dehydrated, and peristaltic waves across a dilated, upper abdomen are visible. The patient undergoes abdominal ultrasonography, which demonstrates a pyloric channel with a thickness of 4 cm and a length of 3 cm. Of the following, which is the best *initial* step in the management of this patient?

**A.** Placement of nasogastric tube for administration of fluids and nutrition

**B.** Consult for emergent surgical pyloromyotomy

**C.** Initiate treatment with a gastric motility prokinetic agent such as erythromycin

**D.** Endoscopic balloon dilatation of the pyloric channel

**E.** Intravenous fluids and correction of any electrolyte imbalances

**20-14.** An 18-month-old female infant presents for a well-child visit. On exam, she has pallor and mild generalized edema. Her mother reports that these findings have been very gradual in onset. She otherwise appears well and does not exhibit any signs of lethargy or tachycardia. She has not been exposed to any sick contacts. The patient's diet consists of 36 to 40 oz. of whole cow's milk daily and some fruits. She does not like eating vegetables or meats. Patient has 1 to 2 nondiarrheal stools daily. She is sent for laboratory studies, which are significant for hemoglobin of 6.2 g/dL, mean corpuscular volume (MCV) of 65 fL per red blood cell (RBC), and albumin of 2.1 g/dL. White blood cell (WBC) count and differential are both within normal limits for age. A stool guaiac test for blood is negative. Of the following, which is the most likely diagnosis?

**A.** Cow milk protein–induced proctocolitis

**B.** Iron deficiency anemia and protein-losing enteropathy

**C.** Food protein–induced enterocolitis syndrome (FPIES)

**D.** Eosinophilic gastroenteritis

**E.** Early-onset Crohn disease

**20-15.** An expectant mother undergoes a routine prenatal ultrasound and severe polyhydramnios is diagnosed. The differential diagnosis of polyhydramnios includes congenital anomalies such as esophageal atresia. Of the following types of esophageal atresia, which is the most common (see following figure)?

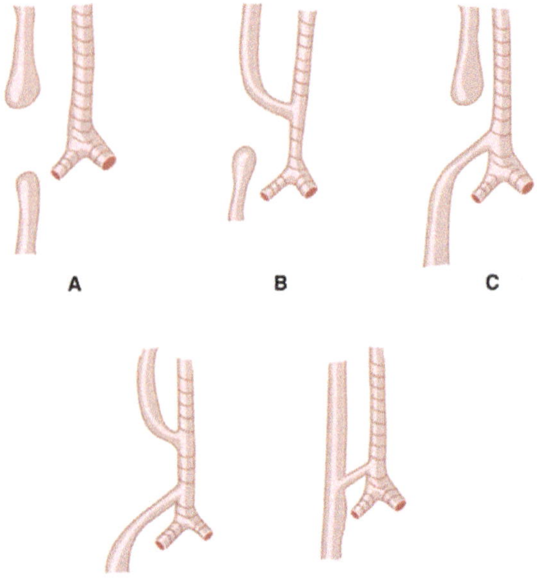


(Reproduced with permission from Lalwani AK. *Current Diagnosis & Treatment in Otolaryngology: Head & Neck Surgery*. 2nd Edition. Copyright © McGraw-Hill Education. All rights reserved.)

- **A.** Esophageal atresia without tracheoesophageal fistula
- **B.** Esophageal atresia with proximal tracheoesophageal fistula
- **C.** Esophageal atresia with distal tracheoesophageal fistula
- **D.** Esophageal atresia with proximal and distal tracheoesophageal fistula
- **E.** Isolated tracheoesophageal fistula without esophageal atresia

**20-16.** A 7-year-old girl with a history of esophageal atresia and distal tracheoesophageal fistula repaired in infancy presents with progressive dysphagia for solid foods. She reports having a previous episode of food impaction while eating a hot dog. She has symptoms of heartburn and acid regurgitation approximately twice weekly. Her parents deny any history of chronic cough or recurrent respiratory tract infections. Of the following, which is the best next step in the management of this patient?

- **A.** Maximize the dosage of proton pump inhibitor medication for treatment of gastroesophageal reflux disease (GERD)
- **B.** Combined esophagoscopy and bronchoscopy to evaluate for recurrent tracheoesophageal fistula
- **C.** Barium swallow examination to evaluate for anastomotic stricture formation
- **D.** Trial of calcium channel blocker medication to help with lower esophageal sphincter relaxation
- **E.** Provide reassurance, since underlying abnormal peristalsis of the lower esophageal segment is common in the natural history of esophageal atresia, even after surgical correction

**20-17.** A 5-week-old boy presents with symptoms of frequent regurgitation following feeds. His mother reports that he "spits up" 4 or 5 times per day. The volume of regurgitated milk varies, but it occurs effortlessly and the patient does not appear to be uncomfortable. He is exclusively breastfed and continues to nurse every 2 to 3 hours. Since regaining his birth weight at 2 weeks of age, he has exhibited appropriate weight gain for age. There is no history of bilious vomiting, abdominal distension, fever, diarrhea, bloody stools, or respiratory symptoms. Of the following, which is the best option for management of this patient?

- **A.** Obtain an upper gastrointestinal contrast study
- **B.** Start patient on empiric proton pump inhibitor therapy
- **C.** Start a prokinetic agent to enhance gastric emptying
- **D.** Switch to a high-calorie formula to compensate for the loss of calories from frequent regurgitation
- **E.** Provide parental reassurance and education

**20-18.** A 15-year-old boy with a history of asthma presents with symptoms of dysphagia, especially with solid foods. He has experienced food impactions, which resolved spontaneously on 2 separate occasions. An upper gastrointestinal contrast study is obtained and is normal. He is started on twice-daily proton pump inhibitor therapy for 6 weeks. Due to continued symptoms of dysphagia, he undergoes esophagogastroduodenoscopy, which reveals linear furrowing and small, white adherent plaques throughout the entire esophagus. Biopsies from the proximal and distal esophagus show increased eosinophils (> 15 eosinophils/high-power field [HPF]) in superficial clusters near the epithelium. Of the following, which is the best option for treatment of this condition?

- **A.** Pneumatic balloon dilatation of the lower esophageal sphincter
- **B.** Referral for allergy testing to identify likely allergic triggers
- **C.** Addition of histamine-2 receptor blocker medication to current proton pump inhibitor therapy
- **D.** A 2-week course of oral fluconazole
- **E.** A 2-week course of oral acyclovir

**20-19.** A 2-year-old girl presents to the emergency department after a witnessed ingestion of a bottle containing liquid oven cleaner. At approximately 1 hour after the time of ingestion, the patient appears irritable but in no acute distress. She is breathing comfortably. There are no visible oral lesions, and the patient is not drooling, but she currently refuses to drink. Of the following, which is the best option for managing this patient?

**A.** Administration of an emetic agent

**B.** Placement of a nasogastric tube for decompression

**C.** Immediate endoscopic evaluation to assess extent of injury

**D.** Admit for observation and intravenous (IV) hydration

**E.** No further treatment is necessary since stomach acid will neutralize the alkali

**20-20.** Which of the following scenarios is most suspicious for a diagnosis of achalasia?

**A.** A 17-year-old girl with symptoms of dysphagia and chest pain, dilated esophagus with distal narrowing on barium swallow, and a nonrelaxing lower esophageal sphincter with complete lack of esophageal peristalsis on esophageal manometry

**B.** A 15-year-old boy with episodic chest pain, normal barium swallow, and evidence of nonperistaltic, prolonged, high-amplitude contractions on esophageal manometry

**C.** A 16-year-old girl with dysphagia, Raynaud phenomenon, normal barium swallow, and abnormally low-amplitude peristaltic contractions and hypotensive lower esophageal sphincter on esophageal manometry

**D.** A 10-year-old boy with symptoms of chest pain and heartburn, normal barium swallow, and normal peristalsis on esophageal manometry

**E.** A 9-month-old girl with gagging and choking on solid-consistency foods and evidence of a short, circumferential narrowing at the level of the cervical esophagus

**20-21.** Which of the following statements regarding congenital imperforate anus is correct?

**A.** Congenital anorectal anomalies usually occur in isolation and are not associated with increased incidence of other lesions.

**B.** Children with "high" anorectal defects are more likely to successfully achieve continence than those with "low" lesions.

**C.** The most common congenital anomaly of the anorectum in males is an imperforate anus with a fistula between the distal anorectum and the urethra.

**D.** All patients with anorectal malformations require a staged repair, including placement of a temporary diverting colostomy.

**E.** Long-term problems with fecal incontinence or constipation are rare.

**20-22.** A 6-month-old girl presents with a history of episodic back arching and rigid posturing, mainly involving the neck, back, and upper extremities. These episodes are generally brief, lasting only 1 to 2 minutes, but occur on a daily basis, usually after feeding. On occasion, the patient's parents have observed visible regurgitation into the mouth during an episode. The patient usually cries after the episode but does not appear to be sleepy or lethargic after the episode. Of the following, which diagnostic test would be best in identifying the cause of these abnormal movements?

**A.** Electroencephalogram

**B.** Upper gastrointestinal radiography

**C.** Upper endoscopy with biopsy of the esophagus

**D.** Nuclear scintigraphy

**E.** Twenty-four-hour esophageal pH-impedance monitoring

**20-23.** A 3-year-old girl presents to your office secondary to vomiting. You had seen her in your office 3 weeks ago for mononucleosis. Mom reports that since her illness she has not had much of an appetite. She will often vomit in the evening, and mom has noticed that the emesis included food she had eaten from breakfast earlier in the day. She has not lost any weight. You suspect she has developed a postinfectious gastroparesis related to her recent infection with the Epstein-Barr virus. You confirm this diagnosis with a scintigraphic gastric emptying study. Your first treatment approach would include which of the following?

**A.** Recommend small, high-fat meals to make sure she meets her caloric needs

**B.** Refer to gastroenterology for endoscopic pyloric Botox® (onabotulminumtoxinA) injections

**C.** Recommend small, frequent liquid meals low in fat to aid in transit

**D.** Initiate a trial of domperidone, a promotility agent

**E.** Initiate nasojejunal feeds until the gastric emptying improves

**20-24.** A 7-day-old male infant with trisomy 21 presents to your office for his first hospital follow-up and weight check. Mom mentions to you that he passed meconium at 72 hours of life after rectal stimulation with a thermometer. He has not had another bowel movement, and mom is concerned that his abdomen appears more distended. He has been spitting up after feeds. Your exam demonstrates a distended but soft abdomen with appropriate bowel sounds. Your rectal exam demonstrates a normally placed anus with a tight anal canal. You are most concerned about which of the following conditions?

**A.** A duodenal web

**B.** Hirschsprung disease

**C.** Milk protein intolerance

**D.** Cystic fibrosis (CF)

**E.** Functional constipation

**20-25.** A 6-week-old, former 29-week premature infant presents to your office with feeding intolerance. She was discharged last week from the hospital and is establishing care with your practice. She had a relatively uncomplicated neonatal course with the exception of some feeding intolerance, which included large-volume vomiting when fed via nasogastric bolus feeds. Prior to discharge, she was transitioned to nasogastric drip feeds. Mom feels this is an inconvenience and asks if you can prescribe a medication to help her infant better tolerate the bolus feeds. You discuss the possibility of starting erythromycin to increase gastric emptying, but you are most concerned about which of the following potential adverse events?

**A.** Dumping syndrome

**B.** Duodenal web

**C.** Dystonic reaction

**D.** Tardive dyskinesia

**E.** Pyloric stenosis

**20-26.** A 4-year-old boy presents to your office secondary to the presence of blood with stooling. You have been following him regularly for chronic constipation, but he has not been taking his stool softener as recommended. He is otherwise healthy. Mom is concerned that there has been bright red blood found on the toilet paper when he stools for the past 2 days. His stools have been large, hard, and difficult to pass. On your exam, you see a small purple mass at the anal verge. It is not painful. The remainder of his rectal exam is normal. What would you recommend?

**A.** Have him be seen by a surgeon for incision and evacuation of the hemorrhoid to prevent further bleeding

**B.** Restart his stool softener and titrate it to daily soft stools

**C.** Refer him to gastroenterology to evaluate for chronic liver disease

**D.** Make a referral to child protective services for concern of sexual abuse

**E.** Refer him to gastroenterology for colonoscopy to rule out other vascular lesions of the colon

**20-27.** A mother brings her 1-year-old infant to your office secondary to a protrusion from his anus. This occurred 30 minutes ago after he passed a hard, large stool. On your exam, you see a red-purple, cylindrical mass from his anus. Your next step is which of the following?

**A.** Ask mom to keep the area moist and proceed to the emergency department for reduction

**B.** Inform mom that the prolapse will spontaneously reduce without further intervention

**C.** Send the patient for an emergent surgical evaluation for surgical reduction

**D.** Prescribe a stool softener to allow the prolapse to spontaneously reduce over the next few days

**E.** Apply gentle pressure to the prolapsed mucosa to manually reduce

**20-28.** A 2-year-old child presents to your office with severe diaper rash. On exam, it appears bright red, well demarcated, and has impetiginous vesicles and honey-colored crusting (Figure 411-7). What is the most appropriate treatment for this rash?

**A.** Oral penicillin

**B.** Topical nystatin

**C.** Topical antibiotics

**D.** Oral nystatin

**E.** Topical cholestyramine

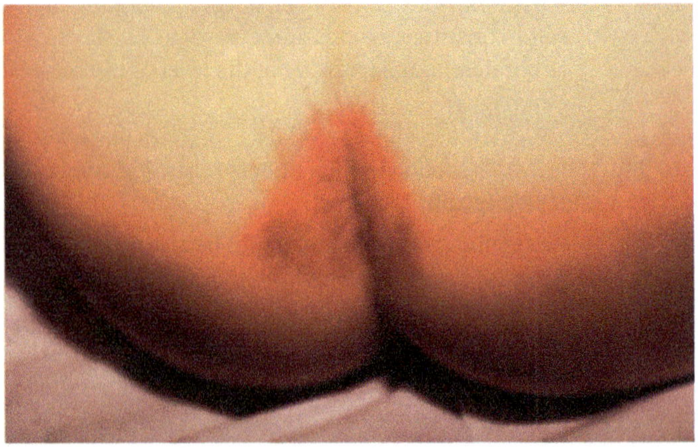

**FIGURE 411-7.** (Reproduced with permission from Knoop KJ, Stack LB, Storrow AB. *Atlas of Emergency Medicine*, 3rd ed. New York: The McGraw-Hill Companies, Inc; 2010. Photo contributor: Raymond C. Baker, MD.)

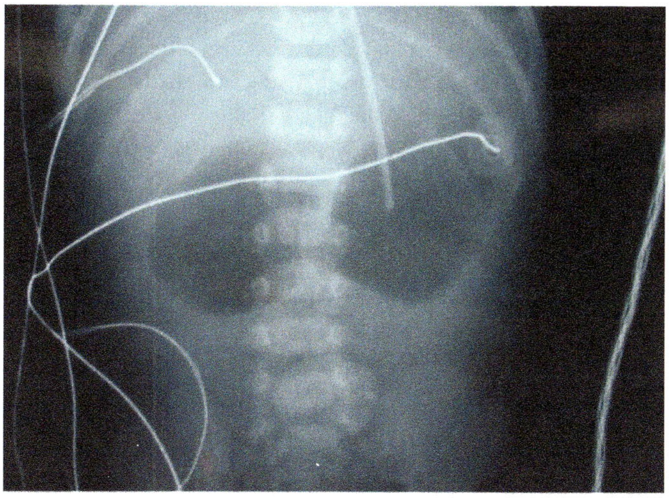

**FIGURE 394-3.** (Mark W. Kline, *Rudolph's Pediatrics*, 23rd Edition. Copyright © McGraw-Hill Education. All rights reserved.)

**20-29.** A 9-month-old female infant with trisomy 21 presents to your office for chronic vomiting. You obtain a plain film abdominal radiograph for further evaluation. You are able to view the film prior to the radiologist's interpretation and you see a "double bubble" in the region of the stomach and first portion of the small intestine (Figure 394-3). This patient most likely has which diagnosis?

**A.** Pyloric stenosis

**B.** Hirschsprung disease

**C.** Annular pancreas

**D.** Antral web

**E.** Choledochal cyst

**20-30.** An 11-year-old boy with a history of epilepsy controlled by valproic acid is admitted to your inpatient hospital service with epigastric abdominal pain and vomiting. His labs, including a complete blood cell count, electrolytes, and liver function tests, were unremarkable.

His serum lipase was 3 times the upper limits of normal. He had an abdominal ultrasound that showed an enlarged pancreas, but was otherwise normal. He plays football but denies any recent abdominal trauma. He has had no other infectious symptomatology including fever, and other than his seizure disorder, he is healthy. What is the most likely etiology of the patient's acute pancreatitis?

**A.** Choledocholithiasis

**B.** Systemic disease

**C.** Viral induced

**D.** Medication induced

**E.** Remote blunt abdominal trauma

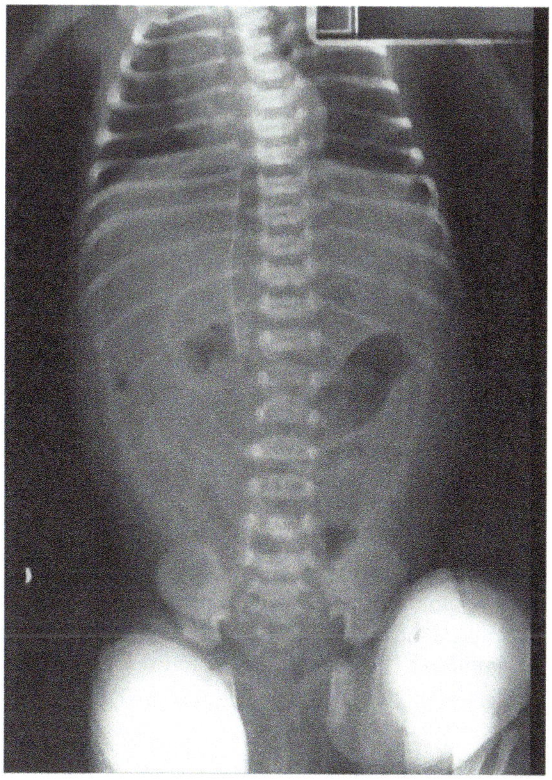

**FIGURE 395-2.** Neonate with massive pneumoperitoneum. (Mark W. Kline, *Rudolph's Pediatrics*, 23rd Edition. Copyright © McGraw-Hill Education. All rights reserved.)

**20-31.** You get called to the bedside of 6-hour-old infant secondary to abdominal distension. The infant had meconium aspiration at birth requiring endotracheal suctioning and bag-mask ventilation. Over the course of the past few hours, she has developed more abdominal distension and lethargy and has fed poorly on 2 attempts. The patient has no respiratory distress and currently has normal blood pressure and heart rate. You obtain an abdominal radiograph and find a large pneumoperitoneum (Figure 395-2). What is your next step in management?

**A.** Transfer to the neonatal intensive care unit (NICU) for nasogastric decompression prior to refeeding

**B.** Transfer to the NICU for nasogastric decompression and sepsis workup

**C.** Transfer to the NICU for nasogastric decompression with a follow-up abdominal radiograph to evaluate for improvement

**D.** Transfer to the NICU for nasogastric decompression, administration of antibiotics, and an operative evaluation and management

**E.** Transfer to the NICU for nasogastric decompression and paracentesis

**20-32.** You are called by the newborn nursery nurse secondary to see a 1-day-old infant vomiting with every feed. The patient takes the formula well, but vomits large amounts soon after his feed. The emesis is nonbilious. The only significant history is polyhydramnios during his mother's pregnancy. You obtain an abdominal radiograph and find a large, dilated stomach. What is the most likely diagnosis?

**A.** Pyloric stenosis

**B.** Duodenal web

**C.** Jejunoileal atresia

**D.** Pyloric atresia

**E.** Duodenal atresia

**20-33.** A 3-year-old boy presents to your office after his mother witnessed him swallowing a button battery earlier that morning. He has normal vital signs. He is asymptomatic, including no respiratory distress, no dysphagia, no drooling, and no complaints of pain. You obtain a chest radiograph and discover the button battery is in the esophagus (Figure 390-1). What is the next appropriate step?

**A.** Because the patient is asymptomatic, provide mom reassurance that it will pass spontaneously

**B.** Observe for symptoms and obtain a repeat chest radiograph weekly to verify progression

**C.** Set up an urgent appointment with gastroenterology to have removal of the battery performed within the next 48 hours

**D.** Refer to the emergency department now for urgent endoscopic removal

**E.** Directly admit for observation and obtain repeat chest radiograph within 6 hours to verify passage

**20-34.** Two healthy siblings are followed in a primary pediatric care clinic. The younger sibling was breastfed until 10 months of age; the older sibling was exclusively formula-fed from birth. Which of the following statements about the siblings during their infancy is true?

**A.** The breastfed infant had significantly higher lactase activity compared to the formula-fed infant.

**B.** The breastfed infant absorbed significantly more dietary lipid than the formula-fed infant.

**C.** Both the breastfed infant and the formula-fed infant secreted pancreatic lipase and bile salt to a greater degree than their adult parent.

**D.** The formula-fed infant absorbed significantly less dietary protein when compared to the breastfed infant.

**E.** The breastfed infant was able to directly absorb medium-chain fatty acids into the portal system, whereas the formula-fed infant was not.

**20-35.** An 11-year-old boy presents to clinic with a complaint of 1 to 2 episodes of vomiting at least 1 time per week over the past 3 months. He reports that vomiting consists of nonbloody, nonbilious food material and is preceded by several minutes of burning substernal pain. His body mass index is in the 80th percentile for age. What is the next most appropriate step in the management of this patient?

**A.** A 2-week trial of $H_2$-receptor antagonist

**B.** Referral to pediatric gastroenterology clinic

**C.** Send blood for complete blood count, aspartate aminotransferase (AST), alanine aminotransferase (ALT), and pancreatic lipase

**D.** Obtain upper gastrointestinal contrast study

**E.** A 2-week trial of ondansetron as needed for nausea

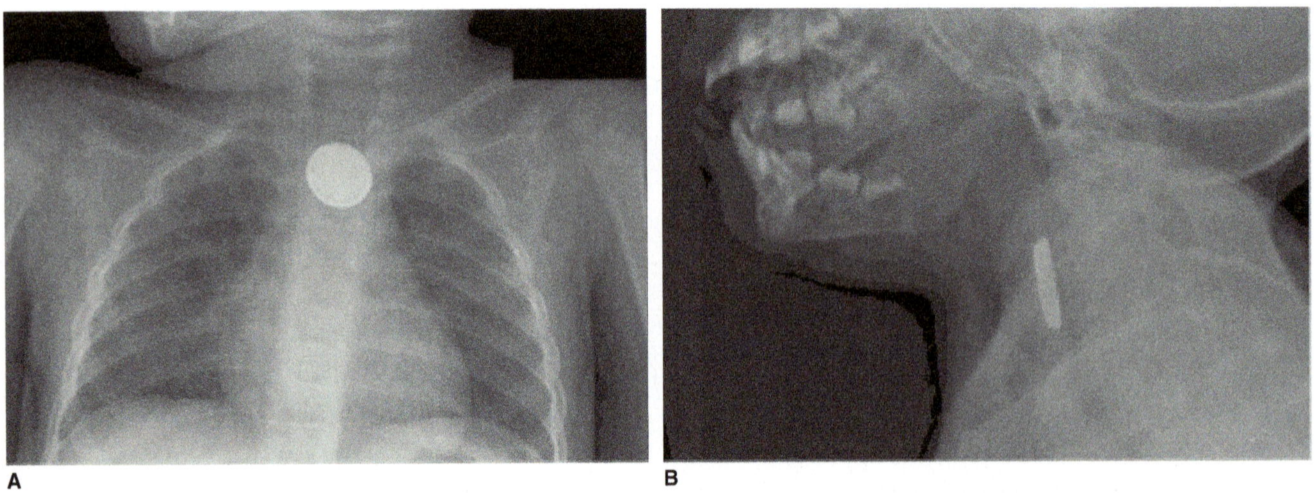


**FIGURE 390-1.** Radiographic image of an esophageal button battery foreign body ingestion. Note double ring in the anteroposterior view (**A**) and "step-off" edge in the lateral view (**B**). (Mark W. Kline, *Rudolph's Pediatrics*, 23rd Edition. Copyright © McGraw-Hill Education. All rights reserved.)

**20-36.** You are examining a 9-year-old boy in the emergency department who complains of severe abdominal pain for the past 6 hours. He said the pain started in the umbilical area and now seems to be "lower down" toward his right side. His temperature is 38.5°C. During physical examination, which of the following signs is associated with acute appendicitis?

**A.** A bluish discoloration of the flank is present.

**B.** When the patient is lying down and the right hip and knee are flexed, pain is elicited when the ankle is rotated away from the body, while the knee is rotated inward.

**C.** When palpating below the right costal margin, pain is elicited with deep inspiration.

**D.** When the thigh is bent at the hip and the knee, pain is elicited with subsequent extension of the knee.

**E.** When the knee is bent slightly and the ipsilateral ankle is dorsiflexed abruptly, pain is elicited in the popliteal area.

**20-37.** A 10-year-old obese child is seen in follow-up at clinic for chronic functional abdominal pain. This patient is most likely to have what other concomitant characteristic?

**A.** Major depressive disorder

**B.** Female gender

**C.** Pain with application of pressure by examiner to point of maximal abdominal tenderness when patient assumes a partial sitting position

**D.** Anxiety

**E.** Resolution of symptoms with antispasmodic medication

**20-38.** A 15-year-old girl complains of daily periumbilical abdominal pain without identifiable trigger for the past 12 months. Review of growth records indicates she has been between the 50th and 75th percentiles for body mass index over the past several years. Physical examination is unremarkable. What additional finding suggests an organic cause for her pain rather than a functional etiology?

**A.** Pain severe enough to cause significant school absenteeism

**B.** History of irritable bowel syndrome in first-degree relative

**C.** Sensation of incomplete evacuation after passage of stool

**D.** Complaint of fatigue and headache in addition to abdominal pain

**E.** Awakening from sleep to pass loose stool at night

**20-39.** A 30-month-old, previously healthy child presents to urgent care clinic in the winter with a 24-hour history of profuse diarrhea. There have been streaks of bloody mucus intermittently mixed in with the stool over the past 8 hours. On examination, the patient has moist mucous membranes, is alert, and is drinking grape juice from a sippy cup. His mother states he is acting hungry but she is concerned about "how fast everything is going through him," so she has not offered him food. Which of the following statements about this patient is true?

**A.** Solid foods should be deferred in favor of clear fluids until the diarrhea has resolved.

**B.** Loperamide is an appropriate treatment for the child's diarrheal illness.

**C.** Stool cultures are not necessary as long as the child is able to maintain adequate hydration with oral intake.

**D.** Stool culture should be sent.

**E.** The most likely etiology of this child's illness is *Rotavirus* infection.

**20-40.** A 20-month-old girl is seen in clinic with a 4-month history of 3 to 5 watery stools per day. She is in the 60th percentile for weight and 75th percentile for height. Her mother describes her as a playful child and has no concerns other than the diarrhea. Dietary history reveals that the girl eats 3 meals and at least 2 small snacks and drinks 2 to 3 cups of apple juice in addition to 12 oz. of cow's milk each day. Which of the following is the next appropriate step in management of this patient?

**A.** Determination of stool electrolytes and osmolality

**B.** Determination of stool pH and reducing substances

**C.** Stool culture

**D.** Two-week trial of lactose-free diet

**E.** Two-week trial of juice-free diet

**20-41.** A previously healthy 8-year-old boy presents to the emergency department with history of passing 3 large bloody stools in the past 6 hours. Initial vital signs show a heart rate of 140 bpm, blood pressure of 76/40 mm Hg, oxygen saturation of 98% on room air, and respiratory rate of 24 breaths/min. He appears pale and sleepy. What is the next most appropriate step in management of this patient?

**A.** Obtain a complete medical history from his parents

**B.** Obtain venous access and infuse normal saline bolus

**C.** Consult pediatric gastroenterology for emergent endoscopy

**D.** Consult pediatric surgery for emergent surgical exploration

**E.** Send for immediate angiography

**20-42.** Which of the following is a cause of painless lower gastrointestinal bleeding in an infant?

**A.** Intestinal duplication

**B.** Infectious colitis

**C.** Malrotation with volvulus

**D.** Anal fissure

**E.** Intussusception

**20-43.** A 2-week-old, term, breastfed infant presents to the emergency department with a 6-hour history of bilious emesis. His father states he had been feeding well and passing soft yellow bowel movements several times a day up until the onset of emesis. Examination reveals a nondistended abdomen; however, the infant cries when you attempt to palpate the abdomen and is somewhat difficult to console afterward. Vital signs are within age-appropriate norms, and the infant has brisk distal capillary refill. What radiologic study has the highest diagnostic yield for this patient?

**A.** Abdominal ultrasound

**B.** Plain abdominal film

**C.** Computed tomography (CT) scan

**D.** Contrast enema

**E.** Upper gastrointestinal contrast study

**20-44.** A 1-day-old infant in the newborn nursery vomits with each attempt at breastfeeding. You are unable to pass a nasogastric tube to the stomach. This child is most likely to have what other coexisting condition?

**A.** Trisomy 21

**B.** Prematurity

**C.** Cystic fibrosis (CF)

**D.** Low birth weight

**E.** Congenital cardiac anomaly

**20-45.** A 10-year-old boy with a history of Fontan procedure for hypoplastic left heart syndrome is admitted with a 4-kg weight gain, peripheral edema, and diarrhea. An echocardiogram done 3 months ago demonstrated elevated right atrial pressures. You suspect protein-losing enteropathy and decide to send fecal $\alpha_1$-antitrypsin as part of the diagnostic workup. Which of the following statements is true?

**A.** Fecal $\alpha_1$-antitrypsin assay is unreliable if the sample is contaminated with urine.

**B.** Fecal $\alpha_1$-antitrypsin assay is reliable for detection of esophageal and gastric protein loss.

**C.** Fecal $\alpha_1$-antitrypsin is stable at room temperature, allowing for ease of specimen transport and storage.

**D.** Fecal $\alpha_1$-antitrypsin assay is preferable to radioisotopic techniques for the diagnosis of protein-losing enteropathy.

**E.** Fecal $\alpha_1$-antitrypsin assay is not affected by meconium, and the test can be used in newborn infants.

**20-46.** Which of the following laboratory findings is most consistent with a diagnosis of Crohn disease?

**A.** Hypoalbuminemia

**B.** Elevated blood urea nitrogen (BUN)

**C.** Elevated mean corpuscular volume (MCV)

**D.** Hyperbilirubinemia

**E.** Hypophosphatemia

**20-47.** You are caring for a 15-year-old patient with Crohn disease who has required complete duodenal resection and bypass due to stenosis and gastric outlet obstruction from her disease. She has developed dumping syndrome characterized by severe diarrhea after eating as a result. The absence of which of the following histologic entities may be contributing to her diarrhea?

**A.** Enterochromaffin cells

**B.** Peyer patches

**C.** Crypts of Lieberkuhn

**D.** Brunner glands

**E.** Chief cells

**20-48.** A 3-year-old boy with Down syndrome presents with abdominal pain, intermittent abdominal distension, and nonbloody, watery diarrhea for the past 3 months. His mother is concerned that he has not gained any significant weight in the past 6 months. On examination, his vital signs are within normal limits for age and he is afebrile. His exam is notable for Down facies and short stature but is otherwise unremarkable. No rash is present. What test would you order next?

**A.** HLA-DQ2/DQ8 genetic typing for celiac disease

**B.** Esophagogastroduodenoscopy

**C.** Sweat chloride test

**D.** Anti-tissue transglutaminase (TTG) IgA and serum IgA levels

**E.** Stool rotavirus assay

**20-49.** Which of the following statements regarding small intestinal bacterial overgrowth (SIBO) is correct?

**A.** SIBO is diagnosed when bacterial counts exceed 1000 organisms/mL on a quantitative culture from a jejunal aspirate.

**B.** Anatomic abnormalities, such as intestinal duplications, bowel dilatation, or small intestinal atresias, are not associated with increased development of SIBO.

**C.** Symptoms of excessive gas formation and abdominal distension are associated with metabolism of carbohydrates by intraluminal bacteria.

**D.** A late rise in breath hydrogen levels on glucose breath hydrogen testing is diagnostic of SIBO.

**E.** Acid-suppressing medications can be used as empiric treatment of SIBO in children.

**20-50.** An 11-month-old infant with history of multiple small bowel atresias has been maintained on total parenteral nutrition via a central venous catheter since birth. He was recently started on trophic enteral feeds via a gastrostomy tube and was discharged from the neonatal intensive care unit (NICU) 1 week ago. He now presents to your office with a 1-day history of lethargy, fever, and vomiting. Serum chemistries reveal chronic, mild elevation of hepatic transaminases and alkaline phosphatase but are otherwise normal. What is the most likely cause of this infant's findings?

**A.** Cholelithiasis

**B.** Fulminant hepatic failure

**C.** Intrahepatic cholestasis

**D.** Infection of the central venous catheter

**E.** D-lactic acidosis

**20-51.** A 3-month-old infant has had diarrhea since the first week of life. The stool is watery and nonbloody. The patient has been exclusively breastfed, and he has not yet started any solid foods. When enteral feeds are held, the diarrhea decreases but does not completely resolve. Findings on physical exam include weight at less than 5th percentile and length at the 10th percentile for age; cachexia; a protuberant abdomen; stool for reducing substances 2+; stool culture negative for enteric pathogens; and sweat chloride of 10 mEq/L. The patient undergoes an esophagogastroduodenoscopy, and biopsies of the small intestine reveal diffuse villous atrophy. These findings are most consistent with which of the following diagnoses?

**A.** Celiac disease

**B.** Cystic fibrosis (CF)

**C.** Congenital chloride diarrhea

**D.** Acrodermatitis enteropathica

**E.** Microvillus inclusion disease

**20-52.** A 14-year-old girl presents to your office with the chief complaint of abdominal pain for 4 months. On further questioning, she admits to very poor appetite, and she has lost 10 lb since her last visit with you. She reports occasional loose stool but no hematochezia. On rectal exam, she is hemoccult positive, and you notice 2 moderate skin tags. The labs that you sent show a hemoglobin of 8.8 g/dL and an albumin of 3.2 g/dL. You are concerned she most likely has which condition?

**A.** Chronic *Giardia* infection

**B.** Crohn disease

**C.** Celiac disease

**D.** Anorexia nervosa

**E.** Irritable bowel syndrome

**20-53.** A 15-year-old boy presents to your office for his yearly well-child exam. Four weeks ago, he had been diagnosed with ulcerative colitis, and he is currently being induced into remission with oral prednisone. The patient's mother is concerned about the consequences of him taking this medication. What side effects of corticosteroids will you discuss with the patient's mother?

**A.** Adrenal insufficiency, hypertension, bone demineralization, and hyperglycemia

**B.** Adrenal insufficiency, weight loss, acne, and hypertension

**C.** Hyperglycemia, hypertension, muscle redistribution, and hirsutism

**D.** Acne, bone demineralization, cataracts, and leukopenia

**E.** Emotional disturbances, bone demineralization, vitamin D deficiency, and adrenal insufficiency

**20-54.** A 10-year-old boy presents to your office with 12 days of bloody diarrhea, abdominal pain, and weight loss. He has been afebrile. His mom has a history of ulcerative colitis, and she is very concerned her son has now developed this condition. What enteric pathogens should be ruled out prior to referral to gastroenterology?

**A.** *Giardia*, *Yersinia*, *Salmonella*, and *Escherichia coli* 0157/H7

**B.** *Yersinia*, *Salmonella*, *Clostridium difficile*, and *Cryptosporidium*

**C.** *C difficile*, *Salmonella*, *Giardia*, and *Campylobacter*

**D.** *C difficile*, *Salmonella*, *Shigella*, and *E coli* 0157/H7

**E.** *Cryptosporidium*, *Giardia*, *C difficile*, and *E coli* 0157/H7

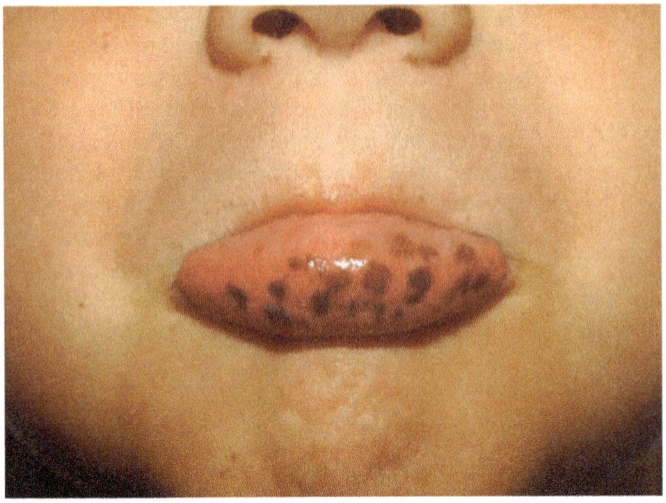

**FIGURE 409-2.** Macular pigmentation of the lips. (Mark W. Kline, *Rudolph's Pediatrics*, 23rd Edition. Copyright © McGraw-Hill Education. All rights reserved.)

**20-55.** A 7-year-old boy presents to your office for the first time with his mother for a routine well-child check. You notice bluish-brown macules on his lips and buccal mucosa (Figure 409-2). You ask his mother if there is any family history of which of the following conditions?

**A.** Tuberous sclerosis

**B.** Peutz-Jeghers syndrome

**C.** Neurofibromatosis

**D.** Familial adenomatous polyposis syndrome

**E.** Juvenile polyposis syndrome

**20-56.** A 2-month-old male infant presents to your office with his mother for a routine well-child check. During the family history, you elicit a strong family history of familial adenomatous polyposis (FAP) syndrome. There has been no gene mutation identified in this family upon testing affected members. At what time should you refer the patient for screening?

**A.** Now to determine if this infant carries an *APC* mutation

**B.** Only upon the development of symptoms such as hematochezia

**C.** During his late teens for an evaluation for colectomy due to the high risk of colorectal cancer

**D.** No referral is necessary given the fact that no gene mutation has been identified

**E.** At 12 years of age or with the development of symptoms for screening colonoscopy

**20-57.** A 3-year-old girl presents to your office for follow-up of her rectal bleeding. You had previously referred her to pediatric gastroenterology for painless rectal bleeding. She was found to have 3 polyps on her colonoscopy that were identified as juvenile polyps on histology. There is no history of juvenile polyps in the family. Which of the following statements is the most appropriate in counseling the parents?

**A.** Juvenile polyps are common in this age group, and she does not need any further follow-up and is not at increased risk of cancer.

**B.** The patient's siblings should be screened for polyps with colonoscopy given her new diagnosis of juvenile polyposis syndrome (JPS).

**C.** The patient should now receive yearly colonoscopy screening to evaluate for recurrence of polyps.

**D.** This patient now has close to a 50% lifetime risk of developing colorectal cancer.

**E.** She should be screened for germline mutations of *SMAD4* and *BMPR1A* to determine if she has JPS.

**20-58.** A 17-year-old girl presents with a 3-week history of recurrent nausea, vomiting, anorexia, and abdominal pain. This is the first time she has had these types of symptoms. She denies dieting or intentional weight loss, but her mother thinks she has lost about 15 lb in the past 3 weeks. She has not had any significant diarrhea or constipation. On exam, her body mass index is now < 5th percentile for age. She has some mild abdominal distension and epigastric tenderness on abdominal exam. Her physical exam is otherwise unremarkable. Serum markers for inflammation (sedimentation rate, C-reactive protein), complete blood cell count, serum albumin, and serum lipase levels are all normal. An upper gastrointestinal contrast study is obtained and demonstrates a dilated stomach and duodenum with abrupt cutoff of the duodenum at the level of the third lumbar vertebra. These findings are most consistent with which of the following?

**A.** Superior mesenteric artery syndrome

**B.** Crohn disease

**C.** Duodenal stenosis

**D.** Chronic pancreatitis (CP)

**E.** Celiac disease

**20-59.** A 3-week-old male infant presents due to several episodes of painless hematochezia. The stool is described as liquid mixed with mucus and flecks of blood. The infant has otherwise been feeding and growing well. He is primarily breastfed. Physical examination, including perirectal exam, is normal. Family history is notable for several family members with asthma and eczema and an older brother with peanut and tree nut allergy. Of the following, which is the best initial step in the diagnosis and management of this condition?

**A.** Maternal dietary restriction of peanuts and tree nuts
**B.** Switch to a soy-based formula
**C.** Obtain hemoglobin level and submit stool sample for bacterial culture
**D.** Referral for flexible sigmoidoscopy
**E.** Switch to a cow milk protein hydrolysate formula

**20-60.** A 4-week-old male infant presents with a mass in the right inguinal region, just superior to the scrotum. His past medical history is significant for premature delivery at 31 weeks' gestation. His mother reports that the mass appears most visible when the patient is crying, while at other times, it is not very noticeable. The patient does not have any symptoms of irritability or pain and has been tolerating feeds well. On exam, a smooth, firm mass is palpable in the right inguinal area. The mass reduces spontaneously when the infant stops crying. Both testes are descended, and the overlying skin appears normal. Of the following, which is the best next step in the evaluation and management of this condition?

**A.** Admission to the hospital for urgent repair of an incarcerated inguinal hernia
**B.** Referral to a pediatric surgeon for elective inguinal hernia repair within the next month
**C.** Referral to a pediatric surgeon for elective inguinal hernia repair, only if the hernia persists beyond 1 year of age
**D.** Referral to the emergency department for an urgent ultrasound for suspected testicular torsion
**E.** Referral to interventional radiology for diagnostic aspiration of the groin mass

**20-61.** Which of the following conditions or complications is *more* likely to be associated with an infant born with gastroschisis than an infant with omphalocele?

**A.** Intestinal dysmotility
**B.** Beckwith-Wiedemann syndrome
**C.** Congenital heart defect
**D.** Trisomy 21
**E.** Intestinal malrotation

**20-62.** A preterm infant born with gastroschisis undergoes primary fascial and skin closure at approximately 24 hours of life. At 12 hours postoperatively, the neonatal intensive care unit nurse first notes increasing abdominal distension. An hour later, there is loss of urine output and decreased pedal pulses. A capillary blood gas is significant for an elevated carbon dioxide level. Of the following, which is the best option for the management of this patient?

**A.** Placement of a nasogastric tube to low intermittent wall suction for gastric decompression
**B.** Initiation of intravenous (IV) antibiotics for empiric coverage of suspected gram-negative bacterial sepsis
**C.** Prompt evisceration of the bowel and placement of a protective silo
**D.** Increased ventilator respiratory rate settings to maximize ventilation
**E.** Abdominal ultrasound with Doppler for evaluation of a vascular thrombus

**20-63.** A 3-year-old girl presents to your office with bloody diarrhea. Her symptoms began with fever, abdominal pain, and diarrhea about 1 week ago. The stools subsequently became bloody, and mom is concerned about her dehydrated and pale appearance. Her brother had similar symptoms; however, his condition resolved without complication. You decide to obtain a stool sample of culture and a complete blood count (CBC) and chemistry. Her CBC shows a hemoglobin of 8.0 g/dL and platelets of 30,000 cells/L. Her creatinine is 2.8 mg/dL. Her stool culture remains pending. What do you advise next?

**A.** Have the patient drink plenty of fluids and repeat labs in 2 days after her hydration improves
**B.** Monitor the patient closely as an outpatient until her infectious colitis resolves
**C.** Prescribe a course of oral antibiotics to shorten the course of her infectious colitis
**D.** Admit the patient to the hospital for supportive treatment of presumed hemolytic-uremic syndrome (HUS)
**E.** Admit the patient to the hospital for workup for ulcerative colitis given her protracted course of bloody diarrhea

**20-64.** A 4-year-old girl presents to your office with 2 weeks of intermittent abdominal pain. Her mother reports that the patient has been having occasional blood in her stool and 2 episodes of vomiting. The past 2 days, she has noticed dark purple-blue lesions on her buttocks and thighs that seem to resemble bruises. Mom reports that over the past 2 hours she has been having episodes of severe abdominal pain where she will draw her legs up and scream. She appears exhausted from the episodes. She had a bowel movement in your waiting room that was loose with more blood than mom has recently observed. What is your next step in management?

**A.** Refer her to the local hospital to rule out intussusception

**B.** Refer her to the local hospital to rule out malrotation with volvulus

**C.** Start a course of oral steroids and have her return to clinic tomorrow to monitor progress

**D.** Recommend ibuprofen treatment for abdominal pain and reassure the mother

**E.** Send a stool culture to evaluate for an infectious colitis

**20-65.** You round on a 12-hour-old male infant for his routine newborn exam. The maternal history is significant for a cystic lesion noted in the newborn's abdomen on a routine prenatal ultrasound at 20 weeks' gestation. It was reported to be consistent with a duplication cyst of the small bowel. What is your recommendation to the family?

**A.** This is an incidental finding, and given the benign nature, no further action is warranted unless symptoms develop.

**B.** Surgical consultation is needed to evaluate for resection of the cyst given the increased risk of obstruction, intussusception, and bleeding.

**C.** The cyst will need to be monitored every 6 months via ultrasound to monitor for any changes.

**D.** Obtain a computed tomography (CT) scan, as surgical intervention is only necessary if the cyst is involving other structures such as the urinary system or spine.

**E.** Obtain a biopsy of the cyst and surgically remove if there are concerning histologic features of malignancy.

**20-66.** A previously healthy 21-day-old male infant presents to the emergency department with lethargy, bilious vomiting, and abdominal distension that have developed over the morning. The upper gastrointestinal contrast study is shown (Figure 397-2A). What is the most likely diagnosis?

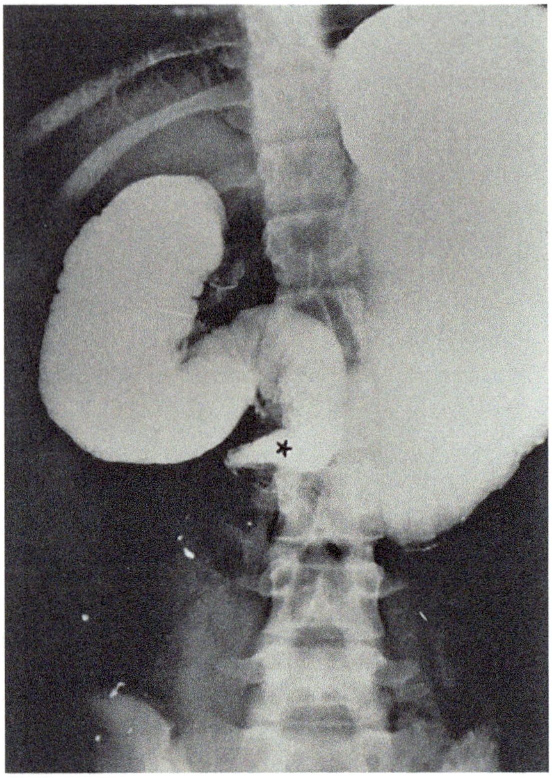

**FIGURE 397-2A.** Upper gastrointestinal contrast study. (Reproduced with permission from Rudolph CD, Rudolph AM, Lister GE, First LR, Gershon AA. *Rudolph's Pediatrics*, 22nd ed. New York: McGraw-Hill; 2011.)

**A.** Pyloric stenosis

**B.** Duodenal atresia

**C.** Jejunal atresia

**D.** Antral web

**E.** Malrotation with midgut volvulus

**20-67.** An 11-year-old boy presents to your office with fever and abdominal pain. Mom reports he was in his usual state of good health last night when he went to bed. He awoke at 3:00 AM with a fever of 101°F and periumbilical abdominal pain. He has associated symptoms of anorexia and 1 episode of nonbloody, nonbilious vomiting. On your exam, he has pain in the right lower quadrant when you palpate either the right or left lower abdomen. You obtain a complete blood count and find an elevated white blood cell count and mild bandemia. What is your next step?

**A.** Obtain stool studies because the patient has likely developed an acute infectious gastroenteritis

**B.** Refer him to the emergency department (ED) for concern of a small bowel obstruction

**C.** Refer the patient to the ED to seek a surgical evaluation for appendicitis

**D.** Discuss with mom that he likely has mesenteric adenitis given the right lower quadrant pain and ask him to return tomorrow for close monitoring

**E.** Obtain an ultrasound of the gallbladder to evaluate for cholelithiasis and acute cholecystitis

**20-68.** You admit a 3-year-old boy who has been passing large amounts of blood per rectum since last night. His hemoglobin in the emergency department was 6 g/dL. He has had no preceding symptoms (eg, no fever, vomiting, diarrhea, or abdominal pain). What is the next most appropriate diagnostic step?

A. Technetium-99m pertechnetate scintigraphy scan
B. Magnetic resonance scan of the abdomen
C. Colonoscopy with biopsies
D. Esophagogastroduodenoscopy with biopsies
E. Stool studies for stool culture and *Clostridium difficile* toxin

**20-69.** A 4-year-old girl presents to your office secondary to recurrent abdominal pain and drainage at her umbilicus. Mom reports that the patient will intermittently complain of abdominal pain. Around these episodes, mom will notice some yellow discharge and crusting at her umbilicus, and her pain appears to be relieved until the next episode. She does not have any fever. You confirm your suspicion of an omphalomesenteric sinus and cyst via a fistulogram. What is your next step in treatment?

A. Long-term antibiotics to clear bacterial contamination of the sinus and cyst
B. Recurrent excision and drainage of the cyst at the time of initial onset of abdominal pain
C. Surgical excision of the omphalomesenteric sinus and cyst
D. No further treatment is necessary given spontaneous drainage
E. Suture placement at the opening of the fistula in the umbilicus to prevent further drainage

**20-70.** A 10-year-old child with severe acute liver failure is being cared for in the intensive care unit. Which of the following laboratory findings best reflects worsening liver function in this patient?

A. Uptrending aspartate aminotransferase (AST)
B. Uptrending alanine aminotransferase (ALT)
C. Hyperglycemia
D. Uptrending total bilirubin
E. Uptrending factor V

**20-71.** A 7-year-old girl is admitted with new-onset elevated serum aminotransferases and jaundice. Gallstones within the gallbladder and dilation of the common bile duct are visualized on initial right upper quadrant ultrasound, as well as a single stone within the common bile duct. Which is the next most appropriate evaluation of the hepatobiliary system to pursue?

A. Computed tomography (CT)
B. Liver biopsy
C. Percutaneous transhepatic cholangiography
D. Hepatobiliary iminodiacetate (HIDA) scan
E. Endoscopic retrograde cholangiopancreatography (ERCP)

**20-72.** A 7-year-old girl is admitted to the pediatric general care floor with jaundice and fatigue. Laboratory evaluation reveals elevated aspartate aminotransferase (AST), alanine aminotransferase (ALT), and bilirubin; prolonged international normalized ratio; IgA deficiency; and a positive anti–liver kidney microsomal type 1 (LKM-1) antibody titer. Which of the following is the most likely diagnosis?

A. Primary sclerosing cholangitis
B. Lupus
C. Type I autoimmune hepatitis (AIH)
D. Type II AIH
E. Intrahepatic cystic biliary dilation (Caroli disease)

**20-73.** A 20-day-old breastfed girl presents to the emergency department with jaundice, vomiting, lethargy, and rectal temperature of 39.0°C. Physical examination is significant for hepatomegaly. Catheterized urinalysis demonstrates reducing substances and white blood cell. Urine Gram stain shows gram-negative rods. What is the most likely diagnosis?

A. Hereditary fructose intolerance
B. Hereditary tyrosinemia
C. Type I glycogen storage disease
D. Type IV glycogen storage disease
E. Galactosemia

**20-74.** A 12-week-old infant with direct hyperbilirubinemia is found to have homozygous deficiency of the protein inhibitor ZZ (PiZZ) phenotype. Which of the following is also likely to be true about this patient?

A. Liver biopsy is likely to show microsteatosis.
B. Liver disease is secondary to decreased proteolytic activity of α1-antitrypsin within the hepatocytes.
C. The patient is at risk for developing renal disease in young adulthood.
D. The PiZZ defect is due to a single amino acid substitution mutation.
E. Liver transplantation is a futile intervention for patients with PiZZ phenotype who progress to end-stage liver disease.

**20-75.** A 6-week-old boy presents to the pediatrician's office for evaluation of "yellow eyes." His parents report that they noticed this 2 days ago. They state that he is otherwise well. He has gained 1 lb since his last visit 2 weeks ago. Physical examination reveals an alert, afebrile, well-appearing infant with icteric sclerae. His liver edge is palpable 1 cm below the right costal margin. There is no stool in the diaper. The pediatrician orders blood work, which reveals a total bilirubin of 9.6 mg/dL, conjugated bilirubin of 3.2 mg/dL, and a γ-glutamyltransferase of 412 U/L. Which of the following is the most appropriate next step in evaluation?

**A.** Blood and urine cultures

**B.** Liver biopsy

**C.** Endoscopic retrograde cholangiopancreatography (ERCP)

**D.** Abdominal ultrasound

**E.** Serum β-carotene level

**20-76.** A 13-year-old boy with ulcerative colitis presents for a routine follow-up visit. He is receiving infliximab infusions every 8 weeks. The last infusion was 5 weeks ago. He reports that he is having 1 to 2 formed bowel movements per day with no visible blood. Physical examination reveals excoriated areas on his arms, legs, and the back of his neck. On further questioning, he admits that he has been itchy for the past 4 weeks and has been scratching these areas. His physical examination is also notable for a yellowish discoloration under his tongue and hepatomegaly. What is the most likely diagnosis?

**A.** Atopic dermatitis

**B.** Allergic reaction to infliximab

**C.** α1-Antitrypsin deficiency

**D.** Primary sclerosing cholangitis

**E.** Scabies

**20-77.** An 18-year-old woman with a history of attention-deficit/hyperactivity disorder returns from her first semester at college and presents for evaluation of fatigue. She reports that she has had difficulty keeping up with her studies due to falling asleep in class and trouble focusing on her work. She denies fever, rash, upper respiratory symptoms, and sore throat. Physical examination reveals a well-nourished female who is mildly jaundiced. Her liver is enlarged and firm. Which of the following tests is most likely to lead to a definitive diagnosis of this patient's liver disease?

**A.** Liver biopsy for copper content

**B.** Serum alkaline phosphatase

**C.** Serum ceruloplasmin

**D.** Heterophile antibodies to Epstein-Barr virus

**E.** Urinalysis

**20-78.** A 17-year-old Hispanic boy presents for a health supervision visit. His only complaint is occasional right upper quadrant pain that usually occurs after eating. His body mass index is 32 kg/m$^2$, above the 95th percentile for age. Physical examination reveals a morbidly obese teenager in no acute distress. He reports mild tenderness on deep palpation of the abdomen in the right upper quadrant. Laboratory evaluation is notable for aspartate aminotransferase of 65 U/L, alanine aminotransferase of 59 U/L, and international normalized ratio of 1.1. Which of the following is a correct statement regarding further evaluation and management of this patient?

**A.** Given his normal international normalized ratio, this patient's elevated transaminases do not require further evaluation.

**B.** A liver biopsy is the gold standard to confirm the diagnosis.

**C.** An ultrasound of the abdomen is sufficient to diagnose this patient's condition.

**D.** This patient's liver disease is unlikely to result in significant liver dysfunction, and no treatment is necessary.

**E.** It is not necessary to exclude other causes of liver disease because this patient is morbidly obese.

**20-79.** A 6-month-old girl presents to the emergency department due to 2 weeks of persistent emesis. On physical examination, she is noted to have mildly icteric sclerae and a palpable mass in the right upper quadrant of the abdomen. Abdominal ultrasound reveals cystic dilation of the common bile duct measuring 6 cm. Which of the following is a correct statement regarding this patient's condition?

**A.** It is recommended that the cystic portion of the bile duct as well as the gallbladder be excised due to the risk of malignant transformation.

**B.** This condition occurs more commonly in males.

**C.** Elevation of serum amylase and lipase is rarely seen in patients with this condition.

**D.** Endoscopic retrograde cholangiopancreatography (ERCP) with biopsy of the bile duct is necessary to confirm the diagnosis.

**E.** Diagnosis of this condition after the age of 2 months is associated with poor survival.

## ANSWERS

**Answer 20-1. B**

The typical patient with CVS presents with recurrent, stereotypic episodes of frequent emesis every 2 to 4 weeks that begin suddenly and last 24 to 48 hours. There is a return to periods of baseline health between episodes. The vomiting cannot be attributed to another disorder. A thorough history and physical examination is important, as specific conditions and symptoms suggest that the diagnosis is not consistent with CVS. These conditions are (1) presentation at < 2 years of age; (2) bilious vomiting, abdominal tenderness, and/or severe abdominal pain; (3) attacks associated with intercurrent illness, fasting, and/or a high-protein meal; (4) abnormalities on neurologic examination; or (5) progressively worsening episodes or a conversion to a continuous or chronic pattern.

The patient in answer choice A had bilious emesis that occurred after a period of fasting or a high-protein meal. These symptoms suggest a partial urea cycle enzyme deficiency, which can occur after such situations. The patient in answer choice C has bilious emesis and abdominal pain. Although CVS can present with similar symptoms, it is important to rule out a surgical condition, such as volvulus or malrotation, as well as pancreatitis. In addition, this child does not have a 3-week cycle with a return to baseline. The patient in answer choice D has neurologic symptoms, which is concerning for increased intracranial pressure or a metabolic disorder. The patient in answer choice E has symptoms consistent with pyloric stenosis.

(Section 21: Disorders of the Gastrointestinal System; Chapter 377: Approach to the Child with Acute, Chronic, or Cyclic Vomiting)

**Answer 20-2. B**

A child who presents with acute vomiting should first be evaluated for the degree of dehydration; if severe (5%–10%) dehydration is present, immediate IV access and fluids should be provided. However, this child is not severely dehydrated.

In addition, there is a high suspicion for CVS. If CVS is suspected in a child without other "alarm" symptoms, such as severe dehydration, shock, abnormal neurologic examination, or severe abdominal pain, it is appropriate to check labs prior to initiation of IV fluids. Serum electrolytes can help assess for the possibility of a metabolic, renal, or endocrine disorder. They can also demonstrate abnormalities such as hypoglycemia or elevated BUN/creatinine that would assist in deciding on appropriate fluid resuscitation.

An abdominal radiograph may be useful in patients with suspected intestinal obstruction; head CT may be useful in patients with focal neurologic findings on exam suggesting increased intracranial pressure as a cause for vomiting. IV proton pump inhibitors are unlikely to be helpful in the immediate treatment of acute recurrent nonbloody, nonbilious vomiting.

(Section 21: Disorders of the Gastrointestinal System; Chapter 377: Approach to the Child with Acute, Chronic, or Cyclic Vomiting)

**Answer 20-3. C**

The management of acute pancreatitis traditionally has consisted of pancreatic rest (no enteral feeding), antiemetics, analgesia, fluid support, and monitoring for complications. These treatments remain the mainstay of therapy, but the approach to pancreatic rest and fluid management has changed. The initial treatment is directed at stabilizing the patient's condition. Limited adult data suggest that aggressive hydration in the first 24 hours decreases the risk of multiorgan system failure. Thus, IV fluid boluses to rehydrate the patient and subsequent fluid administration at 1.5 times maintenance rates are recommended.

Antiemetics and analgesia are necessary to provide comfort and to avoid increased energy expenditure. Opioid analgesics in oral or parenteral forms usually are required for pain control in acute pancreatitis. A careful directed investigation for treatable causes of acute pancreatitis should be conducted.

Perhaps the greatest change in the management of acute pancreatitis is the early institution of nutrition. In patients who have mild acute pancreatitis, oral feedings can be started within 24 to 48 hours after admission. In the past, clear liquids were started, but recent studies in adults show that regular meals can be given. About 10% of patients will have abdominal pain after starting oral intake. Usually, feedings can be resumed in the patients in another 24 hours. An increase in serum levels of pancreatic enzymes is not an indication to stop feedings. Patients who have severe pancreatitis also can be successfully fed early in the treatment course. Typically, these patients are fed through enteral tubes or by using total parenteral nutrition (TPN). Enteral feeding is preferred over TPN because of the complications associated with the IV catheter and the expense of TPN.

(Section 21: Disorders of the Gastrointestinal System, Chapter 412: Disorders of the Exocrine Pancreas)

**Answer 20-4. D**

Pain secondary to pancreatitis localized to the neck and shoulders occurs when the inflamed pancreas causes irritation of the diaphragm, which is in close proximity to the pancreas. Diaphragmatic irritation activates the visceral afferent nerves, which converge in the spinal cord with somatic afferent nerves, leading to well-localized somatic pain. This type of pain is commonly called referred pain.

The pancreas is not in direct contact with the pleural surface; however, pleural irritation due to pneumonia can cause poorly localized lower abdominal pain due to the convergence of pleural somatic afferent nerves with visceral afferent nerves converging in the spine. Parietal peritoneal irritation typically is well localized to the abdomen. There is no reason to believe this patient is a poor historian given that there is a reasonable physiologic explanation for the location of her pain.

(Section 21: Disorders of the Gastrointestinal System; Chapter 378: Acute Abdominal Pain)

**Answer 20-5.** D

It is important to distinguish between the common problem of functional constipation and less common organic causes of constipation, including Hirschsprung disease. A diagnosis of Hirschsprung disease is suggested by small-caliber soft stool, episodes of explosive soft stool preceded by a lack of stool passage and abdominal distension, and history of delayed meconium passage in the first few days of life. If Hirschsprung disease is suspected, suction rectal biopsy should be considered as the next step in evaluation.

Children with functional constipation may have fecal incontinence (encopresis) with soiling of the undergarments due to seepage of liquid stool around impacted rectal fecal mass. Urinary tract infections may also occur due to partial urethral obstruction by pressure from fecal mass in the colon or by ascending infection from soiled undergarments. Many children with functional constipation have a history of large-caliber stools and stool retentive posturing in an attempt to avoid uncomfortable passage of large and/or hard stools.

(Section 21: Disorders of the Gastrointestinal System; Chapter 381: Approach to the Child with Constipation and Fecal Incontinence)

**Answer 20-6.** D

Breastfed infants often pass stools infrequently, up to every 5 days, which may be completely normal if the stool is soft and passage is not painful. It is not unusual for an infant to strain briefly with stooling, but this does not necessarily reflect pain. This child is not constipated, and no specific intervention is required; reassurance should be offered to the mother.

An infant younger than 6 months who is having hard infrequent stools may be constipated and can be offered 2 to 4 oz. of diluted fruit juice initially as treatment. In infants over 6 months of age, lactulose or polyethylene glycol 400 can also be used to treat constipation. There is no reason to believe this otherwise healthy child with no constipation has Hirschsprung disease, so imaging with barium enema is not warranted. Colic is a behavioral diagnosis characterized by frequent inconsolable crying in infants that has not been correlated with a specific gastrointestinal etiology.

(Section 21: Disorders of the Gastrointestinal System; Chapter 381: Approach to the Child with Constipation and Fecal Incontinence)

**Answer 20-7.** D

Acute recurrent pancreatitis (ARP) is defined as at least 2 episodes of acute pancreatitis per year or > 3 episodes over a lifetime in a patient without CP or a pancreatic pseudocyst. With this patient's family history of CP as well as pancreatic cancer, there is a high suspicion for possible genetic factors in his presentation of ARP rather than anatomic abnormality.

In the past 15 years, mutations in several genes have been associated with increased risk for pancreatitis, including *PRSS-1*, *SPINK-1*, and *CFTR* genes.

Several mutations in the *PRSS-1* gene that encodes cationic trypsinogen cause hereditary pancreatitis. Inheritance is autosomal dominant with an 80% penetrance. Patients present in childhood with ARP and later progress to CP with a high likelihood of exocrine and endocrine deficiency. The lifetime risk of pancreatic cancer is 40% or greater in these patients.

The gene product of *SPINK-1* is produced in acinar cells and acts as a defense for premature trypsinogen activation. Several mutations in *SPINK-1* increase susceptibility to ARP and CP; however, *SPINK-1* mutations are considered disease modifiers because most people who have these mutations, even when homozygous, do not develop acute pancreatitis, ARP, or CP. The mechanism of increased risk associated with *SPINK-1* mutations is thought to be related to decreased ability to inactivate trypsin.

As with *SPINK-1* mutations, *CFTR* mutations are considered disease modifiers. Heterozygous, compound heterozygous, and homozygous mutations increase the risk for ARP and CP. These patients often lack other clinical features of cystic fibrosis or have mild disease in other organs and are pancreatic sufficient at presentation, although some will develop pancreatic insufficiency over time.

The anatomy of the biliary and pancreatic ducts can be determined by using magnetic resonance cholangiopancreatography. This study also can identify annular pancreas or congenital pancreatic cysts. Select patients may require endoscopic retrograde cholangiopancreatography to confirm and possibly treat ductal anomalies.

(Section 21: Disorders of the Gastrointestinal System, Chapter 412: Disorders of the Exocrine Pancreas)

**Answer 20-8.** B

Acute and chronic ingestion of NSAIDs has been associated with gastritis and mucosal ulceration that can result in upper gastrointestinal blood loss. The toxic consequences of NSAID use are the result of both direct topical injury and systemic effects, resulting in an imbalance of the gastric mucosal aggressive and protective mechanisms (Figure 404-1). As potent inhibitors of prostaglandin synthesis, NSAIDs decrease mucosal bicarbonate and mucus production, reduce mucosal blood flow, interfere with neutrophil adherence, and inhibit gastric acid production. Enterohepatic recirculation of NSAIDs also may be important in the development of mucosal injury. The effects of NSAIDs on platelet aggregation further potentiate bleeding and may interfere with the normal healing process of the upper gastrointestinal tract.

There appears to be no relationship between the development of NSAID-induced ulceration and infection

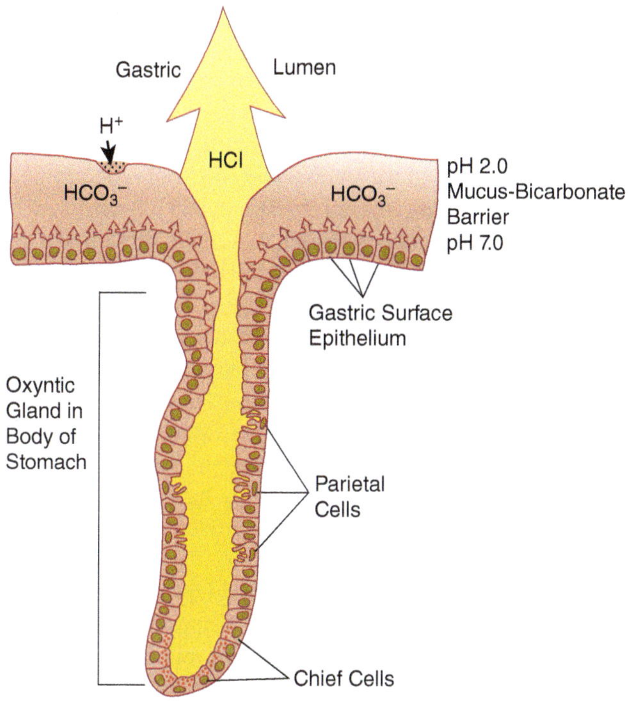


**FIGURE 404-1.** Mucous-bicarbonate barrier. (Mark W. Kline, *Rudolph's Pediatrics*, 23rd Edition. Copyright © McGraw-Hill Education. All rights reserved.)

with *Helicobacter pylori*, so administration of an antibiotic against this pathogen would not be helpful. Aspirin is as toxic as NSAIDs in promoting gastroduodenal inflammation, so substitution of salicylate would not be appropriate. Dyspeptic symptoms are quite common in patients receiving NSAID therapy. However, there are no clinical indicators to differentiate patients who only have dyspepsia from those who have ulcerations. Indeed, patients who have NSAID-associated ulcers are less likely to be symptomatic than patients who have ulcers and have not received NSAID therapy.

Given the efficacy of pharmacologic therapy for peptic ulcer disease, there is little reason to rely on dietary modification as the primary intervention in such patients. A proton pump inhibitor that affords greater suppression of gastric acid, in comparison to an $H_2$ blocker, may be more effective in healing gastric ulcers in patients who must continue NSAIDs. Sucralfate is a mucosal protective agent that is effective in the treatment of gastric ulcers but does not appear to be particularly effective in healing ulcers when the NSAID is continued. The extremely low incidence of gastric malignancy in the pediatric population obviates the need for endoscopy in the initial management of a child suspected of having a gastric ulcer. Endoscopic evaluation of the stomach is reserved for those who fail to respond to an initial course of acid suppression. If endoscopy is performed, assessment for the presence of *H pylori* should be undertaken.

(Section 21: Disorders of the Gastrointestinal System; Chapter 404: Inflammatory Disorders of the Stomach)

**Answer 20-9.** E

*H pylori* is an S-shaped, flagellated, gram-negative rod that colonizes the mucus layer of the stomach and produces urea. The organism's production of urease contributes to its ability to survive in the hostile gastric environment and to penetrate the mucosa of the gastric enterocyte. The pathogenesis of *H pylori* infection remains unclear, but it is likely to include direct penetration through the mucus layer that disrupts the gastric enterocyte and permits back-diffusion of gastric acid. Almost all individuals infected with *H pylori* have some degree of gastritis, but the degree of inflammation and association with complications such as peptic ulcer disease are variable. The most prevalent pattern of gastritis in children in the Western world is an antral-predominant gastritis, with little or no involvement of the body of the stomach. Recent studies have shown an association between long-term infection with *H pylori* and the development of gastric cancer as well as lymphoma arising from mucosa-associated lymphoid tissue. The incidence of gastric malignancy in the pediatric population, however, is extremely low.

If *H pylori* infection is suspected, diagnosis should be made by either positive culture obtained from tissue through upper endoscopy or positive histopathology through upper endoscopy and positive rapid urease test. Therefore, it is recommended that all children with suspected *H pylori* infection undergo upper endoscopy. Noninvasive tests, including the urea breath test and stool antigen test for the *H pylori* antigen, are reliable tests to determine whether *H pylori* has been eradicated following treatment, but these tests should not be used alone for diagnosis. Antibody tests using whole blood, serum, or saliva are not recommended in children for clinical use due to poor sensitivity and specificity. Furthermore, antibody tests often remain positive for years after eradication or resolution of infection, which reduces their clinical utility for diagnosis.

(Section 21: Disorders of the Gastrointestinal System, Chapter 404: Inflammatory Disorders of the Stomach)

**Answer 20-10.** B

Approximately 10% to 20% of newborn infants with CF will present with meconium ileus. The mechanical intestinal obstruction is created by abnormally thick, viscous meconium that results from the relative deficiency of pancreatic proteinases in infants with CF. Patients can present with abdominal distension, feeding intolerance with or without bilious emesis, and failure to pass meconium. The intestinal obstruction associated with meconium ileus is typically located at the level of the terminal ileum. Plain abdominal radiographs are the initial diagnostic test of choice in the setting of most cases of suspected bowel obstruction. In infants with meconium ileus, the inspissated, thick meconium mixed with gas can have a "soap bubble" or "ground glass" appearance in the bowel loops, in addition to evidence of obstruction with proximally dilated loops of bowel. Retrograde contrast enema may be therapeutic as well as diagnostic, showing a patent, unused microcolon with evidence of obstructing meconium in the terminal ileum. Use of hyperosmolar contrast agents or mucolytic agents for the retrograde enema can help mobilize the impacted meconium with the goal of relieving the intestinal obstruction. In patients with persistent obstruction despite retrograde enemas, or those with intestinal perforation or pseudocyst formation, operative exploration may be necessary.

Hirschsprung disease, or congenital aganglionic megacolon, can also present with features of intestinal obstruction in the neonatal period. Failure to pass meconium within the first 48 hours of life is a common feature. Evidence of a cone-shaped transition zone or caliber change in the rectosigmoid area on barium enema examination is highly suspicious for Hirschsprung disease. In the very early newborn period or in infants with total colonic involvement, however, a transition zone may be absent. However, in contrast to infants with meconium ileus, infants with Hirschsprung disease will characteristically show significant amounts of retained barium on a 24-hour postevacuation film.

Infants with cow's milk protein allergy or intolerance are typically healthy in appearance but present with blood-tinged stools. Infants with duodenal atresia, as well as other types of intestinal atresias, also commonly present with abdominal distension and vomiting within the first 48 hours of life. Affected infants may or may not pass meconium. There is often a prenatal history of polyhydramnios. Plain film radiography may reveal a "double-bubble" sign suggesting duodenal atresia, but an upper gastrointestinal contrast study is usually necessary to make the diagnosis and establish the level of obstruction. Malformations of the anorectum, including anal stenosis, can present with abdominal distension and abnormal passage of meconium and stools early in life. These conditions are generally able to be diagnosed on physical exam. Anorectal malformations are often associated with other congenital malformations as well.

(Section 21: Disorders of the Gastrointestinal System, Chapter 398: Meconium Ileus, Meconium Plug Syndrome, and Distal Intestinal Obstruction Syndrome)

**Answer 20-11.** E

Distal intestinal obstruction syndrome (DIOS), formerly known as meconium ileus equivalent, is characterized by an acute complete or partial obstruction of the ileocecum by intestinal contents. By contrast, constipation in patients with CF is characterized by gradual onset of fecal impaction of the total colon. DIOS can occur at any age, but it is more common in older patients and those with pancreatic insufficiency. The most common manifestation of DIOS is crampy abdominal pain, which generally is located in the right lower quadrant. The onset of symptoms usually is acute, and the symptoms tend to become progressively severe over time. Other features include decreased or absent bowel movements, abdominal distension, weight loss, and poor appetite. On examination, a mass may be palpated in the right lower quadrant. Plain abdominal radiographs typically show stool in the distal ileum and proximal colon; signs of small bowel obstruction with air-fluid levels on upright films are also common. DIOS should be distinguished from chronic constipation, in which the onset of symptoms is more gradual and the stool is distributed more evenly throughout the colon. Patients with incomplete (impending) DIOS usually respond to oral rehydration and osmotic laxatives. Those with complete DIOS or signs of peritonitis may require surgery.

Initial management should be aimed at correcting fluid and electrolyte abnormalities. Once electrolyte abnormalities have been corrected, treatment should be aimed at removal of the inspissated plug. This can be attempted using a combination of enemas and laxatives until normal stooling patterns are established. Once the inspissated plug has been eliminated, it is important to initiate or optimize appropriate pancreatic enzyme replacement.

Traditional strategies aimed at treating constipation, such as increased fiber supplementation, rectal suppositories, or stimulant laxatives, may have some benefit, but they do not address the underlying pathophysiology of DIOS. Similarly, although fat-soluble vitamin deficiency is also associated with pancreatic insufficiency, treatment with fat-soluble vitamins will not likely reduce the risk of DIOS recurrence.

(Section 21: Disorders of the Gastrointestinal System, Chapter 398: Meconium Ileus, Meconium Plug Syndrome, and Distal Intestinal Obstruction Syndrome)

**Answer 20-12.** D

IHPS is the most common surgical cause of nonbilious vomiting in infants. The pyloric muscle is not usually hypertrophied at birth, but appears to hypertrophy after birth, leading to gastric outlet obstruction. The typical age of presentation of IHPS is between 3 and 8 weeks old, with the incidence in males being 4 to 6 times higher than females. Typical symptoms include postprandial, projectile, nonbilious vomiting. Despite the persistent vomiting, the infant often remains hungry and appears very eager to feed. In later stages or when the diagnosis is delayed, dehydration, weight loss, and development of a hypochloremic hypokalemic alkalosis can result.

Symptoms of frequent gagging, choking, or coughing with feeds are concerning for possible aspiration. This is often associated with oral aversion and feeding refusal. A history of trisomy 21 and bilious emesis in early infancy should raise suspicions for duodenal atresia or stenosis. Finally, dehydration can occur in infants with severe vomiting and diarrhea secondary to a viral gastroenteritis. The dehydration usually leads to a metabolic acidosis, rather than alkalosis, which is seen in IHPS secondary to loss of secreted hydrogen ion from the stomach.

(Section 21: Disorders of the Gastrointestinal System, Chapter 393: Infantile Hypertrophic Pyloric Stenosis)

**Answer 20-13.** E

Infants with infantile hypertrophic pyloric stenosis (IHPS) commonly present with dehydration and electrolyte abnormalities secondary to persistent vomiting. In the initial phase of management, appropriate fluid/electrolyte resuscitation remains the priority. Placement of a nasogastric tube for feeding or hydration is unnecessary. Pyloromyotomy is the gold standard for treatment but is nonemergent and should be performed only after the patient is stabilized and alkalosis and hypokalemia are corrected. Surgical therapy provides safe and effective treatment, with prompt relief of symptoms. Endoscopic dilatation of the pylorus is not an effective, long-term therapy for IHPS. Enhancement of gastric motility with erythromycin is not beneficial for patients with IHPS. In fact, early exposure to erythromycin in infancy has been linked to the development of IHPS.

(Section 21: Disorders of the Gastrointestinal System, Chapter 393: Infantile Hypertrophic Pyloric Stenosis)

**Answer 20-14.** B

Cow milk protein-induced anemia can present in children between the ages of 1 and 3 years as a result of iron deficiency anemia and protein-losing enteropathy. Key characteristics include a history of excess cow milk intake (typically > 32 oz. of whole milk daily), profound microcytic anemia (hemoglobin 6–8 g/dL), and hypoalbuminemia. Because of the gradual development of anemia and hypoalbuminemia, the child does not develop orthostatic hypotension symptoms. Stools studies are notable for elevated $\alpha_1$-antitrypsin excretion indicating a protein-losing enteropathy. However, stool guaiac test for blood is negative, which is an important distinction from patients with cow milk protein–induced proctocolitis or allergic colitis. The mechanism by which cow milk induces anemia is not completely understood but is likely related to iron deficiency (secondary to excess milk intake) or mucosal toxicity rather than hypersensitivity to cow milk protein.

Cow milk protein–induced proctocolitis typically presents at 4 to 12 weeks of age with symptoms of painless hematochezia mixed with mucus and occasional diarrhea. FPIES is a non–IgE-mediated process that is associated with an anaphylactic-like reaction with rapid onset of symptoms of vomiting and diarrhea as well as systemic manifestations of pallor, hypotension, and shock. Eosinophilic gastroenteritis is characterized by dense eosinophilic inflammation of the gastrointestinal mucosa. Typical symptoms include abdominal pain, vomiting, diarrhea, and growth failure. In more severe cases, iron deficiency anemia and protein-losing enteropathy can develop but are associated with eosinophilia and increased serum IgE. It is rare for Crohn disease to present at this stage in early childhood, but the presenting symptoms include diarrhea and growth failure. With this degree of iron deficiency anemia, a history of diarrhea and hematochezia blood loss would be more likely.

(Section 21: Disorders of the Gastrointestinal System, Chapter 406: Allergic Gastroenteropathies and Eosinophilic Gastrointestinal Diseases)

**Answer 20-15.** C

Congenital atresia of the esophagus and tracheoesophageal fistula are relatively common congenital anomalies, occurring in 1 of every 2500 to 3000 live births. Esophageal atresia has been classified into 5 types based on whether the esophagus is present and the location of fistula to the trachea (see following figure).

The vast majority (85%) of infants born with esophageal atresia have atresia of the esophagus with a distal tracheoesophageal fistula. Also known as type C esophageal atresia, the esophageal fistula typically originates just proximal to the carina in the posterior trachea. The next most common type is a pure esophageal atresia without tracheoesophageal fistula (6%–10%). Once the diagnosis of esophageal atresia is made, a search for associated anomalies is required, including VACTERL association, which includes anomalies of the vertebrae, intestinal atresia, cardiac malformations, tracheoesophageal fistula, renal anomalies, and limb anomalies.

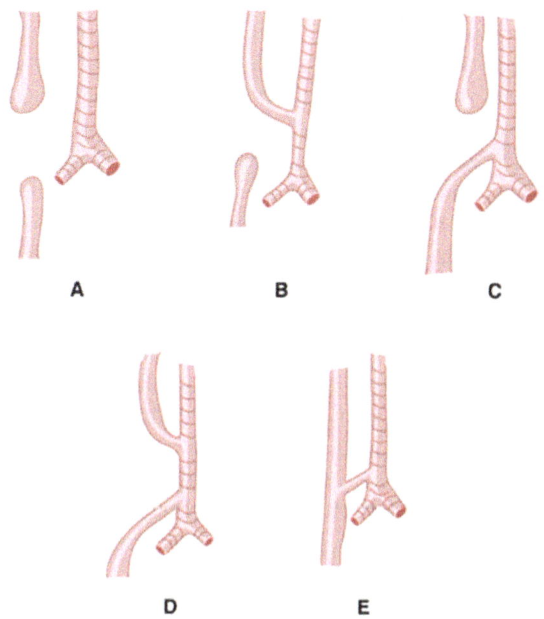

| | Type A | Type B | Type C | Type D | Type E |
|---|---|---|---|---|---|
| **Description** | Esophageal atresia without TEF | Esophageal atresia with proximal TEF | Esophageal atresia with distal TEF | Esophageal atresia with proximal and distal TEF | Isolated TEF without esophageal atresia (H-type fistula) |
| **Abnormal Radiograph** | Gasless abdomen | Gasless abdomen | Distal gas | Distal gas | Distal gas |
| **Incidence** | 6%–10% | 3% | 85% | 1% | 6% |

(Section 21: Disorders of the Gastrointestinal System, Chapter 387: Anatomic Disorders of the Esophagus)

**Answer 20-16.** C

A patient with history of surgical repair for esophageal atresia and symptoms of isolated dysphagia should be evaluated for stricture formation at the site of the esophageal anastomosis. Strictures have been reported to develop in 30% to 40% of patients. Early complications following surgical repair include anastomotic leak, anastomotic stricture, and recurrent fistula. Late stricture development, as in this clinical vignette, is typically attributed to gastroesophageal reflux (GER). Evaluation for stricture formation is performed with a barium swallow esophagram. Anastomotic strictures are usually treated via dilation with a balloon dilator or by progressive bougienage dilatation. Refractory strictures may require steroid injection at the time of dilatation or surgery.

Although GER is exceedingly common in esophageal atresia patients following repair and is likely a causative factor in the formation of an anastomotic stricture, treatment with proton pump inhibitors alone will unlikely lead to resolution of a significant stricture. Patients with severe reflux may require antireflux surgery and should be monitored long term due to the risk of developing Barrett esophagus and esophageal cancer. Recurrent tracheoesophageal fistula is a rare complication following tracheoesophageal fistula repair but typically presents with symptoms of coughing, choking, apnea, and recurrent pulmonary infections, rather than dysphagia. A calcium channel blocker medication such as nifedipine enhances lower esophageal sphincter relaxation and may provide some benefit for patients with dysphagia secondary to esophageal achalasia, but not for patients with a mechanical obstruction secondary to anastomotic stricture. Finally, although the majority of patients with esophageal atresia have some degree of dysmotility or abnormal peristalsis in the lower esophageal segment, even after surgical repair, the presence of an anastomotic stricture must be ruled out first.

(Section 21: Disorders of the Gastrointestinal System, Chapter 387: Anatomic Disorders of the Esophagus)

**Answer 20-17.** E

A thorough history and physical examination is generally sufficient to make a diagnosis of uncomplicated or physiologic gastroesophageal reflux (GER) in infancy. Additional diagnostic testing is usually unnecessary unless there are warning signs, such as forceful or bilious vomiting, abdominal tenderness or distension, gastrointestinal bleeding, diarrhea, constipation, fever, hepatosplenomegaly, seizures, macrocephaly or microcephaly, or onset of vomiting after 6 months of age.

An upper gastrointestinal contrast study is useful for diagnosing anatomic abnormalities that present with recurrent vomiting. The upper gastrointestinal study is not useful for diagnosis of GER because reflux of ingested contrast occurs in healthy individuals.

In uncomplicated GER, characterized by the lack of warning signs or potential complications, such as weight loss, inadequate weight gain, excessive irritability, feeding difficulties, or recurrent respiratory distress, reassurance of the parents is usually sufficient for management. A diagnosis of gastroesophageal reflux disease (GERD) is considered when there are significant complications from GER. Nonpharmacologic options for treatment of GER may be considered for symptomatic infants, including a trial of a hypoallergenic formula or thickening of formula with rice cereal. A high-calorie formula is not indicated for an infant with appropriate growth. Proton pump inhibitor therapy is highly effective for treatment of esophagitis; however, for an infant with uncomplicated GER, acid suppression is unlikely to result in any significant clinical benefit. There are currently no available motility or prokinetic agents that have been proven clearly effective for GERD.

(Section 21: Disorders of the Gastrointestinal System, Chapter 389: Gastroesophageal Reflux and Other Causes of Esophageal Inflammation)

**Answer 20-18.** B

The clinical presentation of eosinophilic esophagitis (EE) varies depending on the age of the patient. Symptoms range from feeding refusal in infants, gagging and solid food aversion in preschool children, to dysphagia and food impaction in adolescents. EE is a clinicopathologic diagnosis that requires histologic evaluation of esophageal biopsies. EE is characterized by an intense eosinophilic infiltrate of the esophageal wall, with evidence of ≥ 15 eosinophils/HPF, and involvement of the entire proximal to distal esophagus. This finding is in contrast with gastroesophageal reflux disease (GERD), in which eosinophilic involvement is typically less intense (< 7 eosinophils/HPF) and limited to the distal esophagus. Endoscopy usually reveals a combination of characteristic features: edema, linear furrowing, ringed appearance (trachealization), and white adherent plaques. EE patients commonly have a personal and family history of atopy. Food allergies may be triggers of EE. Therefore, allergy testing may identify likely causes of EE and guide management of the condition with an elimination diet.

Because the patient in the clinical vignette has already received 6 weeks of high-dose proton pump inhibitor therapy, it is unlikely that the inflammation seen on endoscopy is secondary to GERD. Therefore, further escalation of acid suppression therapy with the addition of a histamine-2 receptor blocker is not indicated. Pneumatic balloon dilatation of the lower esophageal sphincter is an appropriate option for treatment of achalasia, not EE. Infections of the esophagus are rare, except in the immunocompromised host. The typical presenting symptoms of esophageal infection are dysphagia and odynophagia. *Candida albicans* is the usual cause of *Candida* esophagitis and is characterized by evidence of white plaques on endoscopy. Budding yeast and hyphae forms are usually present on histology. *Candida* esophagitis usually responds to treatment with fluconazole. Herpes simplex virus can cause esophagitis in both immunocompromised and immunocompetent hosts. Endoscopically, the infection is usually characterized by discrete ulcers with a surrounding raised edge. If herpes simplex virus is suspected, treatment with acyclovir may shorten the disease course.

(Section 21: Disorders of the Gastrointestinal System, Chapter 389: Gastroesophageal Reflux and Other Causes of Esophageal Inflammation)

**Answer 20-19.** D

Ingestion of strong caustic agents can result in injury to the esophagus and stomach. Acids cause coagulation necrosis of the mucosa and formation of an eschar, whereas alkali substances produce liquefactive necrosis with intense inflammation of the surrounding tissue.

The acid produced by the stomach has limited neutralizing capacity compared with the alkalinity of even small volumes of strong alkalis. Symptoms following caustic ingestion include oral pain, ulcerations, drooling, dysphagia, vomiting, and abdominal pain. Concurrent airway damage is also possible. Symptoms can develop rapidly or be delayed for several hours. Clinical manifestations, such as the presence or absence of oral cavity burns, are generally poor predictors of esophageal injury. Young children with symptoms or an inability to tolerate clear liquids should be admitted for observation and IV hydration.

Emetics and buffers should not be given because of the risk of vomiting and subsequent aspiration. Nasogastric tubes should not be passed in the acute setting because they may perforate a damaged esophagus or stomach. Endoscopic evaluation is recommended between 12 and 36 hours after ingestion to allow evaluation of the degree of esophageal injury. Earlier endoscopy may miss the full extent of injury, since injury may evolve over the first 12 hours. Esophagoscopy after 48 hours is associated with increased risk of perforation.

(Section 21: Disorders of the Gastrointestinal System, Chapter 389: Gastroesophageal Reflux and Other Causes of Esophageal Inflammation)

**Answer 20-20.** A

Achalasia is a motor disorder of the esophagus with characteristic radiographic features on barium swallow (dilated esophagus with "birds beak" appearance secondary to a narrowed gastroesophageal junction) and manometric findings of incomplete relaxation of the lower esophageal sphincter and lack of normal esophageal peristalsis.

Presenting symptoms include dysphagia, regurgitation of undigested food, recurrent pneumonia, weight loss, and chest pain. Diffuse esophageal spasm is rare in childhood but is associated with symptoms of chest pain and evidence of nonperistaltic, prolonged, high-amplitude contractions on esophageal manometry. Patients with systemic scleroderma may present skin findings, such as Raynaud phenomenon, as well as esophageal manifestations. The manometric findings in scleroderma include low-amplitude peristaltic contractions with abnormally low pressures in the lower esophageal sphincter. Gastroesophageal reflux disease (GERD) can also be a cause of a secondary motility disorder. Manometric findings associated with GERD are usually nonspecific, including prolonged esophageal contraction, aperistaltic contractions, and multiple peaked contractions. Mechanical obstruction, such as from an esophageal web or stricture, should always be considered in the evaluation of a patient who presents with dysphagia. Congenital defects are most likely to present when infants are transitioned to solid-consistency foods.

(Section 21: Disorders of the Gastrointestinal System, Chapter 388: Disorders of Esophageal Motility)

**Answer 20-21.** C

The spectrum of anorectal malformations ranges from lesions such as anal stenosis to persistent cloaca. Many of these conditions share a common finding of imperforate anus, or lack of a visible normal anal opening onto the perineum. The most common defect is an imperforate anus with a fistula between the distal anorectum and urethra in boys or the vestibule in girls.

The terms *high* and *low* are used to describe the location of the distal rectum or anal canal relative to the perineum. In high lesions, the rectum ends above the levator muscle. In low lesions, the rectal pouch completely crosses the levator musculature, and a fistula is usually evident on the skin. Congenital anorectal anomalies often coexist with other lesions. Newborns should undergo evaluation for other congenital lesions such as vertebral and sacral anomalies and genitourinary abnormalities. In terms of repair, the newborn infant with anal stenosis, perineal fistula, or an anteriorly displaced anus can usually undergo a primary, single-stage procedure without a colostomy. Patients with more complex anorectal malformations, meconium-stained urine, or other life-threatening anomalies require an initial colostomy as the first part of a 3-stage reconstruction. The most common postoperative complications seen in children with anorectal malformations include constipation, soiling, and incontinence. Patients with "low" lesions and a normal sacrum usually have the best prognosis with regard to continence.

(Section 21: Disorders of the Gastrointestinal System, Chapter 410: Congenital Anomalies of the Anorectum)

**Answer 20-22.** E

In patients with suspected gastroesophageal reflux (GER)-associated Sandifer syndrome, esophageal pH-impedance monitoring (typically performed over 24 hours) is useful in demonstrating GER and in clarifying any temporal association of reflux and posturing.

Other diagnostic tests commonly performed in association with evaluation of gastroesophageal reflux disease (GERD), such as upper gastrointestinal radiography, nuclear scintigraphy, and upper endoscopy with esophageal biopsies, may be helpful in documenting the presence of GER but are not able to temporally correlate reflux events with symptoms.

Sandifer syndrome involves spasmodic torsional dystonia with arching of the back and rigid posturing, mainly involving the neck, back, and upper extremities, associated with symptomatic GER. Spasms are commonly mistaken for seizures, although most patients do not have a clonic component to the movements. An electroencephalogram is usually normal for patients with suspected Sandifer syndrome and is therefore of little benefit unless the clinical presentation is unclear. A relationship with feeding may suggest a diagnosis of Sandifer syndrome, which commonly occurs after feeding. Typically, Sandifer syndrome is observed from infancy to early childhood. Peak prevalence is in individuals younger than 24 months. Children with mental impairment or spasticity may experience Sandifer syndrome into adolescence.

(Section 21: Disorders of the Gastrointestinal System, Chapter 389: Gastroesophageal Reflux and Other Causes of Esophageal Inflammation)

**Answer 20-23.** C

Children may develop delayed gastric emptying after an infection with certain organisms, such as *Rotavirus*, Norwalk virus, herpes zoster virus, or infectious mononucleosis. The symptoms often resolve in time. The gastroparesis can result in symptoms of early satiety, nausea, vomiting, or abdominal discomfort. Children may vomit food hours or even days later.

The goals of treatment are to maintain adequate nutrition and hydration while attempting to control symptoms. With a child with mild postinfectious gastroparesis such as the one presented in this question, conservative initial treatment makes the most sense. This strategy would include introducing small, low-fat meals. Meals lower in fat have a shorter gastric emptying time. Liquid meals also have a shorter emptying time. Meals high in fat will further delay her gastric emptying.

Pyloric injections of Botox® would only be considered if she failed medical management, including altering her diet and failure of promotility drugs.

Domperidone is a prokinetic medication; however, it is not approved for use in the United States by the US Food and Drug Administration and is not readily available for use. Other promotility drugs such as metoclopramide and erythromycin are available for use and could be given to this patient if altering her diet is not effective. Metoclopramide, however, does have a risk of tardive dyskinesia, making its use less popular than erythromycin.

Initiation of nasojejunal feeds may need to be considered in patients with significant delayed gastric emptying and weight loss who have failed more conservative therapy; however, this strategy would not be a first-line treatment.

(Section 21: Disorders of the Gastrointestinal System, Chapter 402: Motor Disorders of the Stomach, Small Bowel, and Colon)

**Answer 20-24.** B

Hirschsprung disease occurs in 1 in 5000 live births. Up to 10% of children with Down syndrome have Hirschsprung disease. Hirschsprung disease is a result of aberrant migration of neural crest cells during colonic development. Ninety-four percent of neonates with Hirschsprung disease do not pass meconium within 24 hours of birth. Other symptoms at presentation may include vomiting, abdominal distension, and enterocolitis. The clues in this case making Hirschsprung disease most likely are his diagnosis of trisomy 21, delayed passage of meconium, and a tight anal canal.

Patients with trisomy 21 are at higher risk of duodenal web. However, although vomiting would be a key symptom related to a web, the patient should not have a tight anal canal or delayed passage of meconium. Milk protein intolerance can be associated with vomiting and constipation in infants; however, one would not expect delayed passage of meconium, and the rectal exam should demonstrate normal tone. Infants with CF may present with constipation or even a small bowel obstruction from meconium ileus; however, again, they should not have an abnormal rectal exam.

Given this patient's history of trisomy 21, delayed passage of meconium, and tight anal canal on rectal exam, functional constipation should not be an initial consideration.

(Section 21: Disorders of the Gastrointestinal System, Chapter 402: Motor Disorders of the Stomach, Small Bowel, and Colon)

**Answer 20-25.** E

Erythromycin is a motilin receptor agonist used to accelerate gastric emptying. There is a caution in using this drug in young infants due to the increased risk of the development of hypertrophic pyloric stenosis. Although erythromycin accelerates gastric emptying, it has not been associated with dumping syndrome. In addition, erythromycin has not been associated with duodenal webs. Tardive dyskinesia and dystonic reactions are both side effects of metoclopramide, which is also a prokinetic medication used in delayed gastric emptying.

(Section 21: Disorders of the Gastrointestinal System, Chapter 402: Motor Disorders of the Stomach, Small Bowel, and Colon)

**Answer 20-26.** B

This patient has an external hemorrhoid. They are generally associated with chronic constipation. Symptoms generally improve with the treatment of the underlying constipation. Incision and evacuation by a surgeon would be considered if the hemorrhoid was thrombosed. Anorectal varices may occur with chronic liver disease; however, in a child with a normal exam and chronic constipation, chronic liver disease would not likely be the etiology. Hemorrhoids may be a sign of sexual abuse; however, with a history of chronic constipation and no other signs of perianal trauma, this diagnosis would not be the most likely etiology. The patient does not need a colonoscopy, as hemorrhoids are not associated with other intestinal vascular lesions.

(Section 21: Disorders of the Gastrointestinal System, Chapter 411: Other Anorectal Disorders)

**Answer 20-27.** E

This patient has a rectal prolapse, likely from his constipation and straining with stooling. Most cases spontaneously resolve. However, in situations where the mucosa does not spontaneously resolve, gentle pressure may be applied to manually reduce the prolapse. This may be done in the home or office setting. If the mucosa does not reduce with gentle pressure, then surgical reduction may be warranted. A stool softener may be needed to treat the underlying condition; however, this treatment would only prevent future prolapses and would not result in resolution of the current prolapse.

(Section 21: Disorders of the Gastrointestinal System, Chapter 411: Other Anorectal Disorders)

**Answer 20-28.** A

This rash is classic for perianal streptococcal infection. Oral penicillin, as opposed to topical antibiotics, is usually effective in treatment. Candidal diaper rash usually has more erythematous plaques with satellite lesions and would be treated with topical nystatin. Topical cholestyramine may be used to bind bile acids in children with a diaper dermatitis related to diarrhea. Neither nystatin nor cholestyramine would be used for a bacterial infection.

(Section 21: Disorders of the Gastrointestinal System, Chapter 411: Other Anorectal Disorders)

**Answer 20-29.** C

Annular pancreas presents with symptoms of a high obstruction including vomiting. Annular pancreas arises from incomplete rotation of the ventral bud off the duodenum during embryonic pancreatic development. It is often associated with a duodenal diaphragm or stenosis.

Pyloric stenosis and antral web are obstructive processes at the gastric outlet. On abdominal radiograph, one would not see the area of duodenal dilation. Hirschsprung disease would present with a more distal obstructive symptomatology such as constipation and infrequent stooling. You may find a lack of air in the rectum on abdominal radiograph with dilated loops of bowel proximal to the affected segment of aganglionosis. A choledochal cyst is found in the hepatobiliary ducts and is seen on other radiologic modalities such as ultrasound, computed tomography scan, or magnetic resonance imaging.

(Section 21: Disorders of the Gastrointestinal System, Chapter 412: Disorders of the Exocrine Pancreas)

**Answer 20-30.** D

The patient is taking a chronic medication, valproic acid, that is known to cause pancreatitis. L-asparaginase, azathioprine, and 6-mercaptopurine are also associated with pancreatitis. All the other conditions are also associated with acute pancreatitis; however, his abdominal ultrasound did not indicate gallstone disease. Epilepsy by itself is not associated with acute pancreatitis, and he did not have any other signs or symptoms of a systemic condition or viral illness. Blunt trauma is associated with acute pancreatitis; however, it would be recent and not a remote event.

(Section 21: Disorders of the Gastrointestinal System, Chapter 412: Disorders of the Exocrine Pancreas)

**Answer 20-31.** D

This neonate has likely experienced a gastric perforation due to trauma from esophageal intubation and bag-mask ventilation. The pneumoperitoneum is confirmed by an abdominal radiograph. Symptoms include poor feeding, lethargy, and abdominal distension. Treatment includes nasogastric decompression, antibiotics, and surgical management.

Refeeding would not occur until surgical repair has occurred. A sepsis workup would not be the first course of action prior to surgical repair. Monitoring with repeated radiographs would not be appropriate, as the diagnosis has already been confirmed. A paracentesis would be the appropriate step preoperatively if the patient is experiencing hemodynamic instability or respiratory compromise, which this patient does not demonstrate.

(Section 21: Disorders of the Gastrointestinal System, Chapter 395: Microgastria and Gastric Perforation)

**Answer 20-32.** D

Neonates with pyloric atresia will present with early onset of vomiting that is nonbilious, as well as a dilated stomach at birth. The mother may also have polyhydramnios during her pregnancy.

Pyloric stenosis is an acquired condition and would not present on the first day of life, nor would it be associated with a large stomach at birth and polyhydramnios. Duodenal webs and atresias would likely present with bilious vomiting. Jejunoileal atresias would also likely present with bilious vomiting and abdominal distension.

(Section 21: Disorders of the Gastrointestinal System, Chapter 394: Congenital Atresias, Stenosis, and Webs)

**Answer 20-33.** D

Twenty percent of foreign body impactions occur within the esophagus. Children may present with a choking episode, respiratory symptoms, coughing, drooling, refusing oral intake, dysphagia, or chest pain. If the child is symptomatic, it warrants urgent endoscopy. Other reasons for an urgent endoscopy include an esophageal impaction with a button battery or sharp object. It is not appropriate to delay removal of a button battery in the esophagus as a button battery may cause a low-voltage burn and corrosive injury of the esophageal mucosa. This injury may occur as early as 4 hours after impaction.

(Section 21: Disorders of the Gastrointestinal System, Chapter 390: Other Esophageal Disorders)

**Answer 20-34.** B

Breastfed infants absorb significantly more dietary lipid when compared to formula-fed infants because they ingest a unique breast milk lipase that assists in the majority (up to two-thirds) of lipid hydrolysis.

Breastfed and formula-fed infants have comparable levels of lactase activity, which peaks at birth and then declines to about 25% of term levels by 1 year of age. Both breastfed and formula-fed newborn infants have relatively lower pancreatic lipase and bile salt secretion overall when compared with adults, with formula-fed infants malabsorbing 10% to 15% of dietary lipids. All infants have efficient protein digestion and absorption; there is no difference between breastfed and formula-fed infants. Both breastfed and formula-fed infants are able to absorb medium-chain fatty acids directly into the portal system, whereas long-chain fatty acids require transport proteins for absorption.

(Section 21: Disorders of the Gastrointestinal System, Chapter 376: Normal Structure and Function of the Gastrointestinal Tract)

**Answer 20-35.** A

This patient has chronic recurrent vomiting, with at least 3 episodes of mild but frequent emesis over a 3-month period. One of the most frequent causes of vomiting in the school-age child and adolescent is gastroesophageal reflux disease (GERD), which may occur after meals and is not typically associated with weight loss. In a child with chronic vomiting without alarm symptoms or other concerning exam findings, the most likely diagnosis is an acid-peptic disorder such as GERD or gastritis that should be initially treated with an empiric 2- to 4-week trial of an $H_2$-receptor antagonist or proton pump inhibitor for acid suppression.

If there is no symptomatic improvement after a time-limited trial of these medications, it may then be appropriate to proceed with laboratory testing, imaging, or consultation with pediatric gastroenterology. Ondansetron may be useful for symptomatic improvement in the setting of acute, rather than chronic, vomiting.

(Section 21: Disorders of the Gastrointestinal System, Chapter 377: Approach to the Child with Acute, Chronic, or Cyclic Vomiting)

**Answer 20-36.** B

Several physical examination signs are associated with acute appendicitis. Answer choice B describes the obturator sign. When the maneuver is performed, the obturator internus muscle can irritate the appendix, causing right lower quadrant pain. Other maneuvers associated with acute appendicitis include the Rovsing sign (left lower quadrant palpation to elicit right lower quadrant pain) and the ileo-psoas sign (pain on passive extension of the right hip).

The tenderness from appendicitis eventually migrates to McBurney's point (located two-thirds of the way lateral on a line from the umbilicus to the anterior superior iliac spine) as peritoneal irritation increases. Abdominal ultrasound may demonstrate inflammation of the appendix and also support the diagnosis. Surgical consultation is appropriate if suspicion for acute appendicitis is high; however, it is appropriate to pursue complete examination and imaging first, if possible, to support the diagnosis.

Answer choice A describes Grey Turner sign, which is associated with retroperitoneal bleeding. Answer choice C describes Murphy sign, which is associated with acute cholecystitis. Answer choice D describes Kernig sign, which is associated with meningitis. Finally, answer choice E describes Homan sign, which is associated with venous thrombosis in the lower extremity.

(Section 21: Disorders of the Gastrointestinal System, Chapter 378: Acute Abdominal Pain)

**Answer 20-37.** D

Up to 80% of children with functional abdominal pain have some form of anxiety; approximately 40% will have a depressive disorder.

Gender has not been shown to be a distinguishing factor for patients with functional versus organic abdominal pain. The examination technique known as the Carnett test, in which the examiner applies pressure to the point of maximal abdominal tenderness and then instructs the patient to assume a partial sitting position, may suggest an organic abdominal wall disorder rather than functional etiology if there is greater tenderness on palpation in partial sitting position compared to relaxed supine position. Antispasmodic medications, such as hyoscyamine, are commonly used in clinical practice to treat functional bowel disorders, but efficacy is controversial.

(Section 21: Disorders of the Gastrointestinal System, Chapter 379: Chronic Abdominal Pain)

**Answer 20-38.** E

Abdominal pain that awakens a child from sleep and/or nocturnal diarrhea should raise the degree of suspicion for an organic etiology of the pain, such as inflammatory bowel disease, and warrants further investigation with laboratory testing and possibly imaging and/or endoscopy.

Children with functional pain frequently miss school due to their discomfort, and once the diagnosis of functional pain is certain, one of the physician's main goals should be to reinstate regular school attendance. Irritable bowel syndrome is one type of functional abdominal pain, and it is known that there is a high frequency of functional disorders among family members. Therefore, history of irritable bowel syndrome in a first-degree relative should support this patient's diagnosis of functional pain rather than refute it. One possible symptom of irritable bowel syndrome is the sensation of incomplete evacuation after passage of stool. Associated symptoms of headache, pallor, and/or fatigue are present in > 50% of patients with functional abdominal pain.

(Section 21: Disorders of the Gastrointestinal System, Chapter 379: Chronic Abdominal Pain)

**Answer 20-39.** D

A stool culture should be performed in every child with bloody diarrhea because bacterial pathogens have been implicated in up to 20% of such cases. It is important to determine which bacterial pathogen is present, because infection with *Shigella* and cholera warrant antibiotic therapy, whereas antibiotic therapy for enterohemorrhagic *Escherichia coli* may increase the risk of subsequently developing hemolytic-uremic syndrome and should be deferred. Stool cultures in children with nonbloody diarrhea are not necessary because they will be unlikely to alter the appropriate therapy.

Patients with acute diarrhea who are able to maintain adequate hydration with oral intake should be offered small frequent volumes of oral rehydration therapy (ORT) solution; there is no contraindication to offering breast milk, formula, or solid feeds in addition to ORT while diarrhea is ongoing. Loperamide is an opiate antimotility agent that is not recommended for management of acute diarrhea in children because it may cause ileus, nausea, and sedation. *Rotavirus* is a common cause of watery diarrhea in the winter months but typically does not cause bloody diarrhea; thus, it is a less likely cause of this patient's diarrhea.

(Section 21: Disorders of the Gastrointestinal System, Chapter 380: Diarrhea)

**Answer 20-40.** E

This patient most likely has chronic nonspecific diarrhea of childhood, also called toddler's diarrhea. She is well grown, has no other symptoms other than diarrhea, and has significant intake of apple juice daily, which has a high fructose-to-glucose ratio and is often implicated in toddler's diarrhea. Toddler's diarrhea is thought to be caused by mild carbohydrate malabsorption and hypermotility; a reasonable first step in treatment of suspected toddler's diarrhea is elimination of juice from the diet with reevaluation.

Determination of stool electrolytes and osmolality can be helpful in distinguishing between osmotic and secretory diarrhea. Stool pH and reducing substances may help in screening for malabsorptive causes of diarrhea. Stool cultures may help identify infectious causes of chronic diarrhea such as protozoal or bacterial infection. However, in an otherwise healthy, well-grown child who has a history consistent with toddler's diarrhea, empiric elimination of juice from the diet is a more reasonable first step in management rather than pursuing laboratory evaluation for less likely causes. Although lactose intolerance/lactase deficiency may be another cause of chronic diarrhea in childhood, excessive juice intake is more likely and should be pursued as a cause prior to trying a lactose-free diet.

(Section 21: Disorders of the Gastrointestinal System, Chapter 380: Diarrhea)

**Answer 20-41.** B

This child is having acute lower gastrointestinal bleeding and is tachycardic and hypotensive, indicative of hemodynamic instability. The most appropriate initial intervention is rapid intravascular volume expansion with crystalloid solution such as normal saline, followed by replacement of blood.

Although it is important to obtain this patient's complete medical history at some point to try to determine what the source of the gastrointestinal bleeding may be, it is more important to stabilize the patient with fluid resuscitation as soon as possible. Performing endoscopy or proceeding with surgical exploration prior to obtaining venous access and addressing this patient's hemodynamic instability initially would be dangerous; once the patient is stabilized, it is more appropriate to consider surgical exploration for lower gastrointestinal bleeding. Angiography is an imaging study that is sensitive with hemorrhage of at least 0.5 mL/min and may also allow embolization of vascular lesions by interventional radiologists; however, it would be unsafe to send this hemodynamically unstable patient for imaging initially.

(Section 21: Disorders of the Gastrointestinal System, Chapter 382: Upper and Lower Gastrointestinal Bleeding)

**Answer 20-42.** A

Painless lower gastrointestinal bleeding in an infant may be caused by Meckel diverticulum, intestinal duplication, or lymphonodular hyperplasia. Other causes of lower gastrointestinal bleeding in infants that typically present with apparent abdominal pain include infectious colitis, malrotation with volvulus, anal fissure, and intussusception.

(Section 21: Disorders of the Gastrointestinal System, Chapter 382: Upper and Lower Gastrointestinal Bleeding)

**Answer 20-43.** E

This infant most likely has volvulus with intestinal malrotation, which most commonly presents in the first week of life but can occur at any age. An infant with volvulus typically has progressive bilious emesis and pain out of proportion to the examination without initial abdominal distension; if the volvulus is not detected and addressed, the patient may later develop abdominal distension and hemodynamic instability. In this hemodynamically stable infant with suspected volvulus, an emergent upper gastrointestinal contrast study should be obtained and is diagnostic if malrotation with volvulus is present.

Abdominal ultrasound is diagnostic for hypertrophic pyloric stenosis. Plain abdominal film can help diagnose various causes of neonatal intestinal obstruction, including necrotizing enterocolitis, meconium ileus, congenital duodenal obstruction, or distal intestinal obstruction. Contrast enema can help diagnose intussusception, Hirschsprung disease, or intestinal stricture. CT scan is rarely useful in initial diagnosis of causes of neonatal intestinal obstruction and will expose the infant to harmful ionizing radiation.

(Section 21: Disorders of the Gastrointestinal System, Chapter 384: Gastrointestinal Obstruction)

**Answer 20-44.** E

A newborn with early feeding intolerance in which the examiner cannot pass a nasogastric tube is suggestive of esophageal atresia. Neonates with gastrointestinal obstruction due to esophageal atresia or anorectal malformations may have these anomalies as part of VACTERL syndrome, which is characterized by multiple associated congenital anomalies that can affect the vertebrae, anus, heart, trachea, esophagus, kidneys, and/or limbs.

Children with trisomy 21 are more likely to have intestinal obstruction due to Hirschsprung disease or congenital duodenal obstruction. Premature or very-low-birth-weight infants are at risk for developing necrotizing enterocolitis. CF is associated with intestinal obstruction due to meconium ileus.

(Section 21: Disorders of the Gastrointestinal System, Chapter 384: Gastrointestinal Obstruction)

**Answer 20-45.** D

Fecal $\alpha_1$-antitrypsin excretion in the stool has largely replaced radioisotopic techniques for diagnosis and evaluation of protein-losing enteropathy.

Among the many advantages of this assay are that it remains reliable even if the sample is contaminated with urine and it is stable at room temperature. One disadvantage of the assay is that $\alpha_1$-antitrypsin is digested in gastric juice, so the reliability of fecal $\alpha_1$-antitrypsin in detecting esophageal or gastric protein loss is questionable. In addition, meconium contains large amounts of $\alpha_1$-antitrypsin. As a result, the test is not valid until after 1 week of age.

(Section 21: Disorders of the Gastrointestinal System, Chapter 385: Protein-Losing Enteropathy)

**Answer 20-46.** A

Fifty to 60% of children with Crohn disease have mild to pronounced hypoalbuminemia.

Elevated BUN, hyperbilirubinemia, and hypophosphatemia are not associated with Crohn disease. MCV may be low in patients with Crohn disease because a microcytic anemia may be present due to chronic gastrointestinal blood loss with associated iron deficiency.

(Section 21: Disorders of the Gastrointestinal System, Chapter 385: Protein-Losing Enteropathy)

**Answer 20-47.** D

Brunner glands are found in the submucosal layer of the duodenum only and secrete bicarbonate to neutralize acidic gastric contents as they enter into the small intestine. In patients lacking Brunner glands (like this patient, who has had a duodenal resection), acidic gastric contents are not properly neutralized prior to entering the remaining small intestine and may precipitate osmotic fluid shift into the intestine, leading to postprandial diarrhea known as dumping syndrome.

Enterochromaffin cells are specialized hormone-secreting cells that are found in the gastric antrum. Peyer patches are a type of lymphoid aggregate that appear in high numbers in the ileum. Throughout the small intestine, crypts of Lieberkuhn appear at the bases of villi and house epithelial stem cells. Chief cells, also called oxyntic cells, secrete pepsinogen and are located mainly in the gastric body.

(Section 21: Disorders of the Gastrointestinal System, Chapter 376: Normal Structure and Function of the Gastrointestinal Tract)

**Answer 20-48.** D

Based on the history and physical examination, this child most likely has celiac disease, an immune-mediated enteropathy secondary to ingestion of gluten. Serologic screening with TTG antibody test is highly sensitive and specific for celiac disease and would be the appropriate lab test to order. This patient's history of Down syndrome places him in a high-risk group for development of celiac disease. Other conditions associated with celiac disease include other autoimmune conditions, type 1 diabetes, Turner syndrome, and Williams syndrome.

The anti-endomysium antibody test (EMA) is also used routinely for screening for celiac disease. A serum IgA level is recommended at the time of testing to identify those who are IgA deficient and who would need IgG-based deamidated gliadin. Celiac disease can present in early or late childhood, adolescence, or even adulthood. Gastrointestinal symptoms such as diarrhea, abdominal pain, distension, and bloating are common in the initial presentation of celiac disease. Nongastrointestinal manifestations include decrease in linear growth velocity, delayed onset of puberty, dermatitis herpetiformis rash (Figure 403-1), and dental enamel hypoplasia.

Histopathologic evidence of celiac disease in the small intestine, such as increased intraepithelial lymphocytes and villous blunting (Figure 403-4), is needed to definitively confirm the diagnosis of celiac disease. An esophagogastroduodenoscopy to perform small intestinal biopsy, however, is usually recommended only after screening tests such as TTG and EMA are found to be positive. Although the presence of genetic markers HLA-DQ2 and/or DQ8 is strongly associated with celiac disease, they are also found in 30% of the general population. Therefore, HLA-DQ2/DQ8 testing is usually not useful in the initial screening evaluation for celiac disease. Given this patient's presentation of chronic diarrhea (symptoms lasting longer than 2 weeks), it is unlikely he has an acute viral gastroenteritis, such as *Rotavirus* infection. A sweat chloride test can be obtained in the evaluation of suspected cystic fibrosis (CF), which can also present with poor growth in early childhood, but is usually characterized by steatorrhea, or fatty foul-smelling stools, as well as pulmonary manifestations.

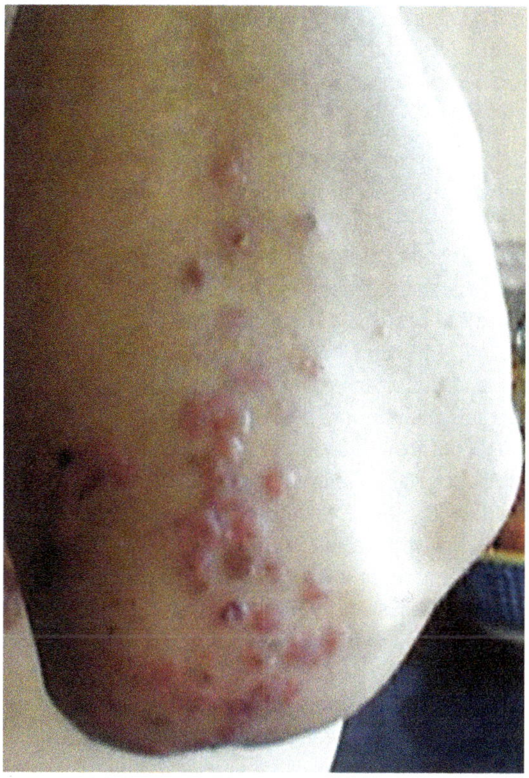

**FIGURE 403-1.** Celiac disease presenting as dermatitis herpetiformis. (Mark W. Kline, *Rudolph's Pediatrics*, 23rd Edition. Copyright © McGraw-Hill Education. All rights reserved.)

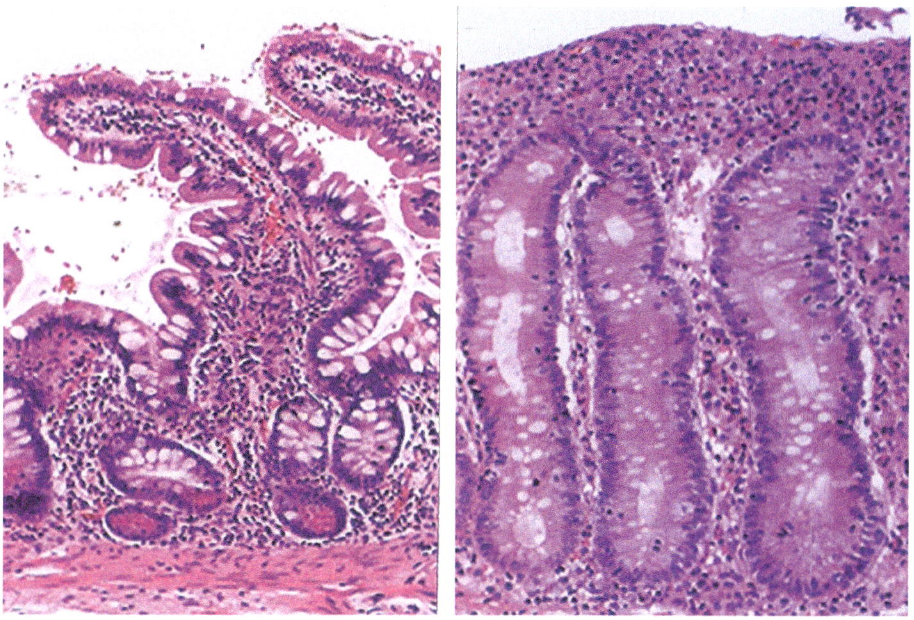

A B

**FIGURE 403-4.** A: Normal small intestinal biopsy. B: Celiac disease showing villous atrophy. (Mark W. Kline, *Rudolph's Pediatrics*, 23rd Edition. Copyright © McGraw-Hill Education. All rights reserved.)

(Section 21: Disorders of the Gastrointestinal System, Chapter 403: Disorders of Digestion and Absorption)

**Answer 20-49.** C

SIBO is characterized by an increased number and/or type of bacteria in the upper gastrointestinal tract. One of the primary mechanisms believed to result in the development of gastrointestinal symptoms such as excessive gas or abdominal distension is metabolism of ingested carbohydrates by intraluminal bacteria. Other processes related to the overgrowth of intestinal bacteria include deconjugation of bile acids leading to secretory diarrhea, fat malabsorption, and direct mucosal injury. The gold standard for diagnosis of bacterial overgrowth is quantitative culture from a jejunal aspirate. A bacterial concentration > $10^5$ organisms/mL fluid is considered diagnostic. A bacterial count of 1000 organisms/mL is considered within normal for the small intestine. A practical alternative to jejunal culture is breath hydrogen analysis. When a patient ingests a test dose of carbohydrate, such as glucose or lactulose, there is an early peak in breath hydrogen level, which corresponds to early metabolism of the carbohydrate by intestinal bacteria. Empiric treatment of SIBO when the index of suspicion is high has been advocated. Antibiotics, such as metronidazole, amoxicillin-clavulanic acid, and trimethoprim-sulfamethoxazole, are the mainstay of therapy. Acid blockade, which results in hypochlorhydria in the stomach, has been associated with increased bacterial counts in the stomach.

(Section 21: Disorders of the Gastrointestinal System, Chapter 403: Disorders of Digestion and Absorption)

**Answer 20-50.** D

Complications associated with short bowel syndrome in children are commonly associated with the use of a central venous catheter as well as total parenteral nutrition. Central line infections are among the most frequent and serious complications. The rate of infection is approximately between 1 and 6 infections per 1000 days of parenteral nutrition and varies with the indication for intravenous nutrition. Ethanol locks of the central line can reduce this risk. Patients who present with fever, jaundice, and lethargy, such as the infant in the vignette, should be evaluated carefully, and blood and site cultures should be obtained. In those with suspected catheter-related infections, empiric antibiotic therapy should be initiated to treat coagulase-negative staphylococci, the most common cause of infections, as well as gram-negative enteric organisms. Because there are limited sites available for placement of central catheters, potential line infections are treated aggressively. However, in some patients who have fungal infection, endocarditis, or persistent positive blood cultures or signs of infection, the central venous catheter must be removed. Thrombotic and thromboembolic catheter problems can also occur. Chronic use of parenteral nutrition can lead to cholestasis and hepatocellular injury that can develop into chronic liver disease and liver failure. Cholelithiasis occurs in 10% to 40% of children receiving parenteral nutrition and is thought to result from stasis and biochemical imbalance in the composition of bile. Jaundice and abdominal pain may occur, but fever and lethargy are unlikely. In some children, cholelithiasis is an incidental finding without symptoms. Cholestasis and bile duct proliferation can often occur in those receiving total parenteral nutrition for > 2 weeks, but life-threatening hepatic cirrhosis rarely presents with acute fulminant hepatic failure. Elevation of serum transaminase and alkaline phosphatase activities without jaundice can result from fatty infiltration of the liver as a result of excessive calories. D-lactic acidosis is another potential complication related to short bowel syndrome, characterized by recurrent episodes of lethargy and ataxia and metabolic acidosis. In this condition, carbohydrates are metabolized by bacterial overgrowth in the colon into D-lactic acid, which then results in recurrent episodes of encephalopathy. Patients usually do not have acute fever.

(Section 21: Disorders of the Gastrointestinal System, Chapter 403: Disorders of Digestion and Absorption)

**Answer 20-51.** E

Given the young age of onset of chronic diarrhea with evidence of villous atrophy on small intestinal biopsy, this clinical scenario is highly suspicious for a congenital enteropathy, such as microvillus inclusion disease. Congenital microvillus inclusion disease is characterized by watery, secretory diarrhea, usually with onset in the first days after birth. Histologically, the small intestine demonstrates diffuse villous atrophy, whereas electron microscopy reveals mucosal surface enterocytes that lack microvilli altogether or show involutions of the apical membrane containing microvilli.

Other conditions that present with early-onset severe diarrhea and evidence of villous atrophy include tufting enteropathy and IPEX syndrome (immune dysregulation, polyendocrinopathy, enteropathy, and X-linkage). Villous atrophy on histologic exam is a nonspecific finding. Although villous atrophy is also classically found in celiac disease, the young age of the patient and lack of exposure to gluten protein in the diet make celiac disease unlikely to be the diagnosis. Patients with CF can present with chronic diarrhea secondary to pancreatic insufficiency, but this patient has had a normal result on sweat chloride testing. Congenital chloride diarrhea and congenital sodium diarrhea are both caused be defects in intestinal transport of electrolytes. They are characterized by large-volume watery stools at the time of birth, which persist even when the infant is given nothing via the enteral route. Both conditions can result in severe dehydration, but congenital chloride diarrhea is associated with metabolic alkalosis, whereas congenital sodium diarrhea is associated with development of metabolic acidosis. Acrodermatitis enteropathica is an autosomal recessive disorder of zinc absorption. Symptoms of zinc deficiency develop in infancy after discontinuation of breastfeeding. Clinical manifestations include dermatitis with bullous and pustular lesions (typically distributed around the mouth), alopecia, diarrhea, and growth retardation. The infant in this clinical vignette is still being breastfed and does not have the characteristic skin findings, which makes acrodermatitis enteropathica unlikely.

(Section 21: Disorders of the Gastrointestinal System, Chapter 403: Disorders of Digestion and Absorption)

**Answer 20-52.** B

Based on the constellation of symptoms of anorexia, loose stools, abdominal pain, weight loss, anemia, hypoalbuminemia, occult blood in stools, and skin tags, the most likely diagnosis is Crohn disease. Presenting symptoms in pediatric Crohn disease include abdominal pain (62%–95%), diarrhea (66%–77%), weight loss (80%–92%), rectal bleeding (14%–60%), growth impairment (30%–33%), perirectal disease (25%), and extraintestinal manifestation (15%–25%). *Giardia* is unlikely given the hemoccult-positive stools, lab abnormalities, and skin tags. Although celiac can result in abdominal pain, anemia, hypoalbuminemia, diarrhea, and weight loss, it would be unusual to have hemoccult-positive stools or skin tags. Anorexia nervosa is unlikely given the other clinical symptoms besides poor appetite and weight loss. Irritable bowel syndrome would not have skin tags, anemia, hypoalbuminemia, weight loss, or hemoccult-positive stools.

(Section 21: Disorders of the Gastrointestinal System, Chapter 405: Inflammatory Bowel Disease)

**Answer 20-53.** A

Side effects of corticosteroids include bone demineralization, adrenal insufficiency, fluid retention, weight gain, striae, acne, fat redistribution, hirsutism, hypertension, hyperglycemia, cataracts, osteonecrosis, myopathy, emotional disturbances, and benign intracranial hypertension. Corticosteroids result in weight gain, not weight loss. They can also result in fat redistribution and muscle mass loss but not muscle redistribution. Corticosteroids can cause leukocytosis, not leukopenia. Corticosteroids do not cause vitamin D deficiency.

(Section 21: Disorders of the Gastrointestinal System, Chapter 405: Inflammatory Bowel Disease)

**Answer 20-54.** D

*Salmonella, Shigella, Campylobacter, Yersinia, E coli* 0157/H7, and *C difficile* can all cause bloody diarrhea and should be excluded before a diagnosis of inflammatory bowel disease can be made. *Giardia* and *Cryptosporidium* can cause chronic diarrhea; however, it is watery and not bloody diarrhea.

(Section 21: Disorders of the Gastrointestinal System, Chapter 405: Inflammatory Bowel Disease)

**Answer 20-55.** B

Peutz-Jeghers syndrome is associated with hamartomas of the small bowel, stomach, and colon. Another characteristic finding is blue-brown macules on the vermillion border of the lips and buccal mucosa. Tuberous sclerosis is associated with hypomelanotic macules of the skin, facial angiofibromas, shagreen patches, and fibrous facial plaques. Neurofibromatosis is associated with café-au-lait spots and freckling of the axilla and inguinal area. There are no unique skin findings for familial adenomatous polyposis syndrome or juvenile polyposis syndrome.

(Section 21: Disorders of the Gastrointestinal System, Chapter 409: Polyps and Tumors of the Gastrointestinal Tract, Hereditary Hamartomatous Polyposis Syndromes)

**Answer 20-56.** E

The patient should begin screening endoscopy by 12 years of age or sooner at the onset of symptoms such as hematochezia, diarrhea, or abdominal pain. If polyps are detected, then patients should undergo yearly screening endoscopies. If the affected family members have been screened for an *APC* gene mutation and none was found, negative genetic testing does not rule out FAP in this patient. The timing of colectomy is determined on a case-by-case basis. It would not be considered in a patient without a diagnosis of FAP. The timing of colectomy is determined based on polyp burden, presence of increasing adenoma dysplasia or adenocarcinoma, and the maturity of the patient. Twenty percent of patients with FAP have no identifiable *APC* gene mutation. Family members still require screening because negative testing does not exclude the possibility of them having FAP.

(Section 21: Disorders of the Gastrointestinal System, Chapter 409: Polyps and Tumors of the Gastrointestinal Tract, Hereditary Hamartomatous Polyposis Syndromes)

**Answer 20-57.** A

Juvenile polyps are a common gastrointestinal disorder. Up to 2% of children under the age of 10 years may have juvenile polyps. JPS is diagnosed when there are 5 or more colonic juvenile polyps, there is a presence of juvenile polyps in the stomach or small intestine, or there is any juvenile polyp and a family history of JPS.

This patient does not meet criteria for JPS; therefore, she is not at increased risk of cancer, nor does she or her family need to undergo yearly surveillance or genetic testing. Patients with JPS may have germline deletions in either *SMAD4* or *BMPR1A*. Once a patient is found to have 5 or more juvenile polyps, genetic testing may prove helpful when counseling family members of their risk. Findings of juvenile polyps do not increase the risk of colorectal cancer; however, the presence of 5 or more polyps suggestive of JPS increases your lifetime risk of colorectal cancer to close to 50%.

(Section 21: Disorders of the Gastrointestinal System, Chapter 409: Polyps and Tumors of the Gastrointestinal Tract, Hereditary Hamartomatous Polyposis Syndrome)

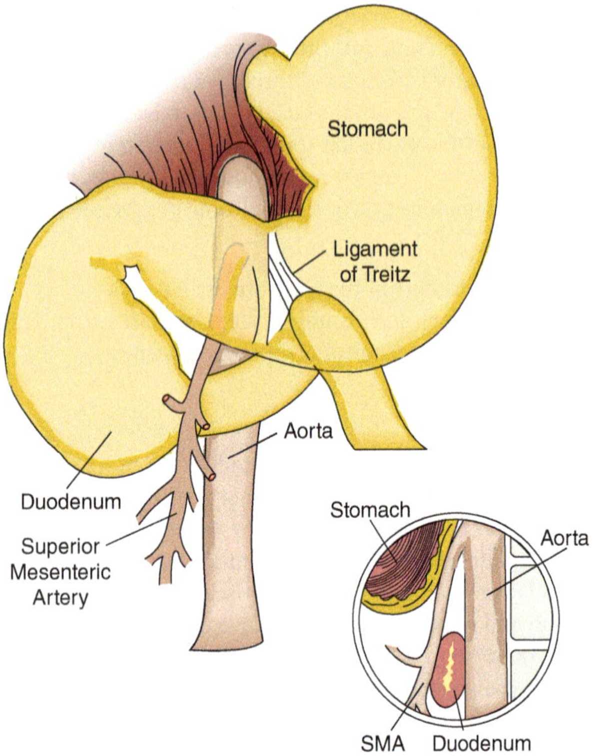


**FIGURE 401-1.** Anterior-posterior and lateral illustration of the anatomic location of the stomach and duodenum in relation to the aorta and the superior mesenteric artery (SMA). (Reproduced, with permission, from Rudolph CD, Rudolph AM, Lister GE, First LR, Gershon AA. *Rudolph's Pediatrics*. 22nd ed. New York: McGraw-Hill, 2011.)

**Answer 20-58.** A

Superior mesenteric artery syndrome (SMAS) is characterized by gastrointestinal obstruction resulting from compression of the duodenum between the abdominal aorta posteriorly and the superior mesenteric artery anteriorly (Figure 401-1).

SMAS is more common in females than males and is associated with acute weight loss. Acute weight loss is thought to result in loss or reduction in size of the anterior mesenteric fat pad, which contributes to the angle between the superior mesenteric artery and the aorta, which is usually between 38 and 65 degrees. In individuals with SMAS, this angle can be significantly reduced. Symptoms of SMAS may be acute or chronic and can include vomiting, nausea, anorexia, abdominal distension, abdominal pain, early satiety, and weight loss. The diagnosis of SMAS is commonly made by upper gastrointestinal contrast radiography, which shows a dilation of the stomach and proximal duodenum, with abrupt cutoff or narrowing of the small bowel at the level of the third vertebra just proximal to the ligament of Treitz. Retrograde peristalsis of contrast is sometimes observed in the proximal dilated segment of small bowel. The diagnosis can also be made by computerized tomography (CT), CT angiography, or magnetic resonance angiography. Treatment of SMAS is primarily aimed at bowel decompression, fluid stabilization, and nutritional support. Small frequent meals may be helpful; in more severe cases, postpyloric feeds with a nasojejunal tube or parenteral nutrition may be necessary.

Crohn disease can also present with nonspecific symptoms of abdominal pain, anorexia, and weight loss. Development of a small bowel stenosis is possible but is usually secondary to chronic inflammation and fibrosis. The patient in this clinical vignette also lacks evidence of systemic inflammation, hypoalbuminemia, and symptoms of diarrhea, which would be more typical in the setting of chronic intestinal inflammation secondary to Crohn disease. Intestinal stenosis and atresia are relatively common congenital anomalies that can affect the duodenum. It would be highly unusual, however, to have a delayed presentation beyond the neonatal period without any other history of intestinal obstruction. CP can present with recurrent episodes of acute pancreatitis or with gradual onset of chronic abdominal pain. Radiographic findings such as calcifications within the pancreas on plain film or CT are suggestive of CP. Obstruction of the duodenum, however, is not a commonly associated finding. Finally, celiac disease is also characterized by involvement of the duodenum resulting in symptoms of abdominal pain and weight loss; however, duodenal inflammation in celiac disease does not typically result in obstruction.

(Section 21: Disorders of the Gastrointestinal System, Chapter 401: Superior Mesenteric Artery Syndrome)

**Answer 20-59.** E

The diagnosis of cow milk protein–induced eosinophilic proctocolitis, also referred to as allergic colitis or cow milk protein hypersensitivity, is made based on the typical symptom presentation and response to removal of the offending antigen. Eosinophilic proctocolitis typically begins at 4 to 12 weeks of age and presents with painless hematochezia mixed with mucus and flecks of blood. Anemia is uncommon at the time of presentation, unless untreated for long periods. The most common protein sensitivities are either to cow milk or soy proteins; therefore, switching to a soy-based formula is not recommended. Maternal restriction of cow milk is effective in > 80% of breastfed cases. In infants with mild symptoms, a cow milk protein hydrolysate or elemental (amino acid) formula should be used for at least 1 month to allow adequate time for mucosal healing. At 1 year, 45% to 50% of infants become fully tolerant to cow milk protein.

Elimination of peanuts and tree nuts from the mother's diet is less likely to result in symptom resolution than elimination of cow milk protein. In patients with typical symptom presentation, further testing is usually not necessary. However, if symptoms persist or do not respond to appropriate dietary management, a full evaluation including hemoglobin, stool cultures, and flexible sigmoidoscopy should be strongly considered.

(Section 21: Disorders of the Gastrointestinal System, Chapter 406: Allergic Gastroenteropathies and Eosinophilic Gastrointestinal Diseases )

**Answer 20-60.** B

The hallmark signs of a nonincarcerated, inguinal hernia on physical examination are a smooth, firm mass in the inguinal region or scrotum that enlarges with increased intra-abdominal pressure (Figure 400-1). The hernia typically reduces spontaneously or can be reduced by gentle, manual pressure along the inguinal canal. In contrast, an incarcerated hernia generally presents with symptoms of irritability, pain in the groin and abdomen, abdominal distension, and vomiting. The mass associated with an incarcerated hernia is usually well defined, tender, and does not reduce. Suppurative lymphadenopathy in the inguinal region can present as a persistent inguinal mass, but skin examination typically reveals a superficial infected lesion with swelling of other affected nodes in the area. Testicular torsion usually presents as a tender, erythematous mass in the groin, with absence of a gonad in the scrotum of the same side.

Inguinal hernias in infants < 1 year of age are unlikely to resolve spontaneously. Due to the high risk of incarceration in the first 6 to 12 months of life, referral to a pediatric surgeon and repair should proceed promptly. In children > 1 year old, the risk of incarceration is less and repair is less urgent. In the case of an incarcerated hernia, failure to treat can lead to strangulation and infarction of the hernia contents. A patient with prolonged history of incarceration (> 12 hours), signs of peritonitis, or small bowel obstruction should not be manually reduced, and surgical consultation should be obtained emergently. Aspiration of a groin mass is discouraged because of the risk of injury to the hernia sac. Ultrasonography can differentiate hernia, hydrocele, and lymphadenitis, as well as identify the presence of testicular torsion. However, as in this case, physical exam generally suggests a diagnosis of inguinal hernia and additional diagnostic studies are not typically required.

(Section 21: Disorders of the Gastrointestinal System, Chapter 400: Abdominal Wall Hernias)

**Answer 20-61.** A

Gastroschisis is a congenital abdominal wall defect through which intraperitoneal contents protrude. The defect typically occurs to the right of the umbilical cord and can range in size from 2 to 5 cm. In contrast, omphalocele is a congenital defect of the midline anterior abdominal wall, where the extruded abdominal organs are covered by a protective membrane.

Intestinal dysmotility is very common in infants with gastroschisis. Many infants have a prolonged ileus after closure of the abdominal wall resulting in delayed achievement of full enteral feeds. In a smaller proportion of gastroschisis infants, intestinal dysmotility can be prolonged for years into childhood. Infants with gastroschisis are also associated with premature delivery, intestinal atresia, and higher risk of developing necrotizing enterocolitis.

Unlike gastroschisis, omphalocele is associated with additional abnormalities, such as structural defects of the heart, kidneys, limbs, and face, in up to 60% of infants. Omphaloceles have been associated with trisomy 13, 14, 15, 18, and 21 as well as other genetic syndromes, such as Beckwith-Wiedemann syndrome. Beckwith-Wiedemann syndrome is associated with macrosomia, macroglossia, hypertrophy of solid organs, and a predisposition for childhood cancers, as well. Unlike gastroschisis, infants born with omphaloceles are relatively protected from heat and fluid loss by the intact membrane covering the viscera and usually do not have impaired gastrointestinal function when the sac remains intact. Omphalocele is associated with variable rotational anomalies of the intestine.

(Section 21: Disorders of the Gastrointestinal System, Chapter 391: Abdominal Wall Defects)

**Answer 20-62.** C

Primary fascial and skin closure of a gastroschisis abdominal wall defect is possible in one-half to two-thirds of infants. Closure of the abdomen may be complicated by abdominal compartment syndrome. After returning the viscera to the abdominal cavity, patients should be monitored for signs of tightness around the viscera. These include evidence of decreased ventilation, loss of pedal pulses, loss of urine output, and discoloration of the intestine. If abdominal compartment syndrome is suspected, immediate evisceration and placement of a protective silo over the intestine are performed. In infants

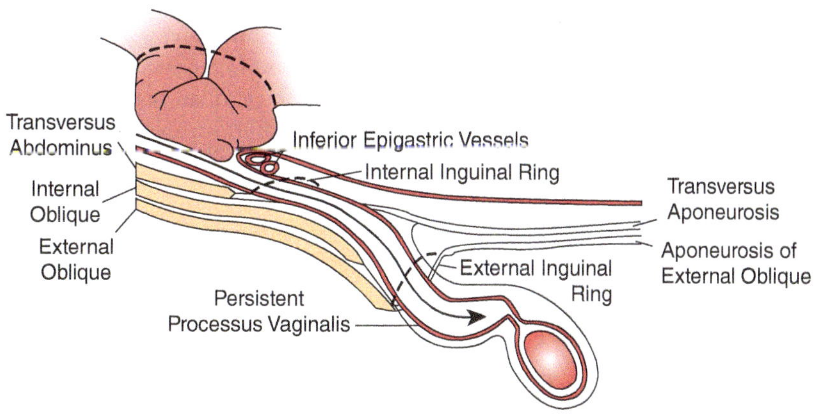


**FIGURE 400-1.** Anatomy of indirect inguinal hernia in boys. (Mark W. Kline, *Rudolph's Pediatrics*, 23rd Edition. Copyright © McGraw-Hill Education. All rights reserved.)

in whom primary closure is not possible, a staged approach may be employed.

Placement of a nasogastric tube for decompression, IV fluid resuscitation, and initiation of antibiotics are all potentially helpful in supporting and stabilizing a patient with abdominal compartment syndrome. However, none of these strategies addresses the underlying problem. Likewise, alterations of ventilator settings and ultrasound evaluation are both inappropriate options in the management of this emergent complication.

(Section 21: Disorders of the Gastrointestinal System, Chapter 391: Abdominal Wall Defects)

**Answer 20-63.** D

With the patient's constellation of signs, including anemia, thrombocytopenia, elevated creatinine, and history of likely infectious colitis, her most likely diagnosis is hemolytic uremic syndrome (HUS). HUS is often preceded by an infection such as *Escherichia coli* 0157:H7, *Shigella*, *Campylobacter*, *Yersinia*, or *Salmonella*. Given her anemia and elevated creatinine, this patient needs to be admitted for supportive care. Although most cases of infectious colitis resolve, given her development of the complication of HUS, it is not appropriate to monitor her as an outpatient.

A course of oral antibiotics will not change the outcome of her HUS and potentially could increase risk for HUS if given during a course of *E coli* 0157:H7, *Shigella*, *Campylobacter*, *Yersinia*, or *Salmonella*. With the patient's symptoms occurring for only 1 week, the history of a sick contact, and now the development of HUS, ulcerative colitis is unlikely.

(Section 21: Disorders of the Gastrointestinal System, Chapter 407: Vascular, Systemic, and Other Disorders Affecting the Gastrointestinal Tract)

**Answer 20-64.** A

This patient is most likely presenting with Henoch-Schönlein purpura (HSP). Approximately 10% of children with HSP and abdominal pain will have intussusception. This patient will need to be evaluated in the emergency department for diagnosis and decompression with a water-soluble enema or surgery.

Her symptoms of abdominal pain and bloody stools could represent malrotation with volvulus; however, the abdominal pain would unlikely come in intermittent waves as it does with intussusception. Also, the purpuric lesions on her legs are not consistent with malrotation with volvulus.

Steroids and ibuprofen can be used in patients with abdominal pain and hemolytic-uremic syndrome; however, this patient is presenting with symptoms suggestive of intussusception, which requires emergent evaluation and treatment to avoid complications.

Given the description of purpuric lesions, an infectious colitis would be much less likely the source of her bloody stools. HSP is a systemic vasculitic disease that results in bowel ischemia, not infection.

(Section 21: Disorders of the Gastrointestinal System, Chapter 407: Vascular, Systemic, and Other Disorders Affecting the Gastrointestinal Tract)

**Answer 20-65.** B

Intestinal duplications are rare congenital anomalies. An enteric duplication is defined by (1) the presence of smooth muscle coat, (2) an intimate association with the alimentary tract, and (3) an inner lining of intestinal epithelium. The treatment for duplication cysts is surgical resection due to the risk of complications such as obstruction and bleeding.

A CT scan may be needed if there is concern that the cyst is involving other organs; however, this test would not determine whether or not surgery is warranted. Duplication cysts are benign lesions and do not require biopsy to determine surgical resection.

(Section 21: Disorders of the Gastrointestinal System, Chapter 396: Duplications and Cysts)

**Answer 20-66.** E

The image shows a complete duodenal obstruction with tapering to the typical "bird's beak" appearance at the site of the volvulus in a patient with malrotation and midgut volvulus. Seventy-five percent of patients with malrotation and midgut volvulus will present in the first week to month of life.

In pyloric stenosis and antral web, the obstruction would be at the gastric outlet and the patient would not present with bilious vomiting. A patient with obstruction due to duodenal or jejunal atresia would not be healthy and tolerating feeds for 3 weeks prior to an acute onset of symptoms as the obstruction is present at birth.

(Section 21: Disorders of the Gastrointestinal System, Chapter 392: Malrotation and Volvulus)

**Answer 20-67.** C

This patient has the classic presentation of appendicitis including fever, anorexia, leukocytosis, and periumbilical abdominal pain evolving to right lower quadrant pain. This patient is also experiencing the Rovsing sign, where palpation of the left lower quadrant results in more pain in the right lower quadrant. A surgical evaluation in the ED is most appropriate to make the diagnosis, administer antibiotics, and obtain surgical intervention.

This patient could have acute infectious gastroenteritis that may be mimicking appendicitis. *Yersinia* is a classic example of this. However, the diagnosis of an infectious gastroenteritis would be considered only after the exclusion of appendicitis. A small bowel obstruction would likely present with bilious vomiting and abdominal distension. Patients presenting with infectious symptoms and right lower quadrant pain may have mesenteric adenitis; however, appendicitis must be ruled out first. Often right lower quadrant lymph nodes are present in the face of a normal-appearing appendix on ultrasound or computed tomography scan imaging. Acute cholecystitis may present with fever, leukocytosis, and pain; however, the pain is typically right upper quadrant in location and character as opposed to a periumbilical pain evolving to a right lower quadrant pain.

(Section 21: Disorders of the Gastrointestinal System, Chapter 408: Acute Appendicitis, Chronic Appendicitis, and Typhlitis)

**Answer 20-68.** A

The most common cause of massive lower gastrointestinal bleeding in children < 4 years of age is a Meckel diverticulum. It is most commonly located 2 feet from the ileocecal valve and presents when the gastric mucosa found in the diverticulum causes ulceration of the adjacent mucosa with subsequent bleeding. The Meckel scan, technetium-99m pertechnetate scintigraphy scan, identifies the gastric mucosa in the diverticulum by concentrating the radiolabeled pertechnetate in gastric epithelium. The test is 85% sensitive after administration of an $H_2$-receptor blocking agent and 95% specific in diagnosing a Meckel diverticulum.

Magnetic resonance imaging is not the imaging of choice to identify Meckel diverticulum. A colonoscopy or upper endoscopy would not be of benefit as the diverticulum is located 2 feet from the ileocecal valve in the small bowel and is not within range of scoping. Given that this patient has no diarrhea, abdominal pain, or fever and has had a significant acute bleeding event, an infectious etiology would be unlikely.

(Section 21: Disorders of the Gastrointestinal System, Chapter 397: Omphalomesenteric Duct Remnants)

**Answer 20-69.** C

The treatment of choice for omphalomesenteric sinuses and cysts is surgical excision, or the patient will continue to experience recurrence of symptoms. Long-term antibiotics are unnecessary given the cyst has drained and the patient has no fever or other signs of infection. Recurrent drainage of the cyst will only treat recurrent symptoms and will not result in resolution of the underlying cyst. Despite the cyst spontaneously draining, the patient is at risk for recurrence of symptoms. Suture placement at the umbilicus opening of the sinus tract will only result in accumulation of fluid with no ability for the cyst to spontaneously drain.

(Section 21: Disorders of the Gastrointestinal System, Chapter 397: Omphalomesenteric Duct Remnants)

**Answer 20-70.** D

A rising total bilirubin in the setting of acute liver failure with loss of hepatic function is an ominous sign that is likely multifactorial in nature. This may be due to reduced hepatic uptake, decreased bile conjugation, and/or decreased biliary excretion as hepatocyte death progresses.

Serum aminotransferase elevation is usually secondary to hepatocellular injury due to inflammation, toxin, or passive congestion, although there are extrahepatic causes of elevated transaminases as well. Aminotransferase levels may remain stable or trend downward even as bilirubin rises as liver failure and hepatocellular death progress, so uptrending AST/ALT levels do not necessarily reflect loss of hepatic function. Hypoglycemia, not hyperglycemia, may occur as hepatic dysfunction progresses due to loss of glycogen stores and gluconeogenesis within the liver. Factor V is a clotting protein synthesized in the liver that, when levels decline to < 10% of normal, may predict fulminant hepatic failure.

(Section 22: Disorders of the Liver and Biliary Tract, Chapter 414: Evaluation of the Infant and Child with Liver Disease)

**Answer 20-71.** E

In a child with cholestasis due to extrahepatic biliary obstruction by gallstones clearly visualized on ultrasound, it is most appropriate to pursue evaluation with ERCP, which not only provides excellent images of the intrahepatic and extrahepatic biliary tree but also allows for endoscopic interventions including stone removal.

CT is useful for 3-dimensional imaging of the hepatobiliary tree but exposes the patient to ionizing radiation and does not offer the therapeutic opportunity that ERCP does. A liver biopsy is useful for evaluation of microscopic hepatic structure and would not be useful for this patient with biliary obstruction of known cause. Percutaneous transhepatic cholangiography allows visualization of the biliary tract by transhepatic injection of contrast into the ductal system and is useful especially for visualization of ducts not accessible by ERCP; it does not offer therapeutic intervention as ERCP does. HIDA scan is useful in evaluating infants with cholestatic liver disease or gallbladder structure and function in older individuals.

(Section 22: Disorders of the Liver and Biliary Tract, Chapter 422: The Biliary Tract)

**Answer 20-72.** D

This patient most likely has type II AIH, which is characterized by positive anti–LKM-1 antibody and/or anti–liver cytosol-1 antibody. Compared with patients with type I AIH, patients with type II AIH tend to present at a younger age and to have a higher incidence of partial IgA deficiency and acute liver failure at presentation (which is suggested by this patient's coagulopathy).

Type I AIH is more common than type II AIH and is characterized by positivity for antinuclear antibody (ANA), anti–smooth muscle antibody (SMA), or anti–F-actin antibodies. Primary sclerosing cholangitis is a disorder resulting in inflammation and obliterative fibrosis of the intrahepatic and extrahepatic bile ducts that may be associated with inflammatory bowel disease in children. Patients with primary sclerosing cholangitis may have a positive ANA, SMA, or LKM-1, which would be suggestive of overlap syndrome, in which AIH and primary sclerosing cholangitis occur together. Patients with lupus may have an elevated ANA titer, which is also seen in patients with AIH, but typically do not present with positive LKM-1 and acute liver failure. Caroli disease is a disease that presents with hyperbilirubinemia that is not associated with positive LKM-1 or IgA deficiency.

(Section 22: Disorders of the Liver and Biliary Tract, Chapter 415: Autoimmune Disorders of the Liver)

**Answer 20-73.** E

Galactosemia is a disorder of carbohydrate metabolism in which early ingestion of galactose, found in breast milk and cow's milk formula, leads to jaundice, lethargy, vomiting, acidosis, cataracts, failure to thrive, and bleeding. Lab abnormalities may include direct hyperbilirubinemia and coagulopathy and urinalysis with reducing substances present but negative glucose on dipstick. Infants with galactosemia commonly present with *Escherichia coli* urinary tract infections or urosepsis, such as in this patient.

Hereditary fructose intolerance is another disorder of carbohydrate metabolism caused by genetic deficiency of fructose-1,6-bisphosphate aldolase. The disease typically presents in infants after they are first exposed to fructose-containing foods (ie, after the introduction of baby food), either with acute onset of vomiting, hypoglycemia, and hypophosphatemia or with subacute development of failure to thrive, irritability, poor feeding, and chronic emesis with eventual development of hepatomegaly, steatosis, jaundice, and ascites. Hereditary tyrosinemia is a protein metabolism disorder characterized by deficiency of an enzyme in the tyrosine degradation pathway that leads to accumulation of toxic metabolites of tyrosine. It may present either acutely in infancy with severe liver dysfunction (jaundice, hepatosplenomegaly, ascites, coagulopathy) or chronically in older children (cirrhosis, renal tubular dysfunction, and rickets). It is not associated with gram-negative rod urinary tract infections. Glycogen storage diseases (GSDs) are disorders of carbohydrate metabolism characterized by the inability to utilize glycogen stores within the liver or other tissues. Glycogen overload causes hepatomegaly in type I and IV GSD; type IV GSD is associated with progressive liver disease that may lead to portal hypertension in early childhood. Both type I and IV GSDs can present with hepatomegaly and hypoglycemia but are not associated with urinary tract infection or acute onset of infantile symptoms.

(Section 22: Disorders of the Liver and Biliary Tract, Chapter 416: Metabolic and Genetic Disorders of the Liver)

**Answer 20-74.** D

The PiZZ phenotype is the most common defect to cause α1-antitrypsin deficiency, a disorder with varying clinical manifestations, including liver and/or lung disease. The PiZZ defect is caused by single amino acid substitution of lysine for glutamate, which leads to misfolding of the protein and retention in the endoplasmic reticulum.

Accumulation of the misfolded protein within the hepatocytes leads to liver injury in patients with α1-antitrypsin deficiency. In addition, patients are at risk for developing lung disease due to an unregulated proteolytic attack on the connective tissue of the lung related to decreased levels of α1-antitrypsin. They are not at risk for developing renal disease.

Giant cell hepatitis is a typical histologic finding in neonates with α1-antitrypsin deficiency; microsteatosis is not a typical finding. Liver transplantation is curative for patients progressing to end-stage liver disease because the recipient assumes the Pi type of the donor organ.

(Section 22: Disorders of the Liver and Biliary Tract, Chapter 416: Metabolic and Genetic Disorders of the Liver)

**Answer 20-75.** D

This infant has jaundice and a conjugated bilirubin level that is > 2 mg/dL or > 15% of the total bilirubin, consistent with a conjugated hyperbilirubinemia.

An abdominal ultrasound is useful to exclude a choledochal cyst or other anatomic abnormalities and should be performed in all infants presenting with conjugated hyperbilirubinemia. A liver biopsy may be performed if other less invasive screening methods do not identify an etiology for the jaundice. ERCP provides detailed imaging of the biliary tree but is invasive and technically difficult in young infants. There are limited data to support its use in the diagnosis of extrahepatic biliary atresia.

Sepsis is a common cause of conjugated hyperbilirubinemia in sick-appearing infants. Because this infant is afebrile and well appearing, the clinical suspicion for sepsis is low. Carotenemia, a condition often seen in children taking a pureed diet containing yellow, carotene-containing vegetables, presents with yellow discoloration of the skin and clear sclera. Infants with carotenemia have normal serum bilirubin levels.

(Section 22: Disorders of the Liver and Biliary Tract, Chapter 414: Evaluation of the Infant and Child with Liver Disease)

**Answer 20-76.** D

Primary sclerosing cholangitis is a chronic condition that results in inflammation and fibrosis of the intrahepatic and extrahepatic bile ducts. This disorder is rare in children. It is most often associated with inflammatory bowel disease, especially ulcerative colitis. The most common presenting symptoms are jaundice, hepatomegaly, and pruritus. Atopic dermatitis and scabies could cause pruritus but would not explain the other findings on physical examination. Allergic reactions to infliximab occur most often during an infusion and may present with symptoms of anaphylaxis. α1-Antitrypsin deficiency is a disorder that results in damage to the liver due to increased deposition of α1-antitrypsin. It may present with jaundice but is not associated with inflammatory bowel disease.

(Section 22: Disorders of the Liver and Biliary Tract, Chapter 415: Autoimmune Disorders of the Liver)

**Answer 20-77.** A

This patient most likely has Wilson disease (hepatolenticular degeneration), an autosomal recessively inherited disorder of copper metabolism. Wilson disease should be considered in any child with an unexplained hepatic, neurologic, or psychiatric illness. Patients with Wilson disease have variable elevation in serum aminotransferase values and in the conjugated and unconjugated serum bilirubin concentrations. Serum alkaline phosphatase levels tend to be normal or even low, but this is not diagnostic of the disease. Serum ceruloplasmin, a protein involved in copper transport, is typically low, although it may also be reduced in other liver diseases. Hepatic copper content remains the gold standard for the diagnosis of Wilson disease. The typical diagnostic concentration is more than 250 μg/g dry weight of liver. Copper toxicity in the kidneys may lead to nephrocalcinosis, hematuria, and aminoaciduria, but urinalysis is not diagnostic of the underlying disorder. Infectious mononucleosis due to Epstein-Barr virus may manifest with fatigue and hepatomegaly but generally does not cause jaundice. This patient has no other signs of infection, and her psychiatric symptoms predate the current illness.

(Section 22: Disorders of the Liver and Biliary Tract, Chapter 416: Metabolic and Genetic Disorders of the Liver)

**Answer 20-78.** B

Nonalcoholic fatty liver disease (NAFLD) is the most common reason for unexplained abnormal liver tests in the pediatric population. Nonalcoholic steatohepatitis (NASH) is a subtype of NAFLD that includes steatosis, ballooning degeneration, and inflammation. NASH-related cirrhosis has been reported in children. The majority of pediatric patients with NAFLD are obese, and many are clinically asymptomatic. Other etiologies of chronic liver disease must be excluded. The diagnosis of NAFLD is a histologic one, and liver biopsy is the gold standard to confirm the diagnosis. Ultrasonography is not completely diagnostic of NAFLD, as it is not sensitive to steatosis < 30%. Lifestyle modification, including dietary changes and exercise, is the mainstay of treatment for NAFLD and NASH.

(Section 22: Disorder of the Liver and Biliary Tract, Chapter 421: Fatty Liver Disease)

**Answer 20-79.** A

This patient most likely has a choledochal cyst, a malformation of the common bile duct that most commonly presents with jaundice and abdominal pain. A combination of jaundice, abdominal pain, and a right upper quadrant mass is also seen in some patients. Patients may also present with fever due to cholangitis, nausea, vomiting, and associated pancreatitis. The etiology of cyst formation is unclear, although there is growing evidence that the dilation results from an anomalous junction of the common bile duct and the pancreatic duct that may allow for the reflux of pancreatic proteases into the extrahepatic biliary tree, resulting in cholangitis and stenosis.

Choledochal cysts are 4 times more likely to occur in females than males, and most present during the first decade of life. These patients may have abnormal serum aminotransferase, bilirubin, and pancreatic enzyme levels. The abnormality is visualized on ultrasound, which is the first-line imaging test. ERCP is reserved for patients with biliary obstruction or in whom an alternative diagnosis is considered. Early treatment is required to prevent hepatic complications including fibrosis. The most worrisome complication of choledochal cyst is the high incidence of associated malignancy. This has led to the recommendation that cysts be completely excised with concurrent removal of the gallbladder.

(Section 22: Disorders of the Liver and Biliary Tract, Chapter 422: The Biliary Tract)

# CHAPTER 21 Nephrology, Fluids, and Electrolytes

Hannah C. Neubauer, Ashley Joshi-Patel, and Stacy B. Pierson

**21-1.** A 4-year-old girl presents to her physician's office with complaints of 1-week history of tea-colored urine and mild edema of the both feet. Current blood pressure is 110/70 mm Hg. Urinalysis is significant for > 10 red blood cells (RBCs)/high-power field (HPF) and 1+ protein. Her mother states that 2 weeks ago she was treated with oral antibiotics for pharyngitis that was associated with abdominal pain and sandpaper-like rash. Subsequent lab workup revealed depressed C3 levels with normal C4 levels, urine protein/creatinine ratio of 1 mg/mg, and lipid levels within normal limits for age. Of the following entities, which is the most likely explanation for this patient's hematuria?

**A.** Immunoglobulin (Ig)-mediated membranoproliferative glomerulonephritis

**B.** Henoch-Schönlein purpura (HSP) nephritis

**C.** Acute poststreptococcal glomerulonephritis

**D.** Infective carditis

**E.** Lupus nephritis

**21-2.** A previously healthy 7-year-old girl presents to the emergency department with a 3-day history of cough, rhinorrhea, and sore throat. Fever, with erythematous rash on bilateral cheeks, started this morning. She was seen by her primary care physician (PCP) 2 days ago and started on penicillin for upper respiratory infection symptoms. Her mother is concerned because she has not had any urine output for 9 hours despite continuing to drink well. She denies any dysuria or myalgia. Based on this history, what urine examination findings are indicative of the underlying cause of her decreased urine output?

**A.** Dipstick – specific gravity of 1.030, no protein or casts seen under microscope

**B.** Dipstick – + blood, no red blood cells (RBCs) seen under microscope

**C.** Dipstick – no protein, 10 RBCs/high-power field (HPF) seen under microscope

**D.** Dipstick – + leukocytes with white blood cell (WBC) casts and eosinophils seen under microscope

**E.** Dipstick – + leukocytes, + nitrites, WBC casts, and bacteria seen under microscope

**21-3.** Which of the following clinical or historical findings is associated with acute kidney injury (AKI)?

**A.** Stunted growth

**B.** Stable elevated blood urea nitrogen (BUN) and creatinine

**C.** Mild anemia

**D.** Small shrunken kidneys

**E.** History of chronic hypertension

**21-4.** Which of the following is a complication of chronic kidney disease?

**A.** Growth impairment

**B.** Mild anemia

**C.** Hypernatremia

**D.** Hypokalemia

**E.** Altered mental status

**21-5.** An 8-year-old boy with Ig-mediated membranoproliferative glomerulonephritis has worsening estimated glomerular filtration rate (eGFR) despite use of systemic steroids. The nephrologist has recommended peritoneal dialysis as the next step in treatment. Prior to committing to peritoneal dialysis, the parents would like to know more about complications of treatment. Of the following clinical findings, which symptoms would be associated with one of the most common complications of peritoneal dialysis?

**A.** Afebrile, diffuse mild abdominal pain with bloody peritoneal fluids
**B.** Fever with rebound and guarding of abdomen
**C.** Nonpurulent fluid drainage from catheter exit site during dialysis
**D.** Respiratory distress with decreased right breath sounds during dialysis
**E.** Soft, nonerythematous, nontender inguinal swelling during dialysis

**21-6.** Chronic dialysis should be considered for initiation in any child with stage 5 chronic kidney disease and/or with which of the following conditions?

**A.** Increasing hypertension responsive to medications
**B.** Uremia controlled with medications
**C.** Serum pH of 7.35
**D.** Pulmonary edema refractory to diuretics
**E.** Tracking along the 10% to 25% weight for age since diagnosis of chronic kidney disease

**21-7.** A previously healthy 6-year-old girl presents to the emergency department (ED) with acute onset of mild bilateral lower extremity edema with no urine output over the past 7 hours. All symptoms were preceded by a 4-day history of bloody diarrhea that was just starting to resolve. Complete blood count (CBC) is significant for hemoglobin of 6.6 g/dL and platelets of $90 \times 10^3/\mu L$ Which of the following additional physical or laboratory findings is associated with the acute cause of this patient's acute kidney injury (AKI)?

**A.** Urine specific gravity > 1.020
**B.** Urine sodium < 20 mEq/L
**C.** Fractional excretion of sodium (FENa) < 1%
**D.** Palpably enlarged bladder
**E.** Urine/plasma creatinine < 20

**21-8.** A 15-year-old healthy girl presents to her primary care physician's office for a sports physical. Other than some muscular soreness from doing resistance training, she has no other complaints at this time. Physical examination is significant for blood pressure of 130/75 mm Hg in the left arm while sitting quietly, using an automated blood pressure measurement device. Height is 62 inches. Of the following actions, which is the next best step in evaluation of this patient?

**A.** Repeat blood pressure measurement in 6 months
**B.** Obtain urinalysis for screening
**C.** Obtain detailed history of over-the-counter medications
**D.** Obtain serum blood urea nitrogen (BUN)/creatinine
**E.** Recheck blood pressure measurement using auscultation

**21-9.** Which of the following is a definite indication for initiating antihypertensive pharmacologic therapy in a child or adolescent?

**A.** Normotensive type 2 diabetes
**B.** Stage 2 hypertension
**C.** Asymptomatic stage 1 primary hypertension
**D.** Persistent stage 1 hypertension despite 4 months of nonpharmacologic therapy
**E.** Prehypertension in child with chronic kidney disease

**21-10.** A 10-year-old boy presents to the clinic with a 4-day history of runny nose, cough, and congestion. During the visit, he also mentions that last night he started having bloody urine. He states that it was bloody this morning also. Urine dipstick in the office shows 4+ blood and 1+ protein. Blood pressure and other vital signs are normal for age. Rest of physical examination is benign. Of the following causes of hematuria, which is most likely the diagnosis for this patient?

**A.** Acute postinfectious glomerulonephritis
**B.** Henoch-Schönlein purpura (HSP)
**C.** IgA nephropathy
**D.** Rapidly progressive glomerulonephritis
**E.** Ig-mediated membranoproliferative glomerulonephritis

**21-11.** A 3-year-old boy presents to the emergency department with a 2-day history of vomiting and diarrhea with decreased oral intake. The father states that he has only had 1 episode of urine output and that was 7 hours ago. Vital signs are significant for a temperature of 98.8°F, pulse of 130 bpm, respiratory rate of 24 breaths/min, and blood pressure of 85/50 mm Hg. Capillary refill is 4 seconds, and skin is cool. A peripheral intravenous (IV) line is placed quickly, and the patient is given a 20 mL/kg normal saline bolus over 1 hour. Pulse is down to 115 bpm after 1 hour, but he still has not had any urine output. Of the following, which would be the next best step in treatment of acute kidney injury (AKI) in this patient?

**A.** Catheterization of the bladder to confirm anuria

**B.** Initiation of continuous renal replacement therapy

**C.** Initiation of diuretics to promote urine output

**D.** Initiation of maintenance IV fluids containing potassium

**E.** Repeat 20 mL/kg normal saline bolus over 60 minutes

**21-12.** Which of the following is the most common complication of hemodialysis?

**A.** Arteriovenous fistula stenosis

**B.** Central venous catheter infection

**C.** Intradialytic hypotension

**D.** Arteriovenous graft thrombosis

**E.** Central line exit site infection

**21-13.** Of the following physical signs, which is more indicative of a postrenal cause of acute kidney injury (AKI)?

**A.** Butterfly rash with joint swelling

**B.** Fever with macular rash

**C.** Palpable purpuric rash on lower extremities

**D.** Palpably enlarged bladder

**E.** Tachycardia with delayed capillary refill

**21-14.** A 3-year-old boy presents to his primary care physician's office with complaints of recurrent episodes of bilateral upper eyelid swelling that has had minimal response to repeated doses of diphenhydramine. On physical examination, he is noted to have mild-moderate pitting edema of the feet and ankles bilaterally. Laboratory evaluation is significant for a spot urine protein-to-creatinine ratio of 2.5 mg/mg, serum albumin of 2.1 g/dL (normal 3.5–5 g/dL), and total cholesterol of 250 mg/dL (normal is < 200 mg/dL). Of the following, which is the most likely diagnosis for this patient?

**A.** Focal segmental glomerulosclerosis

**B.** Ig A nephropathy

**C.** Membranoproliferative glomerulonephritis

**D.** Membranous nephropathy

**E.** Minimal change nephrotic syndrome (MCNS)

**21-15.** A 4-year-old boy presents to the emergency department with acute onset of a papular purpuric rash below his knees bilaterally that was preceded by a 1-week history of recurrent diffuse abdominal pain along with painful swelling of both ankles. Of the following clinical or laboratory findings, which would this patient be most likely to develop in the coming days or weeks?

**A.** Acute kidney injury (AKI) and hematuria with hypertension

**B.** AKI with hemolytic anemia and thrombocytopenia

**C.** Asymptomatic gross hematuria

**D.** Asymptomatic microscopic hematuria

**E.** Proteinuria with edema and hyperlipidemia

**21-16.** Which of the following statements about focal segmental glomerulosclerosis (FSGS) is correct?

**A.** Nephritic syndrome is the most common initial presentation.

**B.** Response to corticosteroid therapy is predictive of prognosis.

**C.** Greater than 50% of patients achieve remission with corticosteroid therapy.

**D.** Kidney biopsy is not needed to make the diagnosis.

**E.** Prognosis for progression to end-stage renal disease (ESRD) is good.

**21-17.** Of the following kidney diseases, which is most likely to be the cause of chronic kidney disease in children?

**A.** Focal segmental glomerulosclerosis (FSGS)

**B.** Hemolytic-uremic syndrome (HUS)

**C.** Lupus nephritis

**D.** Membranous nephropathy

**E.** Posterior urethral valves

**21-18.** Concerning risk factors for progression of chronic kidney disease, which of the following statements is correct?

**A.** Congenital abnormalities of the kidney and urinary tract (CAKUT) are associated with a greater risk of progression to end-stage renal disease (ESRD).

**B.** Pubertal growth spurt is associated with worsening renal function.

**C.** Strict control of hypertension has no effect on progression of kidney function.

**D.** Baseline proteinuria is not predictive of risk of progression.

**E.** Severity of glomerular filtration rate (GFR) at time of diagnosis has minimal effect on risk of progression.

**21-19.** What is the preferred mode of vascular access for hemodialysis in pediatric patients?

**A.** Arteriovenous fistula (AVF)

**B.** Arteriovenous graft

**C.** Percutaneous nontunneled central catheter

**D.** Peripheral intravenous (IV) catheter

**E.** Tunneled central venous catheter

**21-20.** A 4-year-old boy (height of 40 inches) presents to his primary care physician (PCP) for reevaluation of elevated blood pressures. Despite being asymptomatic, on his last 2 previous visits, he has had blood pressure measurements of 115/85 mm Hg and 120/80 mm Hg, both verified by auscultatory measurement. Current blood pressure measurement is 115/80 mm Hg by auscultation. His PCP decides to refer to nephrology and begin workup for stage 1 hypertension. Of the following, which screening test result is most likely to be seen in this patient?

**A.** All screening tests are within normal limits

**B.** 5 to 10 red blood cells (RBCs)/high-power field (HPF) with 3+ protein on dipstick

**C.** Renal mass on ultrasound

**D.** 3+ leukocyte esterase and nitrites on urine dipstick

**E.** Abnormal color Doppler of right renal artery on ultrasound

**21-21.** An 8-year-old girl was diagnosed with asymptomatic stage 1 primary hypertension 7 months ago. Despite therapeutic lifestyle changes, hypertension has continued to persist. Her doctor wants to start pharmacologic therapy. The parents have a lot of questions they want to ask. Which of the following statements is true about pharmacologic therapy in children with hypertension?

**A.** Research has shown that a diuretic agent is the best initial medication for pediatric hypertension.

**B.** Therapy should be initiated with 2 drugs to achieve blood pressure control as soon as possible.

**C.** Poor adherence with medication can be a major contributor to not attaining desired blood pressure goal.

**D.** The goal blood pressure for a school-age child with uncomplicated primary hypertension is < 75th percentile.

**E.** Calcium channel blockers should not be used in children due to their side effect profile in comparison to other agents.

**21-22.** A 9-year-old boy with history of nephrotic syndrome has recently relapsed and was started on systemic corticosteroid 2 weeks ago. This will be his second relapse. He now presents to his pediatrician with acute onset of fever, vomiting, and abdominal pain. Which of the following statements is most likely true for this patient?

**A.** Abdominal pain is due to peritonitis until proven otherwise.

**B.** Avascular necrosis is a common complication due to repeated steroid use.

**C.** Empiric antibiotics should cover gram-positive organisms only.

**D.** Prophylactic penicillin has been shown to decrease the prevalence of pneumococcal peritonitis.

**E.** Use of statins is recommended to help decrease the risk of progression of kidney disease.

**21-23.** On a routine well-child examination, a 9-month-old male infant is found to have hypertension and a left-sided abdominal mass. Urinalysis (UA) reveals hematuria and large (3+) proteinuria. Abdominal imaging reveals a large left renal tumor with local structural destruction and a small right renal tumor, both consistent with Wilms tumor. Given this infant's constellation of findings, which other physical exam finding is most likely to be found?

**A.** Conjunctival telangiectasias

**B.** Cataract

**C.** Deafness

**D.** Nail dysplasia

**E.** Hypospadias with cryptorchidism

**21-24.** A 16-year-old sexually active boy is found to have hematuria on urinalysis (UA). One month later, repeat UA shows 50 to 100 red blood cells, 0 white blood cells, negative protein, and negative nitrites. He fails a vision screen at school and is referred to ophthalmology. When he returns 2 months later, repeat UA continues to show 50 to 100 RBCs. Complete blood count and serum electrolytes are normal. Serum creatinine is 1.3 mg/dL. He reports he was diagnosed with anterior lenticonus by the ophthalmologist. There is no family history of renal failure, hematuria, or deafness. What is the most likely diagnosis?

**A.** Pierson syndrome

**B.** Fechtner syndrome

**C.** Denys-Drash syndrome

**D.** Alport syndrome

**E.** Epstein syndrome

**21-25.** An 8-month-old white female infant is diagnosed with failure to thrive. On examination, there is mild bowing of the lower extremity long bones and widening of the wrist joints. She appears mildly dehydrated with dry mucous membranes and capillary refill of 3 seconds. Her mother reports she is always a vigorous feeder, and she makes > 10 large wet diapers per day. The infant takes a multivitamin and has been formula fed since birth. Radiographs reveal bone findings consistent with rickets. Family history is significant for cystinosis in a maternal uncle. You suspect the infant may have Fanconi syndrome. Which combination of electrolyte abnormalities is most likely to be present in this infant?

**A.** Hyperphosphatemia, hyperkalemia, metabolic alkalosis

**B.** Hypophosphatemia, hyperkalemia, metabolic alkalosis

**C.** Hypophosphatemia, hypokalemia, metabolic acidosis

**D.** Hyperphosphatemia, hypokalemia, metabolic acidosis

**E.** Hypophosphatemia, hypokalemia, metabolic alkalosis

**21-26.** Which of the following statements regarding fetal nephrogenesis and gestational age is correct?

**A.** From 35 to 38 weeks of gestation, new nephrons continue to be formed.

**B.** Nephrogenesis and formation of all nephrons are complete by 32 to 34 weeks of gestation.

**C.** After 34 weeks of gestation, the kidneys remain the same size until birth.

**D.** Branching of the ureteric bud continues until 36 weeks of gestation.

**E.** Renal morphogenesis begins at 12 weeks of gestation.

**21-27.** You are taking care of a 3-day-old newborn male infant born at 39 weeks gestational age. Which of the following statements regarding neonatal renal function is correct?

**A.** Total body water volume in neonates is similar to that in older children.

**B.** In term neonates, plasma creatinine can reflect maternal values for the first 48 hours of life.

**C.** Neonatal urinary concentrating ability is similar to that in older infants.

**D.** Neonates tend to have lower potassium values than older infants.

**E.** Bicarbonate levels in neonates are usually higher than in adults.

**21-28.** A 4-year-old boy with nephrotic syndrome is admitted to the hospital with increased edema noted in the periorbital region, scrotum, and lower extremities. On exam, he is afebrile, heart rate is 130 bpm, blood pressure is 95/52 mm Hg, and respiratory rate is 18 breaths/min. Serum creatinine is 1.2 mg/dL, and albumin is 1.9 g/dL. His weight 2 weeks ago was 16 kg, and weight today is 18 kg. Which of the following best characterizes this patient's fluid status?

**A.** Increased intravascular volume, increased total body volume

**B.** Increased intravascular volume, decreased total body volume

**C.** Decreased intravascular volume, decreased total body volume

**D.** Decreased intravascular volume, stable total body volume

**E.** Decreased intravascular volume, increased total body volume

**21-29.** A 10-year-old girl is diagnosed with Addison disease and is found to have a potassium level of 6.5 mmol/L. Which type of renal tubular acidosis (RTA) is most consistent with this diagnosis?

**A.** Type 4 RTA

**B.** Proximal RTA (type 1)

**C.** Fabry syndrome

**D.** Fanconi syndrome

**E.** Classic distal RTA (type 2)

**21-30.** A 6-month-old female infant presents with 2 days of frequent, large, watery diarrhea. On examination, she appears dehydrated with a sunken fontanelle and dry mucous membranes. Which of the following descriptions of acid-base balance is most consistent with this patient's clinical presentation?

**A.** Increased serum bicarbonate ($HCO_3$) with compensatory decrease in respiratory carbon dioxide ($CO_2$)

**B.** Increased serum $HCO_3$ with compensatory increase in respiratory $CO_2$

**C.** Decreased serum $HCO_3$ with compensatory decrease in respiratory $CO_2$

**D.** Decreased serum $HCO_3$ with compensatory increase in respiratory $CO_2$

**E.** Stable serum $HCO_3$ with compensatory increase in respiratory $CO_2$

**21-31.** A 12-month-old male infant with Bartter syndrome is brought for evaluation due to decreased oral intake and lethargy. His mother reports that the patient was cared for by another family member for the past 3 days and did not receive his regular medications. During the evaluation, you observe the infant drinking 2 oz. of milk. Later you are called back to the patient's room because the patient has a 3-minute generalized tonic-clonic seizure. What is the most appropriate next best step in evaluation?

**A.** Serum sodium and potassium

**B.** Urinalysis (UA)

**C.** Serum phosphate

**D.** Complete blood count (CBC)

**E.** Serum glucose

**21-32.** A 17-year-old boy presents with complaints of muscle pains and brown-colored urine for 1 day. He has been at a summer football camp and lifting weights every day. On examination, he has tenderness to the bilateral upper extremity muscles, with intact distal perfusion and normal pulses. Serum creatinine is 1.2 mg/dL. Which of the following urinalysis (UA) findings are most likely to be found on dipstick and microscopy, respectively?

**A.** 3+ blood, 3+ protein, > 100 white blood cells (WBCs), 0–5 red blood cells (RBCs)

**B.** Negative blood, negative protein, 0–5 WBCs, 0–5 RBCs

**C.** Negative blood, 3+ protein, > 100 WBCs, 0–5 RBCs

**D.** 3+ blood, 1+ protein, 0–5 WBCs, 0–5 RBCs

**E.** 3+ blood, 1+ protein, 0–5 WBCs, > 100 RBCs

**21-33.** A 2-year-old girl presents with failure to thrive and short stature. She is found to have hyperchloremic metabolic acidosis and severe hypokalemia and is diagnosed with distal renal tubular acidosis (RTA). Which of the following would be the appropriate next step in treatment?

**A.** Sodium supplementation

**B.** Furosemide

**C.** Potassium supplementation, then alkali supplementation

**D.** Alkali supplementation

**E.** Calcium supplementation

**21-34.** You are taking care of a 10-day-old neonate born at 30 weeks gestational age, who is receiving total parenteral nutrition. Which of the following statements is true regarding electrolytes and renal function in preterm neonates?

**A.** Sodium requirements are higher (3–5 mEq/kg/d).

**B.** Sodium requirements are lower (1 mEq/kg/d).

**C.** Serum bicarbonate levels are usually high.

**D.** Preterm neonates often require high levels of bicarbonate supplementation.

**E.** Serum creatinine levels reflect maternal levels for the first 48 hours of life.

**21-35.** A 17-year-old boy is newly diagnosed with nephrolithiasis, and his family reports this is his fourth episode in the past 3 years. He is an otherwise healthy, active boy with normal growth, vital signs, and physical exam findings. Serum electrolytes, including calcium and phosphate, are normal. His maternal grandfather had recurrent nephrolithiasis throughout his life for which he took medication, but the family is unsure of his diagnosis. Urinalysis (UA) demonstrates 2+ blood, and on microscopy, hexagonal crystals are seen. What is the most likely diagnosis?

**A.** Adenine phosphoribosyltransferase (APRT) deficiency

**B.** Struvite (magnesium ammonium phosphate) stone

**C.** Distal renal tubular acidosis (RTA)

**D.** Hyperparathyroidism

**E.** Cystinuria

**21-36.** A previously healthy 12-month-old female infant is found to have a left flank mass on routine well-child examination. On imaging, the mass appears as a large cystic nonreniform mass on ultrasonography and is nonfunctional on technetium-99m mercaptoacetyltriglycine (MAG3) radionuclide scanning. The contralateral kidney has normal structure and function on imaging. Voiding cystourethrogram (VCUG) shows no vesicoureteral reflux. What is the most appropriate management of this patient?

**A.** Nephrectomy of the affected kidney

**B.** No special monitoring is required

**C.** Biopsy of the mass

**D.** Renal ultrasound at 6-month intervals

**E.** Repeat VCUG yearly

**21-37.** A 14-year-old boy is diagnosed with peripheral neuropathy and angiokeratoma skin lesions. His maternal grandfather was affected by the same condition, caused by a deficiency of α-galactosidase A. The patient's urinalysis shows 2+ proteinuria and 2+ hematuria, and a renal biopsy is performed. For this patient, what is most likely to be seen on electron microscopy?

**A.** Podocyte foot process effacement

**B.** Diffuse mesangial sclerosis

**C.** Whorls of dense lysosomal inclusions

**D.** Thinning of the glomerular basement membrane

**E.** Moth-eaten appearance of the glomerular basement membrane

**21-38.** An 8-year-old girl complains of polyuria and polydipsia. Urinalysis is significant for 3+ glucose and 1+ ketones. Serum electrolytes are normal, except serum glucose is 285 mg/dL. What is the most likely diagnosis?

**A.** Diabetes insipidus

**B.** Diabetes mellitus

**C.** Renal glucosuria

**D.** Fanconi syndrome

**E.** Glucose-galactose malabsorption (*SGLT1* mutation)

**21-39.** A 15-year-old boy is referred to nephrology for persistent hematuria on urinalysis and was also recently diagnosed with hearing loss affecting the high-frequency wavelengths only. He has no other symptoms. Renal imaging and blood work are obtained. For this patient's most likely diagnosis, which of the following tests should also be performed?

**A.** Ophthalmologic examination

**B.** Echocardiogram

**C.** Brain magnetic resonance imaging (MRI)

**D.** Computed tomography (CT) of the chest, focused on the esophagus

**E.** Dermatologic examination

**21-40.** A 2-year-old boy with normal growth and development presents with hypertension. Serum creatinine is normal, but he is found to have hypokalemic alkalosis. Serum aldosterone level is low. The boy's father has a kidney condition for which he is on a low-sodium diet. Of the following, which is the most likely diagnosis?

**A.** Adrenal hyperplasia

**B.** Fanconi syndrome

**C.** Gitelman syndrome

**D.** Liddle syndrome

**E.** Bartter syndrome

**21-41.** A 13-year-old girl with minimal change disease is admitted to the hospital for intravenous (IV) albumin and furosemide therapy and monitoring of acute kidney injury (AKI). On hospital day 3, she develops a mildly tender area of edema and erythema of the left thigh, although it is not well circumscribed. Bilateral distal pulses are intact, and bilateral ankles and calves have symmetric mild edema. Vital signs are stable, and she is afebrile. What is the next appropriate step in management?

**A.** Urine pregnancy test

**B.** Blood culture

**C.** IV antibiotics for skin infection

**D.** Additional IV furosemide dose

**E.** Ultrasound with Doppler

**21-42.** Which location in the kidney is responsible for absorption of most of the filtered bicarbonate and all of the filtered glucose?

**A.** Collecting duct

**B.** Proximal tubule

**C.** Distal tubule

**D.** Descending loop of Henle

**E.** Thick ascending limb of loop of Henle

**21-43.** During nephrogenesis and development of the glomerulus, mutations of proteins that form the slit diaphragm between podocytes (eg, podocin or nephrin) would likely result in which of the following clinical scenarios?

**A.** A 16-year-old obese boy with hypertension

**B.** A 5-year-old boy with gross hematuria and fever

**C.** A 3-week-old female infant with anasarca

**D.** A 2-year-old boy with hypospadias and bilateral renal tumors

**E.** A 14-year-old girl with facial rash, hematuria, and proteinuria

**21-44.** A 15-year-old boy with chronic renal failure presents to the emergency department with altered mental status after receiving hemodialysis. Which of the following is the correct cellular etiology for his altered mental status?

**A.** Elevated brain urea causes water to move into the brain, leading to elevated intracranial pressure.

**B.** Plasma sodium (Na) levels increase causing intracellular fluid (ICF) hypernatremia and free water to move across the blood-brain barrier.

**C.** Plasma potassium (K) levels decrease, causing a change in atrial natriuretic peptide (ANP), which causes brain edema.

**D.** Damage to the blood-brain barrier occurs during hemodialysis, causing decreased ICF and hypernatremia.

**E.** ANP is secreted in response to hypovolemia after dialysis resulting in decreased water excretion in the brain.

**21-45.** A 5-year-old previously healthy boy who weighs 20 kg presents to the emergency department with 2 days of nausea and vomiting. He has had normal urine output but appears mildly dehydrated. Serum electrolytes are normal. He is given 20 mL/kg of normal saline (NS) with improvement in his dehydration. What is the appropriate maintenance fluid and rate for this patient?

**A.** D5 ½ NS + 2 mEq KCl/L at 60 mL/h

**B.** D5NS + 2 mEq KCl/L at 60 mL/h

**C.** D5 ¼ NS + 2 mEq KCl/L at 60 mL/h

**D.** D5NS + 1 mEq KCl/L at 30 mL/h

**E.** D5NS at 60 mL/h

**21-46.** You are examining a 14-year-old boy with a history of frequent urinary tract infections (UTIs) in the emergency department for respiratory distress. The mother reports they have missed many appointments with their primary doctor due to lack of insurance. Once you stabilize the patient, you notice that he is persistently hypertensive and suspect he has renal disease related to his UTIs. What imaging modality will best assess renal function in this patient?

**A.** Ultrasound

**B.** Computed tomography (CT)

**C.** Technetium-99m mercaptoacetyltriglycine (MAG3)

**D.** Voiding cystourethrogram (VCUG)

**E.** Renal arteriography

**21-47.** You are examining a 10-year-old girl in your office for a well-child exam. Patient reports dysuria and denies sexual activity when interviewed privately. Her exam is unremarkable, and she is Tanner stage 1. A urinalysis (UA) is performed; specific gravity is 1.015, nitrites and leukocyte esterase are negative, and there is trace blood. On further discussion with the patient and her mother, you learn that she has had occasional clots of blood in her urine in the past that have not bothered her. Family history is positive for maternal grandfather with renal stones. Which of the following would be the most appropriate next step in management of this patient?

**A.** Provide reassurance; no further workup indicated

**B.** Obtain urine calcium-to-creatinine (Ca/Cr) ratio

**C.** Obtain renal ultrasound

**D.** Obtain sexually transmitted infection (STI) testing

**E.** Refer to nephrologist

**21-48.** You are examining a 3-year-old boy with right multicystic dysplastic kidney (MCDK) in your clinic for the first time. The patient has been lost to follow-up and returns for the first time since he was 3 months old. What is the appropriate management for this patient with MCDK?

**A.** Immediate referral to nephrologist for nephrectomy

**B.** Genetic testing to determine the etiology of MCDK

**C.** Voiding cystourethrogram (VCUG) to assess for vesicoureteral reflux

**D.** Yearly renal ultrasound

**E.** No further screening labs or imaging

**21-49.** You are rounding on a patient in the neonatal intensive care unit who was born at 34 weeks' gestation due to maternal preeclampsia. On further discussion with the mother, you learn that this is the mom's first child and the mother had oligohydramnios with "abnormal renal imaging." Due to the abnormal renal imaging, both parents themselves had renal images and were normal per mother. On physical examination, you note the infant has low-set ears, a flat nose, and a retracted chin. What potential complications should you educate the family about given their infant's diagnosis?

**A.** Obesity

**B.** Bilateral deafness

**C.** Growth retardation

**D.** Pulmonary fibrosis

**E.** Cardiomegaly

**21-50.** Which of the following is a true statement regarding acute kidney injury (AKI)?

**A.** AKI is a sudden event (within 72 hours) of decreased kidney function that causes an increase in serum creatinine by > 0.3 mg/dL or an increase of > 50% from baseline or oliguria of < 0.5 mL/kg/h for > 12 hours.

**B.** In functional (prerenal) AKI, the renal compensatory mechanisms include dilation of the afferent arterioles along with constriction of the efferent arterioles, leading to an increase in glomerular filtration rate (GFR).

**C.** During initial treatment of functional AKI, protein intake should be limited due to decreased GFR and risk of intrinsic AKI requiring renal replacement therapy.

**D.** In a patient with oliguria and increased serum creatinine for 24 hours due to decreased perfusion, the first step in treatment is high-dose furosemide in order to assess the function of the kidneys.

**E.** In AKI, the decreased circulatory volume leads to activation of the sympathetic nervous system and renin-angiotensin system, causing renal vasodilation and decreased GFR.

**21-51.** You are seeing a 4-year-old boy in your office who you diagnosed with Henoch-Schönlein purpura (HSP). The nurse reports his blood pressure is 90/55 mm Hg, temperature is 99.2°F, and heart rate is 102 bpm. He has continued to gain weight throughout his illness. On exam, he looks well, but you appreciate palpable purpura to his lower thighs and calf. There is no reproducible abdominal pain, and his abdomen is soft. He is able to ambulate but appears to have discomfort in his knees and hips, although he has full range of motion. His urinalysis (UA) shows a specific gravity of 1.012, negative nitrites, negative leukocyte esterase, 3+ protein, and positive red blood cells (RBCs). Based on this patient's clinical course and diagnosis, what recommendations would you make?

**A.** Given this patient's proteinuria, it is important to start steroid therapy daily at 2 mg/kg for 2 to 4 weeks to prevent nephropathy.

**B.** This patient needs admission to the hospital for a renal ultrasound to determine the stage of nephritis and initiation of steroid therapy.

**C.** Close monitoring of renal function and careful use of nonsteroidal anti-inflammatory drugs (NSAIDs) for arthralgia are warranted.

**D.** Complement and IgA levels are necessary to determine the severity of this patient's HSP and renal involvement.

**E.** The majority of patients with self-limiting HSP will develop hypertension over the course of their lifetime, so it is important to initiate antihypertensives within 5 years of diagnosis.

**21-52.** You are seeing a 6-year-old girl in the emergency department (ED) who presents with increased fatigue, polyuria, polydipsia, and weight loss for the past month. Her mother noticed that today she was paler appearing and unable to eat, which prompted her to come to the ED. On exam, she is awake and alert but appears tired and pale. She is very thin and slightly tachycardic but otherwise has an unremarkable physical exam. Initial labs show blood pH of 7.21, serum bicarbonate of 15 mEq/L, sodium of 130 mEq/L, potassium of 7.0 mEq/L, chloride of 100 mEq/L, and glucose of 300 mg/dL. Which of the following is a correct statement about this patient's laboratory results?

**A.** The persistent hyperglycemia causes damage to the Na-K-ATPase pumps in the distal nephron of the kidney, which impacts potassium excretion and causes hyperkalemia.

**B.** Low serum osmolarity drives water from intracellular to extracellular space causing a dilutional hyponatremia.

**C.** Metabolic acidosis is caused by decreased plasma concentration of the acetoacetate and $\beta$-hydroxybutyrate.

**D.** High anion gap is due to the abundance of glucose in the plasma.

**E.** Potassium shifts out of cells when plasma pH is low, causing hyperkalemia; however, the total body potassium is low due to glucose-induced diuresis.

**21-53.** You are seeing a 5-year-old girl who presents to your office with complaints of dysuria, increased urine frequency, and nausea. You are concerned she may have a urinary tract infection (UTI). Mother reports she has never had a UTI in the past, and past medical history is only significant for stable seizure disorder on phenytoin. When obtaining the urine, you notice it is yellow-orange in color and send it for a complete urinalysis (UA). Which of the following statements is correct about urine, urine collection, and testing?

**A.** The yellow-orange urine color is concerning for alkaptonuria, which can lead to chronic renal failure if not treated within the first 5 years of life.

**B.** First morning void is more accurate for testing urine pH in this patient and should be > 8.

**C.** Sensitivity of nitrite dipstick for detecting bacteriuria is highly reliable for UTI if tested within 30 to 60 minutes of collection.

**D.** Hyaline casts and pyuria are pathognomonic of UTI on a UA and warrant initiation of antibiotic therapy.

**E.** Bacteria can resemble urates and phosphates in the UA, so urine culture and UA results should both be analyzed before diagnosing a UTI.

**21-54.** You are teaching medical students about various causes of proteinuria and begin discussing orthostatic proteinuria. Which of the following is an accurate statement about orthostatic proteinuria?

**A.** Dipstick testing of proteinuria has a low false-negative rate, so once it is confirmed that the upright urine has more protein than the recumbent urine, no further testing is indicated.

**B.** The most precise way of measuring for orthostatic proteinuria is to measure the urine protein/creatinine ratio in both the recumbent and upright urine samples.

**C.** Orthostatic proteinuria is associated with hypertension in adulthood, so yearly monitoring is recommended.

**D.** Orthostatic proteinuria should not persist past 2 weeks and warrants further workup including renal function, blood pressure, and complement levels if not resolved within 2 consecutive urine checks.

**E.** Orthostatic proteinuria is the most common cause of proteinuria and can be seen in patients with emotional distress and cold exposure.

**21-55.** You are rounding in the newborn nursery on a 2-day-old former term, previously healthy male infant. The mother reports he has been feeding well, but she is worried because he has only had 1 wet diaper in the past 6 hours, but several since birth. On exam, he is well appearing and alert, and the anterior fontanelle is open and flat. He has moist mucous membranes. His abdomen is soft and nondistended. You obtain the following laboratory values: sodium 141 mEq/L, potassium 3.5 mEq/L, chloride 101 mEq/L, blood urea nitrogen (BUN) 5 mg/dL, creatinine 1.2 mg/dL, magnesium 1.7 mEq/L, and phosphorous 4.0 mg/dL. Which of the following is the next best step in management for this newborn?

**A.** Reassurance, frequent feeding, and monitoring of urine output are appropriate management for this patient.

**B.** Patient needs to be transferred to the neonatal intensive care unit for acute renal failure and oliguria, which warrant further workup and close observation.

**C.** Obtain a more thorough history on the mother's prenatal course and obtain genetic testing to rule out the cause of acute renal failure.

**D.** Collect urine for 24 hours to determine the creatinine clearance for this patient and to more accurately assess renal function.

**E.** Renal ultrasound is indicated to determine the cause of acute renal failure.

**21-56.** You are evaluating a 14-year-old boy who was sent to the emergency department from his primary care physician for concern of lower extremity swelling. Mother denies past medical history, hospitalizations, or recent illness. Exam is only remarkable for 1+ edema to bilateral lower extremities. You are concerned about a primary nephrotic syndrome and obtain lab results. Which laboratory results would be consistent with this diagnosis?

**A.** Microscopic hematuria, elevated proteinuria, elevated antistreptococcal antibody titers, and low complement level

**B.** Normal antistreptococcal antibody titers, normal serum complement, microscopic hematuria, and elevated proteinuria

**C.** Normal antistreptococcal antibody titers, gross hematuria, no proteinuria, and low serum complement levels

**D.** Microscopic hematuria, elevated proteinuria, elevated serum complement level, and elevated antistreptococcal antibody titers

**E.** Normal antistreptococcal antibody titers, normal serum complement levels, no proteinuria, and no microscopic hematuria

**21-57.** You are seeing a 6-year-old girl who presents to your office with her mother for concerns of nocturnal enuresis. The mother reports she has achieved daytime dryness since age 4 but continues to have "accidents" at night. What advice would you provide the mother regarding her daughter's nocturnal enuresis?

**A.** The majority of patients with nocturnal enuresis have organic and functional disease, and the patient needs to have more workup done including a urinalysis (UA) and fasting blood work.

**B.** The best treatment for nocturnal diuresis is desmopressin (DDAVP®) because the relapse rate is so low once the medication is stopped.

**C.** Over time, the patient's nocturnal enuresis will improve as the central ability to inhibit bladder contractions while sleeping improves.

**D.** Limiting fluid intake in the evening has not been shown to change the rate of nocturnal enuresis among healthy patients.

**E.** Most patients with nocturnal enuresis have low urine formation during sleep; however, they have a problem with sleep arousal, which causes bed-wetting.

**21-58.** You are rounding on a 3-day-old, former term, healthy male infant born to a 28-year-old mother with an uncomplicated pregnancy. The nurses report the patient has only had 10 mL of urine since birth despite feeding 30 mL every 3 hours. On exam, the infant is alert, and the anterior fontanelle is soft and flat, not sunken. Moist mucous membranes are present, and regular rate and rhythm are present on the cardiac exam. Abdomen is soft and nondistended, and bladder is not palpable. The patient is uncircumcised with bilateral descended testicles. Based on this patient's history and physical exam, what is the likely etiology of his oliguria?

**A.** Dehydration

**B.** Glomerulonephritis

**C.** Tubulointerstitial nephritis

**D.** Abnormal or absent kidney

**E.** Acute tubular necrosis

**21-59.** You are counseling a mother who is 26 weeks pregnant with her first male child. Her past medical history is significant for severe hypertension, and she has been taking an angiotensin-converting enzyme (ACE) inhibitor under the supervision of her obstetrician. What renal abnormality can be seen in infants born to mothers using ACE inhibitors?

**A.** Renal insufficiency

**B.** Paucity of differentiated proximal tubules

**C.** Renal hypoplasia and cyst formation

**D.** Posterior urethral valves

**E.** Multicystic dysplastic kidneys (MCDKs)

**21-60.** You are seeing a 15-month-old female infant who is new to your clinic and has had limited medical care. Her mother says she was diagnosed with multicystic dysplastic kidney (MCDK) in utero without subsequent follow-up due to lack of funding. Which of the following is the most important first step in caring for this patient with MCDK?

**A.** Refer to oncology to assess for renal cell carcinoma

**B.** Immediate nephrectomy to preserve function of the contralateral kidney

**C.** Begin metoprolol daily to prevent hypertension

**D.** Obtain voiding cysto-urethrogram to assess for vesicoureteral reflux

**E.** Renal ultrasound to measure the size of the dysplastic kidney

**21-61.** You are called to attend the delivery of a male infant with a prenatal diagnosis of a horseshoe kidney. Which of the following malformations may also be noted on your physical exam?

**A.** Developmental dysplasia of the hip (DDH)

**B.** Polydactyly

**C.** Gastroschisis

**D.** Preauricular tags

**E.** Micropenis

**21-62.** You are evaluating a 14-year-old boy with a history of autosomal dominant polycystic kidney disease (ADPKD) in the emergency department (ED) who presents with a headache and blurry vision. Per his parents, he was in his normal state of health and does not have any other chronic medical conditions. His mother also has ADPKD and is now requiring dialysis, but the remainder of the family history is unremarkable. He does not take medications and is a straight A student. His exam is significant for headache localized to frontal lobe and bilaterally dilated pupils with intermittent double vision. His abdomen is soft and tender throughout without peritoneal signs, and he reports nausea. He is dizzy when asked to stand but able to ambulate throughout the room with assistance. Given this patient's history and physical exam, what is the next step in management?

**A.** Fluid resuscitation with normal saline (NS) bolus

**B.** Stat laboratory work to evaluate blood urea nitrogen (BUN) and creatinine

**C.** Computed tomography (CT) of the head

**D.** Complete abdominal ultrasound

**E.** Consult nephrology to assist in starting peritoneal dialysis

**21-63.** A 3-year-old boy is following up in your office for minimal change nephrotic syndrome (MCNS) secondary to severe varicella infection. The parents appear worried about his prognosis. Which of the following statements is true regarding MCNS?

**A.** MCNS is the most severe form of nephrotic syndrome because of the lack of response to steroids.

**B.** MCNS is an antibody-mediated disease and is associated with insulin-dependent diabetes mellitus.

**C.** Patients with MCNS are at risk for hyperthyroidism due to the loss of free and protein-bound thyroid hormone.

**D.** MCNS responds well to steroid therapy and has an excellent long-term prognosis.

**E.** MCNS treatment with immune modulators has been proven to decrease the relapse rate.

**21-64.** You are seeing a 14-year-old boy for the first time for a well-child exam. On exam, you notice the patient is obese, has extra digits on both hands, and is delayed to the level of an 8 years old. During his vision exam, it is determined that he is unable to see anything in his periphery. His mother reports he has had "kidney problems" but is unsure of any further details. What syndrome does this patient have?

**A.** Meckel-Gruber syndrome

**B.** Bardet-Biedl syndrome

**C.** Pierson syndrome

**D.** Frasier syndrome

**E.** Finnish syndrome

## ANSWERS

**Answer 21-1.** C

Acute poststreptococcal glomerulonephritis is the most common acute postinfectious glomerulonephritis. A disease primarily of school-age children, it has been shown to follow infection with specific strains of group A β-hemolytic *Streptococcus* despite appropriate antibiotic treatment. Symptoms of hematuria, edema, and hypertension usually start abruptly about 1 to 2 weeks after having pharyngitis. Symptoms begin to spontaneously improve within a week of onset, with edema and hypertension resolving within 2 to 3 weeks. Urine abnormalities may take several months to years to resolve. Classic laboratory findings include low C3 levels with normal C4 levels. C3 levels usually return to normal within 12 weeks after initial symptoms. Diagnosis is confirmed when the patient has the classic complement findings, combined with a positive streptozyme assay or DNase B.

All of the other choices can cause hematuria or glomerulonephritis but have differences in complement levels. Lupus nephritis and infective carditis usually have low C3 and C4. Ig-mediated membranoproliferative glomerulonephritis is an immune complex–mediated glomerular disease that often follows an acute illness but usually presents with nephrotic syndrome (proteinuria, hypoalbuminemia, and hyperlipidemia) and low C4 levels. HSP presents as a tetrad consisting of papular purpuric rash, abdominal pain, arthralgia, and microscopic hematuria and usually has normal complement levels.

(Chapter 468: Glomerular Diseases)

**Answer 21-2.** D

The 7-year-old patient has acute kidney injury (AKI) as defined by oliguria of < 0.5 mL/kg/h for > 6 hours. Evaluation of a child with AKI starts with a thorough history and physical, followed by careful examination of the urine, which may yield some clues to etiology of the kidney injury. The history of penicillin use is the most important historical revelation because allergic reaction to antibiotics is known to be one of the most frequent causes of acute interstitial nephritis. In turn, acute interstitial nephritis is one of the more common causes of AKI in children. Of the urine examination results given, positive leukocytes with WBC casts and eosinophils seen on microscopic examination are indicative of acute interstitial nephritis; thus, it is the correct choice for this patient. The other choices show typical urine examination findings for other causes of AKI, including hypoperfusion due to hypovolemia (answer choice A), myoglobinuria due to rhabdomyolysis (answer choice B), microscopic hematuria due to lupus nephritis (answer choice C), and classic urine examination findings of pyelonephritis.

(Chapter 467: Acute Kidney Injury)

**Answer 21-3.** C

When a child presents with signs and/or symptoms significant for renal dysfunction, it is important to be able to distinguish AKI from chronic kidney disease because of differences in timing and goals of interventions. In many cases of AKI, prompt treatment of the etiology can result in a return of normal renal function with the main goal being prevention of progression to chronic kidney disease. In comparison, patients with chronic kidney disease have (or will have) renal function monitored over a longer period of time with specific interventions initiated to slow down the progression of their kidney failure and to prevent complications of chronic kidney disease. Clinical or historical features of a child with kidney dysfunction due to AKI may include normal growth, progressive rise in BUN and creatinine, mild anemia, normal or enlarged kidneys, and having a recognizable etiology of AKI.

(Chapter 467: Acute Kidney Injury)

**Answer 21-4.** A

The main goals of the multiple interventions performed on a child with chronic kidney disease are to (1) slow down the progression of disease to eventual end-stage renal disease (ESRD) and (2) prevent complications of chronic kidney disease. Anticipated complications of chronic kidney disease are listed in Table 473-2. Severity and frequency of complications usually increase as the stage of chronic kidney disease increases.

Of the choices presented, growth impairment is a known complication of chronic kidney disease. Fortunately, with appropriate treatment, a normal growth pattern can be reestablished if there is a history of poor growth in the initial stages of chronic kidney disease. Additional treatment with growth hormone is recommended; however, only 1 in 4 children with poor growth and chronic kidney disease are prescribed growth hormone.

(Chapter 473: Chronic Kidney Disease)

**Answer 21-5.** B

Peritoneal dialysis is the preferred mode of dialysis in children < 9 years of age if or when the decision is made to move forward with dialysis. The most common complications of peritoneal dialysis include peritonitis and infection of the catheter exit site. Peritonitis can present as fever with rebound and guarding of the abdomen, whereas catheter exit site infection can present as purulent drainage with erythema, swelling, and/or tenderness around the site.

Noninfectious complications of peritoneal dialysis are less frequent but do occur. These complications include hemoperitoneum, dialysate leaks, hydrothorax, and hernia. Hemoperitoneum can present with mild abdominal pain and bloody peritoneal fluid. Dialysate leaks often occur during the early postoperative period of catheter placement, indicating that the surgical site has not had time to heal adequately. Hydrothorax is caused by leakage of dialysate into the pleural cavity, leading to respiratory issues during dialysis. Finally,

**TABLE 473-2.** Complications of Chronic Kidney Disease (CKD) in Children

| Complication | Management Approach |
|---|---|
| Nutritional disorders | Monitor anthropomorphic data; renal dietician input often needed; optimize caloric intake; no restriction of protein in children with CKD; restrict phosphate, potassium, sodium, and renal solute load diet as required; consider supplemental feeds to ensure appropriate weight gain |
| Growth impairment | Ensure adequate nutrition; treat acidosis and sodium depletion; address mineral bone disorders; consider growth hormone therapy |
| Chronic kidney disease mineral bone disorder | Ensure maintenance of calcium, phosphate, calcium × phosphate product, and parathyroid hormone (PTH); if plasma 25-OH-vitamin D is low, supplement with Calciferol (cholecalciferol 400–800 U/d); correct metabolic acidosis with oral sodium bicarbonate or sodium citrate supplements; consider activated vitamin D analogs (calcitriol) if the calcium level is low and the PTH exceeds the recommended limits; if plasma phosphate is elevated, restrict dietary phosphate and, if ineffective, give phosphate binders |
| Neurocognitive delay, reduced quality of life | Encourage school attendance; recognize importance of daytime fatigue and sleep disturbances; anticipatory counseling of children and parents |
| Anemia | Parenteral erythropoietin (EPO) once or twice weekly or darbepoetin weekly or biweekly; doses are higher in children than adults when corrected for weight; iron supplementation—oral iron 3–6 mg/kg/d, elemental iron twice or three times a day; intravenous iron available in refractory cases |
| Hypertension | Start treatment if blood pressure > 90th percentile for age, gender, and height; treat hypertension with pharmacologic agents to attain blood pressure < 50th percentile for age, gender, and height; preferred agent is angiotensin-converting enzyme inhibitor or angiotensin receptor blockade |
| Hyperlipidemia | Therapeutic lifestyle modifications |
| Metabolic acidosis | Supplemental bicarbonate or citrate solutions |
| Hyponatremia | Salt supplementation, if ensured it is not dilutional hyponatremia |
| Hyperkalemia | Dietary potassium restriction, potassium-binding resins such as Kayexalate or calcium resonium |
| Hypophosphatemia | Phosphate supplementation |
| Hyperphosphatemia | Diet restriction and phosphate binders |

Mark W. Kline, *Rudolph's Pediatrics*, 23rd Edition. Copyright © McGraw-Hill Education. All rights reserved.

leakage of dialysate into the abdominal wall, or inguinal area in infant boys, can lead to development of hernia during dialysis.

(Chapter 474: Treatment of End-Stage Renal Disease: Chronic Dialysis and Renal Transplantation)

**Answer 21-6.** D

There is no absolute indication for the initiation of chronic dialysis using a specific blood urea nitrogen (BUN) or creatinine value cutoff point. In most cases, the decision to start chronic dialysis is made after careful and thoughtful consideration of the patient's clinical condition, laboratory data, and any psychosocial issues. However, there are some relative indications for initiation of chronic dialysis at any stage of chronic kidney disease. These indications include uncontrolled hypertension, volume overload (or signs of volume overload like pulmonary edema) refractory to medical treatment, metabolic issues (acidosis, hyperkalemia, hyperphosphatemia), poor growth, or uremia (or complications of uremia) unresponsive to medical therapy or dietary modification.

(Chapter 474: Treatment of End-Stage Renal Disease: Chronic Dialysis and Renal Transplantation)

**Answer 21-7.** E

The patient in this vignette has historical, physical, and laboratory findings consistent with Shiga toxin–producing *Escherichia coli*–associated (STEC+) hemolytic-uremic syndrome (HUS). HUS is the most common glomerular cause of severe AKI in previously healthy children. Shiga toxin damages glomerular endothelial cells, which induces a thrombotic microangiopathic reaction that ultimately culminates into a hemolytic anemia, thrombocytopenia, and AKI. Because injury occurs at the glomerular level, further laboratory evaluation should be consistent with an intrinsic (renal) cause for the AKI. Additional laboratory values that are consistent with an intrinsic cause of AKI include urine specific gravity $< 1.012$, urine/plasma creatinine $< 20$, urine sodium $> 40$ mEq/L, and FENa $> 2\%$. A palpably enlarged bladder is associated with a postrenal cause of AKI.

(Chapter 467: Acute Kidney Injury)

**Answer 21-8.** E

It is recommended that all children get their blood pressure measured with each medical encounter starting at age 3 years. Regular measurement of blood pressures can lead to earlier detection of hypertension, which could lead to interventions that can lower the risk of hypertensive end-organ damage. The first step in monitoring blood pressures is being able to accurately and correctly measure them. Standardization of blood pressure measurement technique allows for the most accurate readings. Many practices use automated oscillometric devices to measure blood pressures, but measurement by auscultation is the preferred method because all blood pressure measurement data were collected by this technique. Therefore, if a child has an elevated measurement using an automated device, it should be verified by auscultation before being considered true. If the patient has 3 separate visits with hypertensive measurements verified by auscultation, then, and only then, is the patient considered to be hypertensive. Workup and pharmacologic/nonpharmacologic intervention, if needed, can then proceed based on the hypertensive stage.

(Chapter 475: Systemic Hypertension)

**Answer 21-9.** B

Staging of hypertension can assist in identifying children who require more immediate attention and can predict the presence of hypertensive end-organ damage. Stage 1 hypertension is defined as BP levels that range from the 95th percentile to 5 mm Hg above the 99th percentile. Stage 2 hypertension, with BP levels more than 5 mm Hg above the 99th percentile, requires prompt evaluation, and if persistent, is considered to be an indication for institution of antihypertensive therapy. Incorporation of BP staging in the evaluation of the child or adolescent with high BP is essential.

Dietary modification, weight loss, and increased exercise are the recommended initial therapies for all children and adolescents with hypertension. Fortunately, it may be all that is needed to reverse hypertension in children and adolescents with "less severe hypertension, or those with primary hypertension and no hypertensive target-organ disease." Therefore nonpharmacologic therapy should be attempted for a minimum of 6 months in these patients before considering antihypertensive medications.

Although the long-term consequences of untreated or undertreated hypertension in a child or adolescent is unknown, there is a consensus among specialists about when pharmacologic therapy should be initiated. It is believed that blood pressure reduction is likely to be beneficial in reducing the risk of, or slowing the progression of, end-organ damage or chronic kidney disease to end-stage renal disease. Of the choices given, pharmacologic treatment of stage 2 hypertension is a definite indication due to the severity of the hypertension. Currently, there is no recommendation for use of antihypertensive medications to prevent hypertension in normotensive or prehypertensive patients, but studies are ongoing.

(Chapter 475: Systemic Hypertension)

**Answer 21-10.** C

The most common cause of glomerulonephritis in children is IgA nephropathy. Children with IgA nephropathy commonly present with recurrent episodes of painless gross hematuria with onset soon after starting an upper respiratory tract infection. Fortunately, the majority of children with IgA nephropathy have a benign course with no therapeutic intervention needed, but there is a subset of patients that require intervention to prevent development of chronic kidney disease. Optimal treatment for this subset is controversial, but there is some guidance in the medical literature.

The other choices can present with recurrent episodes of gross hematuria, but there are some differences in clinical course and laboratory tests that can help direct further evaluation. Acute postinfectious glomerulonephritis has a similar course as gross hematuria following an acute upper respiratory infection, but hematuria usually occurs 1 to 2 weeks after onset of the upper respiratory infection. HSP is an IgA-mediated vasculitis that is clinically diagnosed based on a tetrad consisting of papular purpuric rash, abdominal pain, arthralgia, and hematuria. This patient has no other features of HSP other than hematuria. Finally, rapidly progressive glomerulonephritis and Ig-mediated membranoproliferative glomerulonephritis can also present after upper respiratory infection, but clinical symptoms are usually much more severe on initial presentation. Both more commonly present with an acute nephritic and/or nephrotic picture and thus need rapid evaluation with kidney biopsy and therapeutic intervention as soon as possible to prevent progression to chronic kidney disease or end-stage renal disease.

(Chapter 468: Glomerular Diseases)

**Answer 21-11.** E

The patient in this vignette has functional, or prerenal, AKI due to hypoperfusion secondary to gastrointestinal losses from acute gastroenteritis and decreased oral intake of fluids. Treatment of functional AKI requires rapid reversal of renal hypoperfusion, with aggressive fluid resuscitation involving up to 3 boluses of normal saline until urine output has been restored. The patient in this vignette has been given only one 20 mL/kg normal saline bolus with a good response; thus, a repeat bolus should be given. In the majority of cases of children with functional AKI, urine output is restored within 4 hours after completion of first bolus. However, if urine output does not return within 4 hours of completion of first bolus, then further treatment depends on the clinical status of the patient at that point.

If the patient has no urine output within 4 hours of completion of first bolus, then the patient should be catheterized to confirm anuria. Once oliguric AKI is confirmed, then fluid management should consist of limiting intake to equal replacement of any output plus insensible losses until kidney function returns or worsens.

If the patient is showing signs of fluid overload, fluid resuscitation should be discontinued. Diuretics should be initiated at this time, and urine output should not be replaced until urine output has been obtained. If the patient fails diuretic challenge, then renal replacement therapy will be required.

A common complication of AKI is hyperkalemia. No matter the cause, no child with AKI should be given potassium-containing fluids until urine flow is reestablished and it is confirmed that potassium levels are within normal limits.

(Chapter 467: Acute Kidney Injury, Treatment)

**Answer 21-12.** C

Hypotension is the most common complication of hemodialysis. Extracellular to intracellular fluid shifts combined with impaired sympathetic activity and vasodilation as a response to warmed dialysate are believed to be the etiology of these intradialytic hypotensive episodes. Symptoms can include nausea/vomiting, cramping, dizziness, and headache. Close monitoring of blood pressure and dry weight while closely monitoring fluid goals can help prevent, or decrease, symptoms of hypotension. Use of an adrenergic agonist and/or dialysate cooling may be needed to meet treatment ultrafiltration goals if hypotension persists.

Access-related complications are a cause of significant morbidity in children maintained on hemodialysis but are not as common as intradialytic hypotension. These complications may include mechanical dysfunction of arteriovenous fistulas, arteriovenous grafts, or central venous catheters due to development of venous stenosis. The presence of the stenosis can also increase the risk of developing thrombosis. Monitoring of the sites with ultrasound can help identify stenosis early, allowing for intervention with revision or angioplasty. If thrombosis is present, treatment can be initiated with thrombin plasminogen activator.

Infection is an access-related complication of hemodialysis that is more prevalent with hemodialysis catheters compared to arteriovenous fistulas or grafts. Infections can present at the catheter exit site, along the tunnel, or within the catheter itself. If infection is suspected, broad-spectrum antibiotics should be initiated as soon as possible to prevent sepsis. In some cases, if infection is not showing signs of improvement with treatment, the catheter may have to be removed. In a patient with an arteriovenous graft site infection, surgical revision may be required to treat a persistent infection.

(Chapter 474: Treatment of End-Stage Renal Disease: Chronic Dialysis and Renal Transplantation, Complications of Hemodialysis)

**Answer 21-13.** D

A detailed history and physical is the first step in evaluation of the patient with AKI. Along with historical elements, physical examination findings can be helpful in deducing the possible cause of AKI. Postrenal AKI, by definition, is due to obstruction of the urinary tract, so physical exam findings should be indicative of urinary tract obstruction. Of the choices given, presence of a palpably enlarged bladder is the only physical exam finding consistent with obstruction.

The other choices show physical exam findings that are consistent with other causes of AKI not related to urinary tract obstruction. Tachycardia with delayed capillary refill is commonly seen in functional AKI due to hypoperfusion from hypovolemia or septic shock. The first 3 choices are physical exam findings seen in classic causes of intrinsic AKI: (1) butterfly rash with joint swelling due to lupus nephritis, (2) fever with macular rash due to acute interstitial nephritis, and (3) palpable purpuric rash on lower extremities pathognomonic for Henoch-Schönlein purpura.

(Chapter 467: Acute Kidney Injury, Clinical Features and Diagnostic Evaluation)

**Answer 21-14.** E

The patient in the vignette has new-onset nephrotic syndrome as defined by proteinuria (a urinary protein-to-creatinine ratio > 2.0 mg/mg), with hypoalbuminemia (serum albumin < 3.0 g/dL) and hyperlipidemia. Nephrotic syndrome is divided into 3 broad categories: congenital/infantile, primary (inherited or idiopathic), and secondary, with primary being the most common. Primary nephrotic syndrome is further divided into MCNS, MCNS with proliferative changes, focal segmental glomerulosclerosis, and membranous nephropathy, with MCNS being the most common form of primary nephrotic syndrome. MCNS is in fact so common that it is the most common cause of nephrotic syndrome in children, accounting for 90% of patients presenting at younger than 10 years of age and 70% to 80% of all pediatric patients with nephrotic syndrome. Systemic corticosteroids induce remission in such a substantial majority of children with MCNS (90%) that it is standard therapy to start corticosteroids in a typical clinical presentation of new-onset nephrotic syndrome without having to undergo kidney biopsy at the time of diagnosis. If after 8 weeks there is no response to corticosteroid therapy, then kidney biopsy is recommended prior to initiating alternative therapies. Children with steroid-resistant nephrotic syndrome are more likely to have one of the other primary nephrotic syndrome entities, more specifically focal segmental glomerulosclerosis.

Nephrotic syndrome is a fairly common (30%–50%) presentation for a child with membranoproliferative glomerulonephritis. Although some may initially respond to corticosteroids, the long-term prognosis for a child with membranoproliferative glomerulonephritis with nephrotic syndrome is poor, and many will develop end-stage renal disease.

IgA nephropathy is the most common primary cause of glomerulonephritis in the world, but in rare instances (< 10%), it can present with nephrotic syndrome that mimics MCNS. However, eventual onset of hematuria usually leads to kidney biopsy showing glomerular IgA deposits. Although treatment of IgA nephropathy is controversial, there is some evidence that corticosteroids can be beneficial in children with IgA nephropathy and nephrotic syndrome.

(Chapter 468: Glomerular Diseases, Nephrotic Syndrome)

**Answer 21-15.** D

The patient in the vignette displays 3 of the classic clinical findings of Henoch-Schönlein Purpura (HSP), which is a self-limited systemic vasculitis characterized by (1) palpable purpuric rash, (2) diffuse abdominal pain, and (3) arthritis/arthralgia. HSP is the most common vasculitis seen in childhood, and all of these features can occur in any order and at any time over a course of days to weeks. However, to meet the criteria for HSP nephritis, the patient has to have some degree of hematuria, which almost always only happens after development of the purpuric rash. In many cases, it may take up to 4 weeks for nephritis to occur after development of the rash. When nephritis does occur, the most common presentation for HSP nephritis is asymptomatic microscopic hematuria. Asymptomatic gross hematuria is the second most common presentation. Approximately 10% of the children with HSP nephritis will present with an acute nephritic syndrome. In rare cases do children with HSP nephritis present with nephrotic syndrome. AKI with hemolytic anemia and thrombocytopenia is the classic presentation for hemolytic-uremic syndrome; this is not a usual presentation for HSP nephritis.

(Chapter 468: Glomerular Diseases, Henoch-Schönlein Purpura Nephritis)

**Answer 21-16.** B

Children with FSGS more commonly present with nephrotic syndrome that is indistinguishable from steroid-sensitive nephrotic syndrome 90% of the time. Although 20% to 25% of these children will respond to steroids, the index of suspicion for FSGS is heightened when this population fails to respond to corticosteroids after a minimum of 8 weeks of therapy. At that time, kidney biopsy is required. Kidney biopsy can help make definitive diagnosis of FSGS histologically and help to determine further therapy if there are any other findings. Unfortunately, the majority of patients with steroid-resistant nephrotic syndrome (approximately 75%) will be found to have FSGS. The single best prognostic indicator in patients with primary nephrotic syndrome is responsiveness to corticosteroid therapy; thus, the decision to obtain kidney biopsy in a child with nephrotic syndrome who is eventually found to have FSGS is highly associated with a poor prognosis; nearly 50% will develop ESRD within 10 years.

(Chapter 468: Glomerular Diseases, Focal Segmental Glomerulosclerosis)

**Answer 21-17.** E

The most common causes of chronic kidney disease in children are congenital abnormalities of the kidney and urinary tract (CAKUT), such as renal hypodysplasia and/or obstructive uropathy. The most common obstructive lesions include posterior urethral valves and prune belly syndrome. Glomerular diseases, such as FSGS, HUS, lupus nephritis, and membranous nephropathy, are very uncommon causes of chronic kidney disease relative to CAKUT. In fact, the presence of a glomerular cause of chronic kidney disease is associated with greater progression of chronic kidney disease to end-stage renal disease compared to CAKUT.

(Chapter 473: Chronic Kidney Disease, Causes of Chronic Kidney Disease in Children)

**Answer 21-18.** B

Researchers have identified certain risk factors that are associated with increased risk of progression of declining kidney function in children with chronic kidney disease. The natural history of chronic kidney disease is gradual deterioration of kidney function after the initial inciting injury, but it does not occur in a linear fashion. Initially, kidney function declines slowly, but as it nears stage 5 chronic kidney disease, the decline begins to accelerate. Fortunately, recognition of these risk factors has been crucial in preventing and/or predicting prognosis of progression of disease. These risk factors include (1) glomerular etiology associated with increased risk of progression, (2) genetic predisposition APOL1 allele associated with increased risk of progression, (3) lower presenting GFR associated with increased risk of progression, (4) baseline proteinuria that starts at 0.5 to 1 mg/mg, with risk increasing as ratio increases, (5) renal functioning worsening with pubertal growth spurt, (6) acceleration of worsening renal function with each episode of acute kidney injury (AKI), (7) acceleration of worsening renal function with each urinary tract infection (UTI), (8) control of hypertension (strict control results in slower decline of renal function), and (9) uric acid and bone mineral metabolism abnormalities.

(Chapter 473: Chronic Kidney Disease, Progression)

**Answer 21-19.** A

Like adults, pediatric patients need appropriate vascular access to accommodate the necessary blood flow needed to adequately remove waste products from the blood during hemodialysis. Although there are several options available to pediatric patients, the best option is AVFs. Compared to tunneled central venous catheters, the second-best choice, AVFs have better survival rates and less rates of infection. However, AVFs are not always a good option. In children < 10 years of age, in children who are expected to get a transplant in < 1 year, and in children who are poor candidates for placement of an AVF, placement of a tunneled central venous catheter is a better option. Arteriovenous grafts are another option for children who are poor candidates for placement of AVF, but due to their higher risk of infection relative to AVFs, they are being used less frequently in children. Peripheral IV catheters are not a good option because they can only be used for a maximum of 3 days and may not be able to manage the necessary blood flow. Although percutaneous nontunneled central catheters should be able to manage the needed blood flow for hemodialysis, these catheters are also at a higher risk of infection relative to AVFs and tunneled central venous catheters.

(Chapter 474: Treatment of End-Stage Renal Disease: Chronic Dialysis and Renal Transplantation, Hemodialysis)

**Answer 21-20.** B

A complete and thorough history and physical examination is the first step in evaluation of a school-age child with confirmed hypertension. If the history and physical is not helpful in determining the etiology of the hypertension or the differential continues to remain broad, screening tests should be obtained to help determine the etiology. Screening tests that are usually obtained include (1) urinalysis (UA), with urine culture if needed; (2) electrolytes, blood urea nitrogen, creatinine, calcium, phosphorus, and uric acid; (3) fasting glucose and lipid panel; (4) complete blood count and platelet count with differential; and (5) a renal ultrasound and should be done on all hypertensive preadolescent patients. Because the most common cause of hypertension (60%–70%) in preadolescent children is renal parenchymal disease, of the choices presented, the UA and urine dipstick are the tests more likely to be abnormal. In a school-age child with primary hypertension, the second most common cause of hypertension, the screening tests are more likely to be normal. Renal ultrasound with Doppler could detect a renal mass (like Wilms tumor) or abnormalities in renal artery flow, but neoplasm and renovascular disease are very uncommon causes of hypertension in school-age children. Hypertension as the final result of repeated episodes of urinary tract infection due to reflux nephropathy can also present at this age, but again, it is an uncommon (5%–10%) cause of hypertension for this age.

(Chapter 475: Systemic Hypertension, Diagnostic Evaluation)

**Answer 21-21.** C

The long-term consequences of untreated, or undertreated, hypertension in asymptomatic children are unknown. For this reason, consensus statements issued in the "Fourth Report on the Diagnosis, Evaluation, and Treatment of High Blood Pressure in Children and Adolescents" by the National High Blood Pressure Education Program (NHBPEP) Working Group on Children and Adolescents state that a "definite indication for initiating pharmacologic therapy should be ascertained before medication is prescribed in a child." One of these indications is persistent hypertension despite nonpharmacologic measures after at least 6 months.

Once the decision has been made to start pharmacologic therapy, the choice of the initial agent is the first hurdle to overcome. Unlike adults, there is very little data that indicate the best initial agent for hypertensive children. Thus, all classes of hypertensive agents can be considered. These classes include diuretics, angiotensin-converting enzyme inhibitors, angiotensin receptor blocker agents, and calcium channel blockers. β-Blockers are another class of agents that can be considered, but they are being less commonly used as first-line agents due to their side effect profile in comparison to other agents.

An individualized stepwise approach in use of antihypertensive medications is recommended by the NHBPEP when initiated. This involves beginning treatment with one drug added to nonpharmacologic therapy. The initial agent is started at a recommended starting dose, and the patient is monitored for side effects and/or efficacy during titration if needed. If there are no adverse effects and blood pressure goal is not met, then another drug can be added or the drug can be switched to another class. If needed, a third drug can be switched to, or added, if blood pressure goal is not met. Always consider poor adherence as a reason for not reaching desired blood pressure goal.

Finally, blood pressure goals for children with uncomplicated primary hypertension are also individualized because there is no evidence existing to help guide treatment goals. The overall consensus is to normalize blood pressure to < 120/80 mm Hg and < 90th percentile for age, gender, and height.

(Chapter 475: Systemic Hypertension, Treatment of Hypertension: Pharmacologic Therapy)

**Answer 21-22.** A

Persistence of nephrotic syndrome can predispose affected children to a multitude of medical complications. The most common of these complications is infections, more specifically primary peritonitis. It is so common, in fact, that any child with nephrotic syndrome with fever and abdominal pain is assumed to have peritonitis until otherwise specified. Prior to routine immunization against pneumococcal organisms, the majority of peritonitis cases were due to *Streptococcus pneumoniae*. Other encapsulated organisms, as well as gram-negative organisms, made up the rest of the culture-positive peritonitis. Consequently, empiric treatment for suspected peritonitis in a child with nephrotic syndrome should cover both gram-positive and gram-negative organisms. Although these patients are predisposed to infection with pneumococcus, prophylactic penicillin has not been shown to be effective in preventing pneumococcal peritonitis.

Recurrent use of systemic corticosteroids in relapsing steroid-sensitive nephrotic syndrome should predispose these patients to common side effects of long-term steroid use, such as avascular necrosis. Fortunately, research has shown that steroid side effects are a rare complication in these patients.

Some controversy still exists about the role statins play in treatment of children with chronic relapsing nephrotic syndrome. The presence of hyperlipidemia could put them at risk of developing premature atherosclerotic disease. Although there are treatment guidelines published by the National Heart, Lung, and Blood Institute to help reduce pediatric cardiovascular risks in children with hyperlipidemia, there are no consensus statements to help guide treatment with statins in children with chronic relapsing nephrotic syndrome. Use of statins in this population is up to the provider, but there is no good evidence that use slows progression of kidney disease.

(Chapter 468: Glomerular Diseases, Medical Complications of Nephrotic Syndrome)

**Answer 21-23.** E

This infant's findings are most consistent with Denys-Drash syndrome, which is characterized by the triad of Wilms tumor, diffuse mesangial sclerosis, and gonadal dysgenesis. Many males present with genital abnormalities, including hypospadias with cryptorchidism. Most females have normal genitalia but may have ambiguous genitalia including labial fusion and/or clitoral enlargement. Children are at high risk for Wilms tumors, which present earlier than sporadic Wilms tumor and are often bilateral. Renal biopsy in affected patients reveals diffuse mesangial sclerosis. Renal disease manifests clinically as early onset of proteinuria, which can be in the nephrotic range. Hypertension and hematuria may also be present. The genetic basis for Denys-Drash is a mutation in the *WT1* gene, which encodes the Wilms tumor suppressor.

Conjunctival telangiectasia can be seen in Fabry disease, which is associated with an onset of proteinuria in young adulthood. Children with nail-patella syndrome may have nail dysplasia, absent or hypoplastic patellae, or dysplasia of the elbows, but this syndrome is not associated with Wilms tumor. Deafness can be observed in Alport syndrome, which is not associated with Wilms tumor or early-onset proteinuria. Cataracts can be seen in Pierson syndrome, a recessive condition associated with congenital nephrotic syndrome, ocular abnormalities, and hypotonia.

(Section 25, Chapter 469: Hereditary Glomerulopathies)

**Answer 21-24.** D

The combination of persistent microscopic hematuria, anterior lenticonus, and renal insufficiency raises suspicion for Alport syndrome complex (ASC). Alport syndrome may be inherited in either an autosomal recessive or X-linked fashion, but 10% to 15% of X-linked cases arise de novo. In inherited cases, family history of hematuria and sensorineural deafness is common.

Sensorineural deafness develops in 80% of patients with X-linked ASC but may not be apparent until late childhood or adolescence. Ocular manifestations occur in 40% of X-linked ASC cases and include anterior lenticonus, posterior polymorphous dystrophy, maculopathy, and recurrent corneal erosions.

Pierson syndrome is a recessive disorder associated with ocular abnormalities such as cataracts, buphthalmos, or microcoria but is associated with proteinuria, which was not present in this patient.

Fechtner and Epstein syndromes are autosomal dominant disorders similar to ASC but additionally manifest with hematologic abnormalities, mainly thrombocytopenia and giant platelets.

Denys-Drash is characterized by the triad of Wilms tumor, diffuse mesangial sclerosis, and gonadal dysgenesis. Patients may have hematuria, but it is not associated with ocular abnormalities.

(Section 25, Chapter 469: Hereditary Glomerulopathies)

**Answer 21-25.** C

Cystinosis is the most common inherited cause of Fanconi syndrome in children. Fanconi syndrome is a disorder that affects the proximal tubule, which is the site of reabsorption for most of the filtered glucose, amino acids, bicarbonate, and phosphate. Therefore, with Fanconi syndrome, patients will develop hypophosphatemia due to excessive loss of phosphate in the urine. This can lead to hypophosphatemic rickets, as in the patient in the vignette. Due to excessive bicarbonate loss, patients also develop metabolic acidosis. The excessive phosphate and bicarbonate in the urine and hyperaldosteronism as a result of dehydration can lead to hypokalemia.

Cystinosis is an autosomal recessive disease that results in accumulation of cysteine in cells, primarily in lysosomes, which eventually causes cellular dysfunction. Children with cystinosis develop symptoms in infancy, usually at or after 6 months of age. They can have failure to thrive, polydipsia, polyuria, dehydration, constipation, and fevers. Hypophosphatemic rickets can develop despite a diet with adequate nutrition and vitamins as described in the vignette.

(Section 25, Chapter 470: Renal Tubular Disorders)

**Answer 21-26.** B

Renal morphogenesis begins at 3 to 4 weeks of gestation, with formation of the pronephros and then the mesonephros. At 5 weeks, the metanephros forms. The ureteric bud forms from the mesonephric duct, and branching is complete by 20 to 22 weeks of gestation. Nephrogenesis and formation of all nephrons are complete by 32 to 34 weeks of gestation. After 35 weeks of gestation, the kidney continues to enlarge in size as the fetus grows. However, this is because of the maturation and enlargement of existing nephrons, not because of the formation of new nephrons.

(Section 25, Chapter 460: Renal Morphogenesis)

**Answer 21-27.** B

Neonatal glomerular filtration rate (GFR) is lower than that in adults, but increases greatly over the first 2 weeks of life. Within 48 hours of birth, serum creatinine is a reflection of the maternal levels. Typically, by 1 week of age, serum creatinine in term neonates is $\leq 0.5$ mg/dL.

The neonate has a much higher total body water volume than older children or adults. The term neonate has a decreased ability to concentrate the urine due to decreased antidiuretic hormone responsiveness and renal tubular immaturity. The neonate also tends to maintain a higher serum potassium as compared to older infants, children, and adults, because a positive potassium balance promotes growth. Neonatal serum bicarbonate levels tend to be lower than in adults because of immature bicarbonate reabsorption and urinary acidification mechanisms.

(Section 25, Chapter 461: Development of Renal Function)

**Answer 21-28.** E

Children with nephrotic syndrome lose albumin and other serum proteins in their urine, which leads to a decreased oncotic pressure within the intravascular space. This promotes the movement of fluid from the intravascular space to the extravascular space (interstitial tissue). In nephrotic syndrome, this manifests as edema, which is most easily seen in the periorbital region, the abdomen, the scrotum or labia, and the lower extremities. The movement of fluid also depletes intravascular volume. The patient in the vignette has tachycardia and an elevated serum creatinine, both indicating intravascular volume depletion. The patient's weight is increased by 2 kg, which is most likely due to retained fluid (in the extravascular space) and indicates an increase in total body fluid volume.

(Section 25, Chapter 468: Glomerular Diseases)

**Answer 21-29.** A

Type 4 RTA is classically associated with hyperkalemia. Sodium reabsorption and potassium secretion are stimulated by mineralocorticoids. A deficiency of mineralocorticoid (as in Addison disease) or an insensitivity to mineralocorticoid can lead to hyponatremia, hyperkalemia, and hyperchloremic metabolic acidosis.

Addison disease results when the adrenal gland does not produce sufficient hormones, including aldosterone, and is one cause of type 4 RTA. Some causes of Addison disease include autoimmunity, hemorrhage, tumors, or tuberculosis. Both proximal and distal RTA are associated with hypokalemia. Fanconi syndrome is associated with hypokalemia and proximal RTA. Fabry syndrome is associated with distal RTA.

(Section 25, Chapter 470: Renal Tubular Disorders)

**Answer 21-30.** C

This patient has acute dehydration due to diarrhea for the past 2 days. $HCO_3$ (a base) is lost with excessive stools, which causes metabolic acidosis and decrease in pH. Respiratory compensation will attempt to reduce acid (and raise pH) by increasing the loss of $CO_2$, most often through increasing the respiratory rate. In contrast, increasing the $CO_2$ (eg, by decreasing the respiratory rate) would make acidemia worse. Finally, the $HCO_3$ is unlikely to be stable in a patient with severe diarrhea and dehydration.

(Section 25, Chapter 462: Fluids, Electrolytes, and Acid-Base Disorders)

**Answer 21-31.** A

Bartter syndrome is a renal tubular disorder that results in loss of sodium, potassium, and magnesium. Dehydration and volume depletion occur and cause a metabolic alkalosis. The patient in the vignette likely takes sodium and potassium supplementation as daily medications. Because there is a history of not taking the medications, this raises concern for hyponatremia and hypokalemia. If severe, hyponatremia can cause seizures.

Some patients with Bartter syndrome have low serum calcium and low serum phosphate, but hypophosphatemia is less likely to cause seizure than hyponatremia. Checking serum glucose on a patient with a seizure is an appropriate step in evaluation, but in this patient who has just recently eaten, hypoglycemia is less likely to be the cause of seizure. UA and CBC may also be appropriate steps to evaluate for infection in a patient with seizure, but checking the serum sodium and potassium is the more appropriate first step.

(Section 25, Chapter 470: Renal Tubular Disorders)

**Answer 21-32.** D

Rhabdomyolysis is the most likely diagnosis in this adolescent patient who presents with a history of possible dehydration, strenuous exercise, and myalgias. Elevated creatine kinase can cause acute kidney injury, as seen with his elevation in serum creatinine. The muscle breakdown in rhabdomyolysis results in excretion of free myoglobin and hemoglobin.

Urinary dipstick for blood will result as positive in the presence of intact RBCs, myoglobin, or hemoglobin. Urinary microscopy will show RBCs if intact RBCs are present (as in glomerulonephritis, nephrolithiasis, or other causes of hematuria). In rhabdomyolysis, however, no RBCs (or WBCs) should typically be seen on microscopy, although sometimes protein is present. If needed, a specific test for urine myoglobin can be sent to test for the presence of urinary myoglobin in rhabdomyolysis.

(Section 25, Chapters 463: Diagnostic Approach to Renal Disease, Chapter 467: Acute Kidney Injury)

**Answer 21-33.** C

Treatment of distal RTA is to provide supplemental alkali, which can be given as sodium bicarbonate, sodium citrate, or potassium citrate. Requirements for children are up to 3 to 5 mEq/kg/d. In contrast, adults require about 1 mEq/kg/d. The goal is to normalize serum bicarbonate levels, which can promote adequate growth in children and prevent other complications, such as hypocitraturia, nephrocalcinosis, and renal insufficiency. With severe hypokalemia, treatment should focus on normalizing potassium prior to increasing bicarbonate. If potassium is not first corrected, it may worsen with alkali supplementation, and more severe complications from hypokalemia can arise.

Sodium supplementation would be appropriate if provided with an alkali (eg, sodium bicarbonate) but not if only provided as sodium chloride. Furosemide is not a treatment for distal RTA and would worsen hypercalciuria. Children with distal RTA can develop rickets and bone demineralization from excessive calcium losses, but calcium supplementation as an initial treatment could worsen hypercalciuria and would not be as appropriate as alkali therapy.

(Section 25, Chapter 470: Renal Tubular Disorders)

**Answer 21-34.** A

Neonates, and especially premature neonates, have a decreased ability to conserve sodium and so are at risk for hyponatremia. The sodium requirements of a premature neonate are higher (3–5 mEq/kg/d) than those of a term neonate (1.5 mEq/kg/d), reflecting the decreased ability of the premature neonate to conserve sodium.

Neonatal serum bicarbonate levels tend to be lower than in adults because of immature bicarbonate reabsorption and urinary acidification mechanisms, but they do not usually require bicarbonate supplementation. In term neonates, serum creatinine is a reflection of the maternal levels within 48 hours of birth. Typically, by 1 week of age, serum creatinine in term neonates is $\leq 0.5$ mg/dL. Due to immaturity in their glomerular filtration rate, in preterm neonates, this process takes much longer, and preterm neonates' serum creatinine reflects maternal levels for > 48 hours of life.

(Section 25, Chapter 461: Development of Renal Function)

**Answer 21-35.** E

Cystinuria is caused by a defect in the transport of amino acids in the renal tubules. As a result, the urinary excretion of lysine, arginine, ornithine, and cystine is increased. Cystine precipitates and forms renal stones. Diagnosis can be made by visualization of hexagonal cystine crystals on urinary microscopy or by measurement of urinary cystine excretion. Cystinuria is commonly inherited in an autosomal recessive fashion and should be suspected in any patient with recurrent nephrolithiasis. Treatment consists of increased fluid intake and urine alkalization.

Under microscopy, APRT deficiency causes round, brown crystals with a Maltese cross pattern. Struvite crystals are elongated with a "coffin-lid" appearance. Patients with both distal RTA and hyperparathyroidism frequently develop nephrolithiasis, but patients with hyperparathyroidism would be expected to have electrolyte abnormalities, which were not present in the vignette.

(Section 25, Chapter 470: Renal Tubular Disorders, Chapter 471: Urinary Tract Stone Diseases)

**Answer 21-36.** D

This patient's lesion is most consistent with multicystic dysplastic kidney (MCDK). This disorder is usually unilateral (bilateral cases are fatal). The contralateral kidney and urinary tract may be normal, but vesicoureteral reflux, positional/anatomic abnormalities, and ureteropelvic junction obstruction can occur.

Commonly, MCDK will gradually reduce in size and can eventually resolve. Often, the contralateral kidney develops compensatory hypertrophy. Current management of MCDK usually involves assessment for reflux, monitoring of blood pressure, and repeat renal ultrasound. Nephrectomy is no longer routinely performed. Renal ultrasound is recommended every 3 months for the first year of life, and then every 6 months up until the mass involutes, or at least up to 5 years of age. Although Wilms tumor and renal cell carcinoma are very rare complications of MCDK, biopsy is not typically performed. VCUG would not need to be repeated unless new findings (hydronephrosis, recurrent urinary tract infection) become apparent. Blood pressure should also be monitored, as hypertension is another rare complication of MCDK.

(Section 25, Chapter 465: Renal Malformations)

**Answer 21-37.** C

The patient and his grandfather have Fabry disease, which is an X-linked condition. It is caused by deficiency of the lysosomal hydrolase enzyme α-galactosidase A (α-Gal A). As a result, glycosphingolipid accumulates in tissues throughout the body. Renal manifestations occur in early adolescence to young adulthood, most commonly starting with proteinuria (hematuria is occasionally seen), and progress to end-stage renal disease in mid-adulthood. Treatment is by enzyme replacement therapy.

Podocyte foot process effacement is seen in nephrotic syndrome. Mesangial sclerosis is seen in Denys-Drash syndrome. Thinning of the glomerular basement membrane can be seen early in Alport syndrome. Moth-eaten appearance can be seen in nail-patella syndrome.

(Section 25, Chapter 469: Hereditary Glomerulopathies)

**Answer 21-38.** B

Diabetes mellitus is the most likely explanation for the patient's symptoms and laboratory findings. Renal glucosuria, in contrast, is not associated with hyperglycemia, polyuria, or polydipsia. It is a benign autosomal recessive disorder resulting from mutation in the *SGLT2* sodium-glucose transporter.

Mutation in a different transporter, the *SGLT1* transporter, instead results in malabsorption of glucose and galactose, and presents in neonates with acidic watery diarrhea, glucosuria, and failure to thrive.

Fanconi syndrome can cause glucosuria but is not associated with hyperglycemia. Diabetes insipidus presents with polyuria and polydipsia, but results in derangements of sodium levels, not glucose.

(Section 25, Chapter 470: Renal Tubular Disorders)

**Answer 21-39.** A

The patient in the vignette has Alport syndrome complex (ASC). Sensorineural deafness develops in 80% of patients with X-linked ASC but may not be apparent until late childhood or adolescence. Hearing loss of high-frequency wavelengths of sound occurs first.

Patients with Alport syndrome should undergo ophthalmologic examination. Ocular manifestations occur in 40% of X-linked ASC and include anterior lenticonus, posterior polymorphous dystrophy, maculopathy, and recurrent corneal erosions.

Alport syndrome does not result in cardiac dysfunction, brain abnormalities, or skin findings, so echocardiogram, brain MRI, and dermatologic examination would not be indicated. Occasionally, Alport syndrome can be associated with smooth muscle tumors (leiomyomata) of the esophagus, pulmonary tree, or external female genitalia, but CT of the chest would not be indicated in this patient without any symptoms.

(Section 25, Chapter 469: Hereditary Glomerulopathies)

**Answer 21-40.** D

Liddle syndrome is a rare autosomal dominant condition that results in hypertension and volume expansion, hypokalemia, and metabolic alkalosis. It is caused by mutations in the epithelial sodium channel and results in increased sodium transport. This leads to increased potassium loss, causing hypokalemic alkalosis. Symptoms of Liddle syndrome resemble hyperaldosteronism, but in Liddle syndrome, aldosterone levels are usually low. Treatment involves a low-sodium diet and triamterene, the sodium channel blocker.

Adrenal hyperplasia can cause hyperaldosteronism, but this patient has low aldosterone. Fanconi syndrome results in metabolic acidosis. Bartter syndrome and Gitelman syndrome also cause hypokalemic alkalosis, but patients are volume depleted and do not have hypertension.

(Section 25, Chapter 470: Renal Tubular Disorders)

**Answer 21-41.** E

Nephrotic syndrome predisposes to thrombosis for several reasons. There are increased serum levels of clotting factors (eg, factors VIII and V and fibrinogen). Urinary protein losses include anticoagulants (antithrombin III and protein S). Finally, there is increased platelet number and adhesiveness. Hypovolemia and immobilization can also add to the risk of developing thrombotic disease. Ultrasound with Doppler is indicated in this patient to immediately evaluate for deep vein thrombosis.

Urine pregnancy test would not be unreasonable in this adolescent patient but would not be the best first step. Erythema and swelling may be signs of skin infection, but there is no fever, and the lesion is not well demarcated or very tender. The asymmetry of the edema suggests it is not from nephrotic syndrome, and therefore, another dose of IV furosemide would not be indicated.

(Section 25, Chapter 468: Glomerular Diseases)

**Answer 21-42.** B

Reabsorption of two-thirds of the glomerular filtrate including 100% of filtered glucose and amino acids, 80% of bicarbonate, and 90% of the filtered phosphate occurs in the proximal tubule. Defects in this reabsorption lead to symptoms of Fanconi syndrome: hypophosphatemia and hypokalemic metabolic acidosis.

The distal tubule and collecting ducts are mostly responsible for water reabsorption, but a small amount of electrolyte reabsorption occurs (about 5% of sodium). After the proximal tubule, in the loop of Henle, further sodium reabsorption occurs. The descending limb is permeable to water, whereas the ascending limb of the loop of Henle is not.

(Section 25, Chapter 470: Renal Tubular Disorders)

**Answer 21-43.** C

Mutation in the *NPHS1* gene, which encodes the podocyte slit diaphragm protein nephrin, can result in congenital nephrotic syndrome. In the first month of life, large proteinuria and anasarca are likely to be caused by this syndrome, which has been described in Finnish families. The proteinuria actually begins in utero. After birth, if it is untreated, this disorder can lead to early death due to malnutrition, infection, and thrombosis. Affected patients can survive infancy and undergo renal transplantation if managed with appropriate therapies.

The other clinical scenarios would not result from mutation in the slit diaphragm proteins. Answer choice D could be consistent with Denys-Drash syndrome, while answer choice E is consistent with a rheumatologic or inflammatory condition such as lupus.

(Section 25, Chapter 469: Hereditary Glomerulopathies)

**Answer 21-44.** A

The patient with chronic renal failure and hemodialysis is at risk of increased intracranial pressure. The equilibrium between the ICF and extracellular fluid (ECF) is dependent on the Na, K, and urea levels. Urea, unlike Na and K, easily crosses most cell membranes; therefore, the ICF and ECF concentrations are typically equal. During hemodialysis, there may be a rapid decline in plasma urea causing the brain urea to remain elevated. This leads to increased water movement into the brain, increased intracranial pressure, and possibly death or coma.

Increased plasma Na concentration (hypernatremia) causes ICF to decrease to maintain osmotic equilibrium, which makes answer choice B incorrect. Hyponatremia is the result of decreased plasma Na levels and subsequent increased ICF cell volume. Damage to the blood-brain barrier may occur during hemodialysis; however, typically it leads to swollen cells (increased ICF) and hyponatremia. ANP acts on the kidney in response to hypernatremia (not hyponatremia) to excrete water and Na and has no effect on potassium levels.

(Section 25: Disorders of the Kidney and Urinary Tract, Chapter 462: Fluids, Electrolytes, and Acid-Base Disorders)

**Answer 21-45.** B

The patient in the vignette appears clinically mildly dehydrated, with normal electrolytes and normal urine output, and responds to the NS bolus. Calculating the rate is based on the Holliday and Seger formula (40 mL/h [for the first 10 kg] plus 2 mL/h for the next 10 kg and 1 mL/h for > 20 kg), this patient's maintenance fluid rate is 60 mL/h. Determining the composition of the fluids is based on the principle that the Na concentration of the fluid should be similar to the plasma Na concentration to reduce the risk of hyponatremia and subsequent complications. The maintenance electrolytes for a well-appearing, clinically stable patient is 3 mmol of sodium and chloride and 2 mmol of potassium for every 100 kcal expended, which is extrapolated to the requirement for each 100 mL of fluid lost (Table 462-1). This amount allows adequate growth of cells in healthy children. Based on this, the patient requires NS fluids. In addition, 50 g/L of dextrose is necessary to avoid ketosis causing protein breakdown, thus making D5NS + 2 mEq KCl/L at 60 mL/h the correct choice.

(Section 25: Disorders of the Kidney and Urinary Tract, Chapter 462: Fluids, Electrolytes, and Acid-Base Disorders)

**TABLE 462-1.** Maintenance Water and Electrolytes

| Measure | Average Value |
|---|---|
| Insensible water (mL/100 kcal) | 40 |
| Metabolic water[a] (mL/100 kcal) | −15 |
| Urinary water (mL/100 kcal) | 75 |
| TOTAL | 100 |
| NaCl (mmol/100 kcal) | 3 |
| K (mmol/100 kcal) | 2 |

[a]"Metabolic" water is water gained during metabolism.

Mark W. Kline, *Rudolph's Pediatrics*, 23rd Edition. Copyright © McGraw-Hill Education. All rights reserved.

**Answer 21-46.** C

This patient has hypertension and a long-standing history of UTIs, which puts him at risk for renal scarring and decreased renal function. MAG3 is the best imaging to identify renal function because it reflects blood flow to each kidney as well as detailed information on the function of the proximal tubules as it excretes the nuclide. Despite being able to accurately access renal function, it is not useful for imaging the ureters or bladder. Renal ultrasound has many benefits because it is painless, is noninvasive, and can determine renal size, position, pelvic dilatation, tumors, cysts, and stones; however, it cannot assess the function of the kidney. VCUG is superior at determining the presence of vesicoureteral reflux and examining the urethra and bladder; however, it has no ability to determine the function of the kidney. CT with intravenous radiocontrast provides superb images of the genitourinary system, which is useful for detecting small renal stones; however, it does not assess renal function. Renal arteriography is useful in examining the renal arterial system such as renal artery stenosis or renal tumors or localizing the site of a renal bleed.

(Section 25: Disorders of the Kidney and Urinary Tract, Chapter 463: Diagnostic Approach to Renal Disease)

**Answer 21-47.** B

Hematuria can be very common in children; however, the characteristics are important in determining the etiology (urinary tract disease vs a benign illness). This patient reports painless, intermittent gross hematuria along with microscopic hematuria noted on UA; therefore, this patient requires further workup. Providing reassurance is not the next appropriate step. Based on the algorithm in Figure 464-1, the UA should be repeated along with evaluation for hypercalciuria given family history of renal stones and painless gross hematuria. Hypercalciuria is defined as > 4 mg of urinary calcium/kg/d, and the Ca/Cr ratio can be used to screen patients. A urinary Ca/Cr ratio > 0.2 is considered abnormal. Imaging and referral to a nephrologist may be warranted in the future but are not the best first steps to diagnosing this patient's renal disease.

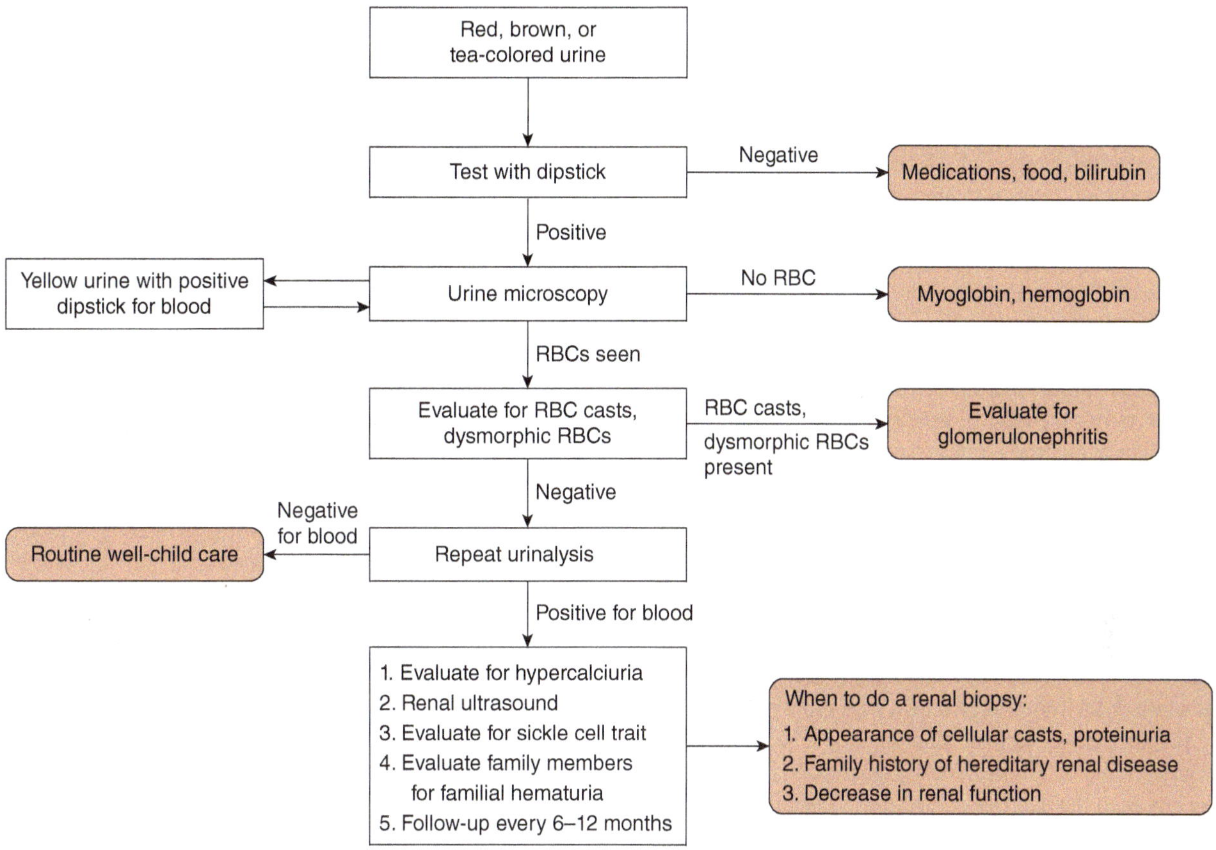


**FIGURE 464-1.** Algorithm for the evaluation of the child with hematuria. RBC, red blood cell. (Mark W. Kline, *Rudolph's Pediatrics*, 23rd Edition. Copyright © McGraw-Hill Education. All rights reserved.)

STI testing should always be considered in a patient with dysuria; however, with a properly conducted HEEADSSS exam (*h*ome, *e*ducation/*e*mployment, *a*ctivities, *d*rugs, *s*ex and relationships, *s*elf-harm and depression, *s*afety and abuse) and premenarchal patient, STIs are less likely the cause for the gross hematuria in this patient, and STI testing is not the next best step.

(Section 25: Disorders of the Kidney and Urinary Tract, Chapter 464: Kidney or Urinary Tract Disorders)

**Answer 21-48.** C

MCDK is described as a large cystic nonreniform mass that is nonfunctional and can be seen on MAG3 or diethylenetriaminepentacetate (DTPA) radionuclide scanning. Although a rare condition, if found to be bilateral, it could lead to death. Commonly, there is reduction in the renal size and, at some point, resolution of the mass. The patient in the vignette has been lost to follow-up, and the size of his mass is unknown. Given the possibility of associated anomalies in the contralateral kidney, vesicoureteral reflux should be assessed with a VCUG as well as close monitoring of blood pressure. Routine renal ultrasound is recommended every 3 months for the first year of life and then every 6 months until the mass shrinks in size, or at least until 5 years old. Immediate nephrectomy is no longer indicated for patients with MCDK, but rather close observation. Genetic testing is not indicated. Lack of routine surveillance imaging would not be acceptable for this patient given the risk of contralateral renal anomalies and associated hypertrophy.

(Section 25: Disorders of the Kidney and Urinary Tract, Chapter 465: Renal Malformations)

**Answer 21-49.** C

The infant in this vignette has autosomal recessive polycystic kidney disease (ARPKD). The history of oligohydramnios and "abnormal renal imaging" (echotexture known as salt-and-pepper appearance) puts intrinsic renal disease high in the differential diagnosis. Oligohydramnios from intrauterine renal failure can lead to insufficient lung development and classic Potter facies, which is described in the vignette (low-set ears, a flat nose, and a retracted chin). In differentiating ARPKD from autosomal dominant polycystic kidney disease, parents should have renal ultrasounds themselves, which this family did and which were reportedly negative. ARPKD has many complications, including chronic renal failure with anemia, growth retardation, osteodystrophy, frequent urinary tract infections, hypertension, nephrolithiasis, bleeding from esophageal varices, and hypersplenism.

Bardet-Biedl syndrome is an autosomal recessive disease that is characterized by obesity, retinitis pigmentosa, infertility, polydactyly, mental retardation and cystic dysplasia of the kidney.

(Section 25: Disorders of the Kidney and Urinary Tract, Chapter 466: Cystic Diseases of the Kidney)

**Answer 21-50.** B

The definition of AKI has changed from the previous definition of a "sudden and rapid decline in GFR leading to accumulation of nitrogenous wastes such as blood urea nitrogen (BUN) and creatinine." The new definition of AKI is defined as "an abrupt (within 48 hours) reduction in kidney function defined as an absolute increase in serum creatinine by > 0.3 mg/dL or a relative increase of > 50% from baseline, or oliguria of < 0.5 mL/kg/h for > 6 hours." The new definition places importance on the time frame of kidney function decline along with the time of oliguria. Research has shown that even small changes in serum creatinine can lead to increased mortality rates. These new findings have led to a greater focus on earlier detection and treatment of AKI.

AKI can be classified into 3 categories: functional (prerenal) due to a response to hypoperfusion; intrinsic due to structural damage to the kidney from ischemia, nephrotoxins, sepsis, or intrinsic renal disease; and postrenal due to obstruction of the urinary tract. In functional AKI, decreased circulatory volume leads to an activation of the sympathetic nervous system and renin-angiotensin axis, resulting in increased production of norepinephrine and angiotensin II. In response to the activation of the renin-angiotensin axis, renal perfusion occurs (vasoconstriction), *not* vasodilation, and GFR decreases; therefore, answer choice E is incorrect (Figure 467-1). The kidney's response to the decreased perfusion causes myogenic autoregulation and increased vasodilatory prostaglandins to dilate the afferent arterioles. The angiotensin effect on the efferent arteriole versus the afferent arteriole leads to increased hydrostatic glomerular arteriole pressure and increased GFR (Figure 467-2).

Treatment of functional AKI begins with aggressive fluid resuscitation (normal saline 20 mL/kg over 30–60 minutes repeated 2–3 times as needed). If no urine output is noted in 4 hours, bladder catheterization should be done to determine if the patient is anuric. Diuretics can be considered for oliguria of < 48 hours if there has not been a response to adequate hydration; however, hydration should be the initial step in treatment of AKI; therefore, answer choice D is incorrect.

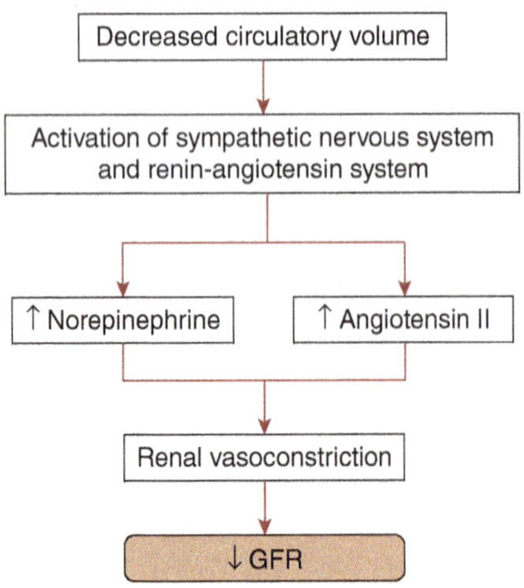


**FIGURE 467-1.** Pathophysiologic mechanisms leading to decreased glomerular filtration rate (GFR) in prerenal acute kidney injury. Baroreceptor-mediated activation of the sympathetic nervous system and renin-angiotensin axis results in afferent renal vasoconstriction and a resultant reduction in GFR. (Mark W. Kline, *Rudolph's Pediatrics*, 23rd Edition. Copyright © McGraw-Hill Education. All rights reserved.)

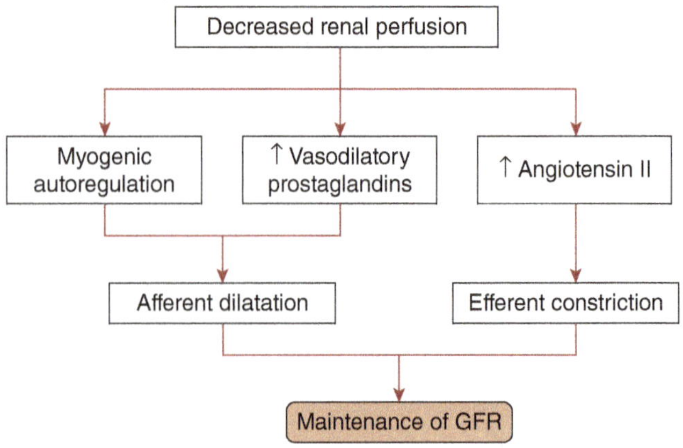


**FIGURE 467-2.** Renal compensatory mechanisms that maintain glomerular filtration rate (GFR) in prerenal acute renal failure. Intrarenal generation of vasodilatory prostaglandins and intrinsic myogenic mechanisms dilate the afferent arterioles. This effect combined with a differential greater constrictor effect of angiotensin on the efferent arteriole versus the afferent arteriole leads to an increased hydrostatic glomerular arteriole pressure with a resultant increase in GFR. Iatrogenic interference with these mechanisms can precipitate a reduction in GFR. (Mark W. Kline, *Rudolph's Pediatrics*, 23rd Edition. Copyright © McGraw-Hill Education. All rights reserved.)

Patients with AKI are at high risk of underfeeding due to fluid resuscitation and false beliefs that protein restriction is necessary to avoid dialysis. To combat this catabolic process, adequate calories should be maintained by oral, enteral, or parental routes. Intake of protein should not be restricted.

(Section 25: Disorders of the Kidney and Urinary Tract, Chapter 467: Acute Kidney Injury)

**Answer 21-51.** C

The patient in this vignette has classic signs of HSP—arthralgia, purpuric rash, and abdominal pain. Although he does not have diagnosed glomerulonephritis, his UA is consistent with asymptomatic hematuria and proteinuria, which is common in patients with HSP. HSP is a self-limited systemic vasculitis that typically resolves in 2 to 6 weeks without definitive medication or testing and has an excellent prognosis. This patient has arthralgia, which can be treated symptomatically with NSAIDs and close monitoring of weekly UAs for the first month, then every 2 weeks for the next 6 months, and then every 6 months for 2 years in the pediatrician's office. If there are signs of worsening proteinuria, then further workup is indicated, including renal biopsy. Steroid treatment appears to decrease the severity of the abdominal pain; however, it is not indicated as first-line treatment of proteinuria without first obtaining biopsy results to determine the grade of nephritis. This patient is well appearing and without signs of dehydration, severe abdominal pain, or worsening proteinuria, so admission to the hospital is not indicated at this time. Complement and

IgA levels are not helpful for diagnosis and, in fact, may be normal or only slightly elevated. Of those with significant renal involvement (3%–4% of patients diagnosed with HSP), 44% will develop hypertension and subsequently need antihypertensive medication to protect their renal function; however, for those with self-limiting HSP and no renal involvement, there is no indication to start antihypertensive medications.

(Section 25: Disorders of the Kidney and Urinary Tract, Chapter 468: Glomerular Diseases)

## Answer 21-52. E

The patient in this vignette is presenting with diabetic ketoacidosis (DKA) This patient has the classic history (polyuria, polydipsia, weight loss, and increased fatigue) along with the supporting laboratory findings (hyperglycemia, hyponatremia, hyperkalemia, and metabolic acidosis). In normal cellular homeostasis, potassium is an intracellular cation. The measured potassium may appear high due to increased entry out of cells in exchange for $H^+$ ion during acidosis as well as decreased insulin levels. Patients with DKA lack insulin, causing metabolic acidosis and apparent hyperkalemia. The total body potassium for these patients is in fact low due to glucose-induced diuresis, and they are at risk for hypokalemia once treatment begins with insulin, thus making answer choice E correct.

Persistent hyperglycemia has not been shown to affect the function of the Na-K-ATPase pumps at time of diagnosis. During DKA when plasma glucose levels are so high, it acts as an osmotic substance, leading to movement of water out of cells and causing a reduction of serum sodium levels, which is dilutional. The hyponatremia associated with hyperglycemia is in fact a pseudo-hyponatremia and an effect of the osmotic pressure of the glucose.

The deficiency of insulin and increase in secretion of counterregulatory hormones causes hyperglycemia and the release of free fatty acids into circulation; this increase in ketoacids in the plasma is the cause of metabolic acidosis in patients with DKA (Figure 537-3).

In metabolic acidosis, the low plasma pH is due to the addition of acid or loss of bicarbonate *not* glucose. The anion gap is used to calculate the unmeasured anions and determine the cause. Using the formula below, this patient's anion gap is in fact elevated to 15 (normal anion gap is < 12). An elevated anion gap indicates there is added acid such as ketones in the plasma causing poor perfusion. Other causes of increased anion gap metabolic acidosis are toxins (methanol, ethylene glycol, salicylate), renal failure, or organic acid production due to inborn errors of metabolism.

$$\text{Anion gap} = \text{measured cations} - \text{measured anions}$$
$$= S_{Na^+} - (S_{Cl^-} + S_{HCO_3^-})$$

(Section 25: Disorders of the Kidney and Urinary Tract, Chapter 462: Fluids, Electrolytes, and Acid-Base Disorders, Section 28: Disorders of the Endocrine System, Chapter 537: Diabetes Mellitus)

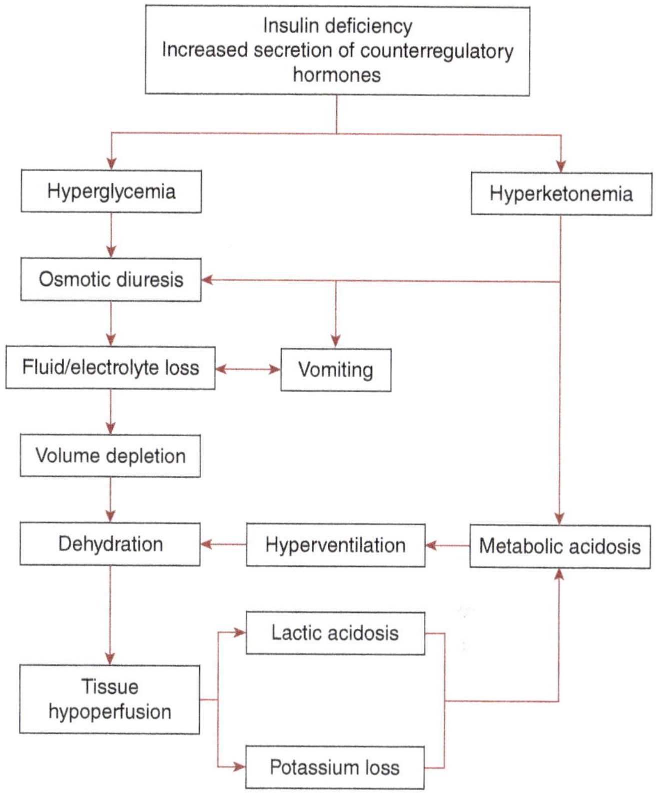


**FIGURE 537-3.** Mechanism of development of diabetic ketoacidosis. (Mark W. Kline, *Rudolph's Pediatrics*, 23rd Edition. Copyright © McGraw-Hill Education. All rights reserved.)

## Answer 21-53. E

The yellow-orange color of the urine is consistent with the use of phenytoin in this patient (Table 463-1); however, if there is concern for causative factors associated with the disease, the most likely would be urobilinogen and bilirubin. If concerned about alkaptonuria, the urine would be dark brown and black in color, not yellow-orange. Furthermore, there has not been evidence that alkaptonuria leads to chronic renal failure if not diagnosed and treated in the first 5 years of life. Urine pH typically ranges from 4.5 to 8 depending on the protein content of the diet (more protein will cause an acidic pH). After an overnight fast, pH is expected to be < 6. Although first morning void is the most accurate way of determining the urine pH on a UA, it is expected to be acidotic, not alkalotic. The nitrite test on the UA is highly specific; however, sensitivity is variable. Gram-negative organisms typically produce nitrates, which are reduced to nitrites over several hours; therefore, if a UA is negative for nitrites, it does not exclude bacteriuria in which a urine culture will be important. It is important for the urine to be analyzed within 30 to 60 minutes of passage to prevent rising pH values, lysing of the red cells, and increase in bacterial counts if the urine is unrefrigerated.

Red blood cells and white blood cells (WBCs) in the urine may originate anywhere along the urinary tract. Normal urine contains < 5 WBCs/HPF. Although increased WBC often indicates infection, pyuria can also be from noninfectious inflammation with more serious renal involvement (eg, glomerulus and

**TABLE 463-1.** Causes of Discolored Urine

| Color | Causative Factors Associated with Disease | Causative Factors Associated with Food or Medications |
|---|---|---|
| Red, pink, rose, brown | Red blood cells, hemoglobin, myoglobin, porphyrins (porphyria), urates in newborn | Aminopyrine, anthocyanin, azo dyes, beets, blackberries, phenolphthalein, rifampin |
| Orange, yellow brown | Urobilinogen, bilirubin | Nitrofurantoin, phenytoin, phenazopyridine |
| Dark brown, black | Homogentisic acid (alkaptonuria), melanin | Methyldopa, metronidazole, phenols, phenothiazines |
| Blue, green | *Pseudomonas* sepsis, blue diaper syndrome | Amitriptyline, methylene blue, methocarbamol |
| White, milky | Chyle, nephritic syndrome, pus, calcium phosphate precipitation | |

Mark W. Kline, *Rudolph's Pediatrics*, 23rd Edition. Copyright © McGraw-Hill Education. All rights reserved.

interstitium involvement) or even nonrenal involvement including fever and dehydration. If there are increased WBCs and clinical symptoms indicative of UTI, antibiotic therapy should be initiated; however, other causes for pyuria should be considered as well. Hyaline casts are commonly seen on normal UA and indicate dehydration and can be seen after exercise; they are not pathognomonic for UTI, and treatment should not be initiated based on hyaline casts or pyuria alone.

Bacteria can be seen on UA but are hard to distinguish from phosphate and urate crystals; therefore, the urine culture results should be obtained prior to diagnosing a UTI.

(Section 25: Disorders of the Kidney and Urinary Tract, Chapter 463: Diagnostic Approach to Renal Disease)

**Answer 21-54. B**

Orthostatic proteinuria is the second most common cause of proteinuria in children and is defined as proteinuria only in an upright position. To diagnose orthostatic proteinuria, the patient should empty their bladder before bed and check the first void for protein upon awakening. Later in the day, a second sample of urine should be checked after being upright for several hours. The most common method of checking for proteinuria is dipstick; however, there is a high false-negative rate, so it is recommended to repeat the dipstick over 5 to 7 days to confirm the diagnosis of orthostatic proteinuria. The most accurate method of determining proteinuria is by measuring the urine protein/creatinine ratio in the recumbent and upright urine samples. The recumbent ratio should be < 0.2, and the upright sample should have an increased ratio.

Orthostatic proteinuria typically is transient; however, it can take some time to resolve, often years. Long-term studies have not shown renal disease (including hypertension) in patients diagnosed with orthostatic proteinuria; however, if persistent proteinuria is noted, renal function, blood pressure, and serum complement levels should be checked yearly to ensure no renal disease is occurring or further workup is necessary.

(Section 25: Disorders of the Kidney and Urinary Tract, Chapter 464: Kidney or Urinary Tract Disorders)

**Answer 21-55. A**

Newborn infants have a higher creatinine level than older children, which subsequently decreases in the first weeks of life as the glomerular filtration rate (GFR) increases (Table 463-2). The newborn in the vignette has had adequate urine output since birth with a 6-hour period of no urine, but the infant is well hydrated. The electrolytes are normal, including the creatinine, which is an appropriate level for a newborn infant in the first week of life. Reassurance, increased feeding, and monitoring of urine output are appropriate for this infant. Most healthy newborns have urine output of 20 mL/d in the first 2 days of life, which subsequently increases in the next few weeks.

The patient is not showing any signs of acute renal failure (anuria for > 24 hours, swelling, poor feeding, confusion) and does not require transfer to the neonatal intensive care unit or any further testing. Although it is always warranted to obtain more history on the prenatal course to ensure this patient is in fact well, there is no indication for genetic testing or further imaging (renal ultrasounds) because the patient does not meet criteria for acute renal failure.

(Section 25: Disorders of the Kidney and Urinary Tract, Chapter 463: Diagnostic Approach to Renal Disease)

**Answer 21-56. B**

The patient in this vignette is presenting with isolated lower extremity edema. Edema in the child with renal disease is seen mostly in areas where the tissue resistance is low (periorbital area, abdomen, scrotum, and labia) and where the hydrostatic pressure is high (lower extremities). There are no signs of congestive heart failure, so further renal workup is indicated. The 4 initial laboratory tests to obtain for workup of renal pathology are antistreptococcal antibody titers, serum complement, urine protein, and urine blood. The patient in the vignette has been well per report, so a normal antistreptococcal antibody titer would be expected (thus eliminating answer choices A and D).

The definition of a primary glomerulonephritis is the combination of nephritic symptoms (hematuria, hypertension, and azotemia) and nephrotic symptoms (proteinuria, low

**TABLE 463-2.** Normal Values for Serum Creatinine, Cystatin C, and Creatinine Clearance by Age

| Age Group | Serum Creatinine (mg/dL ± SD) | Serum Cystatin C (mg/dL ± SD) | Creatinine Clearance (mL/min/1.73 m$^2$ ± SD) |
|---|---|---|---|
| Premature | 1.3 ± 0.1 | 1.56 ± 1.13 | 14 ± 3 |
| Full term | 1.1 ± 0. 2 | 1.34 ± 0.21 | 24 ± 4 |
| 1–2 weeks | 0.4 ± 0.2 | | 50 ± 10 |
| 6 months to 1 year | 0.2 ± 0.2 | 0.94 ± 0.24 | 77 ± 14 |
| 1–3 years | 0.4 ± 0.1 | 0.80 ± 0.19 | 96 ± 22 |
| 4–10 years | 0.5 ± 0.1 | 0.84 ± 0.14 | 118 ± 18 |
| 10–16 years | 0.6 ± 0.2 | 0.82 ± 0.16 | 118 ± 18 |
| > 16 years, female | 0.7 ± 0.2 | 0.82 ± 0.16 | 118 ± 18 |
| > 16 years, male | 0.9 ± 0.2 | 0.82 ± 0.16 | 118 ± 18 |

SD, standard deviation.

Data from Filler G, Priem F, Lepage N, et al. β-Trace protein, cystatin C, β2-microglobulin, and creatinine compared for detecting impaired glomerular filtration rates in children. *Clin Chem*. 2002;48:729-736; Stonestreet D, Oh W. Plasma creatinine levels in low-birth weight infants during the first three months of life. *Pediatrics*. 1978;61:788-789; Nicolino M, Cochat P, Saraidarian B, David L. Valeu dela créatininémie chez l'enfant. *Pediatrie*. 1987;42:393-397; Gordani N, Burghard R, Leititis JU, Brandis M. Serum creatinine and creatinine clearance in healthy neonates and prematures during the first 10 days of life. *Eur J Pediatr*. 1998;148:143-145.

albumin, and edema); therefore, answer choice E is incorrect because all the values are normal and there would be no initial concern for a renal pathology. The laboratory results in answer choice C are consistent with a primary glomerulonephritis that would warrant further workup to include a renal biopsy given the normal antistreptococcal antibody titers, gross hematuria, proteinuria, and low serum complement levels.

The laboratory values in answer choice B are the most consistent with a primary nephrotic syndrome given the hematuria, proteinuria, lack of signs of systemic disease, normal antistreptococcal antibody titers, normal serum complement levels, and edema (Figure 464-3).

(Section 25: Disorders of the Kidney and Urinary Tract, Chapter 464: Kidney or Urinary Tract Disorders)

**Answer 21-57.** C

Enuresis is lack of urine control in a child who one would expect to have bladder control. The majority of enuresis is nocturnal. The patient in this vignette appears to have reached a period of dryness during the day; however, she is having nocturnal enuresis. It is a common problem in 15% of 5 year olds, 7% of 10 year olds, and 1% of adults. The majority of patients do not have an organic or functional disease; however, when working up patients for nocturnal diuresis, it is important to obtain a complete history; assess for psychosocial factors/stressors; consider urinary tract infection (UTI), diabetes mellitus, or diabetes insipidus; complete a careful physical examination; and ensure a normal urine concentration (first morning urinalysis [UA] for specific gravity).

There are 4 main causes of primary nocturnal enuresis: small bladder capacity, excessive urine formation during sleep, problem with sleep arousal, and uninhibited detrusor contractions during deep sleep. Over time, the patient will mature, and the ability to centrally inhibit bladder contracts while asleep will improve similar to the daytime. Patients with nocturnal enuresis have excessive urine formation during sleep, which may be due to the less than normally expected increase in antidiuretic hormone levels at night to concentrate the urine; this leads to excessive urine formation during sleep. Limiting fluid intake in the afternoon and evening is recommended and has been shown to help decrease the occurrence of bedtime wetting. DDAVP® is very effective in reducing bedtime wetting; however, the relapse rate is also quite high (80%) when the medication is stopped. Other techniques to help with bedtime wetting include bed-wetting alarms, treatment of underlying UTI or constipation, limiting fluid intake for several hours prior to bedtime, and imipramine, which has an anticholinergic effect on the bladder to decrease detrusor contractions.

(Section 25: Disorders of the Kidney and Urinary Tract, Chapter 464: Kidney or Urinary Tract Disorders)

**Answer 21-58.** D

Oliguria is defined as low urine flow and typically is due to decreased fluid volume rather than intrinsic renal pathology. In infants, oliguria is defined as < 1 mL/kg/h. The infant in this vignette has had 10 mL since birth at 3 days of life; the normal amount for an infant is 20 mL/d during the first 2 days of life. Per history, the patient is continuing to feed well and does not show any physical examination signs consistent with dehydration. Patients who present with signs of dehydration but do not respond to fluid resuscitation typically have acute tubular necrosis (Figure 464-5). The infant in this vignette does

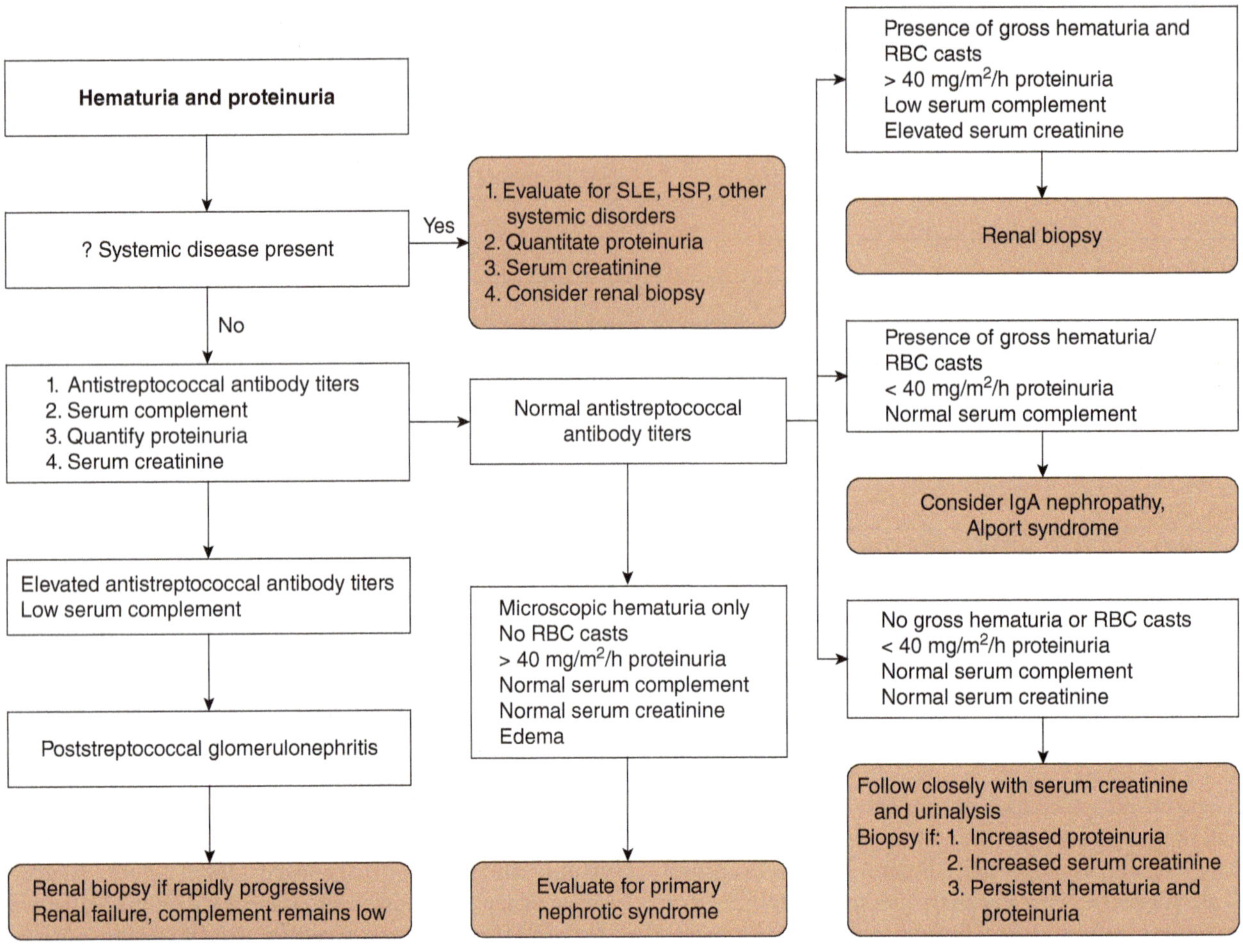


**FIGURE 464-3.** Algorithm for the evaluation of the child with hematuria and proteinuria. HSP, Henoch-Schönlein purpura; IgA, immunoglobulin A; RBC, red blood cell; SLE, systemic lupus erythematosus. (Mark W. Kline, *Rudolph's Pediatrics*, 23rd Edition. Copyright © McGraw-Hill Education. All rights reserved.)

not have signs of dehydration, thus making fluid resuscitation less critical. Glomerulonephritis is less likely given the patient does not have signs of gross hematuria, proteinuria, or cellular casts. The mother in the vignette reports a normal, uncomplicated pregnancy without exposure to nephrotoxins, making tubulointerstitial nephritis an incorrect choice. The patient likely has an abnormal or absent kidney given the poor urine formation and well-appearing clinical status. It is important to also consider obstructive uropathy (although one would expect anuria) as well as arterial or venous thrombosis. In all 3 diagnoses, renal ultrasound is indicated to determine the etiology of oliguria.

(Section 25: Disorders of the Kidney and Urinary Tract, Chapter 464: Kidney or Urinary Tract Disorders)

**Answer 21-59.** B

Patient who are exposed in utero to ACE inhibitors and angiotensin II receptor antagonists have renal tubular dysgenesis (RTD). RTD is a severe perinatal disorder that is associated with early and severe oligohydramnios (secondary to the absence or paucity of differentiated proximal tubules), pulmonary hypoplasia, skull ossification defects, and perinatal death. RTD can also be inherited in an autosomal recessive pattern.

Branchio-oto-renal (BOR) syndrome is an autosomal dominant disorder with external ear anomalies, preauricular tags, unilateral or bilateral renal agenesis, hypodysplasia, disorders of the lower urinary tract (vesicoureteral reflux), obstruction, and ureteral duplication. Interestingly, the father passing down the mutation (*PAX2* mutation) can be found to have a mild renal malformation with late-onset renal insufficiency.

Renal cyst and diabetes syndrome (RCAD) is associated with renal hypodysplasia with cysts and diabetes mellitus. Renal cysts are usually cortical, bilateral, and small and associated with dilatation of the Bowman spaces. Antenatal presentation with enlarged hyperechoic kidneys may be seen. MCDKs can be seen in a variety of genetic disorders (Table 465-2); however, they are not associated with in utero use of an ACE inhibitor.

(Section 25: Disorders of the Kidney and Urinary Tract, Chapter 465: Renal Malformations)

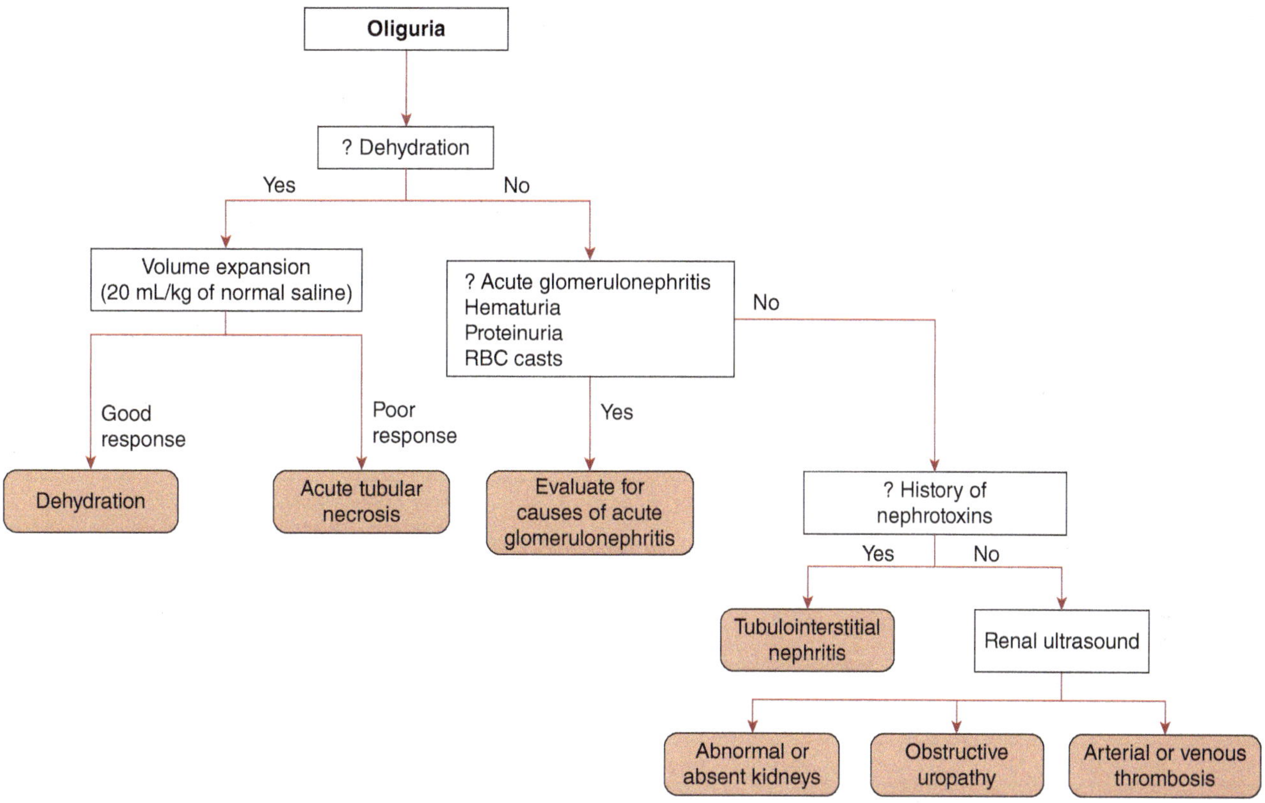


**FIGURE 464-5.** Algorithm for the evaluation of the child with oliguria. RBC, red blood cell. (Mark W. Kline, *Rudolph's Pediatrics*, 23rd Edition. Copyright © McGraw-Hill Education. All rights reserved.)

**Answer 21-60.** D

MCDK is defined as a large cystic nonreniform mass in the renal fossa and can be palpated and felt to be a flank mass. The MCDK is nonfunctioning, which may cause the contralateral kidney to become hypertrophied and increase its workload. The patient in the vignette has been lost to follow-up but requires close examination of the contralateral kidney because of the risk of vesicoureteral reflux and should be evaluated with a voiding cystourethrogram (VCUG). In patients with MCDK, it is important to preserve the function of the contralateral kidney and closely monitor for positional anomalies, renal hypoplasia, and uteropelvic junction obstruction.

In the past, patients with MCDK had routine a nephrectomy; however, the recommendations have changed, and now close monitoring is more appropriate. Complications of MCDK include hypertension (0.01%–0.1%), Wilms tumor, and renal cell carcinoma; however, the incidence is quite low. Although it is important to monitor for hypertension and any signs of renal cell carcinoma, for the patient in the vignette, that would not be the next first step. Renal ultrasound can be helpful in assessing the position of the contralateral kidney, but for this patient, measuring the dysplastic kidney would not be the appropriate first step.

(Section 25: Disorders of the Kidney and Urinary Tract, Chapter 465: Renal Malformations)

**Answer 21-61.** A

The horseshoe kidney is the most common fusion anomaly of the kidney. The fusion occurs near the pole of each kidney, leading to 1 large functioning kidney. The fusion typically occurs between the fourth and ninth weeks of gestation and typically remains low in the pelvis. The majority of patients are asymptomatic; however, nonrenal abnormalities on physical exam can be noted, so it is important to thoroughly examine a patient with a diagnosis of horseshoe kidney. Skeletal defects noted include rib defects, clubfoot, and DDH but not polydactyly. Gastrointestinal tract abnormalities include anorectal malformations such as imperforate anus, malrotation, and Meckel diverticulum; however, gastroschisis has not been associated with horseshoe kidney. Central nervous system involvement includes neural tube defects. Renal abnormalities include frequent urinary tract infections, renal calculi, ureteral duplication, ectopic ureter, and retrocaval ureters. Genital anomalies such as bicornuate or septate uterus, hypospadias, and undescended testes have also been described.

(Section 25: Disorders of the Kidney and Urinary Tract, Chapter 465: Renal Malformations)

**Answer 21-62.** C

This patient has been diagnosed with ADPKD and is having signs consistent with cerebral aneurysm. Patients with ADPKD

**TABLE 465-2.** Human Gene Mutations Exhibiting Defects in Renal Morphogenesis

| Primary Disease | Gene | Kidney Phenotype |
|---|---|---|
| Alagille syndrome | *JAGGED1, NOTCH2* | Cystic dysplasia |
| Apert syndrome | *FGFR2* | Hydronephrosis |
| Beckwith-Wiedemann syndrome | Dysregulation of imprinting in chromosome 11;15.5 | Medullary dysplasia |
| Branchio-oto-renal (BOR) syndrome | *EYA1, SIX1, SIX5* | Unilateral or bilateral agenesis/dysplasia, hypoplasia, collecting system anomalies |
| Campomelic dysplasia | *SOX9* | Dysplasia, hydronephrosis |
| Cenani-Lenz syndrome | *LRP4* | Agenesis, ureteropelvic junction obstruction |
| Duane-radial ray (Okihiro) syndrome | *SALL4* | Unilateral agenesis, VUR, malrotation, cross-fused ectopia, pelviectasis |
| Fraser syndrome | *FRAS1, FREM2, GFIP1* | Agenesis, dysplasia |
| Hypoparathyroidism, sensorineural deafness, and renal anomalies (HDR) syndrome | *GATA3* | Dysplasia |
| Kallmann syndrome | *KAL1, FGFR1, PROK2, PROK2R, SEMA3A* | Agenesis |
| Mammary-Ulnar syndrome | *TBX3* | Dysplasia |
| Meckel-Gruber syndrome | *MKS1, MKS3, NPHP6, NPHP8* | Cystic dysplasia |
| Nephronophthisis | *CEP290, GLIS2, RPGRIP1L, NEK8, SDCCAG8, THEM67, TTC21B* | Cystic dysplasia |
| Okihiro syndrome | *SALL4* | Unilateral agenesis, VUR, malrotation, cross-fused ectopia |
| Pallister-Hall syndrome | *GLI3* | Dysplasia |
| Renal-coloboma syndrome | *PAX2* | Hypoplasia, VUR |
| Renal dysplasia, isolated (cystic or noncystic) | *DACH1, BKC1, CDC5L* | Dysplasia, VUR |
| Renal hypoplasia, isolated | *BMP4, RET, DSTYK* | Hypoplasia, VUR |
| Renal tubular dysgenesis | *RAS* components | Tubular dysplasia |
| Renal cysts and diabetes syndrome | *HNF1b* | Dysplasia, hypoplasia |
| Rubinstein-Taybi syndrome | *CREBBP* | Agenesis, hypoplasia |
| Simpson-Golabi-Behmel syndrome | *GPC3* | Medullary dysplasia |
| Smith-Lemli-Opitz syndrome | *DHCR7* | Agenesis, dysplasia |
| Townes-Brocks syndrome | *SALL1* | Hypoplasia, dysplasia, VUR |
| VACTERL | *TRAP1* | VUR, duplex kidney, cystic dysplasia, agenesis |
| Zellweger syndrome | *PEX1* | VUR, cystic dysplasia |

VUR, vesicoureteral reflux.

Mark W. Kline, *Rudolph's Pediatrics*, 23rd Edition. Copyright © McGraw-Hill Education. All rights reserved.

are at risk for hypertension, urinary tract infections, cerebral aneurysms, diverticulosis, and abdominal or inguinal hernias. This patient does not appear to be dehydrated, so a NS bolus is not the appropriate first step. Laboratory work may be needed at some point during this patient's care; however, starting with renal function testing will not alleviate the mental status changes and headache. Patients with ADPKD are at risk for abdominal hernias, and often a mass can be felt; however, obtaining an abdominal ultrasound to start with is incorrect, especially because the patient does not have any peritoneal signs. Although this patient's mother is on dialysis, this patient is not showing signs of acute renal failure necessitating dialysis (lethargy, shortness of breath, generalized swelling and edema, or weakness).

(Section 25: Disorders of the Kidney and Urinary Tract, Chapter 466: Cystic Diseases of the Kidney)

**Answer 21-63.** D

MCNS is the most common nephrotic syndrome in children and responds very well to steroids (> 90%), has a chronic relapsing course (60%–80%), and also has an excellent long-term prognosis. In fact, it responds very well to steroids as long as it remains steroid responsive. MCNS is idiopathic, although many causes have been identified (Table 468-5). Treatment with corticosteroids induces remission in approximately 90% of patients; however, 60% relapse. Prior to antibiotic and steroid therapy, 40% of patients with MCNS died of infectious complications; today, > 95% of children are alive at age 25 years of life, although infections and thrombotic complications do still occur.

**TABLE 468-5.** Causes of Minimal Change Nephrotic Syndrome

| | Category | Examples |
|---|---|---|
| Primary | Idiopathic | |
| | Inherited | |
| Secondary | Neoplasia | Hodgkin disease, non-Hodgkin lymphoma |
| | | Leukemia |
| | | Thymoma |
| | | Carcinoma |
| | | Kimura disease |
| | Drugs | NSAIDs |
| | | Antibiotics (cefixime, norfloxacin, rifampin) |
| | | Lithium |
| | | Interferon |
| | Infections | Herpes viruses (CMV, EBV, HHV7, VZV) |
| | | Influenza virus |
| | | Human immunodeficiency virus |
| | Allergens | Pollen, dust mites |
| | | Dairy products |
| | | Bee stings |
| | | Poison ivy/oak |
| | Associated with autoimmune disorders | Sarcoidosis |
| | | Graves disease |
| | | Thyroiditis |
| | | Vasculitis |
| | | Myasthenia gravis |
| | | Guillain-Barré syndrome |

CMV, cytomegalovirus; EBV, Epstein-Barr virus; HHV7, human herpes virus 7; NSAIDs, nonsteroidal anti-inflammatory drugs; VZV, varicella-zoster virus.

Mark W. Kline, *Rudolph's Pediatrics*, 23rd Edition. Copyright © McGraw-Hill Education. All rights reserved.

**TABLE 468-8.** Medical Complications of Nephrotic Syndrome

| Timing | Complication |
|---|---|
| Acute | Infections |
| | Thromboembolic events |
| | Hypovolemic AKI |
| Chronic | Vitamin D deficiency (loss of 59-kd vitamin D–binding protein) |
| | Hypothyroidism (loss of free and protein-bound thyroid hormones) |
| | Malnutrition, failure to thrive |
| | Deficiency of trace metal (iron, copper, and zinc due to binding-protein loss) |
| | Steroid toxicity (short stature, cataracts, avascular necrosis, osteoporosis) |
| Long term | Progressive CKD[a] |
| | Accelerated atherosclerotic disease |

[a]Risk depends on the etiology of the nephrotic syndrome (ie, progressive CKD is not a significant risk in children with minimal change nephrotic syndrome).

AKI, acute kidney injury; CKD, chronic kidney disease.

Mark W. Kline, *Rudolph's Pediatrics*, 23rd Edition. Copyright © McGraw-Hill Education. All rights reserved.

Focal segmental glomerulosclerosis (FSGS) is an antibody-mediated disease and therefore can be associated with other immune illnesses such as insulin-dependent diabetes mellitus. A trial of immunosuppressive drugs is recommended for patients with FSGS but not for patients with MCNS. Patients with MCNS are at risk for hypothyroidism, not hyperthyroidism, due to the lack of free and protein-bound thyroid hormone (Table 468-8).

(Section 25: Disorders of the Kidney and Urinary Tract, Chapter 468: Glomerular Diseases)

**Answer 21-64.** B

The patient in the vignette is presenting with obesity, polydactyly, mental retardation, and retinitis pigmentosa, which are all consistent with Bardet-Biedl syndrome. Bardet-Biedl syndrome is an autosomal recessive disease associated with cystic dysplasia of the kidney as well as defects in the function of the primary cilia in many organs (Figure 466-3). Meckel-Gruber syndrome is an autosomal recessive disorder

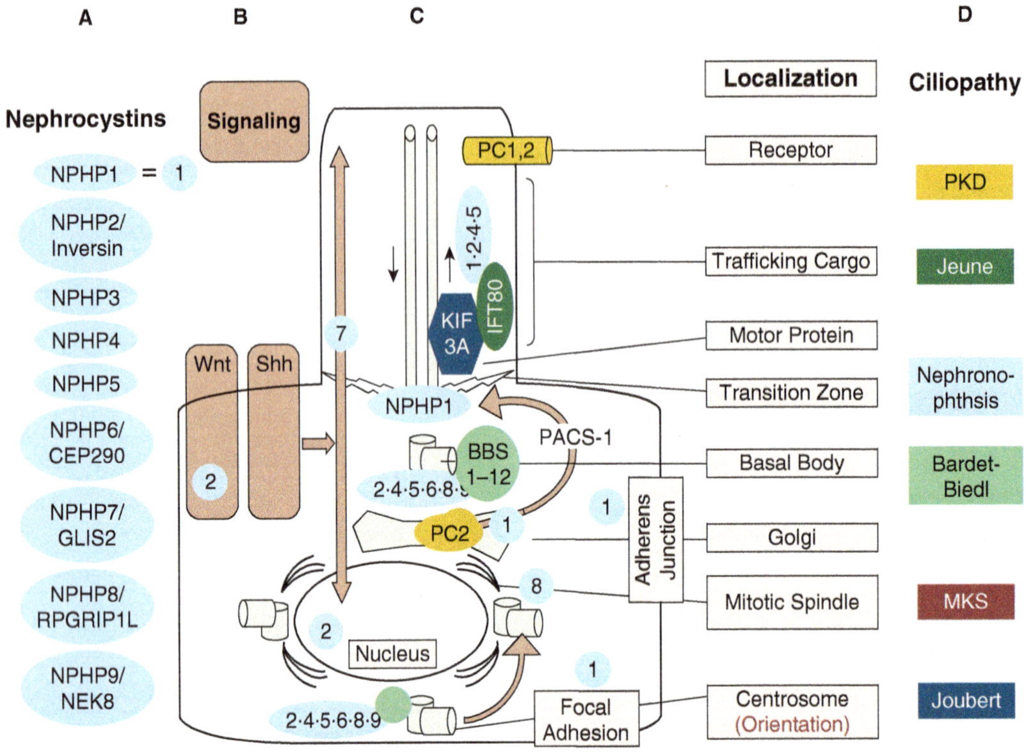


**FIGURE 466-3.** Subcellular localization of nephrocystins (light blue) to subcellular organelles of the cilia/centrosome complex (light pink), specifically to primary cilia, basal bodies, the mitotic spindle, focal adhesions and adherens junctions, and functional interaction with other proteins mutated in renal cystic diseases ("ciliopathies"). Cystoproteins are proteins of genes mutated in cystic kidney diseases. Depending on cell cycle stage, cystoproteins are localized at different subcellular organelles (shown in light gray), including primary cilia, basal bodies, endoplasmic reticulum, the mitotic spindle, centrosomes, adherens junctions, or focal adhesions. Arrows in the primary cilium indicate the direction of anterograde and retrograde transport along the microtubule system, respectively. **A:** Most nephrocystins (light blue) are located at cilia, the basal body, and centrosome in a cell cycle–dependent manner. *NPHP1* is also at the transition zone, focal adhesions, and adherens junctions. **B:** Sensory cilia perceive and process cell external signals, and cystoproteins are involved in signaling mechanisms downstream of cilial signal recognition. Downstream of cilia (dark pink), Wnt signaling and hedgehog signaling play a role in planar cell polarity, which is mediated (**C**) partially through orientation of centrosomes and the mitotic spindle poles. **D:** Cilia-dependent mechanisms of planar cell polarity seem to be central to the pathogenesis of renal cystic diseases, which involve other organ systems due to defects in cilial function (ie, ciliopathies). The most prominent ciliopathies are listed on the right. BBS, Bardet-Biedl syndrome–associated proteins; IFT80, intraflagellar transport protein 80; MKS, Meckel syndrome; NPHP, nephrocystin; PACS-1, phosphofurin acidic cluster sorting protein 1; PC1,2, polycystin-1 and -2; PKD, polycystic kidney disease; Shh, sonic hedgehog signaling pathway; Wnt, Wnt signaling pathway. (Mark W. Kline, *Rudolph's Pediatrics*, 23rd Edition. Copyright © McGraw-Hill Education. All rights reserved.)

with many defects in several organs, usually leading to perinatal death. Diagnosis is based on cystic dysplasia of the kidney, hepatic fibrosis, occipital encephalocele, and postaxial polydactyly. Pierson syndrome is a recessive disorder consisting of congenital nephrotic syndrome with ocular abnormalities (buphthalmos, microcoria, cataracts) and hypotonia, but not retinitis pigmentosa. Frasier syndrome is characterized by male pseudohermaphroditism and renal failure. Patients have normal female external genitalia but a 46,XY karyotype, and often, the condition is not recognized until the patient is evaluated for primary amenorrhea. Proteinuria is present in childhood and progresses to nephrotic syndrome and chronic renal failure by adolescence. Renal abnormalities consist of focal segmental glomerulosclerosis. Finnish syndrome is a type of congenital nephrotic syndrome and presents with proteinuria in the first month of life. Proteinuria actually beings in utero and can be associated with postnatal edema. If left untreated, patients die early in life due to malnutrition, infection, and thrombosis.

(Section 25: Disorders of the Kidney and Urinary Tract, Chapter 466: Cystic Diseases of the Kidney, Chapter 469: Hereditary Glomerulopathies)

# CHAPTER 22 Urology and Genital Disorders

Huay-ying Lo and Rathi Asaithambi

**22-1.** A previously healthy 6-month-old girl is brought to the emergency department (ED) with 3 days of fever and vomiting. Physical examination is significant for fever (39.3°C) and mild dehydration. A catheterized urinalysis shows specific gravity of 1.030, pH of 6.1, 1+ ketones, 3+ leukocyte esterase, 1+ protein, 1+ blood, and positive nitrites. Her urine microscopy shows 50 to 100 white blood cells (WBCs)/high-power field (HPF), < 5 red blood cells (RBCs)/HPF, and bacteria. The urine culture is pending. Her parents would like to know if she has a urinary tract infection (UTI).

Which of the following positive results in this child has the highest sensitivity for presumptively diagnosing UTI?

**A.** Leukocyte esterase on urinalysis
**B.** Nitrites on urinalysis
**C.** WBCs on urine microscopy
**D.** RBCs on urine microscopy
**E.** Bacteria on urine microscopy

**22-2.** You are called to the emergent delivery of a G1P0 mother. Her ultrasound in triage was significant for oligohydramnios. On initial exam, the infant is noted to have mild respiratory distress. His exam is also remarkable for abnormal abdominal musculature and testes that are not palpable. Of the following, which statement is most accurate about the patient's condition?

**A.** This condition is only seen in males.
**B.** Most cases are diagnosed prenatally on ultrasound.
**C.** Vesicoureteral reflux (VUR) is a rare complication.
**D.** Malabsorptive diarrhea is a common complication.
**E.** Bilateral orchiopexy should be completed prior to discharge.

**22-3.** A 13-year-old boy presents to the emergency department with nausea, vomiting, and significant abdominal pain for the past 8 hours. He denies fever, weight loss, penile discharge, dysuria, constipation, diarrhea, and trauma. He and his parents deny any family history of genitourinary or gastrointestinal disorders. Upon chart review, you notice that this is his fourth presentation for similar complaints in the past 18 months. He has never required admission, and with the first 3 presentations, his symptoms spontaneously resolved after a few hours, he was able to tolerate oral intake, and he was discharged home. His vital signs are within normal limits for age, and his abdominal exam is remarkable for right upper quadrant tenderness and a palpable abdominal mass in the right abdomen.

His chemistry (including blood urea nitrogen [BUN] and creatinine), complete blood count (CBC), lipase, and liver function tests are unremarkable. His urinalysis shows specific gravity of 1.020, pH of 7.0, 3+ blood, and no ketones, leukocyte esterase, protein, or nitrites. His urine microscopy shows 50 to 100 red blood cells (RBCs)/high-power field (HPF) and < 5 white blood cells (WBCs)/HPF. No crystals or bacteria are visualized. His imaging is notable for renal ultrasound with hydronephrosis. No cysts are visualized. Which of the following is the most likely cause of this patient's symptoms?

**A.** Wilms tumor
**B.** Autosomal dominant polycystic kidney disease
**C.** Viral gastroenteritis
**D.** Acute appendicitis
**E.** Ureteropelvic junction (UPJ) obstruction

**22-4.** Which of the following is the most common cause of priapism in children?

**A.** Spinal cord injury
**B.** Penile trauma
**C.** Sickle cell disease
**D.** Psychiatric medication
**E.** Leukemia

**22-5.** A previously healthy 16-year-old boy presents to urgent care with testicular swelling. He reports that he woke up and noticed that his left testis was larger than his right testis last week. His swelling is improved in the morning and worsens during the course of the day. He denies fever, dysuria, urgency, hesitancy, frequency, hematuria, abdominal pain, testicular pain, penile discharge, and penile pain. He also denies past or present sexual activity. On physical exam, his vital signs are within normal limits for age. His left testis is swollen in the standing position and has a "bag of worms" appearance, but the swelling improves in the supine position. His testes are nontender to palpation and do not have a significant size discrepancy. The cremasteric reflex is present bilaterally. Which of the following is the most appropriate next step in management?

**A.** Obtain a scrotal ultrasound with Doppler

**B.** Obtain a urinalysis and urine culture

**C.** Obtain a urine nucleic acid amplification test (NAAT) for gonorrhea and chlamydia

**D.** Provide reassurance and observe

**E.** Refer to a urologist for emergent surgical evaluation

**22-6.** A 16-year-old girl presents for her annual wellness exam. She started menstruating 2 years ago and has a 28-day cycle. She has mild intermittent cramping with her cycle but no excessive bleeding. Her review of systems is otherwise negative. She is sexually active and reports consistent condom usage. On physical exam, her vital signs are within normal limits for age. Her breast exam is unremarkable. Her pelvic exam is notable for a right-sided adnexal mass. The remainder of her exam is unremarkable. A pelvic ultrasound with Doppler is ordered and reveals a 4.5-cm anechoic fluid-filled mass in the right ovary and normal blood flow to and from the ovary. Which of the following is the next best step in management?

**A.** Reassurance and anticipatory guidance

**B.** Follow-up pelvic ultrasound in 6 weeks

**C.** α-Fetoprotein testing

**D.** Cystectomy

**E.** Surgical detorsion

**22-7.** A 10-year-old girl presents for a hospital follow-up visit. She has a history of chronic constipation and was admitted overnight for a bowel clean out earlier this week. She has been doing well with decreased abdominal pain and improved stooling, but her mother has noted some bloody spotting on her undergarments.

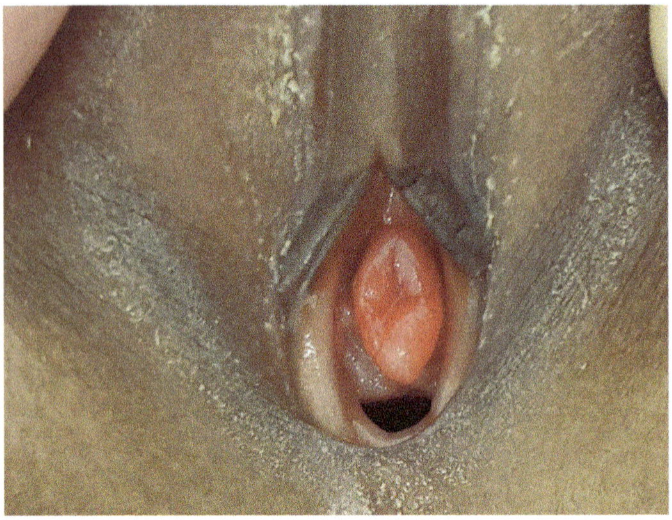

**FIGURE 472-7.** (Mark W. Kline, *Rudolph's Pediatrics*, 23rd Edition. Copyright © McGraw-Hill Education. All rights reserved.)

On physical exam, her vital signs are stable and her genitourinary exam is significant for the finding in Figure 472-7. Which of the following is the most likely diagnosis?

**A.** Sexual abuse

**B.** Ureterocele

**C.** Urethral prolapse

**D.** Rhabdomyosarcoma

**E.** Germ cell tumor

**22-8.** You are asked to examine an appropriate-for-gestational-age newborn male 24 hours after birth. He was delivered at 39 5/7 weeks of gestation by normal vaginal delivery. The pregnancy was unremarkable. He has a circumcision scheduled for later in the afternoon, and his nurse is concerned about an abnormal genital exam. His penile length is 1.8 cm, and she measured the penis with a paper tape measurer on 3 separate occasions, with consistent results. She reports that he is otherwise well appearing with vitals within normal limits for age, and the remainder of his physical exam is normal, including the presence of palpable testes bilaterally. Which of the following is the most appropriate next step in management?

**A.** Remeasure the penile length

**B.** Give clearance to proceed with the circumcision

**C.** Obtain lab work, including a chemistry, complete blood count, and testosterone level

**D.** Obtain a karyotype

**E.** Consult pediatric endocrinology

**22-9.** A 9-year-old girl presents to the emergency department with generalized abdominal pain and dysuria for 2 days. She denies any fever, nausea, vomiting, diarrhea, difficulty breathing, vaginal discharge, vaginal bleeding, or trauma. She has no significant past medical or surgical history and does not take any daily medications. Her vital signs are within normal limits for age, with the exception of mild tachycardia. Her physical exam is only notable for generalized abdominal tenderness to palpation and voluntary guarding. She does not exhibit any rebound. Her bloodwork, including serum electrolytes, ionized calcium, complete blood count (CBC), liver function tests, and lipase, is within normal limits. A urinalysis is performed and reveals 3+ blood. Her urinalysis is negative for ketones, nitrites, leukocyte esterase, and proteinuria. Urine microscopy reveals 50 to 100 red blood cells (RBCs)/high-power field (HPF). Urine culture is pending. A plain abdominal film shows a small calcification in the right midureter. Urine electrolytes are obtained and show elevated urine calcium.

Of the following, what is the most likely cause of her elevated urine calcium?

**A.** Hypervitaminosis D

**B.** Primary hyperparathyroidism

**C.** Adrenal insufficiency

**D.** Medication

**E.** Idiopathic

**22-10.** You are seeing an infant for his routine 6-month visit. He was born at 30 weeks of gestation via normal vaginal delivery. He is breastfeeding well with good urine output and stooling. He is meeting his 6-month developmental milestones. Physical examination reveals a well-appearing and alert infant who is able to sit without support. You are able to palpate his right testis and unable to palpate his left testis. His mother notes that previous providers have also only been able to palpate his right testis. Of the following, what is the most appropriate next step in management?

**A.** Send serum electrolytes and 17-hydroxyprogesterone level

**B.** Send serum $\alpha$-fetoprotein

**C.** Obtain a testicular ultrasound

**D.** Continued outpatient follow-up

**E.** Refer to surgical specialist

**22-11.** A 6-year-old girl is brought by her parents to your office for 1 episode of pink-colored urine the evening prior. She has never had urine discoloration before. She and her parents deny fever, trauma, dysuria, hesitancy, frequency, urgency, abdominal pain, nausea, vomiting, diarrhea, constipation, vaginal discharge, and vaginal bleeding. There is no family history of hematuria or renal disease. Her vital signs and physical exam are unremarkable. You obtain a urine dipstick that shows 4+ blood. Urine microscopy shows 50 to 100 red blood cells (RBCs)/high-power field (HPF). There are no RBC casts or dysmorphic RBCs present. Of the following, what is the next best step in management?

**A.** Routine well-child care

**B.** Close outpatient follow-up with repeat urinalysis

**C.** Obtain a hemoglobin electrophoresis

**D.** Obtain a renal ultrasound

**E.** Refer to nephrology for a renal biopsy

**22-12.** Which of the following is a urologic emergency?

**A.** Physiologic phimosis

**B.** Pathologic phimosis

**C.** Paraphimosis

**D.** Hypospadias

**E.** Nontraumatic urethrorrhagia

**22-13.** A 10-year-old boy is brought by his parents to your office for concerns about abnormal urination. He and his parents report that he typically wets his bed 2 to 3 nights a week, although he is dry during the day. He has never been dry at night. He denies pain with urination, frequent urination, bloody urine, excessive thirst, excessive hunger, constipation, or recent social stressors or significant social changes. No immediate family members have a history of similar symptoms. His vital signs are stable for age, his physical exam is unremarkable, and his screening urinalysis is unremarkable.

When providing anticipatory guidance regarding this condition, which of the following is *most* accurate?

**A.** A short course of desmopressin (DDAVP) leads to a permanent cure in the majority of cases.

**B.** Family history of this condition is uncommon.

**C.** Imipramine is a first-line therapy for this condition.

**D.** Bedwetting alarms can typically be used to achieve dryness within 1 to 2 weeks of initiation.

**E.** Most children spontaneously achieve dryness, regardless of treatment.

**22-14.** You are examining a newborn male infant shortly after birth. He was delivered at 38 weeks of gestation by cesarean section for breech presentation. The patient's mother did not receive any prenatal care. The infant is small for gestational age but appears vigorous. His temperature is 37°C, his heart rate is 145 bpm, his respiratory rate is 55 breaths/min, his blood pressure is 66/44 mm Hg, and his oxygen saturation is 98% on room air. His physical exam is remarkable for an enlarged bladder and palpable kidneys. An ultrasound is ordered, and findings are remarkable for bilateral hydroureteronephrosis with a dilated proximal urethra and bladder. Of the following, what is the most likely cause of the patient's symptoms?

**A.** Renal dysplasia

**B.** Ureteropelvic junction (UPJ) obstruction

**C.** Ureterocele

**D.** Posterior urethral valve (PUV)

**E.** Horseshoe kidney

**22-15.** Which of the following is *most* accurate regarding urinary stones?

**A.** Compared to the general population, patients with bowel disease have a higher prevalence of uric acid stones.

**B.** Cystinuria is an autosomal dominant disorder that can lead to the formation of cystine stones.

**C.** Low urine pH promotes the precipitation of struvite stones.

**D.** Loop diuretics decrease urine calcium and prevent the formation of calcium stones.

**E.** Increased urinary citrate contributes to the formation of calcium stones.

**22-16.** A 16-year-old boy presents with 6 days of right scrotal pain and edema. He denies nausea, fever, abdominal pain, hematuria, urgency, frequency, and dysuria. He has noted some intermittent staining in his underwear but denies any penile discharge or genital lesions. He is sexually active and reports that he always uses condoms and has never had a sexually transmitted infection before. On physical exam, his vital signs are within normal limits for age. His sexual maturity rating is 5 for pubertal development. He has mild right scrotal edema and erythema. His right scrotum is tender to palpation. His cremasteric reflex is intact bilaterally. He does not have any scrotal fluctuance or urethral discharge. Of the following, which organism is most likely responsible for this patient's symptoms?

**A.** *Neisseria gonorrhoeae*

**B.** *Chlamydia trachomatis*

**C.** *Ureaplasma urealyticum*

**D.** *Escherichia coli*

**E.** *Staphylococcus aureus*

**22-17.** You are evaluating a 17-year-old girl for 2 days of vaginal discharge and pruritus. She denies fever, nausea, emesis, abdominal pain, vaginal pain, dysuria, and rash. She is sexually active with one male partner and reports that she has an intrauterine device and intermittently uses condoms. She has never had a sexually transmitted infection before. Her physical exam is remarkable for thin white vaginal discharge with a "fishy" odor. Of the following, which statement is *most* accurate about the patient's condition?

**A.** It is the second most common cause of abnormal vaginal discharge.

**B.** Non–sexually active women cannot develop this condition.

**C.** It is not associated with increased risk of acquiring other sexually transmitted illnesses.

**D.** Treatment of a male partner for this condition will shorten the patient's disease course.

**E.** It is associated with preterm labor.

**22-18.** A 14-year-old girl presents to your office for 2 days of severe abdominal pain. She denies fever, trauma, nausea, vomiting, diarrhea, constipation, dysuria, frequency, urgency, vaginal discharge, and weight loss. Over the past year, she has had roughly 10 episodes of crampy abdominal pain that lasts 3 to 6 days at a time. Her pain is intermittently relieved by anti-inflammatory medications. She is not currently taking any other medications, and her medical history is unremarkable. She denies ever having a menstrual period. She endorses oral sex with one male partner in the past and denies any history of vaginal sex. Her body mass index (BMI) is 18.3, and her vital signs are within normal range for age. Her sexual maturity rating is 4 for pubertal development of breasts and pubic hair. Her vaginal exam is notable for a bulging, bluish discoloration in her perineal region, and her rectal exam is notable for an anterior tender mass. Her bloodwork is notable for normal follicle-stimulating hormone (FSH), luteinizing hormone (LH), and estradiol, and her urine pregnancy test is negative. Which of the following is the most likely etiology of her symptoms?

**A.** Imperforate hymen

**B.** Pregnancy

**C.** Turner syndrome

**D.** Asherman syndrome

**E.** Anorexia nervosa

**22-19.** A 14-year-old girl presents to your office with 4 days of dysuria and gross hematuria. Her urine is described as "bright red with clots." She denies fever, nausea, vomiting, diarrhea, urgency, frequency, hesitancy, abdominal pain, back pain, and flank pain. She has not yet begun menstruating. Her vital signs are within normal limits for age, and her physical exam is unremarkable. Her urinalysis shows a specific gravity of 1.020, pH of 6.2, 4+ blood, 3+ leukocyte esterase, no protein, and no nitrites. Urine microscopy shows > 100 white blood cells (WBCs)/high-power field (HPF) and > 100 red blood cells (RBCs)/HPF. A renal ultrasound is unremarkable. Of the following, what is the most likely etiology of her symptoms?

**A.** Myoglobinuria

**B.** Paroxysmal nocturnal hemoglobinuria

**C.** Cystitis

**D.** Acute pyelonephritis

**E.** Autosomal dominant polycystic kidney disease

**22-20.** Which of the following is most accurate regarding testicular torsion?

**A.** The cremasteric reflex is usually present on physical exam.

**B.** Testicular viability drops to 30% after 24 hours.

**C.** Color Doppler ultrasound has a sensitivity of 85%.

**D.** The "bell clapper" deformity is a predisposing factor.

**E.** It is associated with the "blue dot" sign on physical exam.

**22-21.** You are preparing to perform a circumcision on a 3-day-old male infant. He was born at 39 weeks of gestation via cesarean section for failure to progress. The pregnancy was remarkable for gestational diabetes that was diet-controlled. His vital signs are within normal limits for age. You note on physical exam that his penis curves downward and his urethral meatus opens midway down his ventral shaft. Testes are palpable bilaterally, and penile length is in the 50th percentile for gestational age. The remainder of the physical exam is normal. Of the following, which is the most appropriate next step in management?

**A.** Continue the circumcision and refer to endocrinology for evaluation of disorders of sex development.

**B.** Continue the circumcision and provide reassurance that the child will outgrow the condition.

**C.** Abort the circumcision and consult urology for emergent repair of the condition.

**D.** Abort the circumcision and refer to urology for future repair of the condition.

**E.** Abort the circumcision and advise circumcision after the child outgrows the condition.

**22-22.** A 17-year-old boy presents to your office with testicular swelling. Last night, while showering, he noticed a "small bump" on his right testis. He denies any pain, fever, dysuria, urgency, hesitancy, frequency, hematuria, or penile discharge. He is sexually active with one male partner, engages in oral and anal sex, and uses condoms intermittently. On physical exam, he is afebrile, and the remainder of his vital signs are within normal limits for age. You palpate a smooth, soft, well-circumscribed, 5-cm lesion on the superior aspect of his testis. The lesion transilluminates with light. His testes are both palpable, and his cremasteric reflex is present bilaterally. Of the following, what is the most likely etiology of his symptoms?

**A.** Varicocele

**B.** Spermatocele

**C.** Hydrocele

**D.** Testicular neoplasm

**E.** Scrotal abscess

**22-23.** Which of the following statements is most accurate regarding orchitis?

**A.** Orchitis occurs most commonly in prepubertal males.

**B.** *Neisseria gonorrhoeae* is the most common cause of orchitis.

**C.** Coxsackievirus is the most common viral cause of orchitis.

**D.** Mumps orchitis typically follows parotitis by 4 to 8 days.

**E.** Infertility is a common complication of orchitis.

**22-24.** A 7-year-old girl presents with her guardian for daytime incontinence. She has never fully achieved daytime dryness and has at least 1 episode of daytime incontinence per day. She denies fever, chills, abdominal pain, and pain with urination. Her past medical history is unremarkable, and she does not take any medications. Her vital signs are within normal limits for age, and her physical exam is unremarkable. Which of the following is the most appropriate next step in management?

**A.** Request that the patient and family keep a voiding diary

**B.** Obtain urine electrolytes

**C.** Obtain a renal ultrasound

**D.** Obtain uroflowmetry testing

**E.** Refer to urology for surgical evaluation

**22-25.** Which of the following statements regarding testicular cancer is *most* accurate?

**A.** Testicular tumors represent the second most common solid tumor in males age 15 to 34 years.

**B.** The vast majority of testicular tumors are sex cord stromal tumors.

**C.** Testicular atrophy is associated with testicular cancer.

**D.** All adolescents should be screened for testicular cancer with β-human chorionic gonadotropin and α-fetoprotein.

**E.** The 5-year survival rate for testicular cancer is 75%.

**22-26.** You are seeing a 15-month-old girl in clinic who presents with fever to 103°F, without any concurrent symptoms. Parents deny any upper respiratory symptoms, vomiting, diarrhea, hematuria, or rashes. Her vitals are all within normal limits, and your physical exam is unremarkable. As part of your fever evaluation, you perform a urinalysis, which reveals 3+ protein and is otherwise unremarkable (no hematuria, negative leukocyte esterase and nitrites, 0–4 white blood cells [WBCs] and red blood cells [RBCs]). What is the most appropriate next step in management?

**A.** Prescribe a course of oral antibiotics for urinary tract infection (UTI) while awaiting urine cultures

**B.** Check serum albumin, blood urea nitrogen (BUN), and creatinine to evaluate kidney function

**C.** Order renal ultrasound to evaluate for hydronephrosis or other renal abnormalities

**D.** Perform repeat urinalysis in 1 to 2 weeks

**E.** Refer the parents to a nephrologist for further workup of proteinuria

**22-27.** A 7-year-old boy presents with continued bedwetting at night. He has never had an extended period of time during which he has not wet the bed at night. Which of the following symptoms is frequently associated with children who present with primary nocturnal enuresis?

**A.** Leg weakness

**B.** Dysuria

**C.** Constipation

**D.** Hyperglycemia

**E.** Weak urine stream

**22-28.** An 8-year-old girl presents with primary nocturnal enuresis. Thus far, behavioral changes such as decrease fluid intake in the evening, voiding prior to bedtime, and treating her constipation have not led to resolution of nighttime bedwetting. Which of the following treatment modalities offers the highest likelihood of curing her enuresis with the lowest relapse rate?

**A.** Antibiotic course to treat possible urinary tract infection (UTI)

**B.** Reward chart for remaining dry throughout the night

**C.** Initiation of desmopressin (DDAVP®) to increase urinary water reabsorption

**D.** Bedwetting alarm to awaken the child during voiding

**E.** Imipramine to increase functional bladder capacity

**22-29.** Which of the following metabolic conditions leads to an increased risk for development of kidney stones?

**A.** Hypocalciuria

**B.** Hypocitraturia

**C.** Hypo-oxaluria

**D.** Hypermagnesuria

**E.** Hypouricosuria

**22-30.** A 9-year-old boy who was recently diagnosed with hyperparathyroidism presents with 2 days of abdominal pain and dysuria. He is otherwise previously healthy and does not have any fever, vomiting, diarrhea, or gross hematuria. Urinalysis shows 2+ blood. Of the following tests, which is the most likely to confirm his diagnosis?

**A.** Abdominal computed tomography (CT)

**B.** Urine culture

**C.** Chemistry panel

**D.** Appendix ultrasound

**E.** Kidney-ureter-bladder (KUB) radiograph

**22-31.** Which of the following dietary changes would be helpful in reducing risk for formation of kidney stones?

**A.** Decreased fluid intake

**B.** Decreased protein intake

**C.** Decreased citrate intake

**D.** Increased salt intake

**E.** Increased calcium intake

**22-32.** A 12-year-old girl presents with abdominal pain, hematuria, and dysuria. Urinalysis shows 4+ blood but negative nitrites and leukocytes. Abdominal ultrasound reveals a 2.1-cm radio-opaque kidney stone in the middle renal calyx. Which of the following represents the most appropriate initial treatment modality?

**A.** Open surgery to remove stone

**B.** Percutaneous nephrolithotomy

**C.** Tamsulosin (α-blocker) to expel stone

**D.** Ureteroscopy

**E.** Extracorporeal shockwave lithotripsy

**22-33.** An 8-month-old girl presents to clinic with fever to 102°F and diarrhea. She does not have any upper respiratory symptoms or vomiting and has had normal urine output. Urinalysis shows 2+ leukocytes and positive nitrites, and urine culture ultimately grows pan-susceptible *Escherichia coli*. What additional test(s) would be recommended for this patient?

**A.** Chemistry panel including blood urea nitrogen (BUN) and creatinine

**B.** Renal/bladder ultrasound

**C.** Voiding cystourethrogram (VCUG)

**D.** Renal/bladder ultrasound and VCUG

**E.** Technetium-labeled dimercaptosuccinic acid (DMSA) scan

**22-34.** You are seeing a newborn girl for a 2-week well-child check, during which time her parents inform you that she was diagnosed with mild hydronephrosis prenatally, which was confirmed on postnatal ultrasound. Voiding cystourethrogram (VCUG) revealed grade I vesicoureteral reflux (VUR). The parents are asking what this means for their newborn and whether she needs to be started on any medications. Which of the following statements is the *most* accurate?

**A.** Children < 6 months old who present with first febrile urinary tract infection (UTI) should be started on antibiotic prophylaxis to prevent recurrence, given their young age.

**B.** Children should be continued on antibiotics indefinitely to prevent recurrence of UTIs and associated renal scarring, which can lead to decreased renal function.

**C.** This patient should automatically be started on antibiotic prophylaxis to prevent UTIs given clinical findings of prenatal hydronephrosis and VUR.

**D.** Low-grade VUR typically spontaneously resolves by age 5 and can be followed with serial imaging.

**E.** Antibiotic prophylaxis has been proven to decrease recurrence of febrile UTIs and prevent renal scarring.

**22-35.** You are seeing a 2-month-old boy who recently had endoscopic ablation of posterior urethral valves (PUVs) performed by urology. He is now doing well and has been voiding spontaneously. His parents are asking what they can expect in terms of long-term prognosis. Which of the following statements is the *most* accurate?

**A.** If he continues to do well voiding spontaneously, he will likely not need continued follow-up with urology after his initial postoperative visit.

**B.** Very few patients with PUV go on to develop problems with renal function.

**C.** As he grows older, he may develop bladder dysfunction with impaired emptying of urine.

**D.** There are no effective medications to treat potential complications of PUV.

**E.** In most children, PUV is an isolated finding that is not associated with any other renal or urinary abnormalities.

**22-36.** You are seeing a 2-year-old boy for a well-child check, and the parents state they have noticed frequent white buildup around his penis. They are concerned this may represent an infection and ask whether he needs medications to treat it. Which of the following statements would be the appropriate response and treatment recommendation?

**A.** This finding is physiologically normal, and no medications or procedures are needed.

**B.** This is concerning for a potential bacterial infection of the skin, and you will prescribe a course of antibiotics.

**C.** This represents an infection of the foreskin, and circumcision is recommended to prevent recurrence.

**D.** Parents should fully retract the foreskin to clean the area and remove the white substance to keep the genitalia clean.

**E.** You will send a culture of the substance to help determine the next best step for treatment.

**22-37.** You are rounding on a 1-day-old boy in the newborn nursery, and his parents are currently still undecided about whether they would like to have a circumcision. When counseling them, which of the following statements is the most accurate?

**A.** The American Academy of Pediatrics recommends circumcision as a routine procedure given its potential medical benefits.

**B.** Circumcision only provides medical benefits in the first year of life.

**C.** Complication rates for circumcision are typically around 5%.

**D.** Obstetricians and pediatricians all use the same surgical procedure for performing circumcisions.

**E.** Local and topical anesthesia are analgesic options for boys undergoing circumcision.

**22-38.** Your 4-month-old male patient's parents bring him in due to concern that the right side of his scrotum has become swollen and enlarged compared to the left. After performing a clinical exam, you suspect that your patient has a hydrocele. Which of the following clinical exam findings would *not* be consistent with a diagnosis of hydrocele?

**A.** The scrotum transilluminates.

**B.** The area of swelling seems painless to palpation.

**C.** The swelling seems to change in size depending on the baby's position (upright vs supine).

**D.** The scrotum feels cystlike on palpation.

**E.** The skin overlying the right scrotum is erythematous compared to the left.

**22-39.** You are seeing a 15-month-old girl in clinic who presents with fever and fussiness. She has also had some mild diarrhea but no other significant clinical symptoms. Urinalysis reveals 2+ leukocytes, positive nitrites, and 50 to 100 white blood cells (WBCs)/high-power field (HPF). You inform the parents that she likely has a urinary tract infection (UTI) and start her on empiric antibiotics while awaiting culture results. Which of the following statements about UTIs in children is the most accurate?

**A.** *Klebsiella* is the most common uropathogen that causes UTIs.

**B.** The incidence of UTIs is higher in girls than boys in the first year of life.

**C.** Asymptomatic bacteriuria occurs in 5% of preschool-aged girls.

**D.** The risk of UTIs in children decreases as they begin toilet training.

**E.** The risk of recurrent UTIs is highest 3 to 6 months after initial infection.

**22-40.** Which of the following organisms is not considered a clinically relevant urine isolate?

**A.** *Corynebacterium* species

**B.** *Enterobacter* species

**C.** *Citrobacter* species

**D.** *Staphylococcus saprophyticus*

**E.** *Proteus* species

**22-41.** You are seeing a 7-day-old newborn boy who presents with neonatal fever of 100.8°F. He was born to a G1P1 mom with normal prenatal care, negative serologies, and negative group B *Streptococcus* (GBS) status. A full sepsis workup is done in the emergency center, which reveals peripheral white blood cell (WBC) count of 18,000, cerebrospinal fluid (CSF) WBC count of 2, and urinalysis with 2+ leukocyte esterase and negative nitrites. He is started empirically on intravenous (IV) ampicillin and cefotaxime. Urine culture ultimately grows pan-susceptible *Escherichia coli*. Blood and CSF cultures are negative. When he is ready for transition to oral antibiotics, which of the following would be the most appropriate oral antibiotic option for this patient?

**A.** Trimethoprim-sulfamethoxazole

**B.** Nitrofurantoin

**C.** Cefixime

**D.** Sulfisoxazole

**E.** Ciprofloxacin

**22-42.** The parents of a 4-year-old girl bring her in to see you because she was just diagnosed with her third urinary tract infection (UTI) in the past 6 months. Her previous uropathogens have included *Escherichia coli* and *Klebsiella*. Renal ultrasound was performed after her first UTI, which was normal. Voiding cystourethrogram (VCUG) was done after her second UTI and was also normal, without any evidence of vesicoureteral reflux (VUR) or anatomic abnormalities. She is currently being treated with cefixime empirically while awaiting urine culture results from urgent care. What is the most appropriate next step for management of her recurrent UTIs?

**A.** Referral to urologist for further evaluation due to recurrent UTIs

**B.** Repeat VCUG in 1 to 2 months to evaluate for anatomic abnormalities that may predispose to UTI

**C.** Perform dimercaptosuccinic acid (DMSA) scan to evaluate for renal scarring

**D.** Recommend frequent, timed voiding every 2 to 3 hours for complete voiding

**E.** Begin antibiotic prophylaxis to try to decrease risk of future UTI recurrence

**22-43.** A 15-year-old previously healthy girl presents to the emergency department (ED) with severe, sudden-onset, left-sided lower abdominal pain that began 4 hours ago, with associated nausea. She has tried over-the-counter pain medications including acetaminophen and ibuprofen that have not led to any improvement in her pain. She has not had any fever, upper respiratory symptoms, vomiting, or diarrhea. She denies being sexually active. Physical exam is unremarkable other than an adolescent female with severe pain that localizes to the left lower quadrant. External pelvic exam is unremarkable, and the patient is unable to tolerate an internal exam due to pain. Urine pregnancy test is negative, and complete blood count and electrolytes are normal. What is the most appropriate next step in management?

**A.** Kidney-ureter-bladder (KUB) radiograph

**B.** Abdominal ultrasound

**C.** Computed tomography (CT) of abdomen/pelvis

**D.** Intravenous (IV) fluids for dehydration

**E.** IV antibiotics for infection

**22-44.** A 17-year-old girl presents to your clinic with 1 week of vaginal discharge. Upon further questioning, she reveals that she is sexually active and has had 3 lifetime partners with inconsistent condom use. She reports that she developed some bleeding after sexual intercourse last week, but that it stopped spontaneously. You perform a pelvic exam and note purulent vaginal discharge, which shows many polymorphonuclear cells on Gram stain. Of the following, which is the most appropriate empiric treatment for this patient?

**A.** Metronidazole 2 g orally

**B.** Fluconazole 150 mg orally

**C.** Azithromycin 1 g orally and ceftriaxone 250 mg intramuscularly

**D.** Doxycycline 100 mg orally twice daily for 7 days

**E.** Metronidazole 500 mg orally twice daily for 7 days and ceftriaxone 250 mg intramuscularly

**22-45.** Which of the following statements regarding chlamydia and gonorrhea infections in adolescents is most accurate?

**A.** In sexually active adolescents, screening for chlamydia and gonorrhea is recommended every 6 months.

**B.** Nucleic acid amplification tests (NAATs) are preferred testing for chlamydia and gonorrhea.

**C.** First-catch urine specimens are equivalent to vaginal or cervical specimens in terms of sensitivity and specificity for chlamydia and gonorrhea.

**D.** For patients treated for sexually transmitted infections (STIs), a repeat test should be performed in 2 weeks to confirm treatment success.

**E.** Antibiotic resistance in chlamydia and gonorrhea is rare.

**22-46.** You are seeing a 16-year-old girl in the emergency department (ED) with complaints of right upper quadrant pain that has been present for 2 months but has worsened in the past week. She has been sexually active with 4 partners in her lifetime. Her abdominal exam is benign with no evidence of rebound or guarding, but you note cervical motion tenderness on pelvic exam. Right upper quadrant and appendix ultrasounds are both unremarkable. Which of the following statements about this patient's likely diagnosis is most accurate?

**A.** Liver function tests are typically abnormal.

**B.** Laparoscopy is likely to confirm the diagnosis.

**C.** *Neisseria gonorrhoeae* is the most common cause.

**D.** Hospitalization for intravenous (IV) antibiotic course is standard of care for treatment.

**E.** Intrauterine devices should be removed immediately as part of treatment.

**22-47.** A 16-year-old girl presents to your clinic with a chief complaint of not having begun any menstrual cycles yet. She is otherwise healthy, without any previous hospitalizations or surgeries, although in the past year, she has had several urgent care and emergency department visits for abdominal pain. These episodes always self-resolved. There is no significant family history, and mom reports that she and the patient's sister both had menarche around age 13 to 14. The patient denies any history of sexual activity, and pregnancy test is negative. She and the mom prefer not to have a pelvic examination performed since she is not sexually active. You perform some initial laboratory tests, including serum follicle-stimulating hormone (FSH), luteinizing hormone (LH), estrogen, prolactin, and thyroid function tests. Of the following, which pattern of test results would be consistent with an anatomic cause of this patient's primary amenorrhea?

**A.** Low FSH, low LH, and low estrogen

**B.** High FSH, high LH, and normal estrogen

**C.** Normal FSH, normal LH, and low estrogen

**D.** Normal FSH, normal LH, and normal estrogen

**E.** High FSH, high LH, and low estrogen

**22-48.** You are evaluating a 4-day-old baby boy born at 30 weeks' gestation, and the parents point out an area of right-sided groin swelling that they have noticed in the past day. On exam, you notice an approximately 4-cm mass in the right inguinal area. The mass does not transilluminate, and when you gently push caudally, the mass disappears. Which of the following statements about this patient's likely diagnosis is most accurate?

**A.** The most common cause of this condition is muscle weakness in the internal oblique and transversus abdominis muscles, which form the floor of the inguinal canal.

**B.** This condition typically self-resolves, so observation and continued monitoring are the only indicated treatments.

**C.** Ultrasound is required to confirm your suspected clinical diagnosis.

**D.** This condition is typically seen more frequently in girls than boys.

**E.** The risk of complications resulting from this condition is lower in premature infants.

**22-49.** You are working in the emergency department when a 6-day-old infant presents with vomiting and lethargy. Parents report an uncomplicated newborn period, but over the past 2 days, the patient has begun having vomiting and diarrhea and seems more lethargic today. The patient's vitals show heart rate of 190 bpm and blood pressure of 55/30 mm Hg. On exam, you note delayed pallor and delayed capillary refill. Genitalia exam is notable for hypospadias, chordee, and a bifid scrotum. Lab results include white blood cell (WBC) of 14, hemoglobin of 13.2 g/dL, platelets of 400, sodium of 126 mEq/L, potassium of 6.8 mEq/L, chloride of 96 mEq/L, bicarbonate of 16 mEq/L, blood urea nitrogen (BUN) of 5 mg/dL, creatinine of 0.4 mg/dL, and glucose of 62 mg/dL. Of the following tests, which one is most likely to confirm the patient's underlying diagnosis?

**A.** Cortisol level

**B.** P450 oxidoreductase level

**C.** 17-Hydroxyprogesterone level

**D.** Dehydroepiandrosterone (DHEA) and androstenedione levels

**E.** 11-Deoxycortisol level

**22-50.** You are seeing a 15-year-old girl in clinic who presents with primary amenorrhea. Her mother is concerned because she had menarche at age 11, and the patient has had secondary sexual characteristics including breast development since age 12. The patient is otherwise healthy, with a body mass index (BMI) of 21. She denies any history of sexual activity. On physical exam, you note normal female genitalia, with very sparse axillary and pubic hair. You palpate a small 2-cm mass in her right inguinal canal, but there is no overlying erythema or tenderness to palpation. Given her symptoms, you perform hormonal laboratory evaluation, with the following results: elevated luteinizing hormone (LH) with normal follicle-stimulating hormone (FSH), testosterone, and estradiol levels. What is the most likely diagnosis for this patient?

**A.** XY gonadal dysgenesis

**B.** Prolactinoma

**C.** Turner syndrome

**D.** Primary ovarian insufficiency

**E.** Androgen insensitivity syndrome

## ANSWERS

### Answer 22-1. A

In infants and children who are not toilet trained, the urine sample for urinalysis and urine culture should be obtained via catheterization or suprapubic aspiration. A diagnosis of UTI requires pyuria (≥ 3 WBCs/HPF or ≥ trace leukocyte esterase on dipstick) and at least 50,000 colony-forming units of a single bacterial species per milliliter of urine from a clean catch or catheterized specimen. Results from the urinalysis are typically available before the preliminary urine culture. In a febrile infant with symptoms suggestive of UTI, a urinalysis with leukocyte esterase or nitrites or a urine microscopy with bacteria or WBCs increases suspicion for a UTI. Nitrites have the highest specificity (98%) but result from the conversion of dietary nitrates to nitrites by gram-negative enteric bacteria and require 4 hours in the bladder. A false-negative result may occur from insufficient bladder time in young children who frequently empty their bladders. The highest sensitivity for a diagnosis of UTI is positive results for leukocyte esterase or nitrites (93%), followed by leukocyte esterase only (83%), bacteria on microscopy (81%), WBCs on microscopy (73%), and nitrites only (53%).

(Chapter 233: Urinary Tract Infection; Diagnosis; Table 233-1)

### Answer 22-2. B

The patient in this vignette has clinical findings most consistent with prune belly syndrome (also known as Eagle-Barrett syndrome), which is typically defined by a triad of findings that include deficiency of abdominal wall musculature, anomalies of the urinary tract, and bilateral cryptorchidism in males. Deficiency of abdominal wall musculature can compromise respiratory function and cause constipation due to impaired Valsalva maneuvers. Urinary tract anomalies include megaureter, megacystis, hypoplastic prostate, and megalourethra. Female cases are rare and, instead of cryptorchidism, may present with uterine anomalies or anorectal malformations.

Most cases of prune belly syndrome are diagnosed prenatally on ultrasound, although it may be difficult to distinguish from posterior urethral valves (PUVs). Imaging often shows a dilated bladder and hydroureteronephrosis, and severe cases may be associated with oligohydramnios and pulmonary hypoplasia. Postnatally, patients may present with a significantly distended abdomen or a "pot belly" appearance. Renal ultrasound should be performed to evaluate for urinary tract dilation and possible renal dysplasia. A voiding cystourethrogram (VCUG) will detect vesicoureteral reflux (VUR) in almost 75% of patients.

Initial management in the newborn period focuses on preservation of renal function and pulmonary support. Patients with prune belly syndrome and VUR may require prophylactic antibiotic therapy to prevent end-stage renal disease from recurrent pyelonephritis. Newborns with urinary obstruction may require endoscopic incision or temporizing urinary diversion. Patients who fail conservative management may require urinary tract reconstruction in order to correct VUR or normalize the size of the ureters and bladder. Bilateral orchiopexy can usually be performed at the time of abdominal reconstruction during early childhood.

(Chapter 472: Urologic Abnormalities of the Genitourinary Tract; Prune Belly Syndrome)

**Answer 22-3.** E

The patient in this vignette has a clinical presentation that is most consistent with UPJ obstruction, which is a blockage of normal urine flow passing from the renal pelvis into the ureter. While the majority of cases in infants and children are the result of intrinsic narrowing at the UPJ, older children and adolescents frequently have extrinsic compression of the junction secondary to a crossing vessel.

The majority of UPJ obstructions are diagnosed prenatally, with ultrasound often showing hydronephrosis without ureteral dilation. Postnatal confirmatory ultrasounds are ideally performed after 48 hours of life to minimize false negatives secondary to relative dehydration at birth. A voiding cystourethrogram may also be necessary to exclude vesicoureteral reflux. Infants who are not diagnosed prenatally may be asymptomatic or present with failure to thrive, palpable abdominal mass, or urinary tract infection (UTI). Older children and adolescents may present with UTIs, hematuria, or a Dietl crisis, which is episodic abdominal pain accompanied by nausea and vomiting that occurs when hydronephrosis is acutely worsened. The diagnosis of UPJ in older children and adolescents is often delayed in patients who present with repeat Dietl crises, as their symptoms are often mistaken for gastrointestinal complaints.

The patient in this vignette is presenting with a Dietl crisis. Viral gastroenteritis and acute appendicitis are less likely in the setting of hematuria, hydronephrosis, and multiple self-resolving presentations over 18 months. Autosomal dominant polycystic kidney disease is unlikely in the absence of family history and cysts on renal ultrasound. Wilms tumor is highly unlikely in this patient, given that the majority of cases occur prior to 5 years of age, with the median age at diagnosis being approximately 3.5 years.

(Chapter 472: Urologic Abnormalities of the Genitourinary Tract; Ureteropelvic Junction Obstruction)

**Answer 22-4.** C

Priapism is a prolonged penile erection that lasts 4 hours or longer and is unrelated to sexual stimulus. Priapism can be ischemic or nonischemic, and ischemic priapism is the most common type seen in children, resulting from a veno-occlusive state that causes low-flow ischemia of the corpora cavernosa. Sickle cell is the most common etiology for ischemic priapism, as deoxygenated hemoglobin S aggregates cause microvascular occlusion and impair venous outflow, resulting in the inability for detumescence to occur. Less common causes of ischemic priapism in children include childhood leukemia and antipsychotic medications. Prolonged ischemic priapism can lead to corporal fibrosis and impotence. Workup may include a complete blood count (CBC), reticulocyte count, and sickle cell panel. If sickle cell disease is suspected, standard therapy for sickle cell crises should be initiated. Most ischemic priapism cases will respond to corporal aspiration and irrigation with sympathomimetic injections, such as phenylephrine. If this management fails, surgical creation of a shunt to divert blood flow may be needed.

Causes of nonischemic priapism are often trauma related and occur because of unregulated arterial inflow resulting in a high-flow state of the corpora. Perineal or penile trauma causes aberrant arteriolar-sinusoidal fistulae that can lead to high arterial flow through the corpora, whereas priapism related to spinal cord injury occurs due to a loss of sympathetic input, leading to a relative increased parasympathetic influence resulting in increased arterial flow. Nonischemic priapism may be safely observed but may require further diagnostic testing to guide therapy if the priapism does not resolve over the course of a month.

(Chapter 472: Urologic Abnormalities of the Genitourinary Tract; Priapism)

**Answer 22-5.** D

The patient in this vignette has a varicocele. Varicoceles are dilated and tortuous veins of the pampiniform venous plexus in the spermatic cord. The condition affects about 15% of adolescent boys and is rarely seen before puberty. The process is thought to occur as a result of elevated venous pressure or incompetent venous valves. Of note, only 10% of males with varicoceles have fertility issues.

Most varicoceles are asymptomatic or incidental findings, but patients with varicoceles may present with dull testicular pain that improves with recumbent positioning. On physical exam, the varicocele often subsides in the supine position. Testes should be examined for size discrepancy. Grade I varicoceles can only be palpated when the patient is performing the Valsalva maneuver. Grade II varicoceles are palpable but not visibly apparent. Grade III varicoceles are apparent upon inspection with a "bag of worms" appearance.

The majority of patients can be observed and given anticipatory guidance. Semen analysis can be considered in adolescents who are able to provide a sample. If patients experience pain or have testicular size discrepancy, they may require surgical repair and benefit from an evaluation by urology. A scrotal ultrasound with Doppler is not indicated in this patient but would be helpful for a patient who presents with concern for testicular torsion, with symptoms such as acute-onset testicular pain and absent cremasteric reflex. As this patient has a scrotum with a classic "bag of worms" appearance on exam and no symptoms concerning for urinary tract infection or sexually transmitted infection, a urinalysis, urine culture, and NAAT testing for gonorrhea and chlamydia are not indicated at this time.

(Chapter 472: Urologic Abnormalities of the Genitourinary Tract; Varicocele)

**Answer 22-6.** **B**

In female adolescents, poor reabsorption of an ovarian follicle may lead to the development of a cyst. There should be a follow-up pelvic ultrasound 6 weeks after the diagnosis to evaluate for resolution of the cyst. This testing also helps differentiate simple cysts from cystic neoplasms. Reassurance and anticipatory guidance would therefore not be appropriate for this patient. Given that the patient is currently asymptomatic, cystectomy is also not indicated at this time. With ovarian torsion, the ovary may twist on its vascular pedicle, causing ischemia. Although ovarian torsion may result in a palpable mass in the lower abdomen secondary to congestion from decreased venous return, this patient does not have severe abdominal/pelvic pain or abnormal blood flow to the ovary, making surgical detorsion an inappropriate next step. The differential for adnexal masses also includes tumors of the ovary, such as teratomas, germ cell tumors, sex cord stromal tumors, and surface-epithelial-stromal tumors. The most common ovarian tumor is a teratoma, which would likely be heterogeneous on ultrasound with possible calcifications. Given that the patient's mass is homogeneous and does not have any calcifications, it is likely a simple ovarian cyst that can be followed. If concern for malignancy is greater in the future, based on increased symptoms, a growing cyst, or a cyst with concerning features on ultrasound, laboratory evaluation may include β-human chorionic gonadotropin, α-fetoprotein, and CA-125 levels.

(Chapter 383: Abdominal Masses; Diagnosis and Treatment, Genital Masses)

**Answer 22-7.** **C**

The patient in this vignette has urethral prolapse, with eversion and protrusion of the distal portion of the urethra through the meatus. Although uncommon, the condition typically affects young, prepubertal African American women. Urethral prolapse is thought to be secondary to inherent weakness of the urethral pelvic floor support and increased intra-abdominal pressure from conditions such as chronic cough and constipation. Patients often present with dysuria or bloody spotting. Physical exam reveals a midline, donut-shaped, fleshy urethral mass at the anterior vagina. Differential diagnosis should include vaginal tumors, prolapsed ureteroceles, or sexual abuse, as these conditions may have similar findings. Initial management includes sitz baths, topical estrogen cream, and the treatment of any underlying cough or constipation. If resolution does not occur, surgical excision of the prolapsed tissue may be required.

(Chapter 472: Urologic Abnormalities of the Genitourinary Tract; Urethral Prolapse)

**Answer 22-8.** **A**

This patient's physical exam is concerning for microphallus, which is defined by a stretched penile length < 2.5 standard deviations below the mean for age. In this term newborn male, a stretched penile length < 1.9 cm would be considered microphallus. Proper penile measurement should be done holding a rigid ruler against the pubic symphysis while keeping upward traction on the penis. Given that the patient's measurement was done with a paper tape measurer and it is unclear whether or not the penis was stretched, remeasuring the penile length would be the appropriate first step in management.

If microphallus is confirmed, most cases are the result of fetal testosterone deficiency, caused by a defect of the hypothalamic-pituitary-gonadal axis or local end-organ insensitivity to testosterone. Central causes of microphallus include Kallmann syndrome, Prader-Willi syndrome, and panhypopituitarism. Central defects may cause associated hypoglycemia or failure to thrive. Anorchia, a disorder of in utero vanishing testes, also results in testosterone deficiency. Microphallus with palpable testes and normal scrotal appearance suggests a male karyotype, and abnormal scrotal findings may indicate ambiguous genitalia from disorders of sex development. The conditions of buried penis and webbed penis are frequently diagnosed as microphallus. If microphallus is confirmed in this patient after the appropriate measurement technique is used, the patient may need additional lab work and consultation with a pediatric endocrinologist. Circumcision should be avoided until a full evaluation, gender assignment, and medical therapy are completed.

(Chapter 472: Urologic Abnormalities of the Genitourinary Tract; Microphallus)

**Answer 22-9.** **E**

The child in the vignette has urolithiasis, likely secondary to calcium phosphate or calcium oxalate, the most common stones. Hypercalciuria is one of the most common metabolic risk factors identified in children with renal stones. Most children with hypercalciuria are normocalcemic and have idiopathic hypercalciuria. This is likely the underlying etiology for the patient in this vignette. The exact cause of idiopathic hypercalciuria is unknown and may be a complex disorder of calcium homeostasis characterized by altered calcium transport in the intestine, kidney, and bone due to various combinations of multiple genetic and dietary factors.

Another common cause of normocalcemic hypercalciuria is the use of medications such as corticosteroids and loop diuretics. This patient has no significant past medical history and does not take any daily medications, making this etiology less likely. A less common cause of normocalcemic hypercalciuria is a monogenic defect.

Hypervitaminosis D, primary hyperparathyroidism, and adrenal insufficiency are all causes of hypercalcemic hypercalciuria. These causes are less likely, given that this patient had a serum electrolytes and ionized calcium within normal limits. Other causes of hypercalcemic hypercalciuria include immobilization, hypo- and hyperthyroidism, adrenocorticosteroid excess, osteolytic metastases, milk-alkali syndrome, idiopathic hypercalcemia of infancy, Williams syndrome, and mutation of the calcium-sensing receptor.

(Chapter 471: Urinary Tract Stone Diseases; Etiology)

## Answer 22-10. D

The patient in this vignette has cryptorchidism, the failure of a testis to descend and maintain a scrotal position. Congenital cryptorchidism involves cases noted at birth, whereas acquired cryptorchidism occurs when a previously descended testis is noted to be in an extrascrotal position. Of note, a retractile testis moves easily in and out of the scrotal position but is able to be positioned and remain in the scrotum temporarily.

The descent of the testis through the inguinal canal into the scrotum occurs at 28 weeks of gestation, which explains the higher incidence in premature newborns when compared to term newborns. It is important to note the patient's gestational age at birth, because spontaneous descent of the testis is unlikely to occur beyond 6 months of corrected age. Given that this infant was born at 30 weeks of gestation and is not yet at 6 months of corrected age, continued outpatient follow-up is appropriate. If the testis has not descended by 6 months of corrected age, a surgical specialist referral will be indicated. Congenital cryptorchidism is ideally surgically corrected with orchiopexy between 6 and 18 months of corrected age to maximally preserve spermatogenesis.

A diagnosis of congenital adrenal hyperplasia should be considered for newborns with bilateral nonpalpable undescended testes, but this patient only has one nonpalpable undescended testis, decreasing the utility of evaluation with serum electrolytes and 17-hydroxyprogesterone level. Although potential long-term risks of cryptorchidism include infertility and testicular germ cell tumors, this patient does not have any indication on history or physical exam for serum α-fetoprotein testing at this time. Finally, ultrasounds should not be routinely performed for nonpalpable undescended testes as they do not affect management. Hormonal therapy for inducing testicular descent is also not recommended as it has not been proven to be effective in long term.

(Chapter 472: Urologic Abnormalities of the Genitourinary Tract, Cryptorchidism [Undescended Testes])

## Answer 22-11. B

Hematuria may indicate urinary tract disease but can also occur in otherwise healthy children. The initial presentation may be as discolored red, brown, or tea-colored urine, but can also present as yellow urine with a positive dipstick for blood. History should include a detailed review of systems, including the color of the urine and whether the hematuria is painful or painless, intermittent or persistent, and microscopic or gross. A thorough family history should also be obtained. Brown or tea-colored urine is common in glomerulonephritis, whereas red urine may suggest postglomerular bleeding. Figure 464-1 shows an algorithm for the approach to hematuria.

Gross hematuria is less common than microscopic hematuria and may warrant further evaluation. This patient has no history of trauma, fever, dysuria, or other urinary tract infection symptoms; no abnormalities such as a palpable mass on physical exam; and no casts or dysmorphic RBCs on microscopy. Suspicion for causes such as trauma, renal tumors, glomerulonephritis, hemorrhagic cystitis, sickle cell hemoglobinopathies, or nephrolithiasis is low.

Given her reassuring history, family history, physical exam, and lack of casts or dysmorphic RBCs, she can be closely observed as an outpatient with a repeat urinalysis. If her subsequent urinalysis is negative, routine well-child care can be resumed. If her repeat urinalysis is positive for blood, she may require further evaluation for hypercalciuria, a renal ultrasound, evaluation for sickle cell trait, familial evaluation for familial hematuria, and continued close follow-up. Renal biopsy would be considered if she developed proteinuria or had cellular casts on further evaluations. It would also be considered if she was found to have a family history of hereditary renal disease or a decrease in renal function.

(Chapter 464: Kidney or Urinary Tract Disorders, Approach to the Child with Hematuria)

## Answer 22-12. C

Paraphimosis is a urologic emergency that occurs when the prepuce is left retracted proximal to the glans and becomes edematous, resulting in a tourniquet that impedes blood flow to the glans. Patients often present with significant pain and a constricting band of preputial tissue at the coronal sulcus. This requires prompt reduction. The procedure begins with steady manual compression over the glans and edematous foreskin for 5 to 10 minutes, after which the constrictive ring should be pulled over and distal to the glans.

Almost all newborn males have physiologic phimosis, which describes naturally occurring adhesions that prevent

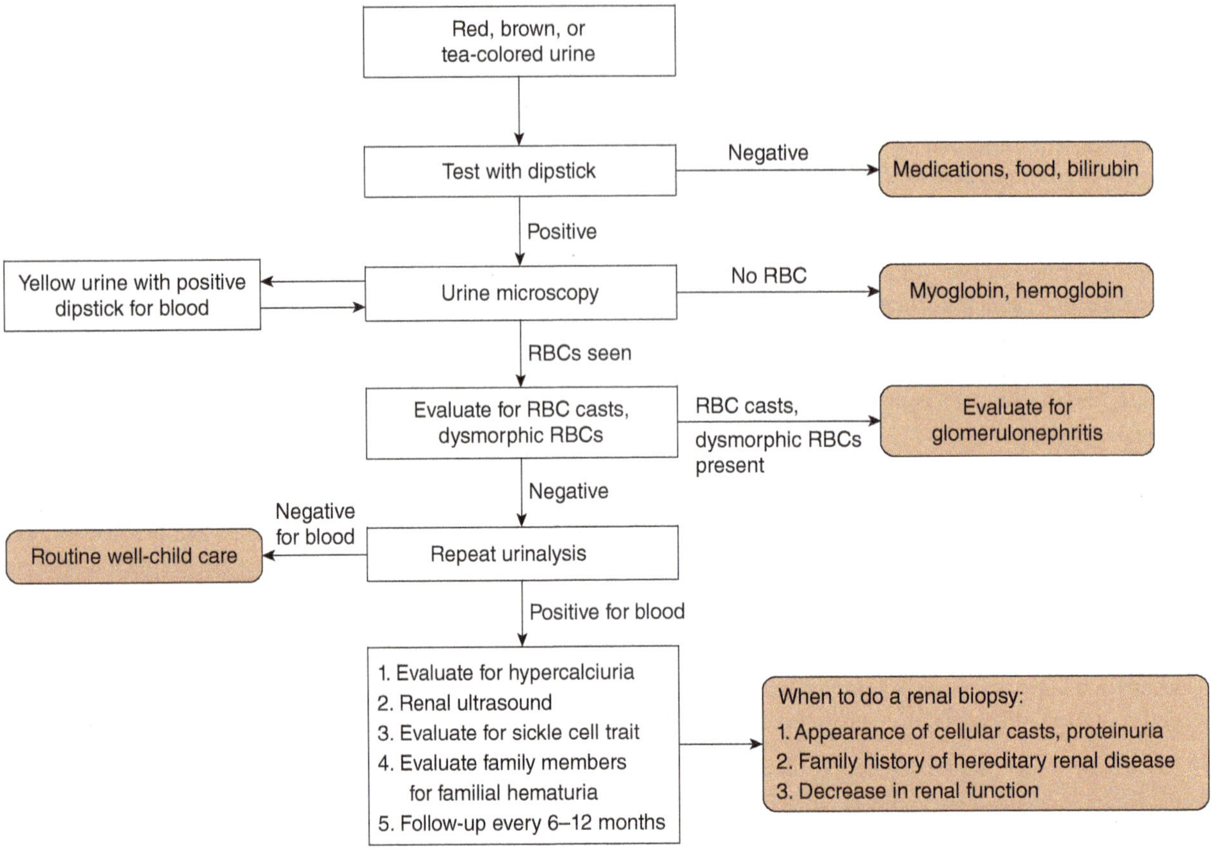


**FIGURE 464-1.** Algorithm for the evaluation of the child with hematuria. RBC, red blood cell. (Mark W. Kline, *Rudolph's Pediatrics*, 23rd Edition. Copyright © McGraw-Hill Education. All rights reserved.)

full retraction of the prepuce and exposure of the glans. The adhesions are gradually loosened by separation of the prepuce from the glans, aided by penile growth and intermittent physiologic erections. Most children are able to fully retract the prepuce by the teenage years. Pathologic phimosis is a true inability to retract the prepuce and can be caused by concentric scarring of the prepuce from infection and inflammation. On physical examination, there is often a fibrous, whitish ring at the edge of the preputial orifice. In severe cases, there may be ballooning of the prepuce with dribbling of urine. Most cases of pathologic phimosis are responsive to a 1-month course of twice-a-day topical corticosteroids. For refractory cases, circumcision may be necessary. Hypospadias is a congenital anomaly that occurs when urethral folds fail to fuse appropriately during penile development, leading to an ectopic location of the urethral meatus. Newborns are usually repaired between 6 and 18 months of age. Urethrorrhagia describes bleeding originating from the urethra. Most cases are idiopathic and self-limited, although urethrorrhagia can also be rarely caused by tumor, trauma, meatal stenosis, or infection. The diagnosis is typically limited to boys and presents with intermittent bloody spotting in the underwear between voids or occurs at initiation or termination of voiding. Most cases are idiopathic and resolve within 1 to 2 years, so reassurance with observation is recommended. If symptoms persist, further workup, such as cystoscopy, can be considered.

(Chapter 472: Urologic Abnormalities of the Genitourinary Tract; Phimosis and Paraphimosis, Hypospadias, and Urethrorrhagia)

**Answer 22-13.** E

The patient in the vignette has nocturnal enuresis, which occurs in roughly 7% of 10 year olds. The majority of children with this problem do not have organic or functional disease. The patient has primary enuresis, as he has never achieved dryness for an extended period of time. Evaluation should include a complete history detailing daytime and nighttime urinary patterns and fluid intake. Additionally, stool history, urinary tract infection (UTI) symptom history, family history, and social history should be obtained. Nocturnal enuresis is commonly familial, with 74% of enuretic males having at least one parent with a history of enuresis. A thorough physical examination and screening urinalysis should also be completed for each patient.

Although a variety of treatment approaches may be helpful, most children become dry with time no matter what approach is used. Initial approaches may include education for the patient and the patient's family, treatment of constipation (if present), limitation of fluid intake, and trial of awakening the child at night to void. Bedwetting alarms work via conditioning and have an initial cure rate of roughly 70%, with only a 10% to

15% relapse rate. Children may initially need to be awakened when the alarm goes off, and use for 3 to 4 months is typically required to achieve dryness. Although DDAVP® is effective in reducing the number of wet nights for most children, the relapse rate exceeds 80% when treatment is stopped. It can be used intermittently for children to participate in short-term activities, such as sleepovers and camp. Imipramine can also be used as a treatment modality, as it combines an anticholinergic effect for increasing functional bladder capacity with a noradrenergic effect to decrease detrusor contractions. The cure rate is between 10% and 60%, and there is a high relapse rate. Given that imipramine has the potential for serious toxicity, it should be used after other methods have failed and only with warnings regarding side effects and risks of overdose.

(Chapter 464: Kidney or Urinary Tract Disorders; Enuresis)

**Answer 22-14.** D

The patient in the vignette has a clinical presentation most consistent with PUV. PUVs are remnant obstructive leaflets of tissue formed during urethral development that result in lower urinary tract obstruction. The condition is almost exclusive to males, and around half of all PUV cases are diagnosed prenatally. This patient's ultrasound showed PUV findings of bilateral hydroureteronephrosis and the pathognomonic "keyhole" sign of a dilated bladder and proximal urethra. Next steps in the management of this patient include immediate bladder decompression, confirmatory voiding cystourethrography (VCUG), and valve resection or ablation.

A ureterocele would be seen on ultrasound as a cyst-like structure at the base of the bladder and may be accompanied by hydronephrosis. UPJ obstruction typically presents on ultrasound as hydronephrosis without ureteral dilation. Although renal dysplasia is strongly associated with PUVs, ultrasonography would also reveal increased renal echogenicity, loss of corticomedullary differentiation, and cortical cysts. Horseshoe kidney is the most common renal fusion anomaly. Fusion typically occurs at the inferior pole of each kidney. On ultrasound, the fused kidney may be located in the midline (symmetric horseshoe kidney) or laterally (asymmetric horseshoe kidney).

(Chapter 472: Urologic Abnormalities of the Genitourinary Tract; Posterior Urethral Valves)

**Answer 22-15.** A

Uric acid stones are relatively uncommon in children but can result from increased uric acid production secondary to hematologic malignancies, gout, or inborn errors of purine metabolism. Other causes of hyperuricosuria and subsequent stone formation are high purine intake, renal tubular disorders, or uricosuric medications. Some patient populations, including those with diabetes mellitus or bowel disease, also have a higher prevalence of uric acid stones.

Cystinuria is a rare autosomal recessive disorder that results in abnormal excretion of amino acids, including cysteine, ornithine, arginine, and lysine. Homozygous mutations typically result in increased excretion of cysteine and stone formation, whereas heterozygous mutations typically result in cysteine excretion that is not usually associated with stone formation. Struvite (magnesium ammonium phosphate) stones are typically associated with urinary tract infections with urea-splitting organisms, such as *Proteus mirabilis*. These organisms hydrolyze urea to generate ammonium and bicarbonate, and the subsequent high urine pH and urinary ammonium concentration promote magnesium and phosphate precipitation. Calcium phosphate and calcium oxalate are the most common stones, and contributing factors include hypercalciuria, hyperoxaluria, or hypocitraturia, in combination or alone. Loop diuretics increase urine calcium excretion and can contribute to stone formation. Low levels of urinary citrate, a natural inhibitor of stone formation, predispose to stone formation.

(Chapter 471: Urinary Tract Stone Diseases; Etiology)

**Answer 22-16.** B

The patient in this vignette has a clinical presentation most consistent with epididymitis, an inflammatory disease of the epididymis. In sexually active adolescents, most cases of epididymitis are attributed to the retrograde extension of *C trachomatis* from the vas deferens. The second most common cause of epididymitis in adolescents is *N gonorrhoeae*. In prepubertal children, epididymitis may be related to underlying genitourinary abnormalities such as posterior urethral valves. Causative organisms are frequently coliform bacteria, such as *E coli*.

Epididymitis is usually clinically diagnosed and may present with gradual scrotal pain and edema. Associated symptoms may include urethral discharge, nausea, fever, and abdominal or flank pain. On exam, the scrotum may be edematous or erythematous and be tender to palpation. Fluctuance or fixation of the scrotal tissue around the epididymitis is concerning for a scrotal abscess. In contrast to patients with testicular torsion, patients with epididymitis should have a cremasteric reflex that is intact. Treatment for the patient in this vignette includes appropriate antibiotic therapy for the patient and his sexual partner(s). Failure to improve with antibiotic therapy within 72 hours should prompt reevaluation for the possibility of an abscess.

(Chapter 78: Scrotal Masses; Epididymitis)

**Answer 22-17.** E

The patient in this vignette has a clinical presentation that is most consistent with bacterial vaginosis (BV). This condition results from the replacement of vaginal *Lactobacillus* species with high concentrations of anaerobic bacteria, including *Bacteroides* species and other bacteria such as *Gardnerella vaginalis* and *Mycoplasma hominis*.

BV is the most common cause of abnormal vaginal discharge. Symptoms may also include pruritus, irritation, and a "fishy" odor, but many patients who meet clinical criteria have no symptoms. On microscopy, vaginal epithelial cells may be studded with adherent coccobacilli and have a "clue cell" appearance. Although rare, BV can be found in non–sexually active women. BV is associated with lack of condom use, multiple partners, and douching. The condition is also associated with increased risk of acquiring sexually transmitted illnesses, such as human immunodeficiency virus (HIV), gonorrhea, chlamydia, herpes simplex virus, and human papillomavirus. In pregnant women, BV is associated with preterm labor. Symptomatic BV may be treated with antibiotics. Male partners of infected women are typically asymptomatic, and treating men does not affect a woman's disease course. There is insufficient evidence to recommend routine screening and treatment in asymptomatic pregnant women to prevent preterm birth.

(Chapter 228: Sexually Transmitted Infections; Bacterial Vaginosis)

**Answer 22-18. A**

This patient presents with cyclic abdominal pain and primary amenorrhea. Her labs (normal FSH, LH, and estradiol) suggest a eugonadotropic state. If primary amenorrhea occurs in a eugonadotropic state, the underlying etiology is often anatomic in origin (Table 79-1). This may include imperforate hymen,

**TABLE 79-1. Differential Diagnoses for Primary and Secondary Amenorrhea, Negative Pregnancy Test**

| | Hypogonadotropic Hypogonadism | Hypergonadotropic Hypogonadism | Eugonadotropic Eugonadism |
|---|---|---|---|
| **Gonadotropin Levels** | Low FSH, normal/low LH, low estradiol | High FSH, normal/high LH | Normal FSH, LH, and estradiol |
| **Differential Diagnosis** | • Constitutional delay of puberty<br>• Chronic disease<br>  • Regional enteritis<br>  • Cystic fibrosis<br>  • Diabetes<br>• Anorexia nervosa/female athlete triad<br>  • Excessive exercise<br>• Stress<br>• Isolated GnRH deficiency (Kallaman Syndrome)<br>• Endocrinopathy<br>  • Hypothyroidism<br>  • CAH<br>  • Cushing disease<br>• Pituitary lesions<br>  • Craniopharyngiomas<br>  • Infiltrative processes<br>  • Infarction/Sheehan syndrome<br>• Pharmacologic agents/drugs<br>  • Contraceptives<br>  • Antiepileptics<br>  • SSRIs<br>  • Phenothiazine derivatives<br>  • Illicit (heroin, cocaine) | • Gonadal dysgenesis<br>• Primary ovarian insufficiency<br>  • Idiopathic<br>  • Infection<br>  • Hemorrhage<br>  • Compromised blood supply<br>  • Trauma<br>• Autoimmune<br>• Radiation<br>• Chemotherapy<br>• Turner syndrome (45,XO)<br>• Androgen insensitivity (46,XY)<br>• Abnormalities of ovarian FSH receptors<br>• Defects in estrogen biosynthesis | • Müllerian duct defects<br>• MRKH syndrome<br>• Uterine scarring<br>• PCOS<br>• Virilizing ovarian and adrenal tumors<br>• Pharmacologic agents/drugs |

CAH, congenital adrenal hyperplasia; FSH, follicle-stimulating hormone; GnRH, gonadotropin-releasing hormone; LH, luteinizing hormone; MRKH, Mayer-Rokitansky-Kuster-Hauser syndrome; PCOS, polycystic ovary syndrome; SSRIs, selective serotonin reuptake inhibitors.

Mark W. Kline, *Rudolph's Pediatrics*, 23rd Edition. Copyright © McGraw-Hill Education. All rights reserved.

vaginal atresia or absence, or other malformations of the cervix and uterus. The patient's physical exam findings of bulging blue membrane on vaginal exam and anterior tender mass on rectal exam are most consistent with hematocolpos (blood-filled vagina) resulting from an imperforate hymen. Her cyclic abdominal pain likely coincides with the timing of her menstrual cycle.

Pregnancy is unlikely in the setting of a negative pregnancy test and the patient's physical exam findings. While Asherman syndrome (uterine synechiae) is also typically associated with normal FSH, LH, and estradiol levels, it is typically a cause of secondary amenorrhea. Uterine synechiae may occur after infection, such as pelvic inflammatory disease or tuberculous endometritis, or after endometrial manipulation, such as pregnancy or dilation and curettage. Turner syndrome may present as primary amenorrhea but is a cause of hypergonadotropic hypogonadism and associated with high FSH and normal/high LH. The patient in the vignette has a low BMI, but primary amenorrhea associated with anorexia nervosa is characterized by hypogonadotropic hypogonadism and associated with low FSH, normal/low LH, and low estradiol.

(Chapter 79: Menstrual Problems; Amenorrhea)

**Answer 22-19.** C

The patient in this vignette has a clinical presentation that is most consistent with hemorrhagic cystitis, particularly in the context of having symptoms of dysuria and gross hematuria and the presence of blood and leukocyte esterase on urinalysis with RBCs and WBCs on microscopy. Other typical symptoms of cystitis include fever, abdominal pain, suprapubic pain, hesitancy, urgency, and frequency. Cystitis is most often caused by infection; other causes include chemotherapy and radiation.

Although acute pyelonephritis may be associated with some lower urinary tract findings, it is less likely the diagnosis in this vignette, given the lack of spiking fevers, chills, nausea, vomiting, abdominal pain, back pain, and flank pain. The presence of RBCs on urine microscopy makes myoglobinuria and paroxysmal nocturnal hemoglobinuria less likely, as these conditions would present with positive findings for blood on urinalysis but lack the presence of RBCs on microscopy. Renal cysts from autosomal dominant polycystic kidney disease occasionally rupture and cause gross hematuria, but a patient with autosomal dominant polycystic kidney disease would likely have findings of cysts on renal ultrasound. Other conditions that should be considered with gross hematuria include genitourinary trauma, renal tumor, glomerulonephritis, sickle cell hemoglobinopathies, nephrolithiasis, hypercalciuria, coagulopathies, and vascular malformations.

(Chapter 464: Kidney or Urinary Tract Disorders; Approach to the Child with Hematuria)

**Answer 22-20.** D

Testicular torsion occurs when the spermatic cord twists, cutting off the testicle's blood supply. It most commonly occurs in adolescent males and is a surgical emergency, given the short window for salvage of the testicle. The "bell clapper" deformity is the most common testicular anatomic abnormality and can predispose to testicular torsion. The tunica vaginalis completely surrounds the testicle, and the absence of the normal posterior anchoring at the gubernaculum testis allows the testicle to twist freely.

Testicular torsion commonly presents as abrupt onset severe testicular pain. Associated symptoms may include nausea, vomiting, fever, and abdominal pain. Patients may describe a history of transient episodes of scrotal pain consistent with intermittent torsion and detorsion. On physical exam, patients may present with a swollen, tender, erythematous scrotum that is difficult to examine. The cremasteric reflex is almost always absent. Conversely, with appendiceal torsion, which results from twisting of the appendix testis or appendix epididymis, the cremasteric reflex is typically present. Physical exam findings for appendiceal torsion may also include tenderness to testicular palpation over the superior or inferior pole of the testis with or without a palpable mass or the "blue dot" sign, which represents the infarcted appendage seen through the scrotal skin.

Diagnosis can be made clinically based on physical examination findings or with the assistance of color Doppler ultrasound, which has a sensitivity of 100% and a specificity of 75%. Treatment consists of emergent surgical exploration and detorsion, given that testicular viability decreases to 0 after 24 hours. In addition, the affected testis and contralateral testis are typically fixed to the scrotum with a scrotal orchiopexy, given the high incidence of retorsion and contralateral testis torsion.

(Chapter 78: Scrotal Masses; Testicular Torsion)

**Answer 22-21.** D

The patient in the vignette has a clinical presentation most consistent with hypospadias. Hypospadias is a congenital anomaly, occurring when the urethral folds fail to fuse appropriately during penile development, resulting in ectopic location of the urethral meatus. The appropriate management is to abort the circumcision and refer to urology for future repair of the condition, as uncorrected hypospadias may result in difficulty with urinary stream control, impaired sexual function, and psychological distress. See Figure 472-10.

Physical exam findings that may be found on neonatal examination include ventral penile curvature, dorsal hooded foreskin, and a displaced urethral meatus. It is important to carefully examine for testicular descent, as patients with hypospadias and cryptorchidism are at higher risk for disorders of sex development. Given that this patient has testes that are palpable bilaterally and penile length within normal limits for age, endocrinology referral is not typically indicated at this time.

If hypospadias is identified, it is imperative that the circumcision be aborted, as the foreskin typically serves as a reconstructive tissue for future hypospadias repair. Hypospadias repairs are generally conducted between 6 and

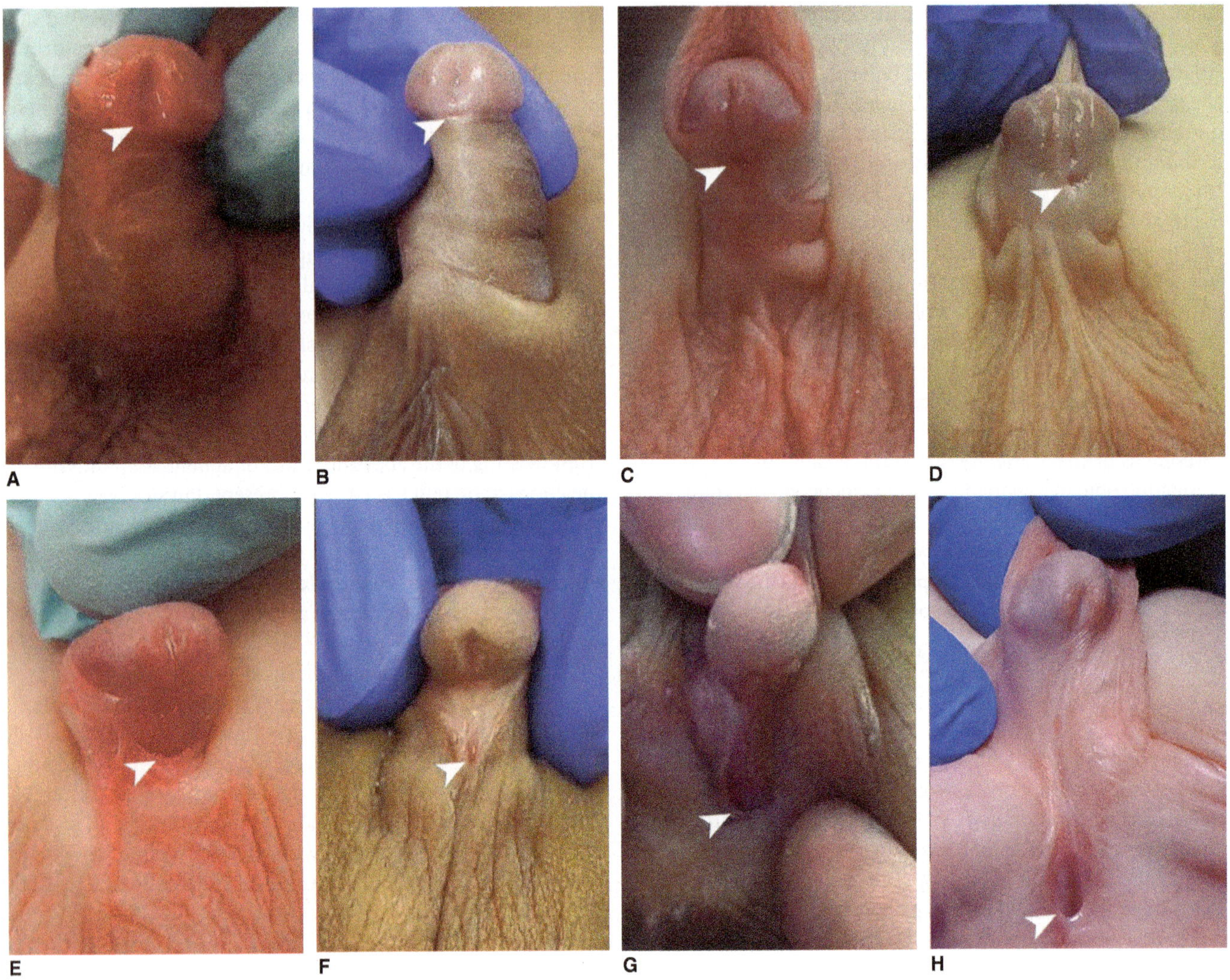


**FIGURE 472-10.** A spectrum of hypospadias based on urethral meatus location: (**A**) glanular, (**B**) coronal, (**C**) distal shaft, (**D**) midshaft, (**E**) proximal shaft, (**F**) penoscrotal, (**G**) scrotal, and (**H**) perineal. (Mark W. Kline, *Rudolph's Pediatrics*, 23rd Edition. Copyright © McGraw-Hill Education. All rights reserved.)

18 months of age, not emergently in the newborn period. Although distal cases can be repaired in a 1-stage procedure, more proximal or severe cases may require a 2-stage approach with potential need for revisions. In the vast majority of cases, children will not "outgrow" this condition.

(Chapter 472: Urologic Abnormalities of the Genitourinary Tract; Hypospadias)

## Answer 22-22. B

This patient has a clinical presentation that is most consistent with a spermatocele, which refers to the accumulation of sperm within the head of the epididymis. These benign cysts are often found by patients on routine physical examination. They are usually smooth, soft, and well-circumscribed, and found on the superior aspect of the testicle. Spermatoceles may transilluminate and generally range in size from 2 to 5 cm. They typically do not require intervention unless the patient is symptomatic with pain and/or pressure. See Figure 78-4.

Varicoceles are dilations of the pampiniform venous plexus within the scrotum and are often diagnosed clinically on physical exam. They may appear or feel like a "bag of worms" on palpation. Small varicoceles may only be detectable when

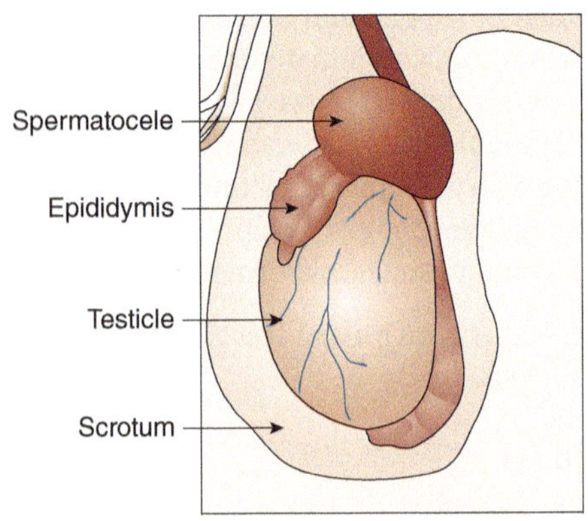


**FIGURE 78-4.** Spermatocele. (Mark W. Kline, *Rudolph's Pediatrics*, 23rd Edition. Copyright © McGraw-Hill Education. All rights reserved.)

a patient performs a Valsalva maneuver or stands. Hydroceles are typically painless on exam. Although communicating hydroceles may shift in size when the patient is upright or performs a Valsalva, noncommunicating hydroceles will not. Hydroceles will often transilluminate and feel like a supple, fluid cyst on palpation. The patient in the vignette most likely has spermatocele rather than a hydrocele given the location of the mass on the superior aspect of his testis. Testicular neoplasms are typically firm, irregular masses that are opaque to transillumination. However, cystic or necrotic areas of the tumor can be soft on palpation. Scrotal abscesses may present with scrotal erythema or edema. Fluctuance or fixation of the scrotal tissue around the epididymis is particularly concerning for the presence of a scrotal abscess.

(Chapter 78: Scrotal Masses; Spermatocele)

**Answer 22-23.** D

Orchitis is an inflammation of one or both testicles. It rarely occurs in prepubertal males and typically presents with edema, erythema, and tenderness of the affected testicle(s). It may be associated with constitutional symptoms such as fever, nausea, and abdominal pain. It is most often unilateral.

The most common cause of orchitis is the mumps virus. Mumps orchitis usually follows parotitis by about 4 to 8 days but can present up to 6 weeks after parotitis. Other viruses that are implicated less frequently are coxsackievirus, echovirus, adenovirus, and varicella. Viral orchitis is treated supportively with rest and nonsteroidal anti-inflammatory drugs. In contrast, bacterial orchitis is often a consequence of contiguous spread from an epididymal infection and is treated with antibiotics and supportive care. Infertility is a rare complication of orchitis and is most commonly associated with bilateral cases.

(Chapter 78: Scrotal Masses; Orchitis)

**Answer 22-24.** A

The patient described in this vignette presents with primary daytime incontinence, as she has never fully achieved dryness for an extended period of time. Wetting problems during the day typically arise as a consequence of the transition from an infantile to an adult voiding pattern. Although infants reflexively empty their bladder when a set volume is reached, most adults cortically inhibit reflex bladder contractions and have increased control of urination.

Organic causes of daytime wetting include urinary tract infections (UTIs), ectopic ureter, neurogenic bladder, and bladder outlet obstruction. Girls may have vaginal reflux of urine when they rise from a toilet. Giggle incontinence, an involuntary emptying of the bladder with giggling, is an uncommon cause of daytime wetting that predominantly occurs in girls. Sudden fright and social stressors, such as the loss of a parent or an abusive home environment, can also be associated with daytime wetting. Toilet training resistance, UTIs, and constipation are also potential contributors to daytime wetting.

Typically, limited evaluation is indicated for children with daytime incontinence. A thorough history and physical exam should be completed. In this patient scenario, a voiding diary may provide valuable information about the daytime wetting. Questions about toilet training, urinary stream, UTI symptoms and history, constipation history, and the family's response to wetting accidents are also helpful to ask. A thorough physical examination should be completed and include evaluation for a distended bladder and possible spinal defects. While observing a urinary stream in boys is helpful, it is more useful to listen to the sound of voiding in girls. Forceful, intermittent streaming or abrupt cessation of voiding may indicate issues with relaxation of the perineum. In general, a urinalysis and, possibly, a urine culture are the only laboratory tests that are useful. Radiographic studies are only typically indicated if there is a presence or history of a UTI, there is constant dampness from a possible ectopic ureter, there is a urinary stream problem in a male, or there are physical exam findings of a neurogenic bladder. Only children who are resistant to conservative measures require uroflowmetry and urodynamic studies. In this case, until further history is obtained, urine electrolytes, imaging, uroflowmetry and urodynamic studies, and subspecialist referral should be deferred.

(Chapter 464: Kidney or Urinary Tract Disorders; Enuresis)

**Answer 22-25.** C

Testicular tumors represent the most common solid tumor in males age 15 to 34 years. Roughly 95% of testicular neoplasms are germ cell tumors (including seminoma, embryonal carcinoma, teratoma, and choriocarcinoma). Sex cord stromal tumors (Leydig and Sertoli cell tumors) are far less common.

Although patients typically present with gradual, painless scrotal swelling, pain may be present if the tumor has hemorrhaged or become necrotic. Adolescents with testicular cancer are more likely to have associated cryptorchidism or testicular atrophy. Physical exam often reveals a firm, irregular mass that is opaque to transillumination. Some areas may be soft on palpation if there are cystic or necrotic areas. There may be accompanying hydroceles or varicoceles. Physical exam should also include evaluation of the contralateral testis, cervical and supraclavicular lymph nodes, and breast tissue.

Tumor markers should not be used for screening. β-Human chorionic gonadotropin and α-fetoprotein are useful tests for evaluation for certain histologic types. β-Human chorionic gonadotropin is elevated in choriocarcinoma, nonseminomatous mixed germ cell tumors, and seminoma with syncytiotrophoblasts, whereas α-fetoprotein is elevated in nonseminomatous germ cell tumors. Imaging of the mass should be done with ultrasound or magnetic resonance imaging, while staging requires chest and abdominal computed tomography (CT). Treatment is dependent upon staging and histology but may include a combination of orchiectomy, retroperitoneal lymph node dissection, radiation, and chemotherapy. The overall 5-year survival rate is > 95%.

(Chapter 78: Scrotal Masses; Testicular Neoplasms)

**Answer 22-26. D**

Isolated proteinuria is not uncommon in otherwise healthy children, particularly in the setting of fever, exercise, cold or heat exposure, or emotional stress. If proteinuria is seen on a urinalysis, other signs of renal disease should be evaluated such as edema, hypertension, or hematuria. In the absence of other clinical signs of renal disease, repeat urinalysis should be performed to determine whether proteinuria is transient or persistent. Some patients may have proteinuria that only presents in the upright position, known as orthostatic proteinuria, which can be diagnosed by checking a urinalysis upon first waking up in the morning and repeating later in the day. Patients who have fixed proteinuria on multiple urinalysis should receive additional evaluation for renal disease.

This patient does not have evidence of UTI, given negative leukocyte esterase, nitrites, and WBC on her urinalysis, so antibiotics would not be indicated. Until the proteinuria is determined to be fixed, additional renal workup such as labs (albumin, BUN, creatinine) or renal ultrasound would not be indicated. Similarly, referral to nephrology would only be warranted if the proteinuria were persistent or evidence of renal disease were found on further workup.

(Chapter 464: Kidney or Urinary Tract Disorders; Approach to the Child with Proteinuria)

**Answer 22-27. C**

Primary nocturnal enuresis is diagnosed when children have never achieved a significant period of dryness at night. It is a more common diagnosis than secondary enuresis, which is defined as enuresis that occurs after a child has had at least 6 months of staying dry. Primary enuresis may be associated with evening fluid intake, constipation, family or behavioral problems, and frequently, a family history of nocturnal enuresis. Constipation may lead to excess stool in the rectum, which can compress the bladder and lead to decreased bladder capacity and bladder overactivity.

Secondary enuresis is more suggestive of an organic cause, such as urinary tract infection (UTI), diabetes mellitus, or diabetes insipidus. Dysuria and hyperglycemia may be associated with UTIs and diabetes mellitus, respectively. Leg weakness may be suggestive of spinal mass or neurologic disorder, which may lead to new onset of urinary incontinence. Weak urine stream may suggest bladder dysfunction, which should not be associated with nocturnal enuresis.

(Chapter 464: Kidney or Urinary Tract Disorders; Enuresis; Chapter 472: Urologic Abnormalities of the Genitourinary Tract; Bladder Bowel Dysfunction)

**Answer 22-28. D**

Primary nocturnal enuresis may have several causes, including small bladder capacity, excessive urine production during sleep, problems with sleep arousal, or bladder contractions during deep sleep. Bedwetting alarms, which condition the child to awaken when voiding, have an initial cure rate of 70% with low relapse rate of 10% to 15%.

Because this child has primary nocturnal enuresis, UTI is unlikely to be the cause, and therefore, antibiotics are not indicated. Children do not voluntarily control their nighttime bedwetting, so reward charts or punishment do not lead to a change in behavior. Although DDAVP is very effective for treatment, the relapse rate is > 80% when stopped, and it is typically most effective when dosed intermittently to allow children to participate in sleepovers. Imipramine has variable cure rates of 10% to 60% and a high relapse rate.

(Chapter 464: Kidney or Urinary Tract Disorders; Enuresis)

**Answer 22-29. B**

Calcium phosphate and calcium oxalate are the most common types of kidney stones and may be associated with hypercalciuria, hyperoxaluria, or hypocitraturia. Low levels of urinary calcium or oxalate decrease the likelihood of stone crystallization and formation. Urinary citrate and magnesium both inhibit formation of calcium-containing kidney stones, so low levels are associated with increased risk of stone formation. Uric acid can lead to formation of calcium oxalate or uric acid stones, so lower urinary levels do not increase risk for stone formation.

(Chapter 471: Urinary Tract Stone Diseases; Etiology)

**Answer 22-30. A**

The patient in the vignette is presenting with a kidney stone, likely due to underlying hyperparathyroidism and increased urinary calcium. Abdominal CT is highly sensitive and specific for diagnosing kidney stones, although in children, abdominal ultrasound should be performed first to limit radiation exposure. Urine culture would be diagnostic for urinary tract infection (UTI), but in this previously healthy boy, UTI would be unlikely. Chemistry panel may reveal electrolyte or kidney function abnormalities but is unlikely to help determine underlying cause. Appendix ultrasound is useful for diagnosing appendicitis, which is not consistent with the clinical picture. Finally, although radio-opaque stones may be visible on an abdominal film/KUB, it is less sensitive and specific for diagnosing kidney stones than CT scan.

(Chapter 471: Urinary Tract Stone Diseases; Evaluation)

**Answer 22-31. B**

Excessive protein intake can lead to increased acid load in the body, which induces bone mineralization and efflux of calcium phosphate, which can predispose to kidney stone formation; reducing protein intake can thus help with reducing risk for kidney stone formation. Fluid intake helps to decrease chance of crystallization and stone formation. Citrate binds calcium and impedes growth of calcium phosphate crystals, and hypocitraturia is a risk factor for stone formation. A salt-restricted diet helps to reduce urinary calcium by promoting reabsorption of sodium and calcium; increased salt intake would not reduce risk for kidney stone formation. The majority of kidney stones are composed of calcium oxalate or calcium phosphate, so increased calcium intake could actually increase risk of kidney stone formation.

(Chapter 471: Urinary Tract Stone Diseases; Therapy)

**Answer 22-32. B**

For patients with stones that are 10 to 20 mm within the ureter, renal pelvis, and upper/middle calyces, lithotripsy to break up the stone to facilitate passing of stone fragments is appropriate management given its minimal invasiveness. Open surgery should be reserved for patients with complex stones, kidney obstruction, or other orthopedic issues that prohibit endoscopic procedures. Percutaneous nephrolithotomy, wherein stones are removed or pulverized under direct visualization during nephroscopy, is typically recommended for stones > 20 mm and located in renal pelvis or calyces. Tamsulosin facilitates medical expulsion of the stone but is generally recommended for smaller ureteral stones < 10 mm. Ureteroscopy is ideal for removing distal ureteral stones > 10 mm.

(Chapter 471: Urinary Tract Stone Diseases; Therapy)

**Answer 22-33. B**

The American Academy of Pediatrics recommends a renal and bladder ultrasound for children 2 to 24 months who present with their first febrile urinary tract infection (UTI). Ultrasound is able to evaluate for hydronephrosis, hydroureter, or bladder abnormalities that may suggest underlying diagnosis such as vesicoureteral reflux or urinary obstruction. VCUG is recommended only if there are abnormalities seen on ultrasound or other atypical or complex clinical situations; otherwise, it is reserved for patients who present with a second febrile UTI.

Chemistry panel to evaluate renal function is not routinely warranted in a patient who presents with febrile UTI with good urine output and is otherwise well appearing. DMSA scans are radionuclide imaging that is able to detect renal function and scarring, which may be a result of recurrent UTIs.

(Chapter 472: Urologic Abnormalities of the Genitourinary Tract; Vesicoureteral Reflux)

**Answer 22-34. D**

VUR is diagnosed via VCUG and graded I to V, with grade I being the most mild (reflux into ureter only) and grade V showing severe dilatation of ureter and pelvicalyceal system. Lower-grade VUR typically resolves by age 5, but higher grades may require surgical intervention such as ureteral reimplantation or injection of bulking agents. See Figure 472-5.

Antibiotic prophylaxis for patients with VUR is controversial but is generally considered for children with higher grade VUR (III–V) who have had at least 1 febrile UTI. A recent large randomized trial (RIVUR study) showed that antibiotic prophylaxis decreases the risk of recurrent UTIs but does not affect renal scarring; it also leads to increase in resistant pathogens. There is no indication to start children < 6 months old with a febrile UTI on prophylactic antibiotics if their renal ultrasound is normal and there is no concern for VUR. For patients who are started on antibiotic prophylaxis, consideration for discontinuation can be made after the child has been toilet trained, particularly if the child is able to communicate UTI symptoms such as dysuria. For this patient who has lowest grade VUR and no history of febrile UTI, there is no automatic indication for initiation of antibiotic prophylaxis.

(Chapter 472: Urologic Abnormalities of the Genitourinary Tract; Vesicoureteral Reflux)

**Answer 22-35. C**

Children with PUV are frequently affected by bladder dysfunction, known as valve bladder syndrome, which leads to poor bladder compliance and impaired emptying. They often require behavioral modifications, such as timed or double voiding, and may need clean intermittent catheterization for complete bladder emptying.

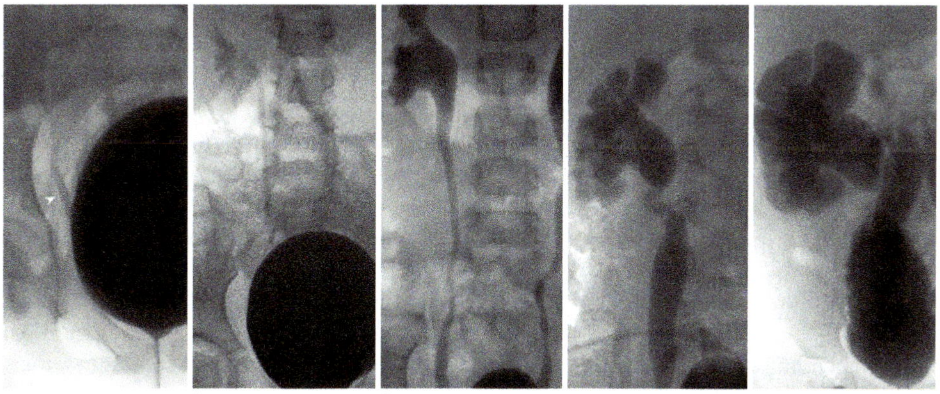


**FIGURE 472-5.** Voiding cystourethrogram studies showing vesicoureteral reflux: (A) grade 1, (B) grade 2, (C) grade 3, (D) grade 4, and (E) grade 5. (Mark W. Kline, *Rudolph's Pediatrics*, 23rd Edition. Copyright © McGraw-Hill Education. All rights reserved.)

Even children who are treated early for PUV will require lifelong follow-up with nephrology and urology due to potential associated complications. About 25% of patients will develop end-stage renal disease in childhood. For patients who do develop bladder dysfunction, anticholinergic or α-blocker medications can potentially be used for treatment depending on urodynamic function. About half of children who have PUV will also be found to have vesicoureteral reflux on voiding cystourethrogram.

(Chapter 472: Urologic Abnormalities of the Genitourinary Tract; Posterior Urethral Valves)

**Answer 22-36.** A

The white substance the parents are noticing between the penis and foreskin is called smegma, and it represents dead skin cells that build up as the foreskin is separating from the penis via desquamation. It is physiologically normal, and no medical intervention is needed beyond typical bathing and hygiene. Smegma does not represent any type of infection, and antibiotics, circumcision, and culture of the substance are not indicated. Parents should never forcibly retract the foreskin in children, as this can cause significant pain or bleeding.

(Chapter 472: Urologic Abnormalities of the Genitourinary Tract; Phimosis and Paraphimosis)

**Answer 22-37.** E

Newborn males undergoing circumcision should receive analgesia in the form of local anesthesia, such as a dorsal penile nerve block or penile ring block, or topical anesthesia, such as lidocaine or prilocaine.

The American Academy of Pediatrics states that the medical benefits of circumcision justify the procedure for families who choose it but are not sufficient to recommend it routinely. Medical benefits of circumcision include decreased risk of urinary tract infection (UTI), penile cancer, and sexually transmitted infections, and its benefits persist into adulthood. Complication rates of circumcision are < 1% and typically include bleeding or infection. There are several techniques and devices that may be used to perform a circumcision, including Gomco or Mogen clamps or PlastiBell device. Different practitioners may have more comfort or expertise with a particular method.

(Chapter 47: Postnatal Care and Observation of Low-Risk Newborns; Circumcision)

**Answer 22-38.** E

Hydroceles form due to congenital abnormalities in the inguinal canal and may be communicating (where fluid tracks down the inguinal canal into the tunica vaginalis, therefore leading to changes in size depending on patient position) or noncommunicating. Hydroceles typically transilluminate, are painless on exam, and feel cystlike on palpation. The scrotum should not be erythematous or warm in patients with hydrocele; scrotal erythema should raise concern for orchitis, epididymitis, or testicular torsion.

(Chapter 78: Scrotal Masses; Hydrocele)

**Answer 22-39.** E

UTI recurrence risk is highest 3 to 6 months after initial infection, so parents should be instructed to seek medical attention and evaluation for UTI if their child has recurrence of fever or other UTI symptoms. *Escherichia coli* is the most common uropathogen, causing 80% of UTIs. The incidence of UTIs is higher in boys (particularly uncircumcised boys) in the first year of life; after the first year, girls have a higher incidence of UTIs than boys. Asymptomatic bacteriuria occurs in 0.8% of preschool girls; this is the reason that a diagnosis of UTI requires positive urine culture as well as evidence of pyuria on urinalysis. Children who are beginning toilet training have a higher risk for UTIs, as they may have uncoordinated relaxation and tightening of the urethral sphincter during this time.

(Chapter 233: Urinary Tract Infection; Pathogenesis and Epidemiology, Diagnosis, Treatment)

**Answer 22-40.** A

*Escherichia coli* is the most common uropathogen, causing about 80% of all urinary tract infections (UTIs). Other gram-negative organisms such as *Klebsiella*, *Proteus*, *Enterobacter*, and *Citrobacter* also frequently cause UTIs. Some gram-positive organisms such as *S saprophyticus*, *S aureus*, or *Enterococcus* may also cause UTIs. Bacterial species that are thought *not* to be significant uropathogens include *Lactobacillus*, coagulase-negative *Staphylococcus*, and *Corynebacterium*.

(Chapter 233: Urinary Tract Infection; Pathogenesis and Epidemiology)

**Answer 22-41.** C

Antibiotic choice for urinary tract infection (UTI) treatment depends on antimicrobial susceptibility profile; typical appropriate options include cephalosporins, amoxicillin-clavulanate, or trimethoprim-sulfamethoxazole. However, sulfonamide antibiotics such as trimethoprim-sulfamethoxazole and sulfisoxazole should be avoided in neonates < 4 weeks old due to risk of hyperbilirubinemia. Nitrofurantoin should also not be used in neonates or patients with renal or liver dysfunction; it is generally not a good antibiotic choice because of low tissue concentrations. Ciprofloxacin may be used to treat *Pseudomonas aeruginosa* UTIs but is not considered first-line therapy, particularly when other treatment options are available. In this patient, cefixime would be the most appropriate antibiotic of the answers listed; other appropriate antibiotic regimens would include amoxicillin or amoxicillin-clavulanate. In general, the narrowest spectrum antibiotic based on culture susceptibilities is appropriate to prevent development of antimicrobial resistance.

(Chapter 233: Urinary Tract Infection; Treatment)

**Answer 22-42.** D

Dysfunctional voiding, or lack of coordination of urethral sphincter relaxation and detrusor muscle contraction in the bladder, is a risk factor for UTIs because inefficient elimination of urine allows for bacterial ascension and adherence to the urethra and bladder. Behavioral modification to encourage frequent, timed voiding, particularly in young children who have recently been toilet trained and may forget to use the restroom while playing, is first-line treatment. Ensuring adequate fluid intake and perineal hygiene are also recommended. Other risk factors for UTIs include constipation, indwelling catheters, and congenital anomalies; treatment of constipation, if present, would also be recommended for this patient.

Referral to urologist is not warranted at this time, since VCUG was normal and did not demonstrate VUR or any other anatomic abnormalities. Repeat VCUG would be low yield, since results would likely be unchanged and not impact management. If the patient continues to have recurrent UTIs despite behavioral modifications and there is concern for renal scarring, then a DMSA scan may be considered to evaluate for renal scarring, but the initial recommendation should be behavioral modifications to decrease risk of recurrent UTIs. Antibiotic prophylaxis would not be indicated in this patient since she does not have any evidence of VUR or anatomic abnormalities for recurrent UTIs.

(Chapter 233: Urinary Tract Infection; Prevention)

**Answer 22-43.** B

This patient is presenting with symptoms of ovarian torsion, where the ovary twists on the vascular pedicle, leading to ischemia. Typical presenting symptoms are severe abdominal or pelvic pain, possibly with associated nausea or vomiting. Sometimes a mass is palpable due to venous congestion. Ultrasound with Doppler is able to detect decreased or absent blood flow to the ovary, and the treatment is surgical detorsion of the ovary, which is a time-sensitive procedure in order to preserve ovarian function.

Although a KUB radiograph may demonstrate bowel obstruction, tumor, or constipation, which may be contributing to abdominal pain, this patient's clinical presentation is concerning for ovarian torsion, which could not be diagnosed via KUB. She has not had any vomiting or abdominal distension suggestive of obstruction. CT of the abdomen/pelvis can be useful in evaluating for other acute abdominal pathologies, such as appendicitis, but is generally not the first-line imaging modality due to radiation exposure. In this patient, ultrasound with Doppler is sufficient to make the diagnosis. There is no indication that the patient is dehydrated and no clear evidence of bacterial infectious process, so IV fluids and antibiotics are not warranted at this time.

(Chapter 383: Abdominal Masses; Diagnosis and Treatment)

**Answer 22-44.** C

This patient's clinical presentation is consistent with sexually transmitted infections (STIs). Chlamydia and gonorrhea are the first and second most commonly reported bacterial STIs in the United States, respectively. Symptoms may include vaginal discharge, bleeding or pain with intercourse, or pelvic discomfort, although the majority of infections are asymptomatic. Twenty-five percent to 50% of women with gonorrhea infection also have a concurrent chlamydia infection. Ceftriaxone 250 mg intramuscularly plus azithromycin 1 g orally would empirically treat both chlamydia and gonorrhea infections.

Metronidazole is the recommended treatment for *Trichomonas vaginalis*, which is typically asymptomatic, although it may occasionally cause frothy vaginal discharge. Fluconazole is used to treat vulvovaginal candidiasis, which typically presents with vaginal pruritus and discomfort or vulvar edema and excoriations; yeast may be seen on wet mount or culture. Doxycycline 100 mg orally twice a day for 7 days is an acceptable treatment for chlamydia, but in this patient whose testing is pending, empiric treatment for both gonorrhea and chlamydia would be warranted. Metronidazole 500 mg orally twice a day for 7 days is used to treat bacterial vaginosis (BV), which typically presents with pruritus, itching, and discharge with "fishy" odor.

(Chapter 228: Sexually Transmitted Infections; Chlamydia and Gonorrhea)

**Answer 22-45.** B

NAATs have been shown to have higher sensitivity and specificity compared to other tests such as immunoassays and serology and thus are the preferred testing modality for both chlamydia and gonorrhea.

Routine screening for STIs is recommended annually, although frequency and extent of testing are dependent on individual risk factors. Although first-catch urine specimens are an acceptable sample on which NAAT testing can be performed, vaginal specimens are the preferred collection site given higher sensitivity. Positive NAATs can persist for up to 3 weeks after successful treatment, so repeat test-of-cure is not routinely recommended. Antibiotic resistance to gonorrhea has become more prevalent in recent years, with strains that are resistant to cephalosporins, tetracycline, and macrolides having emerged; if patients have persistent symptoms 3 to 5 days after receiving therapy, treatment failure should be considered, and culture and antibiotic susceptibility testing should be performed.

(Chapter 228: Sexually Transmitted Infections; Chlamydia and Gonorrhea)

**Answer 22-46.** B

This patient is presenting with Fitz-Hugh-Curtis syndrome, right upper quadrant pain, and liver capsule inflammation due to ascending pelvic inflammatory disease (PID) infection. Findings of cervical motion tenderness, uterine or adnexal tenderness, vaginal discharge, or dyspareunia or vaginal bleeding are suggestive of PID. Laparoscopy typically provides a definitive diagnosis and may demonstrate the pathognomonic finding of "violin-string" adhesions from the liver to the abdominal wall.

Liver function tests are usually normal in these patients. *Chlamydia trachomatis* is the most common causative organism, accounting for 80% of Fitz-Hugh-Curtis syndrome cases.

Treatment of PID and Fitz-Hugh-Curtis syndrome includes empiric antibiotics for chlamydia and gonorrhea. Common outpatient treatment regimens include ceftriaxone and doxycycline, whereas inpatient treatment may consist of cefoxitin and doxycycline or clindamycin and gentamicin. Hospitalization is generally required in certain situations, such as if other surgical emergencies must be ruled out, if pelvic or tubo-ovarian abscess has developed, during pregnancy, if the patient has experienced failure of outpatient therapy, or if the patient has nausea/vomiting or other inability to take oral medications. Serious PID sequelae include ectopic pregnancy and infertility, so empiric and early treatment is recommended for suspected cases.

(Chapter 228: Sexually Transmitted Infections; Pelvic Inflammatory Disease and Fitz-Hugh-Curtis Syndrome)

**Answer 22-47.** D

This patient's clinical presentation is consistent with anatomic abnormality such as imperforate hymen, vaginal atresia or absence, or other cervical or uterine malformations. She is otherwise healthy, with no family history of delayed puberty, and her recent episodes of cyclic abdominal pain may have coincided with menstrual cycles. Amenorrhea can be characterized into 3 categories based on pituitary function in relation to the ovary:

- Hypogonadotropic hypogonadism
  - Inadequate hypothalamic-pituitary stimulation of ovary
  - Characterized by low FSH, LH, and estrogen levels (answer choice A)
- Hypergonadotropic hypogonadism
  - Represents ovarian dysfunction or inability of the ovary to respond to hypothalamic-pituitary hormone signals
  - Characterized by high FSH and LH and low estrogen levels (answer choice E)
- Eugonadotropic eugonadism
  - Represents anatomic causes of primary amenorrhea resulting from defects in the development of the Mullerian duct system (what this patient likely has)
  - Characterized by normal FSH, LH, and estrogen levels (answer choice D)

Answer choices B (high FSH/LH, normal estrogen) and C (normal FSH/LH, low estrogen) do not represent typical hormone patterns for amenorrhea.

Management of amenorrhea typically begins with a progesterone challenge to see if uterine bleeding can be induced; this confirms patency of the reproductive outflow tract and presence of endogenous estrogen. If there is no bleeding after progesterone challenge, then administration of estrogen followed by progesterone challenge is the next step.

(Chapter 79: Menstrual Problems; Amenorrhea)

**Answer 22-48.** E

This premature infant most likely has an indirect inguinal hernia, which has resulted in an opening large enough for intra-abdominal organs (typically intestine) to protrude. The most common complication of indirect inguinal hernias is incarceration, which occurs if the external inguinal ring becomes restricted and cuts off blood flow to the hernia contents, which can become strangulated. If the incarcerated hernia cannot be reduced, it is a surgical emergency. Inguinal hernia incarceration is less common in premature infants because their hernias tend to be larger in size.

Indirect hernias are by far (99%) the predominant type of hernia seen in infants and young children and are secondary to a patent processes vaginalis during embryonic development. Direct hernias are much rarer and are caused by muscle floor weakness of the inguinal canal. Indirect inguinal hernias never spontaneously resolve, so surgical repair is required and is generally scheduled within a few weeks due to higher incarceration risk in infancy. Inguinal hernias are a clinical diagnosis, and ultrasound is not required for diagnosis. Inguinal hernias are 5 to 10 times more common in boys than girls.

(Chapter 400: Abdominal Wall Hernias; Inguinal Hernia)

**Answer 22-49.** C

This patient is presenting with the classic salt-wasting form of congenital adrenal hyperplasia (CAH), which is an inborn error of adrenocortical hormone synthesis. 21-Hydroxylase deficiency is the most common cause of classic CAH, causing up to 95% of cases. The lack of this enzyme leads to inability to convert 17-hydroxyprogesterone (17-OHP) to 11-deoxycortisol, leading to elevated levels of 17-OHP, which is the most useful diagnostic test for CAH and is used to perform newborn screening for this diagnosis. Due to lack of cortisol and aldosterone production, infants may present in initial weeks of life with salt-wasting dehydration characterized by hypovolemia, hypotension, shock, hyponatremia, and hyperkalemia. Female patients usually have virilization of external genitalia due to excess adrenal androgen production.

Cortisol levels would be low in patients with salt-wasting CAH, but the test is not specific for CAH; low cortisol levels may be due to other disorders in steroidogenesis. P450 oxidoreductase deficiency is a rare, autosomal recessive form of CAH that causes partial deficiency of 21-hydroxylase activity; patients typically have virilization of genitalia as well as skeletal malformations. However, this disorder is much less common than classic salt-wasting CAH. Although DHEA and androstenedione levels are expected to be elevated in patients with CAH due to shunting of precursors to the androgen pathway, they are not specific for CAH and cannot confirm the diagnosis. 11-Deoxycortisol is the next step in the cortisol synthesis pathway and may be elevated in patients with 11-hydroxylase deficiency, which may also cause CAH; however, this enzyme defect is much less common than 21-hydroxylase deficiency as a cause of CAH.

(Chapter 532: Disorders of Sexual Development; 46XX Disorders of Sexual Development, Congenital Adrenal Hyperplasia)

**Answer 22-50.** E

This patient's clinical presentation is consistent with complete androgen insensitivity syndrome, which typically results from a mutation in the X-linked androgen receptor. Genital and somatic organs do not respond to circulating testosterone both in utero and at puberty, which leads to external female genitalia and feminization at puberty. Affected individuals have a blind vaginal pouch and absent uterus, so although feminization and breast development occur during puberty, patients present with primary amenorrhea. They typically also have absent or sparse pubic and axillary hair due to impaired response of hair follicles to circulating androgens. These patients have normal testosterone and estradiol levels; FSH is also normal due to feedback from estradiol, but LH is elevated due to insensitivity of the hypothalamic feedback mechanism to circulating testosterone. Testes can frequently be palpated in inguinal canals or labial folds; neoplastic transformation is rare, so gonadectomy is typically recommended after puberty has been completed so that secondary sexual characteristics can fully develop.

Patients with XY gonadal dysgenesis or Swyer syndrome, which is characterized by incomplete or defective testes formation, typically have female external genitalia and present with delayed puberty and primary amenorrhea. Due to lack of functional gonads, secondary sex characteristics do not develop, and LH and FSH levels are both elevated. Prolactinomas are pituitary tumors that secrete abnormally high levels of prolactin; this can lead to galactorrhea and secondary amenorrhea in patients. Gonadotropin levels may be low in patients with prolactinomas due to pituitary compression from the tumor. Patients with 45X Turner syndrome have absent ovaries, which leads to lack of development of secondary sexual characteristics and elevated FSH and LH levels during puberty. Other clinical features of Turner syndrome include atypical facies, shield-like chest, webbed neck, lymphedema, congenital heart defects, and skeletal anomalies. Primary ovarian insufficiency, or premature ovarian failure, may have many different causes, including chromosomal abnormalities, endocrinopathies, infectious processes, or trauma. Lack of ovarian estrogen production leads to amenorrhea and lack of development of secondary sexual characteristics at puberty, and treatment is hormone replacement therapy.

(Chapter 532: Disorders of Sexual Development; 46 XY Disorders of Sexual Development, Androgen Receptor Defects; Chapter 79: Menstrual Problems, Amenorrhea)

# CHAPTER 23 Skin/Dermatology

Lynda Chima Aririguzo, Elisha Acosta,
Jennifer Benjamin, Megan F. Craddock,
Anna Rueda, Omar Jaber, and Grace Liao Lee

**23-1.** A 6-year-old girl was brought to the clinic by her father for concerns that she has lice. There was a case of lice diagnosed in one of the other students in her first-grade class 2 weeks ago. After hearing this, he bought permethrin 1% lotion from the store and applied it as directed in 2 applications 9 days apart. The second treatment was applied 2 days ago. He reports that despite the treatment, he thinks he can still see eggs in her hair. On exam of her hair and scalp under magnification, you see numerous translucent oval-shaped nits attached to her hair shaft approximately 2 inches from her scalp. You see no live adult lice or nymphs. Which of the following is true regarding the exam and treatment for this patient?

**A.** She has an active infection with lice. She should be treated with a second-line agent such as ivermectin 0.5% lotion to completely rid her of the infestation.

**B.** She no longer has an active infection. She needs no further topical treatment, but combing of her hair with a fine-toothed comb can help to remove the empty nits.

**C.** She has an active infection with lice. She should be treated with permethrin 1% lotion again as she failed the first treatment.

**D.** She no longer has an active infection with lice; however, she is at risk of repeat infestation. She should be treated prophylactically with a second-line agent such as ivermectin 0.5% lotion.

**E.** She has an active infection with lice. She should be treated with a second-line ovicidal agent such as lindane 1% lotion to completely rid her of the infestation.

**23-2.** A 10-year-old boy presents with a hairless linear plaque of coalesced yellow-colored papules that has been present and unchanged since birth. On exam, it appears as pictured in Figure 352-7. What is the diagnosis?

**A.** Aplasia cutis congenita

**B.** Alopecia areata

**C.** Nevus depigmentosus

**D.** Sebaceous hyperplasia

**E.** Nevus sebaceous

**23-3.** An 18-year-old high school football player presents to clinic with a new-onset rash on his upper chest and back. He noted the appearance of the rash after starting football practice 2 weeks ago. He noted worsening after swimming in his neighborhood pool yesterday. He has mild pruritus and no other associated symptoms. He is otherwise at his baseline health. On exam, you note hypopigmented macules that are sharply demarcated and have a fine scale overlying the lesions. These macules vary in size from a few millimeters to a few centimeters and are distributed on his posterior neck, upper back, and upper chest only. Which of the following statements is true of this patient's diagnosis?

**A.** The diagnosis can be made by performing a culture of a skin scraping.

**B.** The hypopigmentation resolves with exposure to sunlight.

**C.** Treatment with the appropriate oral or topical medications is equally effective.

**D.** This diagnosis is more common in prepubertal children.

**E.** This rash often starts on the torso and spreads to the inguinal area.

**23-4.** A 13-year-old female presents with lesions in her axilla, shown in Figure 360-4. What is the etiology?

**A.** Keratotic plugs that fill the hair follicle orifice, leading to rough horny follicular papules

**B.** Colonization of the hair follicles by *Propionibacterium acnes*

**C.** Delayed T-cell hypersensitivity reaction

**D.** Inflammatory disorder of the hair follicle with secondary apocrine gland inflammation

**E.** Benign, self-limited eruption of unknown etiology

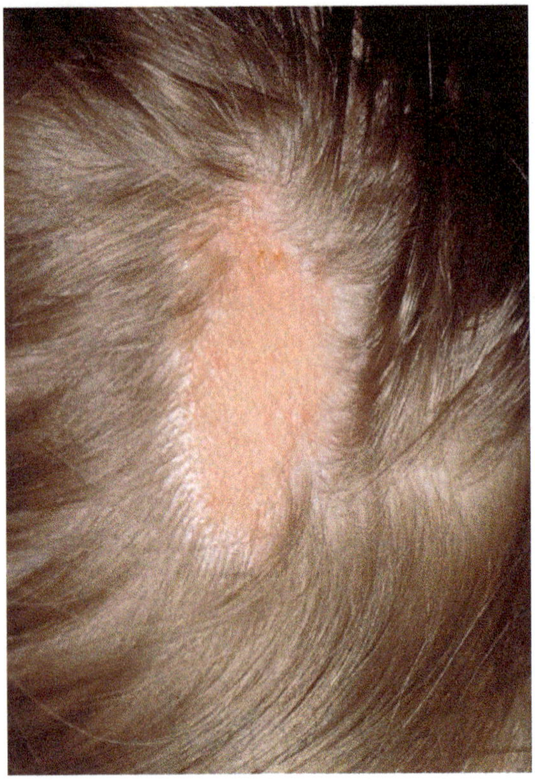

FIGURE 352-7. (Mark W. Kline, *Rudolph's Pediatrics*, 23rd Edition. Copyright © McGraw-Hill Education. All rights reserved.)

**23-5.** A 9-year-old girl presents with hair loss on her scalp and eyebrows for 4 months. She has no significant past medical history, is taking no medications, and has normal growth and development. On exam of her scalp, there are irregularly shaped areas of partial alopecia with broken hairs of varying length. The scalp has no discoloration or lesions seen on exam. She has alopecia on the lateral aspects of her bilateral eyebrows. What is the most appropriate treatment for this patient?

**A.** Behavioral modification

**B.** Oral antifungal

**C.** Topical steroid

**D.** Oral antibiotic

**E.** Dermatology referral

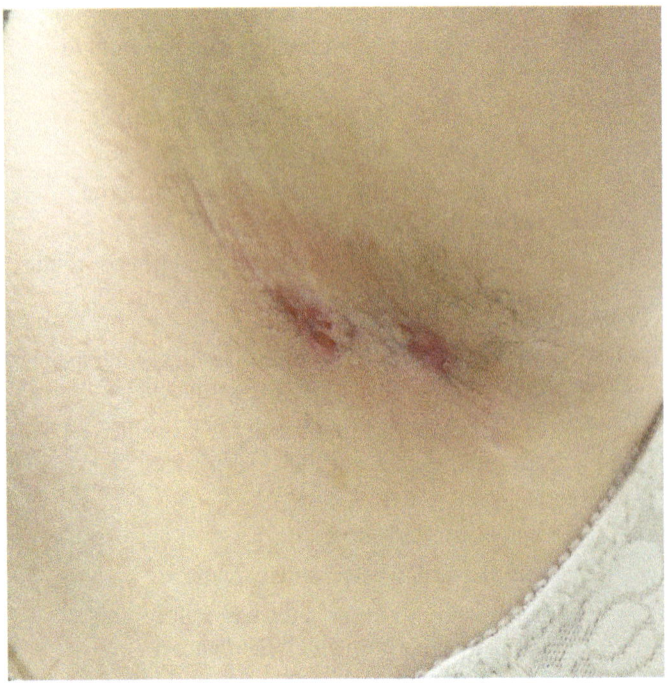

FIGURE 360-4. (Mark W. Kline, *Rudolph's Pediatrics*, 23rd Edition. Copyright © McGraw-Hill Education. All rights reserved.)

**23-6.** An 8-day-old infant presents for a weight check. The mother points out a rash that appeared to start in the diaper but is spreading onto the trunk and axillae. The lesions look like bubbles with straw-colored fluid inside; they rupture easily, and underneath, the skin looks denuded, with a surrounding collarette of residual blister roof. What bacteria would most likely cause this presentation?

**A.** *Candida albicans*

**B.** *Staphylococcus aureus*

**C.** *Streptococcus pyogenes*

**D.** Methicillin-resistant *S aureus* (MRSA)

**E.** Herpes simplex virus (HSV)

**23-7.** A 16-year-old boy who likes to do BMX biking took a bad fall and showed up in clinic today. He has a significant superficial laceration with surrounding bruising on his left lower extremity. His skin is hot to touch, but he has no fever or pus from the lesion. He goes home with a prescription for clindamycin to take orally and mupirocin ointment topically, with instructions for care of his injury. However, he is brought to the emergency department (ED) later that night for fever of 102°F, slight delirium, and extreme swelling of left lower leg. His blood pressure is 90/55 mm Hg, and his heart rate is 120 bpm. X-ray is done of the left lower extremity, and soft tissue gas is seen in the lower extremity x-ray. What is the most likely diagnosis?

**A.** Cellulitis

**B.** Ecthyma gangrenosum

**C.** Necrotizing fasciitis

**D.** Erythrasma

**E.** Staphylococcal scalded skin syndrome (SSSS)

**23-8.** A 15-year-old Latin American boy presents to clinic today with a rash on his chest. He often goes running but lately has been doing so without his shirt on because it is warm outside, and he noticed a hypopigmented, scaly rash on his chest extending to abdomen. Upon exam, you note similar lesions on his back. They are macular and confluent in places. They are somewhat itchy. What is the most likely diagnosis?

**A.** Pityriasis rosea

**B.** Vitiligo

**C.** Psoriasis

**D.** Tinea versicolor

**E.** Seborrheic dermatitis

**23-9.** A 17-year-old girl presents to your emergency department (ED) with high fever after visiting a college campus. She got to stay in one of the dorms for the weekend. However, as soon as she came home, she had a fever of 102°F, complaints of chills, and extreme lethargy per her mother. In the exam room, mom notes a rash of the patient's extremities that was not noted yesterday. Upon examination, there are purpuric, dark reddish-gray macules on the lower legs. Her palms and soles appear to be erythematous and swollen as well. Her vital signs in the ED include temperature of 103°F, blood pressure of 87/55 mm Hg, heart rate of 135 bpm, and oxygen saturation of 95% on room air. She seems "out of it" and cannot seem to answer questions well. What is the most likely diagnosis?

**A.** Rocky Mountain spotted fever (RMSF)

**B.** Henoch-Schönlein purpura (HSP)

**C.** Measles

**D.** Lyme disease

**E.** *Neisseria meningitis*

**23-10.** A 16-year-old boy presents to clinic for acne follow-up. He has multiple deep nodules, tender papules, pustules, and comedones along his face and upper back. He is frustrated because previous therapies, including topical medications and oral antibiotics, have been only minimally helpful, and he continues to develop scarring. After discussion about risks and benefit with him and his father, you decide to start him on oral isotretinoin. Which of the following conditions is he most likely to experience while taking isotretinoin?

**A.** Birth defects in offspring

**B.** Xerosis

**C.** Dyslipidemia

**D.** Depression

**E.** Pancreatitis

**23-11.** You are seeing a 7-year-old girl and her 10-year-old brother for a well-child visit. Their family plans to spend part of their summer vacation hiking in a forested park in Pennsylvania. The parents are concerned about tickborne illness and would like ways to prevent tick bites, including use of repellants. Which of the following repellant recommendations would be most appropriate?

**A.** Apply permethrin-containing products to the skin. Limit permethrin content to no more than 30%.

**B.** Apply DEET-containing products to the skin. Limit DEET content to no more than 30%.

**C.** Apply permethrin-containing products to the skin and clothing. Limit permethrin content to no more than 40%.

**D.** Apply DEET-containing products to the skin and clothing. Limit DEET content to no more than 40%.

**E.** Apply DEET-containing products to the skin. Limit DEET content to no more than 20%.

**23-12.** A 2-month-old female infant of Japanese heritage presents as a new patient for a well-child examination. Her mother is concerned about dark-colored patches on the infant's left eye and face that were first noted shortly after birth. Her physical exam is significant for a well-appearing infant with speckled blue-black patches of the left forehead, left temple, and sclera of her left eye. Her left tympanic membrane also has similar hyperpigmented, speckled lesions. The right side of her face, right eye, and tympanic membrane are spared. Which of the following conditions is she most at risk of developing?

**A.** Glaucoma

**B.** Cataract

**C.** Melanoma

**D.** Acute lymphoblastic leukemia

**E.** Retinoblastoma

**23-13.** A 3-week-old female infant presents to clinic for bumps on her back. The infant was born via spontaneous vaginal delivery at 41 weeks' gestation. Delivery was complicated by meconium aspiration, for which she spent several days in the neonatal intensive care unit (NICU). Although she has been feeding well since discharge, she has developed hard bumps on her back and has become fussier within the last week. On exam, she is well nourished and well hydrated but very fussy and difficult to console. She has several erythematous nodules and indurated plaques on her back. Given her presentation, which of the following laboratory abnormalities is this patient likely to have?

**A.** Hyperglycemia

**B.** Polycythemia

**C.** Hyponatremia

**D.** Hyperkalemia

**E.** Hypercalcemia

**23-14.** A 4-year-old boy is brought to clinic by his grandmother for concern for "weak nails." Over the past week, his finger nails have all started to come off. His grandmother reports that he has sensitive skin and typically uses hydrocortisone for eczema flare-ups. Last month, he contracted hand, foot, and mouth disease from preschool. Since then, she started him on a chewable multivitamin with iron. She reports that their family travels frequently; they went to a beach in Mexico 2 months ago and visited the family ranch in West Texas 10 days ago. At the ranch, he was in contact with cattle, horses, and cats. They also have a dog at home. His exam is significant for proximal separation of the nail plate from each nail bed on both hands. There is no associated erythema, edema, fluctuance, or tenderness to the nail beds, fingers, or hands. He is otherwise well appearing. Which of the following is the most likely event to have triggered the nail findings seen in this patient?

**A.** Regular use of a topical steroid

**B.** Contraction of hand, foot, and mouth disease

**C.** Introduction of a new nutritional supplement

**D.** Travel to a beach abroad

**E.** Physical contact with farm animals

**23-15.** You are seeing a 4-year-old, previously healthy child in clinic for parental concern for nail changes. He is afebrile and well appearing, with exam only notable for horizontal ridges across all 10 fingernails with separation of the distal nail. There is no color change to the nails, and the hands and feet are warm and well perfused. What is the most likely cause for his nail changes?

**A.** Iron deficiency

**B.** Dermatophyte infection

**C.** Psoriasis

**D.** Recent coxsackievirus infection

**E.** Thumb sucking

**23-16.** A 6-year-old boy is presenting for a first visit at your clinic after having been seen by another pediatrician in a neighboring state. There is no family history of diseases, and the child has a healthy older sister. His growth and development are appropriate for his age, although his mother reports that he did receive speech therapy for mild expressive speech delay from age 2 to 4 years old. On your physical exam, you note that he is the 75th percentile for both height and weight and has a normal cardiac and respiratory exam. There are multiple bilateral hamartomas on his irises and 8 café-au-lait spots ranging in size from 2 to 4 cm in diameter. He also has some axillary and inguinal freckling. When you ask the mother, she indicates there are no other family members with notable freckling or skin discolorations like the café-au-lait spots you point out to her. Which of the following is the most likely complication of the disorder you have diagnosed in this child?

**A.** Optic glioma

**B.** Precocious puberty

**C.** Hypertrophic cardiomyopathy

**D.** Hyperthyroidism

**E.** Acoustic neuroma

**23-17.** You are seeing a previously healthy 3-year-old girl who presents for complaints of vulvar pruritus. Mother reports that she has been scratching at her vulvar area for several weeks and complaining of itchiness. She has been afebrile, eating and drinking normally, and attending preschool. She has been toilet trained for about 6 months and has not had any recent changes in bowel or bladder habits. She lives with her parents and 1-year-old baby brother and has no recent travel. On exam, you note white discoloration and atrophy of her labia minora without any vaginal discharge. A urinalysis is within normal limits. What is the most appropriate next step in treatment?

**A.** A course of topical high-potency corticosteroids to the vulva

**B.** Referral to child protective services for concern for sexual abuse

**C.** A course of oral cefdinir

**D.** A course of topical estrogen cream to the vulva

**E.** Daily sitz baths and change of laundry detergent

**23-18.** You are seeing a 6-year-old boy in clinic for follow-up. You saw the patient previously, about 4 weeks ago, for complaint of joint pains, abdominal pain, and rash. The rash initially began as wheals and erythematous maculopapules that progressed to palpable purpura and petechiae on his lower extremities and buttocks. You made the initial diagnosis and provided appropriate treatment. At this follow-up visit, he is afebrile, his rash has completely resolved, and he no longer has any complaints of abdominal pain. You and the family are pleased by how well he is doing, but you remember that patients with this diagnosis can sometimes develop complications months after initial presentation. Which of the following is the most appropriate diagnostic follow-up plan for the next 4 to 6 months?

**A.** Monthly complete blood counts and coagulation studies

**B.** Echocardiogram now and in 6 months

**C.** Weekly erythrocyte sedimentation rate (ESR) and C-reactive protein (CRP) levels

**D.** Monthly abdominal ultrasound

**E.** Monthly urinalysis and blood pressure

**23-19.** A term, 4-day-old baby girl is in clinic for her newborn visit. The baby is doing well and has a normal physical exam, apart from a hemangioma. Which of the following characteristics of the hemangioma would prompt you to do further workup, including imaging and lab testing?

**A.** Segmental (> 5 cm) located on the face

**B.** Small (< 5 cm) located in the axilla

**C.** Large (> 5 cm) on the trunk

**D.** Noncircumferential (> 5 cm) on the leg

**E.** Small (< 5 cm) located on the forehead

**23-20.** A previously healthy 2-year-old boy presents to the emergency department with 2 days of an erythematous rash and fever of 40°C (104°F). The rash is generalized and tender, especially in the flexural and perioral areas. The child is admitted and over the next day develops fissuring and crusting around the eyes, nose, and mouth with desquamation of the skin (Figure 362-9). This child most likely has which of the following?

**A.** Scarlet fever

**B.** Staphylococcal scalded skin syndrome (SSSS)

**C.** Guttate psoriasis

**D.** Acrodermatitis enteropathica

**E.** Ichthyosis

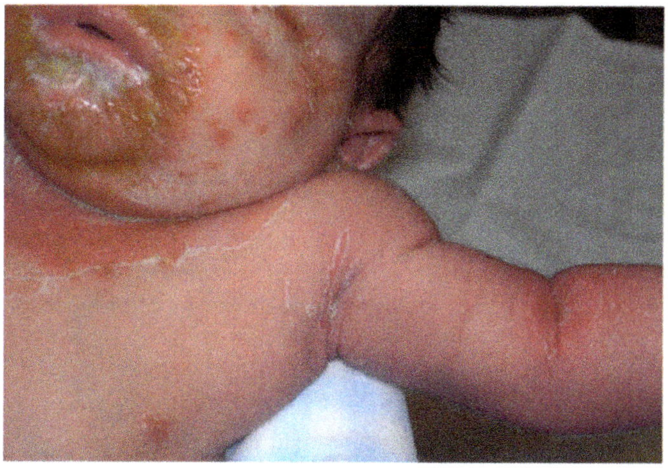

**FIGURE 362-9.** (Mark W. Kline, *Rudolph's Pediatrics*, 23rd Edition. Copyright © McGraw-Hill Education. All rights reserved.)

**23-21.** A 7-year-old boy is brought to the office with a rash on his abdomen. The mother first noticed the rash about 2 weeks ago. The boy has no fever or other symptoms. On examination, there is a well-circumscribed, circular, erythematous, scaly annular patch on his abdomen. The border of the skin lesion is raised and well defined. Which of the following is the most likely diagnosis?

**A.** Erythema nodosum

**B.** Erythema multiforme

**C.** Tinea corporis

**D.** Eczema

**E.** Impetigo

**23-22.** A teenage gardener from Alabama consults a physician about lesions on his hand and forearm. The initial lesion had been a small, nontender papule that slowly expanded and developed a necrotic central area. About a week later, the patient noticed several subcutaneous nodules in his forearm. He did not think they had been there before, but he was not absolutely sure. These nodules continued to enlarge, and he sought medical care when one of them started to ulcerate. Throughout this entire period, the patient had no systemic symptoms. At the time of the physician's examination of the arm, the patient had lesions for approximately 1 month. The physician's examination confirms the patient's observations. It is also noted that the draining nodules are arranged as a chain running proximally up the arm with the most distal lesion being the initial one. Which of the following is the most likely diagnosis?

**A.** Aspergillosis

**B.** Candidiasis

**C.** Cryptococcosis

**D.** Mucormycosis

**E.** Sporotrichosis

**23-23.** One day after sustaining a laceration of the right hand at work, an 18-year-old man comes to the emergency department because of fever, chills, and painful swelling of the right arm. His temperature is 39.4°C (103°F), blood pressure is 110/65 mm Hg, pulse is 110 bpm, and respirations are 20 breaths/min. His right arm is swollen and extremely tender from the elbow up to the shoulder. The skin shows a diffuse dusky erythema. Sensation to touch and pain is reduced in the forearm and hand. A blood sample is immediately taken for cultures. Which of the following is the most appropriate next step in management?

**A.** Supportive measures until culture results are available

**B.** Treatment with clindamycin

**C.** Parenteral treatment with penicillin G

**D.** Parenteral treatment with vancomycin

**E.** Surgical exploration and debridement

**23-24.** A 4-year-old girl presents to your clinic with her mother for a lesion on her cheek. A few weeks ago, the child bumped her face while she was trying to walk under a table. She cried for about 15 seconds and then returned to playing. A few days later, she began bleeding from that area, and her mom noticed a bright red, violaceous nodule (Figure 359-9). She took her to the emergency department, where they took some tests. She received a letter from the pathologist who had mistakenly sent the report to her home. The report states that the lesion is composed of "capillaries and venules with plump endothelial cells separated into lobules by fibromyxoid stroma." Which of the following is the mostly likely diagnosis?

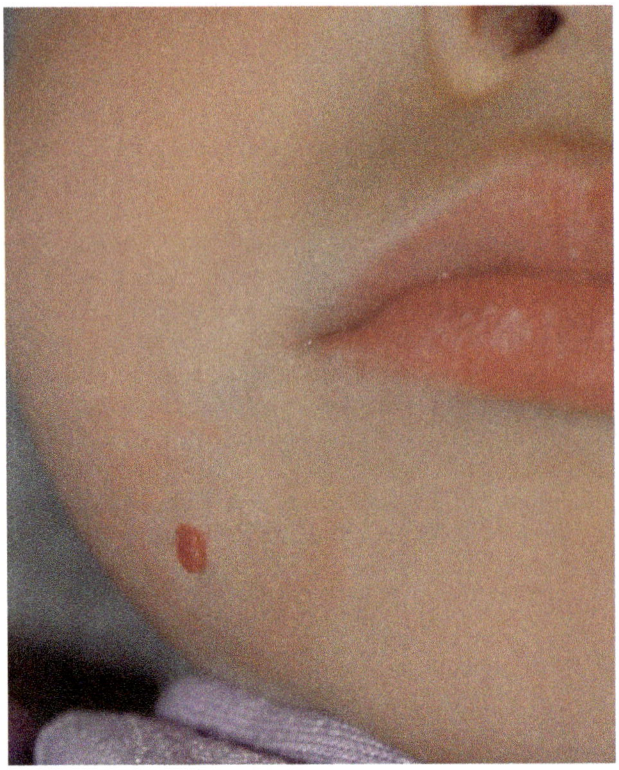

**FIGURE 359-9.** (Mark W. Kline, *Rudolph's Pediatrics*, 23rd Edition. Copyright © McGraw-Hill Education. All rights reserved.)

**A.** Nevus simplex

**B.** Pyogenic granuloma

**C.** Spider angioma

**D.** Kaposi sarcoma

**E.** Gottron papule

**23-25.** A 3-month-old girl presents with a growing bright red papule on the scalp. It was first noted at 1 month of age when it was flatter, but it has since grown in size. Physical exam is otherwise normal for her age. Which of the following statements concerning this child's lesion is *most* correct?

**A.** It will not resolve without immediate surgical intervention.

**B.** The child is likely to develop seizures in the future.

**C.** Topical β-blockers are contraindicated.

**D.** It will continue to grow and then eventually involute as the child gets older.

**E.** Topical antibiotics are recommended to prevent spread of infection.

**23-26.** A 2-month-old girl presents with a dusky purple patch involving the right forehead, upper and lower eyelids, and cheek in a trigeminal nerve ophthalmic branch (V1) distribution. Which of the following is the next best step in management?

**A.** Prescribe oral β-blocker

**B.** Prescribe topical steroid cream

**C.** Refer to ophthalmology and obtain radiologic imaging

**D.** Refer to genetics for testing

**E.** Provide anticipatory guidance and reassurance only

**23-27.** A previously healthy 9-year-old boy presents to your clinic with his mom and a complaint of a worsening rash on his chin. He says that he fell off his bike a week ago and grazed many areas, which have all healed well except the one on his chin, which seemed to get larger and accumulate a yellow crust. On physical examination, his temperature is 37°C, heart rate is 90 bpm, respiratory rate is 16 breaths/min, and blood pressure is 112/68 mm Hg. He is well appearing and does not appear toxic. On his chin, there is a red and inflamed area with many small, fluid-filled vesicles. One small patch on his chin formed a yellow-crusted area, but the majority of the lesions are blistered or weeping. His mucous membranes are moist. The remainder of the physical examination is unremarkable. Of the following, what is the most appropriate antimicrobial therapy for this patient?

**A.** Topical 2% mupirocin ointment twice a day

**B.** Topical 0.05% hydrocortisone ointment twice a day

**C.** Oral amoxicillin twice a day for 7 days

**D.** Oral amoxicillin-clavulanic acid twice a day for 7 days

**E.** Oral clindamycin twice a day for 7 days

**23-28.** A 17-year-old boy develops itchy, small, round, pink macules with a trailing scale on the inner side that coalesce into a large patch on his back in the form of a Christmas tree. He lifts weights at the school gym and is now embarrassed to remove his shirt in the locker room. This patient's symptoms are most likely caused by which of the following?

**A.** A fungus

**B.** A virus

**C.** Bacteria

**D.** A parasite

**E.** An allergic reaction to laundry detergent

**23-29.** A 3-year-old boy with history of atopic dermatitis presents for evaluation of bumps on his arm for several weeks. Yesterday, additional papules appeared on the boy's chin. He has had no fever or irritability, and he is otherwise well. His physical examination is remarkable only for several flat-topped, discrete, dome-shaped, flesh-colored to translucent papules with a central white core distributed across his left antecubital fossa with additional papules on his chin (Figure 362-5). The cause of this rash is most likely due to which of the following?

**A.** *Staphylococcus aureus*

**B.** *Streptococcus pyogenes*

**C.** Poxvirus

**D.** Herpesvirus

**E.** Human papillomavirus (HPV)

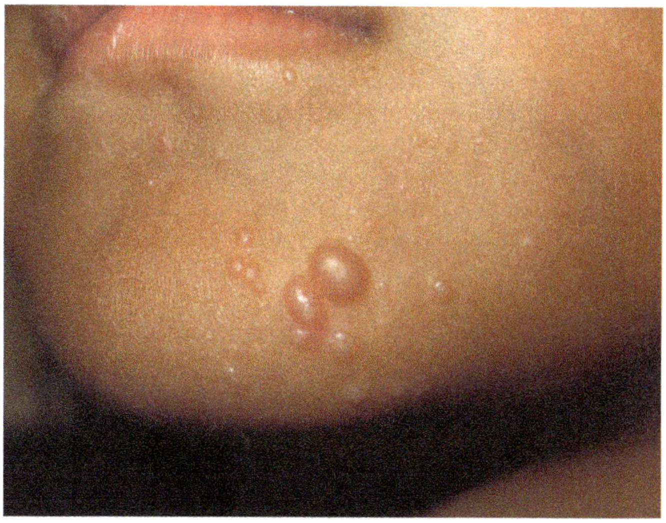

**FIGURE 362-5.** (Mark W. Kline, *Rudolph's Pediatrics*, 23rd Edition. Copyright © McGraw-Hill Education. All rights reserved.)

**23-30.** A 4-week-old infant born after an uneventful pregnancy presents with an intensely pruritic rash on both legs (Figure 352-12). Mother reports no family history of similar rash in the older siblings. She first noticed the lesions around a week ago on her infant's soles, which have spread to her leg. There is sparing of her flexural areas, and no lesions are seen anywhere else on her body. She most likely has which of the following?

**A.** Acropustulosis of infancy

**B.** Eosinophilic pustular folliculitis

**C.** Erythema toxicum

**D.** Miliaria

**E.** Transient neonatal pustular melanosis

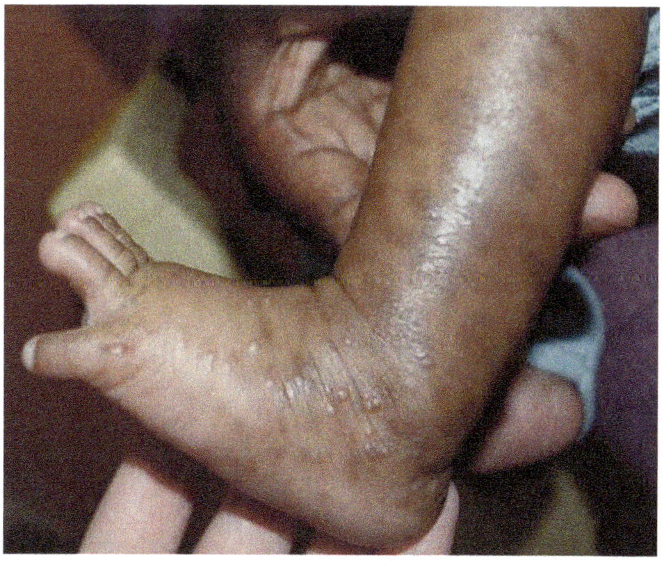

**FIGURE 352-12.** (Mark W. Kline, *Rudolph's Pediatrics*, 23rd Edition. Copyright © McGraw-Hill Education. All rights reserved.)

**23-31.** A 4-week-old infant born after an uneventful pregnancy presents with an intensely pruritic rash on both legs (Figure 352-12). Mother reports no family history of similar rash in the older siblings. She first noticed the lesions around a week ago on her infant's soles, which have spread to her leg. There is sparing of her flexural areas, and no lesions are seen anywhere else on her body. What is the best treatment for the rash?

**A.** Oral prednisolone

**B.** Reassurance

**C.** Permethrin

**D.** Oral acyclovir

**E.** Topical steroids and oral antihistamines

**23-32.** A 2-year-old girl with developmental delay presents with a long-standing rash that appeared as red lines that later developed into fluid-filled puslike lesions (Figure 352-13). These lesions hardened over the next few weeks, and the mother reports that she now has lighter skin in some areas. She is known to have seizure disorder and had previous genetic testing of which the mother is uncertain. What condition does this child have?

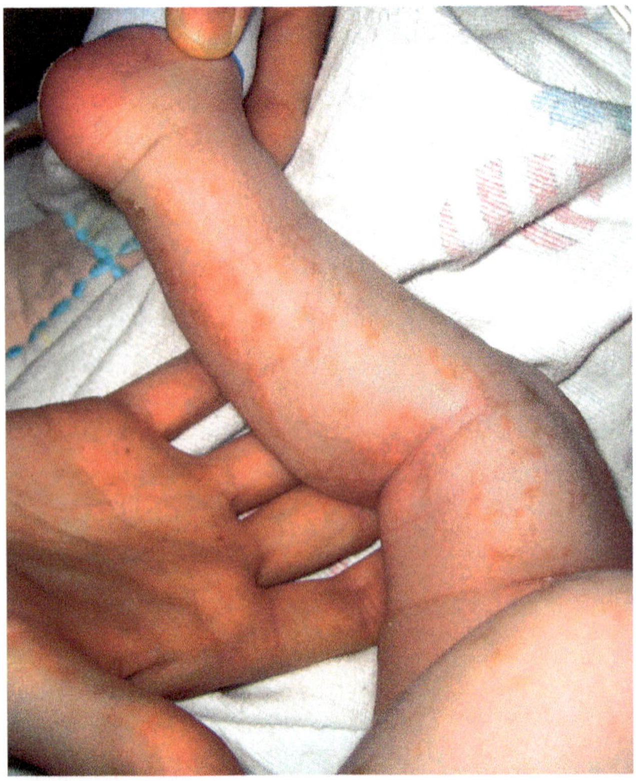

**FIGURE 352-13.** (Mark W. Kline, *Rudolph's Pediatrics*, 23rd Edition. Copyright © McGraw-Hill Education. All rights reserved.)

**A.** Bullous pemphigoid

**B.** Psoriasis

**C.** Epidermolysis bullosa

**D.** Incontinentia pigmenti

**E.** Neurocutaneous melanosis

**23-33.** You notice a newborn with this lesion (Figure 352-7) when performing a well-child check on a 1-month-old infant. What is the best diagnosis?

**A.** Cutis aplasia

**B.** Diffuse hypertrichosis

**C.** Epidermolysis bullosa

**D.** Nevus sebaceous

**E.** Violaceous nodule

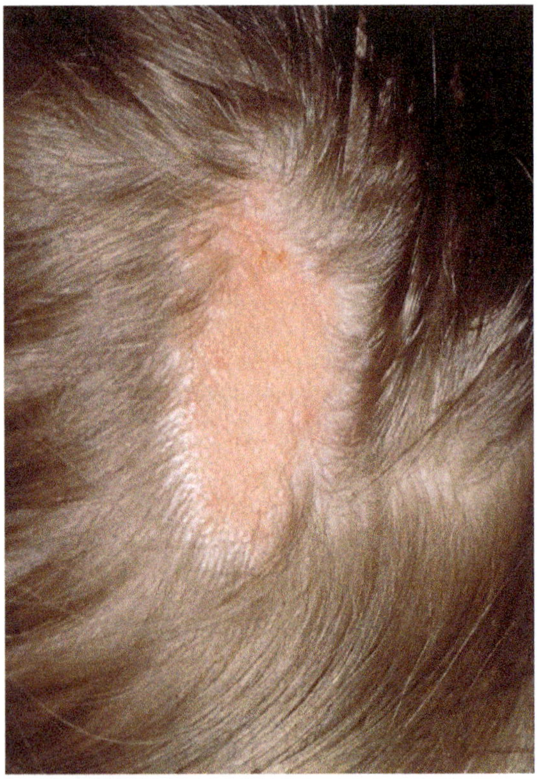

**FIGURE 352-7.** (Mark W. Kline, *Rudolph's Pediatrics*, 23rd Edition. Copyright © McGraw-Hill Education. All rights reserved.)

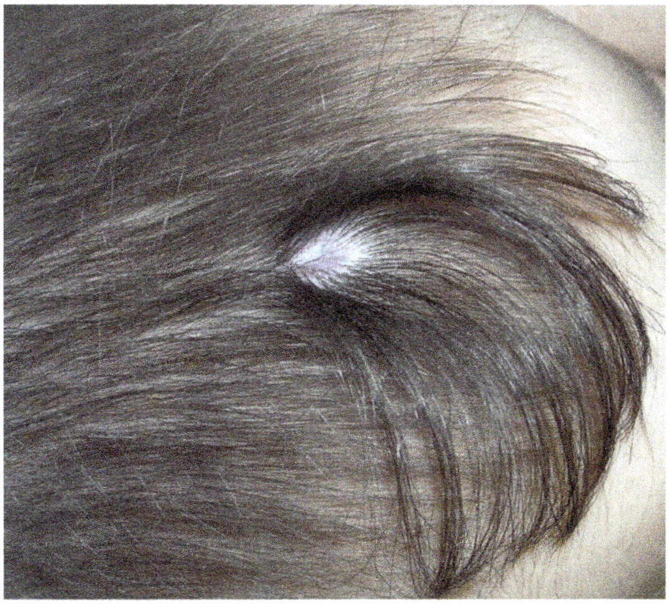

FIGURE 352-1. (Mark W. Kline, *Rudolph's Pediatrics*, 23rd Edition. Copyright © McGraw-Hill Education. All rights reserved.)

**23-34.** You are called to assess a 2-day-old infant in the newborn nursery. She is a healthy 39-week infant born to a G2P1 mother, with no antenatal complications, weighing 3.2 kg. She did not have any scalp electrodes or monitoring done during delivery. You notice this lesion (Figure 352-1) on her newborn examination. What is the next best step in her management?

**A.** Advise topical hydrocortisone

**B.** Look for associated anomalies

**C.** Perform viral cultures

**D.** Oral griseofulvin

**E.** Oral acyclovir

**23-35.** A 16-year-old girl presents for a well-child check. She is doing well in school, with good grades. She has regular menstrual cycles, with normal diet and weight and height in the 50th percentile. Her main concern, however, are the lesions noted on examination (Figure 360-2). Which of the following statements regarding management of this patient's condition is true?

**A.** This patient has moderate acne and warrants oral antibiotics along with a topical retinoid with or without benzoyl peroxide.

**B.** This patient has mild acne that would be best treated with topical retinoid with a keratolytic such as benzoyl peroxide.

**C.** Topical retinoids are useful for comedonal lesions but are not effective against inflammatory lesions.

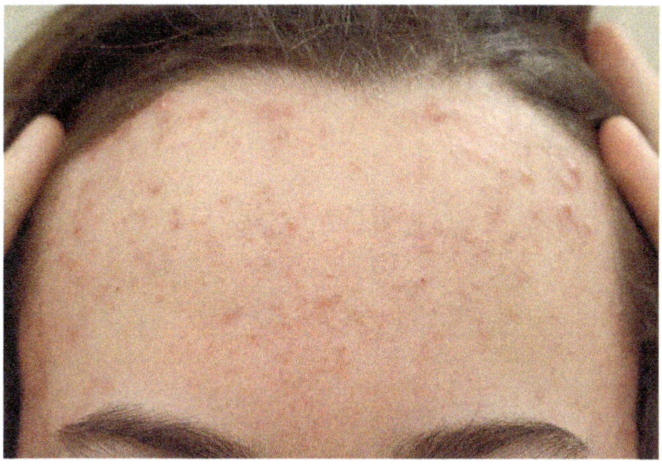

FIGURE 360-2. (Mark W. Kline, *Rudolph's Pediatrics*, 23rd Edition. Copyright © McGraw-Hill Education. All rights reserved.)

**D.** Patients should be advised to use retinoids daily when commencing treatment for better control of symptoms.

**E.** Higher doses of retinoids may be required in a patient with acne fulminans for better control.

**23-36.** A 6-year-old girl presents to clinic for well-child checkup. At the visit, mom also notes recent development of acne lesions on her face. She denies body odor or pubic or axillary hair. There is no family history of severe acne. On physical exam, there are scattered closed comedones and inflammatory papules on her forehead, cheeks, and chin. Which of the following should be the next step in management of this patient?

**A.** Topical benzoyl peroxide-clindamycin gel to affected areas once in the morning

**B.** Avoid high-fat diet

**C.** Oral doxycycline 100 mg twice a day for 3 months

**D.** Topical tretinoin 0.025% cream at bedtime

**E.** Check dehydroepiandrosterone sulfate (DHEAS) and free testosterone

**23-37.** A 10-year-old African American boy presents to clinic for evaluation of hair loss. Patient denies pulling his own hair or associated pruritus. On exam, there is a large focal area of partial smooth alopecia with broken hairs of varying lengths, giving the hair a "moth-eaten" appearance. The eyebrows are not affected, but he also has some loss of eyelashes. Which of the following is the most likely diagnosis?

**A.** Alopecia areata

**B.** Traction alopecia

**C.** Trichotillomania

**D.** Tinea capitis

**E.** Seborrheic dermatitis

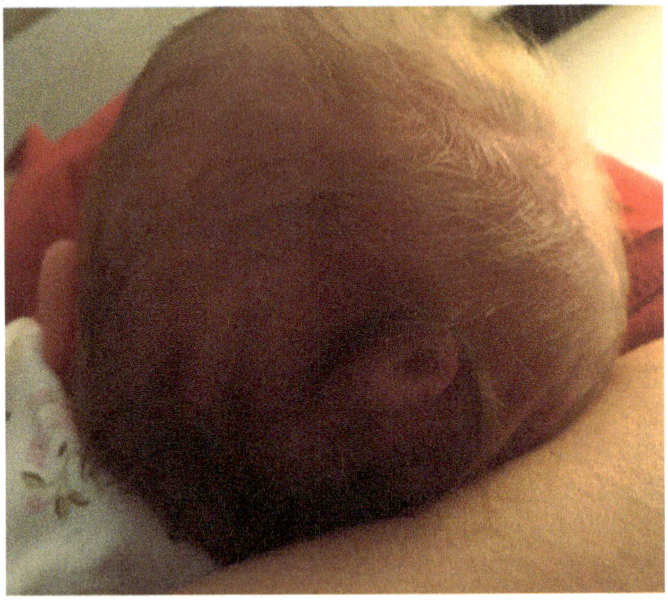

**FIGURE 352-2.** Violaceous nodule on the posterior scalp representing an encephalocele. (Mark W. Kline, *Rudolph's Pediatrics*, 23rd Edition. Copyright © McGraw-Hill Education. All rights reserved.)

**23-38.** A newborn baby was found to have a smooth, well-defined, skin-colored soft nodule on her midline scalp vertex (Figure 352-2). There is no associated hair collar around this nodule. Which of the following is the correct next step in management?

**A.** X-ray of the head

**B.** Skin biopsy of the nodule

**C.** Reassurance and monitor for changes

**D.** Magnetic resonance imaging (MRI) of the head

**E.** Complete surgical excision

**23-39.** A healthy 2-year-old girl presents to clinic for evaluation of skin tags in her genital area. The patient's mother became concerned when this past week she saw 2 skin tags in her perianal region after baths. Her mother has noticed that she has been scratching her private area more. She attends local daycare while parents are at work. She is the younger sibling of 2. There is no other pertinent social history. On physical exam, there are several flesh-colored verrucous papules in her anal verge. Skin exam is otherwise normal. What is the next appropriate step in management?

**A.** Reassurance and prescribe imiquimod

**B.** Skin biopsy and send for human papillomavirus (HPV) typing

**C.** Referral to child protective agency

**D.** Recommend over-the-counter topical salicylic acid

**E.** Workup for possible underlying immune deficiency

**23-40.** A 7-year-old healthy boy presents for evaluation of a chronic rash on his body and extremities. About 6 months ago, he developed pruritic erythematous scaly papules and patches to hands and ankles. His mother tried topical hydrocortisone cream, which helped the itching, but the rash continued to spread to his neck, axilla, trunk, abdomen, scrotum, wrists, and ankles. She has also given him Benadryl as needed with minimal relief. His younger sister has also developed similar rashes. Because of this, his mother is concerned about the possibility of environmental allergies and is requesting allergy workup for the patient. On exam, there are lichenified scaly excoriated papules and plaques on bilateral wrists, dorsal hands, and ankles. There are also small erythematous papules on his palms and finger digits. The rash is also present around his waist, scrotum, and penis. Which of the following is the appropriate treatment for this patient?

**A.** Prescribe a stronger topical steroid ointment to be applied to all affected areas twice a day for 2 weeks

**B.** Cetirizine daily until he can be seen by the allergist for allergy testing

**C.** Oral ivermectin and permethrin 5% cream once and repeat in 1 week

**D.** Oral griseofulvin and check fungal culture for tinea

**E.** Topical mupirocin ointment to all affected areas

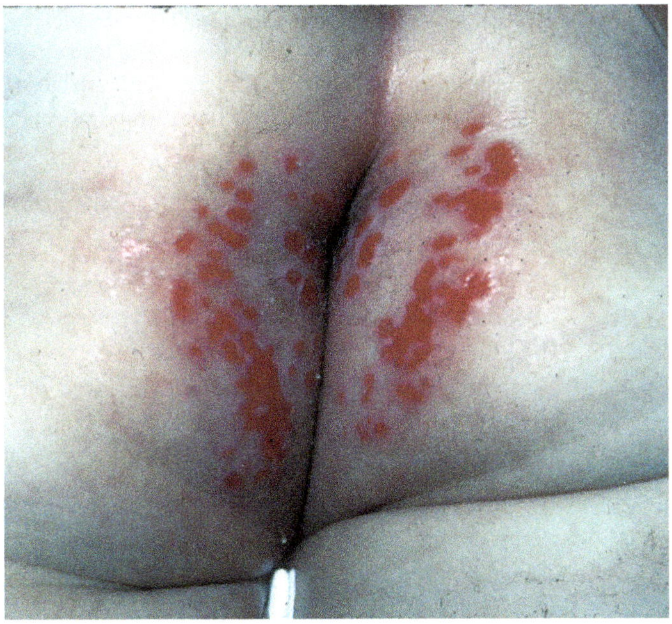

**FIGURE 353-5.** Erosive irritant diaper dermatitis. (Mark W. Kline, *Rudolph's Pediatrics*, 23rd Edition. Copyright © McGraw-Hill Education. All rights reserved.)

**23-41.** A 4-month-old baby boy presents for evaluation of diaper dermatitis. His mother initially started him on breast milk, but he developed redness and erythematous satellite pustules in his diaper area. Nystatin cream was started, and his mother had been applying diaper barrier cream with each diaper change. The rash improved but was persistent. He now has shallow erosions without satellite lesions in the diaper area (Figure 353-5). The mother is concerned that he is having 10 to 15 loose stools daily. Previous herpes simplex virus (HSV) and bacterial cultures taken in the office were all negative. Which of the following is the next appropriate step in management?

**A.** Repeat bacterial and HSV polymerase chain reaction (PCR) and culture

**B.** Initiate workup to determine the underlying cause of frequent stooling

**C.** Start antifungal-corticosteroid combinations such as nystatin and triamcinolone ointment

**D.** Start 5- to 7-day course of oral fluconazole

**E.** Start oral acyclovir

**23-42.** A 3-month-old infant presents for evaluation of rash. She developed sharply demarcated, symmetric, partially erosive, scaly, and crusted plaques on her face, diaper area, dorsal hands, and feet. She was evaluated by an outside dermatologist who prescribed oral antibiotics and oral antifungal therapy. The patient's mother also was instructed to apply hydrocortisone 2.5% ointment twice a day to all affected areas. Despite the topical steroid, her lesions did not improve. Although the infant was recently weaned from breastfeeding, she is otherwise eating well. She has some loose stools. Which of the following is the appropriate next step in management?

**A.** Referral to dermatology for a skin biopsy

**B.** Order a zinc level and start zinc supplement empirically

**C.** Prescribe a more potent topical steroid

**D.** Start oral fluconazole for disseminated tinea corporis

**E.** Referral to gastroenterology for frequent loose stools

**23-43.** A 15-year-old girl is admitted for fever, nausea, vomiting, and cervical lymphadenopathy. She was in her usual state of health until about a week ago, when she developed an itchy rash to her neck, arms, trunk, and legs. The parents also noticed that she has facial swelling. Complete blood count shows eosinophilia. Liver function test is mildly elevated. A month ago, she was started on oral minocycline 100 mg twice daily for acne. She has been otherwise healthy. Which of the following is true regarding her condition?

**A.** Referral to an allergist should be made to confirm her allergy to minocycline.

**B.** Rechallenging the patient with the offending medication can confirm the diagnosis of drug rash.

**C.** Systemic steroids and antihistamines are the first-line treatment for this condition.

**D.** These patients often have concomitant herpes virus infection.

**E.** This type of drug rash has a good prognosis and should resolve within 7 to 10 days after the offending agent is discontinued.

**23-44.** A 10-year-old girl presents for a hyperpigmented rash to her forehead. Her mother noticed the development of a darker band on her forehead about 3 months ago. The rash is not pruritic or painful, but it is slowly spreading. She denies headache and blurred vision. On exam, there is a 2-cm linear hyperpigmented patch on her mid-forehead. Which of the following is correct regarding this condition?

**A.** This type of morphea is at higher risk for progressing into systemic sclerosis.

**B.** Confirmatory diagnosis with skin biopsy is required prior to starting systemic therapies.

**C.** Prognosis is favorable for linear morphea, and skin changes are usually reversible.

**D.** The skin lesions can affect underlying structures causing associated headache, eye abnormalities, or seizures.

**E.** High-potency topical steroid is the first-line treatment for this condition.

**23-45.** A baby girl was born at 30 weeks' gestation and was monitored in the neonatal intensive care unit (NICU) for respiratory distress. At birth, there was an erythematous bruise-like patch to her right side of the forehead. The lesion rapidly became larger and thicker over the next several weeks. At 4 weeks of age, an erythematous plaque covered most of the right side of her forehead to her left upper eyelid. There is no history of skin ulceration or bleeding. The baby was discharged home without issues. The patient's mother brings her to the office to establish care and for her first well-child check. Aside from referral to a dermatologist, which of the following is the correct next step in management?

**A.** Cardiology consult and echocardiogram to rule out underlying coarctation of the aorta

**B.** Reassurance provided to the mother that hemangiomas will resolve with time and there is no indication for treatment at this time

**C.** Empirically start oral propranolol, which is the first-line treatment for large hemangiomas

**D.** Magnetic resonance imaging (MRI) of the lumbosacral spine to rule out tethered cord

**E.** Neurology consult for possible seizures

**23-46.** Which of the following is true of large congenital melanocytic nevi?

**A.** Skin biopsy of satellite nevi is recommended due to concern for increased transformation to melanoma within these satellite lesions.

**B.** Most of the larger congenital melanocytic nevi have a somatic *BRAF* V600E mutation.

**C.** A screening magnetic resonance imaging (MRI) with and without contrast of brain and spine before 6 months of age is recommended if there are associated satellite nevi or multiple medium-sized congenital melanocytic nevi.

**D.** Complete surgical excision is recommended to eliminate the risk of melanoma.

**E.** Neurosurgical referral is required to evaluate underlying central nervous system (CNS) involvement.

**23-47.** A 14-year-old girl presents to the emergency department (ED) with multiple tender, warm, and red nodules on the extensor surfaces of both legs. She reports associated sore throat, fever, malaise, and joint pain in her elbows and knees. She is having difficulty walking due to the pain. She denies dysuria or abnormal vaginal discharges. Rapid strep test was positive. Complete blood count with differential was normal. She was prescribed a course of oral amoxicillin. What would be recommended for the tender nodules in her legs?

**A.** Over-the-counter nonsteroidal anti-inflammatory drugs as needed for pain control and reassurance that these will improve with time

**B.** Reassurance that the amoxicillin will also target the cause of these nodules

**C.** Surgical consultation for excisional biopsy

**D.** Topical mupirocin ointment to the lesions

**E.** Skin scraping of the nodules for bacterial culture to rule out cellulitis

**23-48.** Which of the following skin findings is the first to appear in patients with neurofibromatosis type 1 (NF1)?

**A.** Café-au-lait macules

**B.** Neurofibromas

**C.** Axillary freckling

**D.** Ash leaf spots

**E.** Confetti macules

**23-49.** A 2-year-old boy presents to the clinic for evaluation of a rash. His mother noticed that he developed a skin nodule on his right shoulder 3 months ago. The area occasionally would become swollen, red, and itchy. The lesion looks like a "hive" per the mother's description, and throughout the day, the redness would subside. The lesion has not resolved. On exam, there is a 1.0-cm, single, orange-brown plaque on his right shoulder. After manually rubbing the lesion, the plaque immediately becomes red and swollen. Which of the following is the appropriate management for this lesion?

**A.** Excisional skin biopsy

**B.** Allergy referral for possible allergic reaction

**C.** Topical Benadryl lotion

**D.** Oral antihistamines

**E.** Two-week course of oral prednisone

**23-50.** Which of the following is true of impetigo caused by group A β-hemolytic streptococci (GABHS)?

**A.** The risk of acute glomerulonephritis can be prevented with early initiation of antibiotic treatment.

**B.** GABHS often can cause the bullae also known as bullous impetigo.

**C.** Decolonization regimen with mupirocin ointment to nares is recommended.

**D.** Prognosis is guarded and with typical progression to acute glomerulonephritis.

**E.** Most cases are associated with lymphadenopathy and leukocytosis.

**23-51.** You are called to the bedside of a full-term, 3-day-old female infant prior to hospital discharge due to new-onset rash. The patient has been afebrile and breastfeeding well. Your examination is normal except for scattered erythematous macules and vesiculopustules predominately on the trunk and upper extremities but sparing the palms. To confirm your diagnosis, you perform which of the following?

**A.** Bacterial culture, which is later consistent with *Staphylococcus aureus*

**B.** Wright stain smear, which shows neutrophils

**C.** Viral polymerase chain reaction, which is consistent with herpes simplex virus

**D.** Wright stain smear, which shows eosinophils

**E.** Mineral oil scraping, which shows scybala and eggs

**23-52.** A 2-month-old male infant presents to your clinic for a well-child check. The mother is concerned about an area of hair loss on the right vertex scalp. Upon closer examination, you note a yellow, slightly papillomatous plaque with associated alopecia (Figure 352-7). Which of the following is true regarding this skin lesion?

**A.** There is a high risk of malignant transformation, and it should be surgically excised.

**B.** As the child gets older, the skin lesion will slowly regress with time.

**C.** It is composed of melanocytes and should be clinically monitored.

**D.** It is made up of malformed hair follicles and abundant sebaceous glands.

**E.** Further imaging is required to assess for an intracranial connection.

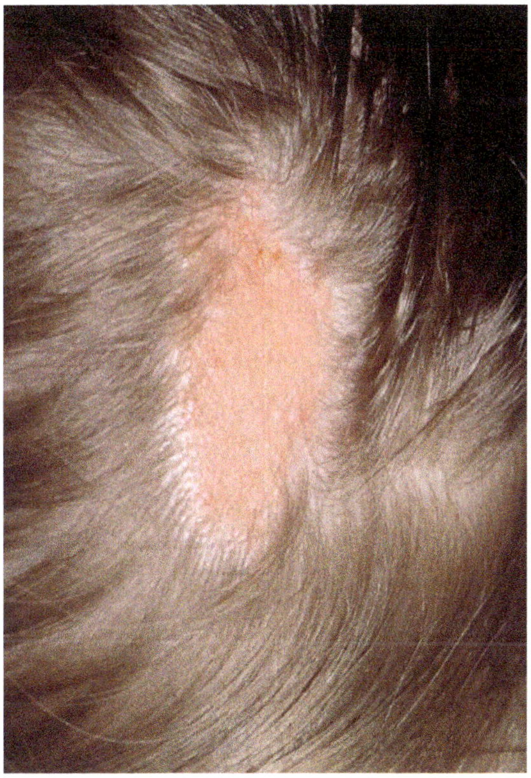

**FIGURE 352-7.** (Mark W. Kline, *Rudolph's Pediatrics*, 23rd Edition. Copyright © McGraw-Hill Education. All rights reserved.)

**23-53.** You are called to the neonatal intensive care unit to examine a premature infant with increased apnea, bradycardia, and temperature instability. On examination, you note vesicles on an erythematous base clustered on the vertex scalp. You are most concerned for herpes simplex virus (HSV) and perform a viral polymerase chain reaction. Which of the following statements is true regarding this infection?

**A.** The majority of infants with neonatal HSV are born to mothers who have recurrent HSV infections.

**B.** The majority of infants with neonatal HSV are born to mothers who were symptomatic at the time of delivery.

**C.** Vesicles or erosions are present at sites in contact with the maternal cervix during delivery.

**D.** Fetal scalp monitoring is not a risk factor for infants acquiring neonatal HSV.

**E.** Women with an HSV outbreak at the time of delivery should avoid breastfeeding.

**23-54.** An 8-year-old girl with asthma presents with a persistent facial rash. The examination shows erythematous papules and pustules surrounding the nose and mouth (see following figure). The rash is asymptomatic and has been present for 3 months. She has been treated with hydrocortisone cream with initial improvement, but the rash always returns. Which of the following is the next best step?

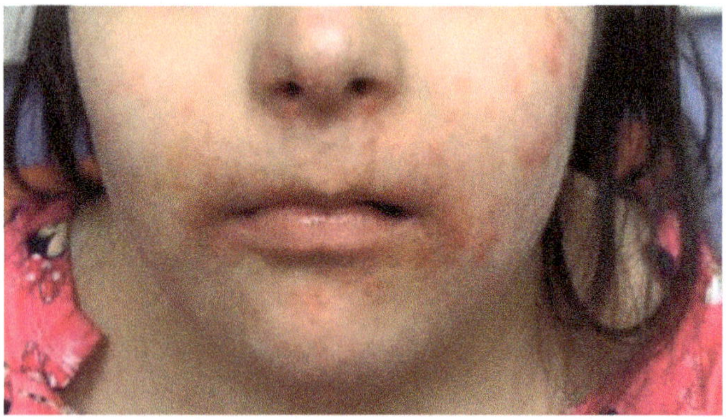

(Paller S, Mancini AJ. Cutaneous disorders of the newborn, in *Hurwitz Clinical and Pediatric Dermatology*. New York, NY: Elsevier; 2016:31-32.)

**A.** Continue hydrocortisone cream twice daily followed by a thick moisturizer until resolved

**B.** Increase to triamcinolone cream twice daily followed by a thick moisturizer until resolved

**C.** Begin benzoyl peroxide gel daily because you are concerned this is acne vulgaris

**D.** Begin metronidazole cream twice daily for approximately 6 to 8 weeks until resolved

**E.** Place referral to allergy because you are concerned this is an allergic contact dermatitis

**23-55.** A 10-year-old boy with atopic dermatitis presents with hair loss of 6 months in duration. He feels that his hair loss is worsening and denies prior treatment. On examination, you see a round alopecia patch with underlying smooth skin (see following figure). There is no evidence of erythema or scale. Which of the following is the next best step?

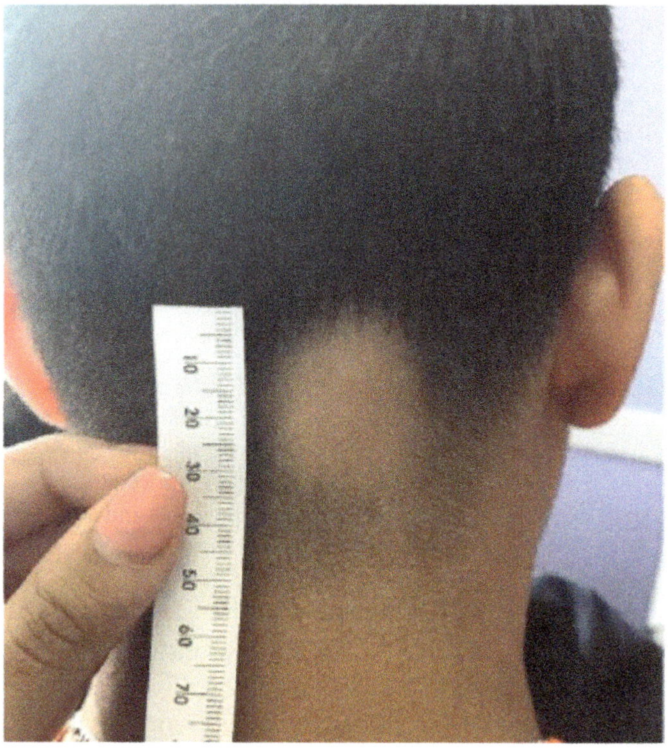

**A.** Diagnose the patient with alopecia areata and begin a high-potency topical steroid

**B.** Perform a fungal culture and begin griseofulvin due to concern for tinea capitis

**C.** Begin ketoconazole shampoo twice weekly due to concern for seborrheic dermatitis

**D.** Have a long discussion with family and place referral to psychology due to concern for trichotillomania

**E.** Perform thyroid testing with referral to endocrinology due to alopecia secondary to thyroid disease

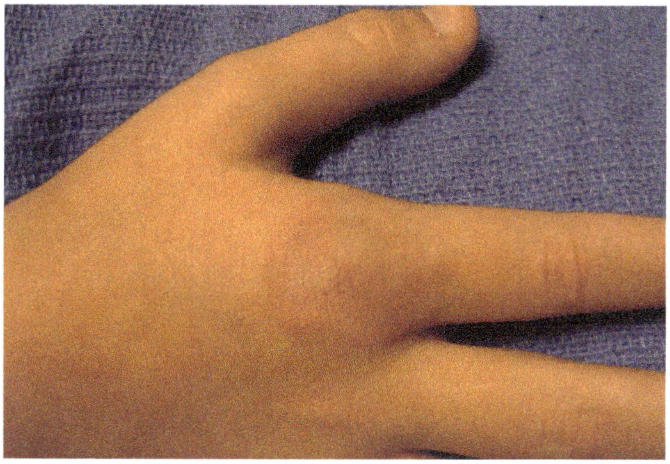

**FIGURE 354-1.** (Mark W. Kline, *Rudolph's Pediatrics*, 23rd Edition. Copyright © McGraw-Hill Education. All rights reserved.)

**23-56.** A 6-year-old boy presents with an asymptomatic annular, nonscaly plaque on the dorsal hand (Figure 354-1). The skin lesion has been present for 6 months and has not improved with topical clotrimazole cream. What is the next best step in management?

**A.** Provide reassurance because this skin lesion will resolve over time without treatment

**B.** Continue topical clotrimazole cream for another month until resolution

**C.** Change to topical terbinafine cream for another month until resolution

**D.** Change to oral terbinafine for a 2-week course until resolution

**E.** Change to oral amoxicillin because you are worried about an underlying tickborne infection

**23-57.** A 6-month-old female infant presents to the clinic for evaluation of a blue-gray patch involving the left side of the face. The skin lesion has been present since birth, is stable in size, and is not bothersome to the patient. What do you tell the parents regarding this birthmark?

**A.** Provide reassurance as this birthmark will fade over time

**B.** Refer to neurology because there is an association with epilepsy

**C.** Refer to ophthalmology because there is an association with glaucoma

**D.** Clinical monitoring because these birthmarks have a high incidence of melanoma

**E.** Refer to cardiology because you are concerned for underlying congenital heart disease

**23-58.** An 8-year-old boy presents with a new hyperpigmented linear patch on his left forearm (Figure 356-4B). The skin lesion is asymptomatic. The family has tried over-the-counter hydrocortisone cream without

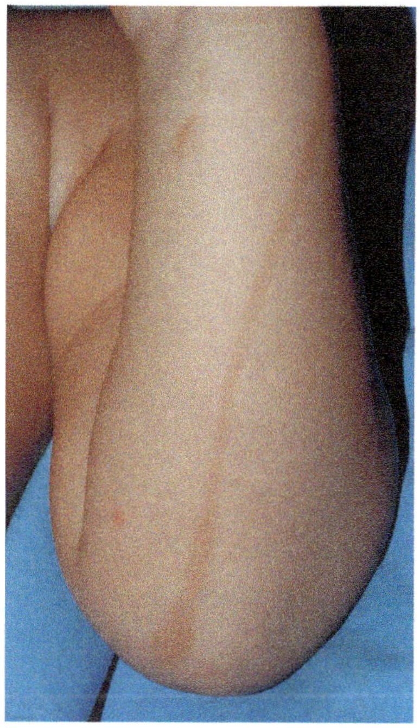

B

**FIGURE 356-4B.** (Mark W. Kline, *Rudolph's Pediatrics*, 23rd Edition. Copyright © McGraw-Hill Education. All rights reserved.)

improvement. Which of the following is a common cause of this acquired skin lesion in children and adults?

**A.** The child had a prior injury to the skin that led to postinflammatory hyperpigmentation.

**B.** This represents delayed-onset pigmentary demarcation line of the upper extremity.

**C.** This is a form of pigmentary mosaicism along lines of Blaschko.

**D.** The child likely had prior contact with lime or another type of citrus fruit.

**E.** The child likely ate a recent meal that contained shiitake mushrooms.

**23-59.** A 17-year-old girl presents with a firm, skin-colored papule on the left posterior earlobe. She states that the papule appeared 4 months after getting her ears pierced. It is tender to palpation, and she would like treatment. Which of the following is false regarding keloids?

**A.** A keloid is secondary to exogenous trauma such as ear piercing.

**B.** A keloid is most commonly seen in persons with lighter skin tones but can be seen in anyone.

**C.** Pathogenesis is secondary to certain growth factors such as transforming growth factor-b.

**D.** Treatments include intralesional or topical steroids, radiation, and surgical excision.

**E.** Common locations for keloids include the ears, shoulders, and upper chest.

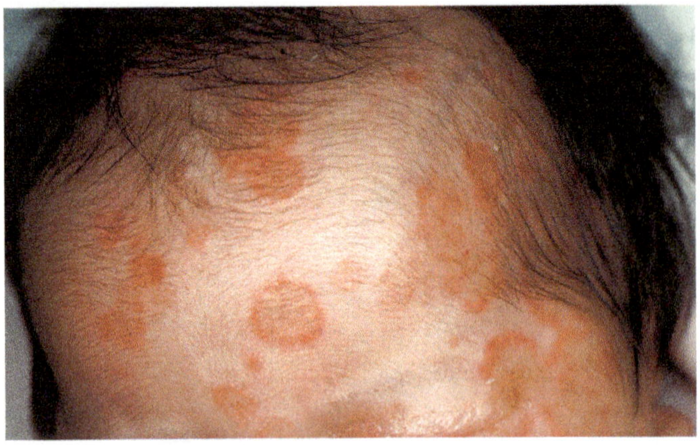

**FIGURE 357-2.** (Mark W. Kline, *Rudolph's Pediatrics*, 23rd Edition. Copyright © McGraw-Hill Education. All rights reserved.)

**23-60.** A full-term 2-month-old male infant presents with new-onset erythematous papules and annular plaques in a periorbital distribution (Figure 357-2). Per history, the pregnancy was uncomplicated and the parents have no medical problems. What is the most appropriate next step in evaluation and management?

**A.** You are concerned for tinea faciei and inquire about pets within the home.

**B.** Order an electrocardiogram (ECG) and advise the mother to have an antinuclear antibody (ANA) profile performed by her obstetrician or primary care physician.

**C.** You are concerned for urticaria and order further blood work to evaluate for an underlying autoinflammatory condition.

**D.** Inquire about recent travel as you are concerned for an underlying tickborne illness.

**E.** Reassure parents that this is a benign skin rash in infants that will resolve without treatment.

**23-61.** A 7-year-old girl presents with pruritus and rash of the genitals (Figure 357-5). The rash has been present for 3 months, and parents deny prior treatment. The patient is otherwise healthy but does suffer from intermittent constipation. What is the next best step in management?

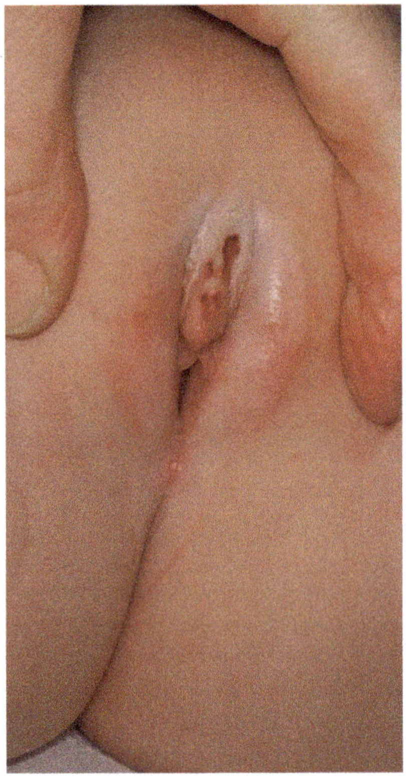

**FIGURE 357-5.** (Mark W. Kline, *Rudolph's Pediatrics*, 23rd Edition. Copyright © McGraw-Hill Education. All rights reserved.)

**A.** Discuss the diagnosis of lichen sclerosus and begin a potent topical steroid.

**B.** Inquire about recent antibiotic use and treat with oral fluconazole.

**C.** You are concerned for child abuse and contact the child protective services.

**D.** Recommend sitz baths and Vaseline ointment because rash is consistent with vulvovaginitis.

**E.** Recommend a low-potency topical steroid twice daily for irritant dermatitis.

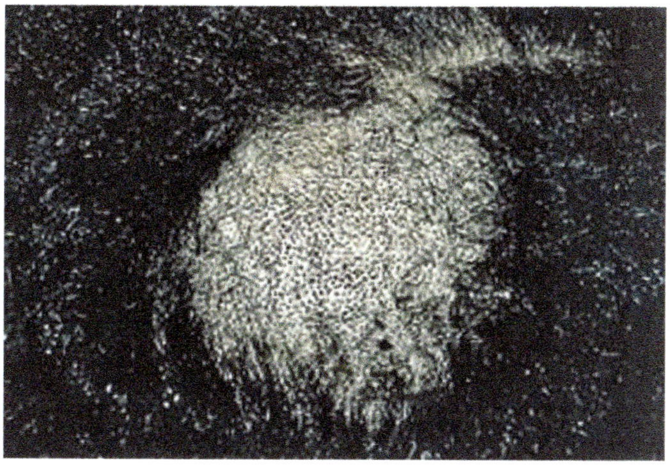

**FIGURE 362-12.** Black dot form of tinea capitis. Black dots demarcate broken hair shafts. (Mark W. Kline, *Rudolph's Pediatrics*, 23rd Edition. Copyright © McGraw-Hill Education. All rights reserved.)

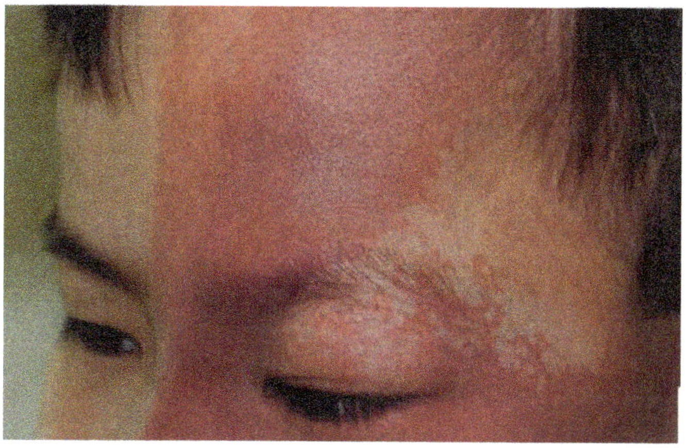

**FIGURE 359-11.** Child with a capillary malformation in the V1 distribution and associated Sturge-Weber syndrome. (Mark W. Kline, *Rudolph's Pediatrics*, 23rd Edition. Copyright © McGraw-Hill Education. All rights reserved.)

**23-62.** A 4-year-old girl presents with a hyperkeratotic plaque with overlying alopecia of the vertex scalp (Figure 362-12). There is associated occipital lymphadenopathy. The skin lesion appeared 1 to 2 months prior and is mildly pruritic. Due to concern for tinea capitis, you perform a fungal culture. What is the most appropriate treatment for this patient?

**A.** Begin topical terbinafine cream twice daily for 6 to 8 weeks followed by repeat fungal culture

**B.** Begin oral griseofulvin daily or divided twice daily for 6 to 8 weeks followed by repeat fungal culture

**C.** Begin topical clotrimazole and betamethasone cream twice daily for 6 to 8 weeks followed by repeat fungal culture

**D.** Begin oral griseofulvin daily or divided twice daily for 2 to 4 weeks followed by repeat fungal culture

**E.** Begin topical clotrimazole cream twice daily for 6 to 8 weeks followed by repeat fungal culture

**23-63.** A 9-year-old boy with known Sturge-Weber syndrome is establishing care at your practice. He has developmental delay and well-controlled epilepsy. He has a port wine stain in a V1 and V2 distribution on his face (Figure 359-11). What do you know to be true regarding this syndrome?

**A.** Port wine stains in Sturge-Weber syndrome commonly fade as the child ages.

**B.** Thirty-five percent of patients with a port wine stain in a V1 distribution have Sturge-Weber syndrome.

**C.** Both sporadic and syndromic port wine stains have a somatic mutation in vascular endothelial growth factor (VEGF).

**D.** These patients need ophthalmologic monitoring due to increased risk of glaucoma.

**E.** These patients need orthopedic monitoring due to bony demineralization under port wine stain.

**23-64.** A 6-year-old girl presents with an intensely itchy scalp. The grandmother states that lice have been reported at the child's school, and she is now concerned her granddaughter has it. On examination, you note scattered nits and lice. Which of the following is true regarding lice treatment?

**A.** Permethrin 1% lotion is a first-line agent because it is cost effective and has low toxicity.

**B.** Benzyl alcohol is an organophosphate and is recommended for children aged 6 months and older.

**C.** Lindane 1% lotion is no longer recommended due to risk of hepatotoxicity.

**D.** Education regarding fomite transmission is not needed because this is a low risk for patients with lice.

**E.** Malathion is an ovicidal organophosphate and carries a risk of neurotoxicity.

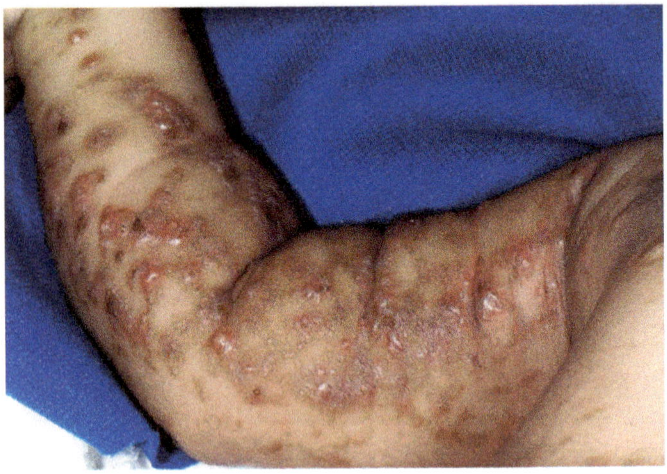

**FIGURE 355-5.** (Mark W. Kline, *Rudolph's Pediatrics*, 23rd Edition. Copyright © McGraw-Hill Education. All rights reserved.)

**23-65.** A 2-week-old female infant presents to your pediatric practice as a new patient. The child was born via spontaneous vaginal delivery, and the pregnancy was uncomplicated. She is breastfeeding and has regained weight to her birthweight. The mother shows you a rash that has been present since birth (Figure 355-5). The rash is asymptomatic, and the mother is applying baby lotion to the area. What are the next steps in evaluation and management?

**A.** Provide reassurance because this is a common rash of neonates and will resolve without treatment.

**B.** You are concerned for herpes simplex virus; perform a viral polymerase chain reaction and instruct the mother to go the emergency department for admission.

**C.** Provide reassurance that this is a form of pigmentary mosaicism and will grow proportionately with the child over time.

**D.** Place referral to ophthalmology and neurology due to risk of eye and neurologic abnormalities.

**E.** Inquire about infestations within the home as you are concerned for arthropod bite.

**23-66.** A 6-month-old girl is brought to the emergency department by her mother due to concern for irritability and rash. Mom notes the infant has had bumps on her hands, feet, arms, neck, and scalp that have been worsening over the past week. She has been fussier than usual over this time but seems somewhat soothed when lotion is applied over the bumps. She has not had any fevers and has been eating and drinking well. Her weight is stable at 6.5 kg. Her 3-year-old sister attends a daycare where there has been a recent scabies infestation, although the 3-year-old was checked by her pediatrician and deemed to not be infected. The patient's vital signs are noted to be within normal limits for her age. Her skin exam is significant for several vesiculopustules on the lateral portions and soles of her feet, as well as on her posterior neck and lower posterior scalp. She has a few, short serpiginous lines on the flexural surface of her elbows and between the webs of her toes. Which of the following treatments would be most appropriate for this rash?

**A.** Permethrin 5% cream applied to the entire body including the face, scalp, and neck

**B.** Urgent referral to dermatology

**C.** Permethrin 5% cream applied from the neck down

**D.** Crotamiton 10% cream applied to the entire body including the face, scalp, and neck

**E.** Oral ivermectin 200 mg/kg/dose, 2 oral doses given 1 week apart

**23-67.** A 12-year-old boy presents to his pediatrician for a recurrent rash on his sacral area and knees that is characterized by papules and vesicles that are intensely pruritic. Multiple courses of topical emollients and steroids fail to improve the rash significantly. Patient and family cannot identify any seasonal or allergic triggers. He is otherwise healthy with normal growth and weight. He denies any fevers, arthritis, diarrhea, constipation, or other concerns. The patient is referred to pediatric dermatology and diagnosed with dermatitis herpetiformis. Which of the following treatments should lead to remission?

**A.** Topical tacrolimus twice daily for 2 weeks

**B.** Acyclovir 40 mg/kg/d divided in 3 doses per day for 10 days

**C.** Ultraviolet (UV) light therapy weekly for 6 weeks

**D.** Prednisone 10 mg/kg/dose once daily for 5 days

**E.** A gluten-free diet

**23-68.** A 12-year-old girl is seen by her pediatrician for sore throat, malaise, and pink, tender nodules on her shins bilaterally. Her pediatrician orders a rapid strep test and a monospot. While waiting, her mother asks the pediatrician about the nodules on her legs and whether they are related to the other symptoms the patient is experiencing. Which of the following statements about erythema nodosum is true?

**A.** Erythema nodosum is most common in patients under the age of 2.

**B.** Erythema nodosum is characterized by tender, red, warm nodules or plaques with overlying scale.

**C.** The most common location for erythema nodosum is the flexor surfaces of the upper extremities.

**D.** Erythema nodosum is the most common panniculitis in children.

**E.** Without appropriate treatment, erythema nodosum lesions will ulcerate and scar.

**23-69.** A 5-year-old boy is brought to his pediatrician by his mother for evaluation of developmental delay. Mom reports the boy has reached age-appropriate gross and fine motor milestones throughout childhood but has struggled in preschool with verbal communication and learning of letters/sounds. The boy is an only child, and his parents are no longer together. Mom is adopted and does not know her biological family or their medical history. She has little contact with dad and does not know his family's medical history either. Mom is healthy and completed college. On exam, the boy is noted to be at the 40th percentile for weight and 60th percentile for height. His skin exam is notable for freckling in his right axilla and 8 sharply demarcated, evenly brown-colored macules over his shoulders and back. Mom also reports recently noting a firm nodule on his forearm. Which mutation may be found on genetic testing of this patient?

**A.** Mutation in *BLM*

**B.** Mutations in the genes encoding hamartin or tuberin

**C.** Deletions of the gene encoding neurofibromin

**D.** Mutations in *STK11/LKB1*

**E.** Mutations in *APC* gene

## ANSWERS

**Answer 23-1.** B

The exam of this child shows that she no longer has an active infection with lice. She has no adult lice or nymphs on exam. She also has empty nits, no longer containing viable nymphs because they are ovoid, translucent, and on the hair shaft away from the scalp. Nits containing viable nymphs are ovoid shape and of brown coloration and are attached firmly within one-fourth of an inch of the base of the hair shaft. Nits are frequently found at the bilateral temples, behind the ears or near the neck. Nits are not a reliable marker of active disease and may appear viable on gross inspection for weeks after hatching or death of the nymph. Permethrin 1% lotion is an over-the-counter product approved for use in children > 2 months old and is recommended by the American Academy of Pediatrics. A second treatment with permethrin 9 days after the first is recommended as it is not ovicidal and nymphs hatch 6 to 10 days after the nit is laid by the adult louse. Prophylactic treatment is not recommended; only treatment of active infections is necessary. Lindane has potential neurotoxic effects and is no longer recommended for treatment.

(Section 18: Disorders of the Skin, Chapter 363: Infestations)

**Answer 23-2.** E

Nevus sebaceous is typically seen on the face or scalp. It presents at birth as a hairless linear plaque of coalesced yellow-colored papules. The diagnosis is made clinically, but a biopsy can be performed if the diagnosis is uncertain. Treatment of a nevus sebaceous is surgical excision, but removal of these lesions is controversial, and observation is appropriate in many cases. Aplasia cutis congenita is a congenital absence of skin, most often seen at the scalp vertex. It can present as single or multiple ulcers, bullae, or scars. Aplasia cutis can have underlying skull, dura, or meninges defects.

Alopecia areata is a common nonscarring alopecia typically characterized by smooth, shiny, round, or oval patches of hair loss on the scalp that appear suddenly over the course of several days. It is an autoimmune disorder and usually first appears in children or young adults, although it can have its onset as early as birth. Nevus depigmentosus is an area of hypomelanosis that may be apparent at birth or detected later in infancy or childhood. Lesions are hypopigmented patches with a polygonal or oval shape and an irregular border. It is rarely associated with extracutaneous abnormalities. Sebaceous hyperplasia is characterized by numerous tiny, pale yellow papules representing hypertrophic sebaceous glands. They are seen on the nose, forehead, cheeks, and upper lip of full-term infants. The condition resolves with waning maternal androgen levels in the first few weeks of life.

(Section 18: Disorders of the Skin, Chapter 352: Neonatal Dermatology)

**Answer 23-3.** C

The patient in this vignette has the diagnosis of tinea versicolor. There are many effective treatment options including both topical and oral medications. Topical treatments include selenium sulfide 2.5% shampoo, ketoconazole 2% shampoo, and terbinafine 1% spray. Oral treatment options are fluconazole or itraconazole. Oral ketoconazole is no longer recommended due to potential toxicity. This rash is caused by a superficial skin infection with the fungus *Malassezia furfur*, also known as *Pityrosporum ovale* and *Pityrosporum orbiculare*. This organism is a lipid-dependent yeast that is part of the normal human skin flora in 90% to 100% of individuals. Most cases occur during the postpubertal period. This infection localizes to areas of skin that are rich in sebaceous glands, including the chest, back, and face. It does not affect the inguinal area. It is caused by factors such as heat, humidity, sweating, and skin occlusion. The hypopigmentation is not improved by sun exposure but is more noticeable after sun exposure due to the uneven tanning of the surrounding unaffected skin. Tinea versicolor can be diagnosed by visual inspection or can be determined by potassium hydroxide (KOH) examination of skin scrapings, which would show numerous clusters of spores and short, stubby hyphae. This classic pattern has been termed "spaghetti and meatballs." Culture is not useful because this organism is a part of the normal skin flora.

(Section 18: Disorders of the Skin, Chapter: 362 Skin Infections and Exanthems)

**Answer 23-4.** D

This patient has mild hidradenitis suppurativa. It is a primary inflammatory disorder of the hair follicle that affects apocrine gland–bearing areas of the body typically involving the axilla, inguinal creases, perineum, and mammary folds. The pathogenesis is primary plugging of the hair follicle with secondary inflammation of the apocrine glands. Mild cases are characterized by cyst or abscess formation without sinus tracts or scarring. Moderate disease has widely separated cysts and abscesses with some tract formation and scarring. Severe cases demonstrate numerous cysts and abscesses that result in multiple interconnected tracts and scarring in the affected area.

(Section 18: Disorders of the Skin, Chapter 360: Acne and Other Disorders of the Pilosebaceous Unit)

**Answer 23-5.** A

This patient's alopecia is due to the diagnosis of trichotillomania. This diagnosis is characterized by compulsive pulling, twisting, or breaking of one's own hair, causing areas of alopecia. Affected areas of the scalp demonstrate irregularly shaped areas of partial alopecia with broken hairs of varying lengths, often described as a "moth-eaten" appearance. Hair is often spared in the frontal area, more inaccessible areas, or painful parts of the occipital scalp. Eyebrows or eyelashes can also be affected. Trichotillomania may be a nervous habit or can indicate a more serious psychopathology, especially in older children. The treatment is behavioral modification techniques such as habit reversal; however, if the problem does not resolve or if other psychiatric concerns are present, a psychiatric evaluation is warranted. A dermatology referral could be helpful if the diagnosis is in question; however, it is not required for treatment. The other treatments, such as steroids, antibiotics, or antifungals, would not be appropriate choices.

(Section 18: Disorders of the Skin, Chapter 360: Acne and Other Disorders of the Pilosebaceous Unit)

**Answer 23-6.** B

*C albicans* is often a cause for diaper rash, especially in infants because they are in diapers and immunocompromised enough that they are often victims of the rash; however, it does not typically spread outside the diaper. The description given in the clinical stem refers to bullae, which are seen in bullous impetigo. Bullous impetigo is caused most often by *S aureus*. *S pyogenes* is also a common skin bacterium that is often a culprit of skin infections but is most likely seen in paronychia versus bullous impetigo. MRSA would likely present more acutely with fever, rapidly spreading erythema, and induration. HSV presents mostly with vesicular lesions rather than bullae, and the lesions are often grouped and in a linear distribution, so this is a less likely answer for this patient.

(Section 18: Disorders of the Skin, Chapter 362: Skin Infections and Exanthems)

**Answer 23-7.** C

Cellulitis presents with swelling, erythema, warmth, and tenderness that may be caused by many different bacterial organisms. The borders of cellulitis are not as well defined as in the more superficial form of erysipelas. Group A β-hemolytic *Streptococcus* (GABHS) and *S aureus* are again the most common etiologic agents, and the lower extremities and feet are the locations most often affected.

Ecthyma gangrenosum is a cutaneous manifestation of *Pseudomonas aeruginosa* bacteremia. Patients are usually systemically ill and have an underlying illness such as hematologic malignancy or immunodeficiency, but a number of healthy children have also been described. They present with 0.5- to 2-cm hemorrhagic papules, nodules, bullae, or ulcers, usually distributed in the genital region. These lesions rapidly progress to necrosis and eschar formation.

Our patient has necrotizing fasciitis, presenting with fever and other systemic signs of serious illness and shock, including low blood pressure, tachycardia, and delirium. Soft tissue gas can be a finding of necrotizing fasciitis on x-ray, but not always. It is important to get a surgery consult for debridement, initiate fluid resuscitation, and start on intravenous (IV) antibiotics.

Erythrasma is a superficial skin infection, primarily occurring in intertriginous zones, caused by *Corynebacterium minutissimum*. The clinical presentation is characterized by well-demarcated reddish-brown patches with mild scaling in the axillae, inframammary creases, groin, gluteal crease, and less commonly interdigital spaces of the toes. It occurs more commonly in individuals who are overweight and diabetic.

SSSS is caused by exfoliative toxin-producing strains of *S aureus* and occurs mainly in children < 5 years old. Patients with SSSS usually present with fever, irritability, and tender erythema of the skin, most marked in flexural areas and around the mouth and nose. Perioral and periocular crusting with radial fissures is a characteristic feature. Within 12 to 24 hours, flaccid blisters and superficial erosions form and may be followed by widespread superficial peeling of the skin in sheets, especially in infants. Superficial separation of the skin after rubbing (Nikolsky sign) is present.

(Section 18: Disorders of the Skin, Chapter 362: Skin Infections and Exanthems)

**Answer 23-8.** D

Pityriasis alba is most common on the face, and patients often have an associated atopic diathesis. Vitiligo results in complete depigmentation and is most common in periorificial regions (around the eyes, mouth, and genitalia) and over bony prominences. Scaling is usually minimal to absent in these 2 disorders. Psoriasis has a more insidious onset and is usually found in older people; lesions are not usually limited to areas with sebaceous glands. Our patient has tinea versicolor due to location and described appearance of the rash. The rash is hypopigmented, especially since he has tanned while running outside. Seborrheic dermatitis presents with yellowish flaky patches, mostly on the scalp and areas with hair follicles, including inner ears and eyebrows.

(Section 18: Disorders of the Skin, Chapter 362: Skin infections and Exanthems)

**Answer 23-9.** E

RMSF also presents with fever, headache, and petechial rash that becomes coalescent and swelling of palms and soles; however, there is no mention of tick exposure, which is how RMSF is spread. This varies as to where in the United States the event is, and the type of tick also differs, but our patient has no mention of tick exposure.

HSP or anaphylactoid purpura is the most common vasculitis in children. It is a self-limited systemic vasculitis syndrome characterized clinically by a tetrad of clinical features that occur in any order and at any time over the course of several days to weeks: a purpuric rash (may initially look urticarial), arthralgias, abdominal pain, and glomerulonephritis. This patient's course is a bit abrupt for HSP, and she is older than the usual patient.

Measles presents approximately 10 days after exposure, and fever and malaise signal the onset of illness. Cough, coryza, and conjunctivitis follow promptly. A gradual worsening of symptoms accompanies a steady rise in fever over the next 4 days. Two days prior to the appearance of the exanthem, Koplik spots develop. With the onset of rash 14 days after infection, the clinical picture attains maximal severity. Constitutional symptoms throughout this 10-day period vary, but headache, abdominal pain, vomiting, diarrhea, and myalgia are frequent complaints. Our patient has no mention of cough, coryza, or Koplik spots, and timing of the rash soon after the fever onset does not follow the usual measles course of rash 4 days after fever starts.

The most common manifestation of early, localized Lyme disease, erythema migrans (EM), appears 3 to 30 days (but typically within 7–14 days) after and at the site of a tick bite (although most often, the bite is not recognized). EM begins as a red macule or papule and usually expands over days to weeks to form a large, annular, erythematous lesion that is at least 5 cm and as much as 70 cm in diameter (median of 15 cm). The rash most often is uniformly erythematous, but it may appear as a "bull's eye" lesion with variable degrees of central clearing. EM is usually asymptomatic but may be pruritic or painful and may be accompanied by nonspecific systemic symptoms such as fever, malaise, headache, myalgia, or arthralgia.

*Neisseria meningitidis* presents with fever, headache, and neck stiffness, and symptoms are sometimes accompanied by photophobia, nausea, and altered mental status. Infants often present with irritability and lethargy and occasionally a bulging anterior fontanel. Bacteria are isolated from the blood in up to 75% of cases. This can present as occult bacteremia in young children being evaluated for fever without a source or as transient bacteremia associated with fever and a nonspecific rash. Meningococcal sepsis occurs in 5% to 10% of patients and is characterized by fever and petechial or purpuric rash. This can progress to fulminant meningococcal septicemia (purpura fulminans) and is associated with rapid growth of meningococci in the bloodstream, resulting in very high concentrations of organisms and endotoxin. Patients present with severe, persistent shock with little or no signs of meningitis. The development of a profound inflammatory response leads to progressive circulatory collapse; severe coagulopathy; and impaired pulmonary, renal, and adrenal function. Disseminated intravascular coagulation results in thrombotic lesions in the skin, limbs, kidneys, adrenals (Waterhouse-Friderichsen syndrome), and choroid plexus and lungs; multiorgan failure ensues. Vascular complications often lead to limb amputation and extensive skin loss. The patient in the clinical stem has vitals consistent with shock and needs immediate attention; *N meningitidis* is very contagious and spreads very rapidly in close quarters and at peer-associated events, such as dorms, army bunks, and concerts. Medical personnel treating the disease should also be provided prophylactic antibiotics.

(Section 18: Disorders of the Skin, Chapter 362: Skin Infections and Exanthems)

**Answer 23-10.** B

This patient has severe nodulocystic acne that is recalcitrant to topical treatments and oral antibiotics. Oral isotretinoin, a synthetic vitamin A derivative, is appropriate therapy for him. The most serious side effect of oral isotretinoin and other oral retinoids is teratogenicity; iPLEDGE is a mandatory US Food and Drug Administration (FDA)-regulated risk management program to prevent pregnancy while on oral isotretinoin. However, the most common side effects of the medication are xerosis, dry mucosa, and cheilitis. Almost all patients develop these conditions. Less common side effects include transient hypertriglyceridemia and transiently decreased high-density lipoprotein. Rarely, severe hypertriglyceridemia causes pancreatitis. Isotretinoin has also been linked to depression and suicide, though the nature of this relationship remains unclear. Patients should be screened for mental illness before and during treatments.

(Section 18: Disorders of the Skin, Chapter 360: Acne and Other Disorders of the Pilosebaceous Unit)

**Answer 23-11.** B

Humans are at risk of encountering ticks from wooded areas, grasses or brush, or household pets. There are about 100 species of ticks that act as vectors for various infectious diseases to humans. It is therefore important to know how to best counsel on prevention of tick bites. A DEET-containing repellant that has no more than 30% DEET is recommended by the American Academy of Pediatrics. DEET-containing repellant can be sprayed onto clothing and exposed skin. Picaridin-containing repellant can also be applied to clothing and exposed skin. Permethrin should not be applied to the skin as a repellant; instead, it can be sprayed on clothing.

(Section 18: Disorders of the Skin, Chapter 363: Infestations)

**Answer 23-12.** A

This infant has hyperpigmented lesions concerning for nevus of Ota. Nevus of Ota (nevus fuscoceruleus ophthalmomaxillaris, oculodermal melanocytosis) manifests as speckled grayish-brown to blue-black patches of the skin, sclera, conjunctiva, tympanic membrane, and/or oral and nasal mucosa along the innervation of cranial nerves V1 and V2. It most commonly occurs in individuals of black or Asian heritage and has a female predominance. More than half of those affected have hyperpigmented areas present at birth or within the first year of life; in others, the hyperpigmented areas become apparent during puberty. Ninety percent of cases are unilateral.

About 10% of those with nevus of Ota develop glaucoma. Therefore, these individuals should have yearly ophthalmologic examinations. Nevus of Ota can also be associated with ipsilateral sensorineural hearing loss. Occasionally, nevus of Ota is associated with melanoma of the uveal tract, central nervous system (CNS), orbit, or skin; this most often occurs in white adults. Nevus of Ota is not associated with cataract, retinoblastoma, or acute lymphoblastic leukemia.

(Section 18: Disorders of the Skin, Chapter 356: Melanocytic Lesions and Disorders of Pigmentation)

**Answer 23-13.** E

This patient's history and physical are consistent with subcutaneous fat necrosis of the newborn (SCFN). SCFN is a self-limited condition of healthy newborns in which erythematous nodules and indurated plaques develop within the first few days to weeks of life. Lesions typically develop on the back. Although the pathogenesis is unclear, a history of meconium aspiration, perinatal trauma, asphyxia, or hypothermia is common. Metabolic abnormalities sometimes occur in children with SCFN. These include hypercalcemia, hypoglycemia, anemia, thrombocytopenia, or hypertriglyceridemia. Hypercalcemia may be severe and can present as irritability (as seen in this patient), lethargy, failure to thrive, nausea, vomiting, renal failure, or cardiac arrest. Unless metabolic abnormalities exist, treatment is not indicated for SCFN. However, frequent monitoring for hypercalcemia is indicated for the first 6 months of life because delayed presentations have been described.

(Section 18: Disorders of the Skin, Chapter 354: Disorders of the Dermis and Subcutaneous Tissues)

**Answer 23-14.** B

This patient presents with complete separation of the nail plates from the nail bed, which is also known as onychomadesis. Onychomadesis is the result of nail matrix arrest and cessation of nail plate growth. In children, common triggers include infection, systemic illness, certain medications, or other stressors. Among infections, the most common culprit is coxsackievirus infection in hand, foot, and mouth disease. Therefore, the most likely triggering event for this patient's onychomadesis is contraction of hand, foot, and mouth disease.

(Section 18: Disorders of the Skin, Chapter 361: Nail Disorders)

**Answer 23-15.** D

This child is presenting with onychomadesis, or matrix arrest and cessation of nail plate growth resulting in complete separation of the nail plate. This is a benign and self-limited condition that can be caused by a variety of triggers, often recent coxsackievirus infection (hand, foot, and mouth disease), other systemic illness, or medication. A less severe presentation can be seen with only raised, horizontal ridges, or Beau's lines.

Dermatophyte infection will typically present with thickened, discolored nails. Iron deficiency does not typically cause skin or nail manifestation but can be associated with koilonychia or "spoon-shaped" nails. Psoriasis can manifest with pitting of nails. Finger sucking can result in onycholysis with white discoloration and distal separation of the nail plate, but it is not typically symmetric because only the sucked fingernails would be affected.

(Section 18: Disorders of the Skin, Chapter 361: Nail Disorders)

**Answer 23-16.** A

This child is presenting with characteristic features of neurofibromatosis type 1 (NF1). The National Institutes of Health consensus diagnostic criteria for NF1 include at least 2 of the following: 6 or more café-au-lait spots > 5 mm in diameter in prepubertal children, 2 or more neurofibromas or 1 plexiform neurofibroma, axillary or inguinal freckling, optic pathway glioma, 2 or more Lisch nodules (iris hamartomas), a characteristic osseous lesion (sphenoid dysplasia or tibial pseudoarthrosis), or a first-degree relative with NF1.

McCune-Albright syndrome is another genetic disease that presents with a triad of café-au-lait spots, polyostotic fibrous dysplasia of the skeleton, and autonomous endocrine dysfunction and could include precocious puberty or hyperthyroidism.

Acoustic neuroma is characteristic of neurofibromatosis type 2 (NF2), which has distinct diagnostic criteria, not usually including café-au-lait spots, Lisch nodules, or freckling.

Hypertrophic cardiomyopathy is a common finding in cases of Noonan syndrome, which can present with café-au-lait spots but also includes short stature and characteristic dysmorphic features.

(Section 18: Disorders of the Skin, Chapter 355: Genetic Disorders of the Skin)

**Answer 23-17.** A

This child is presenting with a case of lichen sclerosis, a common inflammatory condition in prepubertal girls of unknown etiology. It generally presents with pruritus, dysuria, or painful defecation. It may cause labial adhesions and scarring. It generally resolves with puberty and can be treated with topical high-potency corticosteroids.

Adhesions or excoriations can complicate lichen sclerosis and may be confused with child sexual abuse, which would necessitate a report to child protective services. A normal urinalysis excludes the diagnosis of urinary tract infection, which would be treated with oral antibiotics such as cefdinir.

Nonspecific vulvovaginitis is also common in prepubertal girls, but the physical exam would show erythema as opposed to white plaques with atrophy. It would be managed with sitz baths and elimination of any offending agents.

Labial adhesions without lichen sclerosis would be best treated with topical estrogen cream.

(Section 18: Disorders of the Skin, Chapter 357: Immunologic Diseases)

**Answer 23-18.** E

This child has recovered from Henoch-Schönlein Purpura (HSP), or IgA vasculitis. This disease is a systemic leukocytoclastic vasculitis that affects the small vessels of the skin, gastrointestinal tract, and kidneys. The diagnosis is made based on clinical presentation of the characteristic "palpable purpura" rash, most prominent in the lower extremities, and at least 1 of the following: abdominal pain, IgA deposits on biopsy, arthritis or arthralgia, or renal involvement. The rash is nonthrombocytopenic. The gastrointestinal symptoms can include pain, bleeding, and intussusception. Renal manifestations are most commonly nephritis with microscopic hematuria, sometimes with mild proteinuria. Most renal manifestations resolve without long-term nephropathy.

Because the nephritis can present after resolution of other symptoms and up to 3 months after resolution of rash, it is appropriate to check microscopic urinalysis monthly after symptom resolution for at least 3 months.

The rash of HSP presents with normal platelet count and coagulation studies, so following those over time is not indicated. Cardiac manifestations are not a part of HSP but are an important diagnosis in other systemic vasculitides including Kawasaki disease. Inflammatory markers such as ESR and CRP will often be elevated in the acute illness, but it is not necessary to follow them over time for recurrence of HSP.

Abdominal ultrasound would be the appropriate diagnostic test for intussusception in HSP; however, it generally presents with abdominal pain before or during the presentation of the rash, and serial examinations in an otherwise asymptomatic patient are not necessary.

(Section 18: Disorders of the Skin, Chapter 357: Immunologic Diseases [see also Chapter 200])

**Answer 23-19.** A

The infant in this case has an infantile hemangioma. These typically present as flat, erythematous or hypopigmented macules present at birth that rapidly proliferate during the first few months of life and typically involute by 1 year of age. The diagnosis and management is based on risk stratification of the lesion. Large, segmental hemangiomas on the face are a risk factor for visual/airway compromise as well as a potential marker for PHACE syndrome (posterior fossa brain malformations, hemangiomas, arterial anomalies, cardiac lesions, and eye abnormalities). Infants with such hemangiomas should be evaluated with magnetic resonance angiography or magnetic resonance imaging of the brain, cardiac imaging, thyroid studies, and eye exams.

Risk stratification for smaller hemangiomas is based on location. Those that could cause significant scarring or impair vision, respiration, or development may require early treatment. Those that are in intertriginous areas like the axilla or are larger at presentation may have an increased risk for ulceration. Those in the lumbosacral area could indicate spinal anomalies. Multiple lesions across the body can indicate a risk for hepatic involvement, high-output cardiac failure, or hypothyroidism.

(Section 18: Disorders of the Skin, Chapter 359: Vascular Tumor and Malformations)

**Answer 23-20.** B

SSSS is caused by exfoliative toxin-producing strains of *Staphylococcus aureus* and occurs mainly in children < 5 years old. The increased susceptibility of infants and young children may be related to immature mechanisms of renal clearance of the toxin. Predisposing factors in adults, in whom SSSS is rare, include renal failure, immunosuppression, and human immunodeficiency virus (HIV) infection. Most *S aureus* isolates causing SSSS belong to phage group II, types 71 and 55. Patients with SSSS usually have a primary infection at sites other than the skin, such as the nasopharynx, conjunctiva, middle ear, or umbilicus in neonates, and the toxin is hematogenously disseminated. The toxin targets desmoglein 1, resulting in cleavage of the epidermis in a superficial location beneath the stratum corneum or stratum granulosum.

Patients with SSSS usually present with fever, irritability, and tender erythema of the skin, most marked in flexural areas and around the mouth and nose. Perioral and periocular crusting with radial fissures is a characteristic feature. Within 12 to 24 hours, flaccid blisters and superficial erosions form and may be followed by widespread superficial peeling of the skin in sheets, especially in infants. Superficial separation of the skin after rubbing (Nikolsky sign) is present. Subsequent denudation of the skin with a moist, glistening, red surface at sites of prior blistering may lead to significant cutaneous fluid losses and secondary infection with resulting sepsis. Mucosal surfaces are spared. Older children may present with more mild forms of SSSS, with more localization of lesions and less toxicity. The differential diagnosis of SSSS in various stages may include toxic epidermal necrolysis, graft-versus-host disease, scarlet fever, toxic shock syndrome, and Kawasaki disease. In most cases, the history, clinical presentation, and physical examination aid in the differentiation of SSSS from these entities. Although cultures of skin and blister fluid are characteristically negative, recovery of *S aureus* from the blood, nasopharynx, throat, or conjunctiva confirms the diagnosis of SSSS. Although SSSS can be a severe disease, the majority of affected children do well and recover without sequelae, and the mortality rate in children is low, around 3%. Antistaphylococcal antibiotics are a mainstay of therapy for SSSS. Clindamycin has the ability to inhibit toxin production and may therefore be advantageous over penicillin antibiotics. Older children with localized involvement and no toxicity may be managed as outpatients with oral antibiotics, but affected newborns and any patient with severe disease require hospitalization with parenteral antibiotic therapy and aggressive supportive management. Supportive measures include intravenous fluids, electrolyte management, impeccable wound care with minimal handling, and pain control.

(Section 18: Disorders of the Skin, Chapter 362: Skin Infections and Exanthems)

**Answer 23-21.** C

Tinea corporis is caused by dermatophytes, fungal organisms that colonize the most superficial layers of the epidermis. The most characteristic appearance of skin lesions associated with tinea corporis is a ring-like pattern, due to central clearing as the infection spreads in a radial fashion. Potassium hydroxide–treated skin scrapings examined under a microscope allow identification of spores or hyphae.

The description of this skin lesion is consistent with tinea corporis, a very common cutaneous infection in children. It is one of the dermatophytoses (ringworm), which are caused by a group of related fungi including *Microsporum* and *Trichophyton* species. These fungi can invade the stratum corneum, nails, and hairs. The lesions are annular, gyrate, scaling, and discrete. Secondary bacterial infection commonly occurs. Topical antifungal agents are the initial treatment of choice.

Erythema multiforme is characterized by tender erythematous nodules, usually in the pretibial surfaces. It is caused by hypersensitivity reactions to a spectrum of infections, drugs, toxins, and disease states. It is a skin eruption caused by a hypersensitivity reaction to drugs, infections, or toxins. Skin lesions usually appear as macules, papules, wheals, and vesicobullous lesions. There is often central clearing of those skin lesions, which are therefore termed *target lesions*.

Nummular eczema is a highly pruritic idiopathic skin disorder that commonly occurs in association with asthma or allergic rhinitis.

Impetigo is a superficial bacterial infection of the skin usually caused by group A streptococci or *Staphylococcus aureus*. Infection is usually induced by minor trauma or abrasion to the surface of the skin with prior colonization of the bacteria.

(Section 18: Disorders of the Skin, Chapter 362: Skin Infections and Exanthems)

**Answer 23-22.** E

The correct answer is sporotrichosis. A cutaneous infection with sporotrichosis is caused by the fungus *Sporothrix schenckii*. It is commonly referred to as "rose gardener's disease." The fungus is ubiquitous around the world and lives in the soil and on plant matter. Gardening is a common mode of infection with the spores. The fungus will enter the skin through a small break and initially a small, painless nodule forms at the inoculation site. This may occur from 1 to 12 weeks after exposure. As described, the nodule will grow in size and ulceration appears at the center. With the cutaneous infection, there are no systemic symptoms. Sporotrichosis may infect other parts of the body, including the lungs and may disseminate to multiple organs. Most often, sporotrichosis is a clinical diagnosis but a skin biopsy can confirm when sent for fungal culture. Treatment is a 3 to 6 months course of antifungal medications; the most commonly prescribed is itraconazole.

Aspergillosis is another fungal infection occurring in humans. It is typically an opportunistic infection and is caused via respiratory inhalation of the fungal spores. The fungus tends to infect within the respiratory tract (both upper and lower) and is locally invasive and destructive. It does not cause skin findings. The described patient is not immunosuppressed.

Candidiasis is a cutaneous infection by the fungus *Candida albicans*. The common skin findings with candidiasis include a "beefy" red rash with classically described satellite lesions. Infections can occur anywhere, but there is a predilection for moist areas such as skinfolds, the genital area, and oral mucosa.

Cryptocococcosis, a pulmonary or disseminated infection, is caused by the encapsulated yeasts *Cryptococcus neoformans* or *Cryptococcus gattii*. The infection can lead to pneumonia, meningitis, osteomyelitis, or skin and visceral infections. It is usually found in immunocompromised patients and rarely infects immunocompetent patients. The skin findings can manifest as pustular, popular, nodular, or ulcerated. The patient in the clinical scenario is not described as immunocompromised.

Mucormycosis, an infection caused by many different species of fungi, is most common among immunocompromised patients, poorly controlled diabetic patients and those receiving deferoxamine for iron chelation. Cutaneous mucormycosis initially develops with erythema and induration at the inoculation site. The skin quickly becomes necrotic, and an eschar manifests and may progress to necrotizing fasciitis in some patients. The patient will experience rapidly expanding erythema, induration, and significant pain at the site. These clinical symptoms are not consistent with the description given above.

(Section 18: Disorders of the Skin, Chapter 362: Skin Infections and Exanthems)

**Answer 23-23.** E

The acute symptomatology is consistent with necrotizing fasciitis, a severe infection of the subcutaneous tissue and fascia caused by group A *streptococci*. The bacteria gain entry into the subcutaneous tissue through a skin lesion and produce rapidly spreading cellulitis, combined with systemic signs and symptoms of toxemia. Anesthesia/hypoesthesia is a particularly important clue to the diagnosis. As soon as necrotizing fasciitis is suspected, surgical exploration and debridement is mandatory.

Limiting care to supportive measures until culture results are available (answer choice A) may result in rapid necrosis of the affected limb and death due to septic shock.

(Section 18: Disorders of the Skin, Chapter 362: Skin Infections and Exanthems)

**Answer 23-24.** B

Pyogenic granuloma is a vascular tumor that predominantly affects children and young adults. The precise mechanism for the development of pyogenic granuloma is unknown. These lesions can arise spontaneously, in sites of trauma, and within capillary malformations. Pyogenic granulomas have also been associated with medications, including oral contraceptives and retinoids. Most occur as solitary growths, but multiple (grouped) or, rarely, disseminated lesions have been described. These lesions appear as small, vascular papules that grow rapidly over weeks and tend to bleed spontaneously. Histologically, these lesions are composed of capillaries and venules with plump endothelial cells separated into lobules by fibromyxoid stroma. Untreated lesions eventually atrophy, become fibromatous, and slowly regress. Surgery is reserved for problematic lesions. Unfortunately, the risk of recurrence can be as high as 40% to 50%.

Pyogenic granulomas, also known as lobular capillary hemangiomas, are common vascular tumors during childhood. They may develop spontaneously or in response to trauma and vary in size from a few millimeters to 1 to 2 cm. They usually grow rapidly, presenting as a friable red papule or nodule that bleeds profusely and repeatedly despite its small size (Figure 359-9). Over time, lesions often have a black hemorrhagic crust and a peripheral collarette of scale. Pyogenic granulomas also can arise within vascular malformations, particularly port wine stains and arteriovenous malformations. Differential diagnosis includes infantile hemangioma, wart, and Spitz nevus. Spontaneous resolution is rare, but symptomatic lesions may be removed by shave excision or curettage, with light electrocautery of the base. Rarely, recurrences occur despite adequate therapy, and occasionally, multiple "satellite" lesions develop after removal. Topical timolol has recently been reported as another therapeutic option.

Nevus simplexes are the light red macules found over the nape of the neck, upper eyelids, and glabella of newborns. Fifty percent of infants have such lesions over their necks. Eyelid and glabellar lesions usually fade completely within the first year of life. Lesions that occupy the total central forehead area usually do not fade. Those on the neck persist into adult life.

Spider angiomas are common, benign vascular neoplasms in children. They may arise spontaneously or be preceded by a history of trauma, sun exposure, or insect bite. Lesions present as small 2- to 5-mm, brightly erythematous, completely blanchable papules with a central punctum surrounded by radiating vessels and are most often located on exposed areas such as the face and hands. They may involute spontaneously or persist indefinitely. They are completely benign, and unless more than a few are present, they pose no associated clinical concerns and can easily be removed for cosmetic purposes with the pulsed dye laser (treatment of choice) or, if unavailable, electrocautery. This can typically be deferred until later in childhood when it can be tolerated without the need for sedation or anesthesia.

Kaposi sarcoma is a rare malignant vascular tumor associated with a viral etiology (human herpesvirus 8). It is extremely rare in children, although epidemic and iatrogenic forms can result from profound acquired T-cell deficiency resulting from human immunodeficiency virus (HIV) infection or rare immune disorders. A retrospective study investigating the presentation of Kaposi sarcoma in children in endemic areas of Africa found that they usually present with cutaneous lesions, lymphadenopathy, and intrathoracic and oral lesions. Children with Kaposi sarcoma have responded to treatment with chemotherapy.

Gottron papules are erythematous plaques on the extensor surfaces, particularly overlying the small joints of the hands but also frequently over the elbows, knees, and ankles. They are commonly associated with juvenile dermatomyositis.

(Section 18: Disorders of the Skin, Chapter 359: Vascular Tumors and Malformations)

**Answer 23-25.** D

Infantile hemangiomas are the most common benign vascular tumor of infancy, occurring in 3% to 10% of infants. They are not usually present at birth and are most commonly diagnosed by around 3 to 6 weeks of age. These lesions proliferate for an average of 5 months, then stabilize and involute over several years. Hemangiomas, which are more common in females, white non-Hispanic patients, premature infants, and multiple gestations, are associated with advanced maternal age and placental complications.

Although treatment is mainly cosmetic, it is designed to control growth, minimize deformity, and preserve function. Propranolol hydrochloride, a nonselective β-blocker, is the first-line therapy for hemangiomas. Most infantile hemangiomas resolve without the need for surgical intervention. Some hemangiomas are related to complex syndromes (eg, PHACE [posterior fossa malformations, hemangiomas, arterial anomalies, cardiac defects, eye abnormalities] syndrome; PELVIS [perineal hemangioma, external genitalia malformations, lipomyelomeningocele, vesicorenal abnormalities, imperforate anus, skin tag] syndrome); however, this is a rare occurrence. Although the location of certain hemangiomas may predispose children to neurologic complications, for the overwhelming majority, this will not be the case. In 2014, the US Food and Drug Administration approved propranolol hydrochloride for the treatment of proliferating infantile hemangiomas. Other more selective β-blockers, such as atenolol and nadolol, have also been used to decrease side effects of propranolol treatment.

The topical β-blocker timolol maleate has also been used to treat localized cutaneous infantile hemangiomas with good response.

(Section 18: Disorders of the Skin, Chapter 359: Vascular Tumors and Malformations [see also Chapter 458])

**Answer 23-26.** C

Port wine stains, also referred to as nevus flammeus, are capillary malformations that occur in 0.4% of newborns. They are usually pink, red, or violaceous patches that persist throughout life and grow with the child. Port wine stains involving the ophthalmic branch of the trigeminal nerve (V1) can occur with Sturge-Weber syndrome, which is a vascular malformation that can cause neurologic complications like seizures, intellectual disability, hemiplegia, choroid vascular anomalies, and glaucoma. Infants born with port wine stains involving the ophthalmic branch of the trigeminal nerve (V1) should be screened by doing an ophthalmic examination and radiologic studies.

β-Blocker therapy can be useful in accelerating the resolution of hemangiomas, but not for port wine stains. Topical steroid creams have no effect on port wine stains.

Genetic testing may have some benefit in diagnosing specific disorders but is not the next step in management. It is important to first identify if the trigeminal nerve ophthalmic (V1) branch is involved, which would require more immediate intervention.

Anticipatory guidance should be provided, but not in the absence of appropriate ophthalmologic evaluation and radiologic imaging of the head.

(Section 18: Disorders of the Skin, Chapter 359: Vascular Tumors and Malformations)

**Answer 23-27.** A

Impetigo is a highly contagious infection of the superficial epidermis that can occur at any age, but predominantly occurs in infants and preschool-age children during summer months. Exposed areas such as the face, neck, arms, and legs are most commonly affected. Children in daycare and athletes are some of the persons at higher risk, but most patients are young, healthy, and immunocompetent. In general, intact skin is resistant to impetigo, and some form of compromise of the epidermal surface is required to allow for infection such as minor abrasions or lacerations.

Treatment of impetigo can be solely topical when lesions are mild or localized, but when they are more widespread and numerous, systemic antibiotics in addition to topical therapies may be warranted (see Chapter 362, Table 362-1). Steroid cream has shown no benefit for the treatment of impetigo. The use of systemic antibiotics may be warranted in the presence of more widespread disease, but not in the localized infection exhibited by the patient in the vignette. The localized infection exhibited by the patient does not require systemic antibiotics. Clindamycin may be appropriate treatment if there is suspicion for infection due to methicillin-resistant *Staphylococcus aureus* (MRSA); however, there is no reason to suspect MRSA in this patient and systemic administration of antibiotics is not necessary to treat his symptoms.

**TABLE 362-1.** Topical Antibacterial Therapies

| Agent | Regimen | Comment |
|---|---|---|
| Mupirocin 2% ointment | Twice a day | Approved for impetigo, but also useful for folliculitis and minimization of *Staphylococcus aureus* carriage in the nares/rectum |
| Clindamycin 1% lotion | Twice a day | Useful for mild/recurrent folliculitis |
| Retapamulin 1% ointment | Twice a day for 5 days | Approved for MSSA and GABHS skin infections in patients age 9 months and older |
| Antibacterial cleansers (ie, chlorhexidine, triclosan) | Daily–twice a day | Useful for *S aureus* colonization, recurrent infections (eg, folliculitis, furunculosis, impetigo) |
| Sodium hypochlorite (bleach) baths | 1/4–1/2 cup dissolved in full tub (40 gallons), 10 min soak, rinse off. 1–2 times weekly | Useful for *S aureus* colonization of water, recurrent infections (eg, folliculitis, furunculosis, impetigo) |

GABHS, group A β-hemolytic streptococci; MSSA, methicillin-sensitive *Staphylococcus aureus*.

Mark W. Kline, *Rudolph's Pediatrics*, 23rd Edition. Copyright © McGraw-Hill Education. All rights reserved.

(Section 18: Disorders of the Skin, Chapter 362: Skin Infections and Exanthems)

**Answer 23-28.** B

Pityriasis rosea is a common, generalized, and self-limited dermatosis that most commonly presents in adolescence. Pityriasis rosea is characterized by the progressive eruption of numerous round to oval, salmon-colored, 2- to 10-mm flat patches bearing a peripheral ring of scale (Chapter 353). A single, larger, well-circumscribed area of erythema and scale on the trunk or extremities—the herald patch—commonly precedes the generalized rash by 2 to 21 days and may be commonly mistaken for a lesion of tinea corporis or nummular eczema.

The subsequent appearance of the Christmas tree pattern of secondary lesions establishes the diagnosis of pityriasis rosea; alternatively, the "trailing scale" on the inner side of the lesion may distinguish pityriasis rosea from tinea, in which case the scale is usually around the periphery and pointing outward (Chapter 362).

Its cause is unknown, although an infectious trigger has been proposed (human herpesvirus [HHV]-6 and HHV-7). Support for an infectious etiology includes the occasional temporal and geographic clustering of cases, the prodrome of malaise or pharyngitis reported by some patients, and the rarity of recurrences throughout one's lifetime (Chapter 207).

Pityriasis rosea usually resolves in 4 to 6 weeks, and most patients require no treatment. Mild pruritus may be managed with topical antipruritics (calamine lotion, lotions containing menthol and/or camphor, lotions with pramoxine), oatmeal baths, low-potency topical steroids, and oral antihistamines. More severe, symptomatic cases may benefit from phototherapy (Chapter 353).

Pityriasis can be confused with many fungi, particularly tinea from ringworm or *Malassezia*. However, the Christmas tree appearance and herald patch are pathognomonic of pityriasis. The distribution of this boy's rash is consistent with pityriasis, which is not caused by bacteria. Skin parasites can cause rashes that may appear as "trailing" erythema, but the description, distribution, and location of this boy's rash are most consistent with pityriasis. The rash described is not consistent with an allergic rash.

(Section 18: Disorders of the Skin, Chapter 362: Skin Infections and Exanthems)

**Answer 23-29.** C

Molluscum contagiosum is a common cutaneous viral infection caused by the poxvirus *Molluscipoxvirus.* Molluscum lesions typically begin as 3 to 5 mm or larger in diameter, flat-topped, discrete, dome-shaped, flesh-colored to translucent papules, with a central white core, and they umbilicate as they age. Molluscum lesions commonly occur on the trunk, extremities, and face, but may be generalized as well. Molluscum contagiosum is usually asymptomatic, although an eczematous, red, scaling patch can sometimes be seen surrounding the lesions and is termed *molluscum dermatitis.* Scratching of the dermatitis may spread the virus. Molluscum contagiosum is usually diagnosed clinically, based on morphology and distribution. Reassurance that the condition is self-limited and that the lesions may regress spontaneously, as well as controlling the spread of infection, is a reasonable treatment approach. However, treatment may be needed for numerous lesions, to reduce autoinoculation and spread to other individuals, to minimize pruritus or dermatitis, or for cosmetic purposes. Chemical or physical destruction is commonly used to treat molluscum, although there are limited prospective studies to support the various treatment modalities. Although molluscum contagiosum infections usually resolve completely without sequelae, small pitted scars or hypopigmentation may occur spontaneously or secondary to treatment.

*Staphylococcus* infection is usually tender and red and may have pustular drainage. *Streptococcus* infection is usually red and tender and may have crusting. Herpes infections are more painful and generally have a more vesicular quality. HPV is a common cause of warts (verrucae). They present as flesh-colored, hyperkeratotic papules, with interruption of skin tension lines, which may be solitary or multiple. Tiny black dots representing thrombosed capillaries may be visualized centrally, especially after manual debridement of devitalized tissue, and may be a useful diagnostic clue.

(Section 18: Disorders of the Skin, Chapter 362: Skin Infections and Exanthems)

**Answer 23-30.** A

Acropustulosis is an intensely pruritic eruption consisting of vesicles and pustules localized mainly to the palms, soles, and lower extremities. It may be present at birth but usually develops in early infancy and is common in dark-skinned males. It reoccurs in crops every 2 to 3 weeks and fades over the next 7 to 10 days. It closely mimics scabies, but repeated skin scrapings are negative for evidence of mites, and empiric treatment for scabies is ineffective.

Erythema toxicum will present with a rash that is spread all over the body and will present early in the neonatal period (1–2 days) and resolve by 2 weeks, with truncal predominance and palmoplantar sparing; treatment is reassurance.

Transient neonatal pustular melanosis occurs in darker-skinned infants and is always present at birth or within the first 24 hours. Lesions are noninflammatory pustules that rupture, leaving transient collarettes of scale surrounding hyperpigmented macules that may persist for several weeks. The pustular phase is evanescent and may occur in utero, leaving only pigmented macules at birth. The eruption may occur on any part of the skin but usually involves the face, neck folds, hands, and feet. Skin biopsy shows neutrophils.

Miliaria, also called prickly heat, is a common skin finding that results from incomplete canalization of the eccrine ostia with resultant accumulation of sweat droplets within the skin.

A variant of eosinophilic folliculitis occurs in infants and, rarely, neonates. It is characterized by pruritic, recurrent crops of pustules. Unlike acropustulosis of infancy, the lesions are most commonly seen on the scalp and face, although they can occur on the trunk and extremities as well. Skin biopsy reveals a perifollicular infiltrate of eosinophils. The etiology is unknown, but potent topical steroids and oral antihistamines seem to be helpful. The lesions eventually resolve over several months. Neonatal eosinophilic pustulosis is best considered a variant that lacks pruritus and is not folliculocentric.

(Section 18: Disorders of the Skin, Chapter 352: Neonatal Dermatology)

**Answer 23-31.** E

This patient has acropustulosis. Treatment is with potent topical steroids or oral antihistamines. The use of ultrapotent (class I) topical steroids may be justified in severe cases. Severe cases may respond to oral erythromycin or to dapsone.

(Section 18: Disorders of the Skin, Chapter 352: Neonatal Dermatology)

**Answer 23-32.** D

Incontinentia pigmenti is an X-linked dominant disorder affecting mostly females. It may present during the neonatal period or early infancy and affects the skin, brain, and eyes. The incidence may be as frequent as 1 in 10,000. The classic description involves skin lesions transitioning between 4 stages, with the stages often overlapping.

**First stage:** erythema evolving into vesicles and pustules along the lines of Blaschko
**Second stage:** verrucous lesions
**Third stage:** linear hyperpigmentation
**Fourth:** regions of depigmentation in adults

Associated symptoms are as follows:

**Neurologic:** seizures, intellectual disability, cerebral palsy in 20% to 30% of affected individuals
**Eye:** retinal detachment, cataracts, and vision loss
**Appendages:** hair, nails, teeth with alopecia, dystrophic nails, and microdontia
**X-linked:** *IKBKG*, lethal in males

Management is symptomatic with treatment of epilepsy.

(Section 18: Disorders of the Skin, Chapter 355: Genetic Disorders of the Skin)

**Answer 23-33.** D

Nevus sebaceous is a localized lesion on the scalp or face that presents at birth as a hairless linear plaque of coalesced yellow-colored papules. The diagnosis is made clinically, but a biopsy can be considered if the diagnosis is uncertain. Histology reveals absent to malformed hair follicles with an abundance of sebaceous glands. The nevus sebaceous may develop overlying neoplastic growths, most of which are benign, such as syringocystadenoma papilliferum or trichoblastoma.

(Section 18: Disorders of the Skin, Chapter 352: Neonatal Dermatology)

**Answer 23-34.** B

Aplasia cutis is a congenital absence of skin commonly seen on the vertex of the scalp. Inheritance can be autosomal dominant or recessive. They present as sharply demarcated lesions that are single or multiple and can scar. These lesions are also associated with underlying skull or meningeal defects, cleft lip or palate, limb anomalies, epidermolysis bullosa, omphalocele or gastroschisis, and syndromes such as trisomy 13, Johanson-Blizzard syndrome, and Adams-Oliver syndrome. Open defects may be associated with elevated α-fetoprotein levels in the amniotic fluid.

(Section 18: Disorders of the Skin, Chapter 352: Neonatal Dermatology)

**Answer 23-35.** A

Acne is very common in adolescence due to the increase in androgens. It is caused by increased sebum production, abnormal epithelial cell desquamation, microbial proliferation, and inflammation. The formation of closed comedones (whiteheads) and open comedones (blackheads) is initiated by abnormal cornification of the follicular orifice. Monitor for signs of precocious puberty in children who develop acne at < 8 years of age. The goal of treatment is to prevent scarring and to reduce psychological distress from disfigurement, using 3 forms of medications: retinoids, benzoyl peroxide, and antimicrobials (Table 360-2).

Topical retinoids are especially effective in promoting normal desquamation and will benefit patients who have both comedones and inflammatory lesions. All forms of retinoids

**TABLE 360-2.** Acne Treatment Guidelines

| Acne Type | First-Line Therapy | Second-Line Therapy |
|---|---|---|
| Mild comedonal | Topical retinoid | Alterative topical retinoid OR<br>Azelaic acid OR<br>Salicylic acid |
| Mild inflammatory | Topical retinoid + topical antimicrobial | Alternative topical retinoid AND 1 of the following:<br>Alternative topical antibiotic OR<br>Azelaic acid OR<br>Salicylic acid OR<br>Dapsone gel |
| Moderate papulopustular or nodular | Oral antibiotic + topical retinoid<br>+/− Benzoyl peroxide (BPO) | Isotretinoin OR alternative antibiotic + alternative retinoid<br>+/− BPO OR azelaic acid |
| Severe papulopustular or nodular | Isotretinoin<br>+/− Oral steroid | Dapsone OR<br>High-dose oral antibiotic + topical retinoid + BPO |
| Hormonal | Oral contraceptives (OCPs) | OCPs + spironolactone |

Data from Gollnick H, Cunliffe W, Berson D, et al. Management of acne: a report from a Global Alliance to Improve Outcomes in Acne. *J Am Acad Dermatol*. 2003; 49(1 Suppl):S1-37.

should be introduced gradually to decrease the incidence of adverse effects such as drying, irritation, or sun sensitivity. Daily therapy can usually be tolerated after several weeks. It should be applied at night and should not be used at the same time of day as benzoyl peroxide. Acne fulminans is an uncommon severe variant of acne vulgaris seen in adolescent males; presents with systemic symptoms of fever, hemorrhagic crusting of lesions, and increased white blood cell count; and is treated with systemic steroids with slow initiation of retinoids, as higher doses of retinoids may cause worsening of disease.

(Section 18: Disorders of the Skin, Chapter 360: Acne and Other Disorders of the Pilosebaceous Unit)

**Answer 23-36.** E

Acne is a disorder of the pilosebaceous unit involving increased sebum production, abnormal epithelial cell desquamation, bacterial overgrowth, and inflammation. The onset of acne is common during puberty and can occur as early as 8 years of age. While topical benzoyl peroxide, topical retinoids, and oral doxycycline are all considered appropriate treatments for mild to moderate comedonal acne, if onset occurs before age 7, clinicians should monitor for signs of precocious puberty or hyperandrogenism. Currently, there is no study suggesting high-fat diet is linked to the development of acne.

(Section 18: Disorders of the Skin, Chapter 360: Acne and Other Disorders of the Pilosebaceous Unit)

**Answer 23-37.** C

The patient has trichotillomania, which is characterized by compulsive pulling or twisting of one's own hair, leaving irregularly shaped areas of partial alopecia with broken hairs of varying lengths, often described as "moth-eaten" in appearance. Patients with trichotillomania may not be aware of or may fail to disclose their hair-pulling behavior. Alopecia can be categorized into 2 groups: scarring or nonscarring alopecia. Alopecia areata is characterized by smooth, round, shiny, hairless patches on the scalp. Some long hairs can have "exclamation point hairs," but typically the hairs do not have a broken appearance like those seen in hairs that have been pulled out in patients with trichotillomania. Tinea capitis is a common cause of both scarring or nonscarring alopecia in children. It is often pruritic and can have variable inflammation. In severe cases of seborrheic dermatitis, there may be thinning and loss of hair, but alopecia is not a sequela of mild seborrheic dermatitis.

(Section 18: Disorders of the Skin, Chapter 360: Acne and Other Disorders of the Pilosebaceous Unit)

**Answer 23-38.** D

Midline lesions on the scalp can be associated with underlying encephalocele, meningocele, or heterotopic brain tissue. The nodule in Figure 352-2 represents an encephalocele. Therefore, a skin biopsy or surgical excision should be deferred until imaging by computed tomography or MRI is done.

(Section 18: Disorders of the Skin, Chapter 352: Neonatal Dermatology)

**Answer 23-39.** A

Anogenital warts or condyloma acuminata can be seen in sexually active adolescents, but they may occur in infants and prepubertal children. When anogenital warts are seen in children younger than 3 years, typically it is due to nonsexual heteroinoculation, autoinoculation, or vertical transmission. These can occur in healthy children who are not immunocompromised; therefore, immunodeficiency workup is not usually needed. Routine biopsy and HPV typing are also not considered standard management of anogenital warts. Salicylic acid is an effective treatment for common warts on the skin, but it is not typically recommended for anogenital warts. Condyloma acuminata seen in children older than 3 years is unusual, and the American Academy of Pediatrics Committee on Child Abuse and Neglect recommends reporting to the appropriate child protection agency.

(Section 18: Disorders of the Skin, Chapter 362: Skin Infections and Exanthems)

**Answer 23-40.** C

This child has crusted scabies, which can present as hyperkeratotic, lichenified thicken plaques on the dorsal hands and feet and is often mistaken for psoriasis or chronic eczematous plaques. The Centers for Disease Control and Prevention recommends treatment with both oral ivermectin and topical permethrin cream. Scabies reinfestation is common; therefore, all household contacts need to be treated. The infected person's clothing, towels, and bed linens should be decontaminated in hot water and dried at 60°C for 10 minutes or by placing items in a closed container for 5 to 7 days.

(Section 18: Disorders of the Skin, Chapter 363: Infestations)

**Answer 23-41.** B

Diaper dermatitis is one of the most common rashes seen in infants and toddlers. Most diaper dermatitis starts as irritant dermatitis caused by the moist occlusive environment with use of diapers. After infectious etiologies are ruled out, chronic diaper dermatitis can present as erosions or punched-out ulcers. This is also called erosive diaper dermatitis (Figure 353-5). Management includes frequent diaper changes, use of superabsorbent diapers, and application of a barrier cream. Addition of antimicrobial therapy depends on clinical suspicion or after confirmation of an infectious etiology. If bacterial and viral cultures are negative, management includes searching for the cause of frequent stooling.

(Section 18: Disorders of the Skin, Chapter 353: Disorders of the Epidermis)

**Answer 23-42. B**

The baby has an autosomal recessive disorder, acrodermatitis enteropathica, associated with mutation in the *SLC39A4* gene on 8q24.3. The gene codes for a transmembrane protein involved in zinc transport. Symptoms of zinc deficiency often develop in infancy after discontinuation of breast milk. Babies can develop alopecia, bullous or pustular plaques symmetrically distributed on the scalp, face, hands, and feet. Often, treatment with oral zinc is effective, and symptoms typically improve rapidly within 2 to 3 days of zinc replacement.

(Section 21: Disorders of the Gastrointestinal System, Chapter 403: Disorders of Digestion and Absorption)

**Answer 23-43. D**

The patient has developed a drug reaction with eosinophilia and systemic symptoms (DRESS). A typical drug rash can develop within 7 to 10 days of treatment, and the condition improves spontaneously once the offending agent is discontinued. However, a drug rash can progress to DRESS, and patients may have associated facial edema, fever, hepatitis, lymphadenopathy, eosinophilia, atypical lymphocytosis, and variable multiorgan involvement. Due to the severity of the reaction, a rechallenge with the offending agent is not recommended. Patients with DRESS can often have concomitant infection with herpes viruses such as HHV-6, cytomegalovirus, and Epstein-Barr virus.

(Section 18: Disorders of the Skin, Chapter 357: Immunologic Diseases)

**Answer 23-44. D**

Morphea or localized scleroderma is a distinct disease from systemic scleroderma. The patient has the subtype of morphea called linear morphea. When it is located as a linear band on the forehead, it is also called *en coup de sabre*. The prognosis of linear morphea is more guarded and can cause permanent disfigurement and affect underlying structures. Early aggressive systemic treatment can help prevent progression and is recommended.

(Section 18: Disorders of the Skin, Chapter 357: Immunologic Diseases)

**Answer 23-45. A**

The baby has PHACE, a syndrome with *p*osterior fossa brain malformations, segmental *h*emangiomas, *a*rterial anomalies, *c*oarctation of the aorta and cardiac defects, and *e*ye abnormalities. Oral propranolol has become the gold standard for treatment of infantile hemangioma. However, prior to initiating oral propranolol, PHACE should be ruled out because the administration of propranolol can reduce an already compromised cerebrovascular flow in addition to causing hypotension and bradycardia.

(Section 18: Disorders of the Skin, Chapter 359: Vascular Tumors and Malformations)

**Answer 23-46. C**

Congenital melanocytic nevi (CMNs) are present at birth or within the first few months of life. CMNs are categorized based on their expected final size: small (< 1.5 cm); medium (M1 1.5-10 cm, M2 > 10-20 cm); large (L1 > 20-30 cm, L2 > 30-40 cm); and giant (G1 > 40-60 cm, G2 > 60 cm). The large CMNs tend to have activating *NRAS* mutation, whereas the small CMNs have *BRAF* mutation. Large CMNs can be associated with extracutaneous manifestations, specifically neurocutaneous melanosis (NCM); therefore, a screening MRI with and without contrast of brain and spine before age 6 months is recommended. The presence of satellite nevi is also associated with higher risk of NCM. If MRI confirms evidence of CNS melanosis, neurology referral is recommended. Surgical excision of CMNs does not reduce the risk for development of melanoma.

(Section 18: Disorders of the Skin, Chapter 356: Melanocytic Lesions and Disorders of Pigmentation)

**Answer 23-47. A**

The patient has erythema nodosum on her lower legs. This is thought to be a hypersensitivity with variable systemic symptoms of fever, malaise, and arthralgia. In children, the most common association is underlying β-hemolytic streptococcal infection. Other associations may include inflammatory bowel disease, malignancies, and medications. The diagnosis can be made based on clinical presentation, and biopsy can be performed if the diagnosis is unclear. The skin nodules are self-limiting, and symptomatic treatment for pain is all that is needed.

(Section 18: Disorders of the Skin, Chapter 354: Disorders of the Dermis and Subcutaneous Tissue)

**Answer 23-48. A**

NF1 is the most common neurocutaneous disorder. Diagnosis of NF1 can be made by meeting the National Institutes of Health Consensus Diagnostic Criteria for Neurofibromatosis 1. It is important to be aware of the physical findings of NF1. Café-au-lait macules are typically the skin finding to appear by age 2. Axillary freckling typically occurs by late childhood. Cutaneous neurofibromas tend to appear later at the time of puberty. Both ash leaf spots and confetti macules are seen in patients with tuberous sclerosis.

(Section 12: Clinical Genetics and Dysmorphology, Chapter 176: Neurocutaneous Disorders)

**Answer 23-49. D**

The lesion is a solitary mastocytoma. Mastocytosis is a condition where there is an increased number of mast cells infiltrating various organs. Cutaneous mastocytomas are characterized by multiple brown-to-orange macules, papules, or plaques that can have an orange peel–like appearance. When the lesions are rubbed, they can become edematous and bullous-like in urticaria (Darier sign). Treatment for mastocytosis is combination of H1 and H2 antihistamines and avoidance of medications or physical factors that induce mast cell degranulation.

(Section 18: Disorders of the Skin, Chapter: 358 Neoplastic and Proliferative Disorders)

**Answer 23-50.** E

Impetigo can present as nonbullous and bullous impetigo. The nonbullous form can be caused by GABHS and *Staphylococcus aureus*, both methicillin-sensitive *S aureus* and methicillin-resistant *S aureus* (MRSA). The prognosis is good in healthy children, but impetigo caused by GABHS can sometimes lead to acute glomerulonephritis, and the risk of acute glomerulonephritis is not prevented with early treatment. The bullous type is caused by a toxin-producing strain of *S aureus*.

(Section 18: Disorders of the Skin, Chapter 362: Skin Infections and Exanthems)

**Answer 23-51.** D

Erythema toxicum is a benign neonatal rash that occurs in full-term newborns. The exact etiology is not known. It appears several days following birth and regresses within 1 to 2 weeks. The clinical presentation will show a predominate rash on the trunk with erythematous macules, wheals, or vesiculopustules. The eruption spares the perioral and palmoplantar skin. A Wright stain will show eosinophils, but neutrophils are seen in transient neonatal pustular melanosis.

(Section 18: Disorders of the Skin, Chapter 352: Neonatal Dermatology)

**Answer 23-52.** D

Nevus sebaceous is a birthmark that commonly occurs on the scalp or face and is made up of malformed hair follicles and abundant sebaceous glands. As children enter puberty, these birthmarks become raised and verrucous-like and may become a cosmetic concern for patients. Nevus sebaceous may develop secondary benign growths such as syringocystadenoma papilliferum or trichoblastoma and may rarely develop a secondary malignancy such as basal cell carcinoma. Treatment of nevus sebaceous is surgical excision, although due to the low risk of malignant transformation, clinical observation is also appropriate.

(Section 18: Disorders of the Skin, Chapter 352: Neonatal Dermatology)

**Answer 23-53.** C

Neonatal HSV is acquired from an ascending in utero infection or spread during the delivery process. The majority of infants with neonatal HSV are born to mothers with a primary infection and are asymptomatic at the time of delivery. Infants may present with fever, skin lesions, respiratory distress, or central nervous system dysfunction within the first 4 weeks of life. Cutaneous findings include vesicles or erosions at sites in contact with the maternal cervix during delivery. A known risk factor for neonatal HSV includes fetal scalp monitoring, but there is no evidence that breastfeeding poses a risk to the infant.

(Section 18: Disorders of the Skin, Chapter 352: Neonatal Dermatology)

**Answer 23-54.** D

Periorificial dermatitis is a papulopustular eruption on the face that is thought to be a variant of rosacea. Common locations for this rash include periocular, perinasal, and a perioral distribution. Triggers for this rash include oral, topical, or inhaled corticosteroids. Treatment for periorificial dermatitis includes topical antibiotics such as metronidazole, clindamycin, and erythromycin and topical calcineurin inhibitors such as pimecrolimus. Oral antibiotics are used for persistent or severe cases.

(Section 18: Disorders of the Skin, Chapter 360: Acne and Other Disorders of the Pilosebaceous Unit)

**Answer 23-55.** A

Alopecia areata is an autoimmune disorder that leads to nonscarring alopecia. The most common location is the scalp, although other areas can be affected. Although other types of autoimmune disease can be present, such as thyroid disease, diabetes, or vitiligo, this is uncommon. Clinically, patients have round to oval patches of hair loss with underlying smooth skin with no associated erythema or scale. Nails may have associated pitting. Mainstay treatment for alopecia areata includes topical or intralesional corticosteroids.

(Section 18: Disorders of the Skin, Chapter 360: Acne and Other Disorders of the Pilosebaceous Unit)

**Answer 23-56.** A

Granuloma annulare (GA) is a benign inflammatory skin disorder in which the exact etiology is not known. On examination, you see firm annular nonscaly papules or plaques. The most common locations include the dorsal hands, feet, wrists, or ankles. GA is often misdiagnosed as tinea corporis due to the ring-like appearance, but there is no associated scale. Although many treatments have been tried, GA commonly resolves without treatment over several years.

(Section 18: Disorders of the Skin, Chapter 354: Disorders of the Dermis and Subcutaneous Tissue)

**Answer 23-57.** C

Nevus of Ota is a blue-gray patch involving areas innervated by the first and second trigeminal nerve. It may become evident at the time of birth, during the first year of life, or at puberty. Nevus of Ota is secondary to a density of melanocytes in the dermis of the skin. A small percentage of patients may develop glaucoma, ipsilateral sensorineural hearing loss, and rarely melanoma.

(Section 18: Disorders of the Skin, Chapter 356: Melanocytic Lesions and Disorders of Pigmentation)

**Answer 23-58. D**

Phytophotodermatitis is a delayed hyperpigmentation of the skin following exposure to phototoxic furocoumarins. Examples of phototoxic furocoumarins include lime, other citrus fruits, or weeds such as celery, parsnip, or parsley. The hyperpigmentation is commonly in bizarre patterns such as linear streaks or fingerprints (drip mark in Figure 356-4B). Provide reassurance to patient that hyperpigmentation will slowly resolve with time.

(Section 18: Disorders of the Skin, Chapter 356: Melanocytic Lesions and Disorders of Pigmentation)

**Answer 23-59. B**

A keloid is a hypertrophic scar that extends beyond the border of the original insult to the skin. Keloids are most common in darker skinned persons but can occur in anyone. Cytokines and growth factors implicated in the cause of keloids include interleukin (IL)-6, IL-8, IL-10, transforming growth factor-β, and platelet-derived growth factor. Treatments for keloids include topical or intralesional steroids, radiation, surgical excision, and laser therapy.

(Section 18: Disorders of the Skin, Chapter 354: Disorders of the Dermis and Subcutaneous Tissue)

**Answer 23-60. B**

Neonatal lupus erythematosus is secondary to transplacental passage of maternal antibodies, specifically anti-Ro (SSA), anti-La (SSB), and anti-U1RNP. The transient skin lesions of neonatal lupus are commonly erythematous patches and annular plaques predominately on the head and neck with a classic periorbital distribution. Although photodistributed areas are most characteristic, other areas of the body can be involved. Every child with neonatal lupus should be evaluated for conduction system abnormalities with an ECG and blood work performed to evaluate for antibodies, as mentioned earlier, hematologic abnormalities, and hepatitis. The mothers of affected infants should also be evaluated if they do not have known rheumatologic disease.

(Section 15: Rheumatology, Chapter 201: Systemic Lupus Erythematosus, Overlap Connective Tissue Diseases, and Mixed Connective Tissue Disease)

**Answer 23-61. A**

Lichen sclerosus is an autoinflammatory condition of unknown etiology that most commonly affects prepubertal girls and postmenopausal women. When this condition occurs in males, it is termed balanitis xerotica obliterans. Children commonly complain of pruritus, pain, dysuria, or constipation. Clinically, the vulva and the perianal skin are involved and can show a figure-of-8 pattern. The skin may appear pink, hypopigmented, or purpuric and may have associated atrophy. When purpura is present, this condition may be mistaken for child abuse. Potent topical steroids are first-line treatment for vulvar and perianal disease.

(Section 18: Disorders of the Skin, Chapter 356: Melanocytic Lesions and Disorders of Pigmentation)

**Answer 23-62. B**

Tinea capitis is a common dermatophyte infection affecting the scalp of children. The disease is easily spread from person to person as well as by fomites including bedding, clothing, or hairbrushes. Clinical examination can be variable, from mild scaling of the scalp to erythematous papules, pustules, or plaques with overlying alopecia. A kerion may also occur and present as a tender, edematous plaque with adherent crust and associated alopecia. Cervical and suboccipital lymphadenopathy are common. It is important to perform a fungal culture prior to and after treatment to confirm resolution of fungal infection. Treatment should be oral due to involvement of the hair follicle. For appropriate dosing and duration of treatment, see Table 362-3.

(Section 18: Disorders of the Skin, Chapter 362: Skin Infections and Exanthems)

**Answer 23-63. D**

Sturge-Weber syndrome is a neurocutaneous syndrome with a facial capillary malformation, ipsilateral cerebral vascular malformation, and ophthalmologic disease such as glaucoma. Ten percent of patients with a facial capillary malformation (port wine stain) in a V1 distribution have Sturge-Weber syndrome. When other facial dermatomes or bilateral facial involvement is present, this increases the risk of Sturge-Weber syndrome. As children age, facial capillary malformations become thicker and more violaceous in color. Other neurologic manifestations include seizure disorder, developmental delay, migraine headaches, and hemiparesis. Sturge-Weber syndrome is secondary to a *GNAQ* mutation.

(Section 18: Disorders of the Skin, Chapter 359: Vascular Tumors and Malformations)

**Answer 23-64. A**

Pediculosis capitis, also known as head lice, are small wingless insects for which humans serve as the primary host. This commonly affects school-aged children and is easily transmitted via person to person or by fomites such as hair brushes, helmets, hats, or bedding. Scalp pruritus is the most common symptom with associated scalp excoriations. First-line treatment for head lice is permethrin 1% lotion because it is

TABLE 362-3. Treatment of Dermatophyte Infections

| Therapy | Regimen | Comment |
|---|---|---|
| **Tinea Capitis** | | |
| Griseofulvin | | Fat enhances absorption |
| Microsize | 20–25 mg/kg/d, max dose 1000 mg/d for 6–8 wk | |
| Ultramicrosize | 10–15 mg/kg/d, max dose 750 mg/d for 6–8 wk | |
| Itraconazole (OL)[a] | 5–10 mg/kg/d, divided twice a day for 4–6 wk | Potential drug interactions, monitor LFTs, electrolytes |
| Fluconazole (OL) | 6 mg/kg/d, daily for 3–6 wk (up to 12 mg/kg/d for serious infections) | Potential drug interactions, monitor LFTs, electrolytes |
| Terbinafine[b] | < 25 kg: 125 mg daily for 6 wk | Monitor CBC, LFTs; granules cannot be taken with acidic food; some studies document response with 2–4 wk of therapy |
| | 25–35 kg: 187.5 mg daily for 6 wk | |
| | > 35 kg: 250 mg daily for 6 wk | |
| Antifungal shampoo (selenium sulfide 2.5%, ketoconazole 2%) | Use daily | Always used in conjunction with oral treatment; sporicidal may decrease recurrence risk |
| **Tinea Corporis** | | |
| Topicals | | |
| Azoles (econazole, ketoconazole, oxiconazole, clotrimazole [OL], miconazole [OL]) | Apply daily or twice a day for 4–6 wk | |
| Allylamines (naftifine, terbinafine) | Apply daily or twice a day for 2–4 wk | |
| Others (ciclopirox olamine, tolnaftate, butenafine) | Apply daily or twice a day for 4–6 wk | |
| Systemic | | |
| Griseofulvin | Refer to tinea capitis for dosing | Recalcitrant or widespread cases, or in immunocompromised patients. Course of treatment could be shorter. |
| Itraconazole | Refer to tinea capitis for dosing | |
| Fluconazole | Refer to tinea capitis for dosing | |
| Terbinafine [OL] | Refer to tinea capitis for dosing | |
| **Majocchi Granuloma** | | |
| Griseofulvin | Refer to tinea capitis for dosing | |
| Itraconzole [OL] | Refer to tinea capitis for dosing | |
| Fluconazole [OL] | Refer to tinea capitis for dosing | |
| Terbinafine [OL] | Refer to tinea capitis for dosing | |
| **Tinea Pedis** | | |
| Topicals | | |
| Azoles (econazole, ketoconazole, oxiconazole, clotrimazole [OL], miconazole [OL]) | Apply daily or twice a day for 4–6 wk | |
| Allylamines (naftifine, terbinafine) | Apply daily or twice a day for 2–4 wk | |
| Others (ciclopirox olamine, tolnaftate, butenafine) | Apply daily or twice a day for 4–6 wk | |

(Continued)

TABLE 362-3. Treatment of Dermatophyte Infections (*Continued*)

| Therapy | Regimen | Comment |
|---|---|---|
| **Onychomycosis** | | |
| Topicals | | |
| Naftifine [OL] | Apply twice a day | Distal subungual type |
| Ciclopirox 8% nail lacquer[a] | Apply nightly, pare weekly | Superficial white type |
| Systemic | | |
| Itraconazole[a] | See above, pulse 5 mg/kg/d for 1 wk/mo for 2 months (fingernails) or 3 months (toenails) | |
| Terbinafine [OL] | 10–20 kg: 62.5 mg daily for 6 wk (fingernails) or 12 wk (toenails) | Monitor CBC, LFTs |
| | 20–40 kg: 125 mg daily for 6 wk (fingernails) or 12 wk (toenails) | |
| | > 40 kg: 250 mg daily for 6 wk (fingernails) or 12 wk (toenails) | |

[a]US Food and Drug Administration (FDA) approved in patients older than 18 years.

[b]FDA approved in patients older than 4 years.

CBC, complete blood cell count; LFTs, liver function tests; OL, off-label use.

Mark W. Kline, *Rudolph's Pediatrics*, 23rd Edition. Copyright © McGraw-Hill Education. All rights reserved.

easily accessible, has low toxicity, and is cost effective. Second-line agents include ivermectin 0.5% lotion; benzyl alcohol 5% lotion, which leads to asphyxiation of lice; and malathion 0.5% lotion, which is an organophosphate with risk of respiratory depression if ingested. Lindane 1% lotion is no longer recommended due to risk of neurotoxicity.

(Section 18: Disorders of the Skin, Chapter 363: Infestations)

**Answer 23-65.** D

Incontinentia pigmenti is an X-linked dominant disorder primarily seen in females. Because this neurocutaneous disorder is usually lethal in males, affected mothers may report an increased frequency of miscarriages. Incontinentia pigmenti is secondary to a mutation in nuclear-factor-κb essential modulator (*NEMO*). Cutaneous findings present during the first 6 weeks of life commonly as vesicles (blistering) along lines of Blaschko. The 4 overlapping stages of skin manifestations include vesicular, verrucous, hyperpigmented, and hypopigmented. Noncutaneous manifestations of incontinentia pigmenti include dental abnormalities such as delayed dentition, absent or malformed teeth, ophthalmologic abnormalities such as strabismus or retinal neovascularization or detachment, and neurologic abnormalities such as seizure disorder.

(Section 18: Disorders of the Skin, Chapter 352: Neonatal Dermatology)

**Answer 23-66.** A

Scabies is an intensely pruritic mite infestation that is common across age groups. The presentation of scabies in infants can include lesions of the face, scalp, head, neck, palms, and soles—areas that are typically spared in adolescents and adults. Additionally, although papules and excoriations are much more common in older children and adults, vesiculopustules are often present in infants. Permethrin 5% cream is US Food and Drug Administration (FDA) approved for children > 2 months old and first-line treatment due to its high efficacy and low toxicity. In infants, it is important to apply the medication to the entire body including the face, scalp, and neck because there is a high rate of recurrence in infants. Crotamiton 10% is FDA approved for use in adults but not children. Ivermectin is not FDA approved for treatment of scabies and is considered off-label for children weighing < 15 kg. Because the patient is nontoxic appearing and has clinical features consistent with classic scabies, treatment can be started prior to dermatology referral.

(Section 18: Disorders of the Skin, Chapter 363: Infestations)

**Answer 23-67.** E

Dermatitis herpetiformis is a rare blistering disease with direct immunofluorescence of perilesional skin showing granular deposition of IgA within the dermal papillae. In 85% to 90% of patients with this finding, gluten-sensitivity enteropathy can be seen on intestinal biopsy/evaluation, although overt gastrointestinal symptoms are often absent. Treatment focuses on maintaining a gluten-free diet and, sometimes, dapsone. Although used for other skin eruptions, tacrolimus, acyclovir, UV light therapy, and prednisone are not used in the treatment of dermatitis herpetiformis.

(Section 18: Disorders of the Skin, Chapter 357: Immunologic Diseases)

**Answer 23-68.** D

Erythema nodosum is presumed to be caused by a hypersensitivity response, with β-hemolytic streptococcal infection being the most widely recognized etiology in the pediatric population. However, numerous etiologies have been associated including multiple infections, systemic inflammatory disorders (such as irritable bowel disease and sarcoidosis), malignancies, and medications. It is characterized by tender, red, warm plaques or nodules without overlying scale, and the most common site is the extensor surface of the lower legs. Incidence of erythema nodosum peaks in adolescence and is uncommon before the age of 2. Unlike other forms of panniculitis, the lesions of erythema nodosum do not ulcerate.

(Section 18: Disorders of the Skin, Chapter 354: Disorders of the Dermis and Subcutaneous Tissue)

**Answer 23-69.** C

This clinical vignette describes café-au-lait spots, axillary freckling, and concern for a dermal neurofibroma, which are features of neurofibromatosis type 1 (NF1). The most common causative genetic change for NF1 is deletion in the gene encoding neurofibromin, a large tumor-suppressor protein. NF1 is autosomal dominant and, in addition to the features described, is also associated with neurofibromatosis in a first-degree relative and optic gliomas or Lisch nodules. Additionally, one-third of affected patients experience speech and learning disabilities. Mutations in *BLM*, a DNA helicase, are seen in Bloom syndrome. Mutations in the genes encoding hamartin or tuberin are seen in tuberous sclerosis. Mutations in *STK11/LKB1* are seen in Peutz-Jeghers syndrome. Mutations in the *APC* gene are associated with Gardner syndrome.

(Section 18: Disorders of the Skin, Chapter 355: Genetic Disorder of the Skin)

# CHAPTER 24 | Psychosocial Issues

Rachael Keefe, Brent Mothner, and Michelle A. Lopez

**24-1.** More than 70% of children in foster care have been exposed to which of the following?

- **A.** Tuberculosis
- **B.** Venereal disease
- **C.** Child abuse or neglect
- **D.** Drug use
- **E.** Alcohol abuse

**24-2.** Foster children often have experienced significant psychological trauma, which may manifest as a variety of physical, emotional, and behavioral symptoms. Which of the following is an evidence-based trauma therapy that is recommended to treat these symptoms?

- **A.** Trauma-focused cognitive-behavioral therapy
- **B.** Participation in afterschool programs
- **C.** Inclusion in appropriate and varied peer groups
- **D.** Play therapy
- **E.** Frequent exposure to biological family

**24-3.** Children in foster care are prescribed which of the following at a rate 3 times that of other children enrolled in Medicaid?

- **A.** Antibiotics
- **B.** Antipyretics
- **C.** Allergy medications
- **D.** Antacids
- **E.** Psychotropic medications

**24-4.** In foster children, once psychotropic medications are initiated, a clinician should do which of the following?

- **A.** Consider starting other psychotropic medications from a similar class to achieve maximum therapeutic benefit
- **B.** Initiate the medication at a low dose and titrate slowly with close monitoring
- **C.** Involve as many prescribing providers as possible to provide a broad range of expertise
- **D.** Follow up only as needed
- **E.** Discuss only the most common medication side effects so as to avoid unnecessary anxiety in the child and caretakers

**24-5.** A child in foster care may experience fragmented health care due to experiencing multiple foster placements. Which of the following is a recommended strategy to ameliorate this problem?

- **A.** Enroll the child in or provide the child a “medical home” in the primary care provider’s office
- **B.** Advocate that a foster child not be transitioned to another placement at any cost
- **C.** Require that a case worker have all health records available before scheduling a medical appointment
- **D.** Only see those foster children who have an activated and updated “health passport”
- **E.** Provide other sources of continuity such as participation in a team sport or involvement in an afterschool program

**24-6.** The American Academy of Pediatrics (AAP) recommends an initial health screening for children in foster care at what point?

- **A.** Before their next birthday
- **B.** Within 72 hours of placement
- **C.** When they are due for their next well-child appointment
- **D.** Only if they have previous health problems
- **E.** Once all previous health records are made available

**24-7.** After an initial health screening, for whom should a follow-up health assessment be completed within 60 to 90 days of placement?

**A.** Foster children with chronic health conditions

**B.** Foster children with a new placement

**C.** Foster children with exposure to drug/alcohol abuse

**D.** Foster children with a history of child abuse or neglect

**E.** All children and adolescents in foster care

**24-8.** A foster parent of a 4-year-old child reports to your office due to some newly developing behavioral concerns. This child has been with this foster family for 2 weeks. The foster mother tearfully explains to you that her foster son has been acting out aggressively at home and at school over the past week by hitting, kicking, and biting teachers and other children. She is afraid that he might be dismissed from his daycare facility due to his behavior. What measures can you take to reassure this foster mother and direct her to a next course of action?

**A.** Advocate that the child find an alternate placement

**B.** Look into respite care options

**C.** Have the child spend more time with his biological family

**D.** Reframe the child's behavior in the context of trauma and toxic stress and focus on positive parenting principles

**E.** Consider having the patient admitted to a pediatric psychiatric facility

**24-9.** As the number of adverse childhood experiences (ACEs) increases in a child's life, as an adult, he or she is at increased risk for which of the following?

**A.** Alcohol abuse

**B.** Smoking

**C.** Obesity

**D.** Suicide attempts

**E.** All of the above

**24-10.** Children in foster care are more likely than peers to have which of the following?

**A.** Mental health concerns

**B.** Chronic illness

**C.** Developmental challenges

**D.** Dental disease

**E.** All of the above

**24-11.** A foster family contacts you for the initial intake evaluation of their 10-month-old foster daughter within the recommended 72-hour time frame. One of the many purposes of the initial screen is to identify which of the following?

**A.** Signs of child maltreatment

**B.** Appropriate bonding with the foster family

**C.** A stable chronic disease that currently requires no further treatment

**D.** Appropriate sleep habits

**E.** Gaps in foster family parenting knowledge

**24-12.** A 4-year-old foster child comes to your clinic for a comprehensive medical evaluation after entering foster care 60 days prior, in accordance to the American Academy of Pediatrics (AAP) guidelines. You have tried to no avail to locate his immunization records from the biological family, case worker, and state immunization program. What is your next best course of action?

**A.** No further action can be taken.

**B.** Assume he has had all immunizations up to this point.

**C.** Give current and prior immunizations according to the catch-up schedule from the Centers for Disease Control and Prevention (CDC).

**D.** Obtain a court order to mandate that all previous health records be released to you.

**E.** Write a letter to the biological parents asking for his health records.

**24-13.** A 15-year-old girl comes to your clinic for a comprehensive health evaluation 30 days after initially being placed in foster care. You discuss routine anticipatory guidance for an adolescent and complete a HEEADSSS (home, education/employment, eating, activities, drugs, sexuality, suicide/depression, and safety) exam, which reveals no acute concerns. She is reluctant to share personal details of her past medical or social history. What screening measures specific to adolescents should be considered at this time?

**A.** Lead

**B.** Complete blood count

**C.** Body mass index

**D.** Urinalysis

**E.** Gonorrhea, chlamydia, and pregnancy

**24-14.** Independent living skills, educational or career plans, and future support systems should be discussed for the foster child who:

**A.** Will be aging out of the foster system

**B.** Will be returning to their biological family

**C.** Will be transitioning to an alternate placement

**D.** Struggles with developmental delay

**E.** Has been diagnosed with depression

**24-15.** A child who is demonstrating frequent nightmares, enuresis, and food hoarding should be screened for which of the following?

**A.** Psychological or emotional trauma

**B.** Gastrointestinal illness

**C.** Urinary tract infection

**D.** Autism

**E.** Heavy metal poisoning

**24-16.** A foster mother returns to your office with her 5-year-old foster son due to some behavioral concerns. She tearfully recounts to you a scenario in which her foster son was attempting to climb the shelves in the supermarket. When the foster mother gently redirected the child and pulled him off the shelves, he began screaming loudly, threw his body on the floor, and bit the foster mother on the arm. What strategies would be best to give this foster mother?

**A.** Spank her foster son

**B.** Leave the store immediately without buying groceries

**C.** Allow him to climb the shelves so as to avoid making a scene

**D.** Bite him back to demonstrate the discomfort he caused her

**E.** Avoid yelling, give the child words to label his emotions, and demonstrate some breathing techniques to help the child self-regulate his emotions

**24-17.** A 6-year-old boy presents to clinic for a well-child check. During the visit, his parents are frequently arguing and visibly angry. You complete a family functioning screen including asking the parents, "Are there ongoing tensions or arguments within your marriage or family?" The parents reveal that they are in the process of a divorce. Which of the following statements about divorce is incorrect?

**A.** Divorce impacts a child's psychosocial development and how they view relationships.

**B.** Divorce impacts parental functioning, and parents are often less spontaneously available in the home.

**C.** Divorce impacts family finances, and fathers often suffer the more serious financial harm.

**D.** Children may feel decreased self-esteem due to insecurities related to the divorce.

**E.** Divorce rate is highest during child-bearing years.

**24-18.** A 6-month-old infant is seen in clinic for a well-child check, and the parents disclose that they married during pregnancy for the sake of the child. They are fighting all of the time and unhappy. They entered counseling, and they are seriously considering divorce at this point. They would like to know how divorce affects children at different ages. Which of the following developmental reactions to divorce is correct?

**A.** Infants are the most immune to divorce and do not show a response to family conflict.

**B.** Toddlers are influenced by the emotional state of their caregivers and react most overtly when their parents are distressed.

**C.** Children 4 to 5 years of age react less directly and may express psychosomatic complaints.

**D.** Younger school-aged children may develop oppositional behavior and unite parents' attention on their behavior.

**E.** Adolescents have a rich imagination for fantasy and frequently imagine their parents reuniting.

**24-19.** A child with terminal illness is currently admitted to the hospital. The parents ask for help talking with the child about the child's own death. Which of the following is an incorrect approach to talking with children based on their age?

**A.** Under age 2 years, no discussion of death will be understood, and it is best to focus on symptom relief, holding, and hugging the child.

**B.** For children aged 2 to 7 years, death is viewed as temporary or reversible, and it is often necessary to correct misperceptions.

**C.** Around the age of 7 years, children may begin to grasp aspects of death and often ask repetitive questions to understand the details of death.

**D.** For children around age 11 years, there is a strong desire to understand the afterlife, and caregivers/providers need to address this in discussing death.

**E.** Adolescents focus on changes in physical appearance, hair loss, and weakness, and these concerns should be acknowledged and validated.

**24-20.** A 5-year-old boy and his mother present to his primary medical home. The child has experienced speech and motor delays and is currently undergoing physical, occupational, and speech therapies. Results of his intelligence quotient (IQ) test are consistent with intellectual disability. He will be starting kindergarten in a few months. Evidence demonstrates that which of the following factors is the most predictive of limitations in academic advancement for children with intellectual disability?

**A.** Lack of siblings

**B.** Presence of co-occurring mental health condition

**C.** Divorced parental status

**D.** Parents with limited English proficiency

**E.** Coming from black or Hispanic racial/ethnic background

**24-21.** A 13-year-old girl who suffered a hypoxic-ischemic event at birth presents to a complex care clinic for follow-up. She has intractable seizure disorder, gastrostomy tube dependence, a ventriculoperitoneal shunt, and behavioral problems and is followed by multiple subspecialists. You have known the patient and her family for many years and notice an increased level of stress and anxiety in the patient's mother at her visit today. Which of the following statements is correct?

**A.** Disruptive behaviors in children with intellectual disability emerge as early as adolescence.

**B.** Siblings of children with disabilities may exhibit worse physical health than their peers.

**C.** The complex care physician should refer the patient's mother to her own primary care provider to screen for caregiver burnout and provide referrals for respite care if needed.

**D.** Children with intellectual disabilities often suffer from sleep disturbances, and poor sleep may lead to behavior problems.

**E.** Parents of children with disabilities are often in better emotional health than parents of children without disabilities.

**24-22.** A 12-year-old child presents to clinic for a back-to-school physical. During the interview, his mother, who is a single parent, reveals that she was laid off from work. You have been taking care of the patient since he was born and know this family has struggled with poverty cyclically throughout his life. Which of the following is true about poverty?

**A.** The American Academy of Pediatrics (AAP) has a policy statement on screening for poverty-related issues.

**B.** The federal poverty level (FPL)/poverty guidelines are adjusted for the size of the household and regional variations in cost of living.

**C.** Families living in rural poverty have increased exposure to lead and household allergens.

**D.** Support service agencies alleviate the majority of stress for families in poverty.

**E.** Fifty percent of all children live in "poor" households.

**24-23.** Which of the following statements about teen dating violence (TDV) is incorrect?

**A.** TDV includes physical, sexual, and psychological abuse.

**B.** Adolescents with a history of TDV exhibit higher rates of depression, anxiety, and substance abuse compared to their peers.

**C.** Teens with a history of exposure to family or community violence are at increased risk of TDV.

**D.** Females are as likely as males to perpetrate TDV.

**E.** Adolescents with TDV will often present for medical care with bruises or broken bones.

**24-24.** A 4-year-old girl presents to clinic with her grandmother. Her history is significant for exposure to violence in her neighborhood, father being incarcerated, and clinical depression in her mother. You consider the adverse childhood experiences (ACEs) this child has faced. Which of the following is incorrect about ACEs?

**A.** ACEs are linked to poor school performance.

**B.** ACEs include abuse, neglect, and household dysfunction.

**C.** The original study on ACEs found a high prevalence of ACEs in its participants.

**D.** The original study on ACEs found a dose-response relationship between childhood adversity and adult medical outcomes.

**E.** Recent studies demonstrate that 10 years in a stable home ameliorate the effects of ACEs.

**24-25.** Death rates due to homicide in the pediatric population (birth to age 21 years) have followed what trend over the past 15 years?

**A.** Up for white race, up for black race, and up overall for all races

**B.** Up for white race, down for black race, and up overall for all races

**C.** Up for white race, down for black race, and down overall for all races

**D.** Down for white race, up for black race, and down overall for all races

**E.** Down for white race, down for black race, and down overall for all races

**24-26.** A 14-year-old boy presents to the clinic with right hand pain. Social history is significant for the child being a victim of physical abuse, currently being in foster care, and having a history of multiple altercations. The child protective services case worker reveals that the current injury happened when the patient punched a smaller boy. He has been in trouble at school multiple times for bullying. Evidence demonstrates that students who bully others are most at risk for which of the following consequences in adulthood?

**A.** Bipolar disorder

**B.** Drug abuse

**C.** Committing suicide

**D.** Incarceration

**E.** Obesity

**24-27.** A 16-year-old Hispanic girl presents to urgent care with a laceration on her arm. She is accompanied by a police officer and is currently housed in a juvenile detention facility. Which of the following is the most often true of patients in the juvenile justice system?

**A.** They have often been the victim of a traumatic incident such as child abuse.

**B.** They meet criteria for a mood disorder such as depression.

**C.** They meet criteria for posttraumatic stress disorder (PTSD).

**D.** They have problems with substance abuse such as alcohol abuse.

**E.** They often have a learning disability such as dyslexia.

**24-28.** A 3-year-old boy presents to clinic for a sick visit. His mother's primary language is Vietnamese, and she has a poor understanding of English. His aunt accompanied them today and speaks fluent English. Which of the following statements about language barriers is most correct?

**A.** When using an interpreter, the provider should have a brief conversation with the interpreter before starting the encounter.

**B.** With parental permission obtained using an interpreter, the aunt should serve as the interpreter for the encounter.

**C.** When using an in-person interpreter, it is best to position the interpreter slightly behind the provider in order for the parent to maintain eye contact with the provider.

**D.** If the mother requests an interpreter, failure to provide interpreter services is considered fraud.

**E.** If the mother and interpreter need to sign a consent form, the aunt is a better translator option than a phone interpreter.

**24-29.** A 10-year-old girl with Crohn's disease presents to her pediatrician for a routine examine. During the visit, the family discusses her ongoing management plan as directed by gastroenterology, including anti–tumor necrosis factor injections. The family is unhappy about the potential side effects and are planning to stop therapy in favor of changing her diet and starting acupuncture and an herbal supplement. Which of the following strategies is an effective way to discuss integrative therapeutic options with patients and their caregivers?

**A.** Wait for families to bring up complementary or integrative medicine options.

**B.** Use terminology such as *unproven* or *alternative*.

**C.** Do not ask whether change in therapy is consistent with religious, spiritual, or cultural beliefs.

**D.** Avoid asking specific questions about diet therapies, herbal therapies, or involvement of other healthcare providers.

**E.** Do not offer your opinion about the therapies they tried until after you ask whether they think the therapies worked.

**24-30.** Which of the following factors has the strongest association with a child's use of complementary alternative medicine (CAM)?

**A.** Failure of mainstream medicine treatment

**B.** Having dermatologic conditions

**C.** Parent's use of CAM

**D.** Living in the western region of the United States

**E.** Being uninsured

**24-31.** A 3-year-old girl presents to the emergency department (ED) with frequent vomiting, diarrhea, and dehydration. She will require admission for intravenous (IV) antiemetics and IV fluids due to her inability to tolerate oral medication or fluids. She is accompanied by her parents who are worried about the admission because the child does not have insurance. The child and her parents are also undocumented immigrants. Which of the following statements is incorrect about caring for undocumented immigrant families?

**A.** The ED often serves as a point of care for the children of undocumented immigrants.

**B.** The Emergency Medicaid program may provide coverage for uninsured documented and undocumented children with an emergency medical condition.

**C.** The children of undocumented immigrants often lack access to outpatient medical care.

**D.** Fear of the US Immigration and Customs Enforcement agency potentially limits undocumented immigrants' ability to seek care.

**E.** Medical providers are bound by law to provide medical information to the US Immigration and Customs Enforcement agency if requested.

## ANSWERS

**Answer 24-1.** C

The majority of children entering foster care have lived in deprived and chaotic environments for a significant period of time until removal for imminent safety concerns secondary to maltreatment. More than 70% of children in foster care have a documented history of child abuse or neglect, and > 80% have been exposed to significant levels of violence, including domestic violence.

These factors should be kept in mind to deliver the most effective and trauma-informed care to patients in foster care.

While foster children may have been exposed to the other answer choices mentioned, the rates of exposure are not known at this time, and child abuse and neglect remains a significant factor and has a major psychological and health impact in the lives of foster children.

(Chapter 38: Foster Care and Adoption)

**Reference**

US Department of Health and Human Services, Administration for Children and Families, Administration on Children, Youth and Families, Children's Bureau. The AFCARS Report. Preliminary FY 2010 estimates as of June 2011. Available at: www.acf.hhs.gov/programs/cb/resource/afcars-report-18. Accessed October 22, 2014.

**Answer 24-2.** A

Parent-child interaction therapy, child-parent psychotherapy, trauma-focused cognitive-behavioral therapy, and the attachment, self-regulation, and competency model are some recommended evidence-based trauma therapies for children in foster care. There still remains a shortage of mental health professionals with appropriate training or availability to work with foster children.

Although beneficial, the other answer choices are not evidence-based strategies that help ameliorate trauma-associated symptoms.

(Chapter 38: Foster Care and Adoption)

**Answer 24-3.** E

Children in foster care are prescribed psychotropic medications at a rate 3 times that of other children enrolled in Medicaid and have higher rates of polypharmacy. Psychotropic medications, if indicated, should be initiated at a low dose and titrated slowly, with close monitoring for efficacy and adverse effects. Polypharmacy should be avoided if possible. No patient should receive therapy with > 1 psychotropic medication from any given class.

It is important for primary care providers to be aware of the risks of polypharmacy and the frequent use of psychotropic medications in the foster care system.

(Chapter 38: Foster Care and Adoption)

**Reference**

Texas Department of Family and Protective Services and The University of Texas at Austin College of Pharmacy. Psychotropic medication utilization parameters for children and youth in foster care. Available at: https://www.dfps.state.tx.us/Child_Protection/Medical_Services/documents/reports/2016-03_Psychotropic_Medication_Utilization_Parameters_for_Foster_Children.pdf. Accessed November 6, 2020.

Zito JM, Safer DJ, Sai D, et al. Psychotropic medication patterns among youth in foster care. *Pediatrics*. 2008;121(1):e157-e163.

**Answer 24-4.** B

Psychotropic medications, if indicated, should be initiated at a low dose and titrated slowly, with close monitoring for efficacy and adverse effects. Polypharmacy should be avoided if possible. No patient should receive therapy with > 1 psychotropic medication from any given class.

It is important for primary care providers to be aware of the risks of polypharmacy and the frequent use of psychotropic medications in the foster care system.

(Chapter 38: Foster Care and Adoption)

**Answer 24-5.** A

Children entering foster care have often had limited access to preventive and other health services before placement or have sought care from multiple health resources and may continue to receive fragmented care because of transitions in foster care placements. Thus, enrollment in a medical home is imperative to ensure the receipt of high-quality, comprehensive, coordinated health care that is continuous over time, compassionate, culturally competent, family centered, and child focused. The medical home should provide uninterrupted care, regardless of the placement transitions a child may experience.

Answer choice B is not the correct answer because it is at times best and necessary to transition a child out of a previously placed foster home due to safety or emotional concerns. Answer choice C is not correct because often records will not be available at the time of the health evaluation, yet a full evaluation should ensue and not be delayed. Answer choice D is also not correct because many foster children will not have a health passport yet will still require a health evaluation. While giving the foster child as many sources of stability as possible, participating in a sports team will not help ameliorate the fragmentation of care the child has received.

(Chapter 38: Foster Care and Adoption)

**Reference**

American Academy of Pediatrics, The National Center for Medical Home Implementation. What is a family-centered medical home? Available at: www.medicalhomeinfo.org/. Accessed October 22, 2014.

Johnson C, Silver P, Wulczyn F. Raising the bar for health and mental health service for children in foster care: developing a model of managed care. Council of Family and Child Caring Agencies and the New York State Health Foundation. Available at: www.cofcca.org/pdfs/FosterCareManagedCare-FinalReport.pdf. Accessed March 15, 2015.

**Answer 24-6.** B

The AAP recommends an initial health screening within 72 hours of placement. However, younger or preverbal children, any child who is a suspected victim of abuse, or any child with a chronic medical or developmental condition should be seen within 24 hours. Ideally, children should have at least 3 health encounters over the first 3 months of foster care, as they adjust to their new circumstances. It is recommended that children in foster care be seen monthly during the first 6 months of life, every 3 months from 6 to 24 months of age, and then at a minimum of every 6 months to monitor their health, emotional well-being, development, psychosocial stressors, continued adjustment to their foster family, and visitation with birth parents or other relatives. Transitions in placement, changes in visitation, and separation of siblings represent events that indicate a need for even closer monitoring.

(Chapter 38: Foster Care and Adoption)

**Answer 24-7.** E

All children and adolescents should have a follow-up health assessment within 60 to 90 days of placement to help identify acute and chronic health conditions, assess for ongoing stressors, assess "goodness of fit" in the new home, update immunizations, provide health education, and review findings from developmental and mental health evaluations, as well as update and reinforce the treatment plan.

(Chapter 38: Foster Care and Adoption)

**Answer 24-8.** D

Reframing child behavior issues in the context of childhood trauma and toxic stress and focusing on positive parenting principles and the child's strengths and talents can help to defuse caregiver distress and promote resilience.

Finding an alternate placement or reintroducing the child back into the care of the biological family may introduce further volatility, trauma, and a lack of stability and could exacerbate some behavioral or emotional issues in the child.

(Chapter 38: Foster Care and Adoption)

**Answer 24-9.** E

Toxic stress and the presence of multiple ACEs in the absence of support or decreased resiliency place children at increased risk of a multitude of chronic illnesses than can result in early death. An understanding of the effects of toxic stress in childhood is an important public health concept, especially when treating foster children who often come with multiple adverse childhood experiences.

(Chapter 38: Foster Care and Adoption)

**Answer 24-10.** E

Exposures such as insufficient prenatal care, prematurity, or in utero toxins as well as chronic abuse/neglect have direct and indirect effects on the health and well-being of this population. The interplay of chronic or prolonged stress, physiologic response to that toxic stress, and behavioral adaptations to this stress impacts the health of children over the life course. These factors likely contribute to foster children being more likely than their peers to have the disease processes mentioned in the question stem.

(Chapter 38: Foster Care and Adoption)

**Reference**

Leslie LK, Gordon JN, Lambros K, Premji K, Peoples J, Gist K. Addressing the developmental and mental health needs of young children in foster care. *J Dev Behav Pediatr.* 2005;26(2):140-151.

**Answer 24-11.** A

The purpose of the initial screen is to identify health needs that require urgent medical attention such as chronic diseases requiring therapy, acute infections requiring treatment, signs of child maltreatment, immediate nutritional problems, acute mental health needs, or pregnancy.

(Chapter 38: Foster Care and Adoption)

**Reference**

American Academy of Pediatrics. Healthcare of young children in foster care. *Pediatrics.* 2002;109(3):536-541.

Jaudes KP, Champagne V, Harden A, Masterson J, Bilaver LA. Expanded medical home model works for children in foster care. *Child Welfare.* 2012;91(1):9-33.

**Answer 24-12.** C

If records are unavailable by 60 days after entry, immunizations should be commenced using the catch-up schedule from the CDC. It would not be best to deny vaccines due to a delay in obtaining records, as the records may never come. A court order is unnecessary, and the biological parents may not have records.

(Chapter 38: Foster Care and Adoption)

**Reference**

Centers for Disease Control and Prevention. Catch-up immunization schedule for persons aged 4 months through 18 years who start late or who are more than 1 month behind. Available at: https://www.cdc.gov/vaccines/schedules/hcp/imz/catchup.html. Accessed November 6, 2020.

**Answer 24-13.** E

For adolescents in foster care, there are rarely opportunities to discuss the issues of safety, sexuality, and teen risks. A particular focus by the pediatrician on family planning and sexual safety has the potential to make significant impact for an adolescent in foster care. Specifically, teens may need guidance with sexuality/sexual safety, birth control, questions regarding sexual orientation, and partner violence.

Due to their unique risk, adolescents should be screened for all sexually transmitted infections, including chlamydia/gonorrhea, hepatitis C, syphilis, and human immunodeficiency virus (HIV), when coming into foster care. Females should also be screened for pregnancy.

(Chapter 38: Foster Care and Adoption)

**Answer 24-14.** A

Teens aging out of foster care will face their own unique challenges in leaving a previously supportive system to enter a new world where they will be primarily responsible for their finances, educational goals, and workforce potential. They may be facing these challenges alone or with less support from their biological families than their peers. Such subjects such as living skills, education, and support systems should be discussed and monitored before the child exits foster care.

(Chapter 38: Foster Care and Adoption)

**Answer 24-15.** A

Children may show many signs of previous trauma such as difficulty initiating or maintaining sleep, experiencing nightmares, rapid eating, lack of satiety, food hoarding, loss of appetite, toileting issues such as constipation, encopresis, enuresis, and regression of toileting skills. These symptoms could signify significant trauma exposure, and further inquiry should ensue.

(Chapter 38: Foster Care and Adoption)

**Reference**

Forkey H, Szilagvi M. Foster care and healing from complex childhood trauma. *Pediatr Clin North Am.* 2014;61(5): 1059-1072.

**Answer 24-16.** E

Traumatized children need to be redirected, or behavior may start to escalate. Children do not always know how to say what they are feeling. It can be hard for them to find words. Often, they are not told that how they feel is okay. Traumatized children do not have the skills for self-regulation or for calming down once upset. Responding with aggression will trigger the child's brain back into threat mode; therefore, yelling and aggression should be avoided by the caretaker. Give the child words to label his or her emotions, and help develop breathing techniques, relaxation skills, or exercises that the child can do when getting upset. Traumatized children have had to constantly be watchful and hypervigilant for danger. This response has served them well and helped them stay alive in tumultuous environments, but the parts of the brain used for self-regulation and calming have not grown with the child. Caretakers must be able to reframe a traumatized child's behavioral difficulties to understand why they act the way they do in certain situations.

(Chapter 38: Foster Care and Adoption)

**Reference**

American Academy of Pediatrics. Helping foster and adoptive families cope with trauma. Available at: http://www.aap.org/traumaguide. Accessed November 6, 2020.

**Answer 24-17.** C

The impact of divorce can be divided into 3 broad categories including psychological development, parental functioning, and financial strain. The financial effects occur with the spread of family resources over 2 households, legal fees, and so on, and the effects are often more serious for the mother.

Divorce rates are highest during the child-bearing years and common during the first 5 to 10 years of marriage. The long-term effects of divorce, such as child self-esteem issues, can be ameliorated if parents focus on their love for their children during and after the divorce process.

(Chapter 31: Family Discord and Divorce)

**Answer 24-18.** B

Infants and toddlers are heavily influenced by the emotional state of their caregivers and suffer the most overtly when their custodial parent is overwhelmed, clinically depressed, or preoccupied. Additionally, toddlers are less tolerant of long absences and require more frequent visitations. Children 4 to 5 years of age have cognitive limitations that make it difficult to understand the implications of divorce. They also have a rich fantasy life and take responsibility for what happened, causing feelings of guilt. School-aged children have a better understanding of divorce in concrete terms and have loyalty conflicts. They wonder if they could have prevented the divorce by being "better" and frequently wish their parents would reunite. Older school-aged children react less directly with psychosomatic complaints and oppositional behavior to gain their parents' attention. Adolescents are at a vulnerable stage as they are developing their own sense of autonomy and capacity for intimacy. Adolescents may respond to divorce by engaging in young adult behaviors such as substance abuse or early sexual activity. School performance may also decline.

(Chapter 31: Family Discord and Divorce)

**Answer 24-19.** D

For children under the age of 2 years, there is likely no intellectual concept of death, and no discussion is needed. It is more helpful to focus on symptoms, comfort, holding, and hugging. Children aged 2 to 7 years have a self-centered orientation of the world. They initially feel that they can prevent animals and people from dying due to a magical spell that they can cast, and it is often necessary to attempt to correct misperceptions. Parents should also monitor for feelings of fear of separation and abandonment for children aged 2 to 7 years. Around the age of 7 years, children have a better understanding of death as universal and inevitable, and they will try to understand the details of the dying experience. They often ask repetitive questions. Children aged 7 to 11 years have more concrete thinking, and reasoning is based on direct observation. They are often less concerned about the afterlife and other abstract concepts. Adolescents often focus on their appearance and physical changes, and these feelings should be validated.

(Chapter 126: Palliative Care for Children with Chronic Diseases)

**Answer 24-20.** B

Approximately 10% to 60% of children with intellectual disabilities have a co-occurring mental health condition, which is higher than the general population.

Evidence supports the importance of diagnosing and managing behavioral health conditions in children with intellectual disability. Comorbid mental health conditions in children with intellectual disabilities can be more predictive of academic advancement than the severity of intellectual disabilities. It is crucial for providers to screen for and address mental/behavioral comorbidities early in the child's life course. While family support inclusive of parents and siblings is critical in the care of children with intellectual and developmental disabilities, there is limited evidence on the specific impact of this on academic advancement. In addition to family support, appropriate educational services and community inclusion can improve the quality of life for children with disabilities. Race/ethnicity and language proficiency are important factors implicated in numerous health disparities, but there is limited evidence on the degree of the effects of these specific factors on school performance for children with intellectual disabilities.

(Chapter 122: Managing Children with Intellectual and Developmental Disabilities)

**Answer 24-21.** D

Up to 85% of children with intellectual disabilities may have poor sleep, leading to excessive daytime sleepiness, hyperactivity, and aggressive behavior and a decline in overall functioning. Disruptive behaviors in children with disabilities may emerge at the age of 2.5 to 3 years old, which add to family stress at an early child age. The behavior issues in the child in this vignette are likely longstanding. The siblings of children with disabilities often experience worse mental health but not worse physical health than their peers. Siblings contribute to care and often experience frustration surrounding perceived competition for parental attention. Siblings may exhibit negative psychological effects such as anxiety and depression requiring therapy. Evidence demonstrates worse physical and mental health in the parents of children with disabilities, and it is important for the child's medical provider to screen for burnout and depression and make appropriate referrals for respite care, attendant services, parent support groups, and so on. This is not solely the responsibility of the parent's primary care provider.

(Chapter 122: Managing Children with Intellectual and Developmental Disability)

**Reference**

Murphy NA, Carbone PS; American Academy of Pediatrics Council on Children with Disabilities. Parent-provider-community partnerships: optimizing outcomes for children with disabilities. *Pediatrics*. 2011;128(4):795-802.

**Answer 24-22.** A

The AAP has a policy statement on poverty including recommendations for how pediatricians can support the health and well-being of children living in poverty. The FPL/poverty guidelines are adjusted for household size but do not account for regional variations in cost of living. The one caveat is that different poverty guidelines exist for Hawaii and Alaska. The FPL/poverty guidelines are used to determine eligibility for Head Start, Supplemental Nutrition Assistance Program (SNAP), and the National School Lunch Program. Children living in rural poverty have increased difficulty accessing services. Children in urban poverty have increased exposure to violence, household allergens, air pollution, and lead. While generally helpful, support services can also increase stress for families due to the application and bureaucratic process. In 2014, it was estimated that 21% of children lived in poor households (< 100% FPL). Poverty is disproportionately seen in black, Hispanic, and American Indian children.

(Chapter 30: Poverty, Homelessness, and Social Disorganization)

**Answer 24-23.** E

TDV includes physical, sexual, and psychological abuse, and new forms of cyber or electronic abuse contribute to psychological abuse. Universal screening by pediatricians is recommended, but specific patients should always be screened for TDV. These include those who have been exposed to relationship, family, or community violence or adverse childhood experiences (ACEs); those who associate with delinquent or violent peers; those with risky sexual or substance abuse behaviors; pregnant teens; patients with symptoms of depression or anxiety; those who display attitudes dismissive or accepting of violence; and adolescents with irregular medical care histories. Adolescents who have experienced TDV often come to medical attention for depression, stress, anxiety, or psychosomatic symptoms rather than bruises or broken bones. Data show females are at least as likely as males to perpetrate TDV.

(Chapter 33: Teen Dating Violence)

**Answer 24-24.** E

As demonstrated in Chapter 28, ACEs include abuse, neglect, and household dysfunction (substance abuse, mental illness, violence against mother, parental separation/divorce, incarcerated household member, and criminal behavior). ACEs are associated with poor school performance. The landmark Adverse Childhood Experiences Study was done in the late 1990s and demonstrated a high prevalence of ACEs and a dose-response relationship between ACEs and adult medical and psychosocial outcomes. The mechanism by which ACEs expose children to long-lasting negative outcomes appears to be related to toxic stress. While strong social and emotional support can buffer tolerable stress, research currently suggests that toxic stress leads to permanent epigenic alterations. Children who have experienced ACEs should receive treatment focused on therapy.

(Chapter 28: Childhood Adversity and Toxic Stress)

**Answer 24-25.** E

Death rates due to homicide in the pediatric population have been declining since 1999. Overall homicide rates in this age group have fallen > 27% in all races, and declines in homicides were also seen in white and black races. There was a period in the mid-2000s when black homicide rates increased, but these have since declined and are lower than they were in 1999. It is worth noting that homicide remains the third leading cause of death in 15 to 24 year olds, behind unintentional injuries and suicide, and homicide rates remain highest among children of black race.

(Chapter 32: Family and Community Violence)

**Answer 24-26.** D

Bullies often come from disordered homes and have the greatest risk of long-term health consequences. They are unlikely to complete school and are at elevated risk of unemployment, incarceration, and living in poverty as adults. Although there may be concomitant substance abuse and mental health issues, data demonstrate that bullies are particularly at risk of incarceration.

Bullied youth are at greater risk of low self-esteem, disordered eating, anxiety, depression, somatic symptoms, and school absence.

(Chapter 32: Family and Community Violence)

**Answer 24-27.** A

Over 90% of youth in the juvenile justice system have been the victim of at least 1 traumatic incident such as child abuse. The prevalence of mental health disorders in this population is estimated to be two-thirds of males and three-quarters of females and includes mental health conditions other than mood disorders. Nearly half have substance abuse disorders, and approximately 11% of the population in juvenile detention meet criteria for PTSD. The estimated prevalence of learning disabilities ranges from 30% to 80%.

(Chapter 32: Family and Community Violence)

**Answer 24-28.** A

When using an interpreter, the physician should allow time for introductions between patient, physician, and interpreter, and the physician should have a conversation with the interpreter to explain the purpose of the visit before starting the encounter. It is never recommended to use a family member as the interpreter because there can be problems with accuracy and confidentiality. It is especially important that family members not serve as interpreters when a caregiver is consenting to a procedure. It is recommended that the provider maintain eye contact with the patient/caregiver and the interpreter for effective communication, and this can be accomplished by having the patient/caregiver, interpreter, and provider positioned as the points of an equilateral triangle. Whether or not the mother requests an interpreter, if she has limited English proficiency, failure to provide an interpreter can be considered discrimination, rather than fraud, based on national origin, which is prohibited by Title VI of the Civil Rights Act of 1964.

(Chapter 14: Health Disparities in Practice)

**Answer 24-29.** E

Providers should ask how well the family thinks therapies worked or did not work before offering their opinion. It is important to demonstrate an open-minded, nonjudgmental attitude when discussing complementary and integrative therapies. Families are often fearful that providers will disapprove of nonmainstream medical care and may not bring it up on their own. Pediatricians should ask patients and their caregivers about all the therapies they use to treat their illness or promote health even if the families do not initiate the conversation on their own. Providers should also ask about the specific herbal and dietary treatments and other healthcare professionals involved in the treatment. Although the term *alternative* is often used, it is recommended to avoid words such as *unproven* or *unconventional*, which may be perceived negatively and limit the patient/caregiver willingness to discuss therapies. Additionally, it is important to elicit the values, beliefs, and influences that led to the decision, including family members, beliefs, and fear of side effects of mainstream treatment. In this vignette, the family has stopped mainstream medical care for their daughter's Crohn's disease, which has negative implications for her health outcomes. It appears that they have fears related to the side effects of anti–tumor necrosis factor injections, and it is important for them to feel comfortable discussing concerns and having an open dialog with their pediatrician.

(Chapter 13: Complementary and Integrative Pediatrics)

**Answer 24-30.** C

Parent's use of CAM is the most predictive factor of a child's use of CAM. Additional factors with weaker associations are living in the western region of the United States and the patient having chronic conditions including cystic fibrosis, cancer, asthma, cerebral palsy, and dermatologic conditions. Parents and patients do not typically choose CAM due to a dissatisfaction with mainstream medicine; rather, it is more likely that CAM is consistent with their beliefs. Additionally, there is not a known specific association between uninsured or vulnerable populations using CAM. To the contrary, parents of children using CAM are more likely to have a college education.

(Chapter 13: Complementary and Integrative Pediatrics)

**Answer 24-31.** E

EDs often serve as a safety net for undocumented immigrants who may lack primary care providers. The Emergency Medicaid program, which was established in 1986, is an insurance option for eligible undocumented children with an emergency medical condition including conditions requiring hospitalization. There is a reported fear among undocumented immigrants in seeking medical care due to currently rare cases of immigrants being arrested or questioned by US Immigration and Customs Enforcement inside or near healthcare facilities and due to potential for healthcare providers to report undocumented immigrants. Medical providers are bound by the Health Insurance Portability and Accountability Act of 1996 when caring for undocumented immigrants and generally are not required to report protected health information unless there is a warrant. Immigration policies around reporting undocumented immigrants (without disclosure of protected health information) are evolving, and organizations such as the American College of Emergency Physicians currently oppose federal or state initiatives that would require reporting of undocumented immigrants.

(Chapter 152: Ethical Considerations, in *Strange and Schafermeyer's Pediatric Emergency Medicine*, 5th ed)

# CHAPTER 25 | Ethics

Julia T. Shelburne, Judy Kim, Andria Tatem,
Patrick M. Jones, and Lynda Chima Aririguzo

**25-1.** A 10-year-old boy received a diagnosis of osteosarcoma a year ago, and his treatment regimen is no longer effective. The oncology team discusses different treatment plans, including enrollment in phase I trials, and during the conversation, his parents ask the patient if he thinks the benefit of such a trial would outweigh the potential burdens. The patient communicates that he believes there would be benefit and he would like to enroll in the trial. Which concept is being demonstrated in this scenario?

- **A.** The patient is giving informed consent to participating in the trial.
- **B.** The patient is giving assent to participating in the trial.
- **C.** The medical team is providing assent to the patient's participation in the trial.
- **D.** The parents are serving in the role of guardian ad litem and allowing the patient to consent to the trial.
- **E.** The meeting has resulted in collective consent for the clinical trial.

**25-2.** A newborn is found to have sickle cell disease (HbSS) on routine screening. His father asks when, and to what detail, he should eventually tell his son about his medical condition as he gets older. How should you respond?

- **A.** When the child turns 4 years old, an appointment can be set to meet with a child life specialist to help him understand his condition.
- **B.** Discussions about his medical condition should start with the appearance of disease progression or his first hospitalization.
- **C.** Prior to him starting elementary school, conversations about his condition should be limited to him simply knowing that he is sick but there are effective treatments.
- **D.** Discussions vary from child to child based on intellectual development, and a child's own questions can serve as a guide.
- **E.** Initial reading lessons should include basic medical information so as to normalize future conversations about his medical condition.

**25-3.** A 17-year-old girl is scheduled for a new patient visit. The day before, her mother calls to let your office know that she is concerned her daughter might be sexually active and she would like for you to "perform an exam to determine if she is still a virgin." Which choice represents the best response?

- **A.** Explain that your medical practice has a confidentiality policy that guides how you handle sensitive information, including disclosure of sexual activity, and that the policy will be discussed at the first visit.
- **B.** Explain that an exam is unable to confirm or exclude sexual activity because hymeneal tears can be the result of nonsexual activities.
- **C.** Tell the mother that sexual activity disclosed by an adolescent is never disclosed to others because it would be a violation of state law.
- **D.** Take time to better understand why the mother is concerned about her daughter being sexually active and incorporate those concerns into the questions you ask the daughter the next day.
- **E.** Refer the patient to a gynecologist so the family can have this specific issue handled by an expert.

**25-4.** A 15-year-old boy goes to the school nurse because he is concerned that he might have contracted a sexually transmitted infection (STI). On her history and exam, the nurse does not find signs or symptoms of an STI, but she does refer him to your office for testing. In your office, he asks if the nurse will keep his sexual history confidential. Which of the following replies would be accurate?

**A.** The school nurse is held to the same confidentiality standards as your pediatric practice, so his disclosure will remain protected.

**B.** A school nurse would only disclose his sexual history if he was found to have signs and symptoms of an STI.

**C.** Reports made to a school, including the school nurse, may not be held to the same level of confidentiality as your pediatric practice.

**D.** His disclosure to the school nurse is protected by the Health Insurance Portability and Accountability Act (HIPAA).

**E.** The school nurse is required by law to disclose information regarding sexual activity to his parents or guardians.

**25-5.** Which of the following ethical principles refers to the moral obligation to act on the basis of fair adjudication between competing claims?

**A.** Justice

**B.** Veracity

**C.** Beneficence

**D.** Autonomy

**E.** Nonmaleficence

**25-6.** A 17-year-old girl with cystic fibrosis is admitted to the pediatric intensive care unit (PICU) after contracting influenza. After waking up intubated in the PICU, she communicates to her family that she had a near-death experience. Upon discharge from the hospital, she tells her parents that she feels a peace about death and she no longer wants to be admitted to the hospital. Which of the following statements is accurate?

**A.** An advance directive will ensure her decision regarding medical treatment is followed.

**B.** Although rare, some courts have upheld a minor's right to refuse life-sustaining treatments.

**C.** It is illegal to withhold life-sustaining treatment from a minor without a court order.

**D.** The parents may not withhold life-sustaining treatments on their daughter's behalf, but they are able to withdraw futile therapies.

**E.** A mental health evaluation is required for the patient prior to further discussion about treatment decisions.

**25-7.** Which term refers to a person's ability to come to a complete understanding of risks, benefits, and alternatives to a medical decision being offered?

**A.** Veracity

**B.** Judgment

**C.** Nonmaleficence

**D.** Capacity

**E.** Autonomy

**25-8.** A 7-year-old boy is being treated for asthma in the hospital, and his mother signed the consent to medical treatment upon admission. During the hospitalization, his mother falls very ill, and she is admitted to the intensive care unit (ICU) at a nearby hospital. While in the ICU, she requires sedation, and she no longer has the capacity to make medical decisions for her son. No other surrogate decision maker for the child was identified prior to her sudden illness. Which of the following statements accurately reflects the steps that should be taken to continue to provide medical treatment to the 7-year-old child?

**A.** Because the initial consent to medical treatment covers the entire hospitalization, the team should continue to treat as indicated.

**B.** Two attending physicians must agree on the plan of care and sign a new consent to medical treatment on behalf of the surrogate.

**C.** Local statutes should be followed to identify a new surrogate decision maker for the child.

**D.** If the child is able to demonstrate understanding for his medical condition, he should be allowed to consent to his own medical care.

**E.** A bedside nurse with the best knowledge of the patient should be identified as the patient's guardian ad litem.

**25-9.** After finding out that their 5-year-old son's osteosarcoma is no longer responding to treatment, the parents ask you what, if anything, they should tell their son. Which of the following is a proper response?

**A.** A child with a chronic illness often knows more than parents realize; including their son in conversations about hopes, fears, and wishes may help him feel less alone.

**B.** Prior to having a discussion with their son, a child psychologist should evaluate his capacity to understand the medical information discussed.

**C.** If the family reveals that treatments are no longer working, they run the risk of taking away hope and worsening his condition.

**D.** When the patient is a young child, it is best to have the medical information communicated to the child by a specialized pediatric-trained palliative care team.

**E.** The family should remain positive when talking to their son and provide reassurance that he will get better.

**25-10.** A 15-year-old boy is being seen in your busy office for his annual well-child examination. His mother, who has accompanied him today, expresses concern that his grades are falling and that he is becoming more reclusive. When interviewing him privately, he endorses depressed mood and hopelessness after his girlfriend broke up with him. He admits that he often asks himself, "What is the point of life?" He has also considered using his father's gun at home to "end it all." He is worried about what his mother might think and asks you not to disclose this information to her. What would be the most appropriate next step?

**A.** Inform the patient he needs to address his depressed mood and risk of suicide at a follow-up appointment, given the time constraints today.

**B.** Inform the mother about his depressed mood and risk of suicide, but do not inform the patient of this disclosure.

**C.** Inform the patient that adolescents commonly feel depressed after a major social change and offer him reassurance.

**D.** Inform the patient that you all need to discuss his depressed mood and risk of suicide with his mother today.

**E.** Inform the patient that he needs to contact his school counselor to obtain assistance with his depressed mood.

**25-11.** Which of the following patients would most likely have legal authority to make their own medical decisions?

**A.** A 17-year-old girl who attends college out of state

**B.** A 17-year-old boy who is in foster care

**C.** A 17-year-old girl who is cared for by her aging grandparents

**D.** A 17-year-old boy who is considering running away

**E.** A 17-year-old girl who is engaged to be married

**25-12.** A 16-year-old girl presents to the emergency department with her father for abdominal pain and dysuria. When her father is out of the room, she discloses that she is sexually active with her new boyfriend. She is worried about being pregnant because she does not use contraception. She does not want her father to know that she has a boyfriend and is sexually active. On exam, she is afebrile, in no acute distress. Her heart has a regular rate and rhythm. Abdominal exam is significant for mild suprapubic tenderness. Genitourinary exam is significant for white, milky vaginal discharge without tenderness of cervix or adnexa. Lab results reveal the following:

| Urinalysis | | | |
|---|---|---|---|
| **Specific gravity** | 1.010 | **White blood cells** | 5/HPF |
| **pH** | 6.0 | **Red blood cells** | 0/HPF |
| **Leukocyte esterase** | Negative | **Squamous epithelial cells** | Few |
| **Nitrite** | Negative | **Bacteria** | Negative |
| **Protein** | Negative | **Urine human chorionic gonadotropin** | Negative |
| **Glucose** | Negative | **Urine *Chlamydia trachomatis* polymerase chain reaction (PCR)** | **Positive** |
| **Ketones** | Trace | **Urine *Neisseria gonorrhoeae* PCR** | Negative |
| **Urobilinogen** | Normal | **HIV antibody** | Negative |
| **Bilirubin** | Negative | **Rapid plasma regain** | Nonreactive |
| **Blood** | Negative | | |

Which of the following is the most appropriate plan of care for her?

**A.** Provide her with healthy reproductive counseling and treatment with azithromycin once her father returns because she is a minor.

**B.** Provide her with healthy reproductive counseling privately, but explain that her father needs to consent for treatment with azithromycin.

**C.** Treat her with azithromycin and provide healthy reproductive counseling with her father outside of the room. Discuss the details of the visit with her father separately because she is a minor.

**D.** Provide her with healthy reproductive counseling privately, but request that she return at another time without her father so that she can be treated with azithromycin.

**E.** Treat her with azithromycin and provide healthy reproductive counseling with her father outside of the room. Do not disclose details to her father according to her request.

**25-13.** You have been caring for a 12-year-old boy with glioblastoma multiforme that is not amenable to extensive surgical resection. He continues to do poorly despite therapies. He admits that he is tired and would rather focus on comfort care, but his parents insist that they want "everything possible to be done" to save their son. Which of the following would be the most appropriate approach for management?

**A.** Continue aggressive treatment according to the parents' wishes

**B.** Transition to comfort care only according to the patient's wishes

**C.** Transfer care to another medical provider who is more experienced with ethical challenges

**D.** Facilitate a conversation among the family about patient's preferences and parents' concerns

**E.** Exchange some of his aggressive treatments with placebos without the parents' knowledge

**25-14.** A 14-year-old girl presents for a well-child examination. She has a history of acne and would like to discuss treatment options. Her exam is significant for mild open and closed comedones and a few inflammatory pustules along her face and back. As you begin to discuss conventional topical acne medications, she and her mother raise concerns about the chemical content of these medications. They explain that their relatives have recommended topical application of tea tree oil as an alternative acne treatment and prefer the "most natural" treatment possible. Which of the following is the most appropriate management for this family?

**A.** Review the risks and benefits of conventional medications as well as tea tree oil. Discourage the use of tea tree oil, reasoning that the conventional medications will be more effective.

**B.** Review the risks and benefits of conventional medications as well as tea tree oil. Permit use of topical tea tree oil as long as it does not cause unwanted side effects.

**C.** Review the risks and benefits of conventional medications. Because conventional medications have been proven to be efficacious, tea tree oil's risks and benefits do not need to be considered.

**D.** Review the risks and benefits of conventional medications. Ask the family to bring the tea tree oil and articles supporting tea tree oil use at the next follow-up visit for review.

**E.** Explain that tea tree oil use has no place in medical management. Suggest that the family see another provider if they prefer "natural" therapies over conventional medicine.

**25-15.** You are seeing a patient in clinic with a rare, progressive neurologic disorder. His mother asks you about his overall prognosis. Questions regarding prognosis would be best answered by which of the following types of study?

**A.** Systematic review

**B.** Cohort study

**C.** Randomized controlled trial

**D.** Cross-sectional study

**E.** Prospective blinded comparison trial

**25-16.** Which of the following measures are most appropriate for randomized controlled trials (RCTs)?

**A.** Number needed to treat, relative risk, odds ratio

**B.** Relative risk, odds ratio

**C.** Absolute risk reduction, number needed to treat, prevalence

**D.** Absolute risk reduction, number needed to treat, relative risk

**E.** Confidence interval, incidence, relative risk

**25-17.** Which of the following individuals needs parental consent for medical care?

**A.** A 16-year-old girl who was recently married to her 17-year-old boyfriend

**B.** A 17-year-old boy who is in the military

**C.** A 17-year-old girl who is a mother to 2 children

**D.** A 17-year-old boy who has been working and living independently for the past year

**E.** A 17-year-old girl who attends college out of state

**25-18.** A physician's disclosure of medical information regarding a minor can be elective in which of the following scenarios?

**A.** A 17-year-old boy is seen independently and tests positive for gonorrhea. He asks the physician not to share this with anyone.

**B.** A 16-year-old girl is seen independently and discloses that she is in a sexual relationship with her mother's 35-year-old boyfriend. She says she likes having sex and asks the physician not to share this with her mom.

**C.** A 5-year-old boy who is human immunodeficiency virus (HIV) positive is entering kindergarten and has medical history forms to be completed. His mother asks the physician whether disclosure of his HIV status is necessary.

**D.** A 15-year-old boy is seen independently and expresses suicidal thoughts and reports having looked for household medications that can be used for overdose.

**E.** A 13-year-old girl is seen independently and says she wants to harm herself, has a plan, and has access to firearms at home.

**25-19.** The Four Habits Model outlines 4 habits a physician should practice to help organize medical visits in a way that fosters and strengthens interrelationships between the patient, parent, and physician. The 4 habits include all of the following except which?

**A.** Invest in the beginning
**B.** Elicit the patient's perspective
**C.** Provide the patient with information
**D.** Demonstrate empathy
**E.** Invest in the end

**25-20.** A patient presents with a disease process with which you are not familiar. You decide to do literature review to learn more about the prognosis of this disease process. Which study type would be the best to address a question about prognosis?

**A.** Randomized controlled trial
**B.** Systematic review
**C.** Case series
**D.** Cohort study
**E.** Prospective blinded comparison trial

**25-21.** As a pediatrician, you have to communicate with your patients, their parents, and often other family members regularly during the patient care encounter. This requires a variety of verbal and nonverbal communication skills. Using nonverbal communication effectively helps to promote an environment of trust and support. Which of the following nonverbal communication strategies would help to convey this to your patient and their family?

**A.** Stand up during the visit while the family is sitting
**B.** Answer phone calls and beeper pages during the patient encounter
**C.** Address the adult in the room and not the child
**D.** Establish eye contact with the child frequently while talking to the adults
**E.** Pace around the room during your patient encounter

**25-22.** The end of the patient encounter is vital in regard to sharing information, providing education, partnering with the family and child, and including them in choices. Which of the following is the best method to provide closure for the patient encounter?

**A.** Summarize what was discussed and clarify follow-up plans.
**B.** Walk out of the room when your exam is complete.
**C.** Send the nurse into the room to answer the family's questions.
**D.** Ignore the parents' questions.
**E.** Direct your final words to the adults only.

**25-23.** A 17-year-old female patient asks you how she can make all of her appointments confidential from her parents. She would like to know what situations would qualify for her to become an emancipated minor. You explain to her that these laws vary by state but give her a typical example that is accepted by most states. Which of the following scenarios would typically qualify a patient to become an emancipated minor?

**A.** Pregnancy
**B.** Having a part-time job
**C.** Having a child
**D.** Enlistment in the military
**E.** Living with a family member

**25-24.** Patients should be able to communicate with their physicians and trust that the information that they disclose will be shared in confidence. Physicians are obligated to preserve patient confidentiality when information is shared during the patient encounter. There are some situations where the physician is obligated to disclose patient information without the consent of the patient for the safety of the patient or public health safety. Which of the following scenarios would be appropriate for a physician to disclose without consent?

**A.** A 16-year-old girl is requesting contraception.
**B.** A 14-year-old boy discloses that he is homosexual.
**C.** A 17-year-old girl discloses that she is pregnant.
**D.** A 16-year-old boy tests positive for a sexually transmitted infection (STI).
**E.** A 15-year-old girl discloses a sexual relationship with a 15-year-old boy.

## ANSWERS

**Answer 25-1. B**

Minors, defined as persons under the age of 18, typically do not have legal authority to provide consent to medical treatments, although this varies by state and type of medical treatment. The mature minor doctrine may allow children as young as 13 years to provide consent if able to demonstrate understanding, but in this case, the child is 10 years old. This decision-making process represents the team and family seeking the child's assent to participating in the trial.

(Section 1: Foundations in Pediatric Practice and Child Health, Chapter 5: Law, Ethics, and Clinical Judgment)

**Answer 25-2.** D

Discussions with a child about his or her medical conditions should always be guided by the child's intellectual capacity, with longitudinal discussions adjusted to reflect ongoing development. There is no specific age or timing in disease progression that should mark these discussions. Observation of questions asked by a child can serve as an effective gauge for the timing and depth of these discussions, working on the assumption that a child typically does not ask a question unless and until they are capable of processing the answer.

(Section 1: Foundations in Pediatric Practice and Child Health, Chapter 5: Law, Ethics, and Clinical Judgment)

**Answer 25-3.** A

It is strongly recommended that pediatricians have a policy regarding patient confidentiality that conforms to state laws and clearly identifies to patients, parents, and staff how disclosures of sensitive information will be handled. A pediatrician should not promise to never break confidentiality, as there are circumstances (harm to self or others, public health reporting) that may require disclosure. Addressing issues of sexual health for adolescents falls well within the scope of a general pediatrician.

(Section 1: Foundations in Pediatric Practice and Child Health, Chapter 5: Law, Ethics, and Clinical Judgment)

**Answer 25-4.** C

A report made to a school nurse may well not be confidential, and regulations that typically protect medical information (such as HIPAA) do not apply to schools because they are not HIPAA-covered entities. It is important for families to know that medical information submitted to a school may not remain confidential so they can make informed decisions about what information is shared.

(Section 1: Foundations in Pediatric Practice and Child Health, Chapter 5: Law, Ethics, and Clinical Judgment)

**Answer 25-5.** A

The principle of justice is the moral obligation to act on the basis of fair adjudication between competing claims. In healthcare ethics, this can be subdivided into 3 categories: fair distribution of scarce resources (distributive justice), respect for people's rights (rights-based justice), and respect for morally acceptable laws (legal justice). Veracity is a principle that refers to honesty or truth telling. Beneficence underscores the importance of acting on the behalf of others, whereas nonmaleficence means minimizing harm to others. Autonomy refers to "self-rule," or one's right to make decisions and act on them freely and without interference.

(Section 9: Children with Medical Complexity, Chapter 123: Ethical Issues in Pediatric Patients with Medical Complexity)

**Answer 25-6.** B

Although it is rare, some courts have approved a minor's request to forgo life-sustaining treatments. The default, however, is that a minor can only make medical decisions under specific circumstances. For this reason, an advance directive would not ensure her wishes were followed. There are cases where withholding or withdrawing life-sustaining treatments for a child is appropriate, and in those cases, a court order is not required when there is a clear legal guardian. A desire for a child to discuss the burdens and benefits of ongoing treatments should not be conflated with suicidality, but it is important to be aware of signs and symptoms of mental illness because children with chronic health conditions may be at higher risk.

(Section 10: Palliative Care, Chapter 128: Ethics, Law, and Medical Care Near the End of Life)

**Answer 25-7.** D

Capacity is the only term that matches this definition. Judgment simply means the ability to make a decision, while the other terms refer to moral principles.

(Section 10: Palliative Care, Chapter 128: Ethics, Law, and Medical Care Near the End of Life)

**Answer 25-8.** C

In the case of a surrogate decision maker losing capacity to make decisions, the team should quickly work to establish a new surrogate using the process dictated by local statutes, which may vary significantly from state to state. Although the team can continue to provide medically necessary treatment in the absence of a new surrogate, this should not serve as an excuse to ignore the process. While some mature minors are beginning to gain the legal right to consent to medical treatment, a 7-year-old child would not fit into this category. Hospital staff should not be selected as a surrogate, and a guardian ad litem can only be assigned by a court of law.

(Section 10: Palliative Care, Chapter 128: Ethics, Law, and Medical Care Near the End of Life)

**Answer 25-9.** A

Medical providers should encourage parents to include children in discussions about their medical care, especially when treatment is no longer effective. Because children often pick up more information than parents realize, efforts to hide information as a way to protect their child can backfire, creating a sense of distrust or distance at a time when trust and connection are desperately needed. While a child psychologist or pediatric-trained palliative care specialists can help parents communicate, the bulk of the conversation should be between the child and the parent or another trusted figure in his life. There is no evidence that these serious discussions will remove a child's hope or adversely affect his chance at recovery.

(Section 10: Palliative Care, Chapter 128: Ethics, Law, and Medical Care Near the End of Life)

**Answer 25-10.** D

Adolescence is an important developmental stage in which children dependent on their caregivers transition into independent adults. Cognitively normal adolescents, therefore, should generally be afforded confidentiality surrounding their health care. There are exceptions to this general adherence to confidentiality in which the parents' need to know overrides the adolescent's desire for confidentiality. An important example of exception to adolescent confidentiality is when the adolescent may be a danger to himself or herself or to others. In the scenario in this case, the adolescent not only has symptoms of depression and suicidal ideation, but he has also identified a possible method for suicide attempt (his father's firearm). He is at a high risk of suicide and is therefore currently a threat to himself. He needs immediate psychiatric evaluation, which can be done through the emergency department or direct presentation to an inpatient psychiatric facility. His mother needs to be informed of his suicidality and need for emergent psychiatric evaluation. Out of respect for the patient and in an effort to maintain a good doctor-patient relationship while fostering open communication with caregivers, the adolescent should be informed that his mother must know about his depression and risk of suicide because he is a danger to himself. The other answers are inappropriate next steps to take. He needs immediate psychiatric evaluation; any delays in evaluation and treatment (answer choices A, C, and E) could unfortunately result in suicide.

(Section 1: Foundations in Pediatric Practice and Child Health, Chapter 5: Law, Ethics, and Clinical Judgment)

**Answer 25-11.** A

To answer this question, one must have an understanding of emancipated minors. Emancipated minors have the legal authority to make their own decisions for their life, including decisions related to medical care. Although the laws defining an emancipated minor vary from state to state, emancipated minors are generally those who are married, those in the military, and those who support themselves and live away from their families. Students in college who live away from their families (answer choice A) are almost always viewed as emancipated minors, even if their parents pay their college expenses. Some minors who are runaways may be able to show that they are self-supporting and independent. The other answer choices are not emancipated minors. A minor in foster care is still under the care and responsibility of the state. Although it may be difficult for some elderly guardians to care for minors, the minors are still not emancipated if they live with the guardians and are not self-supporting.

(Section 1: Foundations in Pediatric Practice and Child Health, Chapter 5: Law, Ethics, and Clinical Judgment)

**Answer 25-12.** E

This adolescent presents with a sexually transmitted infection (STI): chlamydial infection manifested as uncomplicated cervicitis with vaginal discharge. She needs appropriate care, which includes treatment with single-dose azithromycin and reproductive health counseling. Adolescents are legally allowed to consent to STI treatment without parental/guardian involvement. They should also generally be afforded confidentiality surrounding their health care. The exception to adolescent confidentiality is when they are a danger to themselves or to others (eg, suicidal ideation or homicidal ideation). The patient in this case is not putting herself or others in danger. Therefore, her request for confidentiality regarding STI management ethically should be respected. The correct answer is E. Her father should not be informed of the details of the visit, and his consent for treatment does not need to be obtained. She should be treated promptly, as delays in therapy (answer choice D) increase her risk of complications from untreated chlamydia infection, including pelvic inflammatory disease.

(Section 1: Foundations in Pediatric Practice and Child Health, Chapter 5: Law, Ethics, and Clinical Judgment)

**Answer 25-13.** D

Disagreements between patients and families regarding life-sustaining therapies and aggressive treatment in the setting of a poor prognosis can be ethically difficult. Commonly, a patient may want to focus on comfort care while the family wants to continue aggressive treatment (as in this scenario). The provider should encourage and facilitate discussion between patients and their parents, allowing the patient's preferences to be heard and considered. Although the parents have ultimate decision-making authority, providers can consider limiting therapeutic options offered to those that the provider believes will benefit the patient without significant burden.

Transferring care to another medical provider in this case would break the doctor-patient-family relationship that was already established. A new provider who does not have well-established rapport may find it difficult to facilitate conversations about the patient's preferences; a more appropriate option could be to seek advice or partnership with a provider who has more experience or to consult the ethics council of the institution. Giving the patient fake treatments is not something to which the parents consented and is both ethically and legally wrong.

(Section 10: Palliative Care, Chapter 128: Ethics, Law, and Medical Care Near the End of Life)

**Answer 25-14.** B

Complementary and alternative medicine (CAM) encompasses a wide range of therapies outside of mainstream conventional or Western medicine that are used for medical intervention, health promotion, and disease prevention. Providers should be aware of complementary health approaches, which are common among pediatric populations within the United States. About 12% of children aged 4 to 17 years use some form of complementary health approach, of which the most common are natural products like dietary supplements other than vitamins and minerals. Families that use CAM therapies often do so because they view CAM therapies to be more congruent with their own culture, values, or beliefs. Several medicolegal issues should be considered when using CAM therapies in children. In general, a patient should be permitted to use a CAM therapy if it is safe, will not deter use of necessary or life-saving conventional therapy, and does not pose a financial strain on the family. In this scenario, the family is considering tea tree oil for a CAM therapy for acne. Tea tree oil in general is safe when used topically but can sometimes cause skin dryness, itching, and irritation. The provider should have an open discussion about the risks and benefits of all treatment options, including tea tree oil. Given its low risk, tea tree oil use should be permitted as long as there are no unwanted side effects.

Families who use CAM therapies often do so as an adjunct to conventional therapies. The patient should be allowed to try it as an adjunct if she chooses.

Studies have shown that families want and appreciate their pediatrician's professional guidance regarding CAM. Providers should engage families in open conversations about CAM use. The burden of proof of efficacy of a CAM should not be placed on a family alone; the provider should look for information on safety and efficacy and discuss it with families.

(Section 1: Foundations in Pediatric Practice and Child Health, Chapter 13: Complementary and Integrative Pediatrics)

**Answer 25-15.** B

Questions regarding prognosis are best answered by cohort studies. In a cohort study, 2 groups are studied: one group with a particular exposure and the other without the exposure (Figure 2-1A). Both groups are followed over time to see which individuals within each group develop disease. If a greater proportion of individuals in the exposed group develop the disease, then an association (not causation) can be made between the exposure and disease.

Systematic reviews (answer choice A) and randomized controlled trials (answer choice C) are best suited to answer questions regarding therapy. Cross-sectional studies (answer choice D) are useful for answering questions regarding prevalence.

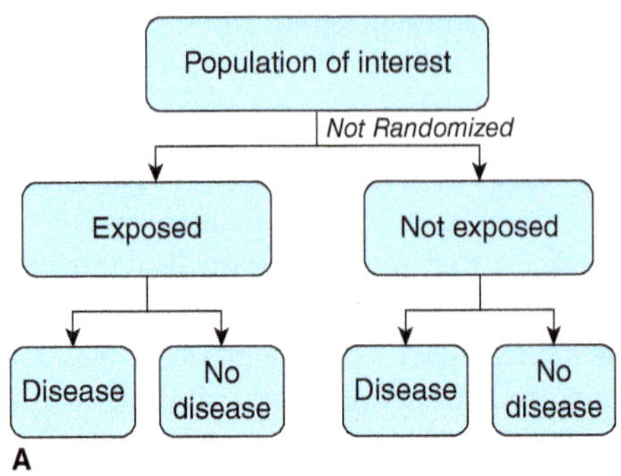


**FIGURE 2-1A.** Design of a cohort study. (Mark W. Kline, *Rudolph's Pediatrics*, 23rd Edition. Copyright © McGraw-Hill Education. All rights reserved.)

(Section 1: Foundations in Pediatric Practice and Child Health, Chapter 2: Decision-Making in Pediatrics: Use of Evidence-Based Medicine)

**Answer 25-16.** D

RCTs are best used to answer questions regarding therapy, and measures used to measure therapy effect include absolute risk reduction (ARR), number needed to treat (NNT), and relative risk (RR). ARR is the difference in outcome rates between the control group versus the treatment group. NNT is the inverse of ARR (NNT = 1/ARR), and it reflects the number of individuals that would need to be treated to prevent one additional bad outcome. RR reflects the degree to which a therapy confers benefit (or harm). It is calculated as the ratio of the probability of outcome in the therapy group to the probability of outcome in the control group. An RR of 1 indicates that the therapy confers no benefit, as the probability of the outcome is equal in both the control and therapy groups. An RR $< 1$ indicates that the therapy is beneficial in reducing probability of the outcome. An RR $> 1$ indicates that the therapy causes harm and is associated with greater probability of the outcome.

Prevalence measures the proportion of a population that has a particular disease or characteristic at a given time. This is best measured through cross-sectional studies. Odds ratio is used in cohort studies and case-control studies, and it measures the odds of an outcome occurring given a particular exposure versus absence of an exposure.

(Section 1: Foundations in Pediatric Practice and Child Health, Chapter 2: Decision-Making in Pediatrics: Use of Evidence-Based Medicine)

**Answer 25-17.** C

In most states, individuals under the age of 18 are considered minors and thus cannot consent to treatment. Emancipated minors, however, have the legal right to make their own decision on all aspects of life, including medical care. While states may vary, emancipated minors usually include individuals who are married, in the military, or self-supporting and living independently from their families.

(Section 1: Foundations in Pediatric Practice and Child Health, Chapter 5: Law, Ethics, and Clinical Judgment)

**Answer 25-18.** C

The promise of confidentiality between a physician and patient (and at times the parent) is of utmost importance to obtain accurate information and uphold the physician-patient relationship. There are, however, scenarios in which disclosure is required. In most states, physicians are required to report to state agencies certain communicable diseases, including sexually transmitted infections (STIs). Therefore, although a physician can treat a minor (such as in answer choice A) for an STI without notifying his or her parents, the physician is obligated to report the infection to the state agency. Physicians are also obligated to report to the police any concerns for possible statutory rape, as is likely in answer choice B. While the physician may not necessarily inform the parent directly, the parent will be informed by the police. The physician may also breach confidentiality if there is a concern that the minor may be a danger to himself or to others (answer choice D). Disclosures of information to schools may not necessarily be confidential. Therefore, parents (and adolescents) should be aware of what information is disclosed to the school, and in most cases, they have the right to decline disclosure (answer choice C). The physician may also breach confidentiality if there is a concern that the minor may be a danger to himself or to others (answer choices D and E).

(Section 1: Foundations in Pediatric Practice and Child Health, Chapter 5: Law, Ethics, and Clinical Judgment)

**Answer 25-19.** C

The Four Habits Model was developed by Frankel and Stein, and the 4 habits are as follows: invest in the beginning, elicit the patient's perspective, demonstrate empathy, and invest in the end.

(Section 1: Foundations in Pediatric Practice and Child Health, Chapter 3: Communication with Children and Families, Table 3-2)

**Answer 25-20.** D

Questions about prognosis are best addressed in cohort studies. Case-control studies and case series studies would be next in line regarding prognosis. Systematic reviews and randomized controlled studies would best address questions regarding therapy. A prospective, blinded comparison trial would be best to determine the efficacy of a diagnostic test.

(Section 1: Foundations in Pediatric Practice and Child Health, Chapter 2: Decision-Making in Pediatrics: Use of Evidence-Based Medicine)

**Answer 25-21.** D

Establishing eye contact with the child while talking to the adults in the room will help the child become more comfortable with your presence and bring the child into the interaction.

Make yourself appear less threatening by positioning yourself at eye level with the child and the adults in the room. Avoid interruptions during patient encounters. This lets the patient and the family know that they are your priority. Acknowledge and interact with the child nonverbally throughout the patient encounter. Be present during the encounter, appear unhurried, and convey interest and caring.

(Section 1: Foundations in Pediatric Practice and Child Health, Chapter 3: Communication with Children and Families)

**Answer 25-22.** A

Answer choice A is the only option that includes the family members in the follow-up plans for the end of a visit. It is inappropriate to walk out of the room at the end of the exam with no follow-up with the patient and family. While the nurse has an important role in the care of the patient, it is important for the patient and family to feel that they are included in the decisions made with the physician. Studies show that involving the patient and family in making decisions corresponds with improved outcomes. The child and the family should be engaged throughout the encounter, particularly in the end.

(Section 1: Foundations in Pediatric Practice and Child Health, Chapter 3: Communication with Children and Families)

**Answer 25-23.** D

State laws vary, but emancipated minors typically include those who are married, those who are in the military, and in most states, those who are self-supporting and living away from their families.

Most states do not recognize pregnancy or being a parent for emancipation of minors. A part-time job is not enough for a minor to support themselves financially. Living with a family member does not typically qualify for emancipation; again, the minor has to be able to self-support living away from their families.

(Section 1: Foundations in Pediatric Practice and Child Health, Chapter 5: Law, Ethics, and Clinical Judgment)

**Answer 25-24.** D

Infectious diseases, particularly STIs, are reportable to the state public health authorities. However, this information should not be disclosed to the patient's parents without the consent of the patient

In order for physicians to obtain honest information from an adolescent patient, they may have to promise confidentiality. It is important to give a disclaimer to the patient that certain conditions are excluded from this promise of confidentiality. State laws determine the excluded conditions. Most states allow confidentiality regarding family planning, sexual orientation, pregnancy, and consensual sexual relationships. Cases of abuse must be reported to the local governing bodies.

(Section 1: Foundations in Pediatric Practice and Child Health, Chapter 5: Law, Ethics, and Clinical Judgment)

# CHAPTER 26 | Research Methods

Michael D. Cabana

**26-1.** The Lentis study is designed to evaluate a new treatment for infantile eczema. Infants with eczema are recruited for the study. After families are recruited and consented, the infants are randomly assigned to receive either the treatment cream or a placebo cream. Parents are instructed to give the assigned cream 3 times a day for the next 10 days. After 10 days, the investigators will reexamine the study patients. The treatment cream and the placebo cream are both identical in terms of appearance, smell, and texture. The Lentis study uses what type of study design?

**A.** Case-control study

**B.** Cohort study

**C.** Observational study

**D.** Randomized controlled trial (RCT)

**E.** Quasi-experimental study

**26-2.** The Lentis study is completed, and the study results are published. A description of the participating infants in the Lentis study by arm is listed in the following table.

What is the most likely reason why there is a greater percentage of Hispanic patients who were randomized to the intervention arm compared to the control arm of the study?

**A.** The difference occurred by chance, as randomization does not guarantee that both groups will be similar in every aspect.

**B.** The difference occurred because too few Hispanic participants were recruited.

**C.** The difference occurred because participants could determine which study arm to join.

**D.** The difference occurred because the study coordinators could determine which study arm to assign.

**E.** The difference occurred because of the use of intent-to-treat analysis.

Lentis Study Participant Characteristics by Study Arm

| | **Control (n = 200)** | **Intervention (n = 200)** |
|---|---|---|
| Male | 104 (52%) | 98 (49%) |
| Infant race | | |
| White | 100 (50%) | 104 (52%) |
| African American | 22 (11%) | 22 (11%) |
| American Indian/Alaskan Native | 8 (4%) | 6 (3%) |
| Asian | 20 (10%) | 20 (10%) |
| Pacific Islander | 26 (13%) | 22 (11%) |
| Other | 24 (12%) | 26 (13%) |
| Hispanic ethnicity | 38 (19%) | 60 (30%) |
| Gestational age, in weeks (standard deviation [SD]) | 38.9 (1.3) | 39.0 (1.4) |
| Birth weight, in grams (SD) | 3440 (442) | 3427 (506) |
| Cesarean section | 50 (25%) | 56 (28%) |
| Mean number of months of breastfeeding in first year of life (SD) | 7.5 (5.1) | 7.7 (4.9) |

**26-3.** In the Lentis study, 10 of the 200 patients (5%) in the intervention group were not adherent to the protocol and did not receive the entire 10-day course of treatment. It was also later discovered that 2 (1%) of the 200 patients in the control group were exposed to a similar medication cream during the 10-day exposure to the placebo. In both cases, the parents had given an "old" medication used for another child in the family on their child who was currently enrolled in the Lentis study. For the analysis of the study results, the investigators conduct an intent-to-treat analysis. In an intent-to-treat analysis, data from which patients are used for analysis?

**A.** Only the data from the 190 intervention patients who used the study medication correctly and the 198 control patients who used the placebo correctly

**B.** Only the data from the 190 intervention patients who used the study medication correctly and all of the 200 control patients

**C.** Only the data from the 200 intervention patients and the 198 control patients who used the placebo correctly

**D.** All the data from the 200 intervention patients and the 200 control patients

**E.** None of the above

**26-4.** The Supplement to Neutralize Asthma Flare-Ups (SNAFU) Study is assessing the effect of a new supplement X in preventing asthma exacerbations. Eight hundred children with asthma are randomized to either the treatment group or the control group. After 1 year, 80 children in the treatment group experience an asthma exacerbation. One hundred children in the control group experience an asthma exacerbation.

| | Exacerbation | No Exacerbation | Total |
|---|---|---|---|
| Treatment | 80 | 320 | 400 |
| Control | 100 | 300 | 400 |

Based on the results of the SNAFU Study, what is the absolute risk reduction for supplement X in decreasing an asthma exacerbation?

**A.** 5%

**B.** 10%

**C.** 15%

**D.** 0%

**E.** 25%

**26-5.** The Supplement to Neutralize Asthma Flare-Ups (SNAFU) Study is assessing the effect of a new supplement X in preventing asthma exacerbations. Eight hundred children with asthma are randomized to either the treatment group or the control group. After 1 year, 80 children in the treatment group experience an asthma exacerbation. One hundred children in the control group experience an asthma exacerbation.

| | Exacerbation | No Exacerbation | Total |
|---|---|---|---|
| Treatment | 80 | 320 | 400 |
| Control | 100 | 300 | 400 |

Based on the results of the SNAFU Study, what is the relative risk reduction for supplement X in decreasing an asthma exacerbation?

**A.** 5%

**B.** 10%

**C.** 20%

**D.** 25%

**E.** 50%

**26-6.** The Supplement to Neutralize Asthma Flare-Ups (SNAFU) Study is assessing the effect of a new supplement X in preventing asthma exacerbations. Eight hundred children with asthma are randomized to either the treatment group or the control group. After 1 year, 80 children in the treatment group experience an asthma exacerbation. One hundred children in the control group experience an asthma exacerbation.

| | Exacerbation | No Exacerbation | Total |
|---|---|---|---|
| Treatment | 80 | 320 | 400 |
| Control | 100 | 300 | 400 |

Based on the results of the SNAFU Study, what is the number needed to treat (NNT) for supplement X in decreasing an asthma exacerbation?

**A.** 20

**B.** 50

**C.** 200

**D.** 400

**E.** 500

**26-7.** The Lucid study is testing the effectiveness of a new antibiotic in treating bacterial conjunctivitis versus a currently available (eg, control) antibiotic. For this study, 20 patients with conjunctivitis are randomized to either the new antibiotic or the control antibiotic treatment. Both treatments are 90% effective in treating the conjunctivitis ($P = 1.00$), and the authors conclude that the new antibiotic is just as effective as the currently available (eg, control) antibiotic. Which of the following statements is true?

**A.** It is possible that a real difference in effectiveness between the intervention and control was missed because the *P* value was not > .05.

**B.** It is possible that a real difference in effectiveness between the intervention and control was missed because the sample size was too small (eg, not enough power).

**C.** It is possible that a real difference in effectiveness between the intervention and control was missed because the sample size was too large (eg, not much power).

**D.** It is possible that a real difference in effectiveness between the intervention and control was missed because an intent-to-treat analysis was not conducted.

**E.** None of the above is correct.

**26-8.** A cross-sectional study is used to assess a new diagnostic test for Disease Z compared to the gold standard test. Four hundred children who present with potential symptoms of Disease Z undergo both tests. Of the 400 patients, 100 are diagnosed with Disease Z based on the gold standard test. The following results are published.

| | Gold Standard Positive for Disease Z | Gold Standard Negative for Disease Z | Total |
|---|---|---|---|
| New Test Positive for Disease Z | 95 | 30 | 125 |
| New Test Negative for Disease Z | 5 | 270 | 275 |
| Total | 100 | 300 | 400 |

Which of the following statements is correct?

**A.** The sensitivity of the new diagnostic test is 0.90.

**B.** The sensitivity of the new diagnostic test is 0.05.

**C.** The specificity of the new diagnostic test is 0.90.

**D.** The specificity of the new diagnostic test is 0.10.

**E.** The positive predictive value of the new diagnostic test is 0.10.

**26-9.** A cross-sectional study is used to assess a new diagnostic test for Disease X compared to the gold standard test. Four thousand children who present for well-child visits undergo both tests. From the 4000 patients, 400 are diagnosed with Disease X based on the gold standard test. The following results are published in the following table.

| | Gold Standard Positive for Disease X | Gold Standard Negative for Disease X | Total |
|---|---|---|---|
| New Test Positive for Disease X | 360 | 80 | 440 |
| New Test Negative for Disease X | 40 | 3520 | 3560 |
| Total | 400 | 3600 | 4000 |

Which of the following statements is correct?

**A.** The sensitivity of the new diagnostic test is 0.10.

**B.** The specificity of the new diagnostic test is 0.90.

**C.** The positive predictive value of the new diagnostic test is 0.99.

**D.** The negative predictive value of the new diagnostic test is 0.82.

**E.** The prevalence of Disease X in this population is 0.10.

**26-10.** You are designing a study to determine whether an intervention is effective in the treatment of a common condition. The treatment has few side effects reported. What is the best study design to determine the effectiveness of a treatment or intervention?

**A.** Case series

**B.** Cohort study

**C.** Cross-sectional study

**D.** Case-control study

**E.** Randomized controlled trial (RCT)

**26-11.** Which of the following study designs is best for determining the relative risk of developing an outcome based on an exposure?

**A.** Case report

**B.** Case series

**C.** Cohort study

**D.** Cross-sectional study

**E.** Case-control study

**26-12.** Which of the following study designs is best for determining the odds of developing a rare outcome?

**A.** Case report

**B.** Case series

**C.** Cohort study

**D.** Cross-sectional study

**E.** Case-control study

**26-13.** On January 1, 2010, the population of the city of Hoboken, New Jersey, was 50,000 persons. Five hundred persons in Hoboken had Disease X. On January 1, 2011, the population of Hoboken, New Jersey, was unchanged at 50,000 persons; however, now 1500 persons have Disease X.

Which of the following statements about prevalence is correct?

**A.** The prevalence of Disease X in Hoboken, New Jersey, on January 1, 2010, was 0.010.

**B.** The prevalence of Disease X in Hoboken, New Jersey, on January 1, 2011, was 0.020.

**C.** The prevalence of Disease X in Hoboken, New Jersey, on January 1, 2010, was 500.

**D.** The prevalence of Disease X in Hoboken, New Jersey, on January 1, 2011, was 1500.

**E.** The prevalence of Disease X in Hoboken, New Jersey, from January 1, 2010, to January 1, 2011, was 0.02 cases/year.

**26-14.** On January 1, 2010, the population of the city of Hoboken, New Jersey, was 50,000 persons. Five hundred persons in Hoboken had Disease X. On January 1, 2011, the population of Hoboken, New Jersey, was unchanged at 50,000 persons; however, now 1500 persons have Disease X.

Which of the following statements about incidence is correct?

**A.** The incidence of Disease X in Hoboken, New Jersey, from January 1, 2010, to January 1, 2011, was 0.01 cases/year.

**B.** The incidence of Disease X in Hoboken, New Jersey, from January 1, 2010, to January 1, 2011, was 0.02 cases/year.

**C.** The incidence of Disease X in Hoboken, New Jersey, from January 1, 2010, to January 1, 2011, was 0.03 cases/year.

**D.** The incidence of Disease X in Hoboken, New Jersey, from January 1, 2010, to January 1, 2011, was 1000.

**E.** The incidence of Disease X in Hoboken, New Jersey, from January 1, 2010, to January 1, 2011, was 2000.

**26-15.** An investigator plans to evaluate a new treatment for juvenile idiopathic arthritis (JIA) in her clinic population. In this study, 120 patients with JIA will be enrolled and randomized. Sixty patients will receive the active agent and 60 patients will receive no new treatment (standard of care) for the next 6 months. The active agent is an oral tablet that is given by the principal investigator to the participants in the intervention group once a month during the study visit. At the end of the visit, the principal investigator assesses the outcome based on a joint examination for all the patients. The principal investigator has been trained and certified in the proper examination technique. Based on the description, which of the following is a major flaw in the study design?

**A.** The principal investigator is the only person who is assessing the outcome.

**B.** The principal investigator is not blinded, and she is also assessing the outcome.

**C.** The principal investigator is recruiting patients from her own clinic.

**D.** All the study participants will have joint examinations.

**E.** Only half of the study participants will be randomized to the intervention group.

## ANSWERS

**Answer 26-1. D**

RCTs are usually the best study designs to answer questions about therapy. In an RCT, after recruitment and consent, the study participants are randomly assigned either to an intervention group or to a comparison group. In the Lentis study, the comparison was a placebo cream. Randomization helps decrease the likelihood of bias in assigning the study participant to a particular group. The study then compares the 2 groups as they move forward in time simultaneously.

In a case-control study, participants are recruited on the basis of an outcome (eg, severe eczema or mild eczema). The investigators then look backward in time to assess for an exposure of interest (eg, daily bathing vs infrequent bathing as an infant). If daily bathing is hypothesized to be associated with severe eczema, then there would be a higher percentage of infants with severe eczema who had a history of daily bathing (compared to infants with mild eczema). The case-control design is useful for evaluating claims of causation.

In a cohort study, participants are recruited on the basis of an exposure (eg, infants who live near freeways vs infants who do not live near freeways). In the cohort study design, the investigators follow a group of participants from a point in time to another point in time to assess if an outcome of interest occurs. The cohort design is useful for studying the effects of rare exposures or for studying the prognosis of a condition.

The term *observational study* is descriptive, but not specific. An observational study can refer to a cohort study, case-control study, cross-sectional study, or even a case series or case study (Figure 2-1). Unlike an interventional study, an observational study usually takes advantage of a "natural" experiment.

A quasi-experimental study usually refers to the before and after evaluation of an intervention without the benefit of a control group. This study design is less useful for assessing causality, as pre-post studies do not have control for other factors that may also be evolving or changing during the observation period. For example, there may be changes in the environment that affect the outcome that also happen to occur at the time of the intervention.

(Chapter 2: Decision-Making in Pediatrics: Use of Evidence-Based Medicine; Retrieving the Evidence)

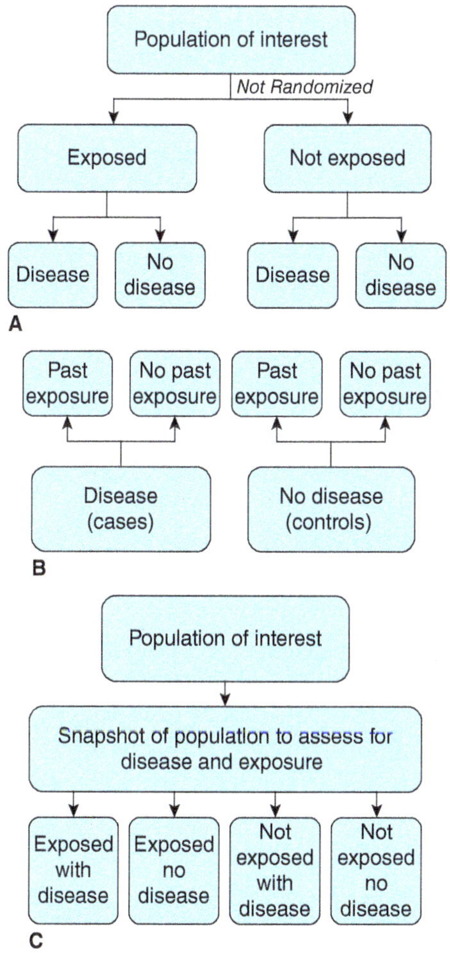


**FIGURE 2-1.** (A) Cohort study. (B) Case-control study. (C) Cross-sectional study. (Mark W. Kline, *Rudolph's Pediatrics*, 23rd Edition. Copyright © McGraw-Hill Education. All rights reserved.)

**Answer 26-2. A**

When reading the results of a randomized controlled trial (RCT), it is not unusual to see some differences in the group characteristics of the intervention group and the control group. In general, the process of randomization tends to balance *both* known and unknown factors between the intervention and control group. However, occasionally the groups may have statistically significant differences just by chance, especially when a large number of different characteristics are compared. When reading the results of an RCT, most studies will provide a table of demographic data and other potentially relevant characteristics of the participants in the different study arms. It is important to assess whether the groups are similar enough to assure that randomization was effective. If there are differences, it is important to assess whether such differences may limit the validity of the results of the study.

The difference in the 2 groups did not occur because too few Hispanic participants were recruited. A total of 98 Hispanic patients were recruited. The issue is that the distribution of the patients was uneven. Just by chance, a greater percentage of Hispanic patients were randomized to the intervention group.

The difference did not occur because participants could determine which study arm to join. Similarly, the difference did not occur because the study coordinators could determine which study arm to assign. After families are recruited and consented, the infants were randomly assigned to receive either the treatment cream or a placebo cream. Although there have been cases of investigators tampering with randomization procedures to manipulate a participant's group assignment, based on the description of the randomization process, the difference was due to chance.

Intent-to-treat analysis refers to the principle that study participants should be left in the treatment group to which they were originally assigned for analysis, even if they received one of the other treatments after the original treatment failed. Intention to treat would not affect the distribution of patients in the control or intervention arms.

(Chapter 2: Decision-Making in Pediatrics: Use of Evidence-Based Medicine; Critical Appraisal of the Evidence)

**Answer 26-3. D**

Intent-to-treat analysis refers to the principle that study participants should be left in the treatment group to which they were originally assigned for analysis, even if they received one of the other treatments after the original treatment failed. As a result, for an intent-to-treat analysis, data from all 200 patients from both groups would be used in the analysis.

In clinical practice, nonadherence is common. As a result, how a potential treatment performs in a real-world situation is clinically important. If the investigators ignore the data from nonadherent participants or control patients who might have accidentally been exposed to a similar intervention, the study design then starts to lose the benefits of randomization. In addition, the reasons for nonadherence may have been related to the intervention (eg, families who noticed the intervention was not working gave up on the intervention medication). An intent-to-treat analysis provides a "real-word" estimate and tends to be the most conservative estimate regarding the effectiveness of the study intervention.

Many studies will conduct an intent-to-treat analysis that includes all patients, as well as a per-protocol analysis that only includes those patients who were completely adherent to the study protocol.

(Chapter 2: Decision-Making in Pediatrics: Use of Evidence-Based Medicine; Critical Appraisal of the Evidence)

**Answer 26-4.** A

The absolute risk reduction is the risk of disease in the control group minus the risk in the treatment group. For the SNAFU Study, the absolute risk reduction = (100/400) – (80/400) = 5%.

(Chapter 2: Decision-Making in Pediatrics: Use of Evidence-Based Medicine; Critical Appraisal of the Evidence)

**Answer 26-5.** C

The relative risk reduction compares the degree to which a new treatment shows benefit (or harm). It is a comparison of the risk of disease in the experimental group (or, in a cohort trial, the exposed children) with the risk in the control group (or the nonexposed children).

The risk of an asthma exacerbation in the experimental group is 80/400 = 0.20. The risk of an asthma exacerbation in the control group is 100/400 = 0.25. The relative risk reduction is thus (0.25 – 0.20)/0.25 = 0.20 or 20%.

(Chapter 2: Decision-Making in Pediatrics: Use of Evidence-Based Medicine; Critical Appraisal of the Evidence)

**Answer 26-6.** A

The number needed to treat (NNT) is the reciprocal (inverse) of the absolute risk reduction. When the absolute risk is extremely low, the NNT is a very large number. Similarly, when the absolute risk is high and the treatment is very effective, then the NNT is very low.

For the SNAFU Study, the number needed to treat = 1/absolute risk reduction = 1/0.05 = 20.

(Chapter 2: Decision-Making in Pediatrics: Use of Evidence-Based Medicine; Critical Appraisal of the Evidence)

**Answer 26-7.** B

The Lucid study was a "negative" study because the results suggested no difference between the control and the intervention. In a negative study (ie, no statistically significant difference between groups), it is possible that a real difference between the study groups was missed (a type II error, or β). In these studies, in order to decide if the sample size was large enough to avoid this error, the clinician must examine the methods section of the study for an explanation of how the sample size was determined. If unrealistic assumptions were made in the sample size calculation, it is possible that the study was inadequately powered to be able to detect a clinically meaningful difference in the 2 groups. As a result, it is possible that a real difference in effectiveness between the intervention and control was missed because the sample size was too small.

A $P < 0.05$ suggests that if the study was repeated multiple times, the likelihood of a value more extreme would only occur 5% of the time. By convention, a $P \leq .05$ is usually accepted. In this case, the $P$ value was > .05. When the $P$ value is > .05, the possibility that a real difference in effectiveness between the intervention and control was missed is not an issue. The $P$ value is a critical issue for "positive" studies (ie, a statistically significant difference between the group occurs and there is a risk that this difference is not actually present).

Finally, an intent-to-treat analysis includes all participants in the study. In an intent-to-treat analysis, all patients are analyzed based on the group to which they were randomized.

(Chapter 2: Decision-Making in Pediatrics: Use of Evidence-Based Medicine; Critical Appraisal of the Evidence)

**Answer 26-8.** C

The specificity of a diagnostic test is the ability of a test to accurately identify those *without* disease. The specificity is the proportion of individuals without the disease in whom the test is negative. In this case, the specificity is the number of patients with "New Test Negative for Disease Z" divided by the number of patients with "Gold Standard Negative for Disease Z" = 270/300 = 0.90.

The sensitivity of a diagnostic test is the ability of a test to accurately identify those *with* disease. The sensitivity is the proportion of individuals with the disease in whom the test is positive. In this case, the sensitivity is the number of patients with "New Test Positive for Disease Z" divided by the number of patients with "Gold Standard Positive for Disease Z" = 95/100 = 0.95.

The *positive predictive value* of a diagnostic test is the likelihood that a positive result represents the identification of an individual who has the disease. In this case, the positive predictive value is the number of patients with "Gold Standard Positive for Disease Z" divided by the number of patients with "New Test Positive for Disease Z" = 95/125 = 0.76.

(Ambroggio L, Schondelmeyer AC. Chapter 6: Infectious diseases epidemiology, in Shah SS, Kemper AR, Ratner AJ (eds.), *Pediatric Infectious Diseases: Essentials for Practice*, 2nd ed. New York, NY: McGraw-Hill; 2018.)

**Answer 26-9.** E

The prevalence of disease is the number of cases of the disease at a single point in time. In this case, 4000 patients were tested and 400 were positive based on the gold standard test. As a result, the prevalence of disease is 400/4000 = 0.10.

The sensitivity of a diagnostic test is the ability of a test to accurately identify those *with* disease. The sensitivity is the proportion of individuals with the disease in whom the test is positive. In this case, the sensitivity is the number of patients with "New Test Positive for Disease X" divided by the number of patients with "Gold Standard Positive for Disease X" = 360/400 = 0.90.

The specificity of a diagnostic test is the ability of a test to accurately identify those *without* disease. The specificity is the proportion of individuals without the disease in whom the test is negative. In this case, the specificity is the number of patients with "New Test Negative for Disease X" divided by the number of patients with "Gold Standard Negative for Disease X" = 3520/3600 = 0.977.

The *positive predictive value* of a diagnostic test is the likelihood that a positive result represents the identification of an individual who has the disease. In this case, the positive predictive value is the number of patients with "Gold Standard Positive for Disease X" divided by the number of patients with "New Test Positive for Disease X" = 360/440 = 0.82.

The negative predictive value of a diagnostic test is the likelihood that a negative result represents the identification of an individual who does not have the disease. In this case, the negative predictive value is the number of patients with "Gold Standard Negative for Disease X" divided by the number of patients with "New Test Negative for Disease X" = 3520/3560 = 0.988.

(Ambroggio L, Schondelmeyer AC. Chapter 6: Infectious diseases epidemiology, in Shah SS, Kemper AR, Ratner AJ (eds.). *Pediatric Infectious Diseases: Essentials for Practice*, 2nd ed. New York, NY: McGraw-Hill; 2018.)

**Answer 26-10.** E

RCTs are usually the best study designs to answer questions about therapy. Unlike observational studies, such as a cohort study or a case-control study, in an RCT, the study participants are randomly assigned either to an intervention group or to a comparison group. Randomization helps decrease the likelihood of bias in assigning the study participant to a particular group.

In a cross-sectional study, all the data are obtained at the same point in time. Although it is possible to observe associations, it is not possible to infer causality in a cross-sectional study.

In a case series, there is no comparison or control group. Thus, it is not possible to determine if the observed outcomes are due to any of the other factors being observed in the series of cases.

(Chapter 2: Decision-Making in Pediatrics: Use of Evidence-Based Medicine; Retrieving the Evidence)

**Answer 26-11.** C

A cohort study is a type of observational study where participants are recruited on the basis of an exposure (eg, children exposed to high altitudes vs children not exposed to high altitudes). In the cohort study design, the investigators follow a group of participants from a point in time to another point in time to assess whether an outcome of interest occurs. The cohort design allows the investigators to determine the relative risk of developing an outcome based on the exposure of interest (Table 2-1).

**TABLE 2-1.** Appropriate Measures in Clinical Trials

| Randomized Control Trial | Cohort Study | Case-Control Study | Cross-Sectional (Prevalence) Study |
|---|---|---|---|
| Absolute risk reduction | Relative risk | Odds ratio | Prevalence |
| Number needed to treat | Odds ratio | | |
| Relative risk | | | |

Mark W. Kline, *Rudolph's Pediatrics*, 23rd Edition. Copyright © McGraw-Hill Education. All rights reserved.

Unlike a cohort study, a case-control study recruits participants on the basis of an outcome (eg, leukemia vs no leukemia). Those with the outcome of interest are cases. These cases are matched with participants without the outcome (ie, controls). In a case-control study design, the investigators then look backward in time to assess for an exposure of interest (eg, exposure to plastic products). If plastic product exposure is hypothesized to be associated with leukemia, then there would be a higher percentage of children with leukemia who had a history of exposure to plastic products (compared to children without leukemia). In a case-control study, the odds ratio can be calculated; however, the relative risk cannot be directly calculated. In situations where the outcome of interest is very rare, the odds ratio can be used to approximate the relative risk.

In a cross-sectional study, a sample of the population is surveyed at a point in time. The prevalence of the disease can be determined. The cross-sectional study design can establish associations between different conditions; however, because the data are collected at the same point in time, it is not possible to make statements regarding causality. Similarly, one cannot estimate a relative risk based on a cross-sectional study.

In a case report or case series, observations are noted regarding an interesting case or cases. In general, case reports or case series studies can give some insight into a condition or disease; however, because there are no control groups, it is difficult to make inferences regarding causality.

(Chapter 2: Decision-Making in Pediatrics: Use of Evidence-Based Medicine; Retrieving the Evidence; Ambroggio L, Schondelmeyer AC. Chapter 6: Infectious diseases epidemiology, in Shah SS, Kemper AR, Ratner AJ (eds.), *Pediatric Infectious Diseases: Essentials for Practice*, 2nd ed. New York, NY: McGraw-Hill; 2018.)

**Answer 26-12.** E

A case-control study design is the best approach for determining the association between a risk factor, or exposure, and a rare outcome. In situations where the outcome of interest is very rare, the odds ratio can be used to approximate the relative risk.

A cross-sectional study surveys a sample of the population at a single point in time. If the outcome of interest is rare, it can be can be difficult to obtain a meaningful result with any power. A similar issue will occur with a cohort study and a rare outcome. However, if the exposure (instead of the outcome) is rare, a cohort study is a better approach.

Case reports or case series studies give some insight into a condition or disease; however, because there are no control groups, it is difficult to make inferences regarding causality.

(Chapter 2: Decision-Making in Pediatrics: Use of Evidence-Based Medicine; Retrieving the Evidence)

**Answer 26-13.** A

Prevalence is calculated based on the number of persons with a condition at a specific point in time, divided by the number of persons at risk for that condition at the same specific point in time. On January 1, 2010, the prevalence of Disease X is (500 persons with disease)/(50,000 persons at risk for disease), or 0.010. On January 1, 2011, the prevalence of Disease X is (1500 persons with disease)/(50,000 persons at risk for disease), or 0.030.

(Chapter 2: Decision-Making in Pediatrics: Use of Evidence-Based Medicine; Retrieving the Evidence)

**Answer 26-14.** B

Incidence is calculated as the number of persons who develop a condition during a specific interval of time divided by the number of persons at risk for the condition at the start of the time interval. In this case, there are 1000 new cases between January 1, 2010 and January 1, 2011. There are a total of 50,000 persons at risk at the start of the time interval. As a result, the incidence (*not* prevalence) of Disease X in Hoboken, New Jersey, from January 1, 2010 to January 1, 2011, was 0.02 cases/year.

(Chapter 2: Decision-Making in Pediatrics: Use of Evidence-Based Medicine; Retrieving the Evidence)

**Answer 26-15.** B

A major potential flaw in the study design is that the principal investigator is not blinded and she is also assessing the outcome. When "blinding" occurs, it prevents someone involved in the study from knowing the participants' assigned group. In this case, it is possible to recognize who is in the control group and who is in the intervention group, as only the intervention group participants are receiving an oral treatment. It is critical to "blind" the person measuring the outcome to the group assignment of the subject for an unbiased result. This step is especially important when the outcome measure is subjective. One way to "blind" the principal investigator is to have the control participants receive a similar oral placebo. The placebo and the intervention drug would have to be administered by an unblinded investigator who is not involved in the outcome assessment.

To make sure there are consistent evaluations, it is helpful that the principal investigator is consistently involved in assessing the outcome. To strengthen this design, it might be helpful to have multiple persons consistently assess the outcome of interest. For consistency, it is important that all the study participants have joint examinations.

It is not unusual for investigators to recruit patients from their own clinic, as long as the patients are appropriately informed and consented. In addition, the study should be approved by an institutional review board.

In many randomized controlled trials, randomization occurs at a 1:1 ratio. As a result, half of the study participants will be randomized to the intervention group.

(Chapter 2: Decision-Making in Pediatrics: Use of Evidence-Based Medicine; Critical Appraisal of the Evidence)

# CHAPTER 27 Patient Safety

Whitney Chadwick

**27-1.** What is the largest single category of adverse events due to medical error experienced by hospitalized pediatric patients?

**A.** Surgical site infections

**B.** Central line–associated blood stream infections

**C.** Catheter-associated urinary tract infections (UTIs)

**D.** Ventilator-associated pneumonia

**E.** Adverse drug events

**27-2.** Kevin, a 6-year-old patient with cerebral palsy and a seizure disorder, is admitted for pneumonia. Shortly after admission, he is found unresponsive in his bed. You discover that he received a dose 5-fold greater than his usual home clonazepam antiepileptic medication. Kevin's father reports that he told the pediatric resident who admitted him that Kevin takes 10 mL of clonazepam 3 times daily; however, the hospital pharmacy formulary only stocks clonazepam at 0.5 mg/mL, but Kevin's outpatient pharmacy compounds clonazepam at 0.1 mg/mL. Which of the following factors contributed most significantly to this error?

**A.** Kevin had already missed his evening medications while waiting to be admitted from the emergency department, and his father asked the team to "rush" to get his medications so he could go to sleep.

**B.** Kevin's bedside nurse did not confirm the dose of the medication with the father prior to administering the clonazepam.

**C.** The pediatric resident did not confirm each aspect of the medication signature with Kevin's father and at least one other source.

**D.** The understaffed inpatient pharmacist quickly verified Kevin's admission medication orders without double checking the clonazepam dose.

**E.** Sound-a-like medications (clonazepam and clobazam) resulted in false reassurance when the pediatric resident mistakenly checked the dose range for clobazam instead of clonazepam in her reference manual.

**27-3.** You are the first physician to respond to a rapid response page placed by the charge nurse on the acute pediatric ward in your hospital. The patient is a 3-year-old girl whose medical history is unknown to you. The child appears unresponsive, with vitals on her bedside monitor showing a heart rate of 154 bpm, blood pressure of 87/43 mm Hg, respiratory rate of 28 breaths/min, and oxygen saturation of 94% on room air. Which structured communication by the bedside nurse should you ask for to aid in the urgent assessment and management of this patient?

**A.** Closed-loop communication

**B.** Situation–background–assessment–recommendation (SBAR)

**C.** Critical language

**D.** Huddle

**E.** Debrief

**27-4.** Lana, a 2-year-old patient with trisomy 21 and congenital heart disease, is hospitalized for failure to thrive and nasogastric tube placement for initiation of supplemental feeding overnight. Rishi, her nurse, is taking care of 3 other patients, one of whom had a prolonged seizure this shift and was transferred to the pediatric intensive care unit. Distracted, Rishi bustles into Lana's room with her evening medication doses in 3 enteral syringes and attempts to interlock the first enteral syringe with Lana's peripheral intravenous (IV) line. He quickly realizes the syringe and IV are not compatible and then correctly administers Lana's medications through her nasogastric tube. Which error prevention strategy most contributed to prevention of Lana receiving her enteral medications through her IV?

**A.** Standardization

**B.** Simplification

**C.** Visual controls

**D.** Forcing functions

**E.** Redundancies

**27-5.** Ryan, a 3-day-old male infant born at 33 weeks and 2 days of gestational age, is under your care in the intermediate care nursery for prematurity and neonatal sepsis due to group B *Streptococcus* bacteremia. You discover on monitoring labs today that he has a serum total bilirubin of 23 mg/dL and immediately start triple bank phototherapy and consult neonatology for exchange transfusion. In reviewing how the patient's bilirubin level had become so elevated, you find the following:

- A total bilirubin was drawn at 6 hours of life with the complete blood count (CBC) and blood culture ordered at the time of Ryan's first fever, instead of at 24 hours of life, your hospital's standard.
- The bilirubin was 6 mg/dL at that time, a concerning level, but it was not "flagged" as abnormal in your electronic health record, which only flags neonatal total bilirubin levels higher than 8 mg/dL.
- The nurse caring for the infant at 24 hours of life spent most of his shift tending to acute issues for 2 other infants and so did not catch that the 24-hour total bilirubin order was missing (as it had already been completed ahead of schedule).
- The nurse practitioner caring for the infant on days of life 2 and 3 was new to the neonatal intensive care unit and unaware of the policy to perform a total bilirubin at 24 hours or that sepsis and prematurity both put the infant at high risk for hyperbilirubinemia.

Which of the following was most significant in causing this adverse event?

**A.** Complex system with multiple latent failures
**B.** Inadequate clinician knowledge
**C.** Inadequate nurse staffing
**D.** Technology failure
**E.** Equipment failure

**27-6.** Dr. Wu, an anesthesiologist, administered a dose of dexmedetomidine to her patient at the end of a simple otorhinolaryngology procedure when she intended to administer dexamethasone for antinausea effect. The large dose of dexmedetomidine resulted in bradycardia, hypotension, and prolonged sedation. Dr. Wu, deeply ashamed, realizes her mistake and submits a safety event report.

On scrutiny of the medication cart, "dexmedetomidine" and "dexamethasone" vials are both in 10-mL clear glass vials with purple labels located next to each other. The chief anesthesiologist reviews the event with the local improvement team, and they determine that any other anesthesiologist working in that room could have just as easily made that mistake, commend Dr. Wu for event reporting, and restructure the medication carts to separate the 2 look-a-like, sound-a-like medications. What leadership strategy most likely contributed to the appropriate accountability displayed in this case?

**A.** Critical language
**B.** Psychological safety
**C.** Transparency and visibility
**D.** Continuous learning
**E.** Substitution test

**27-7.** You are the physician in a multidisciplinary patient safety group focused on improving medication safety in your hospital. You have had a recent spike in admission medication reconciliation errors and have received hospital funding to incorporate pharmacy technicians performing medication histories at admission as an evidence-based intervention to improve medication reconciliation accuracy. What will likely be the most critical step to ensuring success of your new intervention?

**A.** Requiring all hospital staff to complete an online module educating them on the new pharmacy technician medication reconciliation process
**B.** Developing hospital policies and training manuals to use to teach the pharmacy technicians how to perform medication reconciliation
**C.** Obtaining approval and input from key stakeholders in the design and implementation of pharmacy technician medication reconciliation
**D.** Ensuring appropriate access for pharmacy technicians to view and document in the electronic medical record, as well as flags to note when pharmacy medication reconciliation is incomplete, in progress, and completed
**E.** Implementing pharmacy technician medication reconciliation in a single ward while frequently collecting and analyzing data used to make prompt changes in the process

**27-8.** You are a primary care physician in a medium-sized urban practice. Several patient families have recently filed complaints with your office around prolonged wait times before seeing a doctor. You know the clinic has had long wait times for years, and this is a source of frustration for staff and families alike. You form a team with your immunization nurse, a medical assistant who rooms patients, and the front desk clerk to take a closer look at the problem. You also obtain the support of the clinic leadership team to proceed with improvement work. What is the ideal order of the steps below for your improvement project?

1. Show special cause variation on your control chart and sustain improvement for 6 months.
2. Create a key driver diagram.

3. Perform multiple plan-do-study-act (PDSA) cycles.
4. Test your first countermeasure on a small scale.
5. Create a process map of current clinic flow.

**A.** 5, 2, 4, 3, 1
**B.** 5, 4, 3, 2, 1
**C.** 2, 5, 4, 3, 1
**D.** 2, 5, 1, 4, 3
**E.** 1, 5, 4, 3, 2

**27-9.** You are the physician manager in a large pediatric primary care group with 25 physicians. You have sensed some tension from staff about the group's newest hire, Dr. Dunn. Over the course of 6 months, staff inform you of several events, the most recent of which include the following:

- While on call, Dr. Dunn did not respond to repeated pages from the triage nurse for over an hour regarding a patient for whom the triage nurse was concerned. When Dr. Dunn did respond, he said "Sorry. I wanted to catch the end of the inning, and I could tell from your pages it wasn't a real emergency."
- After seeing a family who refuses to vaccinate their 3 small children after their eldest was diagnosed with autism, Dr. Dunn walked out of the room and mumbled to the medical assistant, "Some people are just idiots. How many times do we need to prove that vaccines don't cause autism?"
- Performing a circumcision in the clinic's procedure room, the nurse assisting with the procedure requested to perform a time out before starting. Dr. Dunn said, "For just the two of us? That's overkill," and proceeded to start the procedure without performing a time out.

You are aware that one of Dr. Dunn's colleagues, Dr. Wickrema, has spoken with Dr. Dunn about his behavior informally. You have also spoken to Dr. Dunn briefly to express concern after the circumcision event, but the unprofessional behavior has still continued. What is the next best step in addressing Dr. Dunn's behavior?

**A.** Have an informal, nonjudgmental conversation with Dr. Dunn to make him aware of the reports and to hear his side of the story.
**B.** Schedule a formal meeting to set behavioral expectations, demonstrate prior deficiencies, and develop an accountability plan moving forward.
**C.** Do nothing as long as Dr. Dunn's patients continue to have good outcomes and provide glowing feedback.
**D.** Assign Dr. Dunn extra holiday and weekend calls as punishment for the behavior.
**E.** Terminate Dr. Dunn, effective immediately.

**27-10.** Jasmine is a 4-year-old girl with acute myeloid leukemia admitted for chemotherapy. Weekly electrocardiograms have demonstrated a persistently prolonged QTc interval, which has been documented in her lengthy daily progress note, and attention has been paid to ensuring her serum electrolytes are followed and her cardiac rhythm is monitored.

Tonight, Jasmine's nurse, Jack, is caring for 3 complex oncology patients on his night shift, all of whom are receiving multiple infusions and are on monitors. Jack receives an intravenous (IV) pump or monitor alarm notification every few minutes—most of which signify benign events such as a patient pulling off their monitors to use the bathroom or bending their elbow and kinking off their IV infusion. Jack receives a few alert notifications for "arrhythmia" from Jasmine's room amid the other notifications, but the alarms seem to resolve after a couple minutes, so Jack chalks it up to intermittent sinus tachycardia with vomiting.

Two hours later, the charge nurse calls a code blue to Jasmine's room after noting a sustained run of ventricular tachycardia on the central monitors. On review of her cardiac monitors, the prior alerts Jack received were for intermittent torsades de pointes. What factor played the most significant role in the delayed detection of Jasmine's arrhythmia?

**A.** Automation bias
**B.** Note bloat
**C.** Staff burnout
**D.** Alarm fatigue
**E.** Poor interoperability

## ANSWERS

**Answer 27-1.** E

In 1999, the Institute of Medicine (IOM) estimated in their seminal report, *To Err Is Human*, that between 44,000 and 98,000 deaths occur annually in the United States due to medical errors, with an estimate of 7000 deaths annually attributed to medication errors. In the IOM's 2007 report, *Preventing Medication Errors: Quality Chasm Series*, they estimated that 400,000 preventable adverse drug events occur annually in US hospitals. Medication errors are the most prevalent type of iatrogenic adverse events in US health care.

Medication errors can occur at any point in the manufacturing, prescribing, or administration of a medication to a patient.

Pediatric patients are particularly vulnerable to medication errors because of the calculations required for weight-based dosing, developing organ systems, and decreased ability to report side effects or self-advocate. Some studies have suggested that pediatric patients experience up to 3-fold more adverse drug events compared to adults. In 2010, the Centers for Medicare and Medicaid Services (CMS) estimated the incidence of hospital-acquired conditions in the United States to be as follows: adverse drug events, 1,900,000/year; catheter-associated UTIs, 530,000/year; central line–associated blood stream infections, 40,000/year; surgical site infections, 110,000/year; and ventilator-associated pneumonia, 40,000/year.

(Frush KS, Krug SE. Pediatric medication safety, in *Pediatric Patient Safety and Quality Improvement.* New York, NY: McGraw-Hill; 2015.)

**References**

1. Kohn LT, Corrigan J, Donaldson MS. *To Err Is Human: Building a Safer Health System.* Washington, DC: National Academy Press; 2000.
2. Aspden P, Wolcott JA, Bootman JL, Cronenwett LR. *Preventing Medication Errors: Quality Chasm Series.* Washington, DC: National Academy Press; 2007.
3. Kaushal R, Bates DW, Landrigan C, et al. Medication errors and adverse drug events in pediatric inpatients. *JAMA.* 2001;285:2114-2120.
4. Ferranti J, Horvath M, Cozart H, et al. Reevaluating the safety profile of pediatrics: a comparison of computerized adverse drug event surveillance and voluntary reporting in the pediatric environment. *Pediatrics.* 2008;121:1201-1207.
5. Agency for Healthcare Research and Quality. *2013 Annual Hospital-Acquired Condition Rate and Estimates of Cost Savings and Deaths Averted From 2010 to 2013.* Rockville, MD: Agency for Healthcare Research and Quality; October 2015. AHRQ Publication No. 16-0006-EF. http://www.ahrq.gov/professionals/qualitypatient-safety/pfp/index.htm. Accessed November 18, 2020.

**Answer 27-2. C**

Multiple factors contribute to the complexity of patient care, including staff, workflows, social or psychological environments, physical environments, technology, equipment, patients' family members, and of course the patients themselves. Many obstacles can impact the safe prescribing and administration of medications to hospitalized patients, including fatigue, burnout, understaffing, missed safety checks, and sound-a-like or look-a-like drug names; however, the absence of a complete and accurate medication reconciliation process was the most significant contributor to this patient's overdose.

Admission medication reconciliation is the process by which a clinician obtains a medication history from the patient or guardian, reconciles that history with any existing/available records for the patient, and then decides to continue, hold, or adjust home medications during the patient's ongoing inpatient care. When done properly, a medication history should confirm each aspect of the medication signature (name, formulation, dosage, route, frequency, and indication) with the patient or patient representative and then confirm again with a second source (eg, electronic health record medication list, clinic documentation, pharmacy records, pill bottles brought from home). Medication histories should also probe for easily forgotten medications, such as over-the-counter medications, medications given infrequently, or medications taken by nonenteral routes.

(Frush KS, Krug SE. Pediatric medication safety, in *Pediatric Patient Safety and Quality Improvement.* New York, NY: McGraw-Hill; 2015.)

**Answer 27-3. B**

Effective communication is critical for delivering high-quality care when a patient has an acute deterioration. The SBAR structured communication format rapidly conveys critical information to healthcare workers receiving information about a situation and supports executive thinking by the team member formulating the SBAR, all of which promotes rapid and effective care of the patient.

| SBAR Component | Description |
|---|---|
| Situation | The statement that describes the problem and gets the attention of the receiver |
| Background | The historical and situational context needed to understand the situation |
| Assessment | The team member's analysis of the facts and clinical scenario; however, in complex situations with uncertainty, the team member may simply state what is specifically concerning and that the current situation is unexplained |
| Recommendation | The team member's suggested plan of action for the patient |

Closed-loop communication, or repeat back, is another structured communication tool used to ensure transmission of the correct information between transmitter and receiver. For example, for an actively seizing patient, a physician might verbally request the nurse administer "half a milligram of lorazepam intravenous (IV)," and the nurse could use closed-loop communication to say, "Confirming you want zero-point-five milligrams of lorazepam IV?"

Critical language is a statement used by a healthcare worker, and is understood as a critical signal by staff across the institution, to communicate concern for a perceived or potential risk to a patient's safety. Example phrases include, "I need clarity" and "I have a concern."

Huddles promote situational awareness and contingency planning by bringing teams together to discuss the plan for the shift, unit, or patient, with anticipation of factors such as being short staffed, high-acuity patients, or equipment failures.

Debriefs promote continuous learning by bringing teams together after a routine or emergency event to discuss what went well, what did not go well, and what they should do differently next time.

(Frush KS, Krug SE. The role of leadership in safe and reliable pediatric care, in *Pediatric Patient Safety and Quality Improvement*. New York, NY: McGraw-Hill; 2015.)

**Answer 27-4. D**

Forcing functions are one of the most powerful error-reduction strategies for promoting safe, high-quality care because they make it impossible to do the wrong thing, such as connecting an enteral syringe to a peripheral IV hub. Forcing function examples exist outside of medicine as well, such as not being able to turn on a car engine without having a foot on the brake or automatic teller machines (ATMs) that will not dispense your cash withdrawal until you have removed your ATM card.

Standardization is an important error-reduction strategy in which workflows, roles/responsibilities, or equipment are standardized. Examples include stocking code carts located across the hospital in exactly the same way, such that any respiratory therapist responding to an emergency event anywhere in the hospital will know where in the cart to locate intubation supplies.

Simplification is another important error-reduction strategy. Simplifying workflows to decrease the cognitive strain on clinicians' limited mental resources whenever possible leaves clinicians with more bandwidth to process the many complexities of providing health care that cannot be simplified. A simplification may be to bundle all the necessary supplies for a lumbar puncture procedure into a single kit.

Visual controls, another error-reduction strategy, uses visual cues and signals to bring healthcare worker focus to a goal behavior or process. Examples include brightly colored stations for hand washing or isolation signage on the patient's door indicating mask, gown, and gloves are required before entering.

Redundancies are independent safety measures put in place to ensure critical errors do not occur. For instance, to ensure a hospitalized patient does not receive a medication to which she has had a documented allergic reaction, most electronic health records will alert the provider at the time of prescribing, the pharmacist at the point of dispensing, and the nurse at the point of administering; in addition, the patient may wear a red "allergy" wristband to further alert the nurse to perform manual double checks before administering any medications.

(Frush KS, Krug SE. Medical errors, adverse events, and human factors, in *Pediatric Patient Safety and Quality Improvement*. New York, NY: McGraw-Hill; 2015.)

**Answer 27-5. A**

The question scenario is a perfect example of James Reason's Swiss-cheese model of accident causation. In the Swiss-cheese model, multiple slices of cheese stacked on top of each other represent the layers in a healthcare system that act as barriers to prevent errors from reaching patients and causing harm. The holes in the cheese represent the active and latent failures in these barriers. Latent failures are often routinely present factors, such as poor equipment design, inadequate modes of communication, and budget constraints. Active failures are errors or violations committed by individuals within the system. When the holes align, a triggering event or error can penetrate all the layers of defense, reaching the patient and causing harm.

In this example, inadequate clinician knowledge (trainee new to neonatology), inadequate nurse staffing (nurse with high-acuity patients), and technology failures (electronic health record not "flagging" an abnormal value) were all latent failures. When these latent failures combined with the active failure of the nurse drawing the 24-hour total bilirubin several hours too early, this resulted in patient harm.

(Frush KS, Krug SE. Medical Errors, Adverse Events, and Human Factors, in *Pediatric Patient Safety and Quality Improvement*. New York, NY: McGraw-Hill; 2015.)

**Answer 27-6. E**

The chief anesthesiologist and local improvement team displayed use of the substitution test—asking whether healthcare workers with similar training would have behaved in similar ways or made similar mistakes. When the substitution test demonstrates that other healthcare workers would have acted similarly as the healthcare worker in question (Dr. Wu), it indicates that a simple human error has occurred, attributable in large part to inadequacies in the system surrounding the healthcare worker.

In an organization with a "just culture" or "appropriate accountability," an understanding of system complexity and human factors is used to evaluate healthcare workers involved in medical errors (see following figure). In a just culture, a team evaluating the decision-making of a healthcare worker must determine whether his or her actions were reckless (lack of consideration of risks), risky (flawed decision-making, inappropriate estimation of risk), or a simple error (appropriate clinical decisions made, but a human error occurred). It is important for the team evaluating the staff member involved in the adverse event to primarily evaluate the decisions and actions made by the staff member, without consideration of harm that may (or may not have) come to the patient. Staff with impaired judgement (mental illness, substance use) or malicious intent are excluded from the appropriate accountability algorithm and evaluated separately.

Critical language is a statement used by a healthcare worker, and is understood as a critical signal by staff across the institution, to communicate concern for a perceived or potential risk to a patient's safety. Example phrases include "I need clarity" and "I have a concern."

Psychological safety is established in a team when all team members are willing to speak up or ask questions without fear of psychological injury or negative consequences to current position or future opportunities. Institutions with just culture or appropriate accountability promote psychological safety.

| The fair evaluation and response chart | | |
|---|---|---|
| **How to use this chart:** This chart should be used to categorize an individual caregiver's actions, not groups or systems. Evaluate each factor that influenced the caregiver's actions separately. When determining accountability, consider the context in which the action occurred. | | |
| 1. First, exclude individuals with impaired judgement or whose actions might be malicious. (These cases must be managed using other appropriate avenues, ie, employee assistance programs for substance abuse and psychosocial problems, legal authorities for cases with possible criminal intent) | | |
| **Impaired judgment**<br>The caregiver's thinking was impaired<br>- by illegal or legal substances<br>- by cognitive impairment<br>- by severe psychosocial stressors | **Malicious action**<br>The caregiver wanted to cause harm. | |
| • Discipline is warranted if illegal substances were used.<br>• The caregiver's mindset and performance should be evaluated to determine whether a temporary work suspension would be helpful.<br>• Help should be actively offered to the caregiver. | • Discipline and/or legal proceedings are warranted.<br>• The caregiver's duties should be suspended immediately. | |
| 2. Second, use best judgement to categorize each action as either reckless, risky, or unintentional based on the definitions in the chart. The categorization determines the general level of culpability and possible disciplinary actions; however, these general categories require further analysis as below prior to making a final decision. | | |
| **Reckless action**<br>The caregiver knowingly violated a rule and/or made a dangerous or unsafe choice. The decision appears to be self-serving and to have been made with little or no concern about risk. | **Risky action**<br>The caregiver made a potentially unsafe choice. Their evaluation of relative risk appears to be erroneous. | **Unintentional error**<br>The caregiver made or participated in an error while working appropriately and in the patients' best interests. |
| • The caregiver is accountable and needs re-training. Discipline may be warranted.<br>• The caregiver should participate in teaching others the lessons learned. | • The caregiver is accountable and should receive coaching.<br>• The caregiver should participate in teaching others the lessons learned. | • The caregiver is not accountable.<br>• The caregiver should participate in investigating why the error occurred and teach others about the results of the investigation. |
| 3. Third, perform a substitution test by asking at least three others with similar skills if they, in a similar situation, would act similarly, if the answer is "No" the individual is accountable. If "We do it all the time" system influence is substantial. If the answer are divided, evaluators should assign accountability with a goal to ensure perceptions of fairness by others. | | |
| The system supports reckless action and requires fixing. The caregiver is probably less accountable for the action, and system leaders share in the accountability. | The system supports risky action and requires fixing. The caregiver is probably less accountable for the action, and system leaders share in the accountability. | The system supports error and requires fixing. The system's leaders are accountable and should apply error-proofing improvements. |
| 4. Fourth, evaluate whether the individual has a history of unsafe or problematic acts. If they do, this may influence decisions about the appropriate responsibilities for the individual, ie, they may be in the wrong job. Organizations should have a reasonable and agreed-upon statute of limitations for taking these actions into account. | | |

The fair evaluation and response chart. (Reproduced from Frush KS, Krug SE. The role of leadership in safe and reliable pediatric care, in *Pediatric Patient Safety and Quality Improvement*. New York, NY: McGraw-Hill; 2015.)

**Answer 27-7.** E

While staff education, policies, key stakeholder approval, and technical support can all aid the implementation of a new quality improvement project, rapid cycle testing is critical to success. Starting with a small scope that widens as the intervention is refined through rapid cycle testing is also key to being able to minimize any potential harms caused by an untested intervention and optimize the intervention more quickly and efficiently with a small pilot team.

The model for improvement, developed by Associates in Process Improvement (API), has 2 key components: (1) answering 3 key questions, followed by (2) rapid cycle testing using plan-do-study-act (PDSA) cycles. The 3 questions each improvement team should answer at the start of their improvement journey are "What are we trying to accomplish?" "How will we know that a change is an improvement?" and "What change can we make that will result in improvement?" The team can then test the proposed changes using cycles of planning a change, implementing the change, studying the effects of the change, and then acting on lessons learned from each PDSA cycle to inform subsequent cycles until the team's improvement goal has been reached.

(Frush KS, Krug SE. Quality improvement methods and improvement science, in *Pediatric Patient Safety and Quality Improvement*. New York, NY: McGraw-Hill; 2015.)

**Answer 27-8.** A

The first steps in an improvement project are to identify the process that you would like to improve and form a team to do the improvement work. Improvement teams typically are multidisciplinary, with representation of all of the professions involved in the process targeted for improvement, as well as team members who will likely be integral for developing countermeasures. The team should also identify key stakeholders—those who can help facilitate your improvement work through access to resources and those who could be impacted (positively or negatively) by your improvement work—to collaborate with and support the effort.

The next step in an improvement project is to understand the existing process, also called a current state analysis. This step can involve creating a process map, observing the clinical process in real time from multiple perspectives, collecting data on current error rates or inefficiencies, and speaking with front-line workers to better understand current barriers to achieving a goal process. A process map diagrams out the clinical process in question in an improvement project, showing each step chronologically in fine detail, so that steps with high variability, poor quality, or frequent delays can be readily identified and targeted for intervention.

Following a current state analysis, an improvement team can now begin to brainstorm potential interventions, or countermeasures. Creating a key driver diagram is helpful in this process. A key driver diagram starts with a SMART aim (the specific, measurable, action-oriented, realistic, and time-bound aim of your quality improvement work, which may have been developed before or after your current state analysis) and then details the key drivers, or the factors that need to "go right" to accomplish your SMART aim (eg, patients have vitals complete and placed in clinic room by 5 minutes after appointment start time). Once several key drivers are identified, the team can brainstorm possible countermeasures to try for each one (eg, station a medical assistant at the front desk to perform vitals on patients during check in to the clinic).

Finally, the team is ready to start testing their countermeasures. The model for improvement recommends starting to implement countermeasures on a small scale, such as with just a few patients on one afternoon. The pilot size can be grown as the intervention is shown to be effective through ongoing data collection and analysis on rapid cycle testing (PDSA cycles). The primary outcome metric(s) for the project (clinic wait times in our example) should be mapped on a run chart over time. Statistical process control (SPC) charts are a specific type of run chart that include a mean line, as well as upper and lower control limits at 3 standard deviations above and below the mean. An SPC chart can visually show when the outcome metric displayed has changed significantly, more so than would be expected from usual variation in the process, and this is termed *special cause variation*. Data collection should continue, and the SPC chart should be maintained for months after the team achieves improvements to continue to ensure the improvements are sustained or to identify and address any lapses that may occur.

(Frush KS, Krug SE. Applying quality improvement in practice, in *Pediatric Patient Safety and Quality Improvement*. New York, NY: McGraw-Hill; 2015.)

**Answer 27-9.** B

Professional behavior from all healthcare workers is essential to nurture the mutual respect and trust needed for a team to provide high-quality care. Unprofessional behavior causes team dysfunction and can negatively impact the safety culture; staff may be less willing to report safety events, speak up when they see a safety event in progress, or even be so distracted by workplace tensions that they are more likely to commit errors themselves. The healthcare organization is responsible for ensuring adequate professionalism policies, confidential reporting systems, and a consistent track record of acting in situations of verified unprofessional behavior. Leaders within healthcare organizations are responsible for addressing behavior. The Promoting Professionalism Pyramid (PPP) is a validated model for graduated interventions to address unprofessional behavior. The PPP recommends informal "cup of coffee" conversations to discuss single, unprofessional incidents (see following figure).

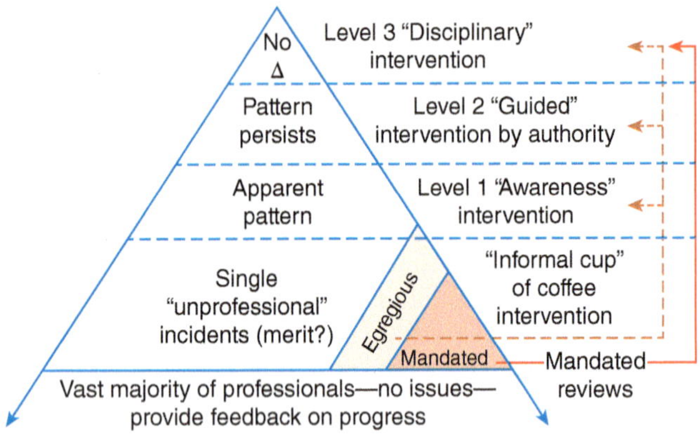


Promoting professionalism pyramid. (Adapted, with permission, from Hickson GB, Pichert JW, Webb LE, et al. A complementary approach to promoting professionalism: identifying, measuring, and addressing unprofessional behaviors. *Acad Med.* 2007;82:1040-1048.)

For persistent unprofessional behavior, the PPP recommends an "awareness" intervention—a formal meeting with a leader or a trained member of the peer review committee to ensure the staff member knows the administration is aware of their unprofessional behavior. When there is an obvious pattern of behavior that does not improve after informal "cup of coffee" or formal "awareness" interventions, a formal "guided" intervention with an authority figure is recommended. In the "guided" intervention, an authority figure sits down with the staff member and reviews the administration's *e*xpectations, reviews the staff member's behavioral *d*eficiencies, creates an *i*ntervention (or accountability action plan) with the staff member, and reviews *c*onsequences for ongoing unprofessional behavior, as well as the *t*imeline for improvement and plan for ongoing *s*urveillance. The acronym EDICTS is useful for remembering the critical components for this meeting structure. Dr. Dunn, having not responded to the "cup of coffee" and "awareness" conversations, currently requires a "guided" intervention for his persistent unprofessional behavior. If Dr. Dunn does not improve following the "guided" intervention, the next step will be disciplinary action. Of course, some unprofessional behavior requires automatic disciplinary action, either as mandated by institutional policies or law (eg, Health Insurance Portability and Accountability Act violations) or if the behavior is truly egregious (eg, physically striking a coworker).

(Frush KS, Krug SE. Professional accountability and pursuit of a culture of safety, in *Pediatric Patient Safety and Quality Improvement*. New York, NY: McGraw-Hill; 2015.)

**Answer 27-10. D**

Jack has become desensitized to the myriad of alarms in his unit, whether from patient monitors, infusion pumps, or the electronic health record. As many alarms are clinically inconsequential, Jack has begun to disregard them in his clinical work, resulting in an inadequate response to an alarm signaling impending patient deterioration. This concept is called *alarm fatigue* or *alert fatigue* and is the most significant factor in the delayed detection of Jasmine's arrhythmia.

Automation bias describes the tendency for humans to over-rely on automatically generated decisions or recommendations, such as a dose recommendation made by the electronic health record for high-dose amoxicillin when treating streptococcal pharyngitis when low-dose amoxicillin is more appropriate.

Note bloat refers to overdocumentation in the clinical setting or the documentation of excess nonessential information. Note bloat has been attributed to autopopulated fields, copy-forwarded text, and bulky note templates created to support the highest level of billing possible. Note bloat can lead to patient harm by perpetuating inaccurate or outdated information and obscuring key/essential information.

Burnout is a syndrome of emotional exhaustion or depletion, depersonalization or cynicism, and a sense of ineffectiveness or lack of achievement. Burnout occurs at high rates in health care, as well as other human service industries (eg, teaching). Burnout occurs more often in work environments with heavy workloads, low autonomy, insufficient recognition, poor relationships or low sense of community, and when work is not felt by staff to be fulfilling or meaningful.

Interoperability refers to the ability of computer systems (particularly electronic health records) to exchange information. Poor interoperability can result in patient harm when multiple providers for a single patient are not able to access all the requisite health records to provide care for the patient.

(Frush KS, Krug SE. The importance of information technology in pediatric patient safety, in *Pediatric Patient Safety and Quality Improvement*. New York, NY: McGraw-Hill; 2015.)

# CHAPTER 28 Quality Improvement

Keith J. Robinson

**28-1.** You would like to conduct a quality improvement project to reduce the wait time for patients to register in your clinic. Before assembling your improvement team, you believe the best way to reduce the wait time is to change the registration process. What is the best approach to ensure that the change is an improvement?

**A.** Test the new registration process on a small number of patients

**B.** Change the registration process for all patients

**C.** Form a team that understands the registration process from various perspectives

**D.** Develop an electronic monitoring system to track wait times

**E.** Observe the current registration process yourself

**28-2.** You are improving the care of children with asthma by using improved education. You realize that changing one component of care may affect other components of care, either positively or negatively. Which of the following outlines the elements of the Institute for Healthcare Improvement (IHI) Triple Aim to help guide the consideration of the effect of other components with any intervention?

**A.** Experience of care, per capita cost, and population health

**B.** Outcome measures, process measures, and balancing measures

**C.** Health outcomes, administrative burden, and public health

**D.** Healthcare utilization, patient satisfaction, and patient safety

**E.** Standardized processes, patient engagement, and medication cost

**28-3.** Your practice is engaging in an accountable care organization (ACO). As a partner in the ACO, you are asked to improve the health of children with asthma in your clinic by completing asthma action plans at health supervision visits. The completion of asthma action plans is an example of which of the following?

**A.** Process measure

**B.** Outcome measure

**C.** Patient experience

**D.** Structure

**E.** Balancing measure

**28-4.** You are reviewing data from an improvement project to increase completion of asthma action plans at well-child visits to a goal of 70%. Which of the following graphs best represents significant and sustained improvement following your intervention during a Plan-Do-Study-Act (PDSA) cycle?

**A.**

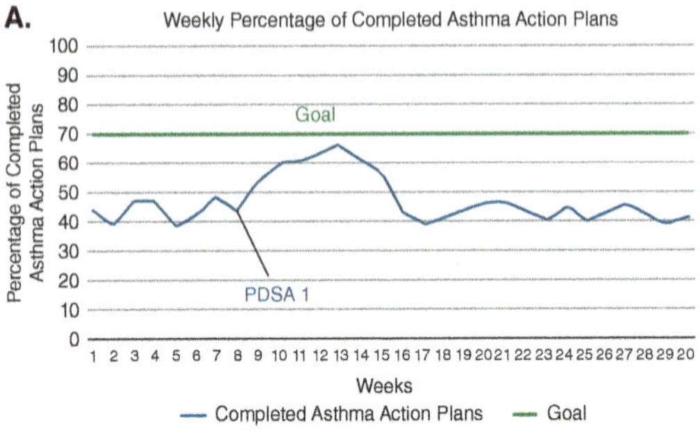


**B.**

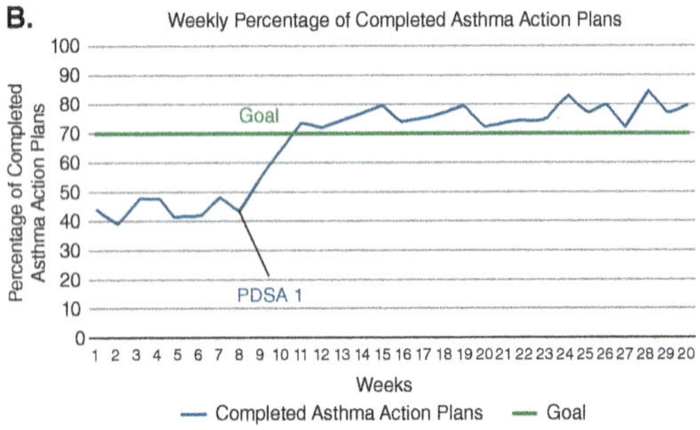


**C.**

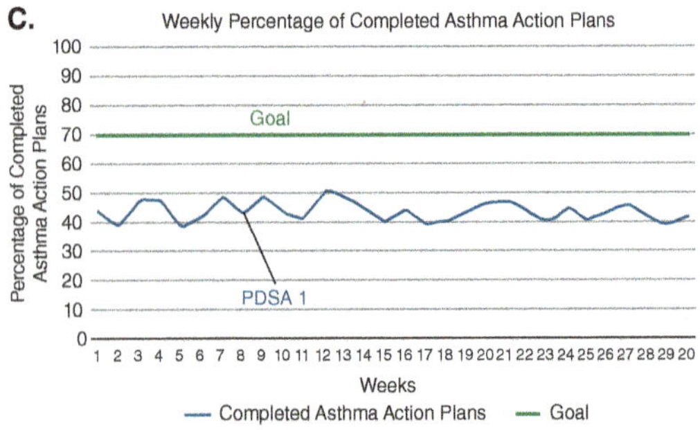


**D.**

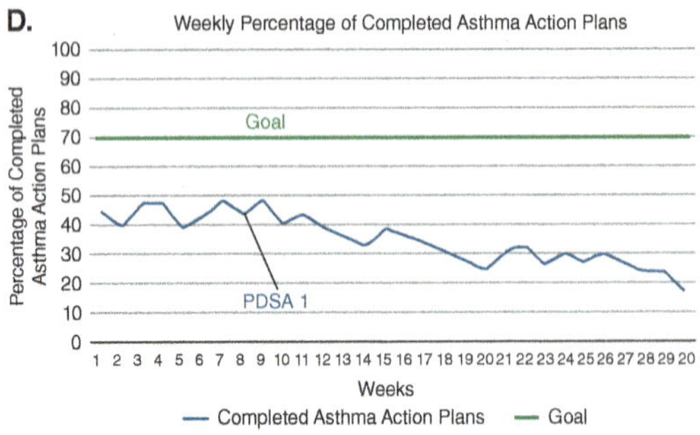


**E.**

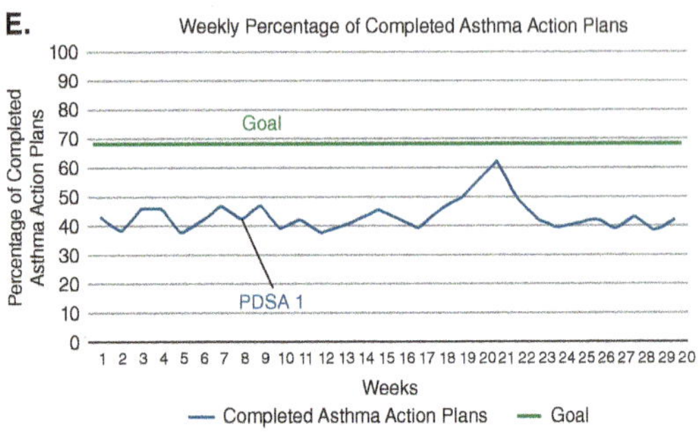


**28-5.** You are conducting a Plan-Do-Study-Act (PDSA) cycle to improve vaccination rates in your clinic. Your team formulates an objective for your next intervention, predicts the result of the intervention, and identifies a data-collection strategy. This work best represents which phase of the PDSA cycle?

**A.** Plan
**B.** Do
**C.** Study
**D.** Act
**E.** Interpret

**28-6.** Your practice is partnering with other practices, local hospitals, and health insurers to improve the health of your community. The partnership is aimed at improving coordination of care and reducing healthcare costs for patients in your health service area. As part of the partnership, your practice will assume part of the financial risk for achieving quality metrics and reducing costs across the service area. This partnership best represents which alternative payment model?

**A.** Value-based purchasing (VBP)
**B.** Accountable care organization (ACO)
**C.** Pay-for-performance
**D.** Hospital network
**E.** Merit-based incentive payment system (MIPS)

**28-7.** Your practice has been asked to transition from a paper medical record to an electronic health record. The goal of the implementation is to promote computer order entry, identify active medications, list drug allergies, and maintain problem lists. Which piece of federal legislation established the criteria for meaningful use of the electronic health record leading to increased payments to providers?

**A.** Children's Health Insurance Program Reauthorization Act (CHIPRA)
**B.** Patient Protection and Affordable Care Act
**C.** American Recovery and Reinvestment Act (ARRA)
**D.** Health Insurance Portability and Accountability Act (HIPAA)
**E.** Health Information Technology for Economic and Clinical Health (HITECH) Act

**28-8.** Your multidisciplinary improvement team would like to implement a new screening tool for social determinants of health for 90% of all well-child visits in the next year. Your practice does not currently screen for social determinants of health and does not have an established process for screening for social determinants of health and offering interventions. When thinking about how to best implement the new screening tool in your practice, what is the next most appropriate step?

**A.** Begin using the screening tool on all patients

**B.** Implement the process from a neighboring practice

**C.** Conduct a Plan-Do-Study-Act (PDSA) cycle using the screening tool on a small number of patients

**D.** Implement the screening tool for certain providers

**E.** Allow each provider to implement their own screening process

**28-9.** You are part of an improvement team to increase use of a standardized admission order set to improve patient safety. Your team is reviewing data from your project after 3 Plan-Do-Study-Act (PDSA) cycles. The chart below is a statistical process control chart (P chart) for your project. Which of the points on the graph below indicates special cause variation?

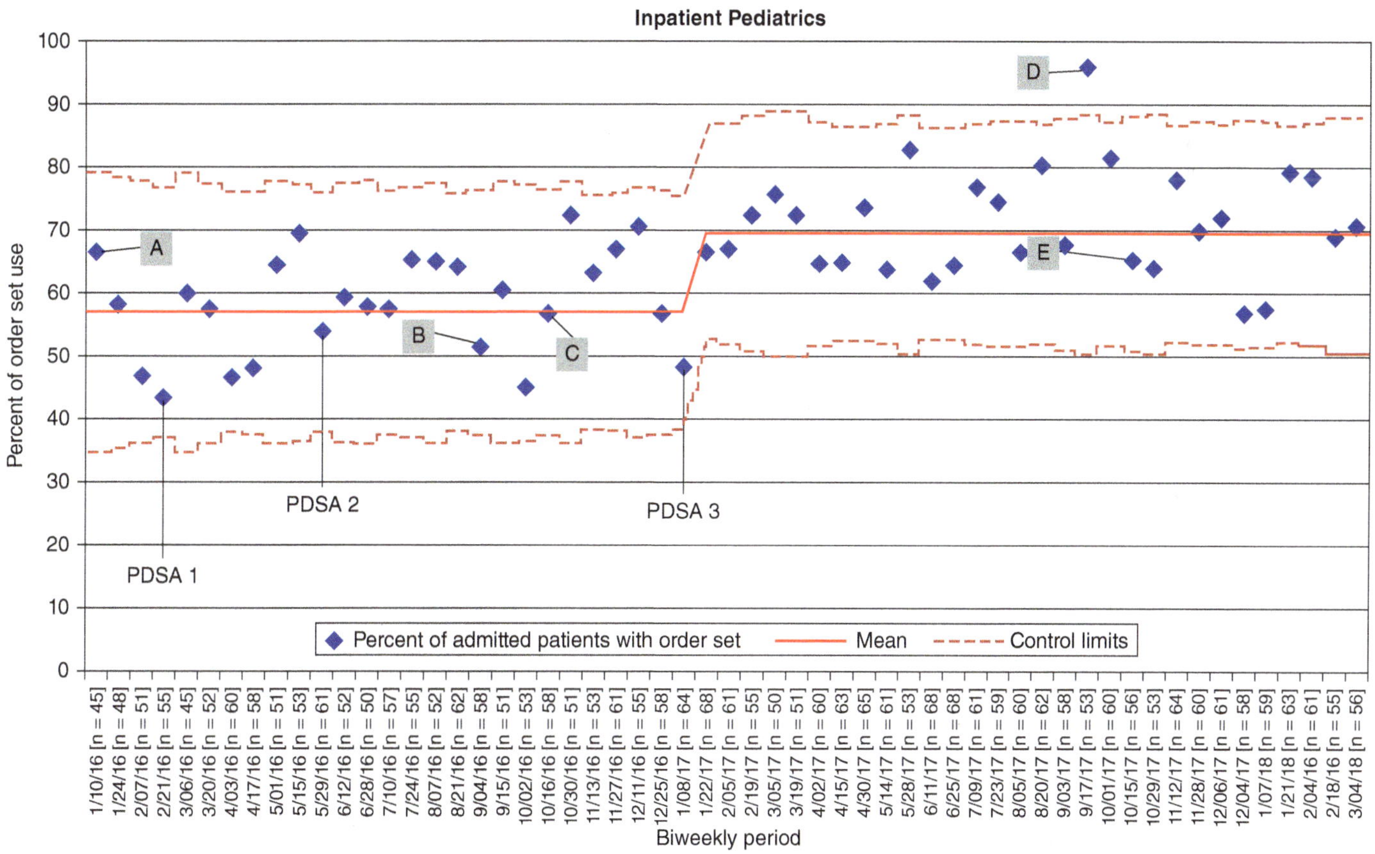


**A.** Point A

**B.** Point B

**C.** Point C

**D.** Point D

**E.** Point E

**28-10.** You are working with your practice administration on an improvement project to increase screening for depression among adolescents. Your project team would like to use the Institute for Healthcare Improvement (IHI) Triple Aim as a framework for your project. Through the course of your project, which of the following would ideally occur that best represents the IHI Triple Aim?

**A.** Cost to treat adolescents with depression decreases

**B.** Provider satisfaction decreases

**C.** A balance of cost per capita, outcome improvement, and population health improvement

**D.** Outcomes for adolescents with depression improve

**E.** Population health measures for adolescents with depression improve

**28-11.** You are leading change in your practice to increase clinical integration to improve the health of the population you serve. Which of the following represents ideal clinical integration for children with asthma?

**A.** Improving your clinic rates of asthma action plans completed at health supervision visits

**B.** Sharing a patient's emergency plan of care with a patient's parent

**C.** Increasing screening for social determinants of health annually

**D.** Working with local emergency medical services to establish a home visiting program for children with recent emergency department visits for asthma

**E.** Completing medication refill history during asthma visits

## ANSWERS

**Answer 28-1.** C

It is important that the project team is certain that a change they make is an improvement in the system. The Institute for Healthcare Improvement (IHI) developed the Model for Improvement (Figure 6-2) that outlines an approach that is analogous to the scientific method.

The first question to ask is "What are we trying to accomplish?" This question provides direction for the improvement team that is further clarified by the question, "How will we know that a change is an improvement?" These 2 critical questions are best answered by an interprofessional team that understands the system to be improved from various perspectives (IHI; Taylor et al, 2014). The power of an interprofessional team should not be underestimated as it frequently leads to more rapid and sustained improvement. Each member of the team involved in the system to be improved will serve as a subject matter expert that will help build the collective knowledge of the system. One should also consider adding a patient and family advisor when conducting improvement projects.

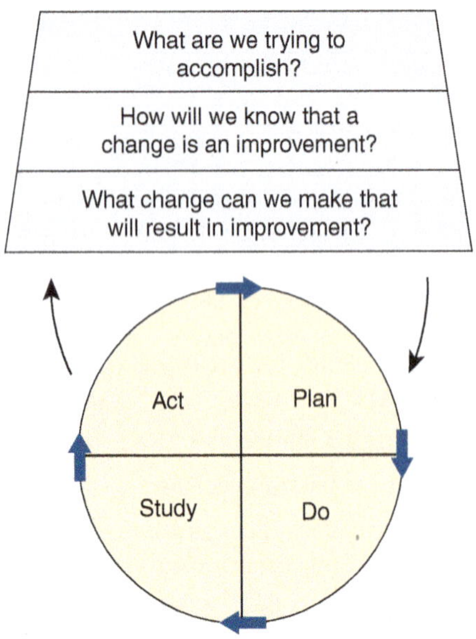


**FIGURE 6-2.** The Plan-Do-Study-Act cycle. (Reproduced with permission from Langley GJ, Moen RD, Nolan KM, et al. *The Improvement Guide: A Practical Approach to Enhancing Organizational Performance*, 2nd ed. San Francisco, CA: Jossey-Bass; 2009.)

The third question is "What change can we make that will result in improvement?" This question leads into the classic Plan-Do-Study-Act (PDSA) cycle. The PDSA cycle or small test of change should occur after a team answers the 3 crucial questions that establish the goals, measurement strategy, and hypothesis development that lead to successful PDSA cycles.

In this vignette, answer choice C is the best answer because the improvement team has not yet been formed to answer the 3 questions in the Model for Improvement and conduct PDSA cycles.

Completing a PDSA cycle (answer choice A) is incorrect because an interprofessional team has not been formed to evaluate the system and develop a set of aims, measures, and a hypothesis for the PDSA cycle. In a similar way, choice B is also incorrect because it represents widespread implementation before thoughtful PDSA cycles have been conducted. In general, interventions should be scaled on a PDSA ramp beginning with a small test of change on a limited number of patients or samples. Data (outcome measures, process measures, balancing measures) should be collected and analyzed by the improvement team to determine if the change is an improvement. The team should then decide if the intervention should be adapted for future tests of change, adopted into the system, or abandoned.

Developing a data strategy is important to the success of an improvement project. However, in this case, it is likely too early to know how to define a "wait time" until a team has been formed and agrees on the goals of the project.

Observing the process (choice E) is critical to success in an improvement project. Ideally, multiple team members would observe the process to gain the richest perspective.

(pp. 20, 21: Part 2: Systems of Care, Chapter 6: US Healthcare System, Efforts to Address Costs and Quality of Care)

**References**

Langley GL, Moen R, Nolan, KM, Nolan TW, Norman CL, Provost LP. *The Improvement Guide: A Practical Approach to Enhancing Organizational Performance*, 2nd ed. San Francisco, CA: Jossey-Bass Publishers; 2009.

Moen RD, Nolan TW, Provost LP. *Quality Improvement Through Planned Experimentation*, 3rd ed. New York, NY: McGraw-Hill; 2012.

Taylor MJ, McNicholas C, Nicolay C, Darzi A, Bell D, Reed JE. Systematic review of the application of the plan-do-study-act method to improve quality in healthcare. *BMJ Qual Saf.* 2014;23:290-298.

**Answer 28-2.** A

The IHI Triple Aim emphasizes the experience of care, per capita cost, and population health (Figure 6-3). Experience of care commonly refers to delivery of care to patients. Often these can be thought of in relation to the Institute of Medicine (IOM) STEEEP measures; the IOM stated that care should be ***s***afe, ***t***imely, ***e***quitable, ***e***fficient, ***e***ffective, and ***p***atient-centered. Examples of these measures include number of central line–acquired bloodstream infections, time to antibiotics for patients experiencing sepsis, access to specialty care, and patient satisfaction questionnaires.

Per capita cost is an important topic for insurance companies, affordable care organizations, and patients. In 2016, the United States spent 17.8% of the gross domestic product on health care. When compared to 10 high-income countries, the United States had similar utilization but spent twice as much to deliver care. Causes for the discrepancy in spending were attributed to administrative costs, labor, and pharmaceuticals.

The definition of population health has been debated for several years. The IHI defines population health as measurable health outcomes for a specific patient population. Examples include mortality, health and functional status, and life expectancy. Kindig and Stoddart (2003) defined population health as "the health outcomes of a group of individuals, including the distribution of such outcomes within the group." Common to both definitions of population health is the idea that we are attempting to define a measurable outcome for a specific group of people that adequately measures their health and well-being.

(pp. 20, 21, Part 2: Systems of Care, Chapter 6: US Healthcare System, Triple Aim)

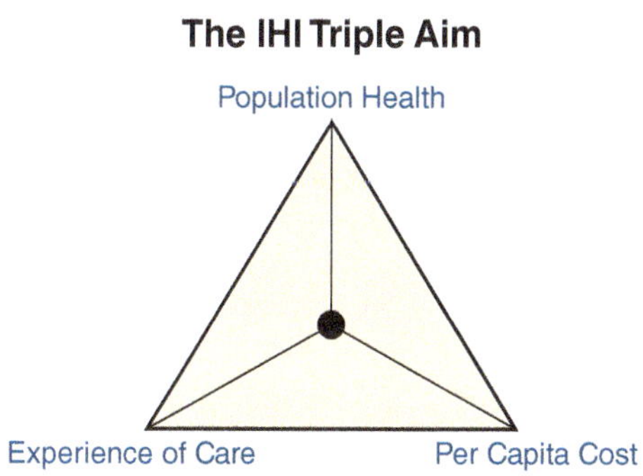


**FIGURE 6-3.** The Triple Aim. (The IHI Triple Aim framework was developed by the Institute for Healthcare Improvement in Massachusetts, USA [IHI.ORG].)

**References**

Institute of Medicine (IOM). *Crossing the Quality Chasm: A New Health System for the 21st Century*. Washington, DC: National Academy Press; 2001.

Kindig D, Stoddart G. What is population health? *Am J Public Health.* 2003;93(3):380-383.

Papanicola I, Woskie LR, Jha AK. Health care spending in the United States and other high-income countries. *JAMA.* 2018;319(10):1024-1039.

Stiefel M, Nolan K. *A Guide to Measuring the Triple Aim: Population Health, Experience of Care, and Per Capita Cost.* IHI Innovation Series white paper. Cambridge, MA: Institute for Healthcare Improvement; 2012.

**Answer 28-3.** A

Process measures assess a step or a procedure that leads to an outcome measure. Process measures are sometimes the "easiest" to achieve because clinicians can often have an immediate and direct impact on them relative to outcome measures. From the provider perspective, examples of process measures include completion of asthma action plans, assessment of asthma control using a validated questionnaire, and education regarding appropriate spacer use. In this vignette, the provider is being asked to complete a step, an asthma action plan, in ideal asthma care according to the National Heart, Lung, and Blood Institute guidelines. Completion of the asthma action plan can measure the provider's individual performance or the clinic system performance relative to this process. In order to construct a meaningful process measure, one must be specific about the attributes of the measure. In this example, the measure only applies to health supervision visits. Consider how the measure would be impacted if the measure also included any acute visit for ankle injuries or headaches. The lack of specificity in the measure would decrease the meaningfulness and usefulness of the measure.

Outcome measures are the result of a system. In the example of a patient with asthma, an example of an outcome measure would be emergency department encounters for asthma exacerbations.

Patient experience can be measured using standardized satisfaction surveys that directly assess a patient's opinion about their healthcare experience. A common example of patient experience surveys is the Consumer Assessment of Healthcare Providers and Systems (CAHPS) program. These anonymous surveys are funded and overseen by the Agency for Healthcare Research and Quality and contain several essential elements of quality such as provider communication and access to health care. Examples can be found at https://www.ahrq.gov/cahps/surveys-guidance/index.html.

Structure is often defined as a change in the system of care or policy.

A balancing measure is an unintended consequence of an improvement project. Balancing measures ensure that our efforts to improve a system do not negatively impact aspects of another system or cause adverse effects. In the example in this question, a balancing measure would be increased time of the physician to complete the asthma action plan. A project team should weigh the increased time to complete the asthma action plan against the value to the patient and care team.

(p. 20, Part 2: Systems of Care, Chapter 6: US Healthcare System, Efforts to Address Costs and Quality of Care)

**References**

Agency for Healthcare Research and Quality. CAHPS Patient Experience Surveys and Guidance. Available at https://www.ahrq.gov/cahps/surveys-guidance/index.html. Accessed December 31, 2019.

Institute for Healthcare Improvement. How to Improve. Available at http://www.ihi.org/resources/pages/howtoimprove/scienceofimprovementestablishingmeasures.aspx. Accessed May 20, 2019.

Langley GL, Moen R, Nolan KM, Nolan TW, Norman CL, Provost LP. *The Improvement Guide: A Practical Approach to Enhancing Organizational Performance*, 2nd ed. San Francisco, CA: Jossey-Bass Publishers; 2009.

Provost LP, Murray SK. *The Health Care Data Guide: Learning From Data for Improvement*. San Francisco, CA: Jossey-Bass Publishers; 2011.

**Answer 28-4. B**

The graphs are examples of run charts, a common tool used to evaluate quality improvement data. Run charts allow an improvement team to display performance data to determine if changes result in an improvement, provide insight into the temporal relationship between interventions and system performance, and to evaluate the sustainability of performance.

The fundamentals of a run chart consist of time on the x-axis and the performance measurement on the y-axis. In this example, weeks are identified on the x-axis, and percentage of completed asthma actions plans are identified on the y-axis. Annotations regarding PDSA cycles and interventions are an important element of run charts that help test theory and identify which interventions have the most impact on the system.

There are several run chart rules that allow improvement teams to determine if the performance changed with statistical significance. The following 2 rules are common examples of a significant change equivalent to a *P* value of .05:

1. 6 or more consecutive points all above or all below the median
2. 5 or more consecutive points all trending in the same direction (eg, all going up in succession)

In this example, answer choice B shows a baseline performance with a median of 45% before the PDSA cycle. After the PDSA cycle, the median performance is 75% and has been sustained for several weeks.

Answer choice A shows a transient improvement that is not sustained because the performance returns to 45%. An improvement team should evaluate why the change could not be sustained and consider adjusting the intervention or pairing the initial intervention with another system change.

Answer choice C does not show any change in performance after the intervention. The improvement team should evaluate why the intervention did not result in an improvement and how it impacts their hypothesis of the PDSA cycle.

Answer choice D demonstrates a decline in performance after the PDSA cycle. The improvement team would certainly want to understand why there was a decline in performance following the PDSA cycle. Although frustrating, valuable information can be learned from failed PDSA cycles that can lead to future successful interventions.

Finally, there is a small random improvement in answer choice E that occurs well after the PDSA cycle. Although the change does not appear to be related to the PDSA cycle, the improvement team would want to understand what happened during that period of time to appreciate potential positive forces on performance. This example also illustrates the importance of evaluating longitudinal data to detect subtle changes that can help system learning.

(p. 20, Part 2: Systems of Care, Chapter 6: US Healthcare System, Efforts to Address Costs and Quality of Care)

**References**

Langley GL, Moen R, Nolan KM, Nolan TW, Norman CL, Provost LP. *The Improvement Guide: A Practical Approach to Enhancing Organizational Performance*, 2nd ed. San Francisco, CA: Jossey-Bass Publishers; 2009.

Perla RJ, Provost LP, Murray SK. The run chart: a simple analytical tool for learning from variation in healthcare processes. *BMJ Qual Saf.* 2011;20(1):46-51.

Provost LP, Murray SK. *The Health Care Data Guide: Learning From Data for Improvement*. San Francisco, CA: Jossey-Bass Publishers; 2011.

**Answer 28-5. A**

Success in quality improvement is often found when the project team appreciates the system to be improved through multiple viewpoints—a multidisciplinary team. After clearly identifying the problem and possible solutions, experimentation must be undertaken to test the changes to confidently know that any changes are measurable improvements.

The Institute for Healthcare Improvement Model for Improvement (Figure 6-2) outlines the architecture of improvement in health care using PDSA cycles. PDSA cycles are an essential quality improvement methodology founded on the scientific method to improve product, systems, or processes. The PDSA cycle and scientific method aim to improve existing knowledge by testing a hypothesis through experimentation and thoughtful analysis of data. The PDSA cycle should begin with a hypothesis or prediction about the

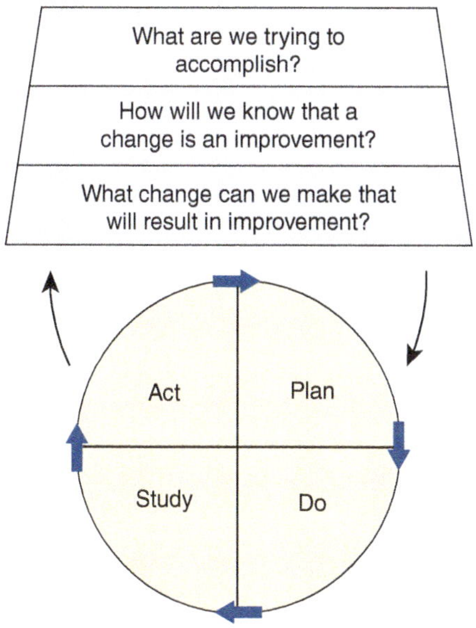


**FIGURE 6-2.** The Plan-Do-Study-Act cycle. (Reproduced with permission from Langley GJ, Moen RD, Nolan KM, et al. *The Improvement Guide: A Practical Approach to Enhancing Organizational Performance,* 2nd ed. San Francisco, CA: Jossey-Bass; 2009.)

experiment to be conducted. The "plan" phase encourages teams to clearly state the objective(s) of the experiment, make predictions, plan the experiment, and identify the data-collection strategy. The do phase involves carrying out the experiment and documenting the results. The study phase evaluates data from the experiment relative to the predictions. Interpretations and decisions about the test of change are completed in the act phase. This is often where teams decide if the change should be scaled up, adopted, implemented, or abandoned.

(p. 20, Part 2: Systems of Care, Chapter 6: US Healthcare System, Efforts to Address Costs and Quality of Care)

**References**

Institute for Healthcare Improvement. How to Improve. Available at http://www.ihi.org/resources/Pages/HowtoImprove/ScienceofImprovementTestingChanges.aspx. Accessed May 20, 2019.

Institute for Healthcare Improvement. Tools. Available at http://www.ihi.org/resources/Pages/Tools/PlanDoStudyActWorksheet.aspx. Accessed January 1, 2020.

Langley GL, Moen R, Nolan KM, Nolan TW, Norman CL, Provost LP. *The Improvement Guide: A Practical Approach to Enhancing Organizational Performance*, 2nd ed. San Francisco, CA: Jossey-Bass Publishers; 2009.

Moen RD, Nolan TW, Provost LP. *Quality Improvement Through Planned Experimentation*, 3rd ed. New York, NY: McGraw-Hill; 2012.

Taylor MJ, McNicholas C, Nicolay C, Darzi A, Bell D, Reed JE. Systematic review of the application of the plan-do-study-act method to improve quality in healthcare. *BMJ Qual Saf.* 2014;23:290-298.

**Answer 28-6.** B

The American healthcare system continues to evolve in an effort to reduce cost while improving quality outcomes. A number of reform efforts have emerged related to the Patient Protection and Affordable Care Act. VBP refers generally to programs aimed at financially rewarding attainment of quality metrics. Pay-for-performance is a model that relies on financial incentives to providers who achieve assigned quality metrics or penalties for failing to reach a goal. ACOs are partnerships between providers, payers, and hospitals that share financial risk to control costs for a patient population through achievement of quality metrics and coordinated care to reduce inefficiency and cost. The example in this question represents the fundamental structure of an ACO.

In comparison, hospital networks may increase engagement with primary care practices with the goal of improving systems of care. However, a hospital network model does not necessarily engage payers and providers with the expressed purpose of achieving quality metrics related through financial incentives. Finally, MIPS is a quality payment program created under the Medicare Access and CHIP Reauthorization Act (2015). MIPS primarily impacts providers caring for Medicare patients and offers financial incentives based on metrics in 4 areas: cost, improvement activities, promoting interoperability, and quality.

(p. 20, Part 2: Systems of Care, Chapter 6: US Healthcare System, Efforts to Address Costs and Quality of Care)

**References**

Centers for Medicare and Medicaid Services. Accountable Care Organization (ACOs): General Information. Available at https://innovation.cms.gov/initiatives/ACO/. Accessed May 14, 2019.

Centers for Medicare and Medicaid Services. Medicare Program; Merit-Based Incentive Payment System (MIPS) and Alternative Payment Model (APM) Incentive Under the Physician Fee Schedule, and Criteria for Physician-Focused Payment Models. Final rule with comment period. *Fed Regist.* 2016;81(214):77008-77831.

Centers for Medicare and Medicaid Services. MIPS Overview. Available at https://qpp.cms.gov/mips/overview. Accessed January 1, 2020.

**Answer 28-7.** E

The correct answer is HITECH Act. The HITECH Act was meant to encourage clinicians to adopt electronic health records in a meaningful way, including incorporation of basic data (eg, demographics, active medications, drug allergies, up-to-date problem lists, and current and active diagnoses), clinical decision support tools, and use of computer order entry. The HITECH Act also requires that meaningful use include electronic reporting of data on the quality of care.

The ARRA was passed in 2009 after the Great Recession to stimulate the economy by investing in health care (Medicaid, community health centers), education, infrastructure, and energy.

The Patient Protection and Affordable Care Act was passed in 2010 and contained several elements including provisions to increase access to health insurance while allowing patients with preexisting conditions to retain health insurance.

CHIPRA, passed in 2009, established several pediatric quality improvement programs and subsequently led to creation of the Pediatric Quality Measures Program.

HIPAA, passed in 1996, outlined rules for sharing protected health information in an age of increased electronic technology to manage claims and document medical encounters. The law defined patient privacy safeguards an agency must achieve while allowing healthcare agencies to adopt new technology.

(p. 20, Part 2: Systems of Care, Chapter 6: US Healthcare System, Efforts to Address Costs and Quality of Care)

**References**

Blumenthal D. Stimulating the adoption of health information technology. *N Engl J Med.* 2009;360(15):1477-1479.

Gold M, McLaughlin C. Assessing HITECH implementation and lessons: 5 years later. *Milbank Q.* 2016;94(3):654-687

Medicaid. CHIPRA. Available at https://www.medicaid.gov/chip/chipra/index.html. Accessed January 2, 2020.

US Department of Health and Human Services. Summary of the HIPAA Security Rule. Available at https://www.hhs.gov/hipaa/for-professionals/security/laws-regulations/index.html. Accessed January 1, 2020.

**Answer 28-8.** C

The vignette presents a common scenario when practices are asked to implement a new screening tool or process. In these cases, it is helpful to use improvement science methodology to ensure success. The Institute for Healthcare Improvement (IHI) Model for Improvement (Figure 6-2) outlines a framework to successfully implement changes while collecting meaningful data.

In this case, the improvement team has an aim; screen 90% of patients at well-child visits for social determinants of health using the new screening tool. In order to efficiently and successfully achieve the goal, the improvement team must be thoughtful about developing and implementing a new process.

Conducting a small test of change allows the improvement team to understand the barriers to full implementation of the new screening process. In quality improvement, a PDSA cycle is a small test of change that involves:

- Planning the intervention and making predictions about the results
- Testing the intervention on a small sample size
- Analyzing the data and interpreting the results
- Deciding if modifications should be made or if the intervention can be scaled up

Ideally, early PDSA cycles involve a small sample size so the improvement team can quickly learn from failure while reducing unintended consequences. As interventions are found to be successful, the sample size can be gradually scaled up based on iterative data collected.

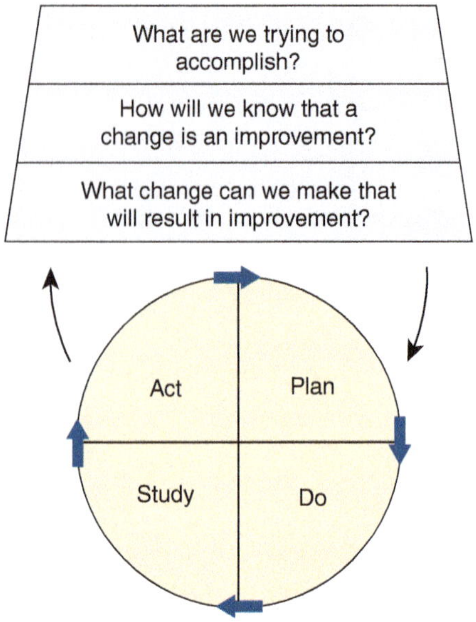


**FIGURE 6-2.** The Plan-Do-Study-Act cycle. (Reproduced with permission from Langley GJ, Moen RD, Nolan KM, et al. *The Improvement Guide: A Practical Approach to Enhancing Organizational Performance,* 2nd ed. San Francisco, CA: Jossey-Bass; 2009.)

In this example, answer choice C is the most appropriate because it encapsulates the best practices of a PDSA cycle.

Immediate full-scale implementation (answer choice A) could create a situation where system learning cannot be achieved and recognizing the negative effects could be delayed. Answer choice D is similar in that there is a larger implementation instead of a small test of change like a PDSA cycle.

Implementing a proven process from another clinic can be helpful to speed the process of improvement. However, an improvement team must be assured the process will be as effective in their clinic by using PDSA cycles. Thus, answer choice B is not ideal.

Answer choice E is suboptimal because it introduces too much variation. However, the improvement team should be thoughtful about how the new process impacts each provider. Soliciting their feedback is essential to success of the project.

(p. 20, Part 2: Systems of Care, Chapter 6: US Healthcare System, Efforts to Address Costs and Quality of Care)

**References**

Langley GL, Moen R, Nolan KM, Nolan TW, Norman CL, Provost LP. *The Improvement Guide: A Practical Approach to Enhancing Organizational Performance*, 2nd ed. San Francisco, CA: Jossey-Bass Publishers; 2009.

Moen RD, Nolan TW, Provost LP. *Quality Improvement Through Planned Experimentation*, 3rd ed. New York, NY: McGraw-Hill; 2012.

Taylor MJ, McNicholas C, Nicolay C, Darzi A, Bell D, Reed JE. Systematic review of the application of the plan-do-study-act method to improve quality in healthcare. *BMJ Qual Saf.* 2014;23:290-298.

**Answer 28-9.** D

Statistical process control charts are powerful quality improvement tools used to display longitudinal data and quickly interpret statistical significance of improvement work. The basic architecture of a statistical process control chart is similar to a run chart. Like a run chart, time is plotted on the x-axis, while the measure of interest is plotted on the y-axis. The mean for a series of data is plotted along with control limits, representing 3 standard deviations above and below the mean. Annotations identifying PDSA cycles or interventions are also made to assess temporality of the data.

Statistical process control charts allow improvement teams to assess the type of variation in a system. There are 2 types of variation, common cause variation and special cause variation. Common cause variation is routine variability in the performance of a system. Common cause variation is often referred to as a stable system operating within normal performance variation. Special cause variation indicates that the system is performing outside of normal variation.

Special cause variation can be identified by using several rules:

1. A single point that is outside the control limit (3 standard deviations)
2. Eight or more consecutive points all above or below the mean (centerline)
3. Six sequential points all descending or ascending

In the example in this question, point D represents special cause variation because it lies outside the control limits from the mean. Identifying the etiology for special cause variation is important for improvement teams so they can quickly identify influences on this system, whether positive or negative.

Points A, B, C, and E represent part of common cause variation. Point B is interesting because it seems like an outlier in a pattern of a small but encouraging data series. It is important to remember the rules for special cause variation because it would be incorrect to overrespond to a data point like point B because it is normal variation.

Data points residing on the mean (point C) are typically omitted when applying the rules to determine special cause variation.

(p. 20, Part 2: Systems of Care, Chapter 6: US Healthcare System, Efforts to Address Costs and Quality of Care)

**References**

Benneyan JC, Lloyd RC, Plsek PE. Statistical process control as a tool for research in healthcare improvement. *Qual Saf Health Care.* 2003;12:458-464.

Brady PW, Tchou MJ, Ambroggio L, Schondelmeyer AC, Shaughnessy EE. Quality improvement feature series article 2: displaying and analyzing quality improvement data. *J Pediatr Infect Dis Soc.* 2018;7:100-103.

Moen RD, Nolan TW, Provost LP. *Quality Improvement Through Planned Experimentation*, 3rd ed. New York, NY: McGraw-Hill; 2012.

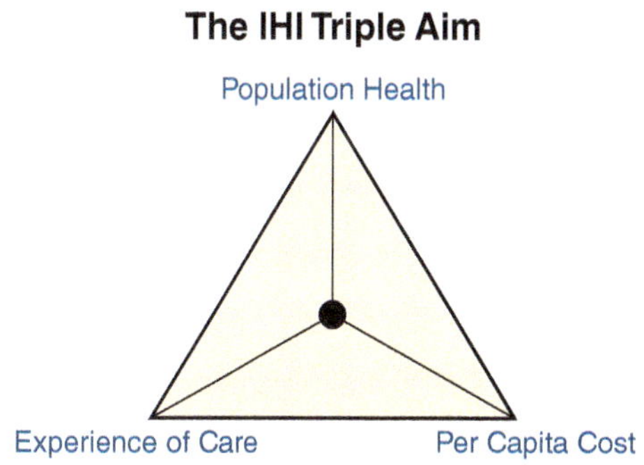


**FIGURE 6-3.** The Triple Aim. (The IHI Triple Aim framework was developed by the Institute for Healthcare Improvement in Massachusetts, USA [IHI.ORG].)

Perla RJ, Provost LP, Murray SK. The run chart: a simple analytical tool for learning from variation in healthcare processes. *BMJ Qual Saf.* 2011;20:46-51.

Provost LP, Murray SK. *The Health Care Data Guide: Learning From Data for Improvement.* San Francisco, CA: Jossey-Bass; 2011.

**Answer 28-10.** C

The IHI Triple Aim (Figure 6-3) consists of 3 arms: population health, per capita cost, and experience of care. It is important to realize that there is an interplay between the 3 main elements of the triple aim. Ideally, an improvement project would lower cost, improve immediate health outcomes, and increase the health of a population. In reality, there is a much more delicate balance between competing priorities. Sometimes, there is a financial cost to improving health outcomes through large system enhancements, redesign, or workforce increases. Each project team must afford equal attention to the arms of the Triple Aim in order to be successful.

On a related note, provider satisfaction has gained attention in the context of reducing fatigue and burnout. Provider burnout is an increasing concern, especially in the changing healthcare landscape. Improvement teams should consider the impact of a project on the care team's well-being.

(p. 21, Part 2: Systems of Care, Chapter 6: US Healthcare System, Triple Aim)

**References**

Bodenheimer T, Sinsky C. From triple to quadruple aim: care of the patient requires care of the provider. *Ann Fam Med.* 2014;12:573-576.

Institute for Healthcare Improvement. How to Improve. Available at http://www.ihi.org/resources/Pages/HowtoImprove/ScienceofImprovementTestingChanges.aspx. Accessed May 20, 2019.

Institute for Healthcare Improvement. Joy in Work. Available at http://www.ihi.org/Topics/Joy-In-Work/Pages/default.aspx. Accessed January 1, 2020.

Langley GL, Moen R, Nolan KM, Nolan TW, Norman CL, Provost LP. *The Improvement Guide: A Practical Approach to*

*Enhancing Organizational Performance*, 2nd ed. San Francisco, CA: Jossey-Bass Publishers; 2009.

Stiefel M, Nolan K. *A Guide to Measuring the Triple Aim:* Population Health, Experience of Care, and Per Capita Cost. IHI Innovation Series white paper. Cambridge, MA: Institute for Healthcare Improvement; 2012.

**Answer 28-11.** **D**

The United States spends more on health care than most other high-income countries, yet medical debt remains the leading cause of bankruptcy in the United States. As the US healthcare system continues to evolve to improve outcomes while reducing cost, providers are being encouraged to engage in the reform effort to improve the health of the population. There are 4 domains (business models, clinical integration, technology, and payment models) that providers can influence to improve population health while working to contain rising cost.

Clinical integration has been a recent focus of several entities including the American Medical Association and the American Hospital Association. At the core of clinical integration is the concept that care is delivered in a continuous fashion rather than in disconnected episodes. Strategies to improve clinical integration may involve case management, increased patient engagement, community paramedicine, and school-based health clinics, among others.

In this vignette, the other choices are examples of good clinical care that may improve outcomes related to asthma. However, they are largely isolated to an episode of care and are not connected to the patient's continuum of care in the spirit of clinical integration and care coordination.

(p. 23, Section 1: Foundations in Pediatric Practice and Child Health, Chapter 7: Population Health Management and Pediatrics)

**References**

American Hospital Association. Clinical Integration: The Key to Real Reform. Available at https://www.aha.org/system/files/research/reports/tw/10feb-clinicinteg.pdf. Accessed January 1, 2020.

Macias CG, Bartley KA, Rodkey TL, Russell HV. Creating a clinical systems integration strategy to drive improvement. *Curr Treat Options Pediatr*. 2015;1(4):334-346.

# INDEX

Note: Page numbers followed by "*f*" denote figures; those followed by "*t*" denote tables.

## B

## H

## N

## Q



## R

## S

## U